MONITORING IN ANESTHESIA AND CRITICAL CARE MEDICINE

THIRD EDITION

EDITED BY

CASEY D. BLITT, M.D.

Old Pueblo Anesthesia, Ltd.
Clinical Professor of Anesthesiology
Department of Anesthesiology
University of Arizona College of Medicine
Staff Anesthesiologist
Department of Anesthesiology
Tucson Medical Center
Tucson, Arizona

ROBERTA L. HINES, M.D.

Acting Chairman and Associate Professor
Department of Anesthesiology
Yale University School of Medicine
New Haven, Connecticut

CHURCHILL LIVINGSTONE

New York, Edinburgh, London, Madrid, Melbourne, Milan, Tokyo

Library of Congress Cataloging-in-Publication Data

Monitoring in anesthesia and critical care medicine / edited by Casey
    D. Blitt, Roberta L. Hines. — 3rd ed.
        p.   cm.
     Includes bibliographical references and index.
     ISBN 0-443-08912-4
       1. Anesthesia. 2. Critical care medicine. 3. Patient monitoring.
    I. Blitt, Casey D., date. II. Hines, Roberta L.
     [DNLM: 1. Anesthesia. 2. Critical Care. 3. Monitoring,
Physiologic. WO 200 M7443 1995]
RD82.M66 1995
617.9′6—dc20
DNLM/DLC
for Library of Congress   94-30518
                                                CIP

Distributed in the United Kingdom by Churchill Livingstone, Robert Stevenson House, 1–3 Baxter's Place, Leith Walk, Edinburgh EH1 3AF, and by associated companies, branches, and representatives throughout the world.

Accurate indications, adverse reactions, and dosage schedules for drugs are provided in this book, but it is possible that they may change. The reader is urged to review the package information data of the manufacturers of the medications mentioned.

The Publishers have made every effort to trace the copyright holders for borrowed material. If they have inadvertently overlooked any, they will be pleased to make the necessary arrangements at the first opportunity.

Assistant Editor: *Ann Ruzycka*
Copy Editor: *Donna C. Balopole*
Production Supervisor: *Sharon Tuder*
Cover Design: *Paul Moran*
Production services provided by Bermedica Productions, Ltd.

Printed in the United States of America

First published in 1995   7 6 5 4 3 2 1

To family, parents, teachers, colleagues, friends, students, and industry:
all have played some part in this educational effort;
to my partners at Old Pueblo Anesthesia,
who teach me amazing things about monitoring;
to my mother and father, Sarah and Aaron,
without whom this would not have been possible;
to my children, Rachel and Joshua,
who understand why I am not always available.
Extraordinary thanks to my wife, Kathryn,
for her patience, encouragement, and understanding.

C.D.B.

To my Grandmother Sadie: in her 90+ years,
she has provided me with immeasurable love, inspiration, and support;
to my parents,
whose patience and understanding are boundless;
to my husband, Jerry,
who has become the local expert on "take-out cuisine,"
I promise you a gourmet dinner.
Finally, I am most grateful to Dr. Casey Blitt
for his encouragement and mentoring
during the preparation of this text.

R.L.H.

Contributors

Hassan H. Ali, M.D.

Professor of Anaesthesia, Harvard Medical School; Anesthetist, Massachusetts General Hospital, Boston, Massachusetts

Paul G. Barash, M.D.

Professor, Department of Anesthesiology, Yale University School of Medicine, New Haven, Connecticut

Robert F. Bedford, M.D.

Clinical Professor, Department of Anesthesiology, University of Virginia School of Medicine; Attending Anesthesiologist, Department of Anesthesiology, University of Virginia Health Science Center, Charlottesville, Virginia

Audrée A. Bendo, M.D.

Associate Professor, Department of Anesthesiology, State University of New York Health Science Center at Brooklyn College of Medicine; Director of Neurosurgical Anesthesia, University Hospital, Brooklyn, New York

Casey D. Blitt, M.D.

Old Pueblo Anesthesia, Ltd., Clinical Professor of Anesthesiology, Department of Anesthesiology, University of Arizona College of Medicine; Staff Anesthesiologist, Department of Anesthesiology, Tucson Medical Center, Tucson, Arizona

Richard Botney, M.D.

Clinical Instructor, Department of Anesthesia, Stanford University School of Medicine, Stanford, California; Staff Anesthesiologist, Anesthesiology Service, Veterans Affairs Medical Center, Palo Alto, California

Amy Caplan, M.D.

Instructor, Department of Anesthesiology and Critical Care Medicine, The Johns Hopkins University School of Medicine; Staff Physician and Director of the Acute Pain Service, Department of Anesthesiology, Johns Hopkins Bayview Medical Center, Baltimore, Maryland

Randall C. Cork, M.D.

Professor, Department of Anesthesiology, Louisiana State University School of Medicine in New Orleans; Clinical Anesthesiologist, Charity Hospital, New Orleans, Louisiana

Marianna P. Crowley, M.D.

Instructor in Anaesthesia, Harvard Medical School; Assistant in Anesthesia, Massachusetts General Hospital, Boston, Massachusetts

John H. Eichhorn, M.D.

Professor and Chairman, Department of Anesthesiology, University of Mississippi School of Medicine; Chairman, Department of Anesthesiology, University of Mississippi Medical Center, Jackson, Mississippi

David M. Feinstein, M.D., M.S.

Instructor in Anaesthesia, Harvard Medical School; Associate Anesthetist, Beth Israel Hospital, Boston, Massachusetts

David M. Gaba, M.D.

Associate Professor, Department of Anesthesia, Stanford University School of Medicine, Stanford, California; Staff Anesthesiologist, Anesthesiology Service, Veterans Affairs Medical Center, Palo Alto, California

Hugh C. Gilbert, M.D.

Assistant Professor, Department of Anesthesia, Northwestern University Medical School; Senior Attending Anesthesiologist, Evanston Hospital, Evanston, Illinois

Mark N. Gomez, M.D.
Assistant Professor, Department of Anesthesia, University of Iowa College of Medicine, Iowa City, Iowa

Betty L. Grundy, M.D.
Professor of Anesthesiology and Pharmaceutics, Department of Anesthesiology, University of Florida College of Medicine, Gainesville, Florida

Benjamin G. Guslits, M.D.
Staff Anesthesiologist, Department of Anesthesiology-Division of Critical Care, and Staff, Critical Care, Departments of Pulmonary and Critical Care Medicine and Surgery-Division of Trauma and Critical Care Surgery, Henry Ford Hospital, Detroit, Michigan

Stuart R. Hameroff, M.D.
Associate Professor, Department of Anesthesiology, University of Arizona College of Medicine; Anesthesiologist, Department of Anesthesiology, University Medical Center, Tucson, Arizona

James V. Harper, M.D.
Assistant Professor, Department of Anesthesiology, Mayo Graduate School of Medicine, Rochester, Minnesota; Chairman, Department of Anesthesiology, Mayo Clinic, Jacksonville, Florida

Eugenie S. Heitmiller, M.D.
Associate Professor, Division of Cardiac Anesthesia, Department of Anesthesiology and Critical Care Medicine, The Johns Hopkins University School of Medicine, Baltimore, Maryland

Michael A. Herzig, M.D.
Assistant Professor, Department of Anesthesiology, George Washington University School of Medicine and Health Sciences, Washington, DC

Roberta L. Hines, M.D.
Acting Chairman and Associate Professor, Department of Anesthesiology, Yale University School of Medicine, New Haven, Connecticut

Linda S. Humphrey, M.D.
Associated Anesthesiologists of Reno, Reno, Nevada

James M. Hynson, M.D.
Assistant Professor, Department of Anesthesia, University of California, San Francisco, School of Medicine, San Francisco, California

Jeffrey A. Katz, M.D.
Professor of Clinical Anesthesia, Department of Anesthesia, University of California, San Francisco, School of Medicine; Chief, Department of Anesthesia, UCSF-Mount Zion Medical Center, San Francisco, California

Daniel J. Kennedy, M.D.
Assistant Professor, Department of Anesthesia, Section on Critical Care, Bowman Gray School of Medicine of Wake Forest University, Winston-Salem, North Carolina

Jacqueline M. Leung, M.D.
Assistant Professor in Residence, Department of Anesthesia, University of California, San Francisco, School of Medicine; Attending Anesthesiologist, Department of Anesthesia, UCSF-Mount Zion Medical Center, San Francisco, California

Joao A. C. Lima, M.D.
Assistant Professor, Department of Medicine, The Johns Hopkins University School of Medicine, Baltimore, Maryland

H. Michael Marsh, M.D.
Chairman, Department of Anesthesiology, Henry Ford Hospital, Detroit, Michigan

William T. Merritt, M.D.
Associate Professor, Department of Anesthesiology and Critical Care Medicine, The Johns Hopkins University School of Medicine, Baltimore, Maryland

J. Stephen Naulty, M.D.
Clinical Professor of Anesthesia in Obstetrics and Gynecology, University of Pennsylvania School of Medicine; Chairman, Department of Anesthesiology, Pennsylvania Hospital, Philadelphia, Pennsylvania

Susan C. Nicolson, M.D.
Associate Professor of Anesthesia, University of Pennsylvania School of Medicine; Director, Cardiac Anesthesia, The Children's Hospital of Philadelphia, Philadelphia, Pennsylvania

Gerard W. Ostheimer, M.D.
Professor of Anaesthesia, Harvard Medical School; Vice Chairman, Department of Anesthesia, Brigham and Women's Hospital, Boston, Massachusetts

Charles W. Otto, M.D., F.C.C.M.
Professor of Anesthesiology and Associate Professor of Medicine, Department of Anesthesiology, University of Arizona College of Medicine; Director of Critical Care Medicine, Department of Anesthesiology, Arizona Health Sciences Center and Veterans Affairs Medical Center, Tucson, Arizona

James H. Philip, M.E.(E), M.D.

Associate Professor of Anaesthesia, Harvard Medical School and Harvard-MIT Division of Health Sciences and Technology; Anesthesiologist and Director of Bioengineering, Department of Anesthesia, Brigham and Women's Hospital, Boston, Massachusetts

Scott Podolsky, M.D.

Clinical Assistant Instructor, Department of Anesthesiology, State University of New York Health Science Center at Brooklyn College of Medicine, Brooklyn, New York

Susan L. Polk, M.D., M.S.Ed.

Associate Professor, Department of Anesthesia and Critical Care, University of Chicago Division of the Biological Sciences Pritzker School of Medicine, Chicago, Illinois

J. Scott Polson, M.D.

Instructor, Clinical Anesthesiology, Department of Anesthesiology, University of Arizona College of Medicine; Anesthesiologist, University Medical Center, Tucson, Arizona

Daniel B. Raemer, Ph.D.

Associate Professor, Department of Anaesthesia (Bioengineering), Harvard Medical School; Director, Department of Clinical Engineering, Brigham and Women's Hospital, Boston, Massachusetts

Michael F. Roizen, M.D.

Professor and Chairman, Department of Anesthesia and Critical Care, and Professor, Department of Medicine, University of Chicago Division of the Biological Sciences Pritzker School of Medicine, Chicago, Illinois

Alan F. Ross, M.D.

Assistant Professor, Department of Anesthesia, University of Iowa College of Medicine; Director of Cardiac Anesthesia, Division of Cardiac Anesthesia, University of Iowa Hospital and Clinics, Iowa City, Iowa

Roger L. Royster, M.D.

Professor and Vice Chairman, Department of Anesthesia, Section on Critical Care, Bowman Gray School of Medicine of Wake Forest University, Winston-Salem, North Carolina

Nitin K. Shah, M.D.

Assistant Professor In-Residence, Department of Anesthesiology, University of California, Irvine, College of Medicine, Irvine, California; Staff, Surgical Intensive Care Unit, Veterans Affairs Medical Center, Long Beach, California

Martin D. Sokoll, M.D.

Professor, Department of Anesthesia, University of Iowa College of Medicine, Iowa City, Iowa

Bruce D. Spiess, M.D.

Associate Professor of Anesthesiology and Chief, Division of Cardiothoracic Anesthesia, Department of Anesthesiology, University of Washington School of Medicine, Seattle, Washington

James M. Steven, M.D.

Assistant Professor of Anesthesia and Pediatrics, University of Pennsylvania School of Medicine; Associate Anesthesiologist, Department of Anesthesiology and Critical Care Medicine, The Children's Hospital of Philadelphia, Philadelphia, Pennsylvania

Judith L. Stiff, M.D.

Associate Professor, Department of Anesthesiology and Critical Care Medicine, The Johns Hopkins University School of Medicine; Attending Anesthesiologist, Department of Anesthesiology, Johns Hopkins Bayview Medical Center, Baltimore, Maryland

John H. Tinker, M.D.

Professor and Head, Department of Anesthesia, University of Iowa College of Medicine, Iowa City, Iowa

Alan S. Tonnesen, M.D.

Professor, Department of Anesthesiology, University of Texas Medical School at Houston, Houston, Texas

Kevin K. Tremper, Ph.D., M.D.

Professor and Chair, Department of Anesthesiology, University of Michigan Medical School, Ann Arbor, Michigan

Leroy D. Vandam, M.D.

Professor Emeritus, Department of Anaesthesia, Harvard Medical School; Anesthesiologist, Department of Anesthesia, Brigham and Women's Hospital, Boston, Massachusetts

Jeffery S. Vender, M.D., F.C.C.M.

Associate Professor, Department of Anesthesia, Northwestern University Medical School; Chief of Anesthesiology and Director, Medical-Surgical ICU, Department of Anesthesiology, Evanston Hospital, Evanston, Illinois

Joyce A. Wahr, M.D.

Assistant Professor, Department of Anesthesiology, University of Michigan Medical School, Ann Arbor, Michigan

David S. Warner, M.D.

Professor, Departments of Anesthesiology, Neurobiology, and Surgery, Duke University School of Medicine, Durham, North Carolina

Richard C. Watt, M.S.E.E.

Director, Advanced Biotechnology Laboratory, Department of Anesthesiology, University of Arizona College of Medicine, Tucson, Arizona

Preface to the Third Edition

The third edition of *Monitoring in Anesthesia and Critical Care Medicine* sports a new, lean look and, more importantly, for the first time the book has a co-editor. Dr. Roberta Hines brings energy, impressive expertise, and new ideas to the book. It is our desire that the third edition should continue to serve as a definitive reference on monitoring of the anesthetized or critically ill patient. We envision the book to be useful to all health care personnel requiring information or knowledge regarding monitoring of these patients. Some chapters from the second edition have been deleted and there are exciting new chapters in this third edition. All chapters have been rewritten to include updating of bibliographic citations when appropriate.

New chapters in this edition include Monitoring and Patient Safety (Ch. 4) focusing on epidemiology and Human Factors Issues in Monitoring (Ch. 3). We have divided the chapter on electrocardiographic monitoring into two chapters, one dealing with arrhythmia (Ch. 8) and the other with detection of ischemia (Ch. 7). A chapter on monitoring coagulation status (Ch. 22) has also been added.

Duplications and overlap of information has, we hope, been minimized by consolidation of some chapters and streamlining of others. Expansion of some chapters has been accomplished to keep up with the changing world of monitoring and technology. The faithful readers of the first two editions will notice that the chapter on precordial and esophageal stethoscopes has been deleted, reflecting the ongoing transition to more sophisticated monitoring modalities. This change is of particular significance to one co-editor (CDB) because in 1983 when the first edition of this book was in progress, it was felt that the precordial and esophageal stethoscopes were important monitoring modalities. However, in 1994, these devices are so overshadowed by pulse oximetry and capnography that current anesthesia practice relegates them to the status of "back-up monitors" or maybe even to historical status.

An important new component of this edition is the inclusion of color plates, which we think will enhance the understanding of transesophageal data collection. We have tried to be responsive to the criticisms of the first two editions and hope that we have been successful in streamlining the book, making it more readable and user friendly without deleting important information.

We thank all the contributors to the third edition for sharing their outstanding expertise and knowledge. We also are extremely indebted to the staff and management at Churchill Livingstone for their tireless efforts in helping to create a truly outstanding work. We also thank our families and colleagues for their support and encouragement in producing this edition.

It is our hope that the third edition of *Monitoring in Anesthesia and Critical Care Medicine* will help improve quality of patient care and improve patient safety as well.

Casey D. Blitt, M.D.
Roberta L. Hines, M.D.

Preface to the First Edition

This book has been written to fulfill several purposes. Foremost was the need I saw for a complete, state-of-the-art text on monitoring, with an emphasis on the fields of anesthesia and critical care medicine. In addition, the book is designed to be a general reference on monitoring, and as such, differs from other publications on the subject of monitoring.

The authors who have contributed to this book are not only experienced and knowledgeable researchers, but also consummate clinicians, familiar with the problems faced by the practicing anesthesiologist. Since one of the purposes of monitoring is to aid the clinician in evaluating the patient, they have approached their topics from the points of view of physiology and clinical experience. They have done their work well. This book assembles a great amount of information of daily importance in the care of the anesthetized patient, and should be useful to the medical student, the clinician, and the medical professor.

Monitoring has become vital in many areas of medicine—internal medicine, surgery, obstetrics and gynecology, emergency medicine, critical care medicine, cardiology, pulmonary medicine, and of course anesthesiology. This book discusses virtually every conceivable monitoring modality, from the simplest to the most complex and from the nontechnical to the highly technical. The text starts with a discussion of some basic principles, then considers the monitoring of major body systems, and finally discusses aspects of monitoring that involve multiple organ systems. The concluding chapter discusses monitoring modalities of the future.

A major reason for writing this book was the thought that it might help improve patient care. If it does, I will indeed have succeeded in my mission. I have devoted a large portion of my career in anesthesiology to the field of monitoring. This book represents the culmination of these efforts.

I would like to thank the contributors to this book for their efforts in producing a fine text. I would also like to thank my family and colleagues for encouragement throughout this endeavor. Only time will tell if this book has fulfilled its goals.

Casey D. Blitt, M.D.

Contents

Color plates appear following page 266.

A Philosophy of Monitoring

Casey D. Blitt

1

Because anesthesia affects all organs, monitoring the anesthetized patient is required. Monitoring provides information to improve the practice of anesthesia with regard to safety, effects of drugs and techniques, and recognition of adverse effects. Appropriate monitoring facilitates timely therapeutic intervention to prevent undesirable outcomes.

Fundamentally, monitoring is data collection. Data may be collected manually, by the senses, or automatically, and must be processed. Automatic data collection methods are most desirable because they provide continual input and unshackle the anesthetist from the tedious task of manual data collection, allowing more time for cognitive decision-making. Automatic data collection devices may also annoy the practitioner with false alarms, incorrect data display, and occasional suboptimal performance in the electrically hostile operating room environment. It is my opinion that the practice of anesthesiology requires the availability of basic automatic data collection devices to ensure safe clinical practice. These basic automatic data collection devices are the pulse oximeter, oscilloscopic electrocardiograph, automatic noninvasive blood pressure instrument, and exhaled carbon dioxide analyzer.

Monitoring enhances vigilance. "Vigilance" is the motto of the American Society of Anesthesiologists, and no other single word best describes the task of the anesthesiologist. The anesthesiologist is the "guardian angel" of the patient.

Anesthesia and surgery are a team effort; all members of the team must communicate to provide the best patient care. Monitoring means many things to many people. Many variables *can* be monitored. The significance of some variables is obvious. For other variables the rationale, data assimilation, and decision-making are much more obscure. The purpose of this book is to provide a comprehensive look at monitoring modalities currently available in anesthesia and critical care medicine. Basic fundamental principles are frequently addressed and some of this book is akin to a textbook of applied physiology. The student in medicine, the physician in training, the practicing physician, and the academic physician should all be able to find some utility in this book. Monitoring and its spin-offs continue to move rapidly forward and, although our goal is to present the state of the art in this book, developments that will have occurred subsequent to the editing and printing process will obviously be omitted—not by choice but by time constraints.

According to Webster's unabridged dictionary, there are many different definitions of a monitor. *Monitor* may be used as both a noun and a verb. The word comes from the Latin *monere*, "to warn." As a noun, a monitor is (1) one who admonishes, cautions, reminds, or advises, (2) a pupil who assists a teacher in routine duties, (3) any device used to record or control a process, (4) an articulated device holding a rotating nozzle used in fire-fighting and mining, (5) a heavily iron-clad warship of the nineteenth century with a low, flat deck and one or more gun turrets; specifically, the first such ship, the Union vessel *Monitor*, which fought the Confederate iron-clad *Merrimack* on March 9, 1862, and (6) any tropical carnivorous lizard ranging in length from several inches to 10 feet, also known as Komodo dragon.

As a transitive verb (including the words *moni-*

tored, monitoring, and *monitors*) *to monitor* means (1) to check (the transmission quality of a signal) by means of a receiver, (2) to test (a surface) for radiation intensity, (3) to keep track of by means of an electronic device, (4) to check by means of a receiver for significant content (message-sending during war), (5) to scrutinize or check systematically with a view to collecting certain specified categories of data, and (6) to keep watch over; supervise (monitoring an examination).

As an intransitive verb, *to monitor* means to act as a monitor.

Can monitoring eliminate critical incidents in anesthetic and critical care areas? Can monitoring eliminate hypoxic accidents, drug overdoses, and equipment failures? Monitoring per se cannot eliminate these events, but it can substantially improve early recognition of esophageal intubation, anesthetic circuit disconnects, errors in gas supply/flow, loss of airway, and anesthetic overdose so as to permit early intervention. Multiple and backup monitoring modalities are desirable. The more systems you have to tell you if your patient is hypoxemic, the greater chance you have to receive input if one system fails.

Many parallels, comparisons, and similarities have been made between the administration of anesthesia and piloting an airplane.[1,2] Repetitive tasks, boredom, fatigue, and the sudden need to act quickly to avoid a disaster are common grounds for the anesthesiologist and the airline pilot. Pilots have backup systems and devices to warn them early of impending problems so that corrective action may be taken. So do anesthesiologists. Pilots have a standardized workplace with which they are very familiar. So *should* anesthesiologists. Pilots are only allowed to fly a certain number of hours without time off. Anesthesiologists should not be allowed to administer anesthesia day and night without rest. Patient safety is a *primary* concern. Accidents will continue to occur. We must have monitors that warn us appropriately so as to avoid undesirable outcomes. A frequently asked question is "How can I obtain the most useful information for the least effort expended?" This is a difficult question to answer. Experience, familiarity, and mastery of various monitoring modalities are excellent sifters and "weeders out" of marginal or nonuseful monitoring modalities. These tools help us separate the "wheat from the chaff" with regard to various monitoring devices. Monitoring modali-

ties and devices are used in direct proportion to their comfort and convenience factor. Monitors that are extremely difficult to use or whose information is extremely difficult to interpret do not achieve widespread usage. Certain monitors over a period of time achieve a designation of "the standard of care," and then not only does it become a professional opinion whether or not to use a monitor, but it becomes a legal one as well. Is blood pressure monitoring more important than an electroencephalogram (EEG)? Is pulmonary artery pressure monitoring better than central venous pressure monitoring? Is transesophageal echocardiography better than an electrocardiogram (ECG)? These questions are difficult if not impossible to answer. It is important to select a monitoring system (with backup) that will tell you what you want to know at an early enough time to keep you out of trouble. Those variables that will allow anesthesia to be administered safely without anesthetic mishaps should be monitored. The ideal is to minimize or eliminate human error, the most common cause of anesthetic catastrophes.[1-3] Monitoring systems that help prevent hypoxic anesthetic accidents, whether they be due to esophageal intubation, circuit disconnect, or anesthetic overdose must be used.

It often has been convenient to categorize monitoring modalities arbitrarily into invasive or noninvasive monitors. Noninvasive monitors do not require penetration of the skin or mucous membranes, whereas invasive monitors do. A noninvasive monitor may unintentionally become an invasive monitor in certain circumstances, such as when a tympanic membrane temperature sensor perforates the eardrum. All monitoring modalities are in a continuum of invasiveness to noninvasiveness, and categorization is always relative to other monitoring modalities.

The cost of monitoring is important simply because economic considerations are important to the practice of medicine. The more sophisticated monitoring devices (regardless of the degree of invasiveness) are more expensive. The cost-benefit ratios for most monitoring devices are not known.

Certain of the more invasive monitoring modalities, such as intra-arterial catheters and pulmonary artery catheters, are definitely here to stay. The practitioner can only ignore the obvious benefits of such monitors for so long before succumbing to their beneficial effects. The burgeoning number of instruments, machines, modalities, and so on that confront the physician, in particular the anesthesiologist or critical care medicine specialist, is at times mind-boggling. Inherent in this tremendous outburst of technology is reliability, maintenance, and the use or operation of the equipment. The physician must not be intimidated, frustrated, or otherwise put off by new techniques, new machines, and new instruments, but must strive to be the master of these modalities.

What monitors should be selected? This is another difficult question to answer. Medical judgment, good medical practice, and personal preference all become factors. Even if we cannot prove conclusively that certain monitors are beneficial, it is clear that certain minimal monitoring guidelines must be set, especially with regard to preplanned anesthetics given in designated anesthetizing locations.[4,5] Monitoring in the labor and delivery suite should be the same as in the operating room. Monitoring for chronic pain management, predelivery labor, sedation/amnesia, or analgesia for various diagnostic and therapeutic procedures should be based on institutional guidelines. If minimum guidelines cannot be met, then appropriate written documentation must be furnished. Minimal monitoring *standards* in anesthesiology have been established.[4,5] It is interesting that all published standards address the issue of "presence" of qualified personnel in the location where the anesthetic is being administered.[4,5] It is clear that the anesthesiologist personally providing anesthesia should be physically present in the operating room or anesthetizing area from the start of the anesthetic to the safe transfer of the patient to the PACU or Intensive Care Unit. "The presence of personnel" statement implies that monitors may not be of great value if there is nobody to observe the information obtained. It must also be appreciated that practicing according to published standards of monitoring cannot guarantee a favorable outcome.[6] The following represents my opinion of what constitutes minimum monitoring guidelines. These guidelines may be exceeded at any time based upon the judgment of the involved anesthesia personnel. Monitoring should be tailored to the specific operative procedure and the patients' risk factors.

The "preflight" check of anesthesia apparatus is important to the safe conduct of anesthesia. I recommend the Anesthesia Apparatus Check Out Procedure endorsed by the American Society of Anesthesiologists, or a reasonable equivalent.[7] This check out procedure is a guideline that users should be encouraged to modify to accommodate differences in equipment, design, and variations in local clinical practice. This anesthesia apparatus check out is periodically updated in conjunction with the FDA, and the most recent update has recently been published. Once the preflight check and the presence of personnel criteria have been satisfied, I recommend the following monitors for patients undergoing general anesthesia:

1. Cardiovascular system
   a. Pulse oximeter
   b. Automatic blood pressure measurement
   c. Oscilloscopic electrocardiogram
   d. Heart rate (any method)
2. Respiratory system
   a. Pulse oximeter
   b. Exhaled gas flow measurement (ventimeter or equivalent) if a circle system is used
   c. Respiratory rate (any method)
   d. Exhaled carbon dioxide analysis
3. Circuit low-pressure alarm if mechanical ventilation is used
4. Oxygen analyzer with low concentration alarm in the circuit (if circle is used)
5. Ability to monitor temperature.

If the patient is undergoing regional anesthesia, I recommend the following monitoring modalities or equivalents:

1. Readily available oxygen source with artificial ventilation support system
2. Cardiovascular system
   a. Pulse oximeter
   b. Automatic blood pressure measurement
   c. Oscillometric electrocardiogram
   d. Heart rate (any method)
3. Respiratory system
   a. Pulse oximeter
   b. Respiratory rate (any method)
4. Ability to monitor temperature

For limited procedures (the practitioner must define limited), I recommend the following modalities:

1. Pulse oximeter
2. Oscillometric electrocardiogram
3. Automatic blood pressure measurement, or continuous precordial stethoscope

Exhaled carbon dioxide measurement is particularly useful in ascertaining tracheal placement of the endotracheal tube in instances where tracheal placement is in doubt. Should monitoring of exhaled/inspired anesthetic gases and vapors be required? As instrumentation for performing anesthetic gas and vapor analysis improves, more and more practitioners will embrace this modality. It will become "standard of care" within five years.

Computers will be playing a larger and larger part of various monitoring systems in the years to come. It becomes imperative, then, that the practitioner live and interact in harmony with computers rather than taking an antagonistic viewpoint toward them. Computers show great promise for producing a fully automated anesthesia record. Systems are now in place to perform this task. A chapter in this edition addresses this issue. If we desire an accurate record, particularly of vital signs, a computer-generated record is desirable because the anesthesiologist is freed from time-consuming record-keeping to concentrate completely on patient care. Additionally, the induction and emergence periods represent times when physicians' concentration and efforts are and should be directed totally toward patient care. Physiologic data collection during these periods is clearly suboptimal if not performed automatically. I am a strong advocate of automated anesthesia data management systems and believe they will be reality for most practitioners within the next five years.

Monitoring in certain areas outside the operating theater has become important recently. Whether this is occurring because patients are cared for by personnel other than anesthesiologists, that is, by nurses, gastroenterologists, pulmonary medicine physicians, pediatricians, and others, or for reasons such as cost, availability of equipment, or as-yet unidentified factors, is difficult to determine. The chapter entitled "Monitoring in Unusual Environments" addresses a portion of this issue. Monitoring modalities should be tailored to the patient with regard to the underlying disease state and the diagnostic or therapeutic procedure being performed. It simply does not make any sense for a patient who is being sedated with intravenous medication in a nondesignated anesthetizing location of a health care facility to be inappropriately monitored. Many health care facilities have developed protocols for monitoring of such patients outside designated anesthetizing locations. Anesthesiologists should be willing to provide input into these monitoring protocols. In my opinion, continuous pulse oximetry, oscillometric

electrocardiography (when indicated), and intermittent noninvasive blood pressure determination (preferably by an automated device) would seem to be of unquestionable value. Since hypoxemia is always a possibility, the use of pulse oximetry would seem to be particularly valuable.

The issue frequently arises as to what should be done if a piece of monitoring equipment is either nonfunctional or unavailable. It is easy to create rationalizations, but in my opinion the prudent health care professional should simply decline to provide care until appropriately functioning equipment is available, except in true emergent conditions. To proceed without appropriate monitoring equipment compromises patient safety and should be avoided despite external pressures to "push ahead."

"Failure to monitor" is increasingly alleged as the reason for failure to achieve a desired outcome (i.e., an undesirable outcome has resulted) and thus becomes an issue in a medical/legal action or lawsuit. In my experience, sometimes the failure-to-monitor allegation is a deserved one and sometimes it is not. It is important to remember that monitoring in and of itself cannot guarantee any given outcome. Some situations where failure to monitor has been alleged to be causative include injuries related to positioning of the patient and the development of peripheral nerve injuries perioperatively. Once a patient has been properly positioned for an operation, it is, in most cases, difficult or impossible to continually monitor the patient to ensure that a position-related injury does not occur. The allegation of "failure to monitor" after a patient has been properly positioned and all the usually accepted clinical precautions taken to ensure that position-related injuries do not occur is simply unreasonable.

Peripheral nerve injuries may be related to improper positioning of a patient, but "failure to monitor" as a causative factor in the development of peripheral nerve injuries is totally unreasonable. Knowledge of potential mechanisms for peripheral nerve injuries and educational strategies to prevent them, particularly outside the operating room are important areas that continually need to be addressed. It is my opinion that most, *but not all,* peripheral nerve injuries that occur in the perioperative period are a result of patient predisposition in combination with other factors that are usually beyond the control or domain of the anesthesiologist.

Central vascular access is commonly performed

for a variety of clinical indications. Because of their expertise, anesthesiologists are frequently consulted to establish central vascular access. Immediate complications or undesirable outcomes relating to central vascular access certainly fall within the realm of the individual placing the catheter or other device. Delayed complications or undesirable outcomes resulting from central vascular access are usually not the responsibility of the anesthesiologist or other individual placing the central vascular catheter. This subject is particularly important in relationship to the "ideal" desired location for the catheter tip of a CVP line. It is my opinion that a right atrial catheter tip location is perfectly acceptable, and leaving a catheter in such a location is in accordance with "standard of care." There are many circumstances (sitting craniotomy, for example) when the tip of the CVP (central venous pressure) catheter is intentionally placed in the right atrium. It is important to avoid perpendicular or close to perpendicular angle impingement of the tip of an intravascular catheter and a vascular side wall. Radiographically, it is difficult, if not impossible, to determine with 100% certainty whether the tip of a central vascular catheter is in the superior vena cava or the right atrium. If the tip of an intravascular catheter is below the pericardial reflection and extravascular migration occurs, the possibility of cardiac tamponade is greater than if the tip of the catheter is proximal to the pericardial reflection. Extravascular migration is such a rare occurrence that manipulation of a central vascular catheter to avoid placing the tip below the pericardial reflection (when you don't know where the pericardial reflection is to begin with) is simply not warranted.

Monitoring has attempted to keep pace with the monumental growth of anesthesiology in the last twenty years. Progress has been made but there needs to be continual growth in the monitoring field. Interfacing of various pieces of monitoring equipment (even by the same manufacturer) is frustrating at best and needs to be addressed, especially by industry. We need to look forward to a complete centralized monitoring array without a spaghettilike gaggle of wires, hoses, and power cords. Alarm sources need to be readily identifiable. The anesthetic workplace needs to be improved and standardized (like an airline cockpit) to minimize human error. Everyone should use standardized color-coded labels for medicines.

Wouldn't it be wonderful if the printing on medicine containers was large enough to read easily? Wouldn't it be wonderful if so many medicine containers didn't look exactly alike? Regardless of our biases, education, or age, we must realize that monitors and complex devices, including intravenous infusion devices, are here to stay; and we must work with them, not against them.

We now know that patients receiving neurally applied opioids can be managed safely in virtually any patient care area if nursing personnel have been appropriately educated and informed.

By continually improving monitoring practices in the operating room, many critical events are now occurring in the postanesthesia care unit (PACU). The PACU should not be ignored once the operating room areas have been "taken care of." Appropriate monitoring in the PACU is important, and all patients should be monitored with a pulse oximeter in the PACU.

Risk management is becoming increasingly important in the field of anesthesia. Aggressive risk management and peer review have the ability to markedly decrease the incidence and severity of anesthesia-related catastrophes. Monitoring and risk management go hand in hand because risk management involves "monitoring" of the practice of anesthesiology. Monitoring and risk management are means to achieve an end; that end is to make anesthesia as safe as possible.

REFERENCES

1. Allnutt MF: Human factors in accidents. Br J Anaesth 59:856, 1987
2. Gaba DM, Maxwell M, DeAnda A: Anesthetic mishaps: breaking the chain of acts and evolution. Anesthesiology 66:670, 1987
3. Deaths during general anesthesia. J Health Care Technol 1:155, 1985
4. American Society of Anesthesiologists: Standards for basic intraoperative monitoring. Am Soc Anesthesiol Newsletter, December 1986, revised 1988, 1992
5. Eichhorn JH, Cooper JB, Cullen DJ et al: Standards for patient monitoring during anesthesia at Harvard Medical School. JAMA 256:1017, 1986
6. Stoelting RK: Standards for minimal intraoperative monitoring; advantages and disadvantages. Literature Scan: Anesthesiology 1:2, 1987
7. American Society of Anesthesiologists: Anesthesia apparatus check out recommendations. Am Soc Anesthesiol Newsletter, October 1986, revised 1993

The Senses As Monitors: The Decline and Fall

2

Leroy D. Vandam

The real value of the inhalation of ether in surgical operations must be mainly determined by the ultimate success of the cases in which it is practiced. A surgical operation is a necessary evil, submitted to for the advantage of a greater good which is expected to result from it: and if the ether added at all to the danger of the operation, or diminished in any way the full advantages to be derived from the operation, it would be the surgeon's duty to recommend his patient to submit to the pain, excruciating as it often would be to him, and distressing to those who have to witness it.
-John Snow[1]

Utilization of the physician's senses—sight, hearing, touch, smell, and even taste—has from the beginning been the mainstay in diagnosis and tracking the course of disease. Indeed no diagnostic device since introduced is useful without the aid of one or more of the senses to interpret the findings. Such observations were empirical, achieving acceptance only because of the extensive clinical experience of the then leaders in medicine. Well into the 1800s the Galenic theory of the origin of disease prevailed, relating to a balance or imbalance among four body humors—blood, phlegm, yellow bile, and black bile. An excess or deficit in any of these qualities might be suggested, among other things, by alterations in body temperature and the degree of moisture or dryness of the skin and mucous membranes. This was the state of the art when surgical anesthesia was demonstrated publicly for the first time in Boston, October 1846. Because of this humoral concept of disease, surgery hardly changed at first, as it remained to be shown that disease, as revealed in pathologic anatomy, had a physical basis, therefore amenable to the scalpel.[2] Auscultatory changes heard via the stethoscope, changes in percussion sounds, and ultimately the revelations of the x-ray not only were authenticated by postmortem examination, but they helped to establish surgery as a medical discipline.

Traditionally, physicians who have relied on contact with patients to diagnose disease have always resented the introduction of devices that would seem to undermine the intrinsic value of physical diagnosis. Lewis Thomas, medical essayist, remarked that when the stethoscope was invented in the nineteenth century, although vastly improving the acoustics of the thorax, it also removed the physician a certain distance from the patient.[3] "It was the earliest device of many still to come—designed to increase that distance." And Comroe[4] wrote, "In the year 1905, when Korotkoff described his new, non-invasive method for measuring both systolic and diastolic blood pressure, a method that at least permitted objective study of the natural course of hypertension and methods to treat it, the British Medical Journal . . . argued that by sphygmomanometry we pauperize our senses and weaken clinical acuity." Similarly, James Mackenzie, England's great cardiologist, was antagonistic toward both the use of x-rays and the electrocardiogram because he was convinced that such aids would "blunt the senses and the acute perception of the clinical observer."

These rather simple mechanical extensions of the senses are still the basic monitoring methods employed in anesthesiology today. The argument is not so much against their practical use but over their credibility and therefore the need to adopt invasive techniques that reach into the physiologic currents of the body. In the light of major extensions of surgical treatment and the precarious state of many a patient operated on, no one can deny the advantages of the information derived from invasive monitoring. The questions relate more to their routine use, cost-effectiveness, and concern over a low but consistent rate of complications associated with their employment. Perhaps one of the reasons why anesthesiologists have surrendered to their lure is that they are no longer adept in physical diagnosis.

Monitoring is merely an extension of the physical examination. Indeed the findings of the preoperative examination influence the choice of anesthesia, suggesting those complications to be anticipated, and the monitoring procedures required during anesthesia. Furthermore, after a simple monitoring plan has been elected, more complex methods must be applied during the operation, as in the treatment of malignant hyperthermia, air embolism, or massive hemorrhage.

Lacking invasive devices, the senses are all the more important and they must be conscientiously and subconsciously at work in addition to any device used. Further, many a complication detectable by the senses is not presently amenable to instrumental detection, or when the monitoring device makes the discovery the warning comes too late to avert a catastrophe.

Although it might seem logical from a didactic standpoint to guide the reader through a typical anesthetic—induction, maintenance, and emergence—in order to depict the use of the senses, the purpose is better served by a system approach.

NEUROLOGY

Although both general and regional anesthesia are neurologic phenomena, quantitative evaluation of the state of anesthesia has been slow to evolve.

The electroencephalogram, with all of the demurrers attached to its interpretation and with the exact source of the brain waves still unknown, has been employed mainly to detect cerebral hypoxia rather than the various planes of anesthesia, which are more readily apparent clinically.[5] Elicitation of sensory-evoked potentials first applied to problems of anesthesia in the late 1940s and 1950s[6] (Fig. 2-1) is now used to measure overall aspects of neural transmission as an index of physical or hypoxic damage to spinal cord or brain. Consequently, in order to monitor depth of anesthesia one may have to rely on those surviving elements of the traditional signs and stages that are partially obscured by the use of neuromuscular blockers, opioids, and other intravenous agents. Few anesthesiologists bother to detect changes in the level of consciousness by employing their senses. Possibly this is why awareness during general anesthesia is a relatively recent phenomenon. Although once pertaining mainly to ether anesthesia, the signs and stages of anesthesia still offer a reasonable guide to depth of anesthesia, even as they are useful in assaying drug overdose and various kinds of coma.

The Traditional Signs of General Anesthesia

Within three months of the introduction of anesthesia, Francis Plomley of Maidstone, England, reported in the *Lancet* on the stages of anesthesia, having breathed ether himself and observed its effects in others.[7]

> [His first stage was characterized as] one merely of a pleasurable feeling of half intoxication, the second as one of extreme pleasure being similar to the sensation produced by breathing nitrous oxide or laughing gas. Also in that stage there was not exactly an insensitivity to pain but rather an indifference. *The third stage, the only one I think for performing operation, is one of profound intoxication and insensibility. The individual is completely lost to pain and to external impressions: the muscles become prostrate, the circulation lessens and the temperature falls.*

Do these criteria differ from those observable today, upon which the concept of minimum alveolar concentration (MAC) is based?

While giving credit to Plomley, John Snow[1] spoke of the third degree whereof,

> the patient may have moved his eyes about in the second degree, but in this degree they are station-

ary, or if they do move, their motions have nothing of a voluntary character. The eyelids may be either open, or partly or tightly closed, but in either case if lifted or moved by the finger, the orbicularis palpebrarum contracts. *The eyelash stroke is not as good a sign of anesthesia. When absent, lid tone is present and the patient will open the eyes on command when lash stroke is negative.*

John Snow had a remarkable record of safety as an anesthetist, even with the use of chloroform, and it is apparent that no small part of his success related to his use of the senses.

Since Snow's time many clinicians have elaborated on the original observations in charting the course of anesthesia. Guedel,[8] for example, emphasized the significance of eyeball position during ether anesthesia, dividing the third stage into four planes. His notes on the changes in respiration are not relevant today because of its early depression caused by the potent halogens and coincident use of neuromuscular blockers. Nevertheless, as we shall see, the anesthesiologist had better observe the respiratory pattern whenever natural breathing is permitted, and during reversal of neuromuscular blockade.

On page 81 of *On Chloroform and Other Anaesthetics*[9] Snow makes this cogent remark about the anesthetized patient. "The surgeon wishes to know

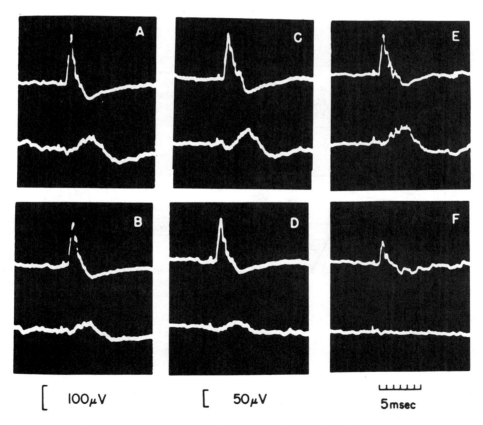

$$\left[\quad 100\mu V \qquad \left[\quad 50\mu V \right. \right.$$

5 msec

Fig. 2-1. Recordings of the changes in evoked responses for each of the three anesthetic gases. The upper tracing of each photograph is from the posteroventrolateral nucleus of the thalamus, the lower from the midbrain tegmental reticular formation. Photographs **A**, **C**, and **E** are controls for the results (photographs shown directly beneath) following 5 minutes administration of nitrous oxide 77 percent-oxygen 23 percent (**B**), ethylene 77 percent-oxygen 23 percent (**D**), and cyclopropane 40 percent-oxygen 60 percent (**F**). The 100 microvolt scale refers to the thalamic tracing; the 50-μV scale to the midbrain. Each division of the time scale equals 5 ms. (From Davis et al.,[6] with permission.)

whether he will lie still under the knife, or whether he will make a resistance and outcry, which he probably would not make in his waking state.'' This was perhaps the first statement on the concept of MAC. Lacking muscle movement, it has been said that the patient speaks to the anesthetist with everything but his voice. In current practice, the reaction to pain of the autonomic nervous system is one such communication: the secretion of tears, a rise or fall in pulse rate or blood pressure, and onset of sweating. These signs may also suggest awareness but not necessarily so. Augmented sympathetic nervous activity is known to be hazardous for the heart with a compromised coronary circulation, the work induced possibly exceeding the available supply of oxygen and leading to ischemia. A report suggests use of the term MAC-BAR, the anesthetic dose (applicable to inhalation or intravenous

agents) that blocks adrenergic stress and the cardiovascular response to the surgical incision.[10]

In 1943, Gillespie, building on Guedel's classification, pointed out that depth of anesthesia could be better ascertained through the manner in which various reflexes are modified[11] (Fig. 2-2).

In addition to the signs of anesthesia, which are no longer as definitive as they were with ether anesthesia, observation of the operative field is ever so much more important, as we shall reiterate in relation to the circulation and respiration. Muscle tone and relaxation can easily be assessed as the surgeon explores and applies retractors to an abdominal incision, thereby eliciting a myotonic reflex. Jaw relaxation also equates well with the degree of neuromuscular blockade. Several kinds of abnormal muscle movement may appear. Muscle contractions may suggest faulty grounding if the

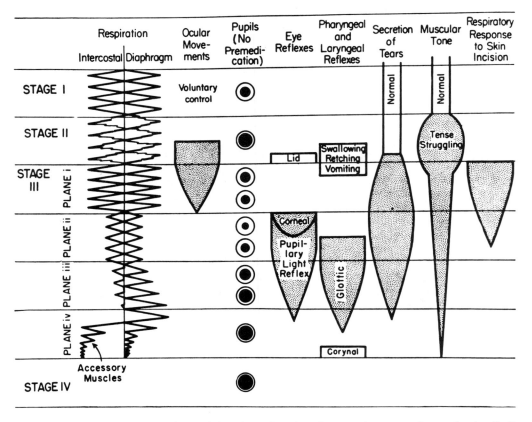

Fig. 2-2. Gillespie's modification of Guedel's chart for the signs and stages of anesthesia. Reflex responses to stimulation are emphasized and their disappearance noted in the plane of the third stage of anesthesia. (From Gillespie,[11] with permission.)

electrocautery is being used. Spontaneous muscle twitching may suggest awareness, but is often an unexplained phenomenon. Generalized convulsions may develop in conjunction with hyperthermia as during ether anesthesia in the febrile child but surprisingly are rare in conjunction with the malignant hyperthermia syndrome. Hyperactive reflexes and clonus are commonly seen on emergence from anesthesia with most potent general anesthetics, apparently a pyramidal tract sign differing from the shivering induced by hypothermia.

Regional Anesthesia

Regional anesthesia calls for other kinds of observation. Upon injection of the test dose of local anesthetic and thereafter, close contact with the patient should be maintained by way of conversation and observation of the face. Slowed verbal responses, slurring of speech, or failure to respond are signs of central depression which may or may not progress to seizures. During spinal or epidural anesthesia, failure to respond suggests that paralysis has affected the respiratory muscles, intercostals, and diaphragm, so that air cannot be moved through the larynx. Blanching of the skin often heralds a vagovagal reflex, the pulse slowing and blood pressure falling; this may be followed by nausea and vomiting. Twitching of the facial muscles is often a prelude to generalized seizures as might occur with unintentional intravenous injection of a local anesthetic during infiltration, during epidural anesthesia, or with deflation of a tourniquet early in the course of intravenous regional anesthesia. In the latter case, blushing of the extremity distal to the tourniquet indicates that the tourniquet no longer occludes the circulation.

A neurologic examination is part of every regional anesthetic. In spinal or epidural anesthesia, the patient first experiences subjective warmth of the part. The skin then feels warm to touch and vasodilation is apparent. Repeated testing for pinprick sensation is the best way to follow the course of a nerve block because the small nerve fibers in that sensation are usually blocked first. Then loss of temperature perception can be shown by application of a cold, wet sponge, followed by loss of position when the part can still be moved and the patient has a phantom image of the original position. Ultimately, motor power and touch disappear. These neurologic signs are not necessarily listed in order of development, their elicitation varying with the type and site of nerve block.

RESPIRATION

The Diagnosis of Respiratory Problems

Observation of respiration begins well before induction of anesthesia, during the physical examination when the pattern of breathing is noted: Is the chest rigid and barrel shaped, mainly with diaphragmatic breathing? Is there restrictive movement associated with arthritis or kyphoscoliosis, or weakness of the muscles as part of a neurologic syndrome? Are the accessory muscles of respiration being used? Will respiratory obstruction occur with loss of consciousness and tracheal intubation be difficult? The latter is predictable when there has been prior difficulty with intubation, when the neck is short and thick, the tongue is large and fills the oral cavity, the jaw is receding with an overbite and precarious incisor teeth; in arthritis, with ankylosis of the temporomandibular joint, rigidity and kyphosis of the cervical spine, and cricoarytenoid joint immobility as suggested by a high pitched voice. Relatedly, is the trachea compressed or deviated, is there tracheal stenosis as might have followed a previous tracheostomy? Forewarned by any of these problems and with several alternate techniques available—blind nasal intubation with the aid of topical anesthesia, use of fiberoptic equipment, and in rare instances preliminary tracheostomy—there may be little excuse for repeated futile attempts at intubation with the accompanying hypoxia, unintentional esophageal intubation, and trauma to tissues of pharynx and larynx. Finally, the extent of pulmonary pathology per se should suggest the extent of monitoring necessary during the perioperative period.

Although most general anesthetics these days begin with a rapid intravenous induction and tracheal intubation, surely the simpler, shorter operations are best handled with a mask and spontaneous respiration. The mask not strapped to the face should be held with one hand while other things are being done. One can both feel and see the onset of respiratory obstruction as manifested by the tug on the jaw, dilation of the alae nasae muscles, and supraclavicular retraction. No subject lying in the supine position is free of some degree of obstruction or increased airway resistance as the jaw muscles begin to relax. It is helpful to observe the lips for their color (use a transparent plastic face mask) and to be sure they are not caught between the teeth and traumatized. With any degree of obstruction, respiratory assistance is essential both to avoid hypoxia and to maintain alveolar ventilation and hasten induction of general anesthesia. If the patient fails to lose consciousness, the intravenous line should be examined to be sure that extravasation of an induction agent has not occurred. In addition, the inhaled mixture should be breathed to be sure that an anesthetic is actually present (e.g., failure to turn on the vaporizer, or an empty vaporizer).

Rigidity of the chest wall muscles may develop after the intravenous sequence of a nondepolarizing neuromuscular blocker then succinyldicholine for rapid intubation—also bringing to mind the possibility of onset of malignant hyperthermia (MH). Rigidity of the chest muscles is not uncommon after induction of anesthesia with large doses of the short-acting opioids: fentanyl, alfentanil, sufentanil. It may be impossible at first to inflate the lungs.

Further Notes on Tracheal Intubation

During tracheal intubation it is important to examine the larynx for presence of pathology, particularly if the patient has recently developed hoarseness or is a heavy smoker. Preoperative, indirect laryngoscopy is indicated if vocal cord paralysis is suspect. If tracheal intubation is performed with the subject breathing spontaneously, it is possible to observe vocal cord movement, the best indicator of paresis or paralysis. Muscle paralysis before intubation eliminates this possibility. Nevertheless one should take a moment to observe the condition of the pharynx, hypopharynx, and structures of the larynx before passing the tracheal tube through the glottis.

As the tracheal tube is inserted, the eye should

follow it full length beyond the vocal cords; otherwise, if placed only at the aditus, it may bounce back into the pharynx or into the esophagus when advanced blindly. If the tube is in the trachea before the balloon is inflated a clear whistling sound will be heard with inflation of the lungs; but a gutteral, regurgitational tone is audible when in the esophagus. Neither sign may be infallible, always calling for confirmation by chest auscultation. Depth of tracheal tube insertion can be determined not only by observing symmetrical movement of the thoraces but by palpation and straddling of the trachea with the fingers at the jugular notch as the catheter balloon is inflated. Thus there are several means available by way of the senses to be sure that an atraumatic tracheal intubation has been successfully accomplished through a normal larynx, and that the tube has progressed just far enough so that the lungs expand equally.

Patterns of Ventilation

Controversy prevails over the efficacy of the so-called educated hand in assuring adequate alveolar ventilation by intermittent manual pressure on the reservoir breathing bag. Immediate attachment of the tracheal catheter to a mechanical ventilator deprives the anesthetist of some essential information. Surely, changes in pulmonary compliance can be detected by the hand, as a manifestation of bronchospasm, breath-holding in response to the surgical incision, tracheal tube obstruction or its displacement, the onset of pulmonary edema or pneumothorax, and the wearing off of neuromuscular blockade.

Egbert and Bisno[12] examined the degree of skill inherent in recognizing changes in pulmonary compliance during manual ventilation, in a blinded fashion, among a group of anesthetists of varied training. By means of deliberately induced alterations in a gas bellows, the resulting pressure and volume changes could be observed apart from the operator's awareness of them. While observing the movement of the bellows, the operators were able to maintain tidal volume at a constant level, also when the view was obscured—so long as compliance did not vary. When compliance was lowered and the view obstructed, the operators sensed the change but manual pressure was not raised sufficiently to maintain tidal volume, so that in most cases the volume fell below 50 percent of the sub-

TABLE 2-1. Comparison of Semiclosed-Cycle and Closed-Cycle Systems

System	Reduction in Tidal Volume*
Semiclosed	193 ml ± 19
Closed	83 ml ± 14

*$P < 0.01$. Data from 7 staff and 10 residents.
(From Egbert and Bisno,[12] with permission.)

jective estimate of ventilatory adequacy (Table 2-1). The error was greater in a semiclosed rather than closed rebreathing system. In the clinical situation, an unconcerned anesthetist not observing chest motion is unaware of the extent to which the tidal volume can escape through an expiratory valve, in semiclosed, semiopen, or open system. In the Egbert experiment, all of the individuals tested made correct statements on changes in compliance while employing a closed system, and they noticed gas leaks in the system more readily than during use of a semiclosed technique. Reservoir bags of smaller volume and shorter conducting tubes made for greater proficiency. Errors were greater if the subjects were distracted by being asked to read aloud (Table 2-2). Just listening to the conducting tubes reduced errors in ventilation and when the subjects watched the bellows their errors approached zero (Table 2-2).

Apparently, watching and listening during manual or mechanically assisted ventilation are essential measures in addition to sensing by the "educated hand." An occasional deep sigh can be heard (and seen) in the patient not too deeply anesthetized or not overdosed with an opioid. In the latter situations, the ventilating hand can make the sigh in order to prevent progressive airway collapse and reduction in residual volume, accompanied by an increase in pulmonary shunting. While there is dispute over the meaning of the sigh, its natural occurrence during spontaneous breathing in the conscious subject suggests its physiologic importance.[13]

Use of a precordial or esophageal stethoscope is simply an economical extension of the senses; a means to observe the respiratory pattern and the quality of the heart sounds and rhythm; and the

event of accidents, such as air embolism, pulmonary interstitial emphysema, and pneumothorax. Harvey Cushing[14] deserves credit for the first description of the precordial stethoscope. In an article on "Some Principles of Cerebral Surgery" he observed:

> **With the patient in the prone position (suboccipital work) it is difficult for the anesthetist to gauge fully the variations in cardiac action, and during the past six months, Dr. Davis has employed in these, as in all operations indeed, a simple device: so satisfactory that one wonders why it has not long since come into general use—namely, the continuous auscultation of cardiac and respiratory rhythm during the entire course of anesthesia.**
>
> **The transmitter of a phonendoscope is secured by adhesive tape over the precordium and connects by a long tube with the anesthetist's ear where the receiver is held by a device similar to a telephone operator's headgear (Fig. 2-3).**

Pathophysiology

Dickinson Richards, Nobel Laureate, once remarked that a stethoscope cannot function without someone at each end. A stethoscope should be a ready resort during the course of anesthesia to test repeatedly the position of a tracheal tube or leakage about the balloon and to find the reason for a change in pulmonary compliance such as atelectasis, bronchospasm, pulmonary edema, and the more unusual complications—pneumothorax, air embolism, and pulmonary interstitial emphysema. Looking into the open chest during thoracotomy can reveal much with regard to development of complications. A lung on the verge of pulmonary edema may show dilated and congested lymphatic vessels. Leakage through a transected bronchus or during lobectomy can be confirmed as the reason for loss of volume in the breathing system. And after deliberate collapse of a lung either with use of a single- or double-lumen tracheal tube, reexpansion of the lungs can be followed by watching aeration as the lobules fill during collateral ventilation, while positive pressure is applied to the airway. Or the trachea may be seen to collapse with inspiration after removal of a goiter when the cartilages have been weakened.[15]

Even without a stethoscope, diagnosis of certain conditions can be made by applying the ear to the chest as the early practitioners must have done.

TABLE 2-2. Reduction of Error When Listening to Breath Sounds

System	Reduction in Tidal Volume*
Listening	91 ml ± 17
Not listening	190 ml ± 24

Increased Error From Distracting Anesthesiologist

System	Reduction in Tidal Volume**
Reading	171 ml ± 22
Not reading	126 ml ± 20

*$P < 0.01$. Data from 12 physicians.
**$P < 0.05$. Twenty physicians using semiclosed system.
(From Egbert and Bisno,[12] with permission.)

W.B. Bean wrote on the precordial noises that can be heard at a distance from the chest.[16] Traumatic pneumothorax, air embolization, pulmonary interstitial emphysema, and pneumopericardium all can produce adventitious sounds that have been described by many a phrase: a paddle wheel on a river, the grinding of gears in a machine, a rustling of leaves, loud crackling noises, or a mill wheel murmur (*Muhlengerausch, bruit de moulin*, Hamman's sign of pulmonary interstitial emphysema), and the pericardial knock and tapping sounds as in the clicking of a telephone receiver. Bowel sounds and borborygmi are also audible with eventration of the diaphragm or trauma, and herniation of stomach or bowel into the thorax. Practically all of these sounds (other than those associated with ruptured heart valves) derive from the presence of air bubbles of various volume in and around the heart or in the mediastinum—as the beating heart agitates them.

Laennec described the pathologic appearance of pulmonary interstitial emphysema as "beads of bubbles along the strands." The Macklins[17] found that such bubbles, originating in rupture of the terminal alveoli adjacent to the septa, are propelled along those pathways either to the mediastinum or subpleural sites, downward retroperitoneally, or into the neck, as subcutaneous emphysema. The pleura, the mediastinum, or the peritoneum may burst with the increased pressure, resulting in pneumothorax or pneumoperitoneum.

Much has been written about the utility of the Doppler effect in recognizing these events, but in the majority of cases a precordial stethoscope would serve the purpose just as well. The use of nitrous oxide during inhalation anesthesia makes every little bubble so much larger by reason of gas diffusion into their lumina.

Hypoxia and Hypoxemia

The blood that flows in operations under the influence of ether is not much altered in color. The blood which spirts [sic] from a divided artery is sometimes of its usual vermilion tint, at the very time when the inhalation is going on: frequently under these circumstances, however, the arterial blood is rather less bright than usual, but the venous blood being at the same time less dark than common, the flow of mixed blood is of the ordinary color of such blood; and the patient's lips remain unchanged in hue.

Thus wrote John Snow[1] in 1847, who could detect hypoxemia and the probable reasons for it, simply by observing the character of bleeding in the operative field. Thus, whenever feasible, anesthetists should examine the color of the blood in the surgical incision to detect hypoxemia, even if

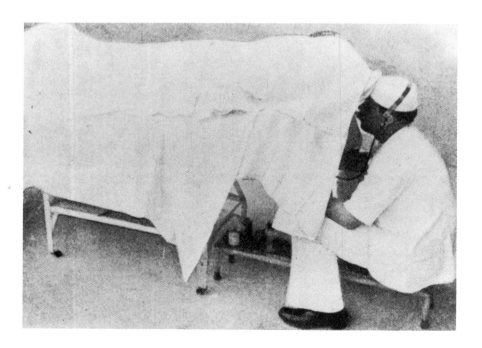

Fig. 2-3. Patient in prone position draped for suboccipital operation. Anesthetist wearing head band with receiver and tube leading from phonendoscope. (From Cushing,[14] with permission.)

the diagnosis causes a false alarm. And so should surgeons view the blood as they work.

Snow commented not only on the color and the force of arterial bleeding but also on the arteriovenous oxygen difference. There is nothing archaic about that observation. An increase in the arteriovenous oxygen difference is easily seen when a skin incision is made during spinal anesthesia. The blood is dark because of stasis and pooling on the capacitance side of the circulation but the arterial blood is bright red—vermilion more aptly describing it. More than a few observers have commented on the appearance of dark venous blood during malignant hyperthermia syndrome where oxygen consumption is high and the arteriovenous oxygen difference is consequently large. Conversely, venous blood is brighter than usual when the mitochondria are poisoned by cyanide as when sodium nitroprusside is given to induce vasodilation and deliberate hypotension.

Cyanosis

Although the routine use during anesthesia of pulse oximeters is now mandated in the United States, it is still important to observe for cyanosis. Interpretation of blood color, though subject to individual variation, may be more accurate than the diagnosis of cyanosis in the skin or mucous membranes. In general, cyanosis may appear without hypoxemia if stasis of capillary flow occurs as in the vasoconstriction of hypothermia or with stasis in the blush area so often observed in the plethoric patient. In order for cyanosis to develop, at least 5 g of hemoglobin must be present in the reduced state in the mean capillary circulation, the equivalent of 7.5 vol% of unsaturated blood.[18] Thus, cyanosis may not develop at all with hypoxemia in the presence of severe anemia, 10 g or less. Conversely, when polycythemia and an increased hemoglobin content pertain, the skin is ruddy in hue despite 95 percent or more of hemoglobin saturated with oxygen. Dark blood and cutaneous cyanosis may also be the result of methemoglobinemia or sulfhemoglobinemia. Basically, the problem in detection lies in the fact that the red plus blue of oxygenated and reduced hemoglobin respectively, give rise to a heliotrope or mauve coloration, which is most pronounced only in areas of high capillary density: the lips, mucous membranes, ear lobes, tips of the digits, and subungual zones. The ap-

pearance also depends on the length and number of capillaries filled with blood plus the thickness and pigmentation of skin overlying those capillaries.[19]

Comroe and Botelho[19] reported on the unreliability of cyanosis in the detection of hypoxemia by selected groups of physicians. With the employment of an ear oximeter to record oxygen saturation, and manipulation, behind a screen, of the oxygen concentration inhaled by a subject who was observed for appearance of cyanosis by the physicians, the accuracy of their diagnoses was recorded. A majority of the observers were unable to detect definitely the presence of cyanosis until the oxygen saturation fell to approximately 80 percent; 25 percent of observers did not note definite cyanosis even at oxygen saturation levels ranging from 71 to 75 percent (Table 2-3). Furthermore, there was wide variation in the ability of any observer to detect cyanosis in different test subjects, even in the same subject at different times. And there were considerable differences in color estimation among five to ten observers as they watched for development of cyanosis in the same subject at the same time. It is worth noting that these experiments were carried out at a controlled, ambient temperature with optimal, natural lighting. Modern fluorescent lighting confuses the issue.

THE CIRCULATION

Of the physiologic systems thus far discussed, the circulation is perhaps least comprehensively and continuously monitored by the senses. We have al-

TABLE 2-3. Highest Level of Arterial Oxygen Saturation at Which Definite Cyanosis Was Noted by Each Observer Who Made One or More Series of Consistent Observations

Oximeter Reading (Arterial O_2 Saturation)	Students	Staff	Total
100–96	1	—	1
95–91	9	2	11
90–86	15	5	20
85–81	19	7	26
80–76	9	2	11
75 or below	18	2	20
Total	71	18	89

(From Comroe and Botelho,[19] with permission.)

ready noted that John Snow could learn much about the circulation by observation of the operative field and the character of bleeding. And so can the modern anesthesiologist!

The Pulse

Snow was also aware of the information to be had by feeling the pulse. In describing the fourth degree of etherization he stated: "The pulse is distinct and of good volume even in patients affected with hectic, in whom just before the inhalation it was small and hard. It is usually accelerated as in all other stages of etherization."[1] During the controversy over the cause of sudden collapse during chloroform anesthesia, many clinicians held the pulse with the finger. Clover's chloroform apparatus with the reservoir of chloroform vapor slung over the shoulder permitted him to apply the face mask and palpate the radial pulse simultaneously (Fig. 2-4). During any anesthetic, the arterial pulse is well within reach: most conveniently and while holding a mask to the face—the external maxillary

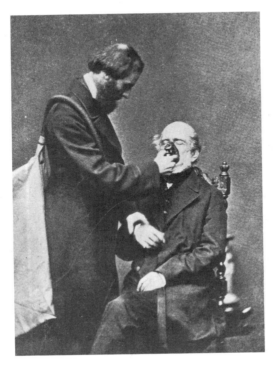

Fig. 2-4. J.T. Clover demonstrating how chloroform was administered with his apparatus. Note finger on the radial pulse. (From Duncum,[27] with permission.)

artery particularly evident in the child, or the superficial temporal just anterior to the tragus of the ear; the carotid over the carotid tubercle when there is a question of adequacy of cerebral circulation; the radial artery because the arm is usually extended on an arm board. Anesthesiologists routinely test for the presence of a pulse in the ulnar artery by means of Allen's test before radial artery catheterization. If the thorax is open, the beating heart is evident and aortic pulsations are accessible to the surgeon, and during laparotomy when question arises the surgeon can always palpate the abdominal aorta. Even the dorsalis pedis, the posterior tibial, the popliteal, and femoral arteries are within reach when the anesthesiologist is working at the patient's side without access to head or neck. The veins in the neck and arms can yield information on elevated pressure, perhaps the result of obstruction within neck or chest or onset of pulmonary edema and congestive heart failure. Elevation of the vasodilated arm above the level of the right auricle can also provide a crude index of venous pressure.

Various patterns of pulse contour are diagnostic of specific circulatory abnormalities: Corrigan's or water hammer pulse with capillary pulsation in severe aortic regurgitation; the slow rise and fall of the pulse wave in aortic stenosis; a rapid rise and runoff in the presence of arteriovenous fistula; and, most commonly, the rapid, thready pulse associated with hemorrhage or diminished blood volume. The commonly held belief that major blood loss is signaled by rapid pulse is erroneous, especially during anesthesia with the circulatory depression caused by the inhalation agents now employed. During World War II when questions arose over the need for blood transfusion, Shenkin et al.[20] bled volunteers progressively larger volumes of blood in an effort to establish reliable diagnostic signs of hemorrhage. The effects of controlled, acute bleeding could be separated into three stages of severity. In the first phase following a 500-ml phlebotomy, there was little alteration in cardiac output as revealed by ballistocardiography, and the subjects while supine were symptom-free with blood pressure and pulse within the normal range. In the second phase, following a 1,000-ml phlebotomy (20 percent of average normal blood volume), there were still no noteworthy abnormalities so long as the subject was recumbent. But an upright position could not be tolerated and syncope arose soon after arising. In the third phase, with a 1,500- to 2,000-ml bleed (40 percent of blood volume), syncope accompanied by bradycardia arose even though the subject was recumbent (Fig. 2-5).

Both palpation of the pulse and recording of blood pressure via auscultation and listening for Korotkoff sounds depend on the character of the pulse wave. The latter is essentially a manifestation of ventricular stroke volume modified by a number of physiologic and physical influences: the quantity of blood returned to the left ventricle during diastole, as assisted by auricular contraction, thus lengthening the ventricular fibers and invoking the Starling effect; the inotropic state of the left ventricle as affected by autonomic tone and the biochemical milieu; and the presence or absence of myocardial dysfunction; the so-called afterload as the ventricle contracts and ejects its contents into an elastic conduit, the aorta. All of these modifiers determine the nature of the propagated wave known as the pulse (Fig. 2-6).

In summary, Bruner[21] depicted the nature of the peripheral pulse as follows:

The pressure pulse begins as a complex phenomenon, subject to marked modifications in traveling from the root of the aorta to the periphery. Broadly arched initially, it increases in amplitude and becomes narrower as it travels. Separate elements show increasing temporal dispersion, some disappear, other undulations are added as the energy package is processed through the systemic arterial tree. Reflections and pressure changes simultaneously occur.

Despite the modifications, however, the pulse as palpated by the finger does yield an index of the cardiac output. Indeed, mathematical formulas have been derived to calculate the stroke volume and cardiac output as measured by the area under the recorded pulse wave. Whether the pulse, as a measure of the mean arterial blood pressure, also connotes adequacy of tissue perfusion is disputable.

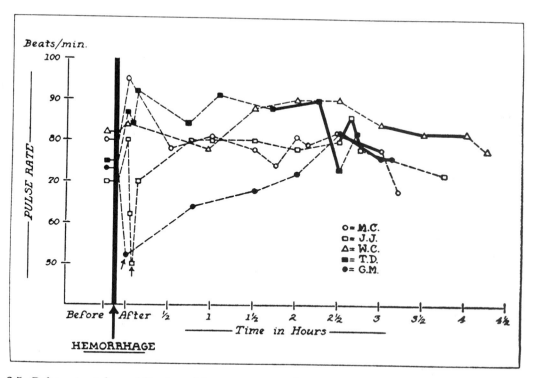

Fig. 2-5. Pulse rates taken while the subjects were recumbent and at rest, in five normal subjects before and after bleeding of approximately 1,000 ml, and after replacement of the blood. The heavy lines connecting the symbols indicate the periods during which the blood was being replaced. The arrows indicate points where some subjects suffered acute symptoms as a result of severe bradycardia. (From Shenkin et al.,[20] with permission.)

The pulse wave as detected by the Riva-Rocci technique is the simplest means of measuring blood pressure, sufficient to allow ready diagnosis of a high or low state and to treat accordingly. Thus the auscultatory technique remains an essential element of circulatory monitoring during anesthesia. Although the pressure is measured routinely at 5-minute intervals (now automatically), there is no reason why the measurement cannot be recorded more frequently in times of trouble. When a question arises and the auscultatory sounds are not heard, pressure can be judged by palpation of the pulse. One should not fault the cuff in such a situation but proceed directly to palpation, then to readjust the cuff if a pressure is indeed present. Devices are now available to measure and visually record the blood pressure at one minute intervals using the principle of the Riva-Rocci technique.

The Nature of Blood Loss

As noted, observation of the character of bleeding in the operative field is an essential means of monitoring both respiration and circulation. When

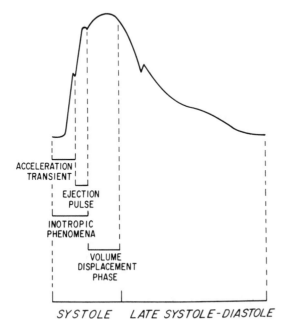

Fig. 2-6. Pressure pulse. The "acceleration transient" (Peterson) is the force that initiates inscription of the upstroke of the pressure pulse. Systolic upstroke is continued as a result of ejection of the first portion of the stroke volume into the aortic root. The other terms are self-explanatory. (From Bruner,[21] with permission.)

a tourniquet is employed on an extremity for a bloodless operation one must be all the more alert to keep track of the circulation elsewhere, by the other means already mentioned. Gillies discussed some of the anesthetic factors that may increase or otherwise influence blood loss during anesthesia.[22] The pattern of intermittent positive breathing, whether manually or mechanically applied, can increase venous pressure and diminish cardiac output, the latter especially in the presence of hypovolemia. Other factors include the position of the patient as it might increase or decrease venous return, carbon dioxide accumulation, overtransfusion or excessive fluid replacement, and the sympathetic stimulation action of certain anesthetics. In using deliberate hypotension for certain kinds of operations, these modifying factors must be controlled in order for the technique to be effective.

No better means exists for routine assessment of blood loss than by observation: the degree of bleeding, either rapid or slow; the saturation of surgical sponges and weighing them; and blood collected in the suction container. These are rough guides but one soon learns to know the approximate amount of blood lost during certain routine operations. It is worth emphasis that excessive oozing in the field may be a manifestation of a mismatched blood transfusion. In hypovolemia not all of the volume lost is blood, for one must take into account the continued loss postoperatively of protein-rich fluid into tissue spaces as well as fluids sequestered in the bowel as a result of intestinal obstruction, plus that recovered by gastric suction. Probably, the most accurate method of measuring blood loss is to rinse all of the sponges and drapes in a washer until clear, then to measure the hemoglobin concentration in the effluent. However, this is a cumbersome, time-consuming technique and can only be completed when the operation is over. Several mathematical equations have been devised to calculate the amount of permissible blood loss before transfusion might be considered necessary.[23] Unfortunately the factors in these equations are little known quantities at the time: the blood volume beforehand, hematocrit before and after, and the degree of hemodilution at the time.

Although urinary output (indirectly an index of blood volume) is a good guide to perfusion of the kidneys, most often output falls because of the antidiuretic effects of the anesthetics given, plus the effects of surgical trauma. In the severely ill and depleted patient, the state of hydration may be estimated by noting skin turgor and condition of the mucous membranes.

BODY TEMPERATURE

The majority of patients are expected to experience a drop in body temperature during anesthesia because of air conditioning in operating rooms, the vasodilation induced by anesthetics, use of semiopen or semiclosed rebreathing systems, the administration of cold fluids intravenously, the heat lost from exposed body cavities and finally the inhibition of thalamic temperature control by anesthetics. Even a degree or two fall in body temperature may be hazardous for the patient with a compromised coronary circulation because postoperative shivering and increase in body metabolism may place large demands on the circulation. Major degrees of hypothermia interfere with the action and metabolism of drugs, delay awakening, and cause difficulty in recording blood pressure via the auscultatory technique.

A rise in body temperature might be anticipated in a patient already febrile with uncontrolled sepsis or in a hot and humid environment where the infant and child might suffer most. Marked and precipitous elevations occur upon transfusion of bacteriologically contaminated bank blood or administration of pyrogen-containing liquids. Most feared, however, is the temperature rise associated with the malignant hyperthermia (MH) syndrome. This is not the place to discuss the development of MH syndrome, its prevention or treatment once recognized. Surely if suspected by reason of a telltale history and physical characteristics of a patient, continuous recording of body temperature is a priority.

Merely feeling the skin of the forehead is a useful guide, and the changes observed may impel the anesthesiologist to record temperature if it is not already being measured. Monitoring of body temperature is rather simply done and, noninvasively, with uncomplicated, reasonable apparatus. With little need for utter accuracy, a pharyngeal, esophageal, or rectal thermistor probe suffices for this purpose. Skin temperature strips have not been reliable in this regard. Tympanic membrane recording, perhaps the closest approximation of all to brain temperature, has not caught on for routine use. Likewise, skin temperature electrodes may be useful for special purposes as in diagnostic and therapeutic nerve blocks.

MISCELLANEOUS OBSERVATIONS

Few if any of the developments noted under this heading can be discovered by technical means. The sense of smell can detect leakage of gases or vapors from the anesthesia machine, the fetor of infection, the occurrence of rectal incontinence during spinal anesthesia, a leaking bowel anastomosis, the uremic odor on the breath of a patient in renal failure, or the smell of smoke or charred material that might suggest a shorted electrical circuit or defective apparatus, or a conflagration elsewhere in the hospital.

No means exist to prevent various kinds of injury to patients other than careful observation: (1) to prevent brachial plexus palsy by assuring that an arm is not hyperabducted, dorsiflexed, or rotated or that the shoulder is not downwardly displaced or the head and neck flexed in the opposite direction; (2) to guard against pressure on the body unknowingly exerted by members of the operating team; to be certain that an arm rest is well padded and arm positioned so as to avoid traction or pressure on ulnar or radial nerves; (3) to watch for extravasation of solutions and blood, particularly when administered under pressure; (4) to be sure that the peroneal nerve is not stretched around the head of the fibula with the legs in stirrups during lithotomy, or that the nerve is not compressed against the uprights of the stirrups; (5) to be certain that the legs are not crossed or that an instrument stand does not dorsiflex the foot; and (6) to watch the hand at the patient's side so that the fingers are not crushed as the foot piece of the operating table is elevated.

Repeated observation is required to be sure that the pressure of a pneumatic tourniquet is not too high and not used over too long a time or allowed to deflate early during intravenous regional anesthesia. Pressure gauges on pneumatic tourniquets should be calibrated from time to time to assure that the gauge reading is correct. And as in the rapid release of a vascular clamp, so must hypotension be anticipated when the pressure of a tourniquet is released.

Ocular injury can largely be prevented by making certain that the lids are closed during operation and that pressure is not unintentionally applied to the orbits by the surgeon, or by pressure of the head in the face-down or occipital positions. With the eyes beyond view, the lids are best taped shut but in ordinary operating positions this need not be done if the lids remain closed. One loses a valuable means of detecting hypoxia and depth of anesthesia if the position of the eyes and the size of the pupils cannot be seen. Lubricants may be instilled into the conjunctival sac to protect the cornea when the conjunctivae are dry but no evidence exists that their routine use prevents damage.

The manner of application of a grounding plate during employment of diathermy apparatus must be checked to avoid burns or electrocution, and the same applies to other kinds of electrodes applied to the skin. Arteriovenous shunts in the patient with renal failure, insulin pumps, cardiac pacemakers, intravenous alimentation lines, and certain kinds of prostheses also merit protective custody during the course of anesthesia.

The skin and mucous membranes are of course observed for appearance of cyanosis, sudden pallor, and the appearance of wheals that might signal the onset of an anaphylactoid reaction.

NOISE IN THE OPERATING ROOM

At one time, operations were performed in an atmosphere of hushed tones and conversation was kept to a minimum so that the procedure might be carried out expeditiously with all the respect due the gravity of the occasion. This philosophy has changed so that excessive noise of various origins is the usual mode: mechanical respirators, drills, saws, suctioning, diathermy apparatus and so on, plus no limit on casual conversation. While it is a good plan to have the conscious patient listen to soothing music via earphones, commonly, today, radios and piped-in taped music blare forth with entertainment of all kinds: classical, jazz, pop, rock, punk rock, and so on. Incidentally, one also worries that the surgeon's hand might be affected in its delicate dissections, but more cogently, noise defeats many of the essentials of monitoring: use of the stethoscope, the alarm that might indicate disconnection of a respirator, the beep of an electro-cardiograph, the warning signal of a low inhaled oxygen concentration, and the many adventitious sounds of importance that come from the patient as previously discussed.

In the journal *Anaesthesia*, Philip Ayre introduced an editorial with the following quotation from Shakespeare's *The Tempest*:

> **The isle is full of noises,**
> **Sounds and sweet airs, that give delight and hurt not.**

There follows, in the opening paragraph, a description of one patient's experience.[24] "A celebrated Scottish opera singer recently complained in a BBC programme that, while waiting in an anaesthetic room before having his hernia repaired, the hospital loudspeaker system played a rousing selection of well-known hymns including, 'Abide with Me,' and 'Nearer My God to Thee,' which he considered highly inappropriate to the circumstances."

Shapiro and Berland[25] noted that modern surgery had discovered the dangers of air and water pollution about a century ago and, as a result, has practiced aseptic antipollution techniques since then. However, they remarked that in our pollution-aware age, surgery has fallen behind in its recognition of what has been called "The Third Pollution." This is noise, defined as unwanted, noxious, or harmful sound. Using a noise-measuring instrument in an operating room, decibel measurements were made on the A scale, which approximates the greater sensitivity of the human physiology to higher frequencies of sound, and the scale used most commonly in noise surveys and establishment of legal controls. Not recorded but omnipresent were the doctors' paging system and a public address system as well as the constant babble of conversation. Recordings revealed that noise in the operating room frequently exceeded that of an automobile freeway, and more frequently approximated that of a kitchen with a food blender in operation, a railway train, or a truck—approximating the 90-dBA maximum permissible noise exposure (for 8 hours) of the United States Federal Occupational Safety and Health Act. The noise worsened during operations in which specialized motorized instruments were employed, and the electrocautery created even more noise. "Surgery," they said, "like other aspects of modern civilization needs a 'Think

Quiet' movement: Working in a pleasantly quiet environment, the surgeon (and anesthesiologist) will suffer less fatigue, fewer psychologic and physiologic effects and greater accuracy; the patient will also benefit.'' And so will the efficiency and efficacy of monitoring.

SUMMARY AND CONCLUSIONS

It is probable that a competent anesthesiologist would be able to give safe anesthesia for most kinds of operations on patients in the better physical status category by simple use of the senses for monitoring purposes, even without the aid of a blood pressure cuff or electrocardioscope. This approach would consist of a continuation of the preanesthetic physical examination throughout operation. To do this, an anesthesiologist would have to stay in close contact with the patient, watching the operative field, feeling for the pulse, observing respiration, listening all the while, and using the other senses to detect more unusual events. In the same context, the anesthesiologist would have to remain at the head of the table to follow the course of operation to anticipate surgical needs and to assess the degree of muscle relaxation and operating conditions in general. With a hand applied to the reservoir bag, most respiratory problems would be diagnosed, with resort to the stethoscope when needed. The state of the circulation would be followed by appraisal of the pulse, the degree of bleeding, and the color of the blood in the operative field. A host of miscellaneous observations would be made that might not be detected in time by mechanical or electrical means to prevent catastrophe.

This kind of approach is not meant to imply that much accessory information of great benefit to the patient might not be gained by the use of more complicated apparatus. But that apparatus must also be monitored by the senses without distracting attention from the patient. Monitoring of the kind envisioned in this chapter applies to general, regional, and local anesthesia: A high degree of dedication and learning is required for success. According to Gillespie,[26] ''Two qualities of the anaesthetist will produce such a result: professional commonsense and skill born of practical experience.''

REFERENCES

1. Snow J: On the Inhalation of the Vapour of Ether. John Churchill, London, 1847
2. Siegrist HE: Surgery before anesthesia. Bull School Med U Maryland 31:116, 1947
3. Thomas L: The Youngest Science. Notes of a Medicine Watcher. Viking Press, New York, 1983
4. Comroe JH, Jr: Retrospectroscope. Insights into Medical Discovery. p. 120. Von Gehr Press, Menlo Park, CA, 1977
5. Galla SJ, Rocco AG, Vandam LD: Evaluation of the traditional signs and stages of anesthesia. Anesthesiology 19:328, 1958
6. Davis HS, Collins WF, Randt CT, Dillon WH: Effect of anesthetic agents on evoked central nervous system responses. Anesthesiology 18:634, 1957
7. Plomley F: Operations upon the eye. Lancet 1:134, 1847
8. Guedel AE: Third stage ether anesthesia: a subclassification regarding the significance of the position and movement of the eyeball. Am J Surg Q Suppl Anesth Analg 53, 1920
9. Snow J: On Chloroform and Other Anaesthetics. Their Action and Administration. John Churchill, London, 1858
10. Roizen MF, Harrigan RW, Frazer BM: Anesthetic doses blocking adrenergic (stress) and cardiovascular responses to incision—MAC BAR. Anesthesiology 54:390, 1981
11. Gillespie NA: The signs of anaesthesia. Anesth Analg Curr Res 22:275, 1943
12. Egbert LD, Bisno D: The educated hand of the anesthesiologist. Anesth Analg 46:195, 1967
13. Gold MI: The present status of sighing. Anesthesiology 30:565, 1970
14. Cushing H: Some principles of cerebral surgery. JAMA 52:184, 1909
15. Mayer EC, Jr: Tracheal collapse during thyroidectomy: a case report. Anesth Analg 30:238, 1951
16. Bean WB: Precordial noises heard at a distance from the chest. Cincinnati J Med 35:121&159, 1954
17. Macklin MT, Macklin CC: Malignant interstitial emphysema of the lungs and mediastinum as an important occult complication in many respiratory diseases and other conditions. Medicine 23:281, 1944
18. Lundsgaard C, Van Slyke DD: Cyanosis. Medicine 2:1, 1923
19. Comroe JH, Jr, Botelho S: The unreliability of cyanosis in the recognition of arterial anoxemia. Am J Med Sci 214:1, 1947
20. Shenkin HA, Cheney RH, Govons SR, et al: On the diagnosis of hemorrhage in man: a study of volunteers bled large amounts. Am J Med Sci 208:421, 1944

21. Bruner JMR: Handbook of Blood Pressure Monitoring. PSG Publishing, Littleton, MA, 1978
22. Gillies J: Anaesthetic factors in the causation and prevention of excessive bleeding during surgical operations. Ann R Coll Surg Eng 7:204, 1950
23. Gross JB: Estimating allowable blood loss: corrected for dilution. Anesthesiology 58:277, 1983
24. Ayre P: Editorial. Anaesthesia 35:233, 1980
25. Shapiro RA, Berland T: Noise in the operating room. N Engl J Med 287:1236, 1972
26. Gillespie NA: Simplicity in anaesthesia. Br J Anaesth 22:192, 1950
27. Duncum BM: The History of Inhalation Anaesthesia. Oxford University Press, London, 1947

Human Factors Issues in Monitoring

3

Richard Botney
David M. Gaba

During World War II numerous aviation mishaps were attributed to *human error*. Many design problems involving the cockpit were discovered and fixed because they were contributing to the likelihood that error would occur. *Human factors,** an applied science with elements of psychology, engineering, physiology, systems analysis, computer science, anthropometry, and other fields, arose out of this work.[1] Its objective is making things easier to use, and tasks easier for a person to accomplish, by optimizing equipment design, tools, the environment, and the task to accommodate human needs and limitations.

Interest in the role of human factors in anesthesia has increased dramatically over the past two decades. It is believed that human factors play a key role in the evolution and prevention of error in anesthesia.[2–4] The importance of human error as a contributing factor in anesthesia safety was emphasized by Cooper and colleagues[5] in their studies of critical incidents in the operating room. Human error was involved in 82 percent of the reported incidents. Furthermore, they found that human factors problems with anesthesia equipment contributed to 12 percent of the incidents that had a "substantive negative outcome."

Monitoring can reduce errors and accidents, and make anesthesia safer, whether it be with a finger on the pulse, or the latest monitoring techniques. However, it has been pointed out that simply introducing monitoring technology into an operating room does not reduce risk.[6] In principle, a significant number of mishaps might be prevented only if the monitors are *applied and used correctly, function continuously, with their outputs assimilated, interpreted, and acted upon correctly.*[6] Some would argue that monitors and alarms, in general, decrease vigilance and distract attention away from patient care.[7–9] Certainly the proliferation of complex monitoring devices, the plethora of alarms, and their potential as distractions add further to the human factors problem in monitoring.

The role of human factors in monitoring is to make monitoring devices that are simple to use, function continuously, and provide accurate information that is easy to interpret and act upon. This goal is accomplished by applying human factors principles to the design of monitors and the workspace, while taking into account that work environments may differ and that workload can vary widely (Table 3-1). A monitor that is poorly designed from a human factors viewpoint may be confusing to use, can increase workload, and is likely to be misinterpreted, thereby increasing the likelihood of mishap. This chapter describes the application of human factors to monitoring in anesthesia and intensive care. It will not address the human factors of devices and techniques that are not involved in monitoring, nor the principles of crisis management, as they are well described elsewhere.[10,11] Please note that specific pieces of equipment may be mentioned as illustrations of some aspect of good or bad human engineering. This in no way

---

*Synonymous terms for human factors, *ergonomics* and *human engineering*, are used interchangeably in this chapter.

constitutes an overall endorsement nor a condemnation of those devices, as every device has both positive and negative features (none is perfect), and each must be evaluated in terms of many attributes. Also please note that the term "anesthetist" will be used to refer to any person administering an anesthetic, whether that person is an anesthesiologist, a physician who is not an anesthesiologist, or a certified nurse anesthetist.

BACKGROUND

Design standards developed in the 1970s and 1980s by the American National Standards Institute (ANSI),[12] and subsequently by the American Society for Testing and Materials (ASTM),[13] began including human engineering specifications for anesthesia equipment. In the mid-1980s, human factors guidelines were published by the Association for the Advancement of Medical Instrumentation for use by designers of medical devices.[14] These standards and guidelines are believed to be beneficial, but it has been recognized that they are limited in their scope and application.[15] In 1986 Eichhorn and others published standards for basic intraoperative monitoring of patients at the Harvard Medical School.[16]

In 1971 Blum described the application of human factors principles to anesthesia monitoring.[17] He was primarily concerned with the human engineering and layout of pressure gauges on the anesthesia machine. In 1973 Drui and coworkers[18] filmed anesthesiologists at work and reported a task analysis of their time in the operating room. Several subsequent time and motion studies have demonstrated that as much as 60 percent of an anesthetist's time is spent observing or monitoring the patient.[19–23]

Further research on the human engineering of anesthesia monitoring devices was performed throughout the 1980s. While much of it, like Blum's original report, concerned "hardware" aspects of device design, making the device physically easier to use, additional human factors problems were also being appreciated. Monitors and the monitoring task have become more sophisticated and complex, with integrated displays, intelligent decision support, "smart" alarms, and automated recordkeepers to help manage the ever-increasing amounts of data presented to anesthetists. Using studies of workload, vigilance, and attention, human factors specialists have begun to address these concerns about making monitoring easier.

HUMAN FACTORS, MONITORING, AND INFORMATION PROCESSING

Human Factors and Usability

The basic principle underlying human factors engineering is that "things" should be designed to assist human beings in simply and safely perform-

TABLE 3-1. Characteristics of Different Anesthesia Work Settings

Characteristic	Routine	Busy	Crisis
Time pressure	Little or no time pressure	Moderate time pressure	Severe time pressure
Resources required	No additional help needed to accomplish tasks	May need assistance	Assistance needed to accomplish tasks
Alarm frequency	Alarms occur infrequently	Alarm frequency is somewhat increased	Alarms sound frequently
Demands on attention	Low; distractions and false alarms are easily managed	Increased; distractions and false alarms impede optimal care but are still manageable	High; distractions, especially from alarms, may impede basic patient management
Task demands	Monitoring is the major activity	Monitoring patient status competes with additional tasks	Additional tasks usurp attention from monitoring and basic patient management
Overall workload	Workload (physical and mental is unremarkable	Workload near capacity	Workload may exceed capacity

ing tasks. Humans should not have to adapt to "things," which may increase a task's difficulty, as well as the potential for error. Originally, changes in the layout and design of hardware, such as the shape, size, and spacing of components, made equipment *physically* easier to use. More recently emphasis has been placed on task support by making equipment *mentally* easy to use. This aspect of human factors in monitoring involves understanding visual and auditory cognition, vigilance and the allocation of attention, decision making, and information processing. Human factors specialists use various methods to evaluate and improve the human-machine *interface* and its *usability* (Fig. 3-1).

A monitor's usability is largely determined by the interface between it and the humans who use it (Fig. 3-2). Much of what is called human error actually results from poor interface design. The interface is more than just the monitor's display and controls, however. It also includes the monitor's alarms, error messages, printouts, user documentation, labels, and on-line help. Nonetheless, this chapter shall focus primarily on the ergonomics of displays, controls, and alarms.

There is no widely accepted, formal definition of usability. However, there are a few attributes that experts seem to agree enhance the usability of an interface. These include ease of learning to use the device, simplicity in using the interface, minimizing of error, speed of use, and performance of the largest number of useful functions. Early applications of human factors in anesthesia dealt primarily with the design of individual components such as gauges, dials, switches, knobs, and other hardware, and their layout on the anesthesia machine. Computer technology has made the user interface much more complex. Instruments now display multiple screens of information and incorporate keys with multiple functions. There are complex interactions between the user and the device, including multiple modes of operation, aspects of which can be relatively hidden from the user. These features have made assessment of the usability and the ergonomics of such devices more complicated than in the past.

The use of contemporary anesthesia monitoring equipment poses ergonomic challenges for several reasons. *First*, the standards for design of monitors and for certain other aspects of the anesthesia work environment are limited in scope.[15] Few ergonomic studies of monitoring have been done. *Second*, a given manufacturer may design only a single piece of equipment, in isolation from other manufacturers, the user, the task, and other equipment. As new instruments become available, they are added to an existing system incrementally, thereby deterring system integration (Fig. 3-3). *Third*, the end

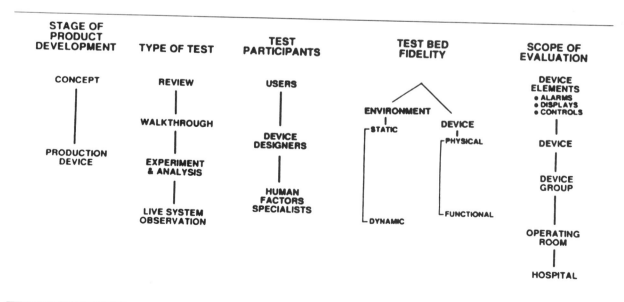

Fig. 3-1. Aspects of human factors evaluations. (From Cook et al.,[15] with permission. Copyright © 1990 by Richard Cook.)

users are usually not involved in the design process. Instruments may be designed by engineers with little knowledge of the user or appreciation for the user's tasks. Error messages often use cryptic language that is unfamiliar to the average user. For example, the SARA mass spectrometer (PPG Industries, Inc., Lenexa, KS) displays the message "SYSERR-01" to indicate a blocked sampling line. *Fourth*, there may be little, if any, prototyping of monitors to see if the users' needs are being met, and if the instruments are indeed usable. The prospective purchaser's evaluation of devices typically takes place under routine conditions of use. However, the operational and usability limitations of a monitoring device may become apparent only during times of high workload or crisis, when the contribution of monitoring to workload should be minimized. *Fifth*, documentation and user manuals for monitors are frequently written using engineering terminology, making them difficult to comprehend. On-line help, a recent development that allows the user to display information relating to the device's operation while the device is in use, tends to be rudimentary. It often provides insufficient assistance to the user, especially in highly time-pressured situations.

Because of all these factors, there is a huge installed base of equipment that suffers from human engineering deficiencies. Methods to improve the usability of this installed base, such as better in-service training and the use of checklists or other cognitive aids, are not widely used at present but are being considered.

Principles of Good Design

The first step in ensuring that monitoring equipment will better support the tasks of anesthetists in the clinical setting is for designers to utilize known principles of good human factors engineering. Guidelines for basic aspects of human factors design of medical equipment have been promulgated by the American Society for Testing and Materials (ASTM)[13] and by the American Association of Medical Instrumentation.[14] These guidelines address mainly the "hardware" aspects of design. They leave much room for interpretation, and there is still much variation in their application. Cook and associates[15] warn that these guidelines "may be only weak filters for identifying deficiencies." Thus, the guidelines represent only the first step in improving the ergonomics of monitoring.

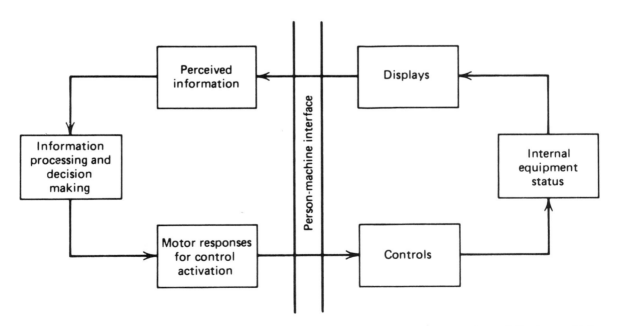

Fig. 3-2. Diagram of a generic human-equipment interface. The interface consists of displays, which provide information to the user, and controls, which permits the user to send information to equipment. (From Kantowitz and Sorkin,[24] with permission.)

In *The Psychology of Everyday Things*, Don Norman,[25] one of the leading figures in applied cognitive science, has enumerated several principles of good design. These are as follows:

Make things visible. Not only should the display and controls be visible, but messages should be easy to understand and the operational mode of the device clearly observable. The function and purpose of a device should be apparent; it should be obvious what actions are possible and how to do them. Furthermore, there should be clear feedback of the user's actions.

Communicate clearly. Labels for controls, displays, and alarms should be clear. The language used in messages, on-line help, in user manuals, and on printouts should be easy to understand (Fig. 3-4).

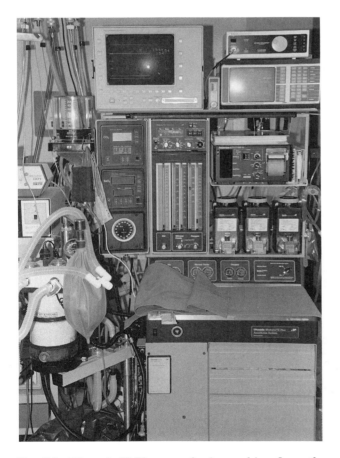

Fig. 3-3. Ohmeda II Plus anesthesia machine from the authors' operating room. Monitors from four additional manufacturers placed upon the machine's shelving form a compact monitoring array.

Provide correct and natural mappings. Mapping describes the relationship between a stimulus and a response. Pushing a button labeled "START" on a noninvasive blood pressure monitor initiates a blood pressure measurement. However, a button that is labeled "START MEASUREMENT" represents a better mapping. The three stages of mapping are (*1*) between intentions and possible actions, (*2*) between actions and the resulting effects, and (*3*) between information about the system and the actual system state. These mappings should each be as clear as possible. Users should be able to determine that the actual system state corresponds to their perception of it.

Don't be arbitrary, be consistent. Guidelines and written or de facto standards should be followed where applicable. Words and actions should have the same meaning in different situations.

Simplify tasks. Whenever possible, tasks should be simply structured. This will minimize the amount of planning or problem-solving required. The appropriate use of technology is to make complex tasks more simple.

Use appropriate constraints. Natural and artificial constraints will limit what the user can and cannot do. An example of this is the O_2/N_2O interlock mechanism that prevents delivery of hypoxic gas mixtures. The user should feel as if there is only one possible thing to do: the right thing. At any step, constraints will reduce the number of alternative actions to very few at most. However, as a recent report illustrates, constraints are not foolproof and can be defeated.[26]

Design for error. Assume that busy users will make errors. Therefore, design clear recovery pathways for all errors that can be imagined. This will require close communication between anesthesiologists, experts in the ergonomics of anesthesia, and manufacturers. Formal research into the human factors of monitoring may be necessary, including the use of simulators to test devices under crisis conditions.

A complementary set of principles for the evaluation and design of usable interfaces has been provided by Molich and Nielsen[27]:

Provide simple and natural dialogues between humans and machines. All information should appear in a logical and natural order. Extraneous information that could compete with relevant information should be avoided (Fig. 3-4). Extraneous information may be irrelevant in all circumstances, or it may be irrelevant only in particular situations. In the latter situation it may be difficult for a device to know what is or is not irrelevant.

Speak the user's language. It is clearly important that dialogue should be expressed in words, phrases, and concepts familiar to the user, rather than in computer-oriented or engineering terms. For example, the Ohmeda 7810 Ventilator Control Module (BOC Healthcare, Inc., Murray Hill, NJ) displays the message "Drive Ckt Open" when the Bag/APL-Ventilator Switch is in the Bag/APL position during mechanical ventilation.

Minimize the user's memory load. The user should not have to remember information from one part of the dialogue to another, for example, the sequence of push buttons to initiate a cardiac output measurement. Instructions for using equipment should be visible or easily retrievable whenever appropriate. Complicated instructions should be simplified as much as possible.

Provide feedback. The equipment should always keep the user informed about what is occurring by providing appropriate status information. For example, the Colin Press-Mate (Colin Medical Instruments Corp., San Antonio, TX) blood pressure monitor gives no indication that a measurement attempt has failed, but instead displays the old reading.

Provide clearly marked exits. The equipment should never trap the user in a situation that has no visible escape. If a mistake is made, it must be clear how to correct it without having to take drastic steps, such as restarting the device.

Provide shortcuts. Appropriate shortcuts can make equipment more useful to the experienced user. These features will make the equipment easier to use, but should remain unseen or unavailable to the novice user. A corollary to this is that the standard operation of a device should be straightforward, while the more esoteric features an experienced user will want to employ can require more effort.

Provide good error messages. Good error messages are precise and constructive. Exact information is provided about the cause of the problem, and meaningful suggestions inform the user what to do about it. The language used should not blame the user for the problem.

Admittedly, there is probably no single best design that applies to all monitors, under all conditions. What is good human engineering for one device or for one work environment (for example, intensive care) may not be so for another (for example, the operating room). There has been a trend to incorporate ever more operational features into devices, which in turn increases their complexity. There is a continual tradeoff between additional features that increase flexibility of use and simplicity of operation. Every new feature re-

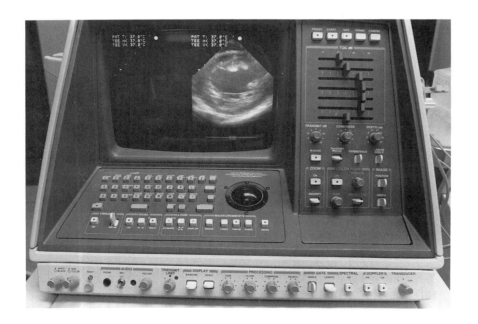

Fig. 3-4. Hewlett-Packard SONOS OR transesophageal echocardiograph. Note the large number of controls, many of which are not typically used by the anesthesiologist. Many keys are labeled with engineering terminology that many anesthetists will not understand.

quires the addition of control functions, whether by adding new switches or knobs or by adding more soft keys and levels of menus (Fig. 3-5A,B). To optimize a device for its intended user, a variety of special techniques are necessary (Table 3-2). In particular, early prototyping with feedback from anesthetists will weed out designs that are clearly deficient. Furthermore, testing of actual devices under a variety of actual or simulated conditions of use will confirm whether design features can actually support the clinician's task.

Monitoring

Monitoring during anesthesia has many definitions, but we prefer the following: monitoring is the *process* by which an anesthetist obtains infor-mation about the course of the anesthetic, and interprets and responds to that information, while continually reevaluating the situation. The information obtained can be about the status of the patient, the status of the equipment, or the status of interventions administered by the anesthetist. Devices such as infusion pumps and patient warming units, with displays, controls, and alarms, also require monitoring.

The monitoring task is an important part of the anesthetist's work. However, the nature of the monitoring task has changed over time. Originally, the anesthetist was the monitor, visually observing ventilation and palpating the pulse. Over the years, instrumentation was added to supplement such direct observation of the patient. However, devices

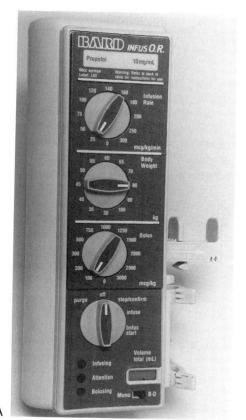

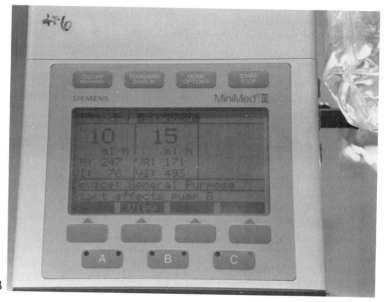

A   B

Fig. 3-5. (A) The BARD INFUS-OR syringe infusion pump uses four knobs to control the infusion. The dedicated controls facilitate straightforward operation. **(B)** The Siemens MiniMed III infusion pump is capable of controlling three separate infusions. Multiple modes of operation for three independent infusions are supported by a small number of controls, using menus and a cursor to indicate the active mode.

TABLE 3-2. Human Factors Techniques for Design and Evaluation of Devices

Technique	Description
Design guidelines and standards, usability specifications, checklists	Starting point for design of usable devices
Questionnaires	Survey users as to what they want or need, or regarding satisfaction with usability of a device
Task analysis	Generic name for a set of observational techniques used to obtain knowledge about the types of tasks and how they are performed
Contextual inquiry	Field research method consisting of observation and interview during ongoing work
Cognitive walkthrough	Evaluation of interface usability by mentally reviewing the steps needed for a typical user to accomplish a task
Interaction analysis	Observational method for the study of videotaped activities that examines the interactions between humans and technology
Link analysis	Study of the flow of activities, including analysis of the probabilities of transition fron one activity to another
Heuristic evaluation	Method of study that looks for properties that, from experience, will lead to usability problems
Controlled experimentation and benchmark testing	Usability testing in which factors influencing usability are systematically manipulated or controlled
Prototyping and simulation	Modeling of devices to evaluate usability prior to production
Iterative design	Design process whereby information on usability is incorporated into redesigns of equipment

like the electrocardiograph (ECG) or instruments for measuring blood pressure were little more than electromechanical replacements for the finger on the pulse. Most recently, with the widespread use of computer technology, monitoring has become much more complex. In addition to monitoring many more parameters than ever before, information is being presented at a higher level, and complex interactions are required to operate the monitors. The anesthetist continues to directly observe the patient, but also uses a wide variety of equipment to obtain information about the anesthetic (Table 3-3).

The above description identifies three important aspects of the monitoring task: (1) the display of information that is acquired by the anesthetist ("input"); (2) information processing; and (3) actions that are taken by the anesthetist ("output"), primarily through the operation of controls, or the administration of drugs.* Another aspect of monitoring is control of the anesthetist's attention, of which alarms are a primary component. Alarms are

designed to attract the anesthetist's attention to certain information on monitors or in equipment.

Monitoring may add to the anesthetist's workload. In periods of high workload the individual's capacity to process information may be exceeded.[28] For example, Gaba and Lee[29] studied the spare capacity of anesthesia residents to respond to addition problems displayed on a computer in the anesthesia workspace. They found that 40 percent of problems were either skipped or were responded to after a long delay because the resident was otherwise occupied. These findings have been confirmed using somewhat different techniques by Weinger and colleagues[23] and by Loeb.[30]

Howard[31] reported a case involving an automated noninvasive blood pressure monitor that illustrates how workload can impair monitoring. In this particular instrument, changing the measurement interval is a two-step procedure. First, the desired interval between measurements is selected. Then the start key must be pressed to enter the change and to restart the measurement cycle. Otherwise, the device remains "in limbo," and does not measure at either the old or the new interval (a design flaw). In the reported case the start key was not pressed (a human error). Because the anesthetists were preoccupied with mixing a nitroglycerin infusion and changing a ventilator bellows,

---

*Please note the following conventions: this chapter refers to devices such as displays as "inputs," because they input information to the user. Similarly, controls are referred to as "outputs." This convention is thus from the view of the anesthetist rather than the device.

they failed to detect that the blood pressure monitor had not cycled for 40 minutes. This design flaw is not likely to be appreciated until an incident such as this occurs.

Thus, monitoring is more than just a vigilance task. It is one of information processing and data management. An important aspect of the anesthetist's task is the conservation of mental capacity and its appropriate allocation during dynamically changing situations. Ideally, the monitoring task is simple, does not increase the anesthetist's workload, and provides accurate information.

Information Processing

Information processing is a generic term referring to the acquisition and manipulation of symbolic data. The typical information-processing model represents human cognitive function as a series of subsystems, each of which performs a different function and has inputs to and outputs from the other subsystems. Many models of human information processing exist that differ in scope and complexity.

Gaba[11] has developed an explicit model of the cognition and information processing involved in the anesthetist's conduct of anesthesia (Fig. 3-6). It depicts the anesthetist as working at five different interacting cognitive levels to implement and control a core process of *observation, decision, action,* and *reevaluation* (Table 3-4). This division of mental activities into cognitive levels follows the work of Jens Rasmussen[32,33] and James Reason.[34,35] Multiple cognitive levels support parallel processing (performing more than one task at a time) and multitasking (performing only one task at a time, but switching very rapidly from one task to another).

Gaba extended Rasmussen's model by adding two more levels of mental activity that provide for dynamic adaptation of the anesthetist's own thought processes. This ability to "think about thinking" in order to strategically control one's own mental activities is called "metacognition" by psychologists and is thought to be an important component of working in complex, dynamic domains.[36,37] *Supervisory control* is concerned with dynamically allocating finite attention between routine and nonroutine actions, between multiple

TABLE 3-3. Devices Requiring Attention in the Operating Room

Routine Equipment Monitors	Routine Patient Monitors	Special Patient Monitors	Additional Devices Requiring Monitoring
Pipeline and cylinder pressure gauges	Automated noninvasive blood pressure	Invasive blood pressures (arterial, central venous, pulmonary artery)	Intraaortic balloon pump
Suction vacuum gauges	Electrocardiograph (ECG)	Cardiac output, PCWP	Infusion pumps
Flowmeters	Capnograph	Electroencephalogram or evoked potentials	Heated humidifiers
Vaporizer dials	Anesthetic agent analyzer	Transesophageal echocardiograph	Forced air warmers
Ventilator controls	Inspired oxygen (F_{IO_2})	Cerebrospinal fluid pressure	Blood/fluid warmers
Ventilator bellows	Airway pressure	Coagulation (activated clotting time)	
Line isolation monitors	Bladder catheter	Fetal heart rate	
CO_2 absorber color and temperature	Esophageal or precordial stethoscope	Continuous blood gases	
	Neuromuscular blockade	Transcranial doppler	
	Pulse oximeter	Cerebral oximeter	
	Temperature	Mixed venous oximeter	
	Spirometer		

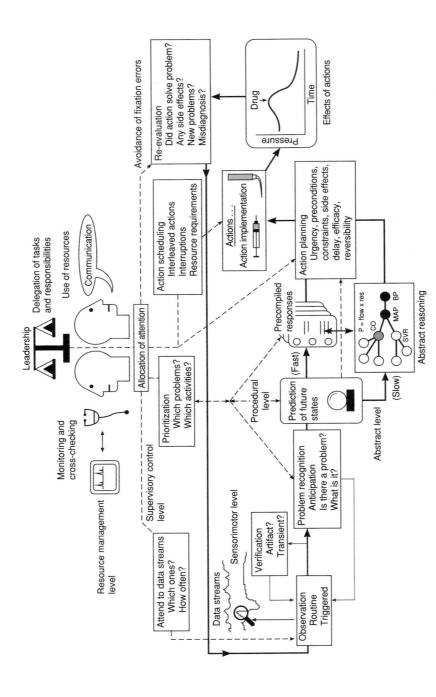

Fig. 3-6. A model of cognition and information processing involved in the conduct of anesthesia. See text for details. (From Gaba et al.,[11] with permission.)

problems or themes, and between the five cognitive levels. *Resource management* deals with the command and control of available resources, including teamwork and communication.

Attention sharing is needed between cognitive levels, between tasks, and often between problems. The intensive demands on the anesthetist's attention could easily swamp the available mental resources. Therefore, the anesthetist must strike a balance between acting quickly on every small perturbation (which requires considerable attention) and adopting a more conservative "wait and see" attitude. This balance must be constantly shifted between these extremes as the situation changes. Erring too far in the direction of "wait and see" can be particularly catastrophic. In addition to the attentional demands of the anesthetist's core tasks, the operating room environment is full of distractions. Routine events, such as turning the operating table or repositioning the patient, distract attention from the main process of conducting the anesthetic. Other distractions include teaching in progress, incoming phone calls, background music, and conversation with operating room personnel. Expert anesthetists *modulate* the distractions, eliminating them when the workload is high, while allowing them to occur when workload is low (in order to improve morale and team building).

Observation

The core process of observation represents the input of displayed information to the anesthetist. A multitude of information sources are present in the operating room. Because the human mind can only attend closely to one or two items at a time, the anesthetist's supervisory control level must decide to what information to attend and how frequently to observe it. Routine aspects of this core process operate primarily at the sensory/motor and procedural levels and are executed repetitively throughout the course of an anesthetic.

Information is obtained by a variety of methods, including scanning or searching, reading text, pattern-matching, and responding to cues that capture our attention. Note that a cue's salient features (e.g., brightness, loudness, flash rate, location in the visual field) may direct attention to that cue out of proportion to its importance. Information is communicated via one or more sensory channels, such as visual, auditory, tactile, or olfactory. Parallel processing improves the human's limited ability to process information from multiple stimuli at one time. Several dimensions of information (e.g., heart rate and rhythm from an ECG tracing) and multiple sensory channels (e.g., heart rate visually from an ECG and auditorily from the pulse oximeter) can be processed simultaneously.

Language factors may affect the anesthetist's comprehension of information. Logical reversals require translation to understand the meaning of a statement.[38] For example, "check to see that the valve is closed" requires less mental processing than "check to see that the valve is not open." Instructions given in the active voice are better understood than those in the passive. Instructions given in a sequence different from the order in which the actions are to be performed are called "order reversal."[38] For example, instructions should read "put probe on finger, then turn on oximeter" rather than "prior to turning on oximeter, put probe on finger."

TABLE 3-4. Description of the Five Cognitive Levels in Gaba's Model of Cognition and Information Processing During the Conduct of Anesthesia

Cognitive Level	Description
Sensory/motor	Activities involving sensory perception or motor actions that take place with minimal conscious control
Procedural	Regular routines, derived and internalized from training and prior work episodes, performed in a familiar work situation
Abstract reasoning	Reasoning from first principles and deep medical knowledge, using abstract causal reasoning in unfamiliar situations for which no well-practiced expertise or routine is available
Supervisory control	Dynamic allocation of finite attention between routine and nonroutine actions, between multiple problems or themes, and between the five cognitive levels
Resource management	Command and control of available resources, including teamwork and communication

Once information has been obtained it must be verified and assessed. If a problem is recognized, decisions must be made about what actions to take in response. In the operating room environment the available information is not always reliable. Most monitoring is noninvasive and indirect, and is therefore prone to *artifacts* (false data). Even direct clinical observations, such as vision or auscultation, can be ambiguous. Brief *transients* (true data of short duration) can occur and will quickly correct themselves. To prevent them from triggering precipitous actions that may have significant side effects, critical observations must be *verified* before they are acted upon. Verification uses a variety of methods, including:

Repeating the observation or observing the short-term trend

Observing an existing redundant channel (e.g., invasive arterial pressure and cuff pressure are redundant)

Correlating multiple related (but not redundant) variables (e.g., heart rate, heart rhythm, and blood pressure)

Activating a new monitoring modality (e.g., placing a pulmonary artery catheter)

Recalibrating an instrument or testing its function (e.g., breathing into a capnometer sampling line)

Replacing an entire instrument with a backup device

Asking for a second opinion from other trained personnel

Anesthetists assess their observations to decide if the patient's course is "on track" or if a problem is occurring. If a problem is found, a decision must be made as to its identity and its importance. Anesthetists and other dynamic decision-makers use approximation strategies to handle ambiguous situations; psychologists term such strategies *heuristics*.[39] Use of heuristics is typical of expert anesthetists and often results in considerable time-saving in dealing with problems.

Decision

Having recognized a problem, how does the expert anesthetist respond? In complex dynamic domains like anesthesia many problems require quick action to prevent a rapid cascade to a catastrophic adverse outcome. For these problems, de-

riving a solution through formal deductive reasoning from "first principles" is too slow. The initial responses of experts to the majority of events stem from precompiled "rules" or "response plans" for dealing with a recognized event.[31–34,40] This is referred to as *recognition-primed decision-making* because once the event is identified the response is well known.[41] However, anesthesia cannot be administered purely by precompiled "cookbook" procedures. Abstract reasoning about the problem utilizing fundamental medical knowledge still takes place in parallel with precompiled responses even when quick action must be taken.

Action

The transfer of information from the anesthesiologist to the anesthesia and monitoring equipment represents the core process of action. A hallmark of anesthesia practice is that anesthetists do not just write orders in a patient chart; they are directly involved in implementing the desired actions. At any time during an anesthetic there may be multiple things to do, each of which is intrinsically appropriate, yet they cannot all be done simultaneously. The anesthetists must consider the following factors:

Preconditions necessary for carrying out the actions (e.g., it is impossible to measure a thermodilution cardiac output if there is no pulmonary artery catheter in place).

Constraints on the proposed actions. Some actions are incompatible with other aspects of the situation (e.g., it is impossible to check the diameter of the pupils when the head is fully draped in the surgical field).

Side effects of the proposed actions. These often play a controlling role in choosing between possible drug therapies.

Rapidity and ease of implementation of proposed actions. Those easily and rapidly performed are preferred to those requiring more time, attention, and skill.

Certainty of success of the actions. This is often traded off against rapidity and ease of implementation. Under some circumstances the higher certainty of success of a set of actions will justify the investment of time, attention, and resources needed to implement them.

Reversibility of the action and the "cost of being wrong." Rapidly reversible actions are preferred to those that cannot be reversed, especially when potential side effects are significant.

"Cost" of the action in terms of attention, resources, and money.

The anesthetist's response involves scanning and searching for the appropriate control to activate, reading to verify that the proper control is being manipulated, and judging the extent of manipulation, such as setting a dial to a precise value. Action implementation can usurp a large amount of the anesthetist's attention. In addition, anesthetists engaged in manual procedures are strongly constrained from performing other manual tasks, as demonstrated in several of the mental workload and vigilance studies described previously.

Reevaluation

In order to cope with the rapid changes and the profound diagnostic and therapeutic uncertainties seen during anesthesia, the core process includes repetitive reevaluation of the situation. Thus, the reevaluation step returns the anesthetist to the "observation" phase of the core process, but with the following specific questions in mind:

Was the initial situation assessment or diagnosis correct?

Did the actions have any effect? (e.g., did the drug reach the patient?)

Is the problem getting better, or is it getting worse?

Are there any side effects resulting from previous actions?

Are there any new problems or other problems that were missed before?

Faulty reevaluation can result in a type of human error termed *fixation error*[42,43] (see below).

Errors in Information Processing

Error is an everyday, unavoidable occurrence in all cognitive activities, including the administration of anesthesia. Monitoring is used to minimize the occurrence of errors, allow their early detection and correction, and mitigate their sequelae. Obviously, not all errors lead to patient morbidity or mortality, and usually the practitioner can recover from an error. In Cooper's[5] study of critical incidents in anesthesia, only 7 percent of incidents actually produced a substantive negative outcome.

Error classification is important because it points the way to corrective action and error prevention (Table 3-5). *Slips* can be prevented by the use of engineered safety devices (e.g., pin-indexed compressed gas cylinders, vaporizer interlocks, O_2/N_2O ratio limiter).[44,45] As previously indicated, errors can still occur if these safety mechanisms are defeated.[26] *Mistakes*, on the other hand, are more difficult to correct, since it is the intention and not the action that is faulty.[44,45] Training, skills, and knowledge appear to be the most important methods for reducing mistakes. *Mode errors* can be prevented by decreasing the number of operational modes, or by indicating the mode extremely clearly. *Fixation error* is best prevented by continued reevaluation of the situation. Three types of fixation error are[42]:

This and only this. The persistent failure to revise a diagnosis or plan. Despite plentiful evidence to the contrary, the available evidence is interpreted to fit the initial diagnosis. A fixation of attention on a minor aspect of a major problem is also an example of this type of error.

Everything but this. The persistent failure to commit to the definitive treatment of a major problem. An extended search for information is made without ever addressing potentially catastrophic conditions. Another example of this type of error occurs when the anesthetist is hypervigilant and too quickly becomes enmeshed in dealing with a number of relatively trivial or transient events.

Everything's OK. The persistent belief that no problem is occurring in spite of plentiful evidence that it is. In such cases abnormalities are attributed to artifacts or transients. This error of denial is also evident when the anesthetist fails to declare an emergency or accept help when facing a major crisis.

TABLE 3-5. Error Classifications

Error Type	Description
Slip	Appropriate action that is improperly executed
Mistake	Inappropriate actions that are executed as planned
Fixation error	Persistent failure to revise a diagnosis or plan despite evidence that it is inadequate or incorrect
Mode error	Action appropriate for one mode of operation that is performed when the device is operating in another mode

Fixation error is an important class of error in dynamic domains such as anesthesiology, and is just beginning to be studied.[46]

DISPLAYS

Task analyses have shown that much of the anesthetist's task consists of gathering information. The display is the interface element by which this information is provided to the anesthetist (Fig. 3-1). This interface between the anesthetist and the equipment provides information to the anesthetist by one or more sensory channels, most commonly visual, although monitoring is performed with our other senses as well. The auditory channel is used for auscultation, for the heartbeat tones emitted by instruments, for alarm tones, and for abnormal noises, such as the sound of blood being suctioned or ventilator operation. Feeling skin temperature, diaphoresis, and CO_2 absorber temperature are examples of monitoring with the sense of touch. The sense of smell can detect volatile anesthetics or fire.

Hardware, software, and cognitive considerations need to be addressed in the design of each individual display, and in the layout and groupings of displays in the workspace. Newer monitors may incorporate multiple monitoring modalities into a single display; this integration of information requires very careful application of human factors principles. The information provided by the display should be clear and unambiguous, and the intended "use" of the display should be self-evident. Good display design will enable rapid and accurate comprehension of the information being displayed. Anything that impedes the processing of information from the display will affect monitoring. For example, messages that are cryptically written require more time to understand.

Visual

The visual display can present information in an alphanumeric or graphic format. The mechanism of display can be mechanical (e.g., dial or counter) or electronic. Which manner of display is best for a particular task usually depends on cost as well as on the task, the person doing the task, and the context in which the task is done. Human factors principles will differ for each type of display, although they share some basic characteristics. Three important properties of visual displays are *visibility*

(can the display be seen), *legibility* (can the displayed characters be distinguished from each other), and *readability* (can the displayed information be understood).[47] However, the overall human factors of visual displays goes beyond these basic features.

The physical characteristics of monitor displays should enable easy acquisition of information by the anesthetist. Such characteristics include character size, font, and style; brightness, contrast, and the effect of ambient lighting; and character and display color. These are generally well described by the available standards and guidelines.[13,14] Other important considerations include display location, type, layout, grouping, format, and how information is coded.

Characters

The appropriate character size for a display will depend on the task at hand. Too small a character will be difficult to read, while too large a character can disrupt normal eye movement patterns and take up scarce display space. The appropriate character height will depend on viewing distance, ambient illumination, and the text's importance. One recommendation is that the minimum character height be 15 minutes of visual angle.[14] At a viewing distance of 24 inches this corresponds to a character height of about 0.10 inches. Most current displays exceed this minimum. Height-to-width ratio, stroke width, and character spacing should also be chosen so as to ensure legibility. Search tasks and reading tasks require characters large enough to be clearly read. For a quick scanning task smaller characters, more densely packed, are satisfactory.

Legibility will also depend on the character font and print style. One essential consideration in assessing fonts is character confusion. In certain fonts, some characters are more easily confused than in other fonts, for example, the "5" and the "S," or the "Y" and the "V." As a rule, the more a character resembles a regular stroke character, the easier it will be to read. Capital letters are preferred to small letters only for short messages.

Brightness and Contrast

Brightness is a subjective sensation associated with a specific luminance of a display. Contrast refers to the difference in luminance between the displayed information and its background (Table 3-6). Generally, the brighter the display and the better the contrast, the more legible the display. Ambient light reflecting off the display will decrease contrast and thus legibility. Various techniques for mitigating the effect of ambient light include reduction of ambient light level, locating the display optimally relative to the ambient light sources, and tilting the display. For example, Ohmeda allows the shelf on its Modulus anesthesia machines to tilt down for this reason, and certain LCD displays allow electronic adjustment of the viewing angle (akin to tilting the display). Other options to improve contrast include the use of nonglare glass on screens or screen filters (which decrease ambient luminance to a greater extent than the luminance of the displayed information, thus increasing contrast). However, the use of tinted goggles, such as those used during laser procedures, may interfere with monitoring. They are generally used in conditions of low ambient light, and their effect on brightness, contrast, and the interpretation of color can affect the visibility and legibility of displayed information.

Color

Color can be used for coding information (see below), but the choice of character and background color can also affect legibility. The use of color is affected by ambient lighting and its effect

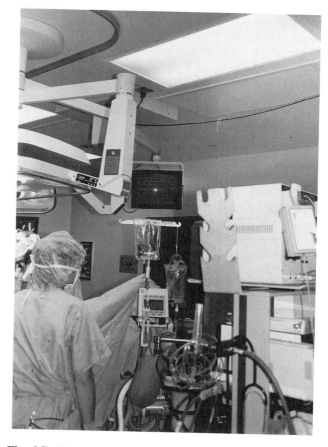

Fig. 3-7. Slave display placed so that the anesthetist can observe it while facing the surgical field.

on contrast, since certain colors have better contrast characteristics than others.

Location

Various methods have been suggested to bring all or some of the visual displays in front of the anesthetist, thereby enabling him or her to view the patient and, at the same time, to observe important monitor information without turning away. *Slave displays* are in use in some operating rooms (Fig. 3-7). A slave display is simply a second display, mounted on the wall or ceiling, that replicates the information from the primary display so that it can be viewed by several personnel, including surgeons. Another alternative is to place the primary display on a boom arm so that it can be brought forward from the machine.

Another suggested method is a *heads-up display*,

TABLE 3-6. Terms Used in the Measurement of Illumination

Term	Definition
Light	Radiant energy in the form of electromagnetic waves, with a wavelength that evokes a visual sensation
Radiant power (flux)	Rate of flow of radiant energy
Luminous power (flux)	Radiant power weighted according to the spectral sensitivity of the eye
Luminance	Luminous power reflected or emitted from a surface in a specified direction
Brightness	Subjective sensations associated with a given luminance
Contrast	Difference (ratio) in luminance between a target and its background

much like those used by fighter pilots. In one attempt at this, the anesthetist wears a headset, which positions the display just above the normal line of sight. To be most useful, the communication between the device and the primary display must be wireless. However, there are important differences between the fighter pilot's tasks and those of the anesthetist. Fighter combat requires intense hand-eye coordination, with the pilot's gaze continuously engaged in tracking the enemy at high speed. Even though the anesthetist's visual channel is highly utilized, the requirement for uninterrupted vision is orders of magnitude lower. Furthermore, the anesthetist is free to move around, and in fact must gaze at a variety of elements in the operating room environment. Thus, although heads-up displays might offer some benefits to the anesthetist, they are likely to be minor compared to those offered to the pilot.

Type

The choice of the appropriate type of visual display to be used for a given monitor will depend on the type of information to be presented, the task for which the information is to be used, the context in which it will be used, and the training and experience of the typical user(s).

Mechanical

Mechanical displays in the operating room are generally limited to pressure gauges, which are used for pipeline and compressed gas cylinder pressures as well as for airway pressure. These use moving pointers with fixed scales. They are best suited for displaying qualitative information, such as whether a gas cylinder is nearly full or nearly empty. Of course, they also provide quantitative information. Important characteristics of mechanical displays of this type include pointer design and scale marking. The pointer should extend to, but not obscure, the scale markings. To readily distinguish between the two ends of the pointer, the "nonactive" end should be shorter in length. The scale should increase in the clockwise direction, and the numbers should be outside the graduation marks so they cannot be obscured by the pointer. There should be an obvious break between the two ends of the scale, for example, to readily distinguish the empty from the full cylinder.

Electronic

The characteristics of electronic displays are more varied. Their readout may be alphanumeric (consisting only of letters and numerals), graphic, or text. The human factors characteristic of electronic displays is consequently more complicated, and depends on factors such as layout and grouping, format, and coding. *Layout and grouping* refers to the arrangement of information on the display, and the arrangement of displays in the workspace. How displayed information is arranged (on a single screen or in the workspace) contributes greatly to its ease of acquisition. The *coding* of information can affect interpretation of a display, as can *compatibility* between different displays. *Format* refers to the manner in which information is displayed. Information can be displayed on separate monitors, or it may be integrated from several sources into a single display. The latter is the current state-of-the-art, and the first generation of these monitors is now being installed in hospitals.

Layout. The layout of displays in the anesthesia workspace should ideally match the anesthetist's visual field. Three areas of attention in the visual field have been described: the stationary field; the eye field, where supplementary movements of the eyes are required for attention; and the head field, where movement of the head is also necessary (Fig. 3-8). Visual targets within a 30 degree angle are within the stationary field. This represents the area of foveal vision wherein multiple displays can be viewed simultaneously. Objects within a visual angle of 30 to 70 degrees are in the eye field, and peripheral vision is used to obtain information. Objects outside this range can be attended to only with head movements.

The relative importance and frequency of use should determine what part of the visual field a display occupies. Critical (primary) displays should preferably be within the stationary field, whereas emergency displays and displays of secondary importance can occupy the eye field. Although these principles are reasonable in the anesthesia work environment, they are not as critical as in other industries. *First*, it is not clear which displays should be considered primary and therefore belong in the central monitoring field. In fact, this may change during different phases of the anesthetic, and for different cases. *Second*, their tasks are rarely dependent on hand-eye coordination. *Third*, the domain is not as visually bound as others. Anesthetists are rarely seated in one position with a constant visual field, and the anesthesia workspace is not (yet) a fixed control panel or cockpit, but an assemblage of targets including the patient, surgeons, nurses, and monitors and equipment.

Grouping. Proper grouping of information elements on a display can enhance its readability, and make the displayed information more meaningful. This requires attention to (1) the overall character density on the screen, (2) the local density of other characters near each character, (3) the number of visual groups of characters, (4) the average visual angle subtended by those groups, (5) the number of labels or data values, and (6) the alignment of screen elements with each other.[49] How information is grouped should reflect its importance, frequency of use, and similarity of function. Gestalt theory is the basis for many grouping arrangements, wherein displays are organized according to innate human perceptual characteristics[47] (Fig. 3-9). Inappropriate or poor grouping can increase the time it takes to find information on the screen. This is especially true when multiple channels of information are viewed simultaneously, or must be mentally integrated. Also, grouping may be deleterious when attention must be focused on a single display element.

Format. Deciding whether an alphanumeric or graphic display format is optimal depends on the

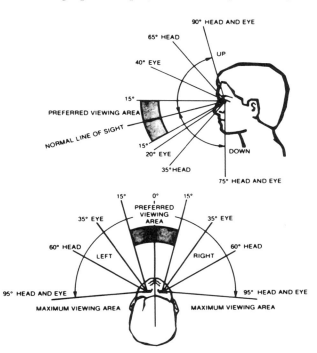

Fig. 3-8. Attention areas in the visual field. (From the Association for the Advancement of Medical Instrumentation,[14] with permission.)

		MAXIMUM*		
	PREFERRED	EYE ROTATION	HEAD ROTATION	HEAD AND EYE ROTATION
UP	15°	40°	65°	90°
DOWN	15°	20°	35°	75°
RIGHT	15°	35°	60°	95°
LEFT	15°	35°	60°	95°

* Display area on the console defined by the angles measured from the normal line of sight.

(Adapted from MIL-STD-1472B)

nature of the information being conveyed. Alphanumeric displays consist of letters and numerals. They are used in almost every electronic device, either for scales and labels, or to convey information. Alphanumeric displays are best for displaying quantitative data and data that are slowly changing. Graphic displays include *waveforms* and static graphics such as trend plots, and *figural* or *object* displays (e.g., bar graphs). Waveform displays are appropriate for rapidly varying data where the shape of the waveform gives specific physiologic information (such as ECG, invasive pressures, capnography). Static graphs are most useful where long-term trends or qualitative relationships between variables are important. Some graphic displays may encourage parallel processing of information (see below).

New display formats that have been recently introduced use dynamically varying graphics to present physiologic relationships in real time. In these techniques, sets of data are arranged to produce

recognizable patterns or "figures." One example is the "bar graph" type of display in which each variable is represented by a bar or an indicator bobbin. When all values are normal the bars or bobbins line up. A slightly different approach presents each "bar" radiating out from the center of the display. When all values are normal a regular polygon or circle is formed. Even newer are displays that represent the data values as attributes of a recognizable object or "glyph." In such a display, multiple attributes (such as color, shape, and size) of a single object can be processed in parallel. Fukui[50] has shown a prototype that uses a cartoonlike human face to represent overall patient status (Fig. 3-10).

Considerable research on such figural displays has been done in applied psychology laboratories and in industrial domains such as aviation and nuclear power. Figural displays appear to be most useful when figural patterns are not arbitrary but represent specific relationships to displayed variables. These displays allow the user to more quickly detect abnormalities, but alphanumeric displays are often superior for identifying the problem and its severity. Additionally, object displays may be best suited to tasks that require integration of information, while separate displays are better when attention must be focused on a single display element. The more abstract object displays have not been formally tested in any realistic setting in anesthesiology.

Coding. Perhaps the most important aspect of display ergonomics is the coding of information. Coding refers to the use of features added to displays that facilitate the interpretation of information by decreasing processing time and by making it easier to understand the displayed information. Displays may be coded by color, size, brightness, flash rate, or by the use of alphanumeric or other symbols.

Color is a common method for coding information that can have a significant effect on a product's usability. Color by itself can communicate information. For example, red constitutes a warning, yellow caution, and green a normal condition. Note that the addition of another coding modality, for example, a flashing red light, indicates an even more serious (life-threatening) condition.[14,47] Other colors can be used for coding, for example, the assignment of red, blue and yellow to arterial, venous, and pulmonary artery blood pressure wave-

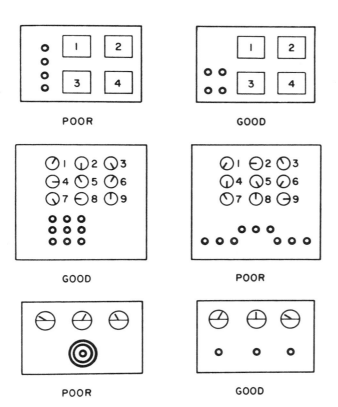

Fig. 3-9. Examples of poor and good groupings, based on Gestalt theory, of displays and their associated controls. (From Helander,[47] with permission.)

forms, respectively. Color coding is especially useful when displays are unformatted, the symbol density is high, or when searching for or tracking specific information.[47] Color can draw the user's attention to certain parts of the interface, for example, finding a specific numeric value that has been high-lighted with color, or discriminating between wave-forms. Functional groupings can be reinforced by using color.

The use of color in an interface depends on the tasks performed by the user and on the flow of information between the device and the user.

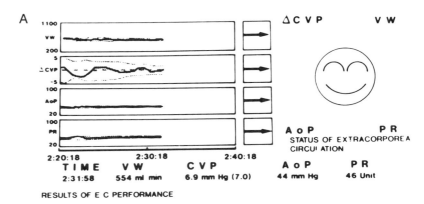

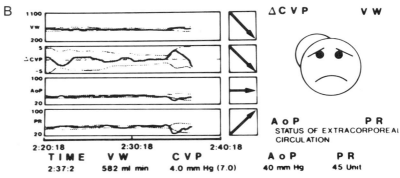

Fig. 3-10. Fukui's display format includes a human face to indicate the overall patient status. (From Fukui,[50] with permission.)

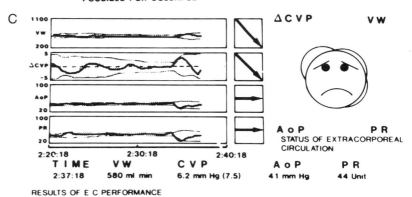

Color selection affects information recognition, discrimination, and legibility. There should be a contrast ratio of at least 7:1 between a colored object and its background.[51] Furthermore, lighting conditions can significantly affect how color is perceived. There is a limit to the number of colors that can be effectively used. More than ten causes visual clutter. Generally, five to seven colors are all that can be readily discriminated.[47,52] Furthermore, color-blind individuals, who constitute about 8 percent of the male population, may not benefit from the color coding of information.[51] Another consideration is the effect of aging on the perception of color. The sensitivity of the eye decreases with age, and some older individuals will experience a loss in their ability to differentiate light intensities and colors.[47,53]

Alphanumeric symbols convey information as text. Other symbols ("pictographs") can also be used (Fig. 3-11). For example, to indicate a disabled alarm, a bell with a line through it can be shown. Such pictographs can make the interface less language-specific and more intuitive. However, simple pictographs may not always convey information comparable to a short text message. For example, does the crossed-out alarm bell indicate that alarms on all variables are disabled, on only some variables, or only the auditory alarms?

When devices require complex interactions between the monitor and the operator, symbolic coding assumes more importance than ever. The symbols used should be simple and easy to understand. Achieving this goal is difficult without testing users under laboratory or carefully controlled field conditions, since the symbols may not be as easily understood by the user as the designer foresees. In a recent study by Forcier and Weinger,[54] American anesthesiologists were tested on their interpretation of the meaning of several proposed European standard graphic warning symbols (Fig. 3-12). In most cases the meaning of the symbols was incorrectly identified by the practitioner.

Auditory

Under certain circumstances, the auditory channel is preferred for the presentation of information to the anesthetist[55] (Table 3-7). For example, auditory displays are preferred for information transfer at low rates, while visual displays are best for high rates of transfer. The auditory channel is better when information occurs randomly or requires the immediate capture of attention. The auditory transfer of information can be used when attention is focused elsewhere. The best known examples of auditory displays include the pulse oximeter and the heart rate tone emitted by the ECG, however, the auditory channel is most commonly used for alarm annunciation (see section on alarms).

An advantage of auditory displays is that they are omnidirectional. However, this is also a disadvantage in that the auditory signal will also be heard

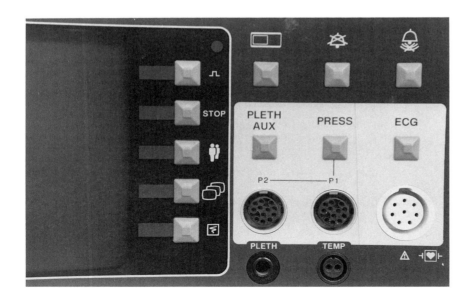

Fig. 3-11. Pictographic symbols on the Hewlett-Packard 78353B patient monitor.

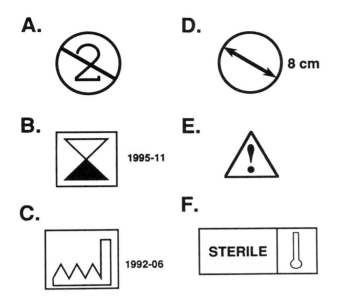

Fig. 3-12. Proposed European standard graphic symbols. The symbols have the following meanings: **(A)** Do not reuse. **(B)** Do not use after November 1995. **(C)** Manufactured in June 1992. **(D)** Internal diameter 8 cm. **(E)** See instruction leaflet(s). **(F)** Must be autoclaved. (From Forcier and Weinger,[54] with permission.)

by other operating room personnel and can be distracting. Furthermore, many individuals will be annoyed by the presence of more than one continuous auditory signal at a time. Because auditory information can be processed in parallel with visual information, using auditory displays can increase the amount of information available to the user. Because it is hard to reliably distinguish more than six different tones, the amount of information available from the auditory channel is limited.[56]

Coding of auditory displays is used to increase their information content, and follows principles similar to those of visual displays. Coding should take advantage of natural or learned relationships. Natural coding utilizes direct relationships between the original information and its displayed component, and is generally easy to decode without training. Methods of coding auditory information include loudness, pitch, duration, and repetition rate.

Pulse oximeter manufacturers frequently encode information about oxygen saturation into the heartbeat tone. The tone's pitch encodes oxyhemoglobin saturation, while the repetition rate displays heart rate. Clearly, this permits the parallel processing of auditory information. Coding of oxyhemoglobin saturation by pitch is an example of natural coding. The higher the pitch, the higher the saturation. However, not all pulse oximeters offer this feature, and some anesthetists are unable to hear the difference in pitch. Currently, the pitch changes 5 Hz for each 1 percent change in oxygen saturation. Schulte and Block[57] found that only 67 percent of volunteer listeners could reliably identify the first pitch change in a simulated pulse ox-

TABLE 3-7. Criteria for Selecting an Auditory or Visual Channel for Presentation of Information

Auditory Presentation	Visual Presentation
The message is simple.	The message is complex.
The message is short.	The message is long.
The message will not be referred to later.	The message will be referred to later.
The message deals with a discrete event in time.	The message deals with location in space.
The message calls for immediate action.	The message does not call for immediate action.
The visual system of the person is overburdened.	The auditory system of the person is overburdened.
The receiving location is too bright or dark-adaptation integrity is necessary.	The receiving location is too noisy.
The person is continually moving about.	The person remains in one position.

(Adapted from Deathridge.[55])

imeter signal; 11 percent of their subjects did not identify a change in pitch until the saturation dropped below 93 percent. They proposed a variety of schemes for improving the detection rate. A larger change in pitch between oxygen saturation tones, and/or a greater frequency range, might result in higher detection rates. A system that plays a "dual tone" is another possibility. However, neither these nor the original scheme have been rigorously tested.

Additional human factors concerns include ambient noise, the hearing-impaired practitioner, the effect of aging on hearing (presbyacusis), and the possible degradation of signal recovery because of these problems. Most pulse oximeters and ECGs make it possible to adjust sound level, thus minimizing the problem of ambient noise ("masking"). However, the effects of aging on pitch recognition are less clear. The earliest and most significant loss in hearing acuity occurs for frequencies above 2,000 Hz. Wallace and coworkers[58] have studied the impact of this hearing loss by measuring the air conduction hearing acuity of a group of anesthesiologist volunteers: 65 percent of the subjects had an abnormal audiogram, as compared with the general population. To assess which alarms would be beyond the hearing of the individuals studied, the abnormal audiograms were compared to frequency spectra that had been measured for 26 operating room alarms. Hearing deficits at high frequencies were found to be of a magnitude sufficient to interfere with alarm detection. Their study suggests that the aging anesthetist may not be capable of accurately detecting some auditory signals in the operating room, and that alarm design should take into account the effects of background noise and loss of hearing acuity. A potential alternative alarm annunciator for such individuals is a vibratory alarm, worn on the anesthetist's wrist.[59]

CONTROLS

Controls are the interface element for information transfer from humans to machines (Fig. 3-1). Controls are actuated by pulling, pushing, sliding, or twisting. Common types of controls in anesthesia include buttons, knobs, levers, switches, cranks, pedals, and keyboards. The type of information conveyed to the anesthetist's equipment may be ei-

ther continuous, discrete (i.e., discontinuous), or alphanumeric. The design of a control will determine the speed with which an action can be taken, the fineness of control, and the frequency with which errors are made. The proper design of controls should ideally support error-free operation of anesthesia equipment, with minimal training and little physical and mental effort. The use of a control, that is, how to manipulate it and what action will result, should be self-evident and unambiguous. Some elements of the human factors of displays, such as coding, layout, and grouping, can be applied to controls, but there are other considerations as well.

Traditionally, there was a single knob or switch for every function, but this is no longer feasible given the proliferation of functions. One strategy is to provide one or two generic buttons or knobs that can actuate multiple different features. For example, on Nellcor pulse oximeters (Nellcor Inc., Hayward, CA), the front panel finger wheel can control the volume of the auditory signal, as well as the settings of alarm thresholds for different variables. A somewhat different strategy frequently employed is to use a fixed set of push buttons or keys to represent different functions, depending on the location within the device's "menus." These are commonly known as "soft keys." Although this allows a nearly infinite variety of control functions, the price to pay is confusion in mastering the navigation of the complex menus. To combat this problem, newer monitors provide a certain number of dedicated keys that return the user to specific points in the menus. Structured dialogue boxes and on-line help screens have also been implemented to simplify user interaction.

The physical characteristics of controls include size, shape, texture, color, location (on the monitor), associated labels, and the type of actuation required (e.g., pushing a switch or turning a knob). Different types of controls and characteristics will be better suited for different types of actions and contexts. Many of these characteristics are addressed in detail by existing standards and guidelines,[13,14] and will not be discussed here. Physical characteristics are also important in the coding of controls, and are discussed in that context. The objective of control coding is to provide rapid and accurate identification of controls. Coding is generally achieved by visual and tactile features.

Size

Controls can be distinguished on the basis of size. Typically, three different sizes can be distinguished by touch, and about a 20 percent size different is required to make that discrimination.[60] Identical size should be used for controls performing similar tasks.

Shape and Texture

Control shape is more effective than size as a coding scheme. Along with size, shape permits control identification without visual contact or when lighting is poor. The shape of a control may be used to reflect the function of the control. In aviation, for example, the landing gear control is shaped like a wheel. Along with shape, texture is used for tactile coding of controls. Controls affecting critical functions should have a special shape. An example of this is the oxygen flowmeter control, which has a fluted knob to distinguish it from the other flowmeter knobs (Fig. 3-13).

Color

As a primary coding scheme, color has limitations, since it is strongly affected by ambient lighting as well as disturbances of color vision in a portion of the population. It is frequently used in combination with other coding methods, however. Color can aid in the search for a control, as in the green assigned to the oxygen flowmeter control. Highlighting a control with color will make it stand out against an array of other controls. This assumes more importance if a control is used frequently or has an important function. Color can also be used to reinforce functional groupings. Certain colors, such as red, yellow, and green, can themselves convey information, as noted in the discussion on displays. It should be noted that color codes are not yet standardized throughout the world. For example, the international color for oxygen is white, not green as it is in the United States.[61]

Layout

The location of controls and their grouping can strongly affect usability (Fig. 3-9). Controls can be grouped sequentially, thereby representing the sequence of steps to be taken. They can be grouped by function, wherein controls of similar function are grouped together. Such grouping arrangements minimize mental processing and the time necessary for multiple-control operations. Certain controls should have standard locations, such as the right-hand position of the oxygen flowmeter knob in the United States (*Note*: both existing European practice and proposed European standards locate this control on the left[62]). If a control is frequently used, or is vital, it should be located within a central actuating range, while infrequently used controls can be placed more peripherally. It should

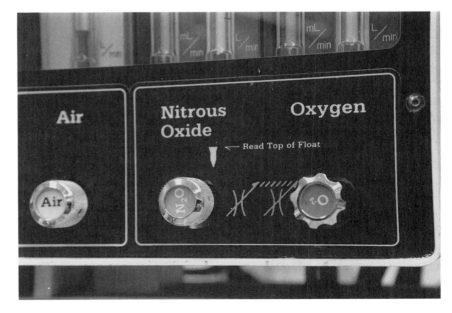

Fig. 3-13. Oxygen flowmeter control on the Ohmeda anesthesia machine, in conformance with ASTM Standard F1161-88. Note that the fluted knob differs from the controls for N₂O and air, and so can be distinguished by feel alone.

be noted that this recommendation is based on studies that may not be completely applicable to the anesthesia work environment, as anesthetists are rarely constrained to a particular position. Controls directly associated with displays are discussed below in the section on stimulus-response compatibility.

Labels and Scales

Labeling provides visual information about a control's function. The considerations discussed for displays apply to control labels, and will not be discussed again here. There are other issues, however. Labels should be clearly associated with controls. Labels and control markings should not be obscured by the control, nor by the operator when using the control. Typically, labels are placed above controls. Labels should be unambiguous as to control function. This is especially important with the increasing use of multiple-function keys. For example, the Marquette 7010 RA Surgical Monitor (Marquette Electronics Inc., Milwaukee, WI) uses the label "ENTER" on a key which has multiple functions. In one mode it is indeed used to enter data. However, it can be used at other times to exit from a screen to the previously displayed screen. Symbols and abbreviations, if used, should be common and easily understood by the user population.

Compatibility

Stimulus-response compatibility is related to the anesthetist's understanding of what action will occur as a result of control actuation. This refers to how a stimulus (i.e., a change in a control) and its response (i.e., what occurs in response to the change) conform to human expectations. By taking movement and population stereotypes into account, mental processing can be decreased. This speeds learning and reduces reaction time. Errors occur less frequently, and the user finds equipment easier to use. Two important types of compatibility are position compatibility and movement compatibility.

Position

Position compatibility refers to the relationship between controls and their associated displays (Fig. 3-9). Controls and displays should be positioned so that there is a clear relationship between them. It should be obvious which display is controlled or affected by what control. This can be accomplished

by placing controls adjacent to their associated display. The display should not be obscured by the user when actuating the control.

Movement

The movement used to adjust a control should conform to the user's mental model of the change produced by that adjustment. These are generally based on existing or acquired human stereotypes (Table 3-8). Typically, clockwise or upward movements represent increases, while counterclockwise or downward movements represent decreases. Again, there may be differences between stereotypes in the United States and elsewhere in the world.

The accepted stereotype for flow control knobs is that the valve is opened and gas flow increases when the knob is turned counterclockwise. This is the "screw" rule. One notable exception to this is in the operation of regulators for E cylinders of oxygen. The flow control on these regulators opens *clockwise*, contrary to convention. Simulator studies have disclosed occasional errors in actuating this control properly during time-pressured crises.[63]

ALARMS

Alarms are the final components of the monitor interface to be discussed. Considerable research has been done regarding alarms in anesthesia, more than has been performed for displays or controls. Some ergonomic considerations of alarms are identical to those already reviewed for displays and controls and will not be repeated.

An alarm is intended to attract the anesthetist's attention to a specific abnormality. This is typically

TABLE 3-8. Recommended Control Movements Based on Population Stereotypes

Function	Control Action
On	Up, right, forward, pull
Off	Down, left, rearward, push
Right	Clockwise, right
Left	Counterclockwise, left
Up	Up, rearward
Down	Down, forward
Increase	Right, up, forward
Decrease	Left, down, rearward

(Adapted from Bullinger et al.,[60] with permission.)

accomplished using an alarm indication on the auditory and/or visual display channel. Thus the alarm first interrupts and directs the user's attention away from the task at hand. The anesthetist must identify the source of the "interrupt." This is done using cues such as the direction the sound is coming from, the nature of the sound made, the clinical context, or a visual message on the device that is alarming. Once the location of an alarm is identified, the exact nature of the alarming condition must be determined. Finally, the alarming condition must be evaluated within the clinical context and any response to it decided upon and carried out. Appropriate responses might include confirming the existence of the alarm condition, disabling the alarm sound, ignoring the alarm, or

specific interventions aimed at correcting the abnormal condition the alarm has identified. Some alarms cease when the abnormality ceases. Others remain active until the user specifically acknowledges the alarm condition ("latched" alarms).

A number of problems have been identified with the way alarms are currently provided. *First*, there are too many alarms. Nearly every monitor and therapeutic device has a variety of alarms. Some warn of serious problems or faults, others warn of problems that are not as serious (Table 3-9). *Second*, alarms use a nonspecific signal to attract the user's attention. This can confuse the user as to the source of the alarm, the nature of the problem, and its importance. *Third*, alarms can be distracting, and in many instances, intrude unpleasantly

TABLE 3-9. Alarms Associated with Operating Room Equipment

Alarm Source	Variable[a]	Comments
Patient conditions		
Cardiovascular system	Heart rate	
	Arterial blood pressure	
	Right heart pressure	
	ST segment	ST-segment depression
	Arrhythmia	
Pulmonary system	Oxygen saturation	Hypoxemia
	Airway pressure	High or sustained pressure, low pressure
	Time between breaths	Apnea, respiratory rate
	End-tidal CO_2	Low/high expired CO_2, high inspired CO_2, apnea
	Spirometry	Apnea, reverse flow, low minute ventilation
Drug administration	Anesthetic gas concentration	
	Infusion pump status	Occlusion, empty syringe
Anesthesia machine	Oxygen supply pressure	Low pressure
	Electrical power supply	Loss of electrical power
	O_2/N_2O ratio	Hypoxic mixture
	Ventilator disconnection	Low pressure, low minute ventilation
	Inspired oxygen concentration (FIO_2)	Low inspired concentration
Environment	Line isolation	Leakage current to ground
Ancillary patient equipment	Tourniquet time/pressure	
	Electrocautery grounding	Ground fault
	Heater/humidifier temperature	
	Blood/fluid warmer temperature	
	TEE probe temperature	
	Cerebral oximeter saturation	

[a]Alarms may activate for variables above or below a threshold value. Alarm annunciation may be audible or visual, and may originate from one or more instruments.

into the work environment. At times of increased workload, when attention may need to be focused in one direction, a noncritical alarm can inappropriately redirect the anesthetist's attention. This is exacerbated markedly when the alarm has a high rate of false annunciations. This often leads to alarms being disabled. *Fourth*, it has also been asserted that the presence of alarms may give the practitioner a false sense of security, and thus may contribute to a decrease of vigilance.[7,8,64]

Sounds

Most devices use alarm sounds to attract the anesthetist's attention to an abnormality. Generally these sounds are a tone or combination of tones. Three aspects of alarm sounds are: *audibility* (can they be heard), *alerting potential* (do they demand and capture the user's attention), and *recognition* (can their source be identified).[65,66] Although an auditory signal is considered best for capturing attention, it carries little information. Other, complementary, sources of information must be used to provide detailed information about the alarm. Existing alarm sounds have some drawbacks: they are nondistinct (sound like other signals), nonspecific (convey little or no additional information), distracting, and frequently unpleasant.

Alarm sounds must be audible above, and distinguishable from, ambient noise. The sound level in the operating room can occasionally approach that of a freeway.[67] However, increasing an alarm's amplitude is not always a good solution, since the operating room is not always noisy, and too loud an alarm is perceived as extremely unpleasant and intrusive by the operating room team. The maximum recommended sound level is 85 dB.[68]

Alarm sounds that are perceived as unpleasant may engender a "make it stop" response, where the primary action is to turn off the alarm, not check the patient.[69] As such they become a distraction more than an aid to management. Stanford and associates[70] studied subjects' affective reactions to a number of alarm sounds in common use. The response to commercially available signals was negative for 71 percent of subjects, provoking aggressive, anxious, and other negative emotions.

There is a limit to the number of alarm sounds that can be effectively used in the operating room. Users will not be able to accurately distinguish more than four to six tones.[56,71] Currently, there

may be more than 20 alarm sounds generated by different devices in the typical operating room. These are often indistinct from each other, and may therefore increase the cognitive workload. At times when the workload is already high, a further increase can be detrimental in managing a situation.

There is, as yet, no standardization of alarm sounds. That is, different instruments made by different manufacturers for different functions may use the same or similar sounds. Conversely, instruments that serve similar functions may have very different sounds. Loeb and colleagues[72] found that anesthetists frequently did not accurately recognize the source of an alarm sound.

The nonspecific nature of an alarm sound does not adequately communicate the reason for the alarm or its urgency. Finley and Cohen[73] examined the perceived urgency of common operating room monitor alarms. Abnormal conditions considered to be very important frequently had alarm sounds that did not convey a sense of urgency. Conversely, abnormal conditions considered to be of low priority were often perceived to be urgent. However, it should be noted that this study was based only upon the alarm sound, and the clinician typically has additional information upon which to base a decision.

One proposed solution, which has already been implemented by North American Drager on its Narkomed 2B, 3 and 4 machines, is an alarm hierarchy using only three specific sound patterns, signaling conditions of high, medium, or low priority[74] (Table 3-10). These alarm annunciators replace the many alarm sounds associated with individual monitors. The anesthetist can then refer to a centralized alarm display, which employs a similar hierarchy, to identify the specific cause of the alarm[74] (Fig. 3-14). Furthermore, only the alarm sound corresponding to the most urgent alarm condition will be annunciated; all other sounds are temporarily suppressed.

A series of general and context-specific alarm sounds, originally described by Patterson[75] for use in civil aviation, have been modified for use in the medical setting. These sounds consist of well-defined, complex sequences of tones that produce distinctive auditory patterns ("signatures"). The alarms consist of six pairs of warning sounds for six "specialized" categories (ventilation, oxygenation, cardiovascular, artificial perfusion, drug administration, and temperature, each with its own unique auditory signature) and one pair of general purpose sounds. Each category has separate emergency and caution alarm sounds. Several objections to the use of ''Patterson sounds'' have been raised.[76] They may no longer be useful in the operating room setting, considering recent progress in monitoring technology. Also, requiring individual devices to generate several complex tones adds cost and complexity. Perhaps most importantly, their use in multiple individual devices will worsen existing problems of noise in the operating room.

Sources

It is necessary to identify the source of an alarm before further assessment and action can be taken. It may be possible to identify the source of an alarm by the direction from which it emanates or from the type of sound emitted. However, as described above, anesthetists frequently cannot identify the instrument with which a particular alarm is associated. The clinical context in which an alarm sounds may aid the user in identifying which instrument is alarming. Perhaps the most common method, however, is the use of visual alarm annunciation, which can take several forms. The alarming instrument may have a flashing light on its panel. Although the flashing light may identify the instrument that is alarming, it provides no additional information on the reason for the alarm. The abnormal variable itself may be flashing on the monitor's display. Text messages describing the alarm condition may be used. As mentioned above, Narkomed

anesthesia machines use a specific message area to display a description of the alarm and the problem that caused it (Fig. 3-14).

Problem Identification

Once the alarming instrument is identified, the user must determine the abnormality that is causing the alarm. Cues similar to those identifying the alarm source are used; that is, the character of the sound, the clinical context, and visual cues. Identifying the abnormal condition is more complicated than simply locating the appropriate piece of equipment. An alarming instrument may not inform us as to which parameter has caused the alarm condition and, in some cases, may not tell us why that condition has occurred. For example, the breathing circuit pressure may be elevated. A simple alarm may inform us that airway pressure is high, but it does not indicate whether it is due to a stuck expiratory valve, an endobronchial intubation, a tension pneumothorax, bronchospasm, or another reason. Systems are being developed to provide more relevant information. Westenskow and colleagues[77] are using neural networks to analyze waveforms from the breathing circuit and provide, in a graphic and text format, details on the cause underlying the alarm.

Another proposed solution by which an alarm can provide additional information is the use of *earcons*.[78] These are the auditory equivalents of (visual) icons, and can be categorized as representational, abstract, symbolic, nomic, and metaphoric.

TABLE 3-10. Proposed Three-level Alarm Hierarchy Similar to That Used by North American Drager

Alarm Priority	Meaning	Desired Response from Operator	Visual Indication	Auditory Indication
High priority	Emergency, warning	Immediate	Flashing red	Complex tone, repeats continually at fast pace
Medium priority	Caution	Prompt	Flashing yellow	Less complex tone, repeats less frequently
	Alert	Increased vigilance	Continuous yellow	No tone or simple tone, repeats infrequently
Low priority	Information, notice, advisory	Awareness	Green or other	None

(Adapted from Loeb et al.,[10] with permission.)

A representational sound such as snoring can indicate that someone is asleep. Symbolic sounds rely on social conventions for meaning, such as applause for approval. An example of nomic representation is the sound of a closing metal cabinet for the closing of a file. Metaphoric sounds use similarities, such as the falling pitch of the pulse oximeter to represent a falling oxyhemoglobin saturation. Earcon attributes can be combined. The pulse oximeter tone is in fact both abstract and metaphoric. Block and coworkers[79] have studied the recognition of musical tones for use as alarms, another example of metaphoric earcons.

Synthesized speech has also been considered for alarm annunciation. It is used in aviation for certain high lethality conditions requiring an immediate response. The speech message is very short and describes the necessary action to be performed (e.g., "pull up" for the ground proximity warning system). However, several potential drawbacks to speech have been identified.[78] Voice output has a tendency to annoy people. A warning in the form of synthesized speech might be difficult to distinguish in the operating room environment, which is already filled with human conversation. Selecting a language suitable to all is another problem. Finally, such messages might be distracting to individuals who don't need to know about them. For example, the surgeon may find it distracting to hear a steady stream of messages emanating from the anesthetist's workspace.

Evaluation and Response

Once the reason for the alarm has been identified the anesthetist must determine what to do about the problem. The priority of the problem must be assessed and possible actions must be evaluated. False alarms are particularly problematic for anesthetists. Kestin and colleagues[80] found that an alarm sounded every 4.5 minutes in a typical operating room and that 75 percent of these were false alarms. To decrease the frequency of false alarms users often widen the alarm thresholds. Unfortunately, this has the drawback of decreasing alarm sensitivity to the point of effectively disabling the alarm. When false alarms occur frequently, practitioners may begin to ignore the alarm (the "cry wolf" syndrome), contributing to the "everything is OK" fixation error. Techniques to automatically modify alarm limits, depending on the phase of the anesthetic or a change in patient status, are being explored to help reduce the problem of false alarms. However, their benefit has yet to be determined.

Abnormal conditions must be evaluated on the basis of several parameters. *First*, the clinical context will help to determine the urgency of the condition. An alarm indicating hypotension when there is obvious extensive and acute blood loss will have much different meaning than the same alarm when all is quiet. *Second*, the veracity of an alarm can be verified using other sources of information.

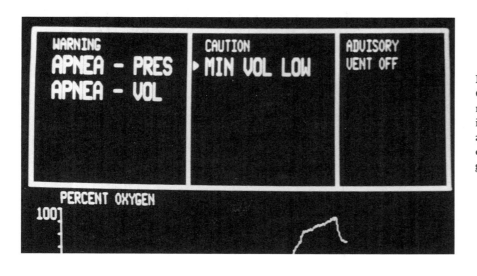

Fig. 3-14. The Narkomed Drager Centralert Display incorporates a message hierarchy to facilitate the identification and location of alarm messages. (Photograph courtesy of North American Drager, Telford, PA)

For example, if the pulse oximeter indicates a low oxygen saturation, it is reasonable to verify the signal integrity by comparing its displayed heart rate with that of the ECG, and by observing the oximeter's plethysmographic waveform. If these are satisfactory, the alarm will have more validity. *Third,* the workload at the time must be factored in, since low-priority alarms may need to be temporarily ignored during situations of high workload. Nonetheless, the burden of proof is always on the anesthetist to ensure that the patient is well before disabling or ignoring an alarm.

SUMMARY

Anesthesia is a complex, dynamic domain. Such domains are characterized by information that changes rapidly and accumulates over time. This results in the need for provisional assessments and plans of action, based on partial and uncertain data, that must be updated and revised as new information is obtained.[42] As such, the performance of anesthesia is prone to human error. Indeed, human error has been implicated as the major cause of most anesthetic mishaps.[5] However, equipment that is poorly designed contributes to and, at times, even encourages the occurrence of such error.

Monitoring technology has progressed considerably over the years. It is generally believed that the changes in monitoring have resulted in improved anesthesia safety. However, monitoring devices have become more difficult to use, and the monitoring task has become much more complex. This chapter has discussed the concepts of human factors and usability as they apply to monitoring in anesthesia. For the most part, little attention has been paid to the human factors design of monitoring instrumentation and the usability of monitor interfaces. Further, even less attention has been paid to integration of monitoring equipment into the anesthetist's work environment. The result has been "clumsy automation."[81] The magnitude of the human factors problem has only recently been appreciated, and research that points the way toward solutions only recently begun. Many different designs have been promoted as solving various human factors problems and making equipment "user friendly." However, there is little solid research to support these claims. The problems are not yet fully understood, and the solutions have not been rigorously tested.

Several other key points are made in this chapter:

1. Monitoring is primarily a task of information processing, the elements of which are data acquisition, interpretation and assessment, and operator response. Although vigilance is necessary, it is not sufficient for good monitoring.
2. The scope of the ergonomics problem in anesthesia, and monitoring in particular, should be appreciated. It should be clear that application of human factors standards and guidelines is not in itself sufficient to solve the problem. Careful evaluations under the dynamic conditions of actual use are vital. Crises are exactly the situations in which good user interface design is most important.[82]
3. While this chapter cannot make the reader an expert in human factors, it does provide an overview of the various human factors issues and the techniques that are applied in evaluating the usability of equipment. Individual anesthetists may be able to apply such principles to their own practice when purchasing equipment and preparing their own work environment.
4. The application of human factors principles depends strongly on the context in which the equipment is used. Contrast the differences between a small community hospital and a tertiary-care facility.
5. There are many sources of information regarding human factors, much of which comes from other domains, such as the aviation and nuclear power industries. However, information from other domains may not always apply to anesthesia. Even those concepts that may apply have not yet been tested in the anesthesia work environment.

The future holds great promise for monitors that will better support information processing by the anesthetist. Integrated monitors with smart alarms, using graphic and alphanumeric display formats to provide higher-level information, are being developed to fulfill this need. However, much remains to be done to design devices and provide monitoring that (1) is indeed easy to use, (2) provides exceptionally clear and accurate information, and (3) truly helps the anesthetist. Improved understanding of the overall anesthesia task, of which monitoring is a part, and very careful attention to the principles of human factors that have been outlined in this chapter, are paramount to achieving this goal.

REFERENCES

1. Mark LS, Warm JS, Huston RL: Ergonomics and Human Factors: Recent Research. Springer-Verlag, New York, 1987
2. Cooper JB, Newbower RS, Long CD, McPeek B: Preventable anesthesia mishaps: a study of human factors. Anesthesiology 49:399, 1978
3. Gaba DM, Maxwell M, DeAnda A: Anesthetic mishaps: breaking the chain of accident evolution. Anesthesiology 66:670, 1987
4. Weinger MB, Englund CE: Ergonomic and human factors affecting anesthetic vigilance and monitoring performance in the operating room environment. Anesthesiology 73:995, 1990
5. Cooper JB, Newbower RS, Kitz RJ: An analysis of major errors and equipment failures in anesthesia management: considerations for prevention and detection. Anesthesiology 60:34, 1984
6. Tinker JH, Dull DL, Caplan RA et al: Role of monitoring devices in prevention of anesthetic mishaps: a closed claims analysis. Anesthesiology 71:541, 1989
7. Hamilton WK: Do we monitor enough? We monitor too much. J Clin Monit 2:264, 1986
8. Moyers J: Monitoring instruments are no substitute for careful clinical observation. J Clin Monit 4:107, 1988
9. Orkin FK: Patient monitoring during anesthesia as an exercise in technology assessment. p. 439. In Saidman LJ, Smith NT (eds): Monitoring in Anesthesia. 3rd Ed. Butterworth-Heinemann, Boston, 1993
10. Loeb RG, Weinger MB, Englund CE: Ergonomics of the anesthesia workspace. p. 385. In Ehrenworth J, Eisenkraft JB (eds): Anesthesia Equipment: Principles and Applications. Mosby Year Book, St. Louis, 1993
11. Gaba DM, Fish KJ, Howard SK: Crisis Management in Anesthesiology. Churchill Livingstone, New York, 1994
12. Minimum performance and safety requirements for components and systems of continuous-flow anesthesia machines for human use, ANSI Z-79.8. American National Standards Institute, New York, 1979
13. Standard specifications for minimum performance and safety requirements for components and systems of anesthesia gas machines, ASTM F-1161-88. American Society for Testing and Materials, Philadelphia, 1989
14. Human factors engineering guidelines and preferred practices for the design of medical devices, AAMI HE-1988. Association for the Advancement of Medical Instrumentation, Arlington, VA, 1988
15. Cook RI, Potter SS, Woods DD, McDonald JS: Evaluating the human engineering of microprocessor-controlled operating room devices. J Clin Monit 7:217, 1991
16. Eichhorn JH, Cooper JB, Cullen DJ et al: Standards for patient monitoring during anesthesia at Harvard Medical School. JAMA 256:1017, 1986
17. Blum LL: Equipment design and "human" limitations. Anesthesiology 35:101, 1971
18. Drui AB, Behm RJ, Martin WE: Predesign investigation of the anesthesia operational environment. Anesth Analg 52:584, 1973
19. Kennedy PJ, Feingold A, Wiener EL, Hosek RS: Analysis of tasks and human factors in anesthesia for coronary-artery bypass. Anesth Analg 55:374, 1976
20. Boquet G, Bushman JA, Davenport HT: The anesthetic machine: a study of function and design. Br J Anaesth 52:61, 1980
21. McDonald JS, Dzwonczyk RR: A time and motion study of the anaesthetist's intraoperative time. Br J Anaesth 61:738, 1988
22. McDonald JS, Dzwonczyk RR, Gupta B, Dahl M: A second time-study of the anaesthetist's intraoperative period. Br J Anaesth 64:582, 1990
23. Weinger MB, Herndon OW, Zornow MH et al: An objective methodology for task analysis and workload assessment in anesthesia providers. Anesthesiology 80:77, 1994
24. Kantowitz BH, Sorkin RD: Human Factors: Understanding People-System Relationships. John Wiley & Sons, New York, 1983
25. Norman DA: The psychology of everyday things. Basic Books, New York, 1988
26. Scamman FL: An analysis of the factors leading to crossed gas lines causing profound hypercarbia during general anesthesia. J Clin Anesth 5:439, 1993
27. Molich R, Nielsen J: Improving a human-computer dialogue. Commun ACM 33:338, 1990
28. Zelcer J: Current issues in integrated monitoring, abstracted. J Clin Monit 7:83, 1991
29. Gaba DM, Lee T: Measuring the workload of the anesthesiologist. Anesth Analg 71:354, 1990
30. Loeb RG: A measure of intraoperative attention to monitor displays. Anesth Analg 76:337, 1993
31. Howard SK: Failure of an automated noninvasive blood pressure device: the contribution of human error and software design flaw. J Clin Monit 9:232, 1993
32. Rasmussen J: Information processing and human-machine interaction: an approach to cognitive engineering. Elsevier Science Publishing, New York, 1986
33. Rasmussen J: Skills, rules, and knowledge: signals,

signs, and symbols, and other distinctions in human performance models. IEEE Trans SMC-13:257, 1983

34. Reason J: Human Error. Cambridge University Press, Cambridge, UK, 1990
35. Reason J: Generic error-modeling system (GEMS): a cognitive framework for locating common human error forms. p. 63. In Rasmussen J, Duncan K, Leplat J (eds): New Technology and Human Error. Wiley, Chichester, UK, 1987
36. Orasanu JM: Decision making in the cockpit. p. 137. In Wiener E, Kanki B, Helmreich R (eds): Cockpit Resource Management. Academic Press, San Diego, CA, 1993
37. Orasanu J: Shared mental models and crew decision making. Princeton University Cognitive Science Laboratory, 1990
38. Wickens CD: Information processing, decision-making, and cognition. p. 72. In Salvendy G (ed): Handbook of Human Factors. John Wiley & Sons, New York, 1987
39. Tversky A, Kahneman D: Judgement under uncertainty: heuristics and biases. Science 185:1124, 1974
40. Orasanu J, Connolly T: The reinvention of decision making. p. 3. In Klein G, Orasanu J, Calderwood R et al (eds): Decision Making in Action: Models and Methods. Ablex Publishing, Norwood, NJ, 1993
41. Klein GA: Recognition-primed decisions. Adv Man-Machine Sys Res 5:47, 1989
42. DeKeyser V, Woods DD: Fixation errors: failures to revise situation assessment in dynamic and risky systems. p. 231. In Colombo AG, Bustamante AS (eds): Systems Reliability Assessment. Kluwer Academic Publishers, Dordrecht, 1990
43. DeKeyser V, Woods DD, Masson M, Van Daele A: Fixation errors in dynamic and complex systems: descriptive forms, psychological mechanisms, potential countermeasures. Technical Report for NATO Division of Scientific Affairs, Brussels, 1988
44. Norman DA: Categorization of action slips. Psychol Rev 88:1, 1981
45. Reason JT, Mycieslka K: Absent-minded? The Psychology of Mental Lapses and Everyday Errors. Prentice-Hall, Englewood Cliffs, NJ, 1982
46. Botney R, Gaba DM, Howard SK, Jump B: The role of fixation error in preventing the detection and correction of a simulated volatile anesthetic overdose, abstracted. Anesthesiology suppl. 79:A1115, 1993
47. Helander MG: Design of visual displays. p. 507. In Salvendy G (ed): Handbook of Human Factors. John Wiley & Sons, New York, 1987
48. Sanders AF: Some aspects of the selective process in the functional visual field. Ergonomics 13:101, 1970
49. Tullis TS: A system for evaluating screen formats. p. 1216. Proceedings of the Human Factors Society, 30th Annual Meeting, 1986
50. Fukui Y: An expert alarm system. p. 203. In Gravenstein JS, Newbower RS, Ream AK, Smith NT (eds): The Automated Anesthesia Record and Alarm Systems. Butterworths, Boston, 1987
51. Wiklund ME: Making color a contributing component of the user interface. Med Design Mater 1:11, 1991
52. Marcus A: Tutorial: the ten commandments of color. Comput Graphics 7:7, 1986
53. Wiklund ME: Designing medical devices for older users. Med Device Diagn Ind 14:78, 1992
54. Forcier H, Weinger MB: An evaluation of proposed graphical symbols for medical devices. Anesthesiology 76:625, 1993
55. Deathridge BH: Auditory and other sensory forms of information processing. p. 124. In Van Cott HP, Kinkade RG (eds): Human Engineering Guide to Equipment Design. American Institutes for Research, Washington, DC, 1972
56. Patterson RD, Milroy R: Auditory warnings on civil aircraft: the learning and retention of warnings. MRC Applied Psychology Unit, Civil Aviation Authority Contract 7D/S/0142, 1980
57. Schulte GT, Block FE: Can people hear the pitch change on a variable-pitch pulse oximeter? J Clin Monit 8:198, 1992
58. Wallace MS, Ashman MN, Matjasko MJ: Hearing acuity of anesthesiologists and alarm detection. Anesthesiology, in press
59. Wallace MS: Silent page: a vibratory alarm for the hearing-impaired anesthesiologist, abstracted. J Clin Monit 8:155, 1992
60. Bullinger H, Kern P, Muntzinger WF: Design of controls. p. 577. In Salvendy G (ed): Handbook of Human Factors. John Wiley & Sons, New York, 1987
61. Dorsch JA, Dorsch SE: Understanding Anesthesia Equipment: Construction, Care, and Complications. 2nd Ed. Williams & Wilkins, Baltimore, 1984
62. Anaesthetic workstations and their modules: essential requirements, CEN TC 215 WG1 N48. European Committee for Standardization, Lübeck, Germany, 1990
63. Botney R, Gaba DM, Howard SK: Anesthesiologist performance during a simulated loss of pipeline oxygen, abstracted. Anesthesiology suppl. 79:A1118, 1993
64. McIntyre JWR: Ergonomics: anaesthetists' use of auditory alarms in the operating room. Int J Clin Monit Comput 2:47, 1985
65. Woods DD: The alarm problem and directed attention in dynamic fault management. CSEL Report 92-TR-05, Cognitive Systems Engineering Laboratory, The Ohio State University, 1992
66. Wilkins PA: Assessing the effectiveness of auditory warnings. Br J Audiol 15:263, 1981

67. Shapiro R, Berland T: Noise in the operating room. N Engl J Med 287:1236, 1972
68. Specifications for alarm signals in medical equipment used in anesthesia and respiratory care (draft), ASTM Subcommittee F29.03.04. American Society for Testing and Materials, Philadelphia, 1991
69. Quinn ML: Semipractical alarms: a parable. J Clin Monit 5:196, 1989
70. Stanford LM, McIntyre JWR, Nelson TM, Hogan JT: Affective responses to commercial and experimental auditory alarm signals for anaesthesia delivery and physiological monitoring equipment. Int J Clin Monit Comput 5:111, 1988
71. Cooper GE: A survey of the status and philosophies relating to cockpit warning systems. NASA-CR-152071, NASA Ames Research Center, Moffett Field, CA, 1977
72. Loeb RG, Jones BR, Leonard RA, Behrman K: Recognition accuracy of current operating room alarms. Anesth Analg 75:499, 1992
73. Finley GA, Cohen AJ: Perceived urgency and the anaesthetist: responses to common operating room monitor alarms. Can J Anaesth 38:958, 1991
74. Schreiber P, Schreiber J: Diagnosis and prevention of operator error and equipment failure. Semin Anesth 8:141, 1989
75. Patterson RD: Guidelines for auditory warning systems on civil aircraft. Civil Aviation Authority Paper #82017, London, 1982
76. Weinger MB: Proposed new alarm standards may make a bad situation worse. Anesthesiology 74:791, 1991
77. Westenskow DR, Orr JA, Simon FH et al: Intelligent alarms reduce anesthesiologist's response time to critical faults. Anesthesiology 77:1074, 1992
78. Wiklund ME: Communicating clinical information with auditory signals. Med Device Diagn Ind 14:74, 1992
79. Block FE: Evaluation of users' abilities to recognize musical alarm tones. J Clin Monit 8:285, 1992
80. Kestin IG, Miller BR, Lockhart CH: Auditory alarms during anesthesia monitoring. Anesthesiology 69:106, 1988
81. Cook RI, Woods DD, McColligan E, Howie MB: Cognitive consequences of "clumsy" automation on high workload, high consequence human performance. Fourth Annual Space Operations, Applications and Research Symposium Proceedings, Albuquerque, NM, 1990
82. Mulligan RM, Altom MW, Simkin DK: User interface design in the trenches: some tips on shooting from the hip. Human Factors in Computing Systems, Computer Human Interactions '91 Conference Proceedings, New Orleans, LA, 1991

Monitoring and Patient Safety

John H. Eichhorn

4

Improved monitoring of both the patient and the anesthesia delivery system over the last several years has significantly helped make anesthesia for surgery much safer. Intraoperative catastrophes solely attributable to problems with anesthesia care causing death, cardiac arrest, and permanent brain damage have been greatly reduced.

The strategies and behaviors associated with attempting to make operative anesthesia safer are referred to as "safety monitoring," a term coined[1] to distinguish this specific program for prevention of major anesthesia accidents from the other types of monitoring best characterized as "physiologic monitoring." This distinction is important. "Monitoring" is often correctly associated with the use of an intraarterial cannula for direct continuous systemic blood pressure measurement, a pulmonary artery catheter for pressure measurements and, now, transesophageal echocardiography for evaluation of left ventricular wall motion (all of which are thoroughly discussed in this volume). These types of monitors allow continuous "fine-tuning" of anesthetic management and physiologic parameters under evolving conditions during surgery. As important as this is, it is secondary in a circumstance of, for example, an unrecognized disconnection of the breathing circuit from the endotracheal tube connector in a patient under full muscle relaxation being mechanically ventilated who, as a result, is *not* ventilated, becomes hypoxemic, and has a cardiac arrest. Such occurrences were alarmingly common relatively recently. Safety monitoring evolved in response to such events.

PURPOSE OF SAFETY MONITORING

"Better monitoring would have prevented this accident!" is the well-meaning but poorly stated conclusion of many investigators and speakers analyzing major anesthesia-related adverse incidents.

This type of pronouncement dramatically illustrates one of the most difficult aspects of the recent revolution in anesthesia practice in general and the safety of intraoperative anesthesia care in particular: the relationship between behavior and technology. Put as simply as possible, technology (in this case, monitoring) *never* "prevents" anything. Behaviors (specifically, the correct response to a much earlier warning of an adverse development during an anesthetic) can and do prevent severe intraoperative anesthesia accidents.

It is well recognized that there is a finite amount of time in the evolution of an anesthesia "critical incident" (a set of circumstances which, left unchecked, will produce patient injury)[2] for the anesthesia provider to recognize that there is a problem, diagnose it correctly, and act definitively to prevent an adverse event. It had been almost a time-honored tradition in anesthesia that the recognition of a severe, even life-threatening, problem came quite late in the development of a clinical scenario with the surgeon calling up over the draped ether screen, "Hey! The blood looks a little dark down here!" Of course, at this point, the patient had become significantly hypoxemic, as evidenced by the hemoglobin desaturation. There was precious little time to intervene before brain and heart ischemia led to injury or even death. The strategic underpinning of safety monitoring acknowledges that critical incidents will *always* occur. Given the nature of the complex technical environment in which anesthesia is administered today and the fallibility of humans functioning in that environment, it is impossible to even suggest than critical incidents will be eliminated, or even dramatically decreased. In spite of all the many advances, breathing system connectors will still become accidently disconnected from endotracheal tubes, esophageal intubations will occur, breathing system tubing and endotracheal tubes will be kinked or internally obstructed, and oxygen supplies will occasionally fail. There will be threats to patient safety during anesthesia.

The central concept of safety monitoring is to provide the earliest possible warning of an untoward development (such as the breathing circuit becoming disconnected from the endotracheal tube), thus maximizing the time available to diagnose and treat the event—and, thus, prevent patient injury. Given the fascination (and investment) of modern medicine in high-level technology, it is not surprising that the emphasis is on the technology, the electronic machines. However, safety monitoring is one of the best examples to illustrate the circumstances in which the machines, the monitors, themselves do nothing but extend the human senses. They facilitate the behaviors—make the behaviors easier. These monitoring behaviors that lead to the earliest possible warning and the maximum time for intervention can be accomplished without electronic machinery. This was clear in the original "Harvard monitoring standards"[3] and must be understood to separate the behaviors from the technology and expose the essence of safety monitoring. It is certainly true that accomplishing the behaviors of safety monitoring is easier when using correctly applied and functioning electronic monitors such as capnography, pulse oximetry, and ECG. It is even legitimate to say in the mid-1990s that effective use of these instruments is the *best* way to implement the behaviors of safety monitoring, particularly the continuous (as opposed to intermittent) nature of the monitoring tasks. This does not diminish the need to emphasize the behaviors first and the technology second. Thus there are two separate but related points regarding the role of safety monitoring. *First*, monitoring does not prevent injury-causing anesthesia accidents. These accidents are prevented by the information generated by the monitoring behaviors leading to earlier identification of untoward developments and consequent correct intervention. *Second*, while sophisticated electronic monitors may be the best way to implement safety monitoring behaviors, precisely how this earliest possible information is obtained is irrelevant as long as there is effective intervention in time to prevent patient injury.

EPIDEMIOLOGY OF CATASTROPHIC ANESTHESIA ACCIDENTS

It would seem relatively simple to be able to collect statistics about adverse outcomes caused by anesthesia care. If a patient has an intraoperative event that clearly or apparently involves the anesthetic rather than the surgery and there is a catastrophic outcome such as cardiac arrest, permanent central nervous system damage, or death, then this would be registered in a data base as an anesthesia accident. Reputable academic investigators could then examine the data collected, assemble information about risk factors and complication rates and try to offer suggestions for improvements in practice. However logical this may sound, it has not happened and likely never will. For a great many years until quite recently, there has been a singular lack of information about even the most basic safety statistics in anesthesia care. Many authors published series of patients experiencing anesthesia complications and these have been reviewed from a historical perspective.[4–6] Prior to the 1980s, virtually all of these reports were anecdotal and retrospective. There was and is extremely little information about rates of major anesthesia complications among large populations undergoing surgery.

The paucity of information about severe anesthesia accidents exists for several reasons. One central factor is the sheer physical difficulty of organizing the collection of such data. Serious adverse anesthesia outcomes were and (even more so now) are very rare. Therefore, meaningful incidence figures require the collection of massive numbers of anesthetics, far more than any one institution or local system of institutions can do in a reasonable period of time. In the United States there never has been any national repository of statistical data about adverse patient outcomes caused by medical care. Even if such a database existed and reporting were mandatory under federal law (both so unlikely as to seem impossible), ensuring full compliance by practitioners and hospitals would be extraordinarily difficult at best. In fact, it is virtually impossible to imagine there could ever be such a system in the United States. Further, definitions of what exactly constitutes an anesthesia accident have varied from study to study, often making the aggregation of statistics from multiple studies impossible. As noted, several papers reporting series of anesthetic mishaps have been published, but each without a valid denominator. Even if the authors believe all the adverse events during a delineated interval have been captured by them and could constitute a valid numerator for an incidence calculation, there is no possible way to even estimate a rate without the total number of anesthetics in that time period as a denominator. Finally, the characteristics of the medical-legal system in the United States virtually guarantee that there will never be widespread reporting of accurate information about adverse medical outcomes, particularly anesthesia catastrophes because these are almost always associated with the potential for very large monetary settlements or awards. Because the financial stakes are so very high, malpractice insurance carriers fiercely guard all information in any way associated with a case that has not been "closed" (come to financial conclusion one way or another). Very often, when a malpractice lawsuit is settled by the insurance company without a trial, one of the very clear stipulations is that the record is sealed and no one will ever know what the testimony would have been—thus preventing academic anesthesiologists from studying the case and potentially gathering valuable information that could help prevent similar accidents in the future. Fortunately, in the mid to late 1980s, there was some modification of the strict denial of access to insurance company files in that the American Society of Anesthesiologists Committee on Professional Liability organized the ASA Closed Claims Study and secured information from several malpractice insurers about claims associated with anesthesia after the files were permanently closed. This was a valuable step, but it constituted only a very limited look at a subset of anesthesia-related accident cases. No incidence data could be generated as no denominators existed. Several very interesting conclusions of this study are subsequently discussed.

From the mid-1950s through the early 1980s, there was a widely accepted axiom in the anesthesiology profession that the death rate associated with anesthesia care was one to two per 10,000 patients.[7] Immediately upon even mentioning such a statistic, problems arise. Does this include all patients, regardless of preoperative physical status and type of surgery? Is this consideration the same from study to study? (The widely differing definitions of anesthesia mortality which were used have been noted.[4]) Should patients with high risks from their surgical conditions be excluded? Should only "healthy" patients (such as ASA physical status I and II) be included in such calculations to focus the attention exclusively on the role of the anesthesia care? What would this do to the resultant calculated rates? However good these questions are, they cannot be answered. There simply is not enough information. Therefore, the "baseline" mortality figures so widely quoted must be interpreted with caution, but the idea of approximately 1/10,000 anesthesia mortality was so widely accepted for so long that it is as reasonable a starting point as any. Then, two questions eventually to be addressed here are: "What has happened to the anesthesia accident rate?" and "How is monitoring and, specifically, safety monitoring involved in this—past, present, and future?"

Refreshingly, certain themes were consistent and meaningful in the earlier reports of anesthesia accidents. Multiple reviews exist,[8] but in searching for a common focus in many reports, it is very clear that unrecognized hypoventilation due to a long list of potential causes is, *by far*, the most common cause of intraoperative anesthesia catastrophes. This reflects back to and correlates with the original critical incident study[2] in which the most common cause of anesthesia critical incidents (events which did cause or would have caused patient injury if left to evolve to their natural conclusion without compensatory intervention) was breathing system disconnection. As noted, the classic list of causes of unrecognized hypoventilation goes on to include esophageal intubation, kinking or obstruction of tubes or tubing, incorrect ventilator settings, and simple inadequate spontaneous or assisted ventilation during anesthesia. A more recent classic study of cardiac arrests due to anesthesia[9] cites "failure to ventilate" as both the most common cause of arrest and one which is completely preventable. Still more recently, the ASA Closed

Claims Study consistently cites "respiratory" causes as the most common for major adverse events and among respiratory causes, "inadequate ventilation" leads the list.[10] A major, though less frequent (yet never to be forgotten) cause of intraoperative anesthesia catastrophe is inadequate delivery of oxygen in the fresh gas flow. [As a parenthetic point, it is relevant to note that this author was introduced to and became involved in the field of anesthesia patient safety by being involved in the investigation of a set of catastrophic anesthesia accidents due to the delivery of an anoxic fresh gas mixture caused by the accidental mistaken attachment of a large tank of the welding gas argon to the central oxygen supply at a small rural hospital in which the anesthesia machine oxygen monitors were not functioning on the day of the event.] Keeping in mind the role and purpose of safety monitoring outlined above, it is not surprising that the monitoring of patient ventilation and oxygenation form the cornerstone of the principles of safety monitoring.

MONITORING STANDARDS AND THEIR IMPACT ON SAFETY MONITORING

The adoption of anesthesia safety monitoring behaviors in the mid- and late 1980s was profoundly accelerated by formal published standards of practice for anesthesia which prescribed safety monitoring principles. Prior to this time, many anesthesia practitioners did already incorporate some of the basic ideas and used precordial or esophageal stethoscopes to auscult breath sounds and heart tones, sometimes even continuously, and applied an ECG monitor to most patients. Formal published standards: (1) codified these behaviors, (2) (and most importantly) promoted the idea of genuinely continuous monitoring—as opposed to the usual intermittent checks, and (3) coincided in time with new technology—the widespread availability of capnography and pulse oximetry (as well as new awareness of oxygen monitors with lower limit alarms and also ventilator disconnect monitors)—thus promoting the synergistic development of new monitoring strategies in a manner unparalleled (past, present, or future) in the history of anesthesia practice.

It is relevant that the original impetus for formal standards of practice grew out of a risk management committee at Harvard Medical School formed in response to a significant concern from Harvard's malpractice insurance company about the great expense of anesthesia-caused patient injury and death claims. Anesthesia patient safety was not good according to the insurance claim statistics. In 1984, the committee reviewed all the claims and incidents on file since the company was founded in 1976. Among healthy patients (ASA Class I and II—patients who should reasonably expect no adverse outcome related to anesthesia), the rate of severe intraoperative accidents was already comparatively low (1/75,700), but the patterns seen in the analysis of the accidents that did occur was unmistakably clear.[1] Unrecognized hypoventilation was, by far, again, the cause most frequently associated with intraoperative catastrophes (cardiac arrest, permanent central nervous system damage, or death). There was, also, a death involving failure of oxygen delivery from an anesthesia machine that did not have an oxygen analyzer. These patterns correlated perfectly with those previously identified in the literature.

Because of the findings and the consequent desire to counteract the problems, the Harvard Anesthesia Risk Management Committee devised the set of simple strategies that later became safety monitoring.[3] Feeling that mere suggestions, guidelines, or even recommendations did not convey the necessary sense of urgency, the group sought a mechanism to make the behaviors mandatory and the concept enforceable. As a risk-management initiative, use of the medical-legal implications of publishing formal standards of practice was chosen. This created an environment in which there was a powerful incentive to adopt the behaviors prescribed by the standards. In early 1985, all nine Harvard teaching hospitals adopted the original standards. There was relatively little opposition, due in large measure to (1) the desirable goal of fewer and less severe patient injuries, (2) the lack of major disruption in that many practitioners already met the standards, and (3) the potential for lowered malpractice premiums if the initiative was successful in saving the insurance company money.

In October 1985, the ASA constituted a Committee on Standards of Care. This was significant because in 1976, a proposal from a few individuals to consider formulating standards for obstetric anesthesia was received with intense negativity. The ASA Standards Committee evaluated all available material, including the Harvard monitoring standards, and sought very broad-based input from the ASA membership. The original ASA "Standards for Basic Intraoperative Monitoring" were adopted unanimously by the ASA in 1986. Whether times had simply changed or there was no opposition due to the inherent reasonableness of the standards cannot be totally known. The ASA monitoring standards paralleled in part the prior effort at Harvard. There have been several key amendments and modifications since then, and the 1993 version is reprinted as an appendix to this chapter.

The original 1986 ASA monitoring standards capture the essence of the concept of safety monitoring. They depend on behaviors to generate information. The standard mandating the presence of qualified anesthesia personnel throughout an anesthetic was questioned by some as so obvious as to be unnecessary. Its inclusion reflected the still extant sad but true circumstances in which patients were left unattended after the institution of regional anesthesia or left fully anesthetized and on a mechanical ventilator during intervals in which the anesthesia provider would "take a break." It was felt that clearly stipulating the unacceptability of these behaviors might not influence the offenders directly but would help create an atmosphere in which all members of the team would assert pressure on negligent anesthesia providers to cease intraoperative absences. Further, the strong emphasis on the provider rather than electronic machines as the central element of safety monitoring set the intended priorities.

Timing figured so prominently in the ASA standards that it was necessary to specifically define the words "continually" and "continuous" in the context of monitoring behaviors. This was felt necessary because of the inevitable medical-legal implications of the interpretation of the document by U.S. plaintiffs' malpractice attorneys. A critical element in these standards was the shift from the often-observed habit of the intermittent check of vital signs and delivery system function with potential lapses of attention in between to a continual process of monitoring that is maintained at a consistently high level of attention. This is the basis for believing that earlier warnings of untoward developments will result from these practices. Specific application of "continuous" use of ECG, an oxygen analyzer with a lower limit alarm, and, during

mechanical ventilation, a disconnect monitor with an alarm are strong illustrations of this thinking.

The modifications since 1986 center on the behavior vs technology considerations. The original ASA standards referred to observation of *qualitative* clinical signs to verify adequate blood oxygenation. Very importantly, there is reference to the desirability of the addition of *quantitative* assessment and pulse oximetry is "encouraged." As the technology of pulse oximetry evolved and became ubiquitously available, it became clear to the ASA Standards Committee and, ultimately, to the ASA membership that this quantitative assessment, applied continuously, was effective and superior. Accordingly, the behavior of assuring adequate blood oxygenation was married to the applicable emerging technology and quantitative assessment (effectively, pulse oximetry) was made mandatory during all anesthetics starting at the beginning of 1990.

Similarly, the original ASA standards "encourage" the use of capnography to verify the correct placement of an endotracheal tube and then to monitor ventilation throughout the anesthetic. In the years following 1986, it was felt by those administering the ASA Closed Claims Study that unrecognized esophageal intubations were the source of catastrophic anesthesia accidents least favorably influenced by the adoption of the standards. Accordingly, the objective identification of exhaled carbon dioxide as verification of correct placement of an endotracheal tube was changed from encouraged to mandatory effective in 1991. Because there is little else other than the filter paper color-change indicator practically possible as a means to do this, the change effectively required the use of a capnograph. Continuous capnography during general anesthesia with an endotracheal tube was upgraded and emphasized as "strongly encouraged" in 1992, but it was not instituted as an official standard. This remains true in 1994. It can be effectively argued that capnography is a "de facto" standard of care.[11] However, it is not an officially published standard because of nagging concerns that capnography may, in certain unusual circumstances, give unreliable information that could conceivably lead the practitioner astray and into an incorrect action. If this point were to become the focus of debate in an anesthesia-related malpractice suit, there would be extremely strong arguments that capnography during general anesthesia has evolved to the status of standard of care despite the absence of the official imprimatur of the ASA. This entire issue again reflects the complex interaction of behavior and technology. It is extraordinarily difficult to argue *against* the thesis that, today, the most efficient and effective way to execute the behavior of ensuring adequate ventilation during general anesthesia is with the continuous use of a capnograph.

It is interesting to note a "reciprocal" of this issue in the case of temperature monitoring. In the original standards, *availability* of a means to continuously measure temperature is mandated and the actual monitoring of temperature is required when "changes in body temperature are intended, anticipated or suspected. . . ." This facilitates the desired behavior of the maintenance of appropriate body temperature. There have been at least three organized attempts to amend the standards to make temperature measurement mandatory during all anesthetics with the principal argument being that this will help identify patients who develop malignant hyperthermia. These proposals for another shift towards requiring technology for the implementation of a mandated behavior have been rejected by the ASA. The reasoning against mandating this additional technology is that it does not involve a primary safety issue. The initial diagnosis of malignant hyperthermia very rarely depends on temperature measurement, especially now with the very extensive use of capnography. Support for the diagnosis by applying the technology that becomes required when temperature change is suspected is appropriate, but depending on mandatory measurements as intraoperative diagnostic screening has not been felt indicated by the ASA, demonstrating thoughtful reliance on behavior of the practitioner rather than reflex adoption of technology because it exists.

Another example of the debate involves volatile anesthetic concentration monitoring. It has been suggested that this be mandated by ASA as a safety standard. This has not happened and it is unlikely that it will. In sharp contrast to the decades of reports chronicling catastrophic anesthesia accidents caused by unrecognized failures of ventilation, there has been no credible evidence to date that vaporizers fail "open" and, thus, accidently and unpredictably deliver toxic doses of a potent inhalation anesthetic. Accordingly, it is not seen as a safety monitoring issue. Certainly, there is practical patient care and also heuristic value in knowing the inspired and expired concentrations of anesthetics,

but this more appropriately fits with physiologic monitoring and patient management than with safety monitoring and specific efforts to prevent major anesthetic accidents.

The role of formal published standards of care in influencing anesthesia outcome has been examined[12] with the monitoring standards studied as the prototypical example. It is very important not to overemphasize the standards themselves. The standards only can initiate behaviors that then must be translated by practitioners into beneficial actions. Further, standards of care represent only one component of the so-called "safety movement" in anesthesia that began in the mid-1980s and continues today.[13] While published standards may be the most visible and widely publicized component, there are many others potentially contributing to safer care: expanded research into patient safety (including newly developed quality assurance/ quality improvement mechanisms); supposed improved "quality" of trainees entering the field of anesthesiology; improved education (longer residency, more and better textbooks and journals, etc.); improved equipment (reliability, design, ergonomics, etc.); improved medications; and increased awareness of anesthesia safety issues by patients and practitioners alike (promoted by the profession itself through its organizations and foundations as well as by the medical-legal and insurance establishments). The monitoring standards have evolved as the most discussed and the best recognized element of the safety movement. This must not obscure the fact that there have been several other components evolving simultaneously, each with its own potential contribution to improved anesthesia patient safety. Dissecting out the exact role of each part may not necessarily be easy.

The published standards both symbolized and prescribed safety monitoring principles and promoted their application through specific mandated behaviors, often now implemented most effectively and efficiently with the technology of modern electronic monitoring devices. It is very important to understand that monitors cannot "prevent" anesthesia adverse events or outcomes. This has been erroneously claimed by many authors and speakers in recent years who glibly state, "Better monitoring would have prevented this accident." There are unstated but critical assumptions in such statements. Monitors themselves do not prevent anything. Monitors can only provide information that allow the actuation of the behaviors of safety monitoring. It is reasonable to hypothesize that the earliest possible warning of an untoward development (such as a disconnection of the breathing system from the endotracheal tube being revealed instantly by the capnogram waveform and signaled in seconds by the associated alarm as well as also by the ventilator disconnect alarm, whether pressure or volume activated) thus alerts the practitioner very early in the evolution of the critical incident and provides the maximum amount of time possible for the practitioner to make the correct diagnosis and intervene appropriately (reconnect the breathing system to the endotracheal tube) and prevent patient injury. The *actions* prompted by safety monitoring, initiated and supported by electronic monitor-generated information, prevent major anesthesia accidents.

HAS SAFETY IMPROVED? DOES SAFETY MONITORING MAKE A DIFFERENCE?

Because safety monitoring is so much associated with publishing standards of anesthesia care, extensive evaluations of the possible impact of the monitoring standards have been carried out.[14,15] The simple answers to the posed questions are: yes, anesthesia safety has improved and yes, it appears safety monitoring does make a difference, although it is somewhat difficult to sort out.

For those traditionalists who demand a clear statistical answer of "$P < .05$" to define truth in all cases, there will be some difficulty in addressing the question. The epidemiology of extremely rare events is not easy to deal with, both conceptually and statistically. Further, the lack of consistent definitions and experimental design among investigations from different times and institutions makes comparisons among different studies very problematic. Finally, it seems impossible that there will ever be a prospective study to "settle" the question once and for all of whether safety monitoring makes a difference. In countries and institutions with institutional review boards or "human experimentation/subjects" committees, there is no logical prospect of justifying a "no monitoring" control group. Because of the evolution of anesthesia practice standards prescribing the principles of safety monitoring as a minimum level of care in

most industrialized countries, proposals to omit this care in the interest of scientific investigation would meet extraordinary opposition and it is unlikely that any reputable investigator would propose such a study in the first place.

Therefore, two additional thinking patterns emerge. The first is that, in regard to this particular type of question, alternative definitions of "truth" must be considered. In spite of the hard-core traditionalists, it is possible that a conclusion may be valid even when there is no means to obtain the $P < .05$ "proof" that physicians have been conditioned to respect and expect since the first day of medical school. Such alternative thinking takes place very frequently in academic anesthesiology departments during case conference presentations. From evaluation of all the available information from all possible sources, the group hearing the case presented discusses what has been heard and eventually comes to a conclusion as to what caused the event being presented, even if there are conflicting accounts from different people involved and gaps in the story. The group comes to a collective definition of the truth with which it is satisfied and upon which it bases recommendations for future action. This is the type of thinking that can be applied when traditional studies and statistics simply do not work for one reason or another. The second point is even more relevant. Even if there were a possible study or other mechanism, it is not necessary to "prove" that safety monitoring in and of itself *alone* has caused a measurable incremental improvement in the outcome of anesthesia care. In fact, to attempt to make such a claim is unrealistic, given all the other factors previously mentioned which have been evolving simultaneously. Of course these other factors have had an impact on anesthesia care. It is not necessary to attempt to isolate improved monitoring as the *only* cause of improved outcome because it would be very difficult or, in fact, impossible to dissect out contributions from the various different components of anesthesia care. Even acknowledging the traditionalists' strong desire for single variable analysis and statistical proof, it may be necessary on this question to recognize a multivariate situation with consensus opinion accepted as the conclusion. It is reasonable to acknowledge safety monitoring as the most dramatic and most visible component of the "safety movement" and the one that best symbolizes what has changed in intraoperative anesthesia care in

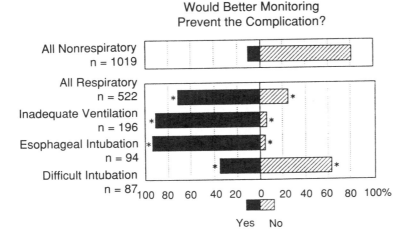

Fig. 4-1. Data from the ASA Closed Claims study as of 1990. Percent of adverse outcomes that the reviewers considered preventable or not with better monitoring in each of the major groups of respiratory events compared with nonrespiratory events at the top. The incidence of "impossible to judge" was 1 to 3 percent in the respiratory groups and 9 percent in the nonrespiratory group. * = *P* < .05 compared with nonrespiratory claims. (From Caplan et al.,[10] with permission.)

the last decade or so. The extremely strong association in time of the development of the ideas for behaviors to make anesthesia safer, the implementation of those behaviors (especially with new and greatly facilitative technology), and the coincident decrease in the number and severity of intraoperative anesthesia catastrophes together can stand as the source of a consensus-derived conclusion that safety monitoring has improved anesthesia care.

It is appropriate to explore this suggestion from several different perspectives. These include: retrospective case analyses, retrospective epidemiologic studies, one prospective epidemiologic study, and insurance industry information.

Among retrospective case analyses, the ASA Closed Claims Study is the most comprehensive. Each case analyzed in this large study was specifically reviewed by independent reviewers who rendered several opinions about the case material, one of which concerned whether "better monitoring would have prevented the adverse outcome." One pass through the data bank yielded a report which focused specifically on respiratory events.[10] Among the adverse outcomes associated with respiratory events, 72 percent were judged by the reviewers as being preventable with better monitoring (see Fig. 4-1) and that nearly all of the "inadequate ventilation" and "esophageal intubation" cases would have been prevented. Recall that this is not the optimal terminology to express this thought. It would be better to state that the information generated from better monitoring would give significantly earlier warning of the untoward development and, assuming a reasonable response from the respon-

sible practitioner, the adverse outcome would have been prevented. In any case, the point is clear that a battery of independent reviewers believed in a retrospective case review that the principles of safety monitoring would have improved anesthesia outcome. Another consideration of the entire ASA Closed Claims data base of which the respiratory events were a subset considered the role of monitoring in mishap prevention.[16] The characteristics of cases classified "preventable with better monitoring" by the reviewers were delineated. The "severity of injury score" averaged at the top of the scale for preventable injuries and near the middle for those judged not preventable. Similarly, the cost of the insurance settlement or judgment for the preventable injuries was over *ten times* that of the nonpreventable ones. Table 4-1 shows the breakdown of this data base by type of negative outcome experienced and shows that over half of *all* (not

TABLE 4-1. ASA Closed Claims Study: Preventability of Complications

Complication	Negative Outcome Considered Preventable by Additional Monitors (no. of cases)	Negative Outcome Considered Not Preventable by Additional Monitors (no. of cases)
Death	241 (57.1%)	158 (37.4%)
Nerve damage	1 (0.6%)	164 (92.1%)
Brain damage	83 (58.4%)	51 (35.9%)

Percentages do not necessarily add to 100 because of cases in which there was insufficient information to judge preventability.
(From Tinker et al.,[16] with permission.)

just respiratory) cases of death and brain damage were considered preventable with better monitoring. Predictably, the "proper use" of the combination of pulse oximetry and capnography was "deemed useful" in preventing the adverse outcome in over half the total cases (Table 4-2).

Analysis of the Harvard data[1] had two purposes, the first of which was a retrospective case analysis. In a manner similar to that later adopted by the ASA Closed Claims Study, a retrospective analysis was carried out of available data relative to all major intraoperative anesthesia accidents (death, permanent CNS damage, cardiac arrest with eventual recovery) among "healthy" (ASA physical status I and II—specifically limited to this population because of the reasonable expectation of no adverse outcome) patients for a 12½ year period through mid-1988. Taking all possible evidence (including confidential insurance files) into account, decisions were made by the author as to whether the events would have been preventable by the application of safety monitoring principles. Of the 11 cases, seven involved unrecognized hypoventilation. These seven and the additional case of the incorrect fresh gas flow setting leading to anoxia were judged preventable via the safety monitoring process (earlier warnings provoking correct responses in time to prevent injury). Again, by implication, this suggests a positive impact on anesthesia outcome from the attitudes and behaviors (including the use of technology) mandated by the monitoring standards. This analysis has been criticized[17] by authors who take a much too narrow view of the intended purpose of these case studies. It is acknowledged that there were "associated issues"

such as the degree of supervision of residents or CRNA's, but it must be emphasized that this in no way diminishes the concept that earlier warning of an untoward development—to any provider with any level of training—should maximize the chance of correct diagnosis and intervention early enough in the evolution of the critical incident to prevent patient injury.

Retrospective epidemiologic studies attack the question of the value of safety monitoring from a slightly different aspect. As noted, it must be accepted that there are associated variables. Several investigators have found associations in time of the advent of safety monitoring with an improvement in anesthesia outcome for various populations. Although there is no specific reference to safety monitoring in the discussion, one of the most impressive studies by far is the mammoth British Confidential Enquiry into Perioperative Deaths.[18] This was the first indication that a change was evolving from the long-accepted idea that the anesthesia mortality rate was 1/10,000 to 1/20,000. In this 1987 publication, Lunn found that the death rate solely attributable to anesthesia was 1/185,000, fully an order of magnitude lower than that previously believed. A different and less rigorous large-scale study of anesthesia death rates in Massachusetts[19] depended on retrospective data gathering from different sources, thus potentially suffering from the potential pitfalls of nonparallel definitions mentioned earlier. Nonetheless, Zeitlin suggests that the anesthesia death rate in that population was 1/4,630 in 1965 and an extrapolated 1/62,500 in 1989. He notes several possible causative factors, but notes the principles of safety monitoring as the most prominent among them.

Another type of retrospective analysis came when Keenan and Boyan (possibly inspired by some earlier ground breaking work[20]) considered intraoperative anesthesia-related cardiac arrest.[21] They compared 107,257 anesthetics in the period 1969 to 1978 with 134,677 anesthetics during 1979 to 1988. In the first interval, the risk of preventable cardiac arrest was 1/6,711 and among those, the rate of arrest caused by respiratory events was 1/11,905. In the second interval, there were statistically significant decreases in both rates to 1/14,925 for preventable arrests and 1/66,666 for arrests with respiratory etiologies. Pulse oximetry was introduced at that institution in 1984 and following that, there had been no arrests from respiratory events.

TABLE 4-2. ASA Closed Claims Study: Monitors Deemed Useful in Cases of Preventable Injuries or Deaths

Monitors	Overall ($n = 346$)[a]	Regional ($n = 51$)	General ($n = 290$)
Pulse oximetry	138 (40%)	41 (80%)	93 (32%)
Capnometry	8 (2%)	1 (1%)	7 (2%)
Pulse oximetry plus capnometry	176 (51%)	8 (16%)	168 (58%)
Other	18 (5%)	0 (0%)	17 (6%)
Not specified	6 (2%)	1 (1%)	5 (2%)

[a]In five cases the type of anesthesia employed was not specified.
(From Tinker et al.,[16] with permission.)

TABLE 4-3. Harvard Medical School Rates for Major Anesthesia Accidents and Deaths Among Healthy Patients Before and After Adoption of Monitoring Standards

Dates	ASA P.S. I and II Patients	Intraoperative Accidents	Associated Deaths
Jan. 1976–June 1985	757,000	10 (1/75,700)	5 (1/151,400)
(*Note*: Original monitoring standards adopted July 1985.)			
July 1985–June 1990	392,000	1 (1/392,000) $P = .08*$	0 0 $P = .12*$

*By Fisher's Exact Test.

These data are cited as suggesting the efficacy of the respiratory (ventilation) monitoring component of safety monitoring. Also, this paper provided the impetus for a discussion of how improvements in anesthesia outcome could be documented.[22]

The other component of the analysis of the Harvard data[1] is a retrospective epidemiologic evaluation. This constituted a functionally prospective examination of the incidence rate of major intraoperative accidents discovered among healthy patients. The Harvard monitoring standards were implemented in July of 1985. As shown in Table 4-3, the rate of major intraoperative anesthetic accidents decreased more than fivefold thereafter through mid-1990. Statistical comparison of extremely rare events (very low rates) is difficult. However, the appropriate two-by-two Fisher exact test reveals that the poststandards rate of 1/392,000 patients with major intraoperative accidents attributable solely to anesthesia care approaches statistical significance with $P = .08$. Importantly, it is fully acknowledged that many positive developments in anesthesiology were occurring simultaneously, with the concept of "safety monitoring" and the associated published standards of care. It is too simplistic to say that safety monitoring alone reduced anesthesia accidents. Rather, these principles and the published standards codifying them are the tangible outward reflection of widespread changes in attitudes and practices. This conclusion is emphasized in an epidemiologic review of potential impact of pulse oximetry and capnography on anesthesia risk.[23] This evaluation includes the French anesthesia risk data,[24] which was generated just before safety monitoring was publicized and used for comparison purposes. The prospect for risk reduction is shown in Table 4-4. The review suggests that anesthesia appears to be safer, but this cannot be attributed to improved monitoring alone as other simultaneous events occurred. The usual plea for more and better epidemiologic studies of anesthesia care and outcome is included.

The only truly prospective trial of any part of the principles of safety monitoring is the Danish study of pulse oximetry in 20,802 patients.[25] This effort focused specifically on pulse oximetry and whether or not there would be any difference in outcome in approximately 10,000 who had pulse oximetry used during and following their anesthetics vs. 10,000 who did not. The rate of diagnosis of hypoxemia, of course, was much higher in the monitored group but, fundamentally, there was no major "statistically significant" improvement in outcome in the monitored group. Does this mean that pulse oximetry is worthless and should be

TABLE 4-4. Estimate of Potential Risk Reduction by Monitoring

Origin	Risk (per 10,000)		Risk Reduction		Number Needed to be Treated[d]
	Control	Treated[a]	Relative[b]	Absolute[c]	
Keenan[19]	0.67	0.00	100%	0.67	14,925
Eichhorn[12]	0.16	0.031	80.6%	0.129	77,519
Tiret[18]	1.25	0.00	100%	1.25	8,000

[a]Assumes that all cardiac arrests are preventable by universal application of monitoring.
[b]Relative risk reduction: the reduction of adverse events achieved by a treatment, expressed as a proportion of the control rate.
[c]Absolute risk reduction: difference in event rates between control and treatment groups.
[d]Number to be treated: The number of patients who must be treated to prevent one adverse event (mathematically equal to the reciprical of the absolute risk reduction).
(From Duncan and Cohen,[23] with permission.)

abandoned, or at least removed from the formal, published standards of care? No. While the work involved in collecting data on over 20,000 patients is massive and admirable, the fundamental difficulty is immediately apparent. An accompanying editorial[26] notes that the authors never expected results oriented toward the question of rate of catastrophic anesthesia outcome because the power analysis done before the study was undertaken showed that demonstrating a difference in the rate of already extremely rare events such as intraoperative anesthesia catastrophes would require patient populations *vastly larger* than used in this study. There were some suggestive points, such as rate of intraoperative cardiac arrest: 12 in the unmonitored group versus 8 in the monitored group. However, the incidence of postoperative coma was higher in the monitored group and this was ascribed to random variations, as probably could be the cardiac arrest data. Critics of technology, safety monitoring, standards, and modern developments in general may seize upon this study, but incorrectly so. While certainly provocative, the Danish study clearly reinforces the previously stated notion that it is physically impossible now to execute a definitive prospective study to evaluate safety monitoring in traditional terms. Alternate definitions of "truth," beyond "$P < .05$" must be sought.

Some of the initial impetus in the United States for the investigations and efforts that led to the concepts of anesthesia safety monitoring came from the insurance industry and its concern about cost and financial loss. It is appropriate to consider the subsequent events regarding anesthesiologists' malpractice insurance losses and premiums. There have been multiple articles in the U.S. lay press concerning the fact that in the last few years, there has been some general reduction in the number and severity of medical malpractice insurance claims—across the board for all specialties. It is equally true, however, that anesthesiology in almost all cases has had the most dramatic of these reductions among all medical specialties. Further, in a great many locations, insurance premiums have been significantly decreased specifically for anesthesiologists, much more so than for any other specialists. Dramatic examples come from the Harvard experience. In the period 1976 to 1985, the insurer's dollar loss per anesthetic was $5.24. In 1986, it fell to $2.00; in 1987, to $1.84; and, in 1988, the insurance loss per anesthetic was $0.78.[27] This rep-

resents a fall of more than sevenfold in a very short period. Another common measure in the insurance industry is the so-called relativity rating, or the degree of insurance risk of a given group of practitioners compared to the lowest-risk medical specialty, usually primary care internal medicine. In 1985 at Harvard, anesthesia's relativity was 5.2. By 1989, it had fallen to 2.5, while that for general surgery decreased slightly from 5.2 to 4.8, and that for obstetrics and gynecology had increased from 7.2 to 7.5. It is extremely unlikely that plaintiffs' attorneys are ignoring cases of major damage allegedly due to anesthesia. Further, malpractice insurance company actuaries and officials are not charitable people; they are not going to reduce their companies' income from premiums unless there is a very good reason. All these data suggest most strongly that there are now fewer and less severe cases of anesthesia-caused injury. Similarly and very importantly, in the period 1986 to 1991, combining the avoidance of increases and actual reductions (including a 32 percent reduction in 1989) malpractice insurance premiums paid by anesthesiologists at Harvard decreased more than 60 percent. Premium reductions specifically for anesthesiologists have also taken place in many other locations across the country. Premiums can be reduced only when there is a surplus of reserves over the need to pay claims. Does this economic evidence indicate that the principles of safety monitoring have improved anesthesia outcome? Not exactly. However, it must be accepted that anesthesia care is safer than only a relatively few years ago. There are fewer and less severe major accidents during anesthesia. It is only logical to again suggest that safety monitoring constitutes one important component (if not the most important—but herein, again, the difficulty of dissecting out one) of the milieu that has led to improved anesthesia care.

Predictably and probably appropriately, there are those who are skeptical about some of the points made here about safety monitoring. Orkin[28] believes that certain of the analyzed accident cases that would have been prevented by correct functioning of the principles of safety monitoring reveal generally poor quality of care and "very poor judgment" on the part of the anesthesia providers. He wonders whether adherence to minimal monitoring standards can compensate for this and, by implication, suggests that it is too simplistic to expect correct responses (even to very early warnings of threatening developments) by the small but definite number of inadequate practitioners who are, in and of themselves, inherently dangerous to patients. Also noted by Orkin is the multifactorial general trend to better care. He suggests that there has been a tendency towards better anesthesia outcome for some time, antedating the development and adoption of the principles of safety monitoring and reflecting the generalized improvements in the many factors related to overall anesthesia care. Because of the general improvements in care and his belief in the importance of nonanesthesia factors to anesthesia outcome, Orkin expects monitoring alone to have a minimal effect. Further, he stresses the already very low rate of events that the monitoring is intended to detect. Because of the unlikely occurrence of preventable events, Orkin suggests that "before and after" statistics supporting a change are more the result of very rare and thus essentially random events rather than an impact on anesthesia outcome by monitoring. Additionally, he notes that the standards codify what in most cases was already routine practice. While this is used as an argument to minimize the potential impact of the standards, he does not address the specific stated intention of the standards to encourage good practice by those already so engaged and to target for improvement the very small minority of questionable practitioners by providing a clear template for action and the requisite peer pressure to force a change of behavior. Orkin incorrectly extracts monitoring out of the larger context outlined previously and functionally sets it up as an isolated "straw man" for him to knock down. This is done effectively but requires his attributing claims for the efficacy of safety monitoring and the associated standards that were never intended in any way by their creators. In conclusion, he makes the universally applicable and appropriate plea for more definitive outcome studies to better evaluate the impact of practice standards and, by implication, safety monitoring.

Keats,[29] on the other hand, gives a sweeping critique of the reasoning (or lack of it) behind many practices in anesthesiology, not limited to just monitoring or the associated standards. Generally, he challenges many modern habits, from electrocardiographic monitoring through scavenging systems and up to pulse oximetry with the fundamental thesis that there is no valid evidence for the efficacy of any of these things. He hypothesizes that there

are many fully accepted standards of care, including for monitoring, that have no demonstrated benefit at all for the patient and that may, in fact, create new risks. Further, Keats states that he believes there is no statistically valid evidence that anesthesia mortality has improved at all in the last several decades. He cites the "error-blame bias" and the common discomfort with saying "I don't know" as the reasons behind what he sees as essentially an irrational drive toward conclusions and actions. His concluding plea for valid data is more specific in that he carefully outlines the desired studies both of the hazards of current "improvements" and of graded outcomes among stratified patient populations. Absent this, he ends, "we will never know, for all our technical sophistication, if we are improving the outcomes of anesthesia care."

As one part of the debate about the efficacy of safety monitoring, it is always interesting to wonder how the critics themselves practice anesthesia. No data are available regarding whether they themselves apply safety monitoring principles when they administer anesthesia or, conversely, what would be their desires if they were patients receiving anesthesia care. While, of course, idle speculation, it does highlight the difference between healthy intellectual debate and the realities of life in the operating room today, where the principles of safety monitoring, as outlined in the ASA standards, have become an integral and inescapable part of modern anesthesia practice.

DISCUSSION

Detractors aside, it is reasonable to attempt to correlate safety monitoring with anesthesia patient safety. In keeping with the analogy to an anesthesia case conference presentation and the resultant consensus definition of truth that shapes future action, the weight of the evidence can be examined.

Until the last few years, major intraoperative anesthesia "critical incidents" (such as an esophageal intubation or the disconnection of the breathing system from the endotracheal tube connector underneath the drapes) often went unrecognized until there was marked cyanosis followed quickly by arrhythmias and preterminal bradycardia. Because the "event" had developed so far by then, this left very little time to diagnose and treat the problem before patient injury occurred. The intention and value of the behaviors of safety monitoring are to create a "system" that dependably alerts the anesthesiologist much earlier in the development of an adverse event and, thus, allows much more time for problem analysis and effective intervention before the patient is damaged. Review of the information presented previously reveals that there can be no doubt that this purpose is accomplished with safety monitoring.

Critical incidents such as esophageal intubations and tubing disconnects will always occur because of both human nature and the nature of mechanical equipment, particularly the complex environment involved in an anesthesia delivery and monitoring workstation. The purpose of safety monitoring is to prevent as many as possible (it is hoped virtually all) of these critical incidents from evolving into anesthesia catastrophes.

The principles of safety monitoring stress *behavior* over technology and this is articulated in the various sets of monitoring standards. The behaviors of genuinely *continuous* monitoring of oxygenation, ventilation, and circulation are the heart of the standards. The utilization of the technologies of pulse oximetry and capnography may, in fact, be the most effective and efficient ways to execute the behaviors of truly continuous monitoring. However, it cannot be emphasized strongly enough that these technologies are not a substitute for human behavior. There is a misperception that both monitoring standards and safety monitoring focus and depend on technology. That simply is not true. The first monitoring standard included in all the sets published (including in the "Recommended Minimal Standards for Anesthesia Care" developed by the International Task Force of Anaesthesia Safety and adopted as world standards by the World Federation of Societies of Anesthesiologists at the Tenth World Congress in June, 1992[30]) always mandates the continuous presence of a qualified anesthesia provider, emphasizing that the continuous vigilance of the person administering the anesthetic is the absolute cornerstone of intraoperative safety.

Consistently, throughout the modern study of intraoperative anesthesia accidents, unrecognized hypoventilation has been identified as by far the most common cause. "Hypoxemia" as the cause of cardiac arrest, central nervous system damage, or death is often listed in reports or reviews, but the actual number of cases of inadequate fresh O_2 are small in number compared to the great many in which failure of ventilation eventually causes injurious hypoxemia. The single most important component of safety monitoring is genuine continuous monitoring of ventilation, including (and perhaps even especially) during regional anesthesia and monitored anesthesia care. Although there have been some persistent warnings that capnography can occasionally give misleading information or can be misinterpreted in various situations (and this has prevented it becoming mandated as an official ASA monitoring standard of care), it is the best way during general anesthesia to verify adequate ventilation. A pretracheal or precordial stethoscope affording attention to breath sounds is valuable, but it is qualitative as opposed to the more definite quantitative nature of capnography. Pulse oximetry is, of course, helpful in a wide variety of situations and it is a very useful safety monitor, but not as much so as many practitioners think. Desaturation is detected before the profound cyanosis and bradycardia are obvious. However, the patient exhibiting definite desaturation (such as to 85 percent when the default alarm sounds) may be quite well along into the downward spiral toward injury when attention is called to the situation by this particular monitor. Reiterating that the goal of safety monitoring is the earliest possible warning of danger and that most serious incidents involve ventilation, a capnograph or other method of continuous ventilation monitoring is the most effective safety monitor.

Reviews suggest a decreasing incidence of intraoperative anesthetic mishaps. One particularly comprehensive and thoughtful review of available published data by Keenan[7] yields the conclusion:

> **To summarize the evidence since 1985, major changes in safety awareness and the widespread adoption of improved monitoring methods (especially of oxygenation and ventilation) during anesthesia, in all likelihood, have led to a substantial reduction in anesthetic mortality and major morbidity. While epidemiologic studies documenting these changes are yet to be published, case collection and critical incident studies have been reported that suggest anesthesia outcome is improving. . . .**

The majority of anesthesia practitioners who have the perspective of at least a decade's experience appear to believe that intraoperative anesthesia is safer today. No one can or should claim that this is *solely* the result of advances in monitoring, but it is reasonable to suggest that the principles of safety monitoring (both in general and as implemented through the standards) contributed significantly to this, along with improvements in the backgrounds and overall quality of anesthesia practitioners, their education, the tools and medications available to them, and the ongoing research on how to best use these.

A very important testimony to the decrement in adverse anesthesia-related occurrences (which has been "caused," as noted, by a great many concurrent factors that are, perhaps, best symbolized by the concepts of safety monitoring) is the specific selective reduction of malpractice insurance premiums for anesthesiologists in almost all locations. Because neither insurance companies nor plaintiffs' attorneys are charitable, this must reflect the fact that there is less patient damage caused by anesthesia today—precisely the goal of safety monitoring. Because the insurance industry is a cyclical one and because attorneys are rather creative and innovative in pursuing medical liability we may expect future increases in malpractice insurance premiums.

It is, of course, understandable that there are some (many?) who believe that almost all in life, if not, in fact, everything is random and there have been no real changes in anything. A thorough examination of all the material presented here, particularly the often repeated qualification that while monitoring may be the most visible and dramatic component, it is not just new and better monitoring that is responsible for the relatively recent improvement in anesthesia outcome, leads to the different belief that anesthesia *is* safer today than it was even relatively recently and that improved monitoring—structured through the principles of safety monitoring—has had a significant role in this improvement.

REFERENCES

1. Eichhorn JH: Prevention of intraoperative anesthesia accidents and related severe injury through safety monitoring. Anesthesiology 70:572, 1989
2. Cooper JB, Newbower RS, Long CD et al: Preventable anesthesia mishaps: a study of human factors. Anesthesiology 49:399, 1978
3. Eichhorn JH, Cooper JB, Cullen DJ et al: Standards for patient monitoring during anesthesia at Harvard Medical School. JAMA 256:1017, 1986
4. Duberman SM, Bendixen HH: Mortality, morbidity and risk studies in anaesthesia, p. 37. In Lunn JN (ed): Epidemiology in Anaesthesia. Edward Arnold, London, 1986
5. Desmonts JM: Outcome after anaesthesia and surgery: epidemiological aspects. In Desmonts JM (ed): Outcome After Anesthesia and Surgery: Bailliere's Clinical Anaesthesiology 6:463, 1992
6. Keenan RL: Anaesthetic mishaps: outcome and prevention. In Desmonts JM (ed): Outcome After Anesthesia and Surgery: Bailliere's Clinical Anaesthesiology 6:477, 1992
7. Keenan RL: What is known about anesthesia outcome. In Eichhorn JH (ed): Improving Anesthesia Outcome: Problems in Anesthesia 5:179, 1991
8. Pierce EC, Cooper JB: Analysis of anesthetic mishaps. Int Anesthesiol Clin 22:190, 1984
9. Keenan RL, Boyan CP: Cardiac arrest due to anesthesia. JAMA 253:2373, 1985
10. Caplan RA, Posner KL, Ward RJ et al: Adverse respiratory events in anesthesia: a closed claim analysis. Anesthesiology 72:828, 1990
11. Eichhorn JH: Are there standards for intraoperative monitoring? Adv Anesth 5:1, 1988
12. Eichhorn JH: The role of standard of care. In Eichhorn JH (ed): Improving Anesthesia Outcome: Problems in Anesthesia 5:188, 1991
13. Eichhorn JH: Risk reduction in anesthesia. In Duncan PG (ed): Anesthetic Risk and Complications: Problems in Anesthesia 6:278, 1992
14. Eichhorn JH: Influence of practice standards on anaesthesia outcome. In Desmonts JM (ed): Outcome After Anesthesia and Surgery: Bailliere's Clinical Anaesthesiology 6:663, 1992
15. Eichhorn JH: Effect of monitoring standards on anesthesia outcome. Int Anesthesiol Clin 31:181, 1993
16. Tinker JH, Dull DL, Caplan RA et al: Role of monitoring devices in prevention of anesthetic mishaps: a closed claim analysis. Anesthesiology 71:541, 1989
17. Ross AF, Tinker JH: Anesthesia risk, p. 625. In Rogers MC et al (eds): Principles and Practice of Anesthesiology. Mosby Year Book, St. Louis, 1993
18. Lunn JN, Devlin HB: Lessons from the confidential enquiry into perioperative deaths in three NHS regions. Lancet 2:1384, 1987
19. Zeitlin GL: Possible decrease in mortality associated with anaesthesia: a comparison of two time periods in Massachusetts, USA. Anaesthesia 44:432, 1989
20. Taylor G, Larson CP, Prestwich R: Unexpected cardiac arrest during anesthesia and surgery: an environmental study. JAMA 236:2758, 1976
21. Keenan RS, Boyan CP: Decreasing frequency of anesthetic cardiac arrests. J Clin Anesth 3:354, 1991

22. Eichhorn JH: Documenting improved anesthesia outcome. J Clin Anesth 3:351, 1991

23. Duncan PG, Cohen MM: Pulse oximetry and capnography in anaesthetic practice: an epidemiological appraisal. Can J Anaesth 38:619, 1991

24. Tiret L, Desmonts JM, Hatton F et al: Complications associated with anaesthesia: a prospective survey in France. Can Anaesth Soc J 33:336, 1986

25. Moller JT, Pedersen T, Rasmussen LS et al: Randomized evaluation of pulse oximetry in 20,802 patients. II. Perioperative events and postoperative complications. Anesthesiology 79:445, 1993

26. Eichhorn JH: Pulse oximetry as a standard of practice in anesthesia. Anesthesiology 78:423, 1993

27. Holzer JF: Liability insurance issues in anesthesiology. Int Anesthesiol Clin 27:205, 1989

28. Orkin FK: Practice standards: the Midas touch or the emperor's new clothes? Anesthesiology 70:567, 1989

29. Keats AS: Anesthesia mortality in perspective. Anesth Analg 71:113, 1990

30. International Task Force on Anaesthesiology: Eur J Anaesthesiol 10 suppl 7:1–44, 1993

31. Directory of Members. p. 735. American Society of Anesthesiologists, Park Ridge, IL, 1994

Appendix
American Society of Anesthesiologists Standards for Basic Anesthetic Monitoring[a]
(Approved by House of Delegates on October 21, 1986 and last amended on October 13, 1993)

These standards apply to all anesthesia care although, in emergency circumstances, appropriate upport measures take precedence. These standards may be exceeded at any time based on the judgement of the responsible anesthesiologist. They are intended to encourage quality patient care, but observing them cannot guarantee any specific patient outcome. They are subject to revision from time to time, as warranted by the evolution of technology and practice. They apply to all general anesthetics, regional anesthetics and monitored anesthesia care. This set of standards addresses only the issue of basic anesthetic monitoring, which is one component of anesthesia care. In certain rare or unusual circumstances, (1) some of these methods of monitoring may be clinically impractical, and (2) appropriate use of the described monitoring methods may fail to detect untoward clinical developments. Brief interruptions of continual[b] monitoring may be unavoidable. *Under extenuating circumstances, the responsible anesthesiologist may waive the requirements marked with an asterisk (*); it is* *recommended that when this is done, it should be so stated (including the reasons) in a note in the patient's medical record.* These standards are not intended for application to the care of the obstetrical patient in labor or in the conduct of pain management.

STANDARD I

Qualified anesthesia personnel shall be present in the room throughout the conduct of all general anesthetics, regional anesthetics and monitored anesthesia care.

Objective

Because of the rapid changes in patient status during anesthesia, qualified anesthesia personnel shall be continuously present to monitor the patient and provide anesthesia care. In the event there is a direct known hazard, e.g., radiation, to the anesthesia personnel which might require intermittent remote observation of the patient, some provision for monitoring the patient must be made. In the event that an emergency requires the temporary absence of the person primarily responsible for the anesthetic, the best judgement of the anesthesiologist will be exercised in comparing the

---

[a]From American Society of Anesthesiologists,[31] with permission.
[b]Note that "continual" is defined as "repeated regularly and frequently in steady rapid succession" whereas "continuous" means "prolonged without any interruption at any time."

emergency with the anesthetized patient's condition and in the selection of the person left responsible for the anesthetic during the temporary absence.

STANDARD II

During all anesthetics, the patient's oxygenation, ventilation, circulation and temperature shall be continually evaluated.

Oxygenation

Objective

To ensure adequate oxygen concentration in the inspired gas and the blood during all anesthetics.

Methods

1. Inspired gas: During every administration of general anesthesia using an anesthesia machine, the concentration of oxygen in the patient breathing system shall be measured by an oxygen analyzer with a low oxygen concentration limit alarm in use.*
2. Blood oxygenation: During all anesthetics, a quantitative method of assessing oxygenation such as pulse oximetry shall be employed.* Adequate illumination and exposure of the patient is necessary to assess color.*

Ventilation

Objective

To ensure adequate ventilation of the patient during all anesthetics.

Methods

1. Every patient receiving general anesthesia shall have the adequacy of ventilation continually evaluated. While qualitative clinical signs such as chest excursion, observation of the reservoir breathing bag and auscultation of breath sounds may be adequate, quantitative monitoring of the CO_2 content and/or volume of expired gas is encouraged.
2. When an endotracheal tube is inserted, its correct positioning in the trachea must be verified by clinical assessment and by identification of carbon dioxide in the expired gas.* End-tidal

CO_2 analysis, in use from the time of endotracheal tube placement is strongly encouraged.
3. When ventilation is controlled by a mechanical ventilator, there shall be in continuous use a device that is capable of detecting disconnection of components of the breathing system. The device must give an audible signal when its alarm threshold is exceeded.
4. During regional anesthesia and monitored anesthesia care, the adequacy of ventilation shall be evaluated, at least, by continual observation of qualitative clinical signs.

Circulation

Objective

To ensure the adequacy of the patient's circulatory function during all anesthetics.

Methods

1. Every patient receiving anesthesia shall have the electrocardiogram continuously displayed from the beginning of anesthesia until preparing to leave the anesthetizing location.*
2. Every patient receiving anesthesia shall have arterial blood pressure and heart rate determined and evaluated at least every five minutes.*
3. Every patient receiving general anesthesia shall have, in addition to the above, circulatory function continually evaluated by at least one of the following palpitation of a pulse, auscultation of heart sounds, monitoring of a tracing of intra-arterial pressure, ultrasound peripheral pulse monitoring, or pulse plethysmography or oximetry.

Body Temperature

Objective

To aid in the maintenance of appropriate body temperature during all anesthetics.

Methods

There shall be readily available a means to continuously measure the patient's temperature. When changes in body temperature are intended, anticipated or suspected, the temperature shall be measured.

Cost-Benefit Analysis in Monitoring

5

Susan L. Polk
Michael F. Roizen

Over 25 million anesthetics are administered every year in the United States. However, anesthesiologists don't just put people to sleep. The practice of anesthesia includes keeping body functions stable even during the variable stresses imposed by the trauma of surgery. It is hard to conceive that human physiological responses can be regulated without monitoring. It is also hard to conceive that the monitoring evolution has not benefited surgical patients. Yet, as we attempt to justify new monitoring devices, we realize that the data are still not plentiful. Three potential benefits from the use of monitoring have been cited. These include (1) reduced morbidity and mortality in monitored patients; (2) a cost benefit in reduction of ICU (intensive care unit) admissions, rule out myocardial infarction protocols, blood gas or other laboratory analyses, or length of hospital stay; and (3) an educational benefit where we learn so much from the patients we monitor that all patients receive some outcome benefit.

The limited resources available to invest in medical care imply that we need some way to determine which choices are best for the well-being of our patients. Unfortunately, data are lacking regarding the most appropriate selection of monitoring strategies to guarantee the best outcome. Prospective studies are difficult to perform. For example, assuming a baseline reinfarction rate of 6 percent, a power analysis[1] indicates that to show an 80 percent benefit at the $P < .05$ level of pulmonary artery catheterization during surgery in patients with previous myocardial infarctions, the experimental de-

sign would require that about 1,000 patients be studied. The logistics of designing such a study are overwhelming. Patients would be required to undergo surgery of similar types by surgeons of similar skill with similar anesthetics administered by anesthesiologists of similar skill and be randomly allocated into a monitored or a control group. Bashein and colleagues[2] have determined that in low-risk patients undergoing cardiac revascularization, more than 6,000 patients would be required in a prospective randomized study to show a positive effect of pulmonary artery catheters in reducing the rate of perioperative infarctions. Similarly, based on information gathered by Moller and colleagues[3] it would take a study of 500,000 to 1,900,000 patients (randomly allocated and blind design) to prove any significant difference in morbidity caused by pulse oximetry. These numbers assume no intervention is allowed in the patients randomized to no monitoring, and that pulse oximetry detects 80 percent of instances leading to morbid events.[4] Perhaps morbidity and mortality are not appropriate endpoints. More importantly, perhaps these studies do not do justice to monitoring because we learn so much from monitoring that we transfer this knowledge to care of the nonmonitored patient as well.

That monitoring has the potential to change outcome is less questioned than before; but the data are still inconclusive. However, monitoring some functions is now a standard, and many malpractice insurance carriers are determining premium scales based in part on the type of monitoring used by the insured.[5,6] This practice arises from the belief that monitoring does change outcome, and is substantiated by indirect data. Data from the ASA Closed Claims Study indicate that 34 percent of the claims involve injuries related to respiratory gas exchange.[7] The ASA Closed Claims analyses have provided expert opinions about percentage of incidents involving inadequate ventilation that could have been prevented with better monitoring. Tinker and coworkers[8] examined claims involving respiratory inadequacy and found that 93 percent of those in adults could have been averted by using and appropriately responding to data obtained from a pulse oximeter and capnograph. In children, 89 percent of these adverse respiratory events could have been prevented.[9] Claims filed as a result of inadequate ventilation resulted in a very high death and permanent brain damage rate: 70 percent death and 30 percent permanent brain damage in children[9] and 70 percent and 15 percent in adults.[7] Eichhorn[10] noted that the rate of death, permanent disability and cardiac arrest from anesthesia in the 12 months after the Harvard monitoring standards (including pulse oximetry) went into effect dropped from .13/10,000 (for the prior 10 years) to .046/10,000. However, this improvement was not statistically significant because of the rarity of such events before these standards were instituted. Keenan and associates[11] reported a 0.67/10,000 incidence of cardiac arrest under anesthesia due to hypoxemia at their institution in the years 1969 to 1985, and an incidence of zero in 31,000 anesthetics after pulse oximetry became a standard in 1984. In contrast, the Canadian four-center study of anesthetic outcomes, which included data on 27,184 inpatients and 6,914 outpatients over a 15-month period, failed to demonstrate a difference in deaths or major events despite a significant difference in utilization of capnography and pulse oximetry.[12–14]

Coté and colleagues[15] used pulse oximeters to monitor 152 pediatric patients but allowed the anesthesiologist to see the monitors only in half the patients unless saturation fell below 85 percent for more than 30 seconds. Major hypoxic events occurred significantly more frequently in the pulse oximeter nonavailable group. This was presumably because the early warning provided by the oximeter (when the anesthesiologist was allowed to monitor it) allowed successful intervention. Of course, the ultimate outcome of those events is only spec-ulative, and so the study really doesn't prove an outcome benefit from oximetry. McKay and Noble[16] detected critical incidents with pulse oximetry in 6 percent of cases. These incidents were serious enough that the authors believed the events would have led to adverse outcomes if intervention had not been achieved. However, we do not know how many of the incidents would have been detected in time and corrected without the use of the technology.[17] Cullen and associates[18] showed that the introduction of pulse oximetry decreased the incidence of postoperative ICU admission for ruling out a myocardial infarction from 19.5/10,000 to 6.05/10,000 and for ventilatory problems from 18.1/10,000 to 9/10,000. However, neither comparison reached statistical significance.

At this time, there are *no* studies demonstrating either an increasing rate of anesthesia accidents or a significant increase in the incidence of accidents due to incorrect monitoring practice. Given our belief that monitors do not cause harm, there are two ways to compare different monitoring strategies with respect to their relative costs and benefits. This chapter explains these analyses and provides several examples. We show how these analyses depend totally on the assumptions one must make about the quality and interpretation of available data, as well as the anesthesiologist's ability to make the changes in management necessary to avert a bad outcome. Our hope is to encourage an understanding of these cost analysis techniques, which can be applied to other monitoring strategies, and to spur the prospective studies that will provide the missing data needed to determine how we should spend our resources.

THE CASE OF RESPIRATORY MONITORING

A cost-effectiveness analysis is used to determine the most efficient or productive use of resources. The costs of different strategies (to achieve the same outcome) are compared, so that the least expensive strategy can be chosen. A cost-benefit analysis, on the other hand, compares strategies with respect to the total economic benefit resulting from their use. The strategy with the highest benefit, regardless of but including the original investment, can then be chosen. The remainder of this chapter will describe these calculations in detail

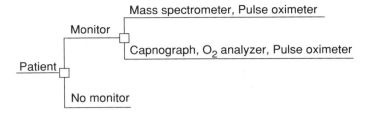

Fig. 5-1. Base of decision tree.

and provide several examples for commonly used monitors.

DETERMINING OUTCOME WITH AND WITHOUT RESPIRATORY MONITORING

For either cost-effectiveness or cost-benefit calculation, the first step is constructing a decision tree, indicating all possible beneficial, harmful, or no effect on outcomes of a particular strategy and the probabilities of each.[19] Decision analysis uses Baysian statistics, or probabilities, at each branch and requires only simple mathematics once the tree is constructed. Decision trees are used extensively in many areas of industry and medicine to allow decision-makers to choose the action with the highest probability of resulting in the desired outcome (highest expected utility).

Let us work through the example of multiplexed mass spectrometry or Raman spectrometry and pulse oximeters ($_M$MSO, $_R$SO) versus capnography, pulse oximeters and oxygen analyzers (COO), versus using no special monitoring strategy for respiratory gases (NM) (Fig. 5-1). The square in the figure represents the decision to monitor or not to monitor. If the decision is made to monitor, then another decision must be made to use either MSO or COO. From this point, branchings of the tree, called *nodes*, represent chance rather than decision opportunities, and are indicated by circles instead of squares. Each possible outcome has a probability of occurring, and at each node all the resultant probabilities add up to 1.0. The simplest branch to develop is that where NM is the strategy (Fig. 5-2).

The possible outcomes of that strategy we will consider are a good outcome [P(G)], a grave disability (indicating permanent brain damage where respiratory accidents are involved) [P(GD)], or death [P(D)]. Grave disability is defined by the National Association of Insurance Commissioners

(NIAC) as quadriplegia, severe brain damage, requirement of lifelong care, or fatal prognosis.[20] Figures for these probabilities are gathered from the older literature, where we assume no monitoring system was used (because none was mentioned and these technologies were not in widespread use). The incidence of grave disability was previously assumed to equal that of death due partially or totally to anesthesia.[21] However, more recent publications from the ASA Closed Claims analysis indicate that the incidence of permanent brain damage in the total database is one-third the incidence of death.[22] Since this estimate is the only number available from the time before routine respiratory gas and pulse oximeter monitoring were in use, we will assume it is accurate. Table 5-1 summarizes estimates for the probability of death under anesthesia before respiratory gas monitoring was in widespread use. It is evident that the more modern the study, the lower the incidence, meaning that many factors other than monitoring or learning from monitoring may be causing the effect. Nonetheless, the figure we will use is the mean, 2.1/10,000 anesthetics. It follows that the incidence we will assume for permanent grave disability is one-third of that, or 0.7/10,000.

Figure 5-3 develops the monitoring branch. Using $_M$MSO, $_R$MO or COO produces either an incident or no incident. P(I), the probability of an incident occurring during anesthesia, was estimated using data reported in the literature, a procedure

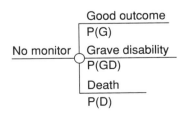

Fig. 5-2. Development of NM (no monitor) branch.

that presents several problems: (1) The accuracy of reporting all incidents is often questionable; (2) there is no mention of which monitoring was in use at the time of data collection; (3) there is often no denominator mentioned, so that the incidence cannot be estimated; (4) we do not know if the incidents leading to death are the same as the incidents leading to [P(GD)]. *Since we are comparing monitoring strategies, however, inaccurate basic assumptions will not affect the relative values if we apply the same assumptions to each strategy.* Table 5-2 summarizes the information used to determine P(I). The mean estimate is used for our calculations, and it is assumed that critical incidents occur in about 9 percent of all cases.

Because all the probabilities at each node of the tree must add up to 1.0, the probability of no incident occurring is [1 − P(I)], or 91 percent of all

anesthetics. Although this is probably a low estimate of all critical incident occurrence, we accept the figure for these calculations because a low occurrence tends to minimize the benefits of monitoring. Cost analyses frequently assume the lowest estimate of benefit because if the strategy is useful under these assumptions it is surely useful under other conditions.

The probability of detecting incidents [P(DET)] once they have occurred can be estimated from older published lists of incidents, although in most cases the information is not detailed enough to allow a estimation that is unbiased to monitoring strategies. We originally assumed that only mass spectroscopy could detect nitrogen leak into the circuit and anesthetic vapor overdoses or delivery mistakes. However, adding pulse oximetry to the two respiratory gas monitoring systems provides a

TABLE 5-1. Incidence of Death Due Partially or Totally to Anesthesia

Incidence[a]	Reference	Comments
67/338,934 to 240/338934 (0.0002 to 0.0007)	Hovi-Viander[66]	100 Finnish hospitals, 1 year, anesthesia totally or partially to blame
67/198,103 (0.00034)	Tiret et al.[24]	Prospective study, French, anesthesia totally or partially to blame
1/10,000 to 1/4000 (0.0001 to 0.00025)	Pierce[21]	Summary of U.S. Estimates
2.2/10,000 (0.00022)	Harrison[67]	One South African Hospital, 1967–77, prospective study
1/10,000 (0.0001)	Minuck[68]	One Canadian hospital, 1957–64, deaths due totally to anesthesia
1/27,500 to 1/30,000 (0.00004 to 0.00003)	Holland[69]	New South Wales, Australia, 1979, deaths due totally to anesthesia
1/10,000 (0.0001)	Lunn and Mushin[70]	Deaths due totally to anesthesia, 1981, England
1.9/10,000 to 2.2/10,000 (0.00019 to (0.00022)	Lunn[71]	Totally or partially due to anesthesia; summary of British, Finnish, and South African studies
2/10,000 (0.0002)	Turnbull et al.[72]	One Canadian hospital, preventable anesthetic deaths
1/3365 (0.0003)	Moller et al.[3]	Prospective randomized study of pulse oximetry in Denmark, 1989–90, 5 hospitals; anesthesia a possible contributor

[a]Range 0.0007 to 0.00003, mean estimate is 2.1 in 10,000.

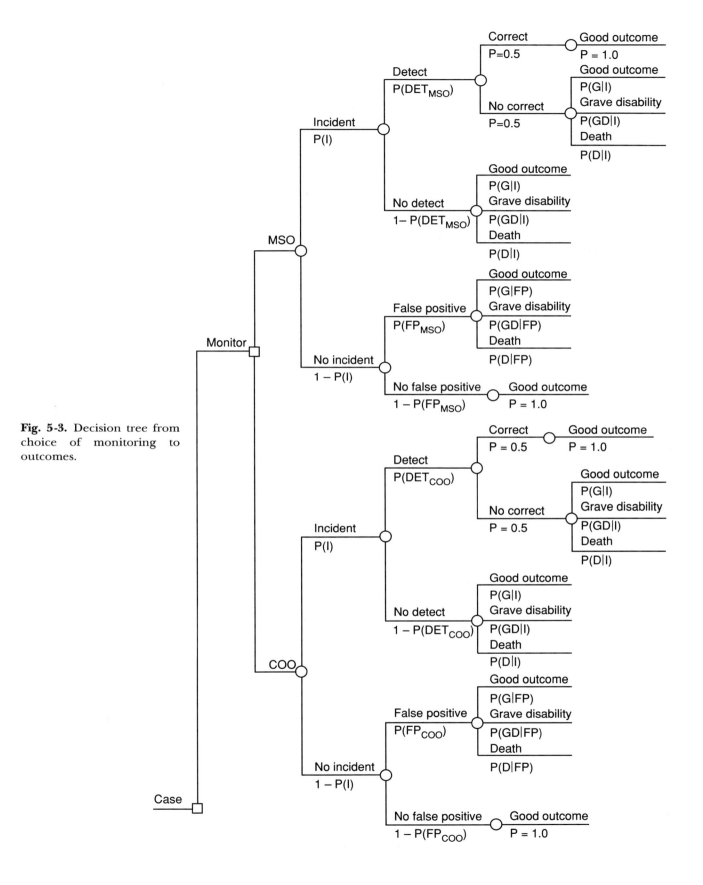

Fig. 5-3. Decision tree from choice of monitoring to outcomes.

TABLE 5-2. Probability of Occurrence of Critical Incidents P (I)

Incidence[a]	Reference	Comments
81/8312 (0.0097)	Craig and Wilson[73]	Reported incidents in 12 hospitals in Bath, UK, over 6 months
1/739 (0.0014)	Tiret et al.[24]	Prospective study of randomly selected French hospitals, 1978–82; major complications
0.18	Cooper et al.[74]	Prospective study, incidents that could or did impact on recovery room care, 1 hospital, some with pulse oximeter monitoring, 12,088 patients, 1985–86
0.106	Cohen et al.[75]	One teaching hospital in Canada, 60,524 patients, 1979–83
0.06	McKay and Noble[16]	Detected by pulse oximeter, prospective study, 1 hospital, 4 months, 1986–87
0.183	Cohen et al.[13]	Canadian 4-center study, major incidents related to anesthesia

[a]Range 0.14% to 18.3%, mean 9% of cases have a critical incident.

warning of hypoxic drug mixture or vapor overdose (if the anesthesiologist is sensitive to a weakening pulse), and so the difference in the two types of monitoring systems becomes negligible in terms of the percentage of incidents detected. Analysis of all the closed claims in the ASA study up to 1989 indicated that 31.5 percent could have been prevented with better monitoring, if properly interpreted and if intervention was appropriate.[8] A survey of many older publications with our estimate of [$P(DET_{MSO})$] and [$P(DET_{COO})$] is presented in Table 5-3. The range for both is 31.5 to 75 percent; the mean estimate is 52.9 percent for both strategies. Since detection of incidents requires a human factor as well as technology, we assumed that only 90 percent of possible detections were picked up by the anesthesiologist. Then we further assumed that only 50 percent of the detected incidents were correctable because that fairly accurately reflects the opinions of adequacy of care presented in the Closed Claims Analysis.[22] This means that with MSO or COO (0.529 × .90 × .50) or 23.8 percent of all deaths and 23.8 percent of all grave disabilities resulting from anesthesia can be prevented. These figures represent the sensitivies of the strategies. These estimates are probably low, the most reasonable figures probably being closer to the higher figures found in the table.

To be even more conservative in estimating the benefit of monitoring, one can assume falsepositive events detected by the monitors, which lead to actions causing death or disability. No figures are available, but let us assume that the bad effect is 25 percent of the good effect to further prejudice the case against monitors and to make them look as expensive as possible. This indicates that for every four detections and corrections of true problems because of the monitoring, there is another detection when in fact there is no incident, which leads to the possibility of a bad outcome. This yields only an 80 percent specificity rate.

Thus COO or MSO prevent [23.8 − (23.8/5)] or 19.2 percent of all deaths and 19.2 percent of all grave disabilities due to anesthesia.

COST-EFFECTIVENESS ANALYSIS OF FOUR STRATEGIES OF RESPIRATORY GAS ANALYSIS

These data and our assumptions indicate that MSO and COO can prevent 19.2 percent of all anesthetic deaths and permanent grave disabilities. After the cost of the technology is calculated per case, the two strategies can be compared with respect to the cost to prevent one death using each.

A pulse oximeter costs about $3,000. Adding 25 percent of that amount over 7 years, and assuming the monitor is used for 3 cases per day × 260 days × 7 years, it costs $1.51 per case. Various probes add to the cost, but if one adult disposable probe at $15 is used for 10 patients, the cost per case is about $1.50 for the probe and $3.00 total.

The cost of COO per case equals the initial investment in capnograph and oxygen analyzer or $6,250 + 25 percent of that cost per year for 7 years for maintenance and depreciation divided by three cases per day × 260 days per year × 7 years or about $3.15 plus $3.00 for the pulse oximeter ($6.15). The cost of a multiplexed MS ($_MMS$) per case equals the initial investment in $_MMS$ + 25 percent of that cost per year over 7 years for upkeep, depreciation, and personnel divided by 16 ORs × 3 cases per day × 260 days per year × 7 years or about $3.15 plus $3.00 for the pulse oximeter, assuming an initial investment of $100,000 ($6.15).

To ensure monitoring ability when the $_MMS$ is "down," half the cost of COO without the oximeter can be added to provide backup abilities, bringing the per-case cost to $7.73. This figure is not fair to $_MMS$, however, because many systems are in use for much longer than the given 7 years and their "down time" does not warrant having the extra capnographs around all the time.

A Raman scattering gas analyzer ($_RSO$) costs about $17,000, and includes the pulse oximeter. They are too new to have established much of a track record, but using our same formula, equipping 16 operating rooms and adding 25 percent of that cost per year over 7 years results in a per-case cost of $8.56.

Table 5-4 compares the strategies. The number of deaths per 100,000 anesthetics that can be averted with each strategy is calculated and divided by the cost of monitoring for those 100,000 cases. The resulting costs per death averted seems quite high at first glance. We have prejudiced the case

TABLE 5-3. Percent of Adverse Outcomes Due to Anesthesia Possibly Preventable by Respiratory Monitoring

Reference	MSO (%)	COO (%)	Comments
Graff et al.[76]	38	38	Study of pediatric patients
Minuck[60]	54	54	Incidents in 1 Canadian hospital, 1 year
Salem et al.[77]	54.2	54.2	12 years, 7 institutions, cardiac arrests in pediatric patients leading to death
Taylor et al.[78]	73.2	73.2	16 years, all cardiac arrests due to anesthesia, CA insurance claims
Harrison[67]	69.8	69.8	1 year prospective study, all anesthetic deaths at 1 South African hospital
Utting et al.[79]	39.4	39.4	All incidents reported to UK Medical Defense Union, which resulted in death or permanent brain damage, 1970–77
Green and Taylor[80]	45	45	All incidents reported to UK Medical Defense Union, which resulted in death, 1977–82
Hovi-Viander[66]	46.3	46.3	1 year, all OR deaths in Finnish hospitals
Rosen[81]	36.7	36.7	British maternal mortality voluntary reports, 1977–78
Cooper et al.[82]	57.1	57.1	Of most frequently reported incidents, prospective study
Davis[83]	72	72	Of major claims to St. Paul's (1976–78)
Solazzi and Ward[84]	47.9	47.9	Of insurance claims, WA, 1971–82
Keenan and Boyan[85]	75	75	Cardiac arrests and deaths due to anesthesia, 1 hospital
Tinker et al[8]	31.5	31.5	Of closed claims analyzed in ASA study, filed 1974–88

Range 31.5–75%, mean 52.9% of incidents could be detected by respiratory monitoring.

TABLE 5-4. Cost Effectiveness Analysis of Respiratory Monitoring Strategies

Strategy	Cost/Case	No. of Cases	No. Deaths Averted	Cost/Death Averted
CO_2 and O_2 monitors and pulse oximetry	$6.15	100,000	21 × .192 = 4.03	($6.15 × 100,000)/4.03 = $152,605
Multiplexed MS and pulse oximetry	$6.15	100,000	21 × .192 = 4.03	($61.5 × 100,000)/4.03 = $152,605
Multiplexed MS with CO backup and pulse oximetry	$7.73	100,000	21 × .192 = 4.03	($7.73 × 100,000)/4.03 = $191,811
Raman spectroscopy	$8.56	100,000	21 × .192 = 4.03	($8.56 × 100,000)/4.03 = $212,407

against the monitors significantly in this analysis because of the low estimates of incident occurrence, detection, and correction, and by including a generous number of false positives leading to harm.

Duncan and Cohen,[23] using recent studies reporting reduction of risk of death or grave outcome since monitoring was routinely incorporated,[10,11,24] figured a pulse oximeter and capnograph would save one life in 8,000 to 77,519 patients treated, so, using these figures and our per-case cost of $6.15, their estimates result in a cost of $49,200 to $476,742 to avert one bad outcome. It has been estimated that it costs $9 million to save one life by routine preoperative hemoglobin testing,[25] so these figures do appear to indicate that monitors are cost effective.

OTHER COST-EFFECTIVENESS ANALYSES

Monitoring for Hypoxic Injury to the Brain

During cardiopulmonary bypass (CPB) the incidence of stroke due to hypoperfusion is 1 to 2 percent, although both hypoperfusion and embolic phenomena are the causes.[26–29] Recent studies of processed EEGs or evoked potential monitoring, (costing $21,000 to $40,000 for compact portable monitors that can be interpreted by properly trained and experienced anesthesiologists) and transcranial Doppler (TCD) (costing $28,000 for unilateral and $34,000 for bilateral monitoring) during CPB have shown no statistically significant effect on outcome, and opinion has been expressed that they are not cost effective in stroke prevention. Nonetheless, we will calculate the cost

effectiveness of these technologies in preventing one stroke.

Bashein and colleagues[2] failed to show a correlation between EEG changes during CPB and postoperative neurologic function in a prospective study of 78 patients, and found the monitoring data inadequate for analysis in 25.6 percent of patients. Other studies have reported repeated difficulties with cerebral function monitors (CFMs) and EEGs.[30] Arom and coworkers[31] found that intervention to improve cerebral perfusion based on data obtained by computerized EEGs resulted in a decrease in global neurologic deficits from 44 percent to 5 percent on postoperative day one, and from 5 percent to 2 percent on later examinations. We do not know the ultimate outcomes of these patients, however. For our calculations we will assume that a processed EEG could detect and enable intervention for cerebral hypoperfusion leading to decreasing strokes by half, or 0.5 to 1 percent of CPB patients. However, accounting for the fact that the data are inadequate for evaluation in 25.6 percent of the patients in which it is used, and that the patients who might develop a stroke are evenly distributed in the adequately monitored and inadequately monitored groups, then the percentage of all coronary artery bypass grafting patients in which the technology is effective becomes (0.744 × 0.005) 0.372 percent to (0.744 × 0.01) 0.744 percent of cases.

For our analysis, we will assume one processed EEG or evoked potential machine costs $30,000. Upkeep and depreciation for 7 years brings the cost of the technology to $82,500. We will assume it is used in one operating room for two cases a day 260 days a year for that 7 years, or for 3,640 patients during its lifetime. The cost per patient for the monitoring therefore is $22.66. Assuming the stroke rate from hypoperfusion during CPB to be 1.5 percent, there would be 1,500 strokes per 100,000 patients. With processed EEG technology we could avert 37.2 percent of those 1,500, or 558 strokes. Therefore it would cost [(100,000 × $22.66)]/558 or $4,060 to avert a stroke with this method.

TCD cannot be used in 5 to 15 percent of patients for anatomic reasons,[30,32,33] but its theoretical advantage in CPB cases is that it monitors more than just superficial electrical activity and can provide an earlier warning of brain hypoperfusion. Unlike the EEG, it is not affected by drugs or temperature changes, but is affected by CO_2 alterations. It is also capable of diagnosing the passage of emboli through cerebral vessels to facilitate intervention if that is possible. Outcome studies using TCD during CPB are missing, but we will assume that it would prevent stroke in half the patients at risk, just as we assumed for EEG monitoring. A bilateral monitor costs $34,000, using our formula for 7 years and one operating room, $25.69 per patient. Since it cannot be used in 5 to 15 percent of patients (we'll say 10 percent),[34] and making the same assumptions as above, that 50 percent of strokes could be averted with it, it costs $3,362 to avert one stroke. It is cheaper than EEG in this analysis because it can be used successfully in a higher percentage of patients, even though we did not take into account its other clinical advantages or disadvantages.

In the case of carotid endarterectomy the incidence of intraoperative hypoperfusion leading to perioperative stroke or death is 1 to 21 percent. Figure 5-4 shows a decision tree comparing monitoring with processed EEG (EEG), transcranial Doppler (TCD), stump pressure (SP), and no monitoring in prevention of a bad outcome from cerebral hypoperfusion.

The International Transcranial Doppler Collaborators[35] performed an 11-center retrospective study of 1,495 carotid endarterectomies monitored with transcranial Dopplers. They found that the incidence of severe cerebral ischemia was 7.2 percent, half of which resolved spontaneously, and the outcome of the other half varied, depending on whether shunting was used as a result of detecting the ischemia. McDowell and colleagues[32] reported very similar results in a study of 238 patients, 9.2 percent of whom developed severe ischemia during carotid clamping. The technology allowed the use of protective measures in patients who were at severe risk and avoided potentially harmful shunting in those who were not. Naylor et al.[30] in a small study, showed that TCD monitoring provided information that allowed intervention to prevent prolonged intraoperative ischemia in 5 of 30 patients. We will assume that it cannot be used in 10 percent of patient. TCD data correlate well with carotid stump pressure monitoring. It remains to be seen whether it provides an advantage over that simple technology, but it is evident that there is an advantage over EEG monitoring because it provides an earlier warning of developing problems[33] and is capable of distinguishing between embolic phenomena and hypoperfusion.[36] Table 5-5 summarizes the figures for stroke rates in the above mentioned situations.

Given our one operating room and two operations per day, EEG monitoring costs $22.66 per case. TCD, because a unilateral monitor can be effective in this situation, costs $21.15 per case and stump pressure monitoring costs about $1.00 per case for the tubing and needle, assuming the transducer, heparinized flush solution, and pressure monitor would already be in use for invasive blood pressure monitoring. Severe ischemia during carotid artery clamping occurs in about 10 to 25 percent of patients. For the purposes of this analysis, we will assume that the TCD and EEG provide the same quality of information in the same percentage of patients, 90 percent. Stump pressures are generally monitored only immediately after clamping, and so might miss later problems like emboli, malfunctioning shunts or decreasing collateral circulation, problems that have occurred at a reported frequency of about 7 percent.[30] Table 5-6 shows that the probability of stroke decreases from 45 percent to zero if a shunt is inserted on the basis of TCD monitoring information. We might assume that in patients who were not ischemic at the time of carotid clamping, the incidence of stroke would decrease to 1.1 percent from the median of 6.8 percent of nonischemic patients who were shunted, a reduction of 5.7 percent. In a population of 1,000 patients, 100 to 250 patients might become severely ischemic on clamping, 45 to 112 might sustain a stroke without a shunt. The other 750 to 900 patients would not be severely ischemic, but if the surgeon were to decide to shunt them, 33 to 51 might sustain a stroke. Of the 750 to 900

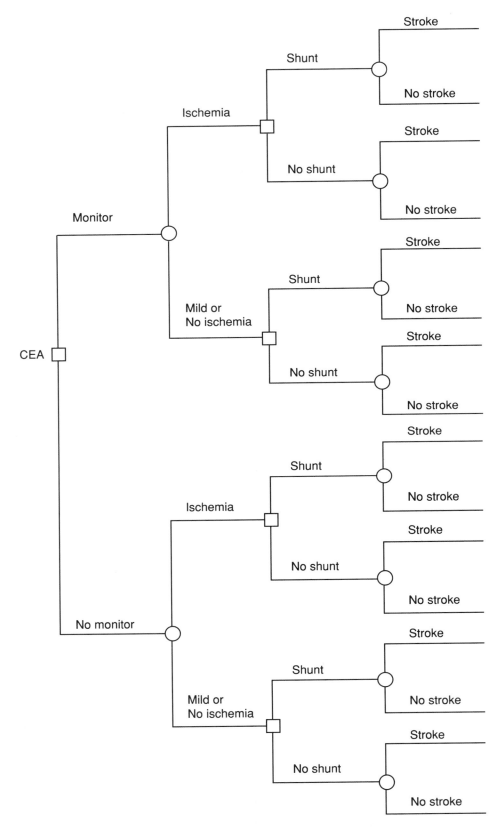

Fig. 5-4. Decision tree for monitoring and shunting in carotid endarterectomy.

TABLE 5-5. Stroke Rate for Carotid Endarterectomy

Reference	Severe Ischemia, Shunt (%)	Severe Ischemia, No Shunt (%)	Mild or No Ischemia, Shunt (%)	Mild or No Ischemia, No Shunt (%)
McDowell et al.[32]	0	44	9.5	1.5
Halsey[35]	0	46	4.2	0.68

patients not ischemic at clamp time and not shunted because of adequate stump pressure, 52 to 63 might develop problems not detected by stump pressure monitoring at clamp time, and go on to sustain a stroke. Therefore, TCD and EEG might prevent 78 to 163 strokes in 1,000 patients, and monitoring stump pressure might prevent 24 to 100 strokes, if the surgeon based his decision to shunt on information from them. Because of anatomic difficulties, however, TCD might not be useful in 10 percent of cases, so for TCD the number of strokes prevented drops to 70 to 147.

In summary, Table 5-6 calculates the cost of each monitor in averting one stroke for carotid endarterectomy (CEA) and coronary artery bypass grafting (CABG) surgery. It is much cheaper to prevent a stroke with stump pressure monitoring than any other technology during CEA, but 7 percent of patients are still at risk. Monitoring brain perfusion during cardiopulmonary bypass (CPB) is extremely expensive because of the rarity of perioperative

stroke, the high percentage caused by phenomena that cannot be reversed, and the sensitivity of cerebral circulation to other factors going on during the procedure. Using expensive technology to monitor during carotid clamping and basing the decision to insert a shunt when severe drops in brain perfusion occur are much more cost effective. Of course, these calculations are relevant only if there is a competent operator to monitor the changes and make the necessary suggestions to reverse them, and if the surgeon agrees with the recommendations.

Monitoring for Myocardial Ischemia

Around 7 to 8 million of the 25 million noncardiac surgery patients undergoing anesthesia yearly in the United States are at risk to develop an adverse cardiac event. In 18 to 45 percent of patients undergoing vascular or cardiac surgery intraoper-

TABLE 5-6. Cost Effectiveness Analysis of Cerebral Perfusion Monitoring Strategies

Strategy	Cost/ Case	No. of Cases	No. Strokes Averted	Cost per Stroke Averted
EEG for CEA	$22.66	1000	78–163	$22,660/78 to 163 ($290.51 to $136.60)
TCD for CEA	$21.15	1000	70–147	$21,150/70 to 147 ($302.14 to $143.88)
SP for CEA	$1.00	1000	24–100	$1000/24 to 100 ($41.00 to $10.00)
EEG for CPB	$22.66	100,000	558	$2,266,000/558 ($4,060)
TCD for CPB	$25.69	100,000	674	$2,569,000/674 ($3,362)

Abbreviations: EEG, electroencephalogram; CEA, carotid endarterectomy; TCD, transcranial Doppler; SP, stump pressure; CPB, cardiopulmonary bypass.

ative myocardial ischemia may occur.[37,38] Pre- and intraoperative ischemia correlate most strongly with the preoperative condition, and the development of postoperative ischemia is the strongest predictor of myocardial infarction.[39] Intraoperative ischemia alone has not been shown to cause adverse outcomes. The value of monitoring for intraoperative ischemia lies in the ability of the anesthesiologist to optimize conditions to prevent further ischemia, since, with Holter-type monitoring, the total time of ischemia has been shown to correlate with outcome.[40] Although no management scheme has yet been proven to improve outcome, our analysis will dwell on the cost of detecting ischemic episodes in high-risk patients undergoing noncardiac surgery; not on the cost of preventing a perioperative myocardial infarction. It seems reasonable that a competent anesthesiologist could manage each individual patient in order to prevent a bad outcome, but the facts show that in many cases patients suffer a bad outcome despite flawless management. This is due to preexisting cardiac disease. This hypothesis has been emphasized by Hollenberg and colleagues,[41] who were able to show that up to 77 percent of postoperative ischemic episodes could be predicted by preoperative cardiac status, and Charlson and colleagues,[42] showed that in high-risk patients, the preoperative ECG predicted 88 percent of postoperative myocardial infarctions and 63 percent of the patients with definite ischemia. Table 5-7 lists several technologies, the percentage of patients with intraoperative ischemia detected with them and the percentage of those who went on to suffer adverse cardiac events. One can see that up to one-third of

patients with intraoperative ischemia go on to suffer adverse outcomes. We do not know what management schemes were practiced as a result of detection of ischemia, but can assume that they were not harmful and may have been helpful. Table 5-8 lists several technologies and their sensitivities (detection of ischemia when ischemia is present) and specificities (no detection of ischemia when ischemia is absent). We will not assign a penalty to the technologies for the lack of specificity (but it is not difficult to imagine that management to optimize hemodynamics taken as the result of a false positive could harm a patient). We will consider the cost effectiveness of the ST-segment trend monitor, continuous 2-lead Holter-type ECG monitor with alarm, transesophageal echocardiography (TEE), and pulmonary artery catheter (PAC) in detecting an episode of myocardial ischemia. We assume that 180 to 450 of 1,000 high-risk patients will become ischemic intraoperatively.[37]

An ST-segment trend monitor costs $300 to $1000. According to the formulas used previously, that comes to $0.15 to $0.50 per case. It cannot be used effectively in patients with pacemaker complexes, LBBB, or LVH (something like one-third of vascular surgery patients and patients who are at risk for perioperative cardiac events). Ischemia might develop in 18 to 45 percent of high-risk patients. ST-segment trend monitor can detect 40 percent of those episodes,[37] but can only be used in 67 percent of high-risk patients because of ECG abnormalities, and thus detects 27 percent of those ischemic episodes, or 48 to 121 episodes in 1,000 patients.

Holter-type continuous ECG monitoring (with

TABLE 5-7. Comparison of Intraoperative Monitoring Technologies in Predicting Postoperative Cardiac Events

Reference	Technology	% of Patients with Intraoperative Ischemia	% of Patients with Intraoperative Ischemia Who Developed Adverse Cardiac Events
Eisenberg et al.[86]	2 lead ECG (Holter)	26	27.4
	TEE	15	32
	12-lead ECG	14	32.6
McCann & Clements[60]	Holter-type	38	12.9
Raby[59]	Holter-type	18	29
Pasternack et al.[40]	Holter-type	37.5–41.2	13.9

Abbreviations: ECG, electrocardiograph; TEE, transesophageal echocardiography.

an alarm that sounds with ST-segment depression or elevation) should provide a better monitor than the ST-segment analyzer attached to the ECG monitor, because continuous surveillance by the anesthesiologist would not be needed. The monitor is more expensive, however. At a cost of $2,000, and our usual formula, the cost comes to $1.01 per patient. An average sensitivity of 50 percent has been reported, but again the monitor cannot be used in a third of patients, so in 1,000 patients 60.3 to 150.8 episodes of ischemia can be detected.

A TEE unit costs $120,000 to $200,000. Its use in the operating room by anesthesiologists may be for detection of various abnormalities, one being ischemia. However, TEE is very sensitive at detecting what we think is ischemia by noting regional wall motion abnormalities, and it also allows intelligent manipulation of volume, contractility and heart rate to optimize cardiac output. Only 6 percent of patients in one study who developed regional wall motion abnormalities (RWMA) actually had an adverse outcome.[43] Studies report that 3 percent of patients could not be monitored because of anatomy and the examinations had to be terminated in 8 percent of cases, for a failure rate of 11 percent.[44,45] Other drawbacks are that the technology to date has not been useful for the critical periods of induction and emergence, and that when used in the operating room, analysis is subjective and discontinuous. Serious complications have been recorded at a rate of 0.2 percent to 0.5 percent.[44–46]

Complications of intraoperative TEE have recently been enumerated, and it appears remarkably safe when used for any surgery except that in the sitting position.[47] Given our usual formula, the technology costs $38.46 to $100.73 (without professional charges) for each patient. Since it has been used as the standard for ischemia in most comparative studies, we will assume it can detect 100 percent of episodes of intraoperative ischemia, but cannot be used in 11 percent of patients because of anatomy or other reasons. Because the anesthesiologist does not look at the monitor continuously, we will assume that only 75 percent of ischemic episodes are noted, and only $.67 \times (180 \text{ to } 450)$ or 90.4 to 301.5 of 1,000 patients benefit. An ST-segment monitor is cheapest, but misses many ischemic episodes. TEE is very expensive but might be best at deciding whom should receive intensive postoperative therapy. Table 5-9 summarizes the cost-effectiveness analysis.

Pulmonary artery catheterization for intraoperative monitoring of patients at risk for myocardial ischemia appears to be ineffective at diagnosing ischemia itself.[42–51] There are myriad ongoing factors that change the wedge pressure (PCWP), and the diagnosis of ischemia is usually made when the PCWP rises ≥3 mmHg.[51] The pulmonary artery catheter should help the anesthesiologist optimize conditions to help prevent permanent damage and a poor outcome, but the evidence showing that it makes a difference is questionable.[52,53]

TABLE 5-8. Sensitivity and Specificity of Various Monitors for Detection of Intraoperative Myocardial Ischemia

Reference	Monitor	Sensitivity (%)	Specificity (%)	Standard
Jain et al.[87]	Marquette MAC-12 (12-lead ECG)	89	94	CK MB >25 IU/L
Ellis et al.[37]	ST-segment analyzer (H-P)	75	69	Continuous 8-lead ECG read-off line by cardiologist
		40	63	TEE, reviewed later
	Continuous 8-lead ECG (ST change and T wave inversion)	40	58	TEE reviewed later
Van Daele[51]	PCWP	25	95	TEE
	12-lead ECG	69	99	TEE
Leung et al.[88]	PCWP	10	NA	TEE
	Holter-type	44	NA	TEE
Eisenberg[86]	Holter	50	75	Adverse outcome

**TABLE 5-9. Cost Effectiveness Analysis of Monitoring Strategies for
Myocardial Ischemia in High-Risk Patients**

Strategy	Cost per Case	No. of Ischemic Episodes Detected	Cost per Detection
ST-segment trend monitor	$0.15–$0.50	48–121 per 1000 patients	$1.24–$10.42
Holter-type	$1.01	60.3–150.8 per 1000 patients	$7.70–$16.75
TEE	$38.46–$100.73	90.4–301.5 per 1000 patients	$127.56–$1114.27

MONITORING FOR POSTOPERATIVE MYOCARDIAL INFARCTION

The use of a pulmonary artery catheter to monitor patients with previous recent myocardial infarction (MI) and to guide normalization of hemodynamics for three days postoperatively has been shown to result in a perioperative MI rate of 1.9 percent with a death rate of 0.7 percent.[54] The results from previous studies in patients over 60 years of age with a history of recent MI, without this type of monitoring, show a perioperative MI rate of 6 percent with a 3 percent mortality. If you assume that you would be using a central venous pressure (CVP) monitor and three days in a regular hospital room otherwise, it costs about $4,200 (more) per patient for the pulmonary artery (PA) catheter, including the equipment to monitor it and three days of postoperative intensive care. Complications of PA pressure monitoring are rare, but potentially severe. Infection and pulmonary infarct and/or necrosis are the most common, occurring at the rate of 2 percent and 1.4 to 8 percent, respectively.[55,56] We will assume a 2 percent incidence of infarct or necrosis since the catheters are now heparin bonded. The cost of a central line infection averages $600 per patient and prolongs hospitalization by an average of 3 days at an additional cost of $400 per day, but these costs occur in both central venous pressure and pulmonary artery groups with equal frequency.[58] Applying figures calculated by Oster and colleagues[57] for a cost effectiveness analysis of prophylaxis against deep

vein thrombosis, a pulmonary thrombosis or infarct might result in $4,179 for diagnosis, intensive care and oxygen or ventilator therapy.[57]

Therefore, using Rao's regime of intensive care and PAC monitoring with hemodynamic normalization for each high-risk patient, in 100 patients over 60 years of age with previous recent MI, 4.1 perioperative MIs can be avoided (6.0 percent − 1.9 percent) at a cost of [($4,200) + ($4,179 × 2 percent)] × 100, and each MI prevented costs [$4283.58/4.1 × 100] or $104,477. At this additional cost of $4284 per case, we can prevent (3 percent − 0.7 percent) or 2.3 deaths in every 100 patients. With intraoperative pulmonary artery pressure monitoring, which is continued for 3 days postoperatively, it costs ($4,283.58 × 100)/2.3 or $186,243 to avert one death.

It has been suggested by many investigators that surveillance for postoperative ischemic episodes is most useful using Holter-type monitoring. It appears that every postoperative ischemic event is preceded by Holter evidence of ischemia. Raby[59] found an 88 percent sensitivity and 91 percent specificity for prediction of cardiac events by postoperative Holter monitoring. Ischemic episodes detected could be treated with more expensive care, but the majority of patients would escape invasive monitoring and intensive care. Holter monitoring for the perioperative period, including in the operating room, would cost $300 to $550 per day. The majority of postoperative myocardial infarctions occur within the first 2 days,[39,42] and so monitoring the day of surgery and 2 days postoperatively would cost $900 to $1,650 per patient. What no one is able to say is that detecting ischemia in the post-operative period allows intervention to prevent the cardiac event. 30.4 to 53.8 percent of high-risk patients[40,59,60] would show ischemia and then need intensive care with or without, but we'll say with a PAC at $1,400 extra per day, or the $4,283.58 we calculated above. Using Holter monitoring for 100 high-risk patients, we might detect 30 to 54 patients at risk for postoperative myocardial infarctions and send them to intensive care with a postoperative myocardial infarction rate of 1.9 percent and a death rate of 0.7 percent. For the 100 patients we incur $90,000 to $165,000 over usual hospital costs to monitor for whom we should put in the ICU and intensively monitor. Of these 100 patients, 30 to 54 need to go on to the ICU. This would cost $4,283.58 per patient, or (30 × $4284) $128,520 to (54 × $4284) $221,336 in addition to the $90,000 to $165,000 [$218,520 to $386,336] instead of the $482,358 we would spend by sending them all for intensive care with PAC and normalization of hemodynamics. So the cost of averting one myocardial infarction using Holter-type monitoring and then putting the ischemic patients in the ICU with intensive monitoring using the logic above, is ($218,520/4.1) $53,297 to ($386,336/4.1) $94,228. The cost of averting one death using this regime is ($218,520/2.3) $95,009 to ($386,336/2.3) $167,972. Avoiding ICU admission and a PAC in patients who do not need it saves $10,249 to $51,180 per myocardial infarction avoided and $18,271 to 91,234 per death avoided.

COST-BENEFIT ANALYSIS: WHAT IS THE TOTAL COST OF A MONITORING STRATEGY?

Another method used to evaluate monitoring strategies and to compare them is to calculate the probabilities and costs of all the possible outcomes using that strategy. Since this is a more complicated procedure, only the example of respiratory gas analysis developed in the first decision tree will be used (Figs. 5-1 to 5-3). The final cost per case includes both the cost of the monitoring technology itself and the cost of the outcome that results from using it.

The costs of the monitoring technologies have been calculated previously (Table 5-4). The initial cost outlay for using NM (no monitors) is zero. For COO and for $_M$MSO the cost is $6.15 a case. For $_M$MSO with CO backup the cost is $7.73 a case and for $_R$SO the cost is $8.56 a case. The cost of the outcomes with monitoring is more complicated. In the ASA Closed Claims Study, which looked at claims from the mid-1970s to the mid-1980s the mean payment for permanent brain damage was $700,000 (range $10,000 to $6,000,000), and for death was $171,000 (range $750 to $4,000,000).[61] However, for claims not meeting the standard of care *at the time of the incident*, the mean payments were higher. We will not use those higher figures because we can't tell if the bad outcomes are avoidable or not. We will assume that one-eighth of all deaths and disabilities result in indemnity, because the Harvard Medical Practice Study of iatrogenic injuries in 30,121 randomly selected patients hospitalized in New York State in 1984 determined that only 12.5 percent filed suit.[62] Table 5-10 shows the calculations for the costs of bad outcomes. We use the average economic loss to society for a death or PGD which reflects medical care and loss of productivity to society. We also use average indemnity from ASA closed claims study not changed to recent dollar amounts. We calculated a low and a high estimate assuming one-eighth of all bad outcomes result in indemnity payment for the low estimate and all bad outcomes result in indemnity payment for the high estimate. Obviously, these numbers are based on many assumptions. For the

TABLE 5-10. Cost of Bad Outcomes from Anesthesia

Outcome	Economic Loss	Indemnity	High Estimate[a]	Low Estimate[b]
Death	$127,148	$176,000	$298,140	$148,523
Permanent grave disability	$542,842	$700,000	$1,242,842	$630,342

[a]High estimate assumes all bad outcomes lead to indemnity.
[b]Low estimate assumes 1/8 of all cases lead to indemnity.

purpose of comparing various strategies, the actual figures are not really as important as are the differences between them. For this example, only the average figures are used, but all are shown so that the tremendous economic losses involved in just one bad outcome can be appreciated.

THE PROBABILITY THAT AN ANESTHETIC INCORPORATING A MONITORING STRATEGY WILL LEAD TO A BAD OUTCOME

Using Baysian statistics and following the decision tree for probability of death or P(GD) using $_M$MSO (with CO backup), $_R$SO, COO, or NM, calculations from the probabilities of outcomes can be used to derive a P(G), P(GD), or P(D) for each strategy. The probability of grave disability following anesthesia is assumed to equal one-third the probability of death, that is P(GD) = 0.7/10,000 and P(D) = 2.1/10,000. The probabilities of death or of grave disability given an incident [P(D|I), P(GD|I)] are calculated by dividing P(D) by P(I) and P(GD) by P(I). We assumed the same figures for death and grave disability given a false positive incident [P(G|FP), P(GD|FP)]. The results are summarized in Table 5-11. Having arrived at overall probabilities of bad outcomes for each strategy, it is simple to calculate the cost of a case in terms of the technology cost and the outcome cost (EC = estimated cost):

$$EC_{monitor} = \text{Cost of Monitor} + [P(D) \times \text{Cost(D)}]$$
$$+ [P(GD) \times \text{Cost (GD)}].$$

$$EC_M\text{MSO with CO backup} = \$7.73 + (.00017 \times \$148,523)$$
$$+ (.00006 \times \$630,342)$$
$$= \$7.73 + \$25.25 + \$37.82 = \$70.80$$

$$EC_M\text{MSO} = \$6.15 + (.00017 \times \$148.523)$$
$$+ (.00006 \times \$630,342)$$
$$= \$6.15 + \$25.25 + \$37.82 = \$69.22$$

$$ECCOO = \$6.15 + (.00017 \times \$148.523)$$
$$+ (.00006 \times \$630,342)$$
$$= \$6.15 + \$25.25 + \$37.82 = \$69.22$$

$$EC_R\text{SO} = \$8.56 + (.00017 \times \$148.523)$$
$$+ (.00006 \times \$630,342)$$
$$= \$8.56 + \$25.25 + \$37.82 = \$71.63$$

$$ECNM = (.00021 \times \$148,523)$$
$$+ (.00007 \times \$630,342)$$
$$= \$31.19 + \$44.12) = \$75.31$$

For each anesthetic delivered without respiratory gas monitoring, the outcome cost averages $75.31. The cost can be reduced by using one of the monitoring strategies utilized here. There is not much difference between the strategies. The difference in costs becomes greater when less conservative estimates of death, incidents, and detection are used. In other words, if there are more deaths, more incidents, and more detections and corrections the monitors become more cost beneficial. If there are fewer deaths and disabilities to be averted, the monitors are not as cost-beneficial.

At least three personal computer programs are available for cost-effectiveness and cost-benefit anal-

TABLE 5-11. Probability of Bad Outcome with Respiratory Gas Monitoring

Strategy	P(D)	P(GD)
MSO multiplexed with or without CO backup	2.1/10,000 − (.192 × 2.1/ 10,000) = .00017	0.7/10,000 − (.192 × 0.7/ 10,000) = .00006
$_R$SO	2.1/10,000 − (.192 × 2.1/ 10,000) = .00017	0.7/10,000 − (.192 × 0.7/ 10,000) = .00006
COO	2.1/10,000 − (.192 × 2.1/ 10,000) = .00017	0.7/10,000 − (.192 × 0.7/ 10,000) = .00006
NM	2.1/10,000 = 0.00021	0.67/10,000 = 0.00007

ysis. These programs will vary any of the individual probabilities over the entire range of the others in a sensitivity analysis and find a threshold value for each probability where one choice costs as much as another, and so can be used to make decisions based on the characteristics of different Hospitals.

OTHER APPROACHES TO COST ANALYSIS

Roizen and colleagues[63] provided a different view of the cost effectiveness of pulse oximetry and capnography when they compared the cost of operating room blood gas analyses in the years before the technologies were widely available in their operating rooms to the five years after. They concluded that introduction of these two monitors resulted in a reduction in cost of providing on site blood gas analysis that more than paid for the monitors and their upkeep. In the year 1985 to 1986, when there were no pulse oximeters and one-third of the rooms were equipped with capnography, arterial blood gas (ABG) costs were $76,880. In the year 1989 to 1990, when every room had pulse oximetry and two-thirds had capnography, ABG costs were $33,300, a savings of $43,580. The number of ABGs had decreased from 7.64 to 4.26 per 100 operating room hours, despite evidence for an increasing severity of illness in the patient mix. They calculated the cost of oximetry to be $33,750 for 1989 to 1990, and for the increased number of capnographs to be $3,975 that year, a total expenditure of $37,725. There was a net profit despite the purchase and upkeep of technology because of the decreased cost of ABG analysis.

Pearson and colleagues[64] performed a prospective cost analysis of CVP, PAC, and oximetric PAC in patients who had undergone cardiac surgery, itemizing and totaling costs *billed to the patient only* for the catheter, professional charges for its insertion, ABGs, cardiac output (CO) measurements, hemoglobin (Hb) and hematocrit (Hct) measurements. The results were somewhat confounded because of a question about a lesser severity of illness in the CVP group and substantial crossover from the CVP group to one of the PAC groups. However, they indicated that it cost the patient twice as much ($1,128 vs $591) to have an oximetric PAC inserted and monitored than a CVP, despite the suggestion that mixed venous oxygen data should decrease the need for laboratory work and cardiac output measurements. The patients with the PACs had charges in the mid-range of the other two groups. There was no difference in outcome between any of the groups.

A different approach to determining the cost savings brought about by monitoring was described by Whitcher and coworkers.[65] They estimated the cost of monitoring one operating room with a standard monitoring package including a pulse oximeter, capnograph, spirometer, halometer, noninvasive automated blood pressure machine, oxygen analyzer, stethoscope, ECG and temperature sensor would require an initial outlay of $22,500. If this monitoring package avoided 50 percent of incidents leading to claims, an assumption different from ours but totally within reason given recent evidence from the Closed Claims Analysis, the savings in insurance premiums for hospital and anesthesiologist would amount to $27,000 for that year, a yearly savings of over five times the annualized cost of the monitoring package.

WHY ARE COST ANALYSES SO DIFFICULT?

Our analyses are made more difficult and less believable by the assumptions one must make. The data backing the assumptions are incomplete. For example, it was assumed that 45 percent of the episodes leading to death (or disability) attributed to inadequate gas exchange will be detected and corrected. Since such episodes are so rare, huge numbers of patients would have to be randomly allocated into control and monitored groups to perform a prospective study that would prove or disprove that assumption. Now that pulse oximetry and oxygen analyzers are the standard of care in most parts of the world, investigators are trying to prove their benefits by the decrease in bad outcomes and indemnity, but the numbers needed for a statistically significant result are so great and the technology is becoming so pervasive, such results will always remain illusive.

On the other hand, specific outcomes that occur with a greater frequency are suitable for randomized controlled trials of monitoring strategies. EEG or TCD monitoring (as they affect the decision to place a shunt) for prevention of strokes and car-

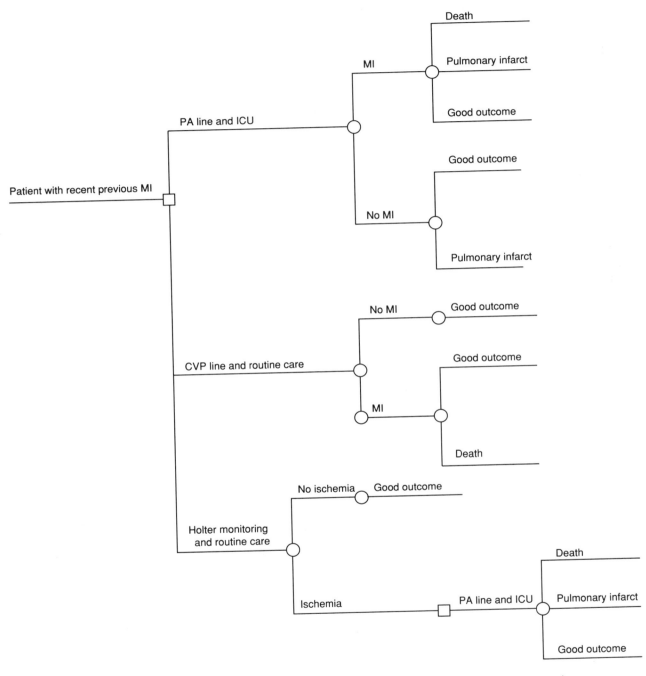

Fig. 5-5. Decision tree for postoperative monitoring for patients with a history of recent previous myocardial infarction.

diac morbidity during carotid endarterectomy is a good example of the kind of monitoring that is being evaluated in this way (Fig. 5-4). Another is comparing various methods of predicting who will have a postoperative myocardial infarction (Fig. 5-5). A third is testing the effects of PAC and oximetric PAC on outcome in surgical and critically ill patients. The latter study is fraught with difficulty as evidenced by the failure of allocation into treatment groups in the Pearson study where if anesthesiologists felt their patient "needed" a PA catheter, the group assignment was altered. No good studies will be easy, but they might eliminate bias introduced by lack of data to support our justification of resource allocation for monitoring. The ASA Task Force on Pulmonary Artery Catheterization[53] and Naylor and coworkers[52] have suggested an agenda for research into the effectiveness of PA catheterization, leading one to hope that some answers about this small part of care for critically ill patients might be forthcoming.

The practice of anesthesiology has evolved from "just putting patients to sleep and waking them up," to the science of disconnecting and then mimicking the regulatory systems of the body so that surgery and recovery can take place. Anesthesiologists provide pain relief, hypnosis, and amnesia, and then take over for the systems inactivated in the process. The data missing in justifying monitoring are the same data that justify this evolution of anesthesiology. These data lie at the very heart of the importance of the role of anesthesia and critical care to surgical patients. Using the assumptions presented in this chapter, monitoring is cost beneficial and cost effective. We believe that if the studies could be performed, they would support these conclusions. It would be ideal to ask for a larger share of the health care dollar with real numbers in hand, but in the meantime the evolution of anesthesiology provides evidence that dollars spent in this way do improve patient care and do result in a net reduction in its cost.

REFERENCES

1. Fleiss JL: Statistical Methods for Rates and Proportions. p. 170. Churchill Livingstone, New York, 1982
2. Bashein G, Johnson PW, Davis KB et al: Elective coronary artery bypass surgery without pulmonary catheter monitoring. Anesthesiology 63:451, 1985
3. Moller JT, Pederson T, Rasmussen LS et al: Randomized trial of pulse oximetry in 20,802 patients, I and II. Anesthesiology 78:436, 1993
4. Orkin FK, Cohen MM, Duncan PG: The quest for meaningful outcomes. Anesthesiology 78:417, 1993
5. Downes JJ, Cohen DF, Raphaelry RC: What difference does pulse oximetry make? Anesthesiology 68:181, 1988
6. Eichhorn JH, Cooper JB, Cullen DJ et al: Standards for patient monitoring during anesthesia at Harvard medical school. JAMA 256:1017, 1986
7. Caplan RA, Posner KL, Ward RJ et al: Adverse respiratory events in anesthesia: a closed claims analysis. Anesthesiology 72:828, 1990
8. Tinker JH, Dull DL, Caplan RA et al: Role of monitoring devices in prevention of anesthesia mishaps: a closed claims analysis. Anesthesiology 89:535, 1989
9. Morray JP, Geiduschek JM, Caplan RA et al: A comparison of pediatric and adult closed malpractice claims. Anesthesiology 78:461, 1993
10. Eichhorn JH: Prevention of intraoperative anesthesia accidents and related severe injury through safety monitoring. Anesthesiology 70:572, 1989
11. Keenan RL, Boyan CP: Decreasing incidence of anesthetic cardiac arrest. Anesthesiology 73:A1022, 1990
12. Cohen MM, Duncan PG, Tween WA et al: The Canadian four-centre study of anaesthetic outcomes: I. Description of methods and populations. Can J Anaesth 39:420, 1992
13. Cohen MM, Duncan PG, Tween WA et al: The Canadian four-centre study of anaesthetic outcomes: II. Can outcomes be used to assess the quality of anaesthesia care? Can J Anaesth 39:430, 1992
14. Cohen MM, Duncan PG, Tween WA et al: The Canadian four-centre study of anaesthetic outcomes: III. Are anaesthetic complications predictable in day surgical practice? Can J Anaesth 39:440, 1992
15. Coté CJ, Goldstein EA, Cote MA et al: A single-blind study of pulse oximetry in children. Anesthesiology 68:184, 1988
16. McKay WPS, Noble WH: Critical incidents detected by pulse oximetry during anesthesia. Can J Anaesth 35:265, 1988
17. Overland PT, Fruend PR, Cooper JO et al: Failure rate of pulse oximetry in clinical practice. Anesth Analg 70:S289, 1990
18. Cullen DJ, Nemeskal AR, Cooper JB et al: Effect of pulse oximetry, age and ASA physical status on the frequency of patients admitted unexpectedly to a postoperative intensive care unit and the severity of their anesthesia-related complications. Anesth Analg 74:181, 1992
19. Weinstein MC, Fineberg HV: Clinical Decision Analysis. WB Saunders, Philadelphia, 1980

20. Sowka MP: Malpractice Claims, Final Compilation. National Association of Insurance Commissioners, Brookfield, WI, 1980

21. Pierce EC: Historical perspectives. Int Anesth Clin 22:1, 1984

22. Cheney FW, Posner K, Caplan RA et al: Standard of care and anesthesia liability. JAMA 261:1599, 1989

23. Duncan PG, Cohen MM: Pulse oximetry and capnography in anaesthetic practice: an epidemiological approach. Can J Anaes 38:619, 1991

24. Tiret L, Desmonts JM, Hatton F, Vourc's G: Complications associated with anaesthesia: a prospective survey in France. Can Anaesth Soc J 33:336, 1986

25. Roizen MF: Routine preoperative evaluation. p. 225. In Miller RD (ed): Anesthesia. 2nd Ed. Churchill Livingstone, New York, 1986

26. Levy WJ: Monitoring of the electroencephalogram during cardiopulmonary bypass. Anesthesiology 76:876, 1992

27. Fessatidis I, Prapas S, Hevas A et al: Prevention of neurological dysfunction: a six year prospective of cardiac surgery. J Cardiovasc Surg 32:570, 1991

28. Kuroda Y, Uchimoto R, Kaieda R et al: Central nervous system complications after cardiac surgery: a comparison between coronary artery bypass grafting and valve surgery. Anesth Analg 76:222, 1993

29. Shaw PJ, Bates D, Cartlidge NEF et al: Neurologic and neuropsychological morbidity following major surgery: comparison of coronary artery bypass and peripheral vascular surgery. Stroke 18:700, 1987

30. Naylor AR, Wildsmith JAW, McClure J: Transcranial Doppler monitoring during carotid endarterectomy. Br J Surg 78:1264, 1991

31. Arom KV, Cohen DE, Strobl FT: Effect of intraoperative intervention on neurological outcome based on electroencephalographic monitoring during cardiopulmonary bypass. Ann Thorac Surg 48:476, 1989

32. McDowell HA, Gross GM, Halsey JH: Carotid endarterectomy monitored with transcranial Doppler. Ann Surg 215:514, 1992

33. Halsey JH, McDowell HA, Gelmon S et al: Blood flow velocity in the middle cerebral artery and regional cerebral blood flow during carotid endarterectomy. Stroke 21:415, 1989

34. Bernstein EF: Role of transcranial Doppler in carotid surgery. Surg Clin North Am 70:225, 1990

35. Halsey JH: Risks and benefits of shunting in carotid endarterectomy. Stroke 23:1583, 1992

36. Spencer MP, Thomas GI, Nicholls SC et al: Detection of middle cerebral artery emboli during carotid endarterectomy using transcranial Doppler ultrasonagraphy. Stroke 21:415, 1990

37. Ellis JE, Shah MN, Briller JE et al: A comparison of methods for the detection of myocardial ischemia during noncardiac surgery: automated ST-segment analysis systems, electrocardiography, and transesophageal echocardiography. Anesth Analg 75:764, 1992

38. Slogoff S, Keats AS, David Y et al: Incidence of perioperative myocardial ischemia detected by different electrocardiographic systems. Anesthesiology 73:1074, 1990

39. Mangano DT, Browner WS, Hollenberg M et al: Association of perioperative myocardial ischemia with cardiac morbidity and mortality in men undergoing noncardiac surgery. N Engl J Med 323:1781, 1990

40. Pasternack PF, Grossi EA, Baumann FG et al: The value of silent myocardial ischemia monitoring in the prediction of perioperative myocardial infarction in patients undergoing peripheral vascular surgery. J Vasc Surg 10:617, 1989

41. Hollenberg M, Mangano DT, Browner WS et al: Predictors of postoperative myocardial ischemia in patients undergoing noncardiac surgery. JAMA 268:205, 1992

42. Charlson ME, MacKenzie R, Ales K et al: Surveillance for postoperative myocardial infarction after noncardiac operations. Surg Gynecol Obstet 167:407, 1988

43. London MJ, Tubau JF, Wong MG et al: The "natural history" of segmental wall motion abnormalities in patients undergoing noncardiac surgery. Anesthesiology 73:644, 1990

44. Daniel WG, Erbel R, Kasper W et al: Safety of transesophageal echocardiography: a multicenter survey of 10,419 examinations. Circulation 83:817, 1991

45. Seward JB, Khandheria BK, Oh JK et al: Critical appraisal of transesophageal echocardiography: limitations, pitfalls and complications. J Am Soc Echocardiog 5:288, 1992

46. Khanderia BK, Seward JB, Bailey K et al: Safety of transesophageal echocardiography: experience with 2070 consecutive procedures. J Am Coll Cardiol 17:20A, 1991

47. Rafferty T, La Mantia KR, Davis E et al: Quality assurance for intraoperative transesophageal echocardiography monitoring: a report of 846 procedures. Anesth Analg 76:228, 1993

48. Cheng DCH, Chung F, Burns RJ et al: Postoperative myocardial infarction documented by technetium scan using single-photon emission computed tomography: significance of intraoperative myocardial ischemia and hemodynamic control. Anesthesiology 71:818, 1989

49. Haggmark S, Hohner P, Ostmann M et al: Comparison of hemodynamic, electrocardiographic, mechanical and metabolic indicators of intraoperative myocardial ischemia in vascular surgical patients with coronary artery disease. Anesthesiology 70:19, 1989

50. Leung J, O'Kelly MB, Browner W et al: Are regional wall motion abnormalities detected by transesophageal echocardiography triggered by acute changes in supply and demand? Anesthesiology 69:A901, 1988

51. Van Daele MERM, Sutherland GR, Mitchell MM et al: Do changes in pulmonary capillary wedge pressure adequately reflect myocardial ischemia during anesthesia? Circulation 81:865, 1990

52. Naylor CD, Sibbald WJ, Sprung CL et al: Pulmonary artery catheterization: can there be an integrated strategy for guideline development and research promotion? JAMA 269:2407, 1993

53. American Society of Anesthesiologists Task Force on Pulmonary Artery Catheterization: Practice guidelines for pulmonary artery catheterization. Anesthesiology 78:380, 1993

54. Rao TLK, Jacobs KH, El Etr A: Reinfarction following anesthesia in patients with myocardial infarction. Anesthesiology 59:499, 1983

55. Elliott CG, Zimmerman GA, Clemmer TP: Complications of pulmonary artery catheterization in the care of critically ill patients. Chest 76:647, 1979

56. Horst HM, Obeid FN, Vij D, Bivins BA: The risks of pulmonary artery catheterization. Surg Gynecol Obstet 159:229, 1984

57. Sise MJ, Hollingsworth P, Brimm JE et al: Complications of the flow directed pulmonary artery catheter: a prospective analysis in 219 patients. Crit Care Med 9:315, 1981

58. Oster G, Tuden RL, Colditz GA: A cost effectiveness analysis of prophylaxis against deep thrombosis in major orthopedic surgery. JAMA 257:203, 1987

59. Raby KE, Barry J, Creager M et al: Detection and significance of intraoperative and postoperative myocardial ischemia in peripheral vascular surgery. JAMA 268:222, 1992

60. McCann RL, Clements FM: Silent myocardial ischemia in patients undergoing peripheral vascular surgery: incidence and association with perioperative morbidity and mortality. J Vasc Surg 9:583, 1989

61. Caplan RA: Closed Claims Studies: relevance to the anesthesiologist. Anesth Analg 74(Supplement Refresher Course Lectures):124, 1993

62. Brennan TA, Leape LL, Laird NM et al: Incidence of adverse events and negligence in hospitalized patients. N Engl J Med 324:370, 1991

63. Roizen MF, Schreider B, Austin W et al: Pulse oximetry, capnography, and blood gas measurements: reducing cost and improving the quality of care with technology. J Clin Mon 9, 1993

64. Pearson KS, Gomez MN, Moyers JR et al: A cost/benefit analysis of randomized invasive monitoring for patients undergoing cardiac surgery. Anesth Analg 69:336, 1989

65. Whitcher C, Ream AK, Parsons D et al: Anesthetic mishaps and the cost of monitoring: a proposed standard for monitoring equipment. J Clin Mon 4:5, 1988

66. Hovi-Viander M: Death associated with anaesthesia in Finland. Br J Anaesth 52:483, 1980

67. Harrison GG: Death attributable to anesthesia: a ten year survey (1967–1976). Br J Anaesth 50:1041, 1978

68. Minuck M. Death in the operating room. Can Anaesth Soc J 14:197, 1967

69. Holland R: Anesthesia-related mortality in Australia. Int Anesth Clin 22:61, 1984

70. Lunn JN, Mushin WW: Mortality Associated with Anaesthesia. Nuffield Provencial Hospital Trust, London, 1982

71. Lunn JN: Anaesthetic mortality in Britain and France. p. 19. In Wickers MD, Lunn JN (eds): Mortality in Anaesthesia. European Academy of Anaesthesiology Proceedings. Springer-Verlag, Berlin, 1982

72. Turnbull KW, Fancourt-Smith PF, Banting GC: Death within 48 hours of anesthesia at the Vancouver General Hospital. Can Anaesth Soc J 27:159, 1980

73. Craig J, Wilson ME: A survey of anesthetic mishaps. Anaesthesiology 36:933, 1981

74. Cooper JB, Cullen DJ, Nemeskal R et al: Effects of information feedback and pulse oximetry on the incidence of anesthesia complications. Anesthesiology 67:686, 1987

75. Cohen MM, Duncan PG, Pope WDB, Wolkenstein C: A survey of 112,000 anaesthetics at one teaching hospital (1975–1983). Can Anaesth Soc J 33:22, 1986

76. Graff TD, Phillips OC, Benson DW, Kelley E: Baltimore anesthesia study committee: factors in pediatric anesthesia mortality. Anesth Analg 43:407, 1964

77. Salem MR, Bennett EJ, Schweiss JF et al: Cardiac arrest related to anesthesia: contributing factors in infants and children. JAMA 233:238, 1975

78. Taylor G, Larson CP, Prestwich R: Unexpected cardiac arrest during anesthesia and surgery: an environmental study. JAMA 236:2758, 1976

79. Utting JE, Gray TC, Shelley FC: Human midadventure in anaesthesia. Can Anaesth Soc J 26:472, 1979

80. Green RA, Taylor TH: An analysis of anesthesia medical liability claims in the United Kingdom, 1977 to 1982. Int Anesth Clin 22:73, 1984

81. Rosen M: Maternal mortality associated with anaesthesia in England and Wales. p. 39. In Wickers MD, Lunn JN (eds): Mortality in Anaesthesia. European Academy of Anaesthesiology Proceedings. Springer-Verlag, Berlin, 1982

82. Cooper JB, Newbower RS, Long CD, McPeek B: Preventable anesthesia mishaps: a study of human factors. Anesthesiology 49:399, 1978

83. Davis DA: An analysis of anesthesia mishaps from medical liability claims. Int Anesth Clin 22:31, 1984

84. Solazzi RW, Ward RJ: The spectrum of medical liability cases. Int Anesth Clin 22:43, 1984

85. Keenan RL, Boyan CP: Cardiac arrest due to anesthesia. JAMA 253:2373, 1985

86. Eisenberg MJ, London MJ, Leung JM et al: Monitoring for myocardial ischemia during non-cardiac surgery. JAMA 268:210, 1992

87. Jain U, Krishnamurthy A: Prognostic significance of S-T elevation during CABG. Anesth Analg 76:S161, 1993

88. Leung JM, O'Kelly B, Browner W et al: Prognostic significance of postbypass regional wall motion abnormality in patients undergoing coronary artery bypass grafting surgery. Anesthesiology 71:16, 1989

Blood Pressure Monitoring: Invasive and Noninvasive

Robert F. Bedford
Nitin K. Shah

6

INVASIVE ARTERIAL PRESSURE MEASUREMENT

History

The first account of invasive blood pressure monitoring was reported in 1733 when the Reverend Stephen Hales cannulated an artery in the neck of a conscious horse and observed that the resulting column of blood rose to a height of 8 feet, 3 inches above the level of the left ventricle. Hales was attempting to disprove the contemporary concept that all the power of the body could be generated from the heart. Hales arbitrarily decided that the zero point for his monitoring system should be the left ventricle and he assumed that power was equal to the product of heart rate and blood pressure. He also noted gross variations in the height of the column of blood depending on the horse's respiratory pattern and its level of anxiety and pain.[1]

Clinical blood pressure measurement continues to utilize several of the principles adopted by Hales: (1) pressure is still determined as the height of a liquid column, that is, millimeters of mercury; (2) derived parameters of cardiovascular performance continue to be calculated from raw blood pressure data; and (3) data acquisition still depends upon an accurate zero reference point.

Blood pressure was not measured in man until 1856 when the French physician Faivre briefly cannulated an artery in the leg of an amputee.[2] It was not until 1947, however, that the use of heparin[3] and the development of electronic and plastic technology permitted Lambert and Wood to use a strain gauge and connecting tubing for clinical measurement of direct arterial pressure.[4] The final link to current clinical practice was the "catheter over needle" cannulation technique described by Barr in 1961.[5]

It was the rapid expansion of cardiovascular surgery in the 1950s and 1960s that necessitated direct blood pressure monitoring as a routine clinical modality. In part, this sprang from the need to measure pressure during the nonpulsatile flow of cardiopulmonary bypass devices, where auscultatory blood pressure monitoring devices are useless, and in part, this was due to the rapid, wide swings in blood pressure that occur regularly in unstable patients undergoing cardiovascular surgery.

Pressure Transducers: Basic Principles and Clinical Caveats

The essential ingredient in direct blood pressure measurement is the device that converts intraarterial pressure into an electrical signal, which in turn can be processed into an intelligible display. We discuss transducers early in this chapter for several reasons: (1) they are probably fraught with the least likelihood of introducing errors into the measurement of blood pressure; (2) accurate blood pressure determinations can only be assured if the clinician understands the intrinsic workings and potential foibles of the pressure-transducer-monitor system; and (3) subsequent discussions on both natural and artifactual changes in blood pressure can be appreciated best by first understanding how the pulse wave gets converted into electrical energy.

Common to all pressure transducing devices is a stiff, low-compliance, pressure-sensing diaphragm capable of bending and creating a small volume change in response to an applied pressure change. Once a pressure differential has been converted into mechanical movement or displacement of a diaphragm, it can be converted into an electrical signal by acting upon an energizing current produced by a monitor's preamplifier.

The principle behind the functioning of resistive transducers is that a stretch force applied to a wire changes the length and cross-sectional area leading to an increase in electrical resistance. Conversely, if a wire is allowed to contract, the electrical resistance will decrease. In an unbonded strain gauge, positive pressure (relative to atmosphere), causes motion of the transducer diaphragm, thus stretching one pair of wires while simultaneously relaxing a second pair of wires.[6] These four wires are variable resistors on the arms of a Wheatstone bridge (Fig. 6-1). The alterations in the small excitation voltage across the Wheatstone bridge change the excitation signal into an output voltage that reproduces the change in pressure applied to the transducer diaphragm.

Contemporary pressure transducers utilize the same principles as the unbonded strain gauge, except that they employ semiconductor technology instead of wires. Silicon crystals, like wires, change resistance in linear proportion to applied pressure. In addition, they can be miniaturized to the point where they can be directly inserted into the arterial tree. Using integrated circuit technology, most manufacturers incorporate a silicon pressure-sensing diaphragm with a Wheatstone bridge etched onto the underside. The entire crystal is then coated with epoxy to produce a "bonded" strain gauge.[6] Contemporary transducers are now available with standardized electronics. Therefore, they can be employed in virtually any monitor preamplifier and display system.

The next step from the transducer to the blood

pressure display is the preamplifier module, which, in addition to providing the energizing signal for the transducer, amplifies the returning blood pressure signal and conditions it for display. The preamplifier contains the controls for the preset electrical calibration of the transducer (electronically unbalancing the Wheatstone bridge to simulate pressure applied to the transducer), and for zeroing the transducer to atmospheric pressure (balancing the Wheatstone bridge resistances so that no current returns to the preamplifier). The advent of solid-state circuitry in blood pressure monitoring hardware has seen the universal adoption

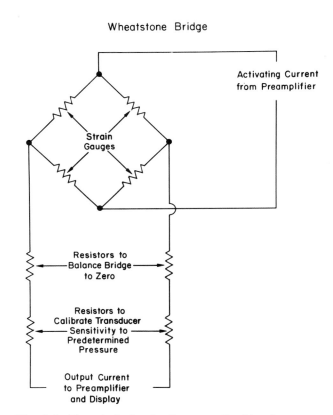

Fig. 6-1. Electrical circuit diagram of a blood pressure transducer based on the Wheatstone bridge. A preamplifier is needed both to supply the activating current for the circuit and also to receive the output current from the transducer. Note that the resistors used to balance the bridge to zero and to calibrate its sensitivity may be entirely within the preamplifier. Thus, the mere presence of a numerical output may not reflect the actual performance of the transducer and, indeed, the display may work even when the transducer is disconnected from the preamplifier.

of transducer-preamplifier sensitivity at 50 μV/10 mmHg. A notable advantage of this convention has been that almost all transducers currently produced can be interfaced with whatever mainframe/ preamplifier a clinician has available and still produce an accurate reading within 1 percent.[7]

After passing through the preamplifier, the electrical analog of the arterial pulse-pressure wave passes to the amplifier section of the monitor. Here, its signal is boosted sufficiently to drive one or more readout devices with a voltage that varies directly with the pressure applied to the transducer. The traditional clinical readout, of course, is the cathode ray tube (CRT), modernized over recent decades by the nonfade scope. Virtually all CRTs are combined with a digital display readout that picks out the highest pressure as the systolic value, the lowest pressure as the diastolic value, and automatically integrates the area under the pulse-pressure wave to determine the mean arterial pressure.

Calibration of the invasive blood pressure monitoring system should be routine, both at the beginning of use and also periodically throughout monitoring. One of the primary advantages of external transducers is their ease of calibration. Ideally, transducers should be checked for baseline drift over a 1-hour period, and any change greater than 1 to 2 percent is clinically unacceptable.[6]

Blood pressure is measured relative to atmospheric pressure, since the atmosphere has an equal effect both on the blood pressure and the transducer. With the stopcock between the transducer and the patient opened to atmosphere, the transducer is balanced electronically and then connected via sterile tubing to a nearby mercury manometer. Usually, the manometer pressure is raised to 50, 100, and 200 mmHg and held constant while the "calibration factor" in the preamplifier is adjusted to reflect these pressures. Then the internal calibration standard in the preamplifier can be used to check the electronic stability of the system.

Like Stephen Hales during the first invasive blood pressure measurement, the clinician must decide the level at which the arterial pressure is to be referenced. For patients in the supine position, the level of the left ventricle is appropriate. For this approach the midaxillary line is usually chosen. The transducer should then maintain the same relationship to the left ventricle whenever the height of the patient's bed is changed. This can be accomplished by affixing the transducer to the bed at a height of 10 cm above the (firm) mattress. For every 15 cm that the patient moves above the level of the transducer, the blood pressure readout will increase by 10 mmHg.

The level of the left ventricle is not always the site of maximum clinical interest. In such situations, the level of the pressure transducer should be raised to the least dependent part of the patient's anatomy. For example, the relatively "normal" mean arterial pressure of 70 mmHg at the left ventricle (in the seated position) means there is only a marginal mean arterial pressure of 50 mmHg in the brain. Conversely, patients in the "high stirrup" position may have impaired perfusion in their legs, while blood pressure at heart level remains "normal."

Once a blood pressure monitoring system has been calibrated for linearity, sensitivity, and baseline stability, the remaining requirement for accurate measurement is adequate frequency response. Most transducers have a flat frequency response. That is, they can accurately reproduce pressure changes up to 150 Hz and many of the intravascular solid-state "micro" transducers can accurately reproduce frequency changes up to 1,000 Hz. As most blood pressure waveforms contain frequency elements only up to 20 to 30 Hz, virtually all transducers are capable of faithfully reproducing the shape of a pulse-pressure wave, since the frequency response of a transducer only needs to be 1.5 times the fastest component wave.[8]

The primary offender in preventing acquisition of accurate data from invasive blood pressure monitoring is not the electronic circuitry. It is the distortion of the pressure waveform caused by the inertia and friction of the column of fluid leading from the artery to the transducer. The length of tubing between artery and transducer and/or the presence of air bubbles within the tubing, stopcocks, dome, and so on, lowers the frequency response of the system so that they approach the frequencies encountered in the pulse-pressure wave. This is particularly true of the inotropic systolic component. The result is distortion of the pressure waveform, with "ringing" and overshooting of systolic pressures. Since the problems of frequency response are related more to the length of the connecting tubing between the artery and transducer than they are to the transducer itself, this topic is covered in greater depth in the section of the coupling system.

Proper maintenance of transducers is essential for accurate, reproducible invasive blood pressure monitoring. In addition, sterility of transducers is an integral part of their maintenance lest they serve as a focus for nosocomial infection[9,10] (Fig. 6-2).

Physiology of the Arterial Pulse-Pressure Wave

The arterial pulse-pressure wave undergoes a series of transformations as it proceeds from the ascending aorta distally through the arterial tree to the sites used clinically for invasive arterial pressure monitoring (Fig. 6-3). These changes in arterial waveform, and particularly those of the systolic component, account in large part (although not entirely) for the disparities observed between cuff pressures measured at the brachial artery and invasive pressures measured at the radial artery. The clinician may wish to derive an approximation of stroke volume, myocardial contractility, and peripheral vascular resistance from observing a peripheral pulse-pressure wave. The fact that the peripheral arterial pulse is very much removed from the central aortic contour makes these assumptions erroneous. The pressure measured at a given point in the circulatory system really only reflects the energy content of flowing blood. An attempt is then made to deduce the condition of the circulation based on these measurements. The purpose of this section is to acquaint the clinician with the changes that may be observed in the normal arterial pressure waveform tracing.

If a miniaturized pressure transducer were placed within the ascending aorta, there would be no artifactual waveforms, and the aortic pulse-pressure wave would look like that in Figure 6-4. As seen on the accompanying diagram, aortic arch pressure increases in response to peak aortic flow acceleration generated by ventricular contraction. Ventricular ejection, then, produces both a true pressure wave and a flow wave in the ascending aorta. It is only aortic arch pressure that can be used to quantitate stroke volume, left ventricular contractility, and systemic vascular resistance. This aortic blood flow is not transmitted to the periphery with the blood pressure wave. It is absorbed by the distensible elastic aortic arch, which Brunner

refers to as a "fixed-capacity, high-pressure reservoir."[7] While the blood flow wave moves out of the aorta at a relatively slow rate (0.5 m/s during aortic elastic recoil, the pulse-pressure wave moves at the rate of 10 m/s.[11] In fact, the dorsalis pedis artery has already started to receive the arterial pulse-pressure wave before ventricular systole is completed. The clinical implication is that what is seen in a peripheral artery pulse-pressure wave may have little to do with actual arterial blood flow.

The initial rapid upstroke of the aortic root pulse reaches a peak that can be viewed as the inotropic component of the pressure-pulse wave. The pressure/flow phenomena at this time cause the upper aorta to expand, producing a higher pressure than would occur if the entire aorta were to distend uniformly. The rounded, sustained portion of the aortic pulse-pressure wave represents a combined effect of (1) ventricular volume ejection, (2) distension of the entire aorta (capacitance), and (3) runoff into the branches of the aorta.

As the pulse-pressure wave moves away from the heart, there is a delay in transmission, the initial upstroke becomes steeper, the high-frequency components, such as the anacrotic and dicrotic notches, disappear, and the systolic maximum becomes progressively more peaked (Fig. 6-3). The dicrotic notch starts out as an incisura and gradually gets lost in transmission, becoming a deep, drawn-out hump or anacrotic wave in the upper extremities, while virtually disappearing into the diastolic pressure within the femoral system. The following characteristics apply to the peripherally measured arterial pressure waveform: the farther into the periphery blood pressure is measured, (1) the narrower the waveform appears; (2) the greater the increase in systolic and pulse pressure; and (3) the lower the diastolic and mean values.

There are several reasons for the changing morphology of the arterial pulse wave trace. Since the arterial tree is usually entered in relatively peripheral arteries, probably the most important factor in modifying the pulse-pressure waveform (particularly the systolic component), is the reflection of waves from the periphery. Just as surface waves are produced by dropping an object in a pool of water, when the waves hit the edge of the pool, they are reflected back, and those reflected waves produce a standing wave that adds to the incident wave (Fig. 6-5). In the arterial tree, the artery-arteriole junction is thought to be the principal site of reflection,[12,13] and standing waves are produced that add or subtract from different portions of the pulse wave. It has been estimated that as much as 80 percent of the incident wave is reflected with normal arterial resistance. When peripheral vasodilation occurs (vasodilator therapy, exercise, arteriovenous fistula), the energy in the pressure pulse is passed on into the periphery and absorbed without reflec-

tion. This results in marked changes in the pulse-pressure contour, particularly a reduction in systolic pressure. Conversely, when a cannulated radial or dorsalis pedis artery is occluded by catheter and/or thrombus, the site of wave reflection is at the catheter tip. In this case, the summation of the reflected and incident waves results in augmentation of the systolic pressure value.[14,15]

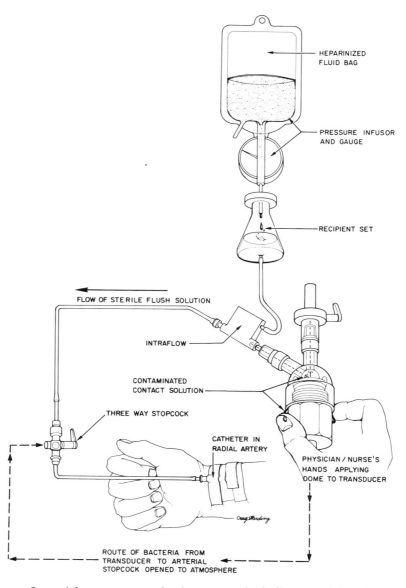

HEPARINIZED FLUID BAG

PRESSURE INFUSOR AND GAUGE

RECIPIENT SET

FLOW OF STERILE FLUSH SOLUTION

INTRAFLOW

CONTAMINATED CONTACT SOLUTION

THREE WAY STOPCOCK

CATHETER IN RADIAL ARTERY

PHYSICIAN / NURSE'S HANDS APPLYING DOME TO TRANSDUCER

ROUTE OF BACTERIA FROM TRANSDUCER TO ARTERIAL STOPCOCK OPENED TO ATMOSPHERE

Fig. 6-2. Diagram of arterial pressure monitoring system including arterial catheter, extension tubes, stopcocks, constant infusion device, disposable pressure dome and transducer. Note the route of bacterial contamination in a sterile system: from the nonsterile transducer to the patient-access stopcock via a health professional's fingers.

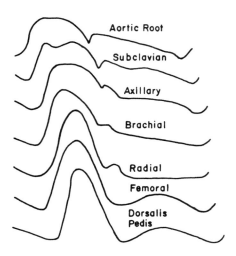

Fig. 6-3. Configuration of the pressure-pulse wave at various sites in the arterial tree. See text for a more complete description of the changes as the arterial pulse wave travels to the periphery.

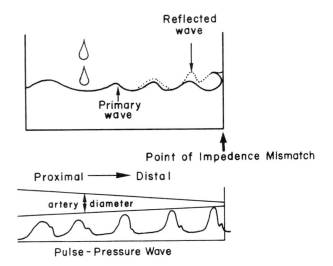

Fig. 6-5. Some factors affecting the arterial pressure-pulse wave shape: Reflection at the artery-arteriole junction and progressive decrease in diameter of arterial lumen. See text for further description.

The radial and dorsalis pedis arteries consistently yield higher systolic pressure than corresponding brachial cuff measurements[16,17] presumably because the site of wave reflection is in close proximity to the site of the arterial cannula. As a result of this wave reflection phenomenon, both radial and dorsalis pedis artery pressures contain higher frequency (dP/dt) components than the central aortic pressure trace. Computer analysis of peripheral arterial waves found frequency components up to 20 Hz in the brachial,[18] which probably means there are still higher components in the radial. The implications of these data will become obvious later on during consideration of the effects of extension

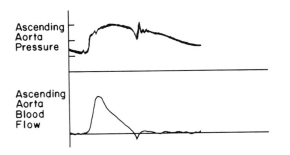

Fig. 6-4. Aortic root pressure pulse wave and the corresponding flow generated in the ascending aorta. See text for explanation.

tubing on the arterial pressure monitoring system frequency response.

Other causes of change in the configuration of the arterial pulse-pressure wave as it moves peripherally relate to such factors as the decreasing content of elastic fibers. As these peripheral arteries become more muscular, the tapering of the vessel diameter acts to amplify arterial waves in a fashion similar to the way an ear trumpet amplifies sound waves (Fig. 6-5) and because high pressure levels of the arterial pulse travel faster than low pressure levels, the peak of the arterial pulse curve summates with earlier pressure components in the peripheral arteries.[19] The observation that older patients have less discrepancy between systolic pressures measured in the aorta and peripherally is thought to be due to less muscle within the vessel wall and a faster pulse-wave velocity with increasing age.[20] Alternatively, the marked augmentation of the dicrotic notch often observed in children's radial arteries, is a function of their greater vessel compliance and greater opportunity for wave reflection and amplification due to slower wave transmission time.

In summary, the arterial system functions as a damped, resonant, transmission line, transmitting various frequencies with different degrees of attenuation. The reshaping of the aortic pulse-pressure wave into the peripheral arterial pressure wave is the result of the attenuation of some frequencies and the augmentation of other frequencies. Although the mean pressure measured in the periphery will be close to the value in the aortic arch, the clinician must dissuade himself from the belief that the peripheral systolic pressure accurately reflects aortic arch systolic pressure.[21]

Arterial Catheters
Caveats for Successful Insertion

Since the early 1960s, the standard technique for percutaneous cannulation for direct arterial monitoring has been the "catheter over needle" approach first described by Barr.[5] Generally, this requires meticulous antiseptic skin preparation, identification of the course of the artery by palpation, and a shallow angle of approach to the vessel. When blood is observed in the flash chamber of the needle, the catheter is advanced into the lumen of the vessel.

Because peripheral arteries are frequently difficult to palpate in hypotensive or vasoconstricted patients, a variety of techniques has evolved to assist in successful cannulation. Among these are use of transillumination to help identify arteries in infants[22] and fine-tip Doppler ultrasound probes to identify weakly palpable arteries in adults. A common clinical problem is that the tip of the needle may enter the vessel but the catheter, being larger, will not "thread" into the lumen. Miniature, flexible guidewire introducers for 20- and 22-gauge catheters have helped to obviate this problem, since the small guidewire usually can be introduced into the vessel lumen and inserted past intima, atheromata, or whatever else has prevented successful catheter passage. Other techniques to rescue cannulation from the "no thread" phenomenon include removing the needle from the catheter and alternately: (1) withdrawing until a flash of blood indicates that the catheter tip is in the middle of the lumen, or (2) attaching an air/fluid-filled plastic extension tube to the catheter and withdrawing the catheter until the air bubble pulsates maximally,[23] again indicating that the catheter tip is in a central location in the vessel lumen. It is hoped that with either of these techniques the catheter can then be advanced up the lumen of the vessel. A variant on these techniques is the "liquid stylet" approach, where a 10-ml syringe is applied to the cannula hub after a "no thread" is encountered.

The cannula is withdrawn while suction is applied to the syringe until blood flows readily; the cannula is then advanced while 1 to 2 ml is injected with the syringe.[24] Since the "no thread" phenomenon usually results from the catheter impinging on the lateral or deep wall of the artery while only part of the needle tip is in the arterial lumen, meticulous identification of the vessel, and stabilization of the extremity, all seem to help to minimize this problem.

Physical Factors

Arterial catheters are manufactured from a variety of plastics, each with different structural properties and tissue reactivity. Most utilize Teflon, polypropylene, polyvinyl chloride, or polyethylene. Although polypropylene catheters were originally popular because they were stiff enough to avoid kinking and could be extruded into a very fine tip, several clinical studies found them to be more thrombogenic than Teflon catheters.[15,25,26] While Teflon catheters are prone to kink, particularly at fine gauges (20–25), Teflon is currently the most widely used plastic catheter material because both in vivo animal testing and clinical use in humans have shown it to be less thrombogenic than polyethylene, polyvinyl chloride, or polypropylene.[15,25–28] Heparin coating or impregnation has been shown to be of short-term value for arterial cannulation, but the heparin leaches out of the plastic after a day or two and no further reduction in thrombogenicity is gained.[29]

The size of an arterial catheter is also an important consideration, both for the monitoring system to perform optimally and for minimizing vascular damage induced by the catheter. In terms of minimizing vascular damage, it appears that the smaller an arterial catheter is relative to the size of the artery, the lower the incidence of vessel thrombosis[30] (Fig. 6-6). Conversely, however, smaller catheters are manufactured with thinner walls and are more prone to kink between the skin and the artery (Fig. 6-7). Within 24 hours of insertion, 20 percent of 20-gauge radial artery catheters kink, resulting in significant degradation of catheter performance.[30] The blood pressure pulse wave becomes damped, and difficulty is encountered in recovery of blood samples. Occasionally, a kinked catheter can be straightened by rotating the catheter through a 180-degree arc, or by applying distal traction and withdrawing it slightly. The temptation to hyperextend the wrist to straighten a kinked radial arterial catheter should be avoided, as this may lead to stretching of the median nerve with subsequent hand numbness.[31] As a last resort, a kinked catheter may be replaced by inserting a sterile, flexible guidewire into the catheter while it is straightened with distal traction, the old catheter is then removed, and a new one is introduced into the vessel over the guidewire.

The size of an arterial catheter also impacts on the ability of the catheter and transducer system to respond to the rapidly changing arterial pulse-pressure wave. Krovetz and Goldbloom[18] found components of the brachial artery pulse pressure wave in the 15- to 19-Hz frequency range. It is assumed that the radial arterial pulse-pressure waves have slightly higher frequencies (between 20 and 25 Hz) because of the proximity to the site of wave reflection at the artery-arteriole junction. If a large catheter occludes an artery or induces thrombotic occlusion, the site of wave reflection will be at the tip of the catheter. In this situation the summated pressure wave will have augmented high-frequency components, resulting in an artificially high systolic pressure.

As discussed in the section on pressure transducers, most of these devices respond accurately to frequencies of 100 Hz or higher, well in excess of the frequency response required for accurate reproduction of peripheral arterial waveforms (i.e., 33 percent higher than the highest frequency in the waveform).[32] The problem with external transducers, however, is that the catheter-extension apparatus induces "ringing" or hyperresonance in response to repetitive pressure waveforms. If the catheter and extension tubing lower the frequency response of the system into the range where the naturally occurring frequencies in the pulse-pressure wave set the monitoring system to oscillating, this results in artificially augmented high-frequency components, such as the systolic pressure peak.

The natural frequency at which a catheter-

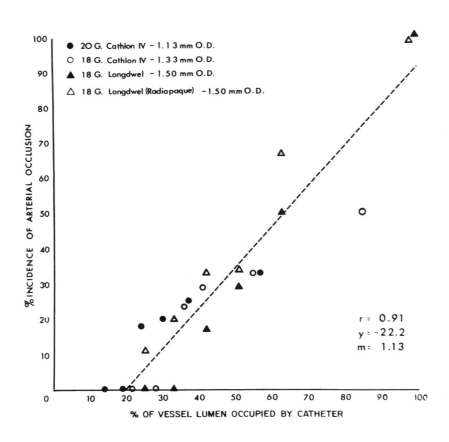

Fig. 6-6. Radial-artery thrombosis, after 24 hours of cannulation. Incidence of radial artery occlusion plotted as a function of the percentage of the vessel lumen occupied by arterial catheter. Small catheters in large vessels tended to induce thrombosis only rarely. Large catheters occupying the entire vessel lumen always induced thrombosis. (From Bedford,[62] with permission.)

extension tubing system tends to "ring" is described by the formula:

$$fn = \frac{1}{2\pi} \sqrt{\frac{\pi D^2}{4\rho L} \cdot \frac{\Delta P}{\Delta V'}}$$

where $\Delta P / \Delta V$ = compliance, D = diameter, L = length and ρ = density of the solution.[33]

In order to keep the natural frequency of a blood pressure monitoring system higher than the frequencies in the arterial pulse-pressure wave, it is desirable to maximize the diameter of the catheter and extension tubing and minimize the length and compliance of the system. The system with the highest frequency response would consist of a heparin-filled, wide-bore, intraarterial catheter directly affixed to a transducer.

Fortunately, large-bore arterial catheters are not needed for invasive blood pressure monitoring. What smaller catheters lose in frequency response,

they make up in damping coefficient which varies as $1/r^3$.[34] Damping is the opposite of resonance. It is the tendency of an oscillation to die down. It is the frictional resistance opposing the movement of a mass. In this case it is composed of the kinetic energy of the blood pressure hitting the end of the catheter[11] and the tendency of the monitoring system to resonate.[7] Damping coefficient (β) ranges downward from a value of 1.0, where there would be no resonance and only mean arterial pressure would be displayed. Examples of overdamping occur with a kinked arterial catheter, a clot lodged in the catheter tip, or a large bubble in the transducer dome. Optimal damping occurs in the range of 0.6 to 0.7, where pressure changes are faithfully reproduced with only a minimal (5 percent) overshoot and there is rapid return to the actual pressure value. Most catheter-extension systems are underdamped, with a β of 0.2 or less. The impact of this underdamping can be appreciated if one recognizes that a β of 0.2 means that only frequencies equal to 20 percent of the system's resonant frequency will be recorded accurately. Thus, even though a system may have an *fn* of 35 Hz, only events up to 7 Hz will be accurately recorded. Early systolic pressure waves may thus be severely augmented in such a system. With a β of 0.6, however, pressure waves with components up to 21 Hz will be reproduced faithfully.[7]

The advantages of small arterial catheters, then, are threefold: (1) they reduce the incidence of vascular complications associated with invasive monitoring; (2) by preventing occlusion of the artery, they help to keep the point of wave reflection distal to the site of pressure monitoring; and (3) they tend to dampen the naturally underdamped catheter-extension tube system so there is less "ringing" in the pulse-pressure wave and systolic pressure is measured more accurately.

The Coupling System: From Catheter to Transducer

External pressure transducers are connected to the arterial cannula by a coupling system that consists of (1) fluid-filled extension tubing, (2) a stopcock for blood sampling and balancing the transducer to atmospheric pressure, (3) a continuous infusion device to prevent accumulation of blood in the catheter, and (4) a dome that covers the transducer diaphragm (Fig. 6-2).

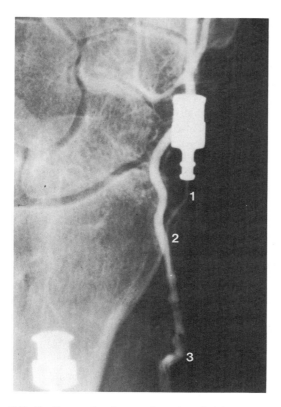

Fig. 6-7. Radiograph of a nonfunctional, 20-gauge radial artery catheter showing three sites of kinking: *1*, above the skin, *2*, between the skin and the artery, and *3*, within the artery lumen.

One of the major sources of pressure measurement artifact is the systolic "ringing," or resonance, induced by extension tubes connecting arterial catheters to the pressure transducer. As indicated by the formula for natural frequency of the catheter-extension tubing system, the longer the length (L) of the system, the lower the natural frequency and the more likely the system is to resonate sympathetically with the pulse-pressure wave measured from a peripheral artery. A Statham P50 transducer without any tubing has an fn of 42 Hz, whereas the fn decreases to 33 Hz with 6 in. of tubing and to 6.45 Hz with 5 ft of tubing. The resultant systolic overshoot in the brachial artery is 16.3 percent higher with 5-ft tubing and would be even worse in the radial artery.[35] Shinozaki, using a pressure simulator set at 150/50, found systolic pressure augmented 7.2 percent with 3 ft of extension tubing, 9.2 percent with 6 ft, and 31.3 percent with 8 ft of extension tubing.[36] With systolic pressure so augmented, calculation of mean pressure as 1/3 × pulse-pressure difference, or rate-pressure product as systolic pressure × heart rate, becomes highly suspect.

Experience has shown that the flush solutions within the coupling system should contain at least some heparin, although the optimal concentration is not known. Absence of heparin results in a far higher incidence of catheter dysfunction and arterial thrombosis as compared with solutions containing 2 U/ml of heparin.[37]

The importance of continuous infusion devices is supported by data from studies using intermittent flush techniques for radial artery catheterization. When an intermittent flush technique was employed, a 23 percent incidence of distal clot embolization was observed using angiography.[29] When continuous flush devices were introduced, the incidence of distal embolization virtually vanished.[30,27,38] Furthermore, continuously flushed arterial catheters have been found to have a lower incidence of nosocomial infection than intermittently flushed catheters.[39] In addition, continuous flush devices have been found not to significantly alter either static or dynamic blood pressure measurement.[38]

The integrated flush mechanism and disposable transducer system has eliminated a host of problems previously associated with nondisposable transducers and their disposable domes. As long as the integrated devices are treated in a sterile fashion, they will not function as a nidus for bacterial growth, nor will they result in artifactual changes in transducer frequency response[40,41] or in the pressure baseline due to accidental unscrewing.[42]

Ideally, transducer domes should be as small as possible, shaped to facilitate removal of air bubbles, and transparent in order to detect bubbles or other foreign matter. At least one opening is required for removal of bubbles, calibrating the transducer with a mercury column, and balancing to atmospheric pressure.

Stopcocks are the weakest link in the invasive blood pressure monitoring system: (1) they permit bacteria to enter[43]; (2) clots can be injected into the circulation[27,44]; (3) they hide air bubbles; (4) they are narrower than connecting tubing, thereby lowering the natural frequency of the monitoring system.

The two major weaknesses in the coupling system are the length of connecting tubing (see above) and the presence of air bubbles. Air bubbles are more compliant than liquid and increase the movement velocity of the coupling solution. This results in a lower frequency response and greater resonance during rapidly changing pressure waveforms (Fig. 6-8). Gross bubbles damp the pulse-pressure wave, whereas small bubbles produce hyperresonance. Adding 0.05 to 0.25 ml of air to an arterial pressure line augmented systolic pressure by 40 mmHg, from 150 to 190 mmHg, while diastolic and electronic mean pressure never changed by more than 3 mmHg.[36]

A practical method for determining the natural frequency and the damping characteristics of a pressure monitoring system in clinical use is outlined in Fig. 6-9.[45] When a continuous-flow flush system is opened to rapid flush and then released, a nearly square-wave pulse of 300 mmHg is applied to the catheter-tubing-transducer system. As the flow is turned off, resonant waves occur in the pulse-pressure contour. Using a strip-chart recorder, the natural frequency of the system can be calculated by dividing the paper speed in millimeters per second by the number of millimeters between resonant peaks. 30 Hz seems to be the minimum desirable natural frequency for an optimally damped blood pressure monitoring system to guarantee accurate values for systolic pressure.

Using the fast-flush test, the damping factor of the system can be calculated by measuring the relative heights of the resonant waves (D_1/D_2) and applying the chart given in Fig. 6-8. By using this maneuver immediately after arterial cannulation and then repeatedly during invasive pressure monitoring, one can determine if the system's frequency response and damping are optimal. One can also readily detect when performance deteriorates during clinical use. Kleinman and colleagues[46] have recently demonstrated that the "fast flush" test accurately portrays the natural frequency and damping characteristics of the entire monitoring system, from arterial catheter to pressure transducer.

In general, a damping coefficient of 0.6 is considered optimal for faithful reproduction of arterial pressure waveforms. A higher damping coefficient is usually associated with a clotted or kinked catheter or a very large air bubble. Most monitoring systems tend to be underdamped, with a damping factor of 0.1 to 0.3 and excessive resonant waves are seen after a fast-flush (Fig. 6-9).

Hazards of Invasive Blood Pressure Monitoring

In general terms, the hazards of invasive arterial pressure monitoring can be summarized as: (1) vascular compromise, (2) disconnection, (3) accidental injection, (4) infection, and (5) damage to nearby nerves. The problems of vascular compromise and nerve damage will be considered in the individual sections discussing the various sites suitable for arterial cannulation.

In a monitoring system exposed to systemic arterial pressures, it should go without saying that a disconnect could potentially result in a patient's rapid exsanguination. Accidental injection of noxious substances into a peripheral artery can be disastrous for an entire limb. The serious complications of intraarterial thiopental and thiamylal injection are well known.[47] Ketamine injected via a dorsalis pedis artery catheter caused severe skin necrosis that extended proximal over the anterior and lateral portion of the leg and foot, and required 5 weeks for the patient to recover.[48] Similarly, retrograde injection of blood clots via a radial artery cannula have resulted in cerebrovascular ischemia,[44] as well as distal embolization and ischemia.[29]

Arterial monitoring catheters may result in nosocomial infection due to either local or systemic sepsis. Local infections are thought to be caused by introduction of cutaneous bacteria at the time of cannulation and are usually of staphylococcal origin. The longer the cannula is in place, the greater the risk of local infection.[49-52] Ointments applied

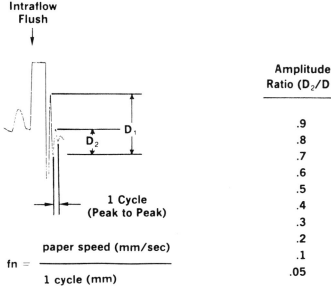

Amplitude Ratio (D_2/D_1)	Damping Coefficient
.9	.034
.8	.071
.7	.113
.6	.160
.5	.215
.4	.280
.3	.358
.2	.456
.1	.591
.05	.690

Fig. 6-8. Calculation of natural frequency (*fn*) and damping coefficient (β) of an arterial pressure monitoring system. The waveforms induced by in Intraflow flush are analyzed in terms of time between cycles and the height of the induced resonant waves.

to intravascular catheter sites reduced the local infection rate from 6.5 percent in nontreated patients to 3.6 percent with iodophor and 2.2 percent with polymyxin, neomycin, or bacitracin ointment. Iodophor ointment is recommended for intravascular cannulation sites.[53] Recently, use of antibiotic-impregnated catheters has been advocated to prevent local infectious complications.[54]

Bacteremia is also associated with use of arterial monitoring systems. This may be the result of contamination of the tubing system[10,43,55] or the catheter itself may become a nidus for infection due to seeding from septicemia. Stopcocks are often the route of access when bacteria are manually trans-

ferred to the tubing system (Fig. 6-2). Maki and Hassemer[56] noted an 11 percent rate of bacterial contamination in transducer domes used for long-term arterial pressure monitoring. As a result, they recommend changing all tubing fluid solutions and transducer domes every 48 hours in patients with long-term arterial cannulas in place. Band and Maki[57] found that 5 of 37 patients with septicemia from a noncannula infection had arterial catheters that grew out identical bacteria. In addition, arterial thrombi induced by monitoring catheters may act as a nidus of infection,[58,59] occasionally requiring surgical removal of the thrombus to treat the infection.[60,61]

6″ Extension Tube Well-Flushed
$fn = 31.25$ Hz (25/0.8)
$\beta = 0.65$ ($D_2/D_1 = 1/13$)

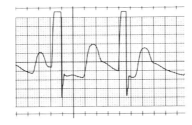

4′ Extension Tube Well-Flushed
$fn = 25$ Hz (25/1)
$\beta = 0.20$ ($D_2/D_1 = 4/8$)

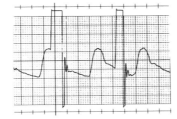

Fig. 6-9. Calculated values of natural frequency (*fn*) and damping coefficient (β) for an arterial pressure monitoring system in a single patient using the same catheter and transducer. Longer extension tubing and air bubbles tend to lower *fn*. Optimal damping and the highest *fn* are achieved with a short extension tube and no air bubbles.

4′ Extension Tube with Bubbles
$Fn = 13.8$ Hz (25/1.8)
$\beta = .25$ ($D_2/D_1 = 11/26.5$)

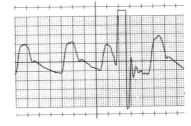

8′ Extension Tube with Bubbles
$fn = 11.3$ Hz (25/2.2)
$\beta = .3$ ($D_2/D_1 = 10/28$)

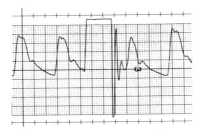

Therefore when arterial monitoring catheters are to remain in place for several days, Band and Maki[57] make the following recommendations:

1. Use sterile gloves during cannulation.
2. Use iodine disinfectant and sterile drapes.
3. If possible, use a percutaneous cannulation technique.
4. Use iodophor ointment both on cannulation site and on stopcocks.
5. Keep stopcocks capped.
6. Inspect puncture site daily.
7. Discontinue catheter if
   (a) local discoloration, pain, or pus develops.
   (b) patient becomes septic (culture catheter).

Radial Artery Cannulation

After Barr's initial description of percutaneous radial artery cannulation,[5] the technique rapidly achieved widespread popularity for invasive blood pressure monitoring. The reasons for this popularity are obvious: (1) the vessel is superficial, easy to identify and cannulate; (2) the cannulation site is accessible; (3) the procedure is reasonably pain-free for the patient; (4) since collateral circulation to the hand is abundant and easy to document, the likelihood of inducing distal vascular ischemia is quite low.

On the other hand, the radial artery is not the ideal cannulation site for acquiring hemodynamic data. The radial pulse-pressure wave is subject to considerable systolic pressure augmentation because it is distal and close to the point of pulse wave reflection. Furthermore, the radial artery lumen diameter is relatively small (2 to 3 mm),[62] and it frequently becomes occluded by either catheter or catheter-induced thrombus. Thus, the site of pulse wave reflection is right at the site of cannulation and systolic pressure becomes augmented with high-frequency pressure wave transients that give a falsely elevated systolic pressure value.

An additional problem with radial arterial pressures has been the observation of pressure gradients as large as 32 mmHg between the aortic and radial arteries associated with separation from cardiopulmonary bypass, particularly during and following rewarming.[63-65] It is thought that these differences may be due to changes in vasomotor tone associated with the wide temperature fluctuations and endocrine responses to cardiopulmonary bypass.

A previous diagnostic catheterization performed in the brachial artery should probably preclude use of the ipsilateral radial artery, since pulse-pressure waves may be markedly damped and a low flow state may tend to induce hand ischemia.[31,66] Other factors that might affect the site of radial artery cannulation include use of the right radial artery for thoracic aneurysm surgery, since the left subclavian is often occluded during surgery, or use of the right radial in premature infants with a patent ductus arteriosus, where the left side would receive desaturated blood from the ductus arteriosus. Finally, cannulation of the radial artery in a hand with inadequate ulnar artery collateral circulation may result in limb ischemia.[67]

There are probably as many techniques for cannulation of the radial artery as there are clinicians performing it. The radial artery is quite tortuous as it passes over the wrist joint (Fig. 6-10). Just palpating a pulse at one point near the wrist does not indicate where the vessel may be when the catheter achieves the depth of the artery, and it does not guarantee that the catheter will be aligned with the vessel lumen when it enters the vessel wall. Accordingly, dorsiflexion and immobilization of the wrist, and identification of the course of the vessel with palpating fingers and/or a skin marking pencil may increase the likelihood of successful cannulation. Cannulation of the radial artery proximal to the wrist joint (where it is straighter) may also improve success rate. Although its greater depth may make it more difficult to palpate, the catheter may slide into the vessel lumen more readily than is the case if it must negotiate twists and turns in the more distal artery. The improved cannulation success rate of the Arrow radial artery catheterization set (Arrow International, Reading, PA), with its built-in flexible guidewire, is possibly due to the propensity of most clinicians to go where the artery is most superficial, rather than where it is straightest.[67] Once the vessel lumen is entered, the flexible guidewire can negotiate turns that a straight needle and catheter assembly cannot manage.

The impact on vessel function of multiple arterial punctures during attempted cannulation is controversial. Some feel that traumatic cannulation is responsible for most ischemic problems related to invasive blood pressure monitoring,[11,68] whereas others have found no evidence for such a claim.[15,69] Transfixion of the radial artery during cannulation does not cause a higher incidence of vascular occlusion than techniques where only the superficial wall of the vessel is punctured during cannulation.[70-72]

Trauma during radial artery cannulation, however, may result in nerve damage at the wrist. Figure 6-11 shows extravasation of radiopaque contrast material outside of a radial artery that had just been cannulated by a transfixing technique. With multiple arterial punctures, considerably more extravasation probably occurs. While the radial nerve lies close to the radial artery, it is the median nerve that has been associated with evidence of neuropathy (pain, weakness, hand-wasting) following multiple radial artery punctures, cutdown cannulation, or traumatic attempted percutaneous cannulation.[73-75] Postmortem examination has shown hematoma from the radial artery extending over the flexor carpi radialis and compressing the median

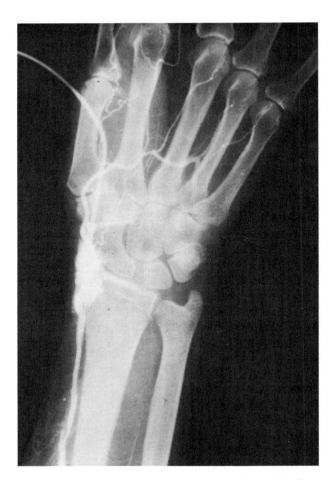

Fig. 6-11. Contrast material extravasating from the deep wall of a radial artery recently cannulated with a transfixing technique. Such extravasation appears to play a role in median nerve dysfunction associated with radial artery cannulation.

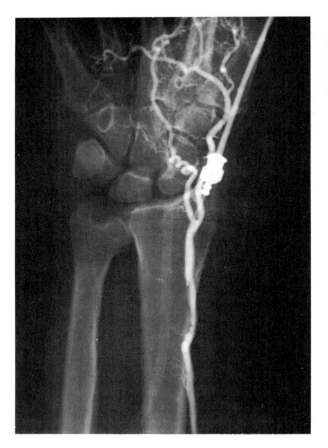

Fig. 6-10. Arteriogram performed by injecting contrast material through a radial artery catheter. Note the tortuosity of the artery as it passes over the wrist joint.

nerve proximal to the transverse carpal ligament.[74] Presumably the median nerve is more susceptible because it is confined within the carpal tunnel and is subject to compression by spreading hematoma. Another possible cause of hand pain after radial artery cannulation is prolonged dorsiflexion of the wrist with stretching of the median nerve.[31,76] Thus, it is probably advisable to return the wrist to a more neutral position after cannulation.

Radial artery thrombosis is a common finding associated with cannulation for blood pressure monitoring. In general, a higher incidence of arterial occlusion results from progressively longer periods of cannulation,[29,69,77-79] and the use of larger catheters[27,30] made of non-Teflon-containing plastics.[25] Current data in adult patients suggest a 10 percent overall incidence of arterial occlusion in adults cannulated with 20-gauge Teflon catheters in place for a period of 1 to 3 days (Fig. 6-12),[77] whereas use of 22-gauge Teflon catheters for 24 hours reduces the risk of arterial occlusion close to zero.[80]

The size of the radial artery lumen relative to the cross-sectional area of the cannula also affects the incidence of vessel thrombosis (Fig. 6-6).[30,62] Women have a higher incidence of radial arterial occlusion than men,[15,26,69,81] and the incidence of radial arterial occlusion in neonates reaches as high as 72 percent when 22-gauge catheters are left in place for up to 10 days.[82] By contrast, adults sustain approximately a 30 percent incidence of occlusion when 20-gauge radial artery catheters remain in place for a similar length of time.[27,77,83]

The pathophysiology of radial artery thrombosis is summarized in Figures 6-13 to 6-16. The presence of a catheter within the radial artery lumen first induces a thickening of the intimal lining which, in turn, is followed by loss of the intima and accumulation of platelet aggregates and fibrinous material. Radial arterial cannulation also causes scarring of the vessel media, and weakness of this layer may result in pseudoaneurysm formation after decannulation.[84]

Thrombotic occlusion of the radial artery after cannulation appears to be a temporary phenomenon (Fig. 6-17), with studies showing a duration up to 75 days.[15,69,83] Smaller arteries remain thrombosed longer than larger arteries,[15] perhaps because they sustain greater anatomic damage while the cannula is in place. As recanalization of radial artery thrombi may take many days, it is not practical to rely on this process for alleviation of distal vascular ischemia should it develop while a cannula is in place. Some thrombi can be removed at the time of decannulation by aspirating vigorously through the catheter while it is withdrawn from the radial artery (Fig. 6-18 to 6-19)[85] and this technique has been used to successfully reinstate flow to pa-

Fig. 6-12. Incidence of radial artery thrombosis plotted against duration of cannulation for 18- and 20-gauge catheters. (From Bedford,[77] with permission.)

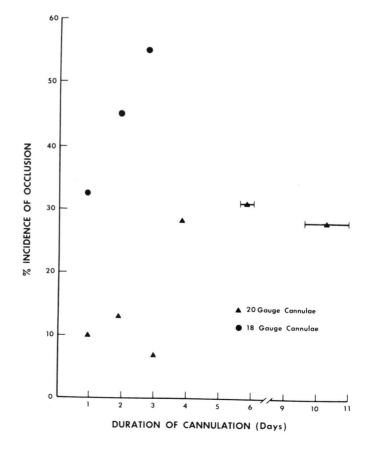

tients' hands that have started to become ischemic during prolonged cannulation. Another approach to remove thrombi from radial arteries with an 18-gauge cannula in place is to perform a surgical cutdown onto the artery and to pass a 3 Fr embolectomy catheter through the arteriotomy created by the 18-gauge cannula. Inflation of the balloon and withdrawal of the embolectomy catheter can remove clot from the artery and reestablish blood flow past the area of occlusion.[28]

The most common complication associated with radial artery cannulation that results in significant morbidity is *not* distal vascular insufficiency, but rather, *ischemic necrosis* of the skin overlying the cannula (Fig. 6-20). This lesion requires several weeks to heal by secondary intention. Originally described as an incidental, isolated finding, this lesion is associated with 0.5 to 3 percent of all cannulations.[86] Bedford found it to occur in 10 percent of all radial arteries that were thrombosed, regardless of the duration of cannulation or the size of the cannula.[77] Arteriography demonstrated occlusion

of the small, cutaneous, perforating branches of the radial artery due to thrombosis around the cannula, and postmortem examination has found thrombus extending into the branches of the radial artery. The incidence of this problem has decreased with the use of smaller catheters, presumably because fewer thrombi are produced.[77]

Given that there is a high incidence of radial artery occlusion associated with percutaneous cannulation, the importance of collateral circulation to the hand should not be underestimated. The elegant anatomic studies of Coleman and Anson[87] in 650 patients demonstrated three arterial arches anastomosing between the radial and ulnar arteries: (1) a superficial volar arch (complete in 86 percent of specimens) formed primarily as a continuation of the ulnar artery; (2) a deep volar arch (complete in 50 percent of specimens) formed from the continuation of the radial artery; and (3) a dorsal arch (complete in 85 percent of specimens) comprised primarily as a continuation of the dorsal radial artery and anastomosing either with

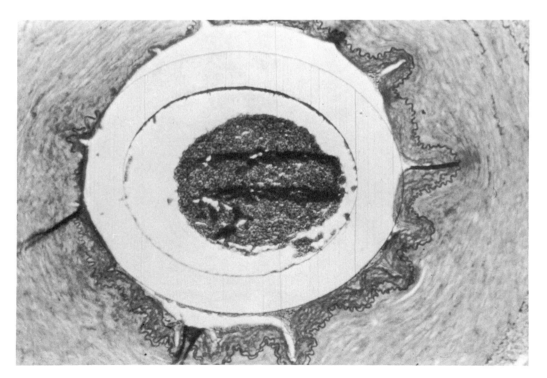

Fig. 6-13. Microscopic section of a radial artery with catheter in situ. There is thickening of the intimal layer as a reaction to the introduction of the foreign body. (Elastic stain).

the interosseus or ulnar arteries. These findings have been verified by radiologic examinations, such as that seen in Fig. 6-21, where collateral flow from the ulnar artery supplies blood to the entire hand and radial artery distal to a cannula-induced, occlusive lesion. Digital blood flow, in turn, radiates from the palmar arches, such that if occlusion of the radial artery is caused by a monitoring cannula, it rarely results in distal vascular ischemia of the hand because of the abundant collateral circulation from the ulnar and median interosseus arteries.

Accurate assessment of ulnar collateral circulation seems warranted because the anatomic studies of Coleman and Anson[87] predict that approximately 3 to 6 percent of patients should have incomplete palmar arterial arches. These findings have been verified by Husum and Palm[88] who found that 6 percent of 259 patients undergoing cardiovascular surgery had inadequate ulnar flow unilaterally (determined by a systolic blood pressure less than 40 mm in the thumb during radial artery occlusion) and 4 percent had inadequate ulnar flow bilaterally. Furthermore, several studies

have found markedly impaired radial artery flow soon after cannulation such that the hand is entirely perfused by collateral flow.[66,89] In patients with acromegaly, where ulnar artery flow is often comprised by ligamentous hypertrophy at the wrist, it has been recommended that either radial artery cannulation be avoided or that particular attention be given to documenting adequate ulnar collateral circulation before the radial artery is cannulated.[90]

Allen's test, devised in 1929 as a method for diagnosing occlusive arterial lesions at the wrist caused by thromboangiitis obliterans,[91] has achieved both popularity and controversy as a technique for documenting adequate collateral circulation from the ulnar artery to the entire hand. Allen described having the patient alternately squeeze and relax his hand in order to exsanguinate it while the examiner occluded both the radial and ulnar arteries with fingertip pressure. Patency of the ulnar artery was indicated by a "prompt return to color" in the hand when pressure over the ulnar artery was released. Allen did not intend to document blood

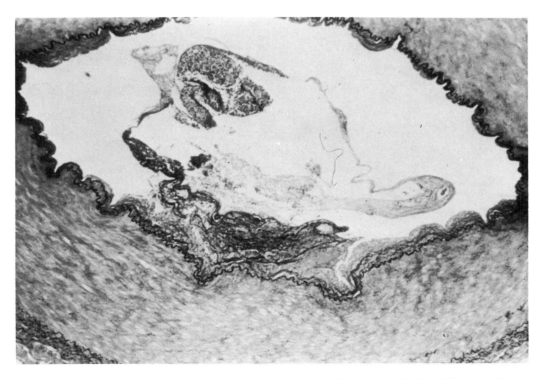

Fig. 6-14. Continued presence of the catheter results in denuding of the intimal lining with accumulation of platelets and thrombotic material on the exposed internal elastic layer.

flow to the entire hand, but only to diagnose arterial occlusion at the wrist.

When used to document collateral flow, Allen's test "return to color" has been a source of controversy. Some clinicians have mistaken a blush in the center of the palm as indicative of blood flow passing all the way from the ulnar artery to the thumb and thenar eminence. Others thought that a 15 second "return to color" indicated satisfactory collateral circulation.[69,92] The result of these misinterpretations was a 10 percent incidence of cold, white thumbs associated with radial artery occlusion. More recent studies using a 5-s limit on complete return to color of the hand, particularly the thumb and thenar eminence, have found Allen's test to be a satisfactory technique for documenting patency of ulnar collateral circulation,[62] although Husum and Berthelson found a 1 percent chance of inadequate thumb flow with a 6-second "return to color" time from the ulnar artery while the radial artery was occluded.[92]

Additional problems with Allen's test are: (1) the patient must be awake and cooperative; (2) it is difficult or impossible to interpret in patients who are burned, pale, or jaundiced; and (3) hyperextension of the digits may give a false pallor, resulting in misinterpretation of the test.[92] Because of the problems in interpreting Allen's test, others have devised more sophisticated techniques for documenting ulnar collateral circulation, including Doppler examination, pulse pressure measurement or pulse oximetry distal to an occluding finger over the radial artery.[93–96] Slogoff and coworkers[81] concluded that Allen's test was not useful because they found no episodes of distal vascular ischemia after cannulating the radial arteries of 16 patients with markedly impaired flow to the hand.[81] As the authors failed to document the duration of the cannulation, the size of the catheters used, and what proportion of the patients were men (with presumably large radial arteries) the results remain controversial.

Despite apparent evidence of satisfactory ulnar collateral circulation, many case reports of severe distal vascular ischemia and gangrene of the hand have been associated with radial artery cannula-

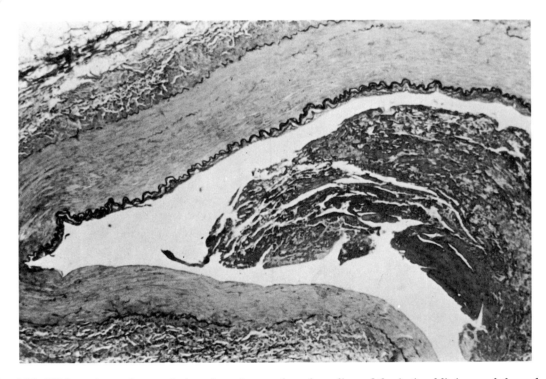

Fig. 6-15. With prolonged cannulation there is complete denuding of the intimal lining and thrombotic occlusion of the vessel lumen.

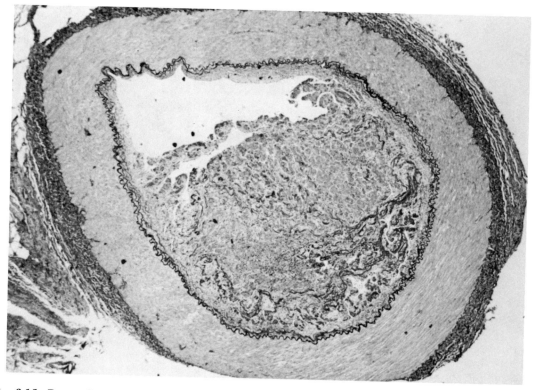

Fig. 6-16. Recanalization of an occluded radial artery occurring several weeks after decannulation.

tion.[97–100] To date, only one such case has been definitely associated with thromboembolic phenomena from the heart.[101] More commonly, however, hand gangrene is associated with low flow states, high-dose vasopressor therapy and no documentation of ulnar collateral flow.[26,44,51,68,73,102–104] Although distal vascular ischemia has been relieved in some of these cases by thrombectomy, sympathetic blockade, intraarterial local anesthetics or papaverine, many others were totally refractory to therapy and went on to require amputation of fingers, hands, or forearms. The overall incidence of severe vascular compromise has been estimated at 0.01 percent for all radial artery cannulations.[7,105] Since these catastrophes usually begin with radial arterial thrombosis, and thrombus around the catheter often causes catheter dysfunction in the form of damped pulse-pressure waves or difficulty in obtaining samples, it has been recommended that evidence of catheter dysfunction probably should be a signal for decannulation.[26] This should be performed preferably with vigorous aspiration

on the catheter as it is withdrawn in an attempt to remove intraarterial thrombus.[85] Attempts at relieving catheter dysfunction by vigorous flushing, however, may only result in cerebral ischemia due to retrograde flow of clot and flush solution to the carotid or vertebral circulation,[44] and has been shown to cause acute hypertension in neonates.[106]

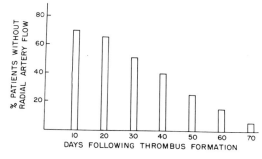

Fig. 6-17. Duration of arterial occlusion in patients whose radial arteries had thrombosed after cannulation. (From Bedford and Wollman,[69] with permission.)

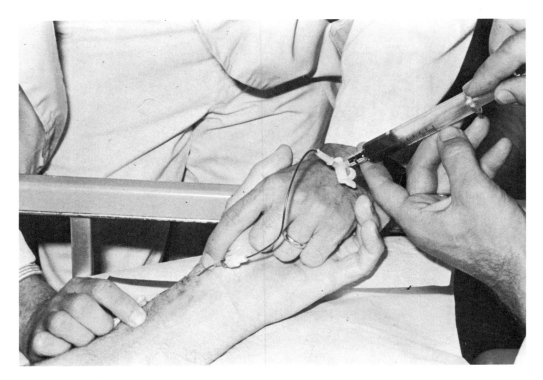

Fig. 6-18. Attempted recovery of thrombus from a radial artery at decannulation. As the catheter is withdrawn, vigorous continuous suction is applied while digital pressure occludes the artery. Thrombus is aspirated into the syringe. (From Bedford,[85] with permission.)

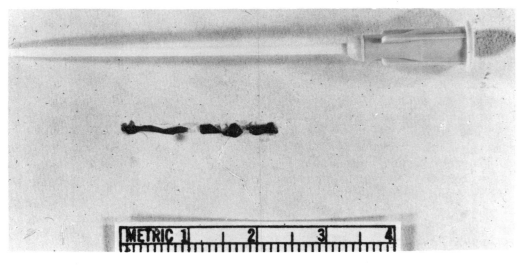

Fig. 6-19. Thrombotic material recovered from a radial artery catheter during decannulation. (From Bedford,[85] with permission.)

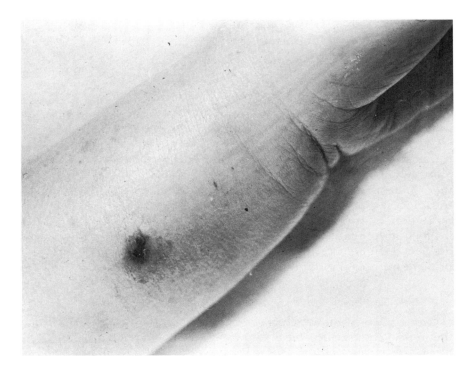

Fig. 6-20. Skin necrosis overlying a segment of radial artery thrombus. The cannula puncture site is seen distal to the lesion.

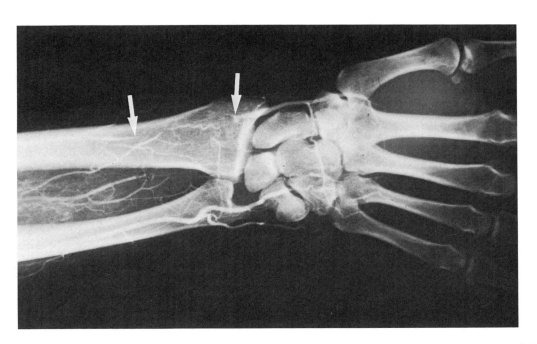

Fig. 6-21. Brachial arteriogram of a patient with an occluded radial artery (*arrows*). Collateral circulation to the hand is supplied via the ulnar artery and two of the three palmar arterial arches described by Coleman and Anson.[87]

Alternative Sites for Arterial Pressure Monitoring

The Ulnar Artery

Ulnar artery cannulation is performed in a fashion similar to cannulation of the radial artery, although it is somewhat more difficult because the vessel is not as superficial as the radial artery and it tends to be quite tortuous as it passes the wrist joint (Fig. 6-21). Several studies have referred to the radial and ulnar arteries as interchangeable sites for peripheral arterial cannulation.[15,66,88,107] Since dominant collateral flow to the hand can be from either the radial or ulnar artery, it seems prudent to document collateral flow from the radial prior to cannulating the ulnar artery.

The Brachial Artery

Cannulation of the brachial artery offers several theoretical and practical advantages over radial and ulnar artery cannulation. It is a larger vessel and, thus, can accommodate a larger catheter with a higher natural frequency. Furthermore, it is more proximal and, therefore, less subject to systolic pressure augmentation due to reflection of the pulse-pressure wave from distal artery-arteriole junctions. As with other sites, however, the incidence of complications increases with duration of cannulation.[11,107–111]

In addition to vascular lesions, damage to the median nerve has also been reported with brachial artery cannulation, either associated with traumatic arterial puncture or hematoma formation.[112,113] From a practical standpoint, brachial artery catheters work well when a patient is anesthetized but tend to be a problem in conscious patients in the intensive care unit in whom the elbow joint becomes more difficult to immobilize than the wrist.

The Axillary Artery

There are several desirable aspects to cannulation of the axillary artery. The vessel is large, it can tolerate relatively large-bore catheters with a low incidence of thrombotic complications and it leaves the patient's arms relatively unencumbered. The axillary artery is often palpable in shock states when more peripheral vessels are faint or absent, and its pulse-pressure trace is a close representation of that in the aortic arch.[114–117]

As the axillary arterial catheter is close to the central circulation, meticulous attention must be directed at preventing the entry of air bubbles or clots into the cerebral circulation during catheter flushing or blood sampling. The left axillary artery is the preferred site, since the tip of a 6-inch catheter in the right axillary artery may lie in the innominate artery, with ready access to the cerebral circulation. Another disadvantage of the axillary artery is its location within a neurovascular sheath, where hematoma formation may result in neurologic consequences.[114,118,119]

The approach to the axillary artery is similar to that for an axillary nerve block. Once the vessel lumen is punctured, cannulation can be performed using either a 3-in. catheter-over-needle device or a 6-in. pediatric CVP catheter advanced into the vessel over a guidewire.

The Dorsalis Pedis Artery

Cannulation of the dorsalis pedis artery is indicated in clinical situations where the arteries of the upper extremities are inaccessible, such as in extensive burns, trauma, or previous arterial catheterizations.[17] Due to its distal location, however, systolic and diastolic pressure readings are subject to considerable resonance and mean arterial pressure is the only value that approximates aortic pressure values. Because it is a small vessel, there is a high incidence of both unsuccessful cannulation and postcannulation arterial occlusion. Fortunately, there is an arterial arcade in the foot that usually supplies collateral circulation from the posterior tibial circulation in the event of occlusion of the dorsalis pedis artery. However, wedge-shaped distal infarcts and impaired toe perfusion have been reported.[120,121] To assess collateral circulation, Kaplan[31] suggests occluding both the dorsalis pedis and posterior tibial pulses with digital pressure, then blanching the patient's great toe with direct compression. If the toe color does not promptly (greater than 5 seconds) return to normal when the posterior tibial artery pressure is released, another site should be selected for arterial cannulation.

The Femoral Artery

When used for blood pressure monitoring the femoral artery is reported to be no more risky than radial artery cannulation.[122,123] It is a large artery and should be relatively free from catheter-induced thrombosis. However, it is also subject to atheroma formation which may make passage of a catheter difficult or which may either break off and embolize distally, or may lead to vascular occlusion. Several reports list an approximate incidence of 0.5 percent for ischemia requiring embolectomy after femoral artery cannulation,[117,124,125] whereas transient self-limited vascular insufficiency occurs in approximately another 0.5 percent.[122,124,126] In these studies, catheter sizes ranged from 14 to 20 gauge with no obvious relationship between catheter diameter and the incidence of occlusive lesions. These data suggest that atheromata may act as a prime cause of occlusion while femoral arterial catheters are in place.

Hematoma formation is also a prominent problem with femoral artery cannulation, occurring in 8 to 13 percent of patients and probably related to placement of catheters through larger needles or via a transfixing cannulation technique.[122,124,126]

As is the case with other intravascular catheters, the incidence of infection increases with the duration of femoral artery cannulation. A 1- to 3-day period appears to be safe, whereas longer periods (4 to 12 days) produce catheter-related infections at a rate of 8 to 17 percent.[117,122,124]

Indications for cannulation of the femoral artery include thoracic aortic surgery where the patency of a Gott shunt can be monitored by femoral artery pressure,[127] patients in shock where other peripheral pulses may be nonpalpable, or those suffering from burns or multiple trauma where other sites are inaccessible.

NONINVASIVE BLOOD PRESSURE MONITORING

Considerable effort has been expended in refining the technology for noninvasive blood pressure (NIBP) measurement. Ever since 1903, when Cushing[128] first advocated clinical use of blood pressure measurement, most arterial pressure monitoring has been done noninvasively, either with a manually operated sphygmomanometer or with an automated noninvasive device. Currently there are approximately 200,000 automated noninvasive BP devices in clinical use worldwide, both in operating rooms and critical care units.

One of the problems with NIBP measurement is the considerable variance in blood pressure data, both within and between the different techniques available.[129] Common to nearly all the contemporary methods for noninvasive arterial pressure measurement is an inflatable circumferential cuff which is placed about an extremity and inflated to a pressure which exceeds systolic pressure and stops either blood flow or arterial wall motion. However, there is little standardization for the estimation of NIBP and there are multiple techniques available for measuring changes in systolic, diastolic, mean arterial, and pulse pressures.

The lack of standardization is further complicated by the multiplicity of sites available for NIBP measurement. As discussed in the section on invasive blood pressure monitoring, the intraarterial pressure changes as it moves away from the aortic root, a consequence of changes in vessel diameter, vessel wall elasticity and the state of arteriolar tone. It is because of these limitations and the observed inconsistencies in NIBP measurement that Brunner and colleagues[16] concluded, "Blood pressure is a function of the way it is measured."

History

Although the circulation of blood in the human body had been known since first described in 1628 by William Harvey, it was 1876 when Von Basch developed a technique for occluding a peripheral artery using hydraulically applied pressure over a bone.[130] The pressure was increased until pulsations in the artery disappeared; this point was taken as the systolic pressure. A variation of this technique of arterial occlusion was undertaken in 1876 by E. J. Marey, who inserted a subject's arm through a seal into a cylinder of water that could have its pressure recorded as well as changed.[130] Marey also developed a somewhat less bulky method using a cylinder that fit tightly around one finger, but this method did not win clinical acceptance, perhaps because of the low amplitude of the oscillations in the manometer.

The use of a pneumatic cuff around the arm was first described in 1896 by Riva-Rocci and in 1897 by Hill and Barnard.[131] Using palpation of the radial artery (the so-called palpatory method) the cuff was gradually inflated until the radial pulse first disappeared; the cuff was then deflated and the pressure at which the pulse then reappeared was recorded. These two readings were averaged to give the systolic pressure.

The auscultatory method of BP determination

was first proposed in 1905 by Korotkoff.[130] He believed that the sounds which were heard through a stethoscope placed over the brachial artery distal to an occluding cuff were caused by the breakthrough of a pulse wave and that the subsequent lessening and then disappearance of the sounds was caused by the passage of an unobstructed pulse wave. He noted that the first sound occurred at a higher pressure than was obtained with palpation of the radial artery and concluded that more of the pulse waveform had to pass down the artery before the pulse was palpable.

Methods of Measurement

Noninvasive blood pressure measurement is currently performed either manually or with a variety of automated electromechanical devices employing techniques such as auscultation, oscillometry, blood flow detection, and photometric pulse wave delay.[7] The following is a partial list of techniques and/or devices used in contemporary medical practice. Each will be discussed in some detail:

Auscultation
Oscillometry
Blood flow detection: palpation, ultrasonic, and photoelectric
Ultrasonic detection of arterial wall movement
Infrasonde (Puritan Bennett)
Finapres
Arterial tonometry
Photometric wave velocity

Auscultation

The auscultatory or Riva-Rocci method for NIBP monitoring has been, and continues to be, the most commonly used NIBP measurement technique.[132] It relies upon Korotkoff sounds, a complex series of audible frequencies that are produced by turbulent flow, instability of the arterial wall, and shock wave formation created as external occluding cuff pressure on a major artery is reduced.[133] The pressure at which the first sound (phase I) is heard is usually taken as the systolic value. The sound character changes (phases II and III), then becomes muffled (phase IV) and finally absent (phase V). Diastolic pressure is recorded at phase IV or V, although phase V may never occur in certain pathophysiologic states, such as aortic regurgitation.[134]

As familiar as the standard BP cuff may be, a number of caveats should be considered in its use. It is of paramount importance to match the size of BP cuff to the size of the patient's arm. Too small a cuff, or one that is wrapped too loosely, will result in falsely elevated BP readings because of the excessive cuff pressure required to occlude a deep artery (Fig. 6-22). Other causes of falsely elevated BP include the extremity's being placed below heart level or uneven cuff compression transmitted to the underlying artery. Falsely low estimates result when cuffs are too large, when the extremity is above heart level, or if the cuff is deflated too rapidly to detect appropriate Korotkoff sounds.[135]

Geddes[130] states that the width of the BP cuff

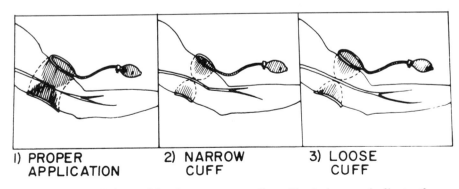

1) PROPER APPLICATION   2) NARROW CUFF   3) LOOSE CUFF

Fig. 6-22. The effect of cuff fit on blood pressure reading. Shaded areas indicate the magnitude of tissue pressure (=cuff pressure). **(1)** With a proper fit the pressure of the cuff is transmitted undiminished to the artery and compresses it. **(2)** A cuff that is too narrow requires greater pressure and results in a higher blood pressure reading. **(3)** A loose cuff also results in artifactual elevation of the blood pressure. A cuff that is too wide is merely bulky and does not distort readings. (From Rushmer,[177] with permission.)

should be 40 percent of the circumference of the arm. The pneumatic bladder should span at least one-half of this circumference and should be centered over the artery. One of the cuffs described in Table 6-1 will be accurate in most cases.

Consideration should also be given to placement of the stethoscope over the brachial artery. Loose fitting diaphragm-type stethoscopes, a poor seal with a bell-type stethoscope or motion of either type will result in the attenuation of the Korotkoff sounds. The Diasyst stethoscope bell is particularly helpful for achieving good skin contact over the brachial artery.

Cuff deflation rate should be slow enough for the sensing process to detect appropriate Korotkoff sound changes and to assign them to the pressure of the cuff. Failure to do so will result in falsely low pressures. A deflation rate of 3 mmHg/s limits this source of error. Coupling of the deflation rate to heart rate (2 mmHg/beat) has been found to further improve accuracy.[136]

Oscillometry

The oscillometric method of NIBP monitoring senses variations in the pressure within a blood pressure cuff during deflation. The cuff is pressurized until no oscillations are seen and is then allowed to deflate until sudden fluctuations in the pressure of the cuff are noted on a pressure gauge. At this point, the cuff pressure is at or near the systolic pressure.[130] The inflation pressure is then allowed to fall further, until the oscillations are seen to reach a maximum and begin to decrease. This point has been shown to be near the *mean* arterial pressure, not the diastolic pressure as had been previously thought (Fig. 6-23).

TABLE 6-1. Commonly Available Blood Pressure Cuff Sizes

Cuff	Arm Circumference (cm)	Bladder Size (cm)
Newborn	6–11	2.5 × 5
Infant	10–19	6 × 12
Child	18–26	9 × 18
Adult	25–35	12 × 23
Large arm	33–47	15 × 33
Thigh	46–66	18 × 36

(Courtesy of WA Baum Co., Inc., Copiague, NY)

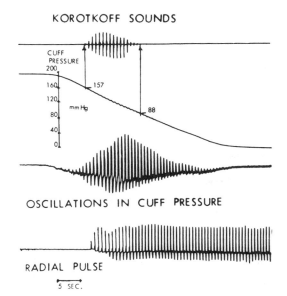

Fig. 6-23. A comparison between Korotkoff sounds, cuff pressure oscillation, and radial pulse. There is a good correlation between the onset of the first Korotkoff sound, the onset of oscillations in the cuff pressure, and the radial pulse wave. By contrast, there is no correlation with the disappearance of the cuff oscillations. (From Reitan and Barash,[178] with permission.)

The first commercially produced automatic oscillometric BP monitor, the Dinamap, entered routine clinical use in 1976.[137] Initially, it determined only mean arterial pressure (MAP), primarily because a change in MAP is easier to interpret than changes in systolic or diastolic pressure, which can often move in opposite directions. Also, at the capillary bed level, most of the pulsation caused by the oscillations of systolic and diastolic pressure has been damped out by the resistance and compliance of the proximal vascular bed. In addition, MAP measurement is less affected by changes in vascular tone than systolic or diastolic pressure measurement because it is determined when the oscillations of cuff pressure reach the greatest amplitude. This property allows MAP to be measured reliably even in cases of hypotension with vasoconstriction and diminished pulse pressure.[138]

The technique for ideal oscillometric NIBP measurement is illustrated in Fig. 6-24. All three pressures are determined individually, and, in contrast to the manual auscultatory method, there is little effect on the accuracy of the measurement when venous engorgement from cuff inflation is not allowed to subside.

Difficulties in blood pressure measurement by oscillometry may arise due to (1) incorrect cuff size, (2) incorrect cuff application, (3) undetected leaks in the cuff, hoses, or connectors, (4) not keeping cuff at heart level, (5) arm movement, and (6) inadequate pulse pressure waves due to shock or vascular compression proximal to the cuff.[138]

In spite of these potential difficulties, numerous reports attest to the accuracy and reliability of the Dinamap monitor in both neonates and adults.[136–156] Most of these studies have shown there is less than 5 mmHg mean error with a standard deviation of less than 8 mmHg when a Dinamap is compared to a centrally placed arterial catheter. The current models of the Dinamap display systolic, mean and diastolic blood pressure as well as heart rate (Fig. 6-25).

Blood Flow Detection

There are three commonly used techniques for measurement of systolic blood pressure by detection of blood flow distal to an occlusive cuff. There is *no* way to measure the mean or the diastolic pressure using this technique.

Palpation

The first method utilizes palpation of the arterial pulse distal to a pneumatic cuff. In brief, an arm cuff of sufficient width is inflated to a point 30 mmHg higher than the point of disappearance of the pulse. The cuff is deflated at a rate of 2 to 3 mmHg per heartbeat. The point of return of the radial pulse denotes the systolic pressure. Patients with irregular heart rates such as those in atrial fibrillation will demonstrate a wide range of systolic pressures, particularly if the cuff is allowed to de-

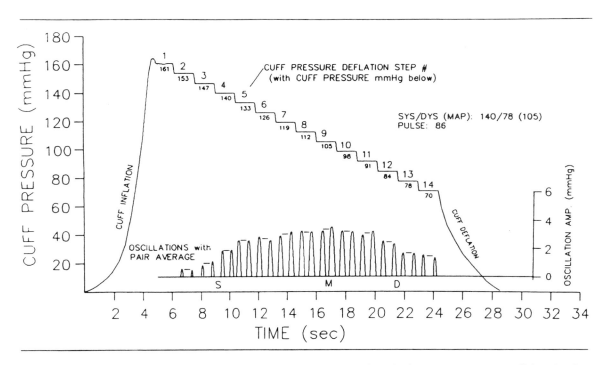

Fig. 6-24. Blood pressure measurement technique illustrating the ideal measurement condition in the absence of artifact. The cuff pressure and oscillation amplitude (*AMP*) are plotted on the same axis with the cuff pressure amplitude axis on the left and the oscillation amplitude axis on the right. Mean arterial pressure (*MAP, M*) is calculated from systolic (*SYS, S*) and diastolic (*DYS, D*) pressures. In this subject, cuff pressure is considerably above systolic pressure and no cuff pressure oscillations are visible either in the figure or the microprocessor. (From Ramsey,[138] with permission.)

flate rapidly. Whenever two systoles occur in close proximity, there is less time for filling of the left ventricle and both stroke volume and blood pressure are lower during the second beat. It is thus possible to miss a beat or two and interpret the blood pressure as lower than it actually is. If the palpated vessel is some distance from the cuff, flow transmission time will delay sensing of systolic pressure slightly (flow velocity is approximately 8 to 10 m/s).[157] Overall, systolic blood pressure measurements by palpation are lower than those determined with Korotkoff systems. This technique has been found useful in neonates, infants, obese patients, and those in whom Korotkoff sounds are inconsistent.[158]

Ultrasonic

More sensitive than the palpation method of measurement of blood flow, an ultrasonic blood flow detector employs an ultrasonic Doppler unit placed over a distal artery. The Doppler transceiver monitors blood flow in the artery by sensing the velocity of erythrocytes.[159] As the ipsilateral upper arm cuff is inflated above systolic blood pressure, the audio output from the unit becomes silent as arterial erythrocyte movement ceases. Systolic pressure is signaled by the cuff pressure at which ''chirps'' from the Doppler unit indicate blood flow which rhythmically follows the heartbeat. Diastolic pressure is signified by the point at which full pulsatile flow occurs. This method is particularly useful when the peripheral pulse is faint or absent such as cold, shocky patients and in infants or obese patients whose Korotkoff sounds may be absorbed by fatty tissue.

A significant disadvantage of ultrasonic blood flow detectors is that electrosurgical equipment produces audible interference which can be annoying or even render blood pressure determination impossible. Newer Doppler flow detectors employ circuits to eliminate this problem by automatically shutting off the external speaker circuit when the electrosurgery unit is activated.

Photoelectric

This technique measures the absorption of light from a source placed against the skin, most conveniently on a finger. The pulsatile changes in blood volume associated with blood flow produce changes in absorption of infrared light. If a cuff is inflated above arterial pressure and then allowed to deflate, a sudden small oscillation in the output of the blood flow detector is seen which is equivalent to the systolic pressure. When the pulse volume amplitude no longer increases, diastolic pressure is reached.

The technique fails, however, if the blood vessels in the finger become constricted due to either hypothermia or hypotension. Furthermore, the constant light source produces a moderate amount of heat which, in combination with poor blood flow under the transducer may lead to thermal injury.

Ultrasonic Detection of Arterial Wall Movement

In addition to detecting flow of erythrocytes, the Doppler principle can be used to indirectly measure blood pressure by detecting motion of an arterial wall distal to an occlusive pneumatic cuff. (Arteriosonde 1216, Roche Medical Electronics Di-

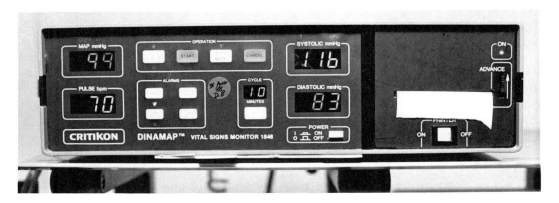

Fig. 6-25. Dinamap (Courtesy of Critikon, Tampa, FL)

vision, Cranbury, NJ). A dual piezoelectric crystal ultrasonic transducer is placed over the artery. One crystal acts as the transmitter of an ultrasonic signal (commonly 2 to 10 MHz), while the other receives the reflected sound wave. With no target (artery) movement, the receiver crystal senses a constant signal frequency. When the cuff pressure falls just below systolic pressure, the vessel opens and then quickly closes as the peak (systolic) pressure wave subsides. This sudden movement of the arterial wall causes a Doppler frequency shift, which is noted by the receiving crystal. The initial arterial opening is taken as the systolic pressure reading. Diastolic pressure is determined when cuff pressure falls to the point where the artery is open throughout the pulse cycle so that the rhythmic arterial opening and closing is no longer present. Several studies have compared NIBP measured by ultrasound to direct intraarterial pressures in both adults and infants with results which are satisfactory for most clinical applications.[160–165]

Infrasonde

The Infrasonde (Puritan-Bennett) uses the auscultatory method to automatically determine systolic and diastolic pressures. Like the Dinamap, the Infrasonde provides for automatic inflation of an arm cuff. Two crystal microphones are positioned over the brachial artery and are used to determine the point at which the Korotkoff sounds first appear. The cuff deflates at a rate selected by the operator; a determination is then made of the systolic, mean and diastolic blood pressures. Accuracy is ensured by a display of the signal strength, a useful feature which aids the operator both in accurately positioning the cuff and for indicating the signal-to-noise ratio under which the machine is operating. As one might infer, the leading disadvantage of the Infrasonde is that it must have its sensors placed accurately over an artery. If the sensors shift away from the artery, the signal strength drops and the machine is unable to give a satisfactory NIBP reading. Unlike the Dinamap, the Infrasonde cannot be placed easily over any portion of an extremity. It thus trades convenience of cuff placement for rapidity of BP determination.[166]

Finapres

First described by Penaz in Czechoslovakia, the Finapres (finger arterial pressure) consists of a small cuff placed over a patient's finger. The cuff is connected to a very rapidly responding solenoid that inflates and deflates the cuff, keeping the volume of the finger constant as pulsatile blood flow increases or decreases. When the instrument senses that finger volume is expanding due to inflow of blood under the constricting cuff, the solenoid pressurizes the cuff just enough to prevent further blood flow. Thus, the device tends to track the mean arterial blood pressure in digital arteries underlying the cuff by nulling the transmural pressure under the cuff. A waveform that closely approximates arterial blood pressure in the finger is displayed on the screen.[11]

The accuracy of the Finapres has been the subject of considerable study. Stokes and coworkers[167] compared Finapres values with invasive arterial pressures and concluded that while providing useful beat-to-beat information on arterial pressure trends, the Finapres could not be recommended as a universal substitute for invasive arterial pressure monitoring. Gorback and associates[168] compared the Finapres with the Dinamap and found that readings by both correlated well for diastolic and mean arterial pressures, while the accuracy of the Finapres appeared to be slightly superior for systolic pressure. Epstein and coworkers[169] compared Finapres and Dinamap measurements with intraarterial pressures. They found that the Finapres had a significantly higher bias than the Dinamap for diastolic and mean blood pressure when compared to intraarterial pressure. They therefore concluded that the Finapres monitor could not be relied upon to accurately measure blood pressure (without a second method of blood pressure) in patients undergoing general anesthesia.

Additional studies comparing NIBP and invasive arterial pressure readings were performed by Brunner and colleagues[16] and are summarized in Figures 6-26 to 6-28. In their series of patients, they found that the correlation between invasive and automated noninvasive measurements was not very good for systolic pressures and that the correlation for diastolic pressures was even worse. In contrast, the correlation between Riva-Rocci systolic pressure and intraarterial catheter occlusion pressure was found to be quite good.

Arterial Tonometry

The technique of arterial tonometry utilizes a pressor sensor positioned over a superficial artery and records arterial wall displacement, which is

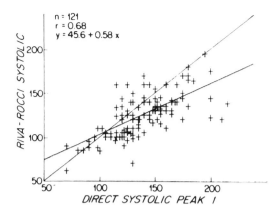

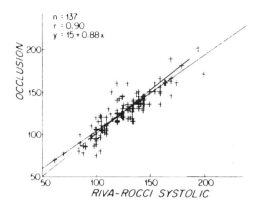

Fig. 6-26. Comparison between systolic blood pressure determined by the Riva-Rocci method and blood pressures determined by direct intraarterial monitoring. Note the large scatter in the data. (From Brunner et al.,[16] with permission.)

Fig. 6-28. Comparison between systolic blood pressures determined by the Riva-Rocci method and by the occlusion method of observing an intraarterial trace from a catheter in the radial artery while a proximal cuff is inflated above systolic pressure and then deflated. The point of appearance of the pulse wave is taken as the systolic pressure. These two methods show the best correlation. (From Brunner et al.,[16] with permission.)

then converted into an electrical signal.[170–172] It requires an adequately sized, superficial artery that is supported by a bony structure. The sensor exerts pressure on the artery, partially flattening against the underlying bone (Fig. 6-29). The force exerted by the blood vessel is then transmitted through the skin with near perfect fidelity. The technique is based on the following assumptions: (1) the skin thickness is insignificant compared to the arterial diameter; (2) the arterial wall behaves essentially as an ideal membrane; and (3) the sensor is smaller

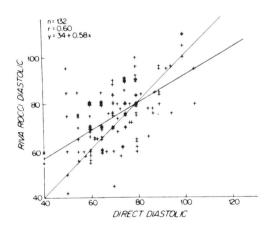

Fig. 6-27. Comparison between diastolic blood pressures determined by the Riva-Rocci method and by direct intraarterial monitoring. There is even more scatter in the data than that in Figure 6-26. (From Brunner et al.,[16] with permission.)

than the flattened area of the artery and is centered above the flattened area. It has been shown that the electrical output signal of the generated force is directly proportional to the intra-arterial blood pressure.

The CBM-3000 (Colin Medical Instruments Corp.) is a multiparameter monitor that employs the newly developed transducer array for tonometric blood pressure monitoring. The transducer array is incorporated into a sensor that is placed over the radial artery just proximal to the wrist joint. The sensor assembly is formed to hold the wrist with the proper degree of extension. A microcomputer analyzes the signal from each transducer of the sensor array and selects the transducer that is properly positioned based on maximum pulse amplitude of the signal. Hold-down pressure is set via microprocessor control of a pneumatic bladder that is incorporated into the sensor assembly. The tonometric blood pressure readings require calibration to oscillometer cuff measurements at user-selected intervals of either 5 or 10 minutes.

Several studies have compared tonometric blood pressure measurements against invasive radial artery pressure tracings in anesthetized patients.[173–176] A good correlation was found between the two techniques, with identical pressure waveforms

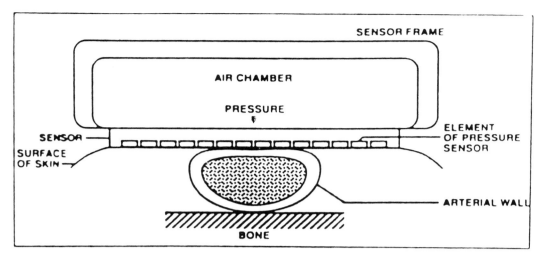

Fig. 6-29. Diagram of the multisensor arterial tonometer in use. The tonometer is placed over the artery and secured with sufficient force to partially flatten the artery. The arterial waveform is then recorded with near-perfect fidelity. (From Eckerle,[172] with permission.)

found in both tonometric and intraarterial BP recordings.

Photometric Wave Velocity Technique

The refinement of pulse oximetry technology has led to advances in photometric sensor development and signal processing techniques that permit NIBP measurement without use of artery occlusion. Instead, systolic and diastolic blood pressure values are determined by measuring arterial pulse wave velocity and changes in local blood volume. The ARTRAC 7000 monitor uses two photometric sensors similar to those used by pulse oximeters, one of which is placed on the ear and the other on a finger. The pulse oximeters sense each heartbeat, with the proximal (ear) pulse arriving before the distal (finger) pulse. The difference in arrival time is called the pulse transit time. The proximal sensor also senses changes in microvascular volume. The pulse wave velocity is a relative measure of diastolic pressure, so that an initial calibration with a traditional blood pressure cuff is necessary to obtain absolute pressure values.

When compared to NIBP data obtained with a blood pressure cuff, the ARTRAC has been found to be within the American Association of Medical Instrumentation (AAMI) and American National Standards Institute (ANSI) standards. When compared to invasive arterial pressures, the bias was within standards for systolic and mean pressures and within a mean value of 7 mmHg for diastolic pressures (DH Wong and DR Bogard, personal communication).

CONCLUSIONS

Will indirect measurement of blood pressure ever replace direct intraarterial blood pressure monitoring? Probably not, since an arterial catheter also functions as a site for drawing multiple blood samples, when this is needed. On the other hand, the rapid development of noninvasive CO_2 and O_2 analysis, in combination with reliable noninvasive blood pressure measurements, have probably reduced the overall need for arterial catheterization.

It must always be remembered, however, that invasive arterial pressure monitoring and noninvasive blood pressure measurement reflect two different phenomena. When a catheter is placed in a patient's artery, the systolic, diastolic, and mean pressures can be obtained even when there is no blood flow in the vessel. In contrast, when an occluding cuff is wrapped around patient's arm and inflated, detection of the systolic, diastolic, and mean pressure is possible only because of blood flow under the cuff. Thus, one technique measures pressure directly whereas the other detects flow and tries to infer pressure indirectly.

Should we resolve these differences? We believe probably not. Attempts to make the direct and indirect methods of blood pressure measurements correspond can lower the accuracy and repeatability of both methods. One should be content with the fact that each method has its particular advantages; comparisons between them, except in the most general terms, should be avoided. The important feature of blood pressure monitoring is that the equipment gives a value which, in turn, should cause the clinician to think about what is happening to the patient and to act accordingly.

REFERENCES

1. Hales S: Vegetable staticks. p. 361. In Innys W, Manby R (eds): Statikal Essays. Vol 1. 3rd Ed. London, 1738. Cited in Geddes LA: The Direct and Indirect Measurement of Blood Pressure. Year Book Medical Publishers, Chicago, 1970
2. Faivre I: Etudes experimentales sur les lesions organique du coerir. Gaz Med Paris, p. 727, 1856
3. McLean J: The discovery of heparin. Circulation 19:75, 1959
4. Lambert EH, Wood EH: The use of resistance wire strain gauge manometer to measure intraarterial pressure. Proc Soc Exp Biol Med 64:186, 1947
5. Barr PO: Percutaneous puncture of the radial artery with a multipurpose Teflon catheter for indwelling use. Acta Physiol Scand 51:343, 1961
6. Hill DW: Physics Applied to Anesthesia. 4th Ed. Butterworth, London, 1980
7. Brunner JMR: Handbook of Blood Pressure Monitoring. PSG Publishing, Littleton, MA, 1978
8. Hunter FP, Eastwood DW: Manometry. In: Instrumentation and Anesthesia. FA Davis, Philadelphia, 1964
9. Buxton AE, Anderson RL, Klimek J et al: Failure of disposable domes to prevent septicemia acquired from contaminated pressure transducers. Chest 74:508, 1978
10. Donowitz LG, Marsik FJ, Hoyt JW et al: *Serratia marcescens* bacteremia from contaminated pressure transducers. JAMA 242:1749, 1979
11. Prys-Roberts C: Measurement of intravascular pressure. In Saidman LJ, Smith NT (eds): Monitoring in Anesthesia. Churchill Livingstone, New York, 1978
12. Brunner JMR, Krenis LJ, Kunsman JM et al: Comparison of direct and indirect methods of measuring arterial blood pressure. Part I. Med Instrum 15:11, 1981
13. O'Rourke MJF: Pressure and flow waves in systemic arteries and the anatomical design of the arterial system. J Appl Physiol 23:139, 1967
14. Brunner JMR, Krenis LJ, Kunsman JM et al: Comparison of direct and indirect methods of measuring arterial blood pressure. Part II. Med Instrum 15:97, 1981
15. Kim JM, Arawaka K, Bliss J: Arterial cannulation: factors in the development of occlusion. Anesth Analg 56:603, 1977
16. Brunner JMR, Krenis LJ, Kunsman JM et al: Comparison of direct and indirect methods of measuring arterial blood pressure. Part III. Med Instrum 15:182, 1981
17. Johnstone RE, Greenhow DE: Catheterization of the dosalis pedis artery. Anesthesiology 39:654, 1973
18. Krovetz LJ, Goldbloom SD: Frequency content of intravascular and intracardiac pressures and their time derivatives. IEEE Trans Biomed Eng BME 21:498, 1974
19. Berne RM, Levy MN: Peripheral arterial pressure curves. p. 110. In: Cardiovascular Physiology. CV Mosby, St. Louis, 1977
20. O'Rourke MF, Taylor MG: Vascular impedance of the femoral bed. Circ Res 18:126, 1966
21. Brunner JMR: Invasive Pressure Monitoring: Practical Application and Pitfalls. American Society of Anesthesiologists Annual Meeting, Refresher Course Lecture, 1982
22. Pearse RG: Percutaneous catheterization of the radial artery in newborn babies using transillumination. Arch Dis Child 53:549, 1978
23. Edelman JD: An aid in arterial cannulation. [Letter]. Anesthesiology 53:79, 1980
24. Stirt JA: Liquid stylet for percutaneous radial artery cannulation. Can Anaesth Soc J 29:492, 1982
25. Bedford RF: Percutaneous radial-artery cannulation: increased safety using Teflon catheters. Anesthesiology 42:430, 1977
26. Davis FM, Stewart JM: Radial artery cannulation: a prospective study in patients undergoing cardiothoracic surgery. Br J Anaesth 52:41, 1980
27. Downs JB, Rackstein AD, Klein EF et al: Hazards of radial-artery catheterization. Anesthesiology 38:283, 1973
28. Feeley TW: Reestablishment of radial artery patency for arterial monitoring. Anesthesiology 46:73, 1975
29. Downs JB, Chapman WL, Hawkins IF: Prolonged radial-artery catheterization: an evaluation of heparinized catheters and continuous irrigation. Arch Surg 108:671, 1974
30. Bedford RF: Wrist circumference predicts the risk of radial-arterial occlusion after cannulation. Anesthesiology 48:377, 1978

31. Kaplan JA: Hemodynamic monitoring. p. 183. In Kaplan JA (ed): Cardiac Anesthesia. 2nd Ed. Grune & Stratton, Orlando, 1987

32. Lee AP: Biotechnological principles of monitoring. Int Anesthesiol Clin 19:204, 1981

33. Gravenstein JS, Paulus DA: Arterial pressure. p. 43. In: Clinical Monitoring Practice. 2nd Ed. JB Lippincott, Philadelphia, 1982

34. Browning DH, Graves SA, Van de Aa J: Catheters for arterial pressure monitoring in pediatrics. Anesthesiology 55:A131, 1981

35. Boutros A, Albert S: Effect of the dynamic response of transducer-tubing system on accuracy of direct blood pressure measurement in patients. Anesthesiology 57:A149, 1982

36. Shinozaki T, Deane RS, Mazuzan JE Jr et al: The dynamic responses of liquid-filled catheter systems for direct measurement of blood pressure. Anesthesiology 53:498, 1980

37. Bedford RF, O'Brien TE: Comparison of bovine lung and porcine intestinal heparin for arterial thrombosis in man. Am J Hosp Pharm 34:936, 1977

38. Gardner RM, Bond EL, Clark JS: Safety and efficacy of continuous flush systems for arterial and pulmonary artery catheters. Ann Thorac Surg 22:534, 1977

39. Davis FM: Bacterial contamination of radial artery catheters. NZ Med J 89:128, 1979

40. Fox F, Morrow DH, Kacher EJ et al: Laboratory evaluation of pressure transducer domes containing a diaphragm. Anesth Analg 57:67, 1978

41. Hunziger A: Accuracy and dynamic response of disposable pressure transducer-tubing systems. Can J Anaesth 34:409, 1987

42. Sisko F, Hagendal M, Neufeld GR: Artifactual hypotension without damping: a hazard of disposable diaphragm domes. Anesthesiology 51:263, 1979

43. Shinozaki T, Deane RS, Mazuzan JE et al: Bacterial contamination of arterial lines: a prospective study. JAMA 249:223, 1983

44. Lowenstein E, Little JW III, Lo HH: Prevention of cerebral embolization from flushing radial-artery cannulas. N Engl J Med 285:1414, 1971

45. Gardner RM: Direct blood pressure measurement: dynamic response requirements. Anesthesiology 54:227, 1981

46. Kleinman B, Powell S, Kumar P, Gardner RM: The fast flush test measures the dynamic response for the entire pressure monitoring system. Anesthesiology 77:1215, 1992

47. Dotii S, Naito H: Intraarterial injection of 2.5 percent thiamylal does cause gangrene. Anesthesiology 59:154, 1983

48. Zweibel FR, Monies-Chas I: Accidental intraarterial injection of ketamine. Anaesthesia 31:1084, 1976

49. Bedford RF: Long-term radial artery cannulation: effects on subsequent vessel function. Crit Care Med 6:64, 1978

50. Pinella JC, Ross DF, Martin T et al: Study of the incidence of intravascular catheter infection and associated septicemia in critically ill patients. Crit Care Med 11:21, 1983

51. Gardner RM, Schwartz R, Wong HC et al: Percutaneous indwelling radial artery catheters for monitoring cardiovascular function. N Engl J Med 290:1227, 1974

52. Norwood SH, Cormier B, McMahon NG et al: Prospective study of catheter-related infection during prolonged arterial catheterization. Crit Care Med 16:836, 1988

53. Maki DG, Band JD: A comparative study of polyantibiotic and iodophore ointments in prevention of vascular catheter-related infections. Am J Med 70:739, 1981

54. Kamai GK, Pfaller MA, Rempe LE et al: Reduced intravascular catheter infection by antibiotic bonding: a prospective, randomized, controlled trial. JAMA 265:2364, 1991

55. Stamm WE, Colella JJ, Anderson RL et al: Indwelling arterial catheters as a source of nosocomial bacteremia: an outbreak caused by flavobacterium species. NM Engl J Med 292:1099, 1975

56. Maki DG, Hassemer CA: Endemic rate of fluid contamination and related septicemia in arterial pressure monitoring. Am J Med 70:733, 1981

57. Band JD, Maki DG: Infections caused by arterial catheters used for hemodynamic monitoring. Am J Med 67:735, 1979

58. Rose HD: Gas gangrene and clostridium perfringens septicemia associated with the use of an indwelling radial arterial catheter. Can Med Assoc J 121:1595, 1979

59. Michaelson ED, Walsh RE: Osler's node: a complication of prolonged arterial cannulation. N Engl J Med 283:472, 1970

60. Fanning WL, Aronson M: Osler node, Janeway lesions and splinter hemorrhages: occurrence with an infected arterial catheter. Arch Dermatol 113:648, 1977

61. Cohen A, Reyes R, Kirk M, Fulks RM: Osler's nodes, pseudoaneurysm formation and sepsis complicating percutaneous radial artery cannulation. Crit Care Med 12:1078, 1984

62. Bedford RF: Radial arterial function following percutaneous cannulation with 18 and 20 gauge catheters. Anesthesiology 47:37, 1977

63. Stern D, Gershon J, Allen F et al: Can we trust the direct radial artery pressure immediately following cardiopulmonary bypass? Anesthesiology 62:557, 1985

64. Pauca A, Hudspeth A, Wallenhaupt S et al: Radial artery to aorta pressure difference after discontinuation of cardiopulmonary bypass. Anesthesiology 70:935, 1989

65. Mohr R, Lavee J, Goor D: Inaccuracy of radial artery pressure measurements after cardiac operations. J Thorac Cardiovasc Surg 94:286, 1987

66. Ryan JF, Raines J, Dalton BC et al: Arterial dynamics of radial artery cannulation. Anesth Analg 52:1017, 1973

67. Mangar D, Thrush DN, Connell GR et al: Direct or modified Seldinger guide wire-directed technique for arterial catheter insertion. Anesth Analg 76:714, 1993

68. Schwander D, Schwander A: Arterial trauma in anesthesia and in the intensive care unit: surgical treatment. Z Gafaesskranhh 2:330, 1973

69. Bedford RF, Wollman H: Complications of percutaneous radial artery cannulation: an objective prospective study in man. Anesthesiology 38:228, 1973

70. Cronin KD, Davies MJ, Domaingue CM et al: Radial artery cannulation: the influence of method on blood flow after decannulation. Anaesth Intens Care 14:400, 1986

71. Davis FM: Methods of radial artery cannulation and subsequent arterial occlusion. [Letter]. Anesthesiology 56:331, 1982

72. Jones RM, Hill AB, Nahrwold ML et al: The effect of method of radial artery cannulation on postcannulation blood flow and thrombus formation. Anesthesiology 55:76, 1981

73. Hayes MF, Morello DC, Rosenbaum RW et al: Radial artery cannulation by cutdown technique. Crit Care Med 1:151, 1973

74. Koenigsberger MR, Moessinger AC: Iatrogenic carpal tunnel syndrome in the newborn infant. J Pediatr 91:443, 1977

75. Marshall G, Edelstein G, Hirschman CA: Median nerve compression following radial arterial puncture. Anesth Anagl 59:953, 1980

76. Ward RJ, Green HD: Arterial puncture as a safe diagnostic aid. Surgery 57:672, 1963

77. Bedford RF: Long-term radial artery cannulation: effects on subsequent vessel function. Crit Care Med 6:64, 1978

78. Palm T: Evaluation of peripheral arterial pressure in the thumb following radial artery cannulation. Br J Anaesth 49:819, 1977

79. Shenoy PNF, Leaman DM, Field JM: Safety of short-term percutaneous arterial cannulation. Anesth Analg 58:256, 1979

80. Abadir AR, Ung K-A, Chaudhry MR: Complications following radial artery cannulation with 22 gauge cannula. Abstracts of Scientific Paper, American Society of Anesthesiologists Annual Meeting, p. 523, 1978

81. Slogoff S, Keats AS, Arlund C: On the safety of radial artery cannulation. Anesthesiology 59:42, 1983

82. Barne PA, Summers J, Wirtschafter E et al: Percutaneous peripheral arterial cannulation in the neonate. Pediatrics 57:1058, 1977

83. Cederholm I, Sorensen J, Carlson C: Thrombosis following percutaneous radial artery cannulation. Acta Anaesth Scand 30:277, 1986

84. Wolf S, Mangano DT: Pseudoaneurysm, a late complication of radial-artery cannulation. Anesthesiology 52:80, 1980

85. Bedford RF: Removal of radial artery thrombi following percutaneous cannulation for monitoring. Anesthesiology 46:430, 1977

86. Wyatt R, Glaves I, Cooper DJ: Proximal skin necrosis after radial-artery cannulation. Lancet 2:1135, 1974

87. Coleman SS, Anson BJ: Arterial patterns in the hand based upon a study of 650 specimens. Surg Gynecol Obstet 113:409, 1991

88. Husum B, Palm T: Arterial dominance in the hand. Br J Anaesth 50:913, 1978

89. Kurki TS, Sanfor TJ Jr, Ty Smith N et al: Changes in distal blood flow during radial artery cannulation. Anesthesiology 65:A121, 1986

90. Campkin TV: Radial artery cannulation: potential hazard in patients with acromegaly. Anaesthesia 35:1008, 1980

91. Allen EV: Thromboangiitis obliterans: methods of diagnosis of chronic occlusive arterial lesions distal to the wrist with illustrative cases. Am J Med Sci 178:237, 1929

92. Husum B, Berthelson P: Allen's test and systolic arterial pressure in the thumb. Br J Anaesth 53:635, 1981

93. McSwain GR, Ameriks JA: Doppler-improved Allen's test. South Med J 72:1620, 1979

94. Ramanathan S, Chalon J, Turndorf H: Determining patency of palmar arches by retrograde radial pulsation. Anesthesiology 42:756, 1975

95. Brodsky JB: A simple method to determine patency of the ulnar artery intraoperatively prior to radial artery cannulation. Anesthesiology 42:626, 1975

96. Raju R: The pulse oximeter and the collateral circulation. Anaesthesia 41:784, 1986

97. Cartwright GW, Schreimer RL: Major complications secondary to percutaneous radial artery catheterization in the neonate. Pediatrics 65:139, 1980

98. Johnson FE, Summer DS, Shandness DE Jr: Extremity necrosis caused by indwelling arterial catheters. Am J Surg 131:375, 1976

99. Mangano DT, Hickey RF: Ischemic injury following uncomplicated radial artery catheterization. Anesth Analg 58:55, 1979

100. Mayer T, Matlak ME, Thompson JA: Necrosis of the

forearm following radial artery catheterization in a patient with Reye's syndrome. Pediatrics 65:141, 1980

101. Vender JS, Watts DR: Differential diagnosis of hand ischemia in the presence of an arterial cannula. Anesth Analg 61:465, 1982

102. Dalton B, Laver MB: Vasospasm with an indwelling radial artery cannula. Anesthesiology 34:194, 1971

103. Cannon BW, Meshier TW: Extremity amputation following radial artery cannulation in a patient with hyperlipoproteinemia Type V. Anesthesiology 56:220, 1983

104. Baker RJ, Chunpraph B, Nybrus LN: Severe ischemia of the hand following radial artery catheterization. Surgery 80:449, 1976

105. Wilkins RG: Radial artery cannulation and ischaemic damage: a review. Anaesthesia 40:896, 1985

106. Butt WW, Gow R, Whyte H et al: Complications resulting from use of arterial catheters: retrograde flow and rapid elevation in blood pressure. Pediatrics 76:250, 1986

107. Barnes RW, Foster EJ, Janssen GA et al: Safety of brachial arterial catheters as monitors in the intensive care unit: prospective evaluation with the Doppler ultrasonic velocity detector. Anesthesiology 44:260, 1976

108. Moran F, Lorimer AR, Boyd G: Percutaneous arterial catheterization for multiple sampling. Thorax 22:253, 1967

109. Bell JW: Treatment of post-catheterization arterial injuries: use of survey plethysmography. Ann Surg 155:591, 1962

110. Bjork L, Enghoff E, Grenvik A et al: Local circulatory changes following brachial artery catheterization. Vasc Dis 2:283, 1965

111. Comstock MK, Ellis T, Carter JG et al: Safety of brachial vs. radial arterial catheters. Anesthesiology 51:A158, 1979

112. Littler WA: Median nerve palsy: a complication of brachial artery cannulation. Postgrad Med J 52:110, 1974

113. Luce EA, Futrell JW, Wilgris EFS: Compression neuropathy following brachial arterial puncture in anticoagulated patients. J Trauma 16:717, 1976

114. Adler DC, Bryan-Brown CW: Use of the axillary artery for intravascular monitoring. Crit Care Med 1:148, 1973

115. Brown M, Gordon LH, Brown OW et al: Intravascular monitoring via the axillary artery. Anaesth Intens Care 13:38, 1984

116. De Angelis J: Axillary arterial monitoring. Crit Care Med 4:205, 1976

117. Gurman GM, Kriemerman S: Cannulation of big arteries in critically ill patients. Crit Care Med 13:217, 1985

118. Gordon LJ, Brown M, Brown OW et al: Alternative sites for continuous arterial monitoring. So Med J 77:1498, 1984

119. Brown M, Gordon LH, Brown OW et al: Intravascular monitoring via the axillary artery. Anaesth Intens Care 13:38, 1984

120. Husum B, Palm T, Eriksen J: Percutaneous cannulation of the dorsalis pedis artery. Br J Anaesth 50:913, 1979

121. Youngberg JA, Miller ED Jr: Evaluation of percutaneous cannulation of the dorsalis pedis artery. Anesthesiology 44:80, 1976

122. Ersoz CJ, Hedden M, Lain L: Prolonged femoral arterial catheterization for intensive care. Anesth Analg 49:160, 1970.

123. Soderstrom CA, Wasserman DH, Denham CM et al: Superiority of the femoral artery for monitoring: a prospective study. Am J Surg 144:309, 1982

124. Colvin MP, Curran JP, Jarvis D et al: Femoral artery pressure monitoring. Anaesthesia 32:451, 1977

125. Russell RA, Joel M, Hudson RJ et al: A prospective evaluation of radial and femoral catheterization sites in critically ill patients, abstracted. Crit Care Med 9:144, 1981

126. Puri VK, Carlson RW, Bander JJ et al: Complications of vascular catheterization in the critically ill: a prospective study. Crit Care Med 8:495, 1980

127. Kopman E, Ferguson TB: Intraoperative monitoring of femoral artery pressure during replacement of aneurysm of descending thoracic aorta. Anesth Analg 56:603, 1977

128. Cushing H: On routine determinations of arterial tension in operating room and clinic. N Engl J Med 148:250, 1903

129. Davis RF: Clinical comparison of automated auscultatory and oscillometric and catheter-transducer measurements of arterial pressure. J Clin Monit 1:114, 1985

130. Geddes LA: The direct and indirect measurement of blood pressure. Year Book Medical Publishers, Chicago, 1970

131. Hill L, Barnard H: A simple and accurate form of sphygmomanometer for arterial pressure gauge contrived for clinical use. Br Med J 2:904, 1897

132. Kirkendall WM, Burton AC et al: American Heart Association: recommendation for human blood pressure determination by sphygmomanometers. Circulation 9:80, 1967

133. Gorback MS: Considerations in the interpretation of systemic pressure monitoring. In Lumb PD, Bryan-Brown CW (eds): Complications in Critical Care Medicine. Year Book Medical Publishers, Chicago, 1988

134. Goldstein S, Killip T: Comparison of direct and indirect arterial pressures in aortic regurgitation. N Engl J Med 267:1121, 1962

135. Simpson JA, Jamieson G, Dickhaus DW, Grover RF: Effect of size of cuff bladder on accuracy of measurement of indirect blood pressure. Am Heart J 70: 206, 1965

136. Young PG, Geddes LA: The effect of cuff pressure deflation rate on accuracy in indirect measurement of blood pressure with the auscultatory method. J Clin Monit 3:155, 1987

137. Ramsey M: Non-invasive automatic determination of mean arterial pressure. Med Biol Eng Comput 17:11, 1979

138. Ramsey M: Blood pressure monitoring: automated oscillometric devices. J Clin Monit 7:56, 1991

139. Yelderman M, Ream AK: Indirect measurement of mean blood pressure in the anesthetized patient. Anesthesiology 50:253, 1979

140. Park MK, Menard SM: Accuracy of blood pressure measurement of the Dinamap monitor in infants and children. Pediatrics 141:908, 1987

141. Wareham JS, Haugh LD, Yeager SB, Horbar JD: Prediction of arterial blood pressure in the premature neonate using the oscillometric method. Am J Dis Child 141:1108, 1987

142. Debru JL, Doyon B, Morin B et al: Mesure automatique de la pression arterialle par methode oscillometrique (Dynamap 845). Arch Mal Coeur 74: 125, 1981

143. Pessenhoefer H: Single cuff comparison of two methods for indirect measurement of arterial blood pressure: standard auscultatory method versus automatic oscillometric method. Basic Res Cardiol 81:101, 1986

144. Silas JH, Barker AT, Ramsey LE: Clinical evaluation of the Dinamap 845 automated blood pressure recorder. Br Heart J 43:202, 1980

145. Cullen PM, Dye J, Huges DG: Clinical assessment of the neonatal Dinamap 847 during anesthesia in neonates and infants. J Clin Monit 3:229, 1987

146. Hutton P, Dye J, Prys-Roberts C: An assessment of the Dinamap 845. Anaesthesia 39:261, 1984

147. Johnson CJH, Kerr JH: Automatic blood pressure monitors; a clinical evaluation of five models in adults. Anaesthesia 40:471, 1985

148. Van den Broeke JJ, Karliczek GF: Labor-Und Kontrollverfahren, DINAMAP: eine neue automatische Blutdruckmessung; Ergebnisse von Vergleichsmessungen. Anesth Intensivther Notfallmed 14:533, 1979

149. Loubser PG: Comparison of intra-arterial and automated oscillometric blood pressure measurement methods in postoperative hypertensive patients. Med Instrum 20:255, 1986

150. Dellagrammaticas HD, Wilson AJ: Clinical evaluation of the Dinamap non-invasive blood pressure monitor in pre-term neonates. Clin Phys Physiol Meas 2:271, 1981

151. Milsom I, Svahn SO, Forssman L, Silverton R: An evaluation of automated indirect blood pressure measurement during pregnancy. Acta Obstet Gynecol Scand 65:721, 1986

152. Hutton P, Dye J, Prys-Roberts C: An assessment of the Dinamap 845. Anaesthesia 39:261, 1984

153. Kimble K, Darnall RA, Yelderman M et al: An automated oscillometric technique for estimating mean arterial pressure in critically ill newborns. Anesthesiology 54:423, 1981

154. Baker LK: Dinamap monitor versus direct arterial blood pressure measurements. Dimens Crit Care Nurs 5:228, 1986

155. Borow KM, Newburger JW: Noninvasive estimation of central aortic pressure during the oscillometric method: a comparative study of brachial artery pressure with simultaneous central aortic pressure measurements. Am Heart J 103:879, 1982

156. Nystrom E, Keid KH, Bennett R et al: A comparison of two automated indirect arterial blood pressure meters: with recordings from a radial arterial catheter in anesthetized surgical patients. Anesthesiology 62:526, 1985

157. Eliakim M, Sapoznikov D, Weinman J: Pulse wave velocity in healthy subjects and in patients with various disease states. Am Heart J 82:448, 1971

158. Ghanassia MD, Huynh KH, Rosenberg S, Delegue L: Blood pressure during pediatric anesthesia: four methods of preoperative indirect measurement. Anesth Analg (Paris) 37:399, 1980

159. Lowry RL, Lichti EL, Eggers GWN: The Doppler: an aid in monitoring blood pressure during anesthesia. Anesth Analg 52:531, 1973

160. Gundersen J, Ahlgren I: Evaluation of an automatic device for measurement of the indirect systolic diastolic blood pressure, Arteriosonde 1217. Acta Anesthesiol Scand 17:203, 1973

161. Poppers PJ: Controlled evaluation of ultrasonic measurement of systolic and diastolic blood pressure in pediatric patients. Anesthesiology 38:187, 1973

162. Massie HL, Ziedonis JG, Black I: Ultrasonic measurement of infant blood pressure. Med Instrum 7: 240, 1973

163. Dweck HS, Reynolds DW, Cassady G: Indirect blood pressure measurement in newborns. Am J Dis Child 127:492, 1974

164. Gordon LS, Johnson PE, Penido JRF et al: Systolic and diastolic blood pressure measurements by transcutaneous Doppler ultrasound in premature infants in critical care nurseries and at closed-heart surgery. Anesth Analg 53:914, 1974

165. George DF, Lewis PJ, Petrie A: Clinical experience with use of ultrasound sphygmomanometer. Br Heart J 37:804, 1975

166. Reitan JA: Noninvasive monitoring. p. 85. In Saidman LJ, Smith NT (eds): Monitoring in Anesthesia. John Wiley & Sons, New York, 1978

167. Stokes DN, Clutton-Brock, Patil C et al: Comparison of invasive and non-invasive measurement of continuous arterial pressure using the Finapres. Br J Anesth 67:26, 1991

168. Gorback MS, Quill TJ, Lavine ML: The relative accuracies of two automated noninvasive arterial pressure measurement devices. J Clin Monit 7:13, 1991

169. Epstein RH, Huffnagle S, Bartkowski RR: Comparative accuracies of a finger blood pressure monitor and an oscillometric blood pressure monitor. J Clin Monit 7:161, 1991

170. Pressman GL, Newgard PM: A transducer for the continuous external measurement of arterial blood pressure. IEEE Trans Biomed Electron 10:73, 1963

171. Drzewiecki GM, Melbin J, Noodergraaf A: Arterial tonometry: review and analysis. J Biomech 116:141, 1983

172. Eckerle JS: Arterial tonometry. p. 2770. In Webster JG (ed): Encyclopedia of Medical Devices and Instrumentation. John Wiley & Sons, New York, 1988

173. Kemmotsu O, Ueda M, Otsuka K et al: Evaluation of arterial tonometry for non-invasive, continuous blood pressure monitoring during anesthesia. Anesthesiology 71:A406, 1989

174. Kemmotsu O, Ueda M, Otsuka K et al: Blood pressure measurement by arterial tonometry in controlled hypotension. Anesthesiology 71:A407, 1989

175. Kemmotsu O, Yokota S, Yamamura T et al: A noninvasive blood pressure monitor based on arterial tonometry. Anesth Anal 68:S145, 1989

176. O'Flynn RP, Siler JN: The CBM-3000 tonometric blood pressure monitor. Anesthesiol Rev 29:33, 1992

177. Rushmer RF: Cardiovascular Dynamics. 3rd Ed. p. 157. WB Saunders, Philadelphia, 1976

178. Reitan JA, Barash PG: Noninvasive monitoring. p. 124. In Saidman LJ, Smith NT (eds): Monitoring in Anesthesia. 2nd Ed. Butterworth, London, 1984

Electrocardiographic Monitoring for Myocardial Ischemia

7

Jacqueline M. Leung

Since its introduction over a 100 years ago by Willem Einthoven,[1] electrocardiography (ECG) has been one of the primary noninvasive techniques used by clinicians as a marker for heart disease. The number of intraoperative monitors of heart function has proliferated over the past 30 years to include invasive systemic and pulmonary arterial pressure monitoring, noninvasive cardiac output measurement, and transesophageal echocardiography. In the perioperative setting, the ECG remains the standard cardiac monitor because it is one of the few inexpensive techniques that can be used to monitor the electrical activity of the heart continuously to evaluate coronary blood flow, anatomy, and metabolic effects. Specifically, the ECG allows perioperative detection of myocardial ischemia, arrhythmias, and hemodynamic abnormalities. This chapter reviews the role of the ECG in perioperative monitoring of myocardial ischemia, examining the following areas: the physiologic basis of ECG changes as markers of myocardial ischemia; localization of myocardial ischemia; experimental and clinical evidence validating ECG changes as markers of ischemia; characteristics of perioperative ECG ischemia; types and characteristics of ECG monitors; and future development.

PHYSIOLOGIC BASIS OF ECG CHANGES AS MARKERS OF MYOCARDIAL ISCHEMIA

Within 30 to 60 seconds after experimental ligation of a major coronary artery, ST-segment elevation was detected via unipolar epicardial ECG leads placed in the center of the cyanotic area.[2,3] The ST changes followed the regional loss of contraction and reached a maximum in 5 to 7 minutes. The electrophysiologic basis of such changes during myocardial ischemia is altered ion transport across the myocardial cell membrane. That is, increases in potassium concentration in the venous effluent were observed during ischemia and believed to indicate loss of intracellular potassium coupled by an increase in intracellular sodium ions.[4] One theory describing the potential mechanism for ST-segment changes during myocardial ischemia suggested that the injured region was depolarized at rest, becoming electronegative relative to the normal regions. Thus, the current of injury flowed during electrical diastole and disappeared with depolarization of the entire heart during electrical systole. An alternative theory suggested that changes in the ST-segment occurred because the injured area failed to depolarize during electrical systole. Although polarized at rest, this failure of the injured area to depolarize normally permitted current flows during electrical systole, resulting in an injured area that was electropositive relative to normal zones.

LOCALIZATION OF MYOCARDIAL ISCHEMIA

Electrodes and Leads

To record the electrical activity of the heart, it is essential to complete an electrical circuit between the heart and the ECG machine. Electrodes are placed at more than one site on the body. Depending on the site of placement (lead), different views of the cardiac electrical impulse can be recorded.

Three standard limb leads have been in use for 90 years (Fig. 7-1). Lead 1 connects the patient's right and left arms, lead 2 connects the right arm with the left leg, and lead 3 connects the left arm with the left leg. Each lead records the potential between the two connected limbs. All three standard limb leads are in the frontal plane of the body. Additional chest leads (precordial leads) may be applied to obtain different views of the heart (Fig. 7-2).

When one electrode is placed in the limb and the other at a precordial position, the limb lead is called the "indifferent" electrode and the precordial lead is called the "exploring" electrode. The standard limb leads are *bipolar*, since they represent the potential between two points. The precordial

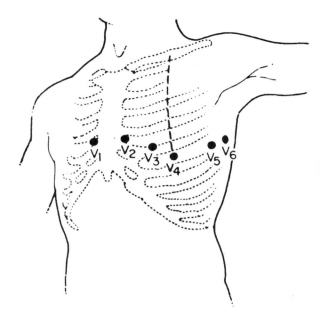

Fig. 7-2. The location of the six precordial leads is depicted. The three standard limb leads are in the frontal plane of the body; the additional "precordial" leads are applied to the chest to obtain different views of the heart. Electrode placement points when using six precordial leads: are *1*, right of the sternum in the 4th intercostal space; *2*, left of the sternum in the 4th intercostal space; *3*, midway between points 2 and 4; *4*, midclavicular line, 5th intercostal space; *5*, anterior axillary line, 5th intercostal space; *6*, midaxillary line, 5th intercostal space. (From Thys,[68] with permission.)

leads are *unipolar* because they are more influential than the limb leads which are more distally located. Unipolar limb leads are created by reversing the standard electrode positions, placing the exploring electrode on the limb and the indifferent electrode on the chest. Depending on the limb to which the exploring electrode is connected, the leads are labeled VR, VL, and VF. Because the amplitude in these leads is small, the potential is augmented by a device, as indicated by the prefix "a," giving rise to leads aVR, aVL, and aVF.

Leads to Monitor for Myocardial Ischemia in the Perioperative Setting

Localization of myocardial ischemia is influenced by multiple factors, including the following:

Coronary anatomy
Lead selection (type and number)

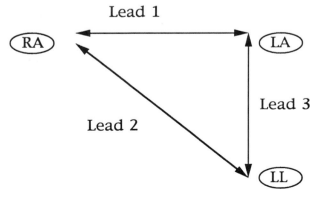

Fig. 7-1. The standard limb leads (I, II, and III) are shown schematically.

Types of monitors used
Criteria used to define ischemia
The severity of ischemia (e.g., transmural *vs* circumferential extent of ischemia)

The specific ECG manifestation of ischemia also is important in localization. That is, different ECG waveforms localize ischemia variably. ST-segment elevation localizes ischemia by its correlation with regional dysfunction.[5,6] In contrast, ST-segment depression localizes ischemia poorly, perhaps because subendocardial ischemia manifests more diffusely than transmural ischemia.

Until only recently, the optimal lead number and location for intraoperative monitoring were not well defined. Work by Blackburn and colleagues[7] in the late 1960s demonstrated that 85 percent of ST-segment depression during exercise treadmill testing occurred in leads II or V_5. Subsequently, Chaitman and colleagues[8] demonstrated that a 14-lead ECG system improved the predictive value of the treadmill test, especially in patients with multivessel disease. Fuchs and coworkers[9] then demonstrated that leads V_5 and V_6 have the highest sensitivity but also showed that 12 percent of all positive stress tests were negative in these leads.

However, the lead-localization data provided by exercise stress testing in ambulatory patients may not be applicable to the intraoperative setting. For example, during exercise stress testing, myocardial oxygen consumption is increased multiplefold, primarily due to an increase in heart rate and, therefore, cardiac output. Systemic vascular resistance generally decreases. In contrast, major hemodynamic changes during anesthesia and surgery usually are related to vascular resistance, with only moderate increases in heart rate and blood pressure. In fact, most intraoperative ischemic episodes are infrequently precipitated by changes in hemodynamics.[10]

To determine which leads best detect ischemia in the perioperative setting, London and associates[11] studied 105 patients with or at risk for coronary artery disease (CAD) undergoing noncardiac surgery. Using microprocessor-assisted continuous 12-lead ECG, they found 51 episodes of ischemia (45 manifest as ST-segment depression, and six as concurrent ST elevation in some leads and ST depression in others). Lead V_5 demonstrated the highest single-lead sensitivity (75 percent) (Fig. 7-3). Lead II alone had very low sensitivity (33 percent),

but, when combined with lead V_5 (the most widely used 2-lead system intraoperatively), increased sensitivity to 80 percent. The use of leads II, V_4 and V_5 permitted detection of 96 percent of intraoperative ischemic episodes. These data indicate that it is important to monitor several carefully chosen and precisely placed leads to enhance the ability of intraoperative ECG for detecting ischemia.

PROGNOSTIC SIGNIFICANCE OF ELECTROCARDIOGRAPHIC CHANGES AS MARKER OF MYOCARDIAL ISCHEMIA

Sensitivity and Specificity of ECG Abnormalities

The sensitivity and specificity of any ECG abnormality are dependent on the setting in which the ECG is recorded, the recording technique, sequencing of the tracings (continuous versus intermittent), and the criteria and skill with which the ECG is interpreted. In addition, the various waveforms within an ECG complex vary in their clinical significance. An example of the low specificity of an ECG waveform is that of T-wave changes. T-wave

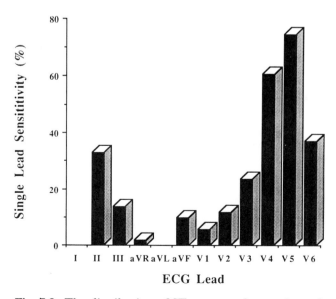

Fig. 7-3. The distribution of ST-segment changes in each of 12 leads is shown (see text for details). (Adapted from London et al.,[11] with permission.)

changes are the most common ECG abnormalities, seen in 50 percent of all abnormal tracings and 2.4 percent to 4.5 percent of all tracings.[12] A decrease of only 12 to 18 ms in the duration of the monophasic action potential in a small area of the myocardium (≤8 percent) will alter the T-wave.[13] However, abnormal T-waves may be detected in the absence of heart disease during pharmacologic and physiologic interventions and extracardial disorders. Similarly, factors other than ischemia can affect ST-segments. Ventricular hypertrophy, altered electrical activity, changes in body temperature, serum electrolytes (especially potassium), ventilatory changes, or administration of drugs such as quinidine and digitalis are known to affect the ST-segments. Additionally, electrical stimulation of the right stellate ganglion can produce ST-segment elevation and T-wave inversions, while converse changes have resulted from left sympathetic stimulation.[14]

ECG Response to Exercise in Predicting Coronary Artery Disease

Exercise stress testing using ECG is a major noninvasive method for diagnosing ischemic heart disease.[15] Numerous epidemiologic studies have reported the prognostic value of exercise ECG stress testing in predicting subsequent ischemic events such as angina pectoris, myocardial infarction, or coronary death.[16-19]

In the perioperative setting, preoperative exercise treadmill testing is valuable as a diagnostic test in patients with chest pain of unknown etiology and for quantitation and prognosis in patients with known coronary artery disease. New-onset chest pain that is ischemic in origin may markedly increase the risk of perioperative morbidity and mortality. Thus, for anesthesiologists, certain stress test results are particularly important, including a diagnosis of coronary artery disease, the magnitude, onset and duration of ST response changes, and the associated hemodynamic effects. The therapies used during exercise stress testing to reverse ischemia and dysrhythmias also may be useful for treatment of perioperative ischemia and dysrhythmias. Similarly, the heart rate and blood pressure values at which ischemic events occur during stress testing may serve as guidelines for perioperative control of these variables.

Incidence, Time Course, and Significance of ECG Changes in the Perioperative Period

Intraoperatively, myocardial ischemia occurs in 20 to 80 per cent of patients monitored using ECG, suggesting the importance of detecting ischemia perioperatively. The wide range of reported incidence of myocardial ischemia is attributable to multiple factors, such as the number and type (bipolar vs unipolar) of leads, the duration of monitoring (intermittent vs continuous), and the patient population studied.

Noncardiac Surgery and ECG Monitoring

Raby and colleagues[20] found that preoperative Holter ischemia predicted perioperative cardiac morbidity in patients undergoing vascular surgery. Subsequently they found that preoperative ischemia in this same cohort also predicted late adverse cardiac outcome.[21]

Mangano and coworkers[22] further explored the predictive value of ECG ischemia in a study of 474 men undergoing noncardiac surgery (both vascular and major nonvascular procedures) with either documented coronary artery disease or at least two risk factors for coronary artery disease. Patients were monitored using continuous 2-lead Holter ECG for up to 2 days preoperatively, intraoperatively, and up to 2 days postoperatively. The presence of postoperative myocardial ischemia was associated with a 9.2-fold increase in ischemic outcomes (cardiac death, myocardial infarction, unstable angina, congestive heart failure) by multivariate analysis. The occurrence of ischemia before or during surgery was not associated with perioperative cardiac morbidity.

Given the link between adverse outcome and postoperative ischemia following noncardiac surgery, subsets of these 474 patients were examined more closely in order to define characteristics of perioperative ischemia. The first study focused on 100 patients at risk for perioperative cardiac morbidity who were monitored with 2-lead Holter ECG during surgery and for 2 days before and after.[23] The second study focused on patients monitored with single-lead (CM5), continuous solid-state ECG for 7 days following surgery.[24] The incidence and severity of ischemia were similar during the preoperative (28 percent) and intraoperative (27 percent) periods. Relative to these, the postoperative period manifest almost twice the incidence of ischemia and a four- to five-fold greater severity (as measured by the product of ST-segment shift and duration of the ischemic episode). Again, only postoperative ischemic episodes were harbingers of adverse cardiac outcome—neither intraoperative nor preoperative ischemia were associated with perioperative cardiac morbidity. Also, the incidence of ischemia in patients with risk factors alone was similar to that in patients with documented coronary artery disease.[23] Postoperative ischemia was most severe on the third postoperative day, and 8 percent of patients experienced severe ischemic episodes as late as day 6.[24]

Cardiac Surgery and ECG Monitoring

The value of ECG monitoring for predicting adverse cardiac outcomes in at-risk patients undergoing noncardiac surgery is clear, given the well-documented high incidence of ischemia in this population. The incidence of ischemia and the value of monitoring in cardiac surgical patients who have been revascularized was less well-defined until the appearance of several recent studies.

Slogoff and Keats[25] used intermittent 2-lead ECG (II, V5) to determine whether intraoperative ischemia during coronary artery bypass graft surgery was predictive of postoperative Q-wave myocardial infarction. Of 1,023 patients, 377 had myocardial ischemia. Myocardial ischemia was surprisingly common upon arrival to the operating room (present in 18 percent of patients). More striking was the finding that new ischemia (ST depression ≥ 0.1 mV) following anesthetic induction prior to cardiopulmonary bypass significantly enhanced the probability of postoperative myocardial infarction (7.4 percent myocardial infarction compared with 2.5 percent in patients who did not have intraoperative ischemia). Slogoff and Keats subsequently confirmed these findings in a similar study of 495 patients.[26] None of these studies, however, examined the period after revascularization.

In contrast, other investigators have found postoperative rather than intraoperative ischemia to be more important. Using continuous Holter ECG monitoring to study patients undergoing myocardial revascularization, Knight and colleagues[27] found that intraoperative ischemia recapitulated the preoperative ischemic pattern, and was of

shorter duration than postoperative ischemic episodes. Similarly, we found that the highest incidence of ECG ischemia occurred in the period immediately following revascularization.[28] Adverse outcomes, however, correlated with new regional wall-motion abnormalities detected by transesophageal echocardiography, and not ECG ischemia. Using a longer period of ECG monitoring, Smith and coworkers[29] confirmed the high incidence of postrevascularization ischemia using continuous solid-state QMED ECG (Qmed, Clark, NJ). They recorded a total of 3,409 ischemic minutes over 10 perioperative days in 50 patients. The incidence of ischemia in the preoperative period was 12 percent (93 percent symptomatically silent), intraoperatively 10 percent, and 48 percent postoperatively—peaking in the first 2 hours. Postoperative ischemia occurred as late as days 3 to 7 in 24 percent of patients. All adverse outcomes occurred immediately following surgery in patients who had early postrevascularization Holter ischemia. A subsequent study by Mangano and associates[30] reconfirmed that peak incidence of ischemia occurred during the first 0 to 8 hours postbypass in patients undergoing coronary artery bypass graft surgery.

Thus, in patients undergoing myocardial revascularization, myocardial ischemia as determined by ECG is prevalent in the period immediately following revascularization. Although there is some evidence that these changes may be harbingers of subsequent adverse outcome, definitive data are lacking to show whether the elimination of these postbypass ECG changes will lead to improved surgical outcome.

CHARACTERISTICS OF PERIOPERATIVE ELECTROCARDIOGRAPHIC ISCHEMIA

Relationship of ST-Segment Changes to Hemodynamic Indices of Supply and Demand

Previous studies of ECG ischemia indicate that a substantial percentage of such episodes are preceded by changes in heart rate or blood pressure.[25,26,31,32] Using intermittent assessment of hemodynamics and ECG, Slogoff and Keats[25,26,31] concluded that approximately 50 percent of ECG ischemic episodes were temporally related to heart rate and blood pressure abnormalities. In contrast, our study found only 25 percent of ECG-ST changes to be associated with abnormalities in heart rate and blood pressure.[10] One possible explanation for the discrepancy in results may be the different degree of hemodynamic control between the two studies. Slogoff and Keats[26] defined hemodynamic abnormality as systolic blood pressure ≥180 mmHg or ≤90 mmHg and/or heart rate ≥90 beats per minute, and they found such abnormalities in 86 percent of their patients. In our study, only 25 percent of our prebypass heart rate values were >60 beats per minute, and only 6 percent of our prebypass systolic blood pressure values were >140 mmHg. Thus, heart rate and blood pressure values during the prebypass period were higher in their patients than in ours, and these marked hemodynamic fluctuations may have precipitated a higher incidence of prebypass ECG ischemia in their patients (28 to 43 percent) *vs* 7 percent in our study.[25,26,31] If intraoperative ischemic changes are not usually precipitated by hemodynamic changes except when they are substantial, this hypothesis would, in part, explain why most of our ECG ischemic episodes tended to be unrelated to hemodynamic change. Furthermore, differences in patient characteristics (such as degree of coronary occlusion), sensitivity of ECG monitors in detecting ischemia, and ECG detection techniques (continuous *vs* intermittent recording) would contribute to the difference in findings.

Etiologies of Nonhemodynamically Related Ischemia

The relatively poor correlation of most regional wall-motion abnormalities and ECG ischemic episodes with hemodynamic changes suggests that intraoperative myocardial ischemia usually is not triggered by acute increases in myocardial oxygen demand. A more important etiology may be a primary decrease in myocardial oxygen supply. This hypothesis is supported by animal[33] and clinical studies[34] which demonstrate that ischemic regional ventricular dysfunction frequently occurs despite stable systemic hemodynamic parameters and normal left ventricular function. Multiple hypotheses have been proposed to account for these hemodynamically silent ischemic changes. First, Maseri[35] has postulated that coronary flow reserve may be

reduced and variable in patients with silent myocardial ischemia. Changes in coronary resistance at the site of a fixed stenosis may produce dramatic reductions in myocardial blood flow that result in ischemia when oxygen demand is low. Proof of the dynamic nature of coronary stenoses was provided by Brown and colleagues[36] who demonstrated a 35 percent change in the luminal area of stenotic vessels during isometric exercise and nitroglycerin treatment; even more dramatic changes in transstenotic coronary resistance have been reported. Thus, coronary stenoses likely are dynamic rather than a fixed-flow limitation, suggesting that changes in stenosis size and vessel resistance may not be limited to patients with classic coronary spasm, but also typical of the majority of coronary stenoses.[37] In fact, α-receptor-mediated adrenergic coronary vasoconstriction persists even in the presence of coronary artery stenosis.[38] Some investigators suggest that, even without hemodynamic changes, localized spasm and thrombus formation concurrent with a significant coronary stenosis also may be an important cause of myocardial ischemia.[39–41]

An additional explanation for the poor correlation between regional wall-motion abnormalities and hemodynamic changes is that measurements of gross indices of myocardial oxygen supply and demand such as heart rate and blood pressure may be insensitive indicators of more subtle imbalances between supply and demand. This hypothesis is supported by studies in patients undergoing percutaneous transluminal coronary angioplasty.[41] During balloon occlusion, peak negative and peak positive dP/dt occurred during the first few seconds, followed by abnormalities of systolic fractional shortening and increases in left ventricular end-diastolic pressure, but heart rate and blood pressure were unchanged. Left ventricular pressure is therefore an earlier indicator of ischemic dysfunction than heart rate or blood pressure measurements. A study by Smith and coworkers[42] suggests that increases in wall stress derived from transesophageal echocardiographic measurements are more frequently associated with regional wall-motion abnormalities than are hemodynamic changes. Patients undergoing carotid endarterectomy who received higher anesthetic concentrations supplemented with phenylephrine demonstrated higher wall stress and a threefold greater incidence of regional wall-motion and wall-thickening abnormalities than those given lower anesthetic concentrations to maintain similar systolic blood pressures and stump pressures. Therefore, reliance on hemodynamic monitoring alone in predicting myocardial ischemia probably is inadequate, especially in high-risk patients.

Comparison of ECG Monitoring with Other Modalities in the Detection of Myocardial Ischemia

Regional wall-motion and wall-thickening abnormalities are thought to be more sensitive and earlier indices of myocardial ischemia than ECG changes in both animals and humans. In 1935, Tennant and Wiggers[43] demonstrated that, with coronary artery ligation, regional contractile failure occurred almost immediately.[43] The earliest changes appear to be biochemical: oxygen deprivation causing insufficient ATP production (anaerobic glycolysis), a decrease in ATP turnover, cellular acidosis and entrapment of calcium. Mechanical dysfunction results, manifest by the inability of the myocardial wall to thicken, followed by wall-motion abnormalities progressing from hypokinesis to akinesis to dyskinesis. Endocardial ECG-ST-segment changes occur, and are followed by surface ECG changes. In previously compromised hearts, or in those which develop global ischemia, diastolic compliance then decreases, filling pressure increases, and systolic dysfunction occurs. Although a number of sensitive techniques are available for detection of ischemia, including magnetic resonance imaging, radiolabeled lactate determinations, or direct measurement of end-diastolic pressure, they are impractical. The most sensitive detector of intraoperative ischemia to date appears to be transesophageal echocardiography. In patients undergoing coronary angioplasty, wall-motion abnormalities are more sensitive and earlier indices of myocardial ischemia than surface ECG changes.[5] In humans undergoing either cardiac or noncardiac surgery, transesophageal echocardiographic wall-motion and thickening abnormalities, consistent with ischemia, are two- to fourfold more common than ECG changes,[28,44,45] even when continuous 12-lead ECG is used.[45]

In a study of 285 patients monitored by simultaneous transesophageal echocardiography, 12-lead ECG and 2-lead Holter ECG, the concordance among the different monitoring techniques was compared.[46] Overall, concordance between transesophageal echocardiography and 2-lead Holter ECG was 78 percent and that between 12-lead and 2-lead ECG was 85 percent. Various explanations may account for the lack of concordance among different monitoring techniques. First, echocardiographic monitoring of the ventricle at one plane (short-axis) may fail to detect ischemic changes occurring at another part of the ventricle such as the left ventricular apex. It is conceivable that the concordance between *multiplane* transesophageal echocardiography and ECG may be higher. Second, there is evidence that ECG is relatively poor in its ability to detect ischemic changes occurring in the posterior and lateral quadrants of the left ventricle.[8,47] If, as reported, a majority of echocardiographic ischemic changes occur in these areas,[28] then discordance between ECG and echocardiographic monitoring is likely.

Since ECG and echocardiography are fundamentally different, whether the true incidence of intraoperative myocardial ischemia is the sum total of ischemia recorded by different modalities remains to be further defined.

TYPES AND CHARACTERISTICS OF ELECTROCARDIOGRAPHIC MONITORS

Operating Room ECG Monitors

The ECG monitor in the operating room should be properly calibrated so that any ECG abnormality is not magnified or diminished. Additionally, the monitor should be placed in the "diagnostic" rather than "monitoring" mode. The monitoring mode filters the ECG signal to eliminate high-frequency noise such as 60-cycle interference from power cords and lights, and to diminish baseline shift that may result from changes in electrode contact and respiration. An *apparent* ST-segment depression may occur which is actually due to a change in baseline from excessive low-frequency filtering.

Continuous Holter ECG Monitor

Transient ST-segment changes have been noted since the introduction of continuous Holter ECG monitoring of ambulatory patients. Since the initial report demonstrating that patients with angina pectoris and coronary artery disease have frequent, asymptomatic episodes of ST-segment depression, we now know that these patients can have silent or painful episodes of myocardial ischemia while some have both silent and symptomatic episodes. On average, the silent ischemic episodes occur three to four times more commonly than the painful ones, as demonstrated by the frequency of ST-segment changes recorded during ambulatory ECG monitoring. That these silent ST-segment changes represent myocardial ischemia is indicated by studies performed with hemodynamic monitoring (demonstrating elevation of left ventricular filling pressure), two-dimensional echocardiography and radionuclide and contrast angiography (demonstrating left ventricular regional dysfunction), and myocardial perfusion imaging with thallium or positron emission tomography (demonstrating perfusion defects occurring with the onset of ST-segment changes).[48–51]

The prognostic significance of silent ST-segment changes detected by ambulatory Holter ECG monitoring is demonstrated by the increased rate of complications over a 1-month and subsequent 2-year period in patients with unstable angina who, despite treatment, continued to have episodes of silent myocardial ischemia after discharge from a coronary care unit.[52,53]

Ambulatory Holter ECG monitoring was first used perioperatively by Knight and coworkers[27] in patients undergoing myocardial revascularization. Typically, two to three bipolar leads are used. The electrical signal being captured is converted to an analog signal which is then recorded onto cassette tape. Each complete ECG recording on Holter tape is then scanned visually using sophisticated computer programs for ST-segment analysis which recognize and quantitate the ST-segment changes automatically. Prior to performing the ST-segment analysis, all abnormal QRS complexes (e.g., ventric-

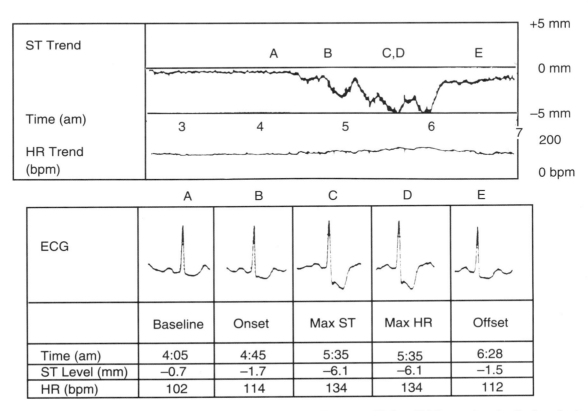

Fig. 7-4. The intraoperative ST-segment trend recorded from a Holter ECG monitor is displayed. *A*, baseline; *B*, onset of an ischemic ST-segment depression; *C*, maximum ST-segment depression; *D*, ST-segment depression when maximum heart rate occurs, and *E*, resolution of ischemic episode.

ular ectopic beats and conduction abnormalities) must be excluded. Figure 7-4 provides an example of the ST trend recorded during the intraoperative period. Typically, the ST-segment is measured at J + 60 ms. The time after the J point can be adjusted by the operator to exclude T-wave abnormalities during tachycardia. However, these computer-generated analyses tend to generate false-positive readings. Most research groups, therefore, still rely on visual validation of hard copies of ischemic episodes after performing the semi-automated ST-segment analysis.

Real-Time ECG Monitor

Another way to store ECG information is in digital form with real-time analysis. These are microprocessor-based devices which are not subject to the technical and time constraints of cassette tape analysis, as are Holter ECG data. A solid-state ECG recorder has been shown to have high sensitivity and specificity (100 percent and 92 percent, respectively) during exercise for detection and quantitation of episodes of ischemic ST-segment depression.[54] In addition, the device can be programmed to produce a tone at the onset of ischemic ST-segment depression to alert the clinician to the onset of a potential ischemic event.

Although the solid-state ECG monitor has automated ST-segment analysis and is capable of collecting large amounts of ST-trend data continuously over a long period of time, there are limitations. Selection of an ischemic event threshold is one important limitation. The risk of false-positive results exists if the ST baseline drifts downward during the monitoring period, the cause of such drift possibly due to slowly changing physiologic variables (electrolyte levels, changes in ECG conduction, body temperature, or response to drug therapy) and not to ischemia. The risk of false-negative results exists if the patient is ischemic at the time of initial testing. The ischemic threshold would then be too low, and subsequent ischemic episodes might go undetected. Since the monitor's ischemic event threshold can be set only in 1.0 mm increments (Fig. 7-5), a conservative way to remedy the situation is to increase specificity at the expense of sensitivity, and set the threshold at 1.0–1.9 mm below the most depressed ST-segment observed during preoperative positional testing.[29]

The other limitations of a solid-state ECG monitor include the lack of full disclosure, that is, only limited samples of baseline ECG hard copy can be retrieved from the monitor. Although the ST-segment analysis algorithm has been validated in several studies,[55–57] it may incorrectly identify primary T-wave changes as ST-segment changes if they cause depression of the latter part of the ST-segment. This can occur if conduction abnormalities, T-wave inversion, or tachycardia are present, because the ECG monitor analyzes the ST-segment at a fixed point.

Monitors with Automatic ST-Segment Analysis

Because most ischemic episodes go undetected in the perioperative setting, high-resolution, multilead, continuous ST-segment monitoring devices have been introduced to most operating room and critical care bedside monitors in an attempt to in-

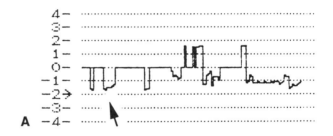

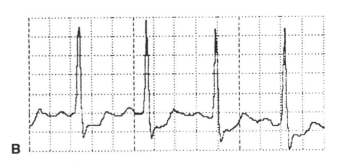

Fig. 7-5. The intraoperative ST-segment trend recorded from a real-time ECG monitor is displayed. **(A)** Note that the ST-segment is measured in 1.0-mm increments. The *arrow* indicates one of the numerous ischemic ST-segment changes recorded from this patient. **(B)** The hardcopy ECG, which provides further validation of the ischemic changes.

crease the ability to detect ischemic episodes. Using signal processing, these monitors create a "mean beat" from, for example, a 10-second analog acquisition that is digitalized during a subsequent 10 to 20 seconds. An internal microprocessor is preprogrammed to superimpose each new ECG recording on the patient's baseline ECG, thus analyzing ST-segment deviation in reference to baseline every 30 seconds in real time during the monitoring period (Fig. 7-6). Krucoff and colleagues[58] monitored 338 patients for 8,331 hours with real-time multilead ST-segment analysis after percutaneous transluminal coronary angioplasty. They found that standard coronary care unit monitoring of patient symptoms and rhythms underestimates transient ischemic activity in 87 percent of patients who experience ischemia after interventions. Although definitive data validating the usefulness of these ST-trending monitors are lacking, they may be useful to act as an alarm to alert the physician to examine the ECG more closely.[59]

When Should Surgical Patients be Extensively Monitored After Surgery?

While there is no disagreement that all patients who are at risk for developing myocardial ischemia should be monitored intraoperatively with ECG, until recently, it was not clear which types of patients should be monitored after surgery. Although there are data demonstrating that myocardial is-

chemia occurring after noncardiac surgery is more prevalent and associated with an increased risk of adverse cardiac events, monitoring all at-risk patients postoperatively is unfeasible and expensive. In a report by Hollenberg and colleagues,[60] five major preoperative predictors of postoperative myocardial ischemia were identified: (1) left ventricular hypertrophy by ECG; (2) history of hypertension; (3) diabetes mellitus; (4) coronary artery disease; and (5) use of digoxin. More interestingly, the risk of postoperative myocardial ischemia increased progressively with the number of predictors present: 22 percent of patients with no predictors, 31 per cent of patients with one predictor, 46 per cent with two predictors, 70 percent with three predictors, and 77 percent with four predictors. Thus, a detailed preoperative assessment may enable the identification of at-risk patients who should be monitored for myocardial ischemia in the postoperative period.

FUTURE DEVELOPMENT

In part, improving outcome relies on improving clinical real-time detection of ischemia during and after surgery so that appropriate clinical intervention can be initiated. It is discouraging that most perioperative ischemic episodes (50–100 percent) identified by ECG criteria appear to be unnoticed

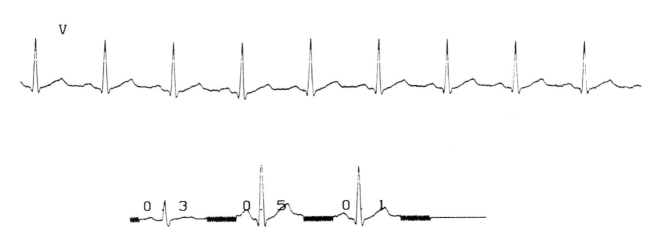

Fig. 7-6. An example of automated ST-segment analysis is shown. Leads I, II, and V are being analyzed for ST-segment changes. The numerical values represent the ST-segment change for each lead, respectively. Lead V5 is being displayed in real-time.

in real time by clinicians.[28,29,61,62] To rectify this requires improving the acuity of detection of both anesthesiologists in the operating room and nurses in the postanesthesia care unit. Thus, maximizing the use of current ECG equipment might increase real-time ischemia detection by multiplefold, based on the percentages of episodes unnoticed by clinicians as reported in the literature, for example, 80 percent,[61] 87 per-cent,[29] and 100 percent.[28] The addition of threshold alarms to automated ST-trend analysis also might improve real-time detection of ischemia.[55,57,59,63–65]

Studies of existing ECG systems designed to determine limitations[66] which might thereby improve current systems, or the development of more invasive lead systems (e.g., esophageal, cardiac, tracheal) to optimize ischemia detection, also might increase real-time detection. Given the relationship of postoperative ischemia to poor long-term outcome in noncardiac surgical patients,[67] more effort and resources need to be directed at the early recovery period. Monitoring all patients at risk is likely to remain prohibitively expensive but it may be possible to select subsets of at-risk patients who can most benefit from more intensive monitoring than currently practiced.[60]

CONCLUSION

Despite the differences among studies, ECG ischemia has been linked to adverse cardiac outcomes following both cardiac and noncardiac surgery. Following noncardiac surgery, patients with two or more risk factors for CAD are equally likely to have perioperative ischemia and adverse cardiac outcomes as those with definite CAD. In cardiac surgical patients with adequate preoperative anti-ischemia management and rigorously controlled intraoperative hemodynamics, the incidence of intraoperative myocardial ischemia is no worse than that occurring preoperatively. Postoperatively, despite apparent myocardial revascularization, myocardial ischemia is prevalent and appears to be related to adverse cardiac outcome.

With the aging of the population, the prevalence of cardiac disease will continue to increase in our surgical population. Perioperative cardiac morbidity will therefore continue to be an important health care problem. Because perioperative myocardial ischemia may have an impact on postoperative outcome, early detection and treatment of ischemia is important. As a result of recognition of this problem, there is a proliferation of intraoperative cardiac monitoring devices. The selection of the appropriate monitors requires a thorough understanding of the advantages and limitations of each. Ultimately, the appropriate choice and use of intraoperative monitoring modalities should lead to better patient care and contribute to a decrease in perioperative cardiac morbidity.

ACKNOWLEDGMENT

I am grateful to Winifred Von Ehrenburg for her excellent editorial assistance. Supported in part by an Anesthesiology Young Investigator Award from F.A.E.R. and the Burroughs Wellcome Fund.

REFERENCES

1. Einthoven W: Un nouveau galvanometre. Arch N Sc Ex Nat 6:625, 1901
2. Rakita L, Borduas J, Rothman S, Prinzmetal M: Studies on the mechanism of ventricular activity. XII. Early changes in the RS-T segment and QRS complex following acute coronary artery occlusion in experimental study and clinical applications. Am Heart J 48:351, 1961
3. Ekmekci A, Toyoshima H, Kwoczynski J et al: Angina pectoris. IV. Clinical and experimental difference between ischemia with S-T elevation and ischemia with S-T depression. Am J Cardiol 7:412, 1961
4. Prinzmetal M, Toyoshima H, Ekmekci A et al: Myocardial ischemia: nature of ischemic electrocardiographic patterns in mammalian ventricles as determined by intracellular electrocardiographic and metabolic changes. Am J Cardiol 8:493, 1961
5. Wohlgelernter D, Cleman M, Highman H et al: Regional myocardial dysfunction during coronary angioplasty: evaluation by two-dimensional echocardiography and 12 lead electrocardiography. J Am Coll Cardiol 7:1245, 1986
6. Alam M, Khaja F, Brymer J et al: Echocardiographic evaluation of left ventricular function during coronary artery angioplasty. Am J Cardiol 57:20, 1986
7. Blackburn H, Taylor H, Okamata N: Standardization of the exercise electrocardiogram: a systemic comparison of cheat lead configurations employed for monitoring during exercise. In Maroven M, Barry AJ (eds): Physical Activity and the Heart. p. 101. Charles C Thomas, Springfield, IL, 1967

8. Chaitman B, Bourassa M, Wagniart P et al: Improved efficiency of treadmill exercise testing using a multiple lead ECG system and basic hemodynamic exercise response. Circulation 57:71, 1978

9. Fuchs R, Achuff S, Grunwald L et al: Electrocardiographic localization of coronary artery narrowings: studies during myocardial ischemia and infarction in patients with one-vessel disease. Circulation 66:1168, 1982

10. Leung J, O'Kelly B, Mangano D, SPI Research Group: Relationship of regional wall motion abnormalities to hemodynamic indices of myocardial oxygen supply and demand in patients undergoing CABG surgery. Anesthesiology 73:802, 1990

11. London M, Hollenberg M, Wong M et al: Intraoperative myocardial ischemia: localization by continuous 12-lead electrocardiography. Anesthesiology 69:232, 1988

12. Friedberg C, Zager A: "Nonspecific" ST and T wave changes. Circulation 23:655, 1961

13. Autenrieth G, Surawicz B, Kuo C, Arita M: Primary T wave abnormalities caused by uniform and regional shortening of ventricular monophasic action potential in dog. Circulation 51:668, 1975

14. Ueda H, Yanai Y, Marao S et al: Electrocardiographic and vector-cardiographic changes produced by electrical stimulation of the cardiac nerves. Japan Heart J 5:359, 1964

15. Redwood D, Epstein S: Uses and limitations of stress testing in the evaluation of ischemic heart disease. Circulation 46:1115, 1972

16. Froelicher V, Yanowitz F, Thompson A: The correlation of coronary angiography and the electrocardiographic response to maximal treadmill testing in 76 asymptomatic men. Circulation 48:597, 1973

17. Robb G, Marks H: Postexercise electrocardiograms in arteriosclerotic heart disease: its value in diagnosis and prognosis. JAMA 200:918, 1967

18. Doyle J, Kinch S: The progress of an abnormal electrocardiographic stress test. Circulation 41:5454, 1970

19. Bellet S, Roman L, Nichols G: Detection of coronary-prone subjects in a normal population by radioelectrocardiographic exercise test: follow-up studies. Am J Cardiol 19:783, 1967

20. Raby K, Goldman L, MA C et al: Correlation between preoperative ischemia and major cardiac events after peripheral vascular surgery. N Engl J Med 321:1296, 1989

21. Raby K, Goldman L, Cook E et al: Long-term prognosis of myocardial ischemia detected by Holter monitoring in peripheral vascular disease. Am J Cardiol 66:1309, 1990

22. Mangano D, Browner W, Hollenberg M et al: Association of perioperative myocardial ischemia with cardiac morbidity and mortality in men undergoing noncardiac surgery. N Engl J Med 323:1781, 1990

23. Mangano D, Hollenberg M, Fegert G et al: Perioperative myocardial ischemia in patients undergoing noncardiac surgery. I. Incidence and severity during the four-day perioperative period. J Am Coll Cardiol 17:843, 1991

24. Mangano D, Wong M, London M et al: Perioperative myocardial ischemia in patients undergoing noncardiac surgery. II. Incidence and severity during the first week following surgery. J Am Coll Cardiol 17:851, 1991

25. Slogoff S, Keats A: Does perioperative myocardial ischemia lead to postoperative myocardial infarction? Anesthesiology 62:107, 1985

26. Slogoff S, Keats A: Further observations on perioperative myocardial ischemia. Anesthesiology 65:539, 1986

27. Knight A, Hollenberg M, London M et al: Perioperative myocardial ischemia: importance of the preoperative ischemic pattern. Anesthesiology 68:681, 1988

28. Leung J, O'Kelly B, Browner W et al: Prognostic importance of postbypass regional wall-motion abnormalities in patients undergoing coronary artery bypass graft surgery. Anesthesiology 71:16, 1989

29. Smith R, Leung J, Mangano D, SPI Research Group: Postoperative myocardial ischemia in patients undergoing coronary artery bypass graft surgery. Anesthesiology 74:464, 1991

30. Mangano D, Siliciano D, Hollenberg M et al: Postoperative myocardial ischemia. Therapeutic trials using intensive analgesia in the intensive care unit. Anesthesiology 76:342, 1992

31. Slogoff S, Keats A: Does chronic treatment with calcium entry blocking drugs reduce perioperative myocardial ischemia? Anesthesiology 68:676, 1988

32. Montejo L, Coriat P, Godet G et al: Hemodynamic predictors of myocardial ischemia in patients undergoing vascular surgery: at last we can measure them! Abstracted. Anesthesiology 69:A279, 1988

33. Lowenstein E, Foëx P, Francis C et al: Regional ischemic ventricular dysfunction in myocardium supplied by a narrowed coronary artery with increasing halothane concentration in the dog. Anesthesiology 55:349, 1981

34. Distante A, Picano E, Moscarelli E et al: Echocardiographic vs. hemodynamic monitoring during attacks of variant angina pectors. Am J Cardiol 55:1319, 1985

35. Maseri A: Role of coronary artery spasm in symptomatic and silent myocardial ischemia. J Am Coll Cardiol 9:249, 1987

36. Brown B, Lee A, Bolson E, Dodge H: Reflex constriction of significant coronary stenosis as a mech-

anism contributing to ischemic left ventricular dysfunction during isometric exercise. Circulation 70: 18, 1984

37. Brown B, Bolson E, Dodge H: Dynamic mechanisms in human coronary stenosis. Circulation 70:917, 1984

38. Feigl E, Buffington C, Nathan H: Adrenergic coronary vasoconstriction during myocardial underperfusion. Circulation 75 suppl I:I-1, 1987

39. Willerson J, Campbell W, Winniford M et al: Conversion from chronic to acute coronary artery disease: speculation regarding mechanisms. [Editorial]. Am J Cardiol 54:1349, 1984

40. Willerson J, Hillis L, Winniford M, Buja L: Speculation regarding mechanisms responsible for acute ischemia heart disease syndromes. [Editorial]. J Am Coll Cardiol 8:245, 1986

41. Sigwart U, Grbic M, Payot M et al: Ischemic events during coronary artery balloon obstruction. p. 29. In Rutishauser W RH (ed): Silent Myocardial Ischemia. Springer-Verlag, Berlin, 1984

42. Smith J, Roizen M, Cahalan M et al: Does anesthetic technique make a difference? Augmentation of systolic blood pressure during carotid endarterectomy: effects of phenylephrine versus light anesthesia and of isoflurane versus halothane on the incidence of myocardial ischemia. Anesthesiology 69:846, 1988

43. Tennant R, Wiggers C: The effect of coronary occlusion on myocardial contraction. Am J Physiol 112: 351, 1935

44. Smith J, Cahalan M, Benefiel D et al: Intraoperative detection of myocardial ischemia in high-risk patients: electrocardiography versus two-dimensional transesophageal echocardiography. Circulation 72: 1015, 1985

45. London M, Tubau J, Wong M et al: The "natural history" of segmental wall motion abnormalities in patients undergoing noncardiac surgery. Anesthesiology 73:644, 1990

46. Eisenberg M, London M, Leung J et al: Monitoring for myocardial ischemia during noncardiac surgery: a technology assessment of transesophageal echocardiography and 12-lead electrocardiography. JAMA 268:210, 1992

47. Berry C, Zalewski A, Koyach R et al: Surface electrocardiogram in the detection of transmural myocardial ischemia during coronary artery occlusion. Am J Cardiol 63:21, 1989

48. Chierchia S, Lazzari M, Freedman B et al: Impairment of myocardial perfusion and function during painless myocardial ischemia. J Am Coll Cardiol 1:924, 1983

49. Deanfield J, Shea M, Ribeiro P et al: Transient ST-segment depression as a marker of myocardial ischemia during daily life. Am J Cardiol 54:1195, 1984

50. Levy R, Shapiro L, Wright C et al: The hemodynamic significance of asymptomatic ST segment depression assessed by ambulatory pulmonary artery pressure monitoring. Br Heart J 56:526, 1986

51. Cohn P: Silent myocardial ischemia and infarction. Marcel Dekker, New York, 1989

52. Gottlieb S, Weisfeldt M, Ouyang P et al: Silent ischemia as a marker for early unfavorable outcomes in patients with unstable angina. N Engl J Med 314: 1214, 1986

53. Gottlieb S, Weisfeldt M, Ouyang P et al: Silent ischemia predicts infarction and death during 2 year follow-up of unstable angina. J Am Coll Cardiol 10:756, 1987

54. Barry J, Campbell S, Nabel E et al: Ambulatory monitoring of the digitized electrocardiogram for detection and early warning of transient myocardial ischemia in angina pectoris. Am J Cardiol 60:483, 1987

55. Levin R: Potential for real-time processing of continuously monitored electrocardiogram in the detection, quantitation, and intervention of silent myocardial ischemia. Cardiol Clin 4:00, 1986

56. Levin R: Quantitation of transient myocardial ischemia by digital, ambulatory electrocardiography. Am J Cardiol 61:13B, 1988

57. Jamal S, Mitra-Duncan L, Kelly D, Freedman S: Validation of a real-time electrocardiographic monitor for detection of myocardial ischemia secondary to coronary artery disease. Am J Cardiol 60:525, 1987

58. Krucoff M, Jackson Y, Kehoe M, Kent K: Quantitative and qualitative ST segment monitoring during and after percutaneous transluminal coronary angioplasty. Circulation 81 suppl IV:20, 1990

59. Ellis J, Shah M, Briller J et al: A comparison of methods for the detection of myocardial ischemia during noncardiac surgery: automated ST-segment analysis systems, electrocardiography, and transesophageal echocardiography. Anesth Analg 75:764, 1992

60. Hollenberg M, Mangano D, Browner W et al: Predictors of postoperative myocardial ischemia in patients undergoing noncardiac surgery. JAMA 268: 205, 1992

61. London M, Tubau J, Wong M et al: The "natural history" of segmental wall motion abnormalities detected by intraoperative transesophageal echocardiography: a clinically blinded prospective approach, abstracted. Anesthesiology 69:A7, 1988

62. Coriat P, Daloz M, Bousseau D et al: Prevention of intraoperative myocardial ischemia during noncardiac surgery with intravenous nitroglycerin. Anesthesiology 63:193, 1984

63. Dodds T, Delphin E, Stone J et al: Detection of perioperative myocardial ischemia using Holter monitoring with real-time ST-segment analysis. Anesth Analg 63:343, 1988

64. Kotrly K, Kotter G, Mortara D, JP K: Intraoperative detection of myocardial ischemia with an ST segment trend monitoring system. Anesth Analg 63:343, 1984

65. Probst S, Wiederspahn T, Dudziak R: Automated, continuous ST segment analysis in the ECG as a monitor of myocardial ischemia during aortocoronary bypass surgery. Anaesthetist 40:380, 1991

66. Slogoff S, Keats A, David Y, Igo S: Incidence of perioperative myocardial ischemia detected by different electrocardiographic systems. Anesthesiology 73: 1074, 1990

67. Mangano D, Browner W, Hollenberg M et al: Long-term cardiac prognosis following noncardiac surgery. JAMA 268:233, 1992

68. Thys DM: The normal ECG. In Thys DM, Kaplan JA: The ECG in Anesthesia and Critical Care. Churchill Livingstone, New York, 1987

Electrocardiographic Monitoring for Arrhythmias

8

Daniel J. Kennedy
Roger L. Royster

Electrocardiographic (ECG) monitoring of patients in the operating room and intensive care setting has become standard practice. Cardiac arrhythmias occur frequently in patients undergoing surgery and in patients with serious illness in the intensive care unit. The many arrhythmogenic influences in this setting and the high prevalence of cardiac disease in these patients puts them at substantial risk for developing an arrhythmia. Arrhythmias may be innocuous or may have profound hemodynamic consequences. Therefore, a thorough understanding of the incidence, genesis, and diagnosis of specific arrhythmias is of critical importance for individuals caring for patients in the operating room or intensive care unit.

INCIDENCE OF ARRHYTHMIAS

The true incidence of arrhythmias is difficult to know. Studies often assign arbitrary classifications, evaluate certain arrhythmias while excluding others, or do not use continuous beat by beat monitoring. Other studies have looked only at patients undergoing cardiac surgery, patients with cardiac disease undergoing noncardiac surgery, and patients with respiratory failure.

The first large series of the use of ECG monitoring in operative patients undergoing surgery was reported by Kurtz[1] in 1936. This study revealed a high incidence of sinus arrhythmias, premature ventricular contractions (PVCs) and junctional rhythms. In 1968, Vanik and Davis[2] reported a 34 percent incidence of intraoperative arrhythmias in patients with cardiac disease undergoing halothane anesthesia, and interestingly found arrhythmias in 16 percent of otherwise healthy patients. Kuner and colleagues[3] reported a 62 percent incidence of arrhythmias in relatively healthy patients, with sinus tachycardia being most common, while junctional rhythms were seen in 20 percent and PVCs in 15 percent of patients.

Certain subgroups have repeatedly been found to be at increased risk for the development of arrhythmias during surgery (Table 8-1). Bertrand and colleagues[4] reported a 60 percent incidence of ventricular arrhythmias in patients with known cardiac disease, compared with an incidence of 37 percent in patients without known heart disease. In this same study, 92 percent of patients with cardiac disease developed either a supraventricular or ventricular arrhythmia during surgery and anesthesia. Arrhythmias were most common at times of endotracheal intubation and extubation. In a study of patients undergoing cardiac surgery, Angelini and coworkers[5] reported 58 percent of patients undergoing valve surgery and 45 percent of patients undergoing coronary artery bypass surgery developed significant postoperative arrhythmias.[5] More importantly, the arrhythmias tended to correlate with

TABLE 8-1. Incidence of Arrhythmias During Anesthesia and Surgery

Study	Year	Number	Arrhythmia (%)	Monitoring	Monitoring Incidence Related to
Vanik and Davis[2]	1968	5013	17.9	Intermittent	Age Intubation Heart disease
Kuner et al.[3]	1967	154	61.7	Holter	Neurologic, head and neck, thoracic surgery Intubation Surgery >3 hours
Bertrand et al.[4]	1971	100	84.0	Holter	Intubation Extubation Heart disease
Angelini et al.[5]	1974	128	50.0	Holter	Severity of heart disease

(Modified from Royster,[68] with permission.)

the severity of the heart disease, led to a prolonged hospital stay, and were responsible for up to 80 percent of the surgical mortality in the series.

Arrhythmias are relatively common in otherwise healthy people as well. Fifty male medical students without heart disease were followed with 24-hour continuous ECG monitoring. Sinus arrhythmia occurred in 50 percent, sinus pauses in 28 percent, atrial extrasystoles in 56 percent, and ventricular premature beats in 50 percent of students.[6] In a more recent study, arrhythmias were seen in more than 60 percent of patients undergoing anesthesia and surgery when continuous methods of monitoring were used.[7]

Therefore, during ECG monitoring, the physician must be aware of the incidence of arrhythmia in healthy individuals as well as those with cardiac disease. The individual must be familiar with situations when arrhythmias are most common. And most importantly, the physician must realize that a change in cardiac rate or rhythm may be a warning signal that something extracardiac is abnormal, such as hypoxemia or hypercarbia.

ELECTROPHYSIOLOGY

Normal Action Potentials

An electrical potential difference exists across the cell membrane in excitable tissue and is maintained by the active pumping of sodium out of, and potassium into, the cell, against their concentration gradients (Table 8-2). As a result, the resting cellular transmembrane potential is maintained at −60 to −90 mV. The time course of the cell membrane potential actively changing during depolarization and repolarization is called the action potential[8] (Fig. 8-1). As the cardiac cell membrane slowly depolarizes to its threshold potential (−45 to −65 mV), a conformational change in membrane sodium channels allows for a rapid, massive increase in sodium permeability. Phase 0 of the action potential begins as sodium rushes into the cell and the transmembrane potential quickly becomes less negative. Phase 1 (early repolarization) begins as the sodium channels quickly inactivate, and increased potassium permeability allows for an outward flow of potassium. An inward chloride flux may also occur during phase 1. Slower calcium currents entering the cell inhibit repolarization and are responsible for the sustained depolarization known as phase 2 (plateau phase) of

TABLE 8-2. Major Ion Movement During Phases of the Cardiac Action Potential

Phase	Ion	Movement Across Cell Membrane
0	Na^+	In
1	K^+	Out
	Cl^-	In
2	Ca^{2+}	In
	K^+	Out
3	K^+	Out
4	Na^+	In

(From Stoelting,[69] with permission.)

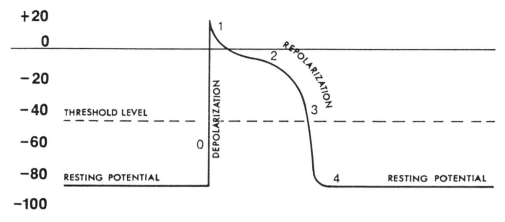

Fig. 8-1. Cardiac action potential from a nonpacemaking cell. The resting potential, threshold potential, and phases of depolarization and repolarization are illustrated. (Adapted from Mangiola and Ritota,[70] with permission.)

the action potential. During phase 3 (rapid repolarization) the inward calcium current diminishes, while potassium continues to flow rapidly out of the cell, thus restoring the electrical gradient across the cell membrane (Table 8-2). Phase 4 of the action potential represents resting membrane potential in nonpacemaking cells. In cells with pacemaker potential, phase 4 represents slow diastolic depolarization due to an inward movement of sodium and possibly calcium, allowing resting membrane potential to slowly approach threshold potential.

This ability to spontaneously generate action potentials is known as automaticity.[8] The rate of depolarization of a pacemaker cell is dependent on the slope of phase 4 depolarization, the resting membrane potential, and the threshold potential (Fig. 8-2). Normally, cells in the sinoatrial (SA) node have the steepest slope of phase 4 depolarization, the least negative resting membrane potential (-60 mV) and threshold potential (-40 mV). They are capable of the most rapid rate of depolarization, allowing them to act as the predominant pacemaker cells controlling the heart rate. Other potential pacemaker cells, including cells near the atrioventricular (AV) node, Purkinje cells, and certain ventricular myocytes, exhibit slower rates of spontaneous phase 4 depolarization. These cells can function as secondary pacemakers if the rate of depolarization from the SA node decreases or their own rate of depolarization increases. Sympathetic stimulation increases the rate of phase 4 depolarization. Vagal stimulation slows the rate of pacemaker

depolarization by making the resting membrane potential more negative (hyperpolarizing the cell) and slowing the rate of phase 4 depolarization.

The sodium channels which are activated during the upstroke are rapidly inactivated and remain so until the membrane potential has been restored to threshold potential (-60 mV). During this time, known as the absolute refractory period, the membrane is completely unexcitable.[8] The sodium channels are gradually reactivated by the increasingly negative membrane potential. As the action potential voltage falls below threshold potential, an action potential can only be generated by a greater than normal electrical stimulus. This is known as the relative refractory period.[8] Cell membrane refractoriness to depolarization prevents rapid repetitive stimulation and allows for completion of me-

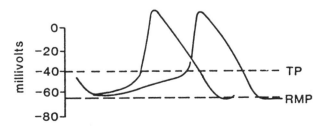

Fig. 8-2. The rate of pacemaker discharge is dependent upon the slope of spontaneous phase 4 depolarization, negativity of the resting membrane potential (RMP) and the threshold potential (TP). (From Stoelting,[69] with permission.)

chanical contraction prior to the onset of the next action potential.

The action potential generated in the SA node spreads through adjacent conducting tissues in the atria to the AV node, and then through the His-Purkinje system to the ventricular myocardium. The P wave and QRS complexes of the surface ECG are generated by phase 0 depolarization of millions of atrial and ventricular muscle cells respectively, while the T wave is generated by phase 3 repolarization of the ventricular cells. Repolarization of the atria occurs in a similar fashion and direction as does depolarization. However, repolarization of the human His-Purkinje system occurs last in the first cells to depolarize (the proximal bundle branches) and vice versa. This phenomena explains aberrant ventricular conduction with premature atrial beats and the positive deflection of the ventricular T wave.

Mechanisms of Arrhythmias

Arrhythmias occur when there is disruption of the normal sequence of depolarization of the SA node, atrial tissue, AV node, His-Purkinje system, and ventricular muscle. Arrhythmias may result from normal physiologic mechanisms which enhance or depress the normal automaticity of pacemaking cells (sinus tachycardia, sinus arrhythmia, etc.). If the rate of impulse generation from a secondary pacemaker such as an AV nodal cell becomes more rapid than the depolarization rate of the SA node, the secondary pacemaker will assume primary control of the heart rate and rhythm (escape rhythm, AV dissociation, etc.). An arrhythmia arises from one of many possible clinical scenarios involving reentry as with accessory AV pathways. Specific therapy for arrhythmias may depend on deciding which of the following mechanisms is its cause: abnormal automaticity, triggered automaticity, or reentry.

Abnormal Automaticity

Abnormalities in the action potential, such as a decrease in the resting membrane potential, an increase in threshold potential, or an increase in the slope of phase 4 diastolic depolarization will increase the depolarization rate for any cell with pacemaker potential.[9] Abnormal automaticity is usually the result of a movement of the resting membrane potential toward the threshold poten-

tial (less negative) which makes the cell more likely to depolarize. Less negative membrane potentials occur most frequently in areas of ischemia and infarction.[10] Abnormal automaticity with spontaneous depolarization of nonpacemaker cells may occur when the resting membrane potential is −60 mV.

Triggered Automaticity

Depolarization of the cell membrane which is triggered by the preceding action potential during or after repolarization is termed afterdepolarization. Early afterdepolarizations occur during phase 3 of repolarizations, whereas late afterdepolarizations occur during phase 4, after repolarization is complete.

Early afterdepolarizations occur because of a change in movement of K^+ out of the cell or an abnormal increased movement of Na^+ or Ca^{2+} into the cell. Conditions which cause early afterdepolarizations include hypokalemia, excess catecholamines, acidosis, hypoxia, delayed repolarization, and slow heart rates.[10] Delayed afterdepolarizations are primarily the result of enhanced calcium entry into the cell. Digitalis toxicity, hypomagnesium, myocardial ischemia, catecholamine excess, and Ca^{2+} administration all can precipitate delayed afterdepolarizations.[10] Triggered activity may be initiated by premature stimuli or rapid pacing, and may terminate spontaneously with rapid pacing or with spontaneous or programmed premature stimuli.

Reentry

The classic mechanism for arrhythmia generation involves reentry of a stimulus into the conducting system.[11] Anatomically contiguous but functionally diverse myocardial tissue is required for reentry to occur. Three conditions must exist: (1) an area of unidirectional block of impulse propagation, (2) a pathway with slow conduction velocity, and (3) distal recovery of excitability in the area formerly blocked (Fig. 8-3).

Reentry has been found to be involved in the generation of many arrhythmias. Supraventricular tachycardia can be caused by reentry occurring in the sinus node, the atrium, the AV node, or via an accessory pathway.[12] Reentrant arrhythmias tend to start and stop abruptly, are frequently precipitated by premature beats, and can be terminated with programmed insertion of premature stimuli.[13]

Elongation of conducting pathways, as seen with dilation of the heart (especially left atrial dilatation associated with mitral stenosis) and decreased conduction velocity from myocardial ischemia, create a situation in which reentry via the Purkinje fibers can occur.

ARRHYTHMOGENIC INFLUENCES IN THE INTENSIVE CARE UNIT AND OPERATING ROOM

Critically ill patients are constantly exposed to a number of factors that can precipitate arrhythmias in the emergency department, operating room, and intensive care unit. Failure to maintain temperature during trauma surgery, anesthesia, and exposure to cold hospital environments may lead to hypothermia. Electrolyte disturbances such as hypokalemia, hypomagnesemia, and metabolic alkalosis may occur from diuretic use,[14] intravenous

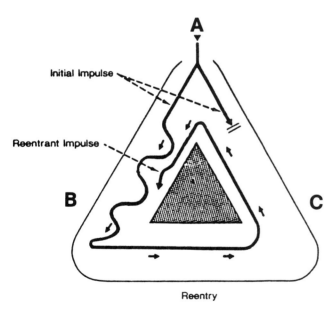

Fig. 8-3. The essential requirement for initiation of a reentry circuit is a unidirectional block preventing anterograde propagation of the cardiac impulse. A premature impulse arriving at A finds pathway C refractory. Conduction in pathway B is slowed because of incomplete repolarization. The impulse travels retrograde via pathway C which has repolarized during the time required for the impulse to traverse pathway B, thus setting up the reentry circuit. (Adapted from Fozzard and Arnsdorf,[71] with permission.)

fluid administration, or acid-base shifts. Hypocalcemia can result from rapid administration of albumin or blood products that contain citrate as an anticoagulant.[15] The presence of an indwelling central venous or pulmonary artery catheter may increase risk of arrhythmias in certain patients.[16] Transient right bundle branch block, frequent ventricular ectopy, or nonsustained ventricular tachycardia are common with insertion of a pulmonary artery catheter.[17] Medications such as digitalis, theophylline,[18] tricyclic antidepressants,[19] anesthetic agents, and antiarrhythmic agents may generate or enhance arrhythmias. Sympathetic stimulation occurs with hypoxia, hypercarbia, endotracheal intubation, surgical incision, pain, sepsis, or catecholamine infusions. This may lead to tachycardia, increased myocardial oxygen consumption, myocardial ischemia, and ventricular ectopy in patients with preexisting coronary artery disease. Parasympathetic stimulation occurs with pain, distension of a hollow viscus such as the bladder, and certain medications. Electrical microshock hazards exist due to the myriad monitoring devices used in the critical care setting and may also precipitate arrhythmias.

ELECTROCARDIOGRAPH LEAD SYSTEMS

Surface Leads

The standard leads system consists of three bipolar limb leads (leads I, II, III), which measure potential differences between two points, and three unipolar limb leads (aVR, aVL, and aVF), also known as augmented leads, which measure the potential between a common negative pole and the positive electrode on the limb. The electrical axes of the unipolar limb leads are perpendicular to the axes of standard limb leads (Fig. 8-4). There are also six standard unipolar chest leads, designated leads V_1-V_6. Leads placed on the right chest at locations corresponding to V_1-V_6 are labeled V_{1R}-V_{6R} (Fig. 8-5). Many modern ECG monitors allow use of all of the six primary limb leads (leads I, II, III, aVR, aVL, and aVF) as well as one or more V leads.

Modified chest leads (MCL) have the negative electrode just below the left clavicle at the midclavicular line, the ground electrode below the right clavicle, and the positive electrode placed in the precordial position corresponding to V_1-V_6. MCL

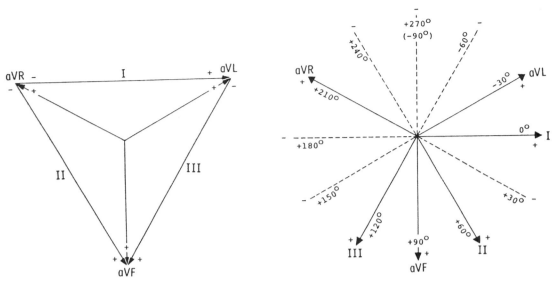

Fig. 8-4. Einthoven's triangle, composed of the standard bipolar limb leads and the augmented limb leads. The Hexaxial Reference System is a modified Einthoven's triangle, and is more useful for rhetorical axis determinations. (From Chung,[72] with permission.)

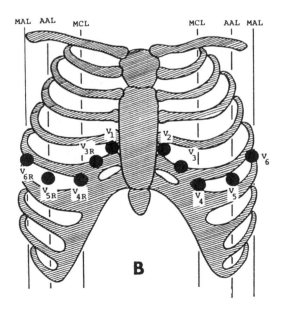

Fig. 8-5. Precordial lead system showing standard V and right-sided VR chest lead positions. (MAL, mid-axillary line; AAL, anterial axillary line; MCL, midclavicular-line). (From Chung,[72] with permission.)

leads are bipolar leads, which stimulate unipolar chest leads and offer similar electrocardiographic information. MCR leads are similar to MCL leads, but the negative electrode is below the right clavicle and the ground electrode is below the left clavicle. Central back leads, such as CBL_5, a bipolar lead with the negative electrode over the right scapula posteriorly and the positive electrode at the usual V_5 site, offer good P-wave morphology and ischemia detection.[20] Central manubrial leads, such as CM_5 where the negative electrode is over the manubrium and the positive electrode is at the V_5 site, have excellent ischemia detection.[21]

Leads I, II, and aVF offer excellent P wave detection and morphology, as do MCL_1-MCL_2, MCR_1, and CBL_5. Lead II, frequently monitored in the operating room and intensive care unit, is inadequate for detecting bundle branch blocks, aberrancy, and is not helpful in evaluating wide-complex tachycardia. Leads V_1, V_6, MCL_1, and MCL_6 are the best leads for detecting bundle branch block and aberrancy or for evaluating wide complex tachycardia.[22] With a dual channel monitor and a four lead system, it is possible to simultaneously monitor MCL_1 and MCL_6 (Fig. 8-6). This lead combination allows for easy P wave recognition and is most effective at arrhythmia diagnosis.

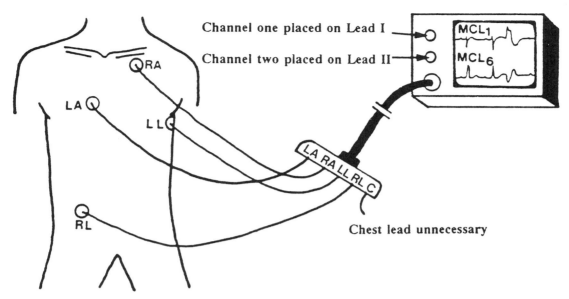

Fig. 8-6. Electrode placement for simultaneous monitoring of MCL$_1$ and MCL$_6$ with a four lead system. With selector dial for channel one placed on lead I, left arm (LA) is the positive and right arm (RA) is the negative electrode. Bipolar precordial lead MCL$_1$ is displayed. With selector dial for channel two placed on lead II, left leg (LL) is the positive and RA remains the negative electrode. The resultant lead on channel two is bipolar chest lead MCL$_6$. The right leg (RL) electrode is a reference or ground electrode, and may be placed anywhere on the body. (From Drew,[22] with permission.)

Esophageal Leads

In situations when the P wave is not detected or the relationship of the P wave to the QRS complex is unclear on surface leads an esophageal electrode may be used. The P waves are much larger in this lead due to the proximity of the esophagus to the left atrium[23] (Fig. 8-7). Using esophageal leads, posterior myocardial ischemia is easily detected and cardiac pacing via the esophagus is feasible.[24] One commercially available esophageal stethoscope has external electrodes placed 7 cm and 20 cm from the distal end, which are connected to standard ECG lead wires. In a study by Katz, a 3 French balloon-tipped temporary transvenous pacing electrode, used as an esophageal electrode, correctly identified the rhythm in 10 of 12 patients when the surface ECG was nondiagnostic.[25] If a commercial esophageal lead is not available, a J guidewire inserted through an 8-F red Robinson catheter taped to an esophageal stethoscope can be used.[26] However, using this system, care must be taken to avoid esophageal burns when electrocautery units are in use.[27]

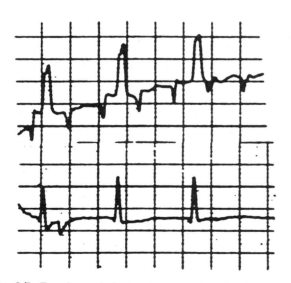

Fig. 8-7. Esophageal electrode recording showing prominent atrial activity (downward deflections), which is not seen on the simultaneous surface ECG. (Adapted from Kaplan and Thys,[73] with permission.)

Epicardial Leads

Many patients have temporary transcutaneous pacer wires sutured to the atrium and ventricle during cardiac surgery to overcome transient postoperative bradycardia or AV block. These leads allow monitoring of electrical activity directly from the surface of the heart in the operating room or cardiac surgical intensive care unit. Atrial electrograms (AEGs) are unsurpassed in detecting atrial activity in situations where the surface ECG fails to detect P waves or establish their relationship with the QRS complex.[28] Ventricular epicardial electrograms are of little value, since the QRS complex is usually readily detected on standard surface ECG.[29]

Unipolar and bipolar AEGs can be obtained. Unipolar AEGs best establish the relationship between atrial and ventrical activity and are obtained by attaching one atrial epicardial lead to one of the limb leads[30] (Fig. 8-8). A bipolar AEG is obtained when both atrial epicardial wires are connected using alligator clips to the positive and negative leads of a standard bipolar lead, such as lead I (Fig. 8-9). Bipolar AEGs enhance while, avoiding masking, atrial activity within simultaneously occurring ventricular complexes. Attaching both epicardial wires to the right and left arm leads allows monitoring of the bipolar AEG by selecting lead I, while selection of lead II or III displays a unipolar AEG.

Appropriate electrical grounding and insulation must be used to prevent electrical injury when recording AEGs. The direct contact of the leads with the heart places the patient at risk for microshock, which can lead to atrial extrasystoles, atrial flutter, or atrial fibrillation. Extreme caution is advised to avoid microshock, which can precipitate ventricular fibrillation when ventricular pacing leads are in use. Rubber gloves should be worn whenever handling the epicardial leads, which should be kept dry and coiled inside a rubber glove to insulate the exposed wires when not in use.[31]

Intracardiac Leads

Recording of intracardiac electrical potentials via temporary transvenous pacemaker leads yields information similar to that obtained with epicardial leads.[32] However, intraventricular electrograms are of little use, as noted above. Intraatrial electrograms may be recorded through a fluid-filled cen-

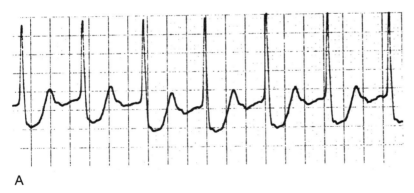

A

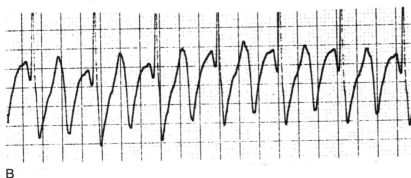

B

Fig. 8-8. Simultaneous recording of an ECG surface lead **(A)** and unipolar atrial electrocardiogram (AEG) **(B)** in patient with new onset tachycardia and hypotension following cardiopulmonary bypass surgery. Surface ECG suggests sinus tachycardia, but AEG **(B)** clearly shows atrial activity at a rate of 270 beats per minute (downward deflections) with 2:1 ventricular response (upward deflections) thus establishing atrial flutter as the diagnosis.

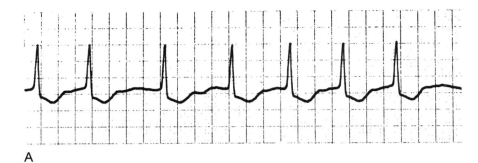

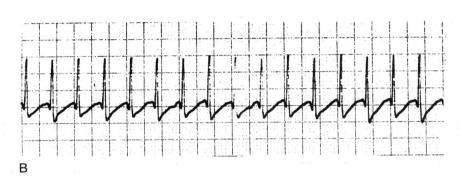

Fig. 8-9. Simultaneous recording of surface ECG (**A**) suggesting atrial fibrillation at approximately 100 beats per minute, but a bipolar AEG (**B**), demonstrating atrial tachycardia at 200 beats per minute with variable A-V conduction.

tral venous[33] or a pulmonary artery catheter,[34] or by inserting a flexible pacing wire through the catheter.[35] Concerns about electrical safety and microshock avoidance are the same as for epicardial leads.

DIAGNOSTIC VERSUS MONITORING MODE

Many monitors are equipped with a bandwidth filter that removes signals above or below a certain frequency. The high-frequency filter removes 60 Hz and other electrical interference, such as from electrocautery units (1×10^6 Hz).[36] In the diagnostic mode, the lower frequency response of most monitors is 0.14 Hz, below which signals are attenuated by the low-frequency filter.[36] Monitor mode involves an additional low-frequency filter which removes all signals below 0.5 Hz.[36] Low-frequency signals are often associated with respiratory movements or the movement of ECG lead wires and can lead to wandering baselines and difficulty in interpretation of the cardiac rhythm. However, distortion of the ST segment and T waves, mimicking ischemic ECG changes, often occurs when the low-frequency filter is used (Fig. 8-10). Thus, when

monitoring for myocardial ischemia, either the diagnostic mode must be used, or the monitor must be calibrated in the monitoring mode. The amplitude and morphology of the P wave may be altered by the low-frequency filter leading to difficulty in interpretation of arrhythmias.

RISKS OF ELECTROCARDIOGRAPHIC MONITORING

The risks of ECG monitoring include electrical shock injury, burns, and institution of inappropriate therapy as a result of misdiagnosis of arrhythmias.

Electrical Hazards

A basic appreciation of the principles of electricity is essential to understanding the risks of ECG monitoring. Ohm's law ($V = I \times R$) describes the relationship between current (I), resistance to current flow (R), and the voltage potential (V). For a given voltage, the current will vary inversely with the resistance. In order for current to flow, a circuit must be completed from the voltage source, through the resistance(s) and back to the voltage source. Current flows from the potential source through a hot wire to the resistance, and returns via a neutral wire.[36] A ground wire connects the neutral side of the circuit to an object with zero voltage potential, such as the earth. Current (units are amperes) divided by the cross-sectional area of flow is the current density. Power (watts) is the product of volts and current, and energy (joules or watt-seconds) is the product of energy and time. If a person contacts a nonisolated circuit at two points, current can flow through the individual and lead to injury or death. Since the earth is the usual ground source for electrical circuits, contact with the circuit at only one point will complete the circuit.

A line-isolation transformer is a device which isolates the power source from the ground, such that connecting one of the two power contacts to the ground does not complete the circuit (Fig. 8-11). In an isolated system, since there is no contact between the power supply and the ground, contact at one point does not complete the circuit, and no current flows.[36] A line-isolation monitor (LIM) measures current flow between the isolated circuit and the ground, allowing for detection of abnormal ground connections (short circuits), indicating that the circuit has become nonisolated.[37] When the LIM alarms indicating a current flow greater than 2 mA, each electrical device attached to the circuit must be investigated to determine where the short circuit is located.[36] Each monitor should be sequentially unplugged until the LIM alarm ceases, starting with the device plugged in most recently. The LIM ceases alarming when the device unplugged contains the short circuit, and this device or monitor should not be used until thoroughly evaluated by the biomedical engineering department.

Electricity applied to the surface of the body travels by the path of least resistance, namely, via the great vessels, muscles, nerves, and connective tissues. This is termed macroshock, and, if greater than 100 to 200 mA, may result in ventricular fibrillation.[38,39] Smaller currents applied directly to the heart via pacemaker wires, fluid-filled intracardiac catheters, or directly during surgery are termed microshock, and the fibrillatory threshold is approximately 50 to 100 μA (0.05–0.1 mA).[38] Extreme care must be taken to ensure all instruments

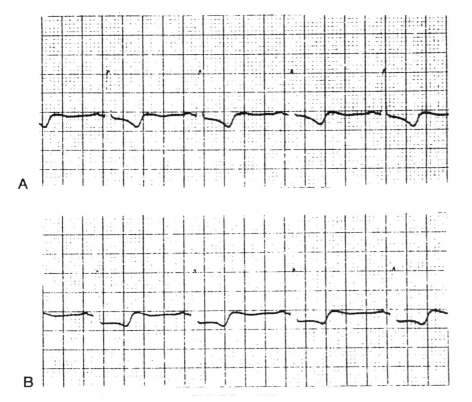

Fig. 8-10. Apparent ST segment depression in a patient with T wave inversion produced by switching from diagnostic mode (A) to monitor mode (B). (From Kaplan and Thys,[73] with permission.)

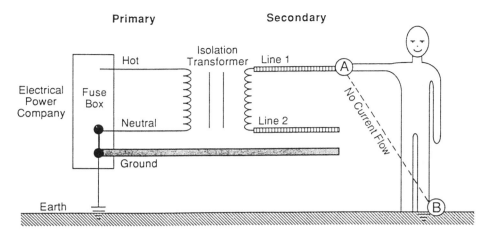

Fig. 8-11. This diagram illustrates a safety feature of the isolated power system. An individual contacting one side of the isolated power system (point A) and standing on the ground (point B) will not receive a shock. The individual is not contacting the isolated circuit at two points and thus not completing the circuit. Point A is part of the isolated circuit, while the ground (point B) is part of the primary or grounded side of the circuit. (From Ehrenwerth,[36] with permission.)

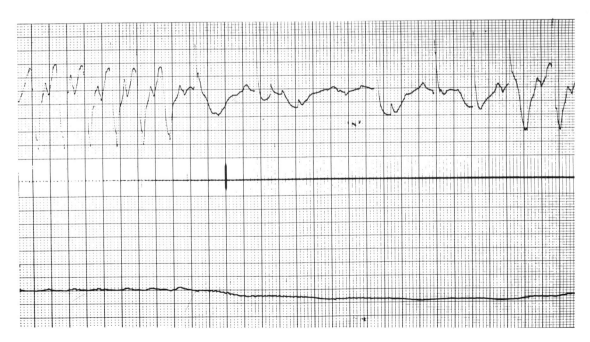

Fig. 8-12. Artifact produced by the arterial roller pump head during cardiopulmonary bypass, mimicking ventricular tachycardia. The pump was briefly turned off revealing an underlying slower cardiac rhythm.

are safely grounded and isolated, as this microshock current is below the threshold for perception (approximately 1 mA) by most personnel working in the operating room or intensive care unit.

Burns

Heat is generated whenever current passes through a resistor, and is proportional to the resistance and the current density. Electrocautery units utilize a large surface area dispersive plate, which decreases the current density as the electrocautery current exits the body.[40] If the grounding pad is poorly applied, the current may exit the patient via an ECG lead with a significantly smaller surface area, in which case the heat generation will be greater, and cutaneous burns can result.[40] Nuclear magnetic resonance (NMR) units employ shifting magnetic fields, which can generate electrical currents in metallic items such as ECG monitor leads.[41,42] The current density exiting via these leads, if significantly large, can generate sufficient heat to cause burns. The use of nonferromagnetic ECG leads eliminates this hazard.[43]

Artifacts

The ECG is subject to many external influences which may generate false signals or interfere with rhythm interpretation. Electrocautery units may completely distort ECG tracings, and patient movements such as shivering or hiccupping may create artifacts resembling P waves, atrial fibrillation, or even ventricular tachycardia. The arterial pump roller head in use during cardiopulmonary bypass often mimics myocardial electrical activity (Fig. 8-12).

COMMON ARRHYTHMIAS

Normal Sinus Rhythm

Normal sinus rhythm is characterized by

1. Regular atrial activity originating in the SA node with a rate between 60 and 100 beats per minute
2. Upright P waves in leads I, II, and aVF and V_2 through V_6
3. A PR interval between 120 and 200 ms
4. A P wave preceding each QRS complex
5. A QRS complex following each P wave.

The rate of sinus node discharge is dependent upon the balance between sympathetic and parasympathetic tone.

Sinus Tachycardia

Sinus tachycardia is essentially sinus rhythm occurring at a rate greater than 100 beats per minute in adults or 140 beats per minute in children.[44] Sinus tachycardia may be caused by many medications, including aminophylline, caffeine, isoflurane, ketamine, and quinidine.[44] Increases in sympathetic tone may result in rates of up to 160 to 200 beats per minute in adults, and greater than 220 beats per minute in children. Hypermetabolic states such as exercise, fever, sepsis, thyrotoxicosis, and malignant hyperthermia are associated with increased oxygen consumption and tachycardia. Inhibition of vagal tone occurs with anticholinergic medications such as atropine or glycopyrrolate. Sinus tachycardia is a physiologic sign of systemic perturbations, and one should attempt to identify and correct the underlying causes.

Sinus Bradycardia

Sinus bradycardia is a sinus rhythm with a rate below 60 beats per minute in adults, or below 100 beats per minute in infants.[45] It is commonly seen in healthy young adults and well-trained athletes. Sinus bradycardia may be due to inhibition of sympathetic activity with drugs such as beta blockers, narcotics, and other anesthetic agents. Augmentation of parasympathetic tone with cholinergic agents such as pilocarpine, succinylcholine, or the anticholinesterases edrophonium or neostigmine, reduces heart rate. Intraoperative traction on the peritoneum or mesentery, manipulation of the ca-

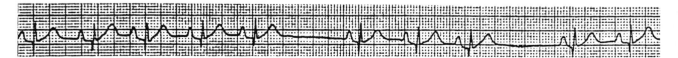

Fig. 8-13. Sinus node exit block. Note the absence of a P wave (following the 5th and 8th QRS complexes), and subsequent P waves occurring at the anticipated time. (From Zipes,[74] with permission.)

Inspiration   Expiration   Inspiration

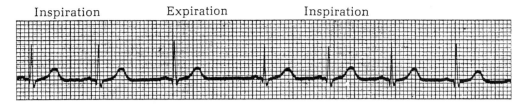

Fig. 8-14. Sinus arrhythmia associated with respiration in a young, healthy adult. Note the constant PR interval and P wave and QRS complex morphology, with varying R-R intervals. (From Conover,[75] with permission.)

rotid sinus, or distension of a hollow viscus can cause a vagally mediated bradycardia. Traction on the extraocular muscles or compression of the globe triggers the oculocardiac reflex, with pronounced bradycardia or, occasionally, asystole. Increased intracranial pressure leads to systemic hypertension, reflex bradycardia, and respiratory irregularities, a phenomenon known as Cushing's reflex. Hypoxia and hypothermia may also lead to sinus bradycardia.

Inferior wall myocardial ischemia or infarction is frequently associated with sinus bradycardia. The blood supply to the SA node most commonly arises from the right coronary artery, and may be compromised during inferior ventricular wall ischemia. Chest pain may initiate a vagally mediated bradycardia. Cardiac sensory fibers may cause a systemic vagotonia resulting in nausea, hypotension, bradycardia, and occasionally varying degrees of heart block (Bezold-Jarisch reflex).

Sinus Node Exit Block, Sinus Arrest

Occasionally, the SA node generates impulses that cannot escape the node to trigger the atrium. This is designated a SA node exit block, and is occasionally a cause of bradycardia. Characteristics of SA exit block (Fig. 8-13) include the absence of a P wave in any lead, with the next P wave occurring at the anticipated time. This is different than a si-

nus arrest, where the SA node fails to form an impulse, and the subsequent P wave usually occurs earlier than anticipated.

Sinus Arrhythmia

Sinus arrhythmia is a benign, rhythmic variation in the sinus rate, usually occurring as a result of changes in vagal tone associated with respiration (Fig. 8-14). The heart rate slowly increases during inspiration, and slowly decreases during exhalation. A nonrespiratory variant of sinus arrhythmia may be seen with digitalis toxicity, hypothyroidism, calcium channel-blocking medications, and with myocardial infarction,[46] or may occur in young, healthy individuals. In sinus arrhythmia, the PR interval and P wave and QRS morphologies do not vary.

Wandering Atrial Pacemaker

The term wandering atrial pacemaker is applied when two or more supraventricular pacemaker foci are competing for control of the heart rhythm (Fig. 8-15). The cycle length is regular, while P wave morphology and PR intervals change with each pacemaker focus. This rhythm rarely requires treatment or deteriorates into a more significant arrhythmia. It must not be confused with an AV node reentrant tachycardia with a retrograde P wave occurring immediately before the QRS complex.

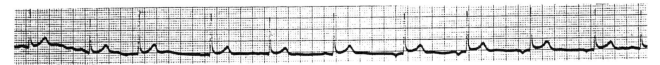

Fig. 8-15. Wandering atrial pacemaker. The first three beats are sinus; then the pacemaking shifts to another pacemaker focus. Note the different P wave morphology, but no significant change in the rate. (From Zipes,[74] with permission.)

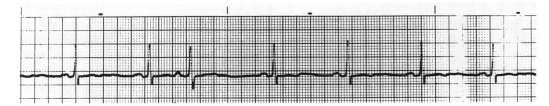

Fig. 8-16. The third beat arrives early and has a different P wave morphology than the preceding beats, identifying it as a premature atrial contraction (PAC).

Premature Atrial Contraction

When the atrial impulse originates from a focus other than the SA node, the P wave has a different morphology than the sinus-generated P wave. If this occurs before the next sinus P wave, it is called a premature atrial contraction (PAC) (Fig. 8-16). An ectopic focus located high in the atrium will generate an ectopic P wave closely resembling the normal sinus P wave. The ectopic P wave will be inverted in leads I, II, and aVF if the focus is low in the atrium. Often, the ectopic P wave is hidden in the T wave of the preceding complex. The ectopic PR interval may be shorter than normal with a low atrial focus, or may be prolonged due to partial refractoriness of the AV node. The pause following the PAC is equal to or slightly longer than the sinus cycle length, if the sinus node is depolarized by the PAC and reset, causing a noncompensatory pause. However, the SA node may depolarize in a normal sequence without interference from the PAC, but not conduct due to atrial refractoriness. The next sinus node beat occurs at the normal interval, and the resulting pause between complexes is fully compensated.

PACs occurring very early in diastole may find the AV node refractory, and depolarization will not spread to the ventricles. This is known as a blocked PAC (Fig. 8-17). Alternatively, the AV conduction system may be only partially repolarized, and the PAC is conducted aberrantly[47] (Fig. 8-18). This usually results in a right bundle-branch block (RBBB) pattern, since the right bundle frequently has a longer refractory period than the left bundle. Aberrant conduction of a PAC combined with the absence of a noncompensatory pause can lead to the erroneous diagnosis of a ventricular premature beat. (See section on premature ventricular contractions.) A PAC may trigger other supraventricular arrhythmias, such as supraventricular tachycardias, atrial flutter or fibrillation, and this is the most frequent reason for treating PACs in the operating room or critical care setting.[48]

Premature Nodal Complexes

The AV node consists of three regions according to cell types: transitional, midnodal, and lower nodal. The transitional zone, also known as the AN region, is the gradual merging of atrial and nodal fibers. The midnodal region or N region, accounts

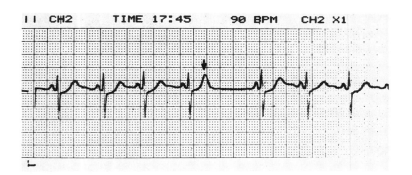

Fig. 8-17. Sinus rhythm with a nonconducted PAC. The blocked PAC marked by the arrow (↓) distorts the T wave morphology compared with the other T waves.

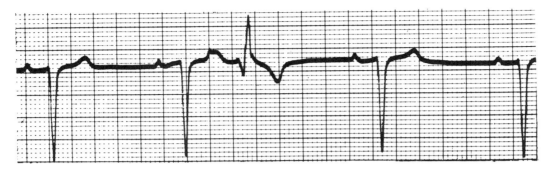

Fig. 8-18. After two normally conducted beats, a PAC arises and is conducted abberrently with a RBBB pattern. A P wave, identifiable in the preceding T wave, distinguishes this from a ventricular premature beat. (From Marriott,[76] with permission.)

for most of the physiologic delay in AV conduction. The lower nodal or NH zone, where nodal and His-Purkinje fibers merge, is the usual focus for nodal pacemaker activity.

The AV node normally acts as an escape pacemaker whenever the atrial rate slows below the intrinsic nodal rate. However, early depolarization of this tissue leads to premature nodal complexes (PNCs). Retrograde conduction to the atrium is possible and is evident by an inverted P wave in leads I, II, and aVF. The retrograde P wave may precede, follow, or be buried within the QRS complex (Fig. 8-19).

The AV node may become the primary cardiac pacemaker if the nodal rate exceeds the sinus rate. Nodal rhythm is regular at the intrinsic rate of 45 to 60 beats per minute. The term accelerated nodal rhythm is used when a nodal rhythm occurs at a rate between 60 and 100 beats per minute, and nodal tachycardia when the rate exceeds 100 beats per minute. PNCs and nodal rhythms may result from the same etiologies as PACs.

Paroxysmal Supraventricular Tachycardia

Paroxysmal supraventricular tachycardia (PSVT) is a generic term encompassing all tachycardias originating in cardiac tissue other than ventricular tissue. The common characteristic is the sudden onset of this arrhythmia. PSVT includes SA node and AV nodal reentry, atrial tachycardias, and atrioventricular reentry tachycardias using an accessory pathway. AV nodal reentrant tachycardia (AVNRT) is the most common—greater than 50 percent—of all PSVT in adults.[12] AVNRT is often precipitated and terminated physiologically by a premature atrial contraction or retrograde conduction of a PVC. The AV node consists of two separate pathways, conventionally named alpha (slow conduction velocity and short refractory period) and beta (fast conduction velocity and long refractory period). Reentry is possible when a PAC is blocked in the beta pathway with the longer refractory period and travels slowly through the alpha pathway. Electrocardiographic diagnosis reveals a rate of 140 to 200 beats per minute, regular rhythm with a narrow QRS complex without visible P waves (Fig. 8-20). Retrograde P waves may be seen preceding or following the QRS complex, but most commonly are obscured in the QRS complex due to almost simultaneous activation of the atria and ventricles. An atrial or esophageal electrogram may document atrial activity in a 1:1 relationship to ventricular activity. At faster rates, widening of the QRS complex due to rate related bundle-branch block may make differentiation from ventricular tachycardia difficult.

Paroxysmal atrial tachycardia (PAT) may result either from an automatic or reentry focus.[49] Electrocardiographic diagnosis reveals a narrow-complex tachycardia with a rate of 150 to 200 beats per minute. P waves usually precede the QRS complexes, but with a morphology different than normal sinus P waves. Depending on heart rate the P waves may be hidden in the T wave of the preceding QRS complex (Fig. 8-21).

Atrial tachycardia, which may be associated with varying degrees of AV block, is seen with digitalis toxicity, catecholamine excess, and critical illness involving hypoxia, acidosis and electrolyte disturbances (Fig. 8-22). This rhythm may reflect underlying sinus node dysfunction, and may be seen as

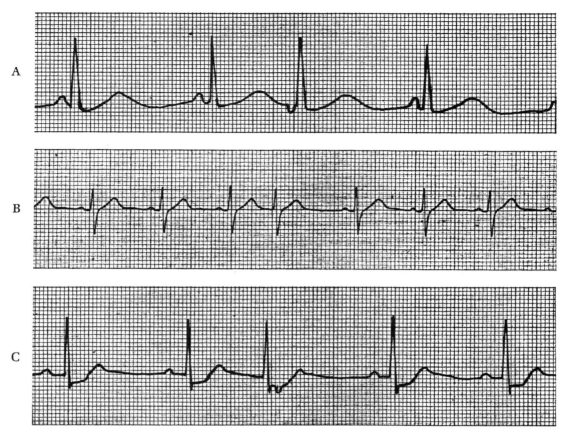

Fig. 8-19. Junctional premature complexes. **(A)** In this tracing the retrograde P wave precedes the QRS complex; **(B)** in this strip it is buried within the QRS; and **(C)** in this strip the retrograde P wave follows the QRS complex. (From Conover,[75] with permission.)

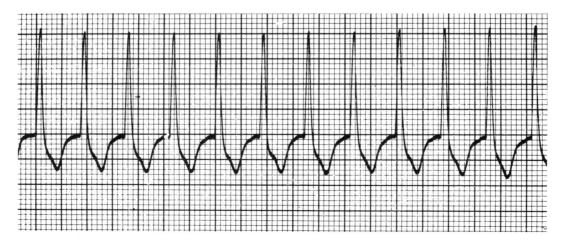

Fig. 8-20. Paroxysmal supraventricular tachycardia. The retrograde P waves are lost within the QRS-T complex and are not definitely discernible. This is typical of AV nodal reentry tachycardia.

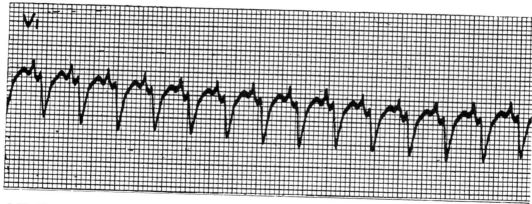

Fig. 8-21. Paroxysmal atrial tachycardia at a rate of 188 beats per minute. The P waves have a different morphology than sinus P waves. (From Mangiola and Riotota,[70] with permission.)

part of the sick sinus syndrome (SSS). This clinical syndrome of abnormal sinus node function is caused by abnormalities in SA node automaticity, SA conduction, and occasionally AV node dysfunction.[50] Sinus node ischemia, mitral valve prolapse, inflammatory and infiltrative diseases, and atrial trauma may all be associated with SSS. It usually manifests as bradycardia, but is often associated with recurrent episodes of tachycardia alternating with bradyarrhythmias (Fig. 8-23). In this context, it is known as tachycardia-bradycardia syndrome.

Multifocal atrial tachycardia, also known as chaotic atrial tachycardia, is characterized by three or more morphologically distinct P waves at a rate greater than 100 beats per minute, with varying P-P and PR intervals (Fig. 8-24). It is most commonly seen in critically ill patients with underlying pulmonary disease,[51] and theophylline has been implicated as the inciting factor in this arrhythmia.[52]

Accessory AV connections are the second most common cause of PSVT (25 to 30 percent) of patients.[53] Wolff-Parkinson-White syndrome (WPW) is

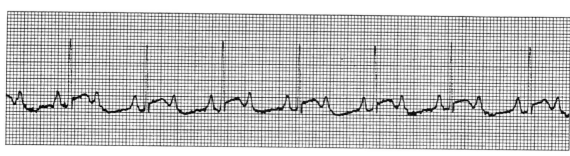

Fig. 8-22. Atrial tachycardia with 2:1 AV block, in a patient with digoxin toxicity. (From Conover,[75] with permission.)

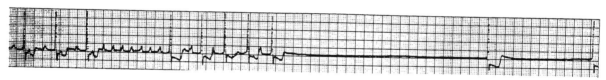

Fig. 8-23. Sick sinus syndrome manifesting as the tachycardia-bradycardia syndrome. Irregular atrial tachycardia is followed by prolonged sinus pause. A junctional escape rhythm begins after 4.8 seconds. (From Zipes,[74] with permission.)

MAT   10 a.m.   Aminophyllin stopped

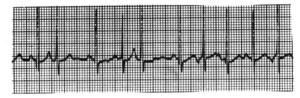

NSR   3 p.m.

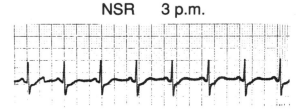

Fig. 8-24. Multifocal atrial tachycardia (chaotic atrial tachycardia) with several different P wave morphologies evident in a patient with chronic obstructive pulmonary disease. Normal sinus rhythm (NSR) is restored after aminophylline is discontinued. (From Royster,[68] with permission.)

associated with an accessory pathway (Bundle of Kent). This abnormal connection between the atrial and ventricular myocardium bypasses the normal delay imposed by the AV node. Electrocardiographic diagnosis reveals a short PR interval and delta wave when the patient is in sinus rhythm (Fig. 8-25). The accessory pathway (James fibers) in the Lown-Ganong-Levine syndrome connects the atrium to the AV node or His-bundle. A shortened PR interval without a delta wave is seen on surface ECG. Reentry occurs with anterograde (atria to ventricle) AV nodal conduction and retrograde (ventricle to atria) conduction through the accessory pathway. This results in a narrow-complex tachycardia with QRS morphology similar to normally conducted beats. The inverted P wave usually follows closely or is hidden within the preceding QRS complex (Fig. 8-26). Occasionally, anterograde conduction is via the accessory pathway with retrograde conduction through the AV node, resulting in a wide QRS complex due to the delta wave of preexcitation.[54] The morphology and QRS-P interval will depend upon the location of the accessory pathway.[55] PSVT, atrial flutter or atrial fibrillation may result in extremely rapid ventricular rates (>300 beats per minute) because of the very fast conduction velocity and short refractory period of the accessory pathway.

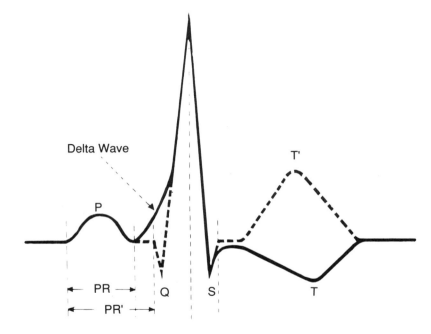

Fig. 8-25. The solid line indicates the anomalous conduction in the Wolff-Parkinson-White syndrome, and the dotted line indicates normal conduction. The PR interval is shortened because of the delta wave. The T wave is inverted because of secondary T wave changes. (Modified from Chung,[72] with permission.)

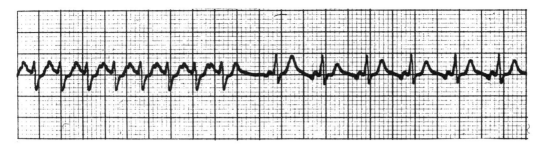

Fig. 8-26. Narrow complex reentrant tachycardia in a child with Wolff-Parkinson-White syndrome. The tachycardia terminates abruptly with the ensuing normal sinus rhythm characterized by a short PR interval and a nondistinct delta wave.

Sinus node reentry is an uncommon form of PSVT, and is characterized by abrupt onset of a narrow complex tachycardia, with P waves identical to normal sinus P waves. As with most reentrant tachycardia, sinus node reentry may be terminated by carotid sinus massage, calcium channel blockers, or programmed insertion of a premature beat.

Atrial Fibrillation

Atrial fibrillation is characterized by a rapid, irregular, disorganized atrial activity representing multiple foci firing simultaneously. Microreentry is likely the predominant mechanism. On surface ECG, no discernible P waves are seen, but the baseline may show very fine or coarse fibrillatory activity (Fig. 8-27). The AEG reveals complexes having a myriad of shapes, sizes, polarities, and amplitudes.[30] Ventricular activity is irregular, reflecting the constant bombardment of the AV node with impulses which traverse the AV node in a variable fashion. The ventricular rate in untreated, healthy patients may vary between 120 and 200 beats per minute. Aberrant conduction, often with a right bundle branch block pattern, is common in atrial fibrillation. Accessory AV pathways allow very rapid conduction of impulses to the ventricles, and may lead to ventricular tachycardia or fibrillation.

The ventricular response is slowed with digitalis, beta blockers, and/or calcium channel blockers.[56] Conversion of acute atrial fibrillation to sinus rhythm is often successful with procainamide,[57] esmolol,[56] and intravenous amiodarone. Cardioversion is indicated for hemodynamically unstable patients with acute atrial fibrillation or if the arrhythmia persists for several days. Cardioversion of acute atrial fibrillation after 5 to 7 days requires anticoagulation.[58]

Atrial Flutter

Atrial flutter is commonly seen in cardiac disease states, especially mitral valve disease. Atrial flutter

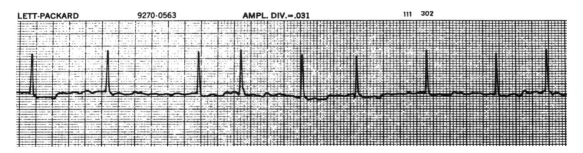

Fig. 8-27. Atrial fibrillation with a slow ventricular response. Note the total irregularity of R-R intervals with a fine fibrillatory baseline.

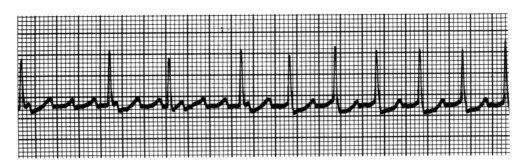

Fig. 8-28. Type I atrial flutter at a rate of 300 beats per minute, with classic sawtooth flutter waves and variable AV block.

is categorized on the basis of atrial rate and the susceptibility to overdrive pacing.[59] Type I (classical) atrial flutter occurs at a rate of 300 beats per minute, with typical sawtooth or biphasic flutter waves (F waves) seen in the inferior leads (Fig. 8-28). Rapid overdrive pacing is usually successful in terminating type I atrial flutter.[60] Type II atrial flutter is characterized by a flatter baseline with positive flutter waves in the inferior leads, at a rate of 350 to 400 beats per minute (Fig. 8-29). Overdrive pacing usually fails to capture the atria in the presence of type II flutter, although conversion to type I flutter may occur with pharmacologic therapy. Ventricular rate depends upon the state of the AV node, with conduction ranging from 2:1 to 8:1. The ventricular response is frequently 150 beats per minute to 2:1 AV block. Carotid sinus massage will increase the block, and the flutter waves will become more readily discerned. Atrial electrograms are useful for defining atrial activity when clear flutter waves are not present on the surface ECG (see Fig. 8-8). Control of ventricular response is obtained by increasing the AV block with digitalis, beta blockers, and/or calcium-channel blockers. Esmolol is very effective in rate control, and appears to convert acute atrial fibrillation or flutter to sinus rhythm in a high percentage of patients (Table 8-3).[61]

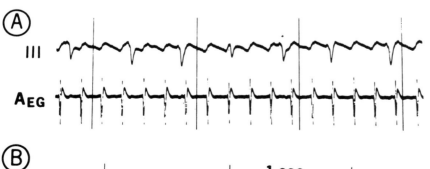
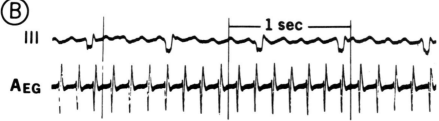

Fig. 8-29. Simultaneous surface ECG (lead III) and atrial electrogram (A$_{EG}$) demonstrating type I atrial flutter **(A)** with classic sawtooth flutter waves at a rate of 300 beats per minute, and type II atrial flutter **(B)** with atrial activity at a rate of 400 beats per minute, and absence of discrete sawtooth flutter waves. (From Waldo and Kaiser,[30] with permission.)

TABLE 8-3. Results of Pharmacologic Therapy Versus Placebo One Hour After Initiation of Therapy in Patients With Recent-Onset Atrial Fibrillation or Flutter

	Converted to NSR	VR (bpm mean ± SEM)
Esmolol $n = 21$	10/21*	151±6 → 104±3**
Verapamil $n = 20$	4/20	147±6 → 94±3**
Digoxin $n = 20$	3/20	139±5 → 135±4
Placebo $n = 18$	2/18	137±4 → 135±4

Abbreviations: NSR, normal sinus rhythm; VR, ventricular response; bpm, beats per minute; SEM, standard error of the mean.

Drugs were administered as follows: Esmolol 10–20 mg bolus followed by infusion 2–16 mg/h; Verapamil 10–20 mg bolus in 2 titration steps; Digoxin 0.5 mg single bolus; Placebo = saline.

*$P < 0.5$ vs V,D,P.

**$P < .05$ vs D,P.

(Adapted from Platia et al.,[61] with permission.)

Arrhythmias Due to Atrioventricular Block

Delayed or blocked impulse propagation between the atria and ventricles may occur in the atrium, AV node, or His-bundle system. First-degree AV block is a delay in A-V conduction, almost invariably occurring in the AV node. The PR interval is greater than 200 ms, with normal P wave and QRS complexes, and with each P wave resulting in a QRS complex. First-degree AV block is usually benign.

Second-degree AV block is defined as failure of some but not all P waves to be transmitted to the ventricles, and occurs in two types. Mobitz type I AV block, also known as Wenckebach block, is characterized by progressive lengthening of the PR interval followed by a blocked beat (Fig. 8-30). The site of this block is usually in the AV node, so it is sometimes referred to as a "proximal block." This rhythm is usually temporary, and does not progress to complete heart block. It is a result of reflex slowing of AV conduction. Proximal AV block is usually

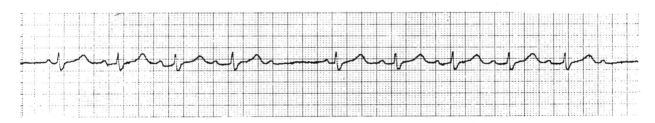

Fig. 8-30. Second-degree Mobitz type I (Wenckebach) AV block. Note progressive PR prolongation, and nonconduction of the P wave before each pause.

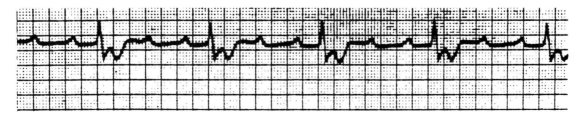

Fig. 8-31. Second-degree Mobitz type II AV block. The PR interval remains constant.

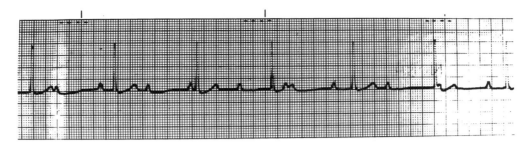

Fig. 8-32. Third-degree or complete heart block, with junctional escape focus at a rate of 45 beats per minute. Note complete dissociation of atrial and ventricular activity.

responsive to atropine. Mobitz type II second-degree AV block, or "distal block," is less common but more severe than type I. The ECG shows fixed PR intervals and intermittent nonconducted P waves (Fig. 8-31). This type of AV block is frequently associated with intraventricular conduction delays such as bundle-branch blocks, and often progresses to complete heart block. Seen more commonly with anterior myocardial infarctions, it is less responsive to atropine than proximal block, and may require permanent pacemaker insertion. When the P to R ratio is 2:1 (every other P wave blocked), it is difficult to differentiate type I from type II AV block. If the PR interval of the conducted beats is prolonged, and there is no bundle-branch block, then it is more likely a type I or Wenckebach block.

Third-degree AV block, or complete heart block, occurs when no P waves are transmitted to the ventricles. The atria and ventricles each are beating independently (Fig. 8-32). The ventricular rate is determined by the site of the escape pacemaker. An AV nodal focus results in narrow QRS complexes (junctional escape rhythm), while a focus within the ventricular myocardium generates wide QRS complexes (idioventricular escape rhythm).

Premature Ventricular Contractions

Premature ventricular contraction (PVCs), also known as ventricular premature beats, originate from the ventricular myocardium. Conduction through the myocardium occurs without the specialized His-Purkinje conduction system, and thus the QRS duration is therefore widened (>0.12 second), and the QRS morphology is significantly altered. The QRS is wide and slurred, with ST segments sloping the opposite direction to the main QRS deflection (Fig. 8-33).

Differentiation between PVCs and PACs with aberrant conduction can be difficult.[47] Obviously, the

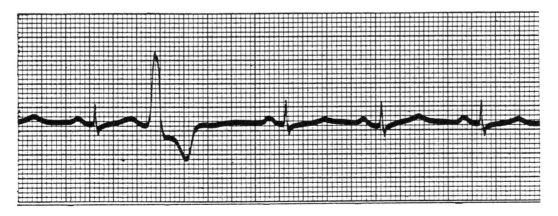

Fig. 8-33. Premature ventricular contraction, demonstrating a fully compensatory pause. (From Mangiola and Riotota,[70] with permission.)

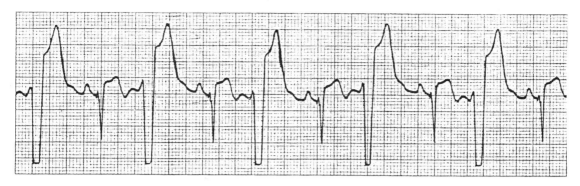

Fig. 8-34. Ventricular bigeminy with a fixed coupling interval. Note the interval between the sinus beat and the PVC is constant. (From Conover,[75] with permission.)

presence of P waves before the QRS complexes favors PACs, although their absence does not rule them out. Retrograde P waves may be seen following a PVC when conduction through the AV node is slowed significantly. PVCs tend to have a fixed coupling interval, that is, the time between the normal QRS and the PVC tends to be constant (Fig. 8-34). The coupling interval is more variable with PACs. Fusion beats, where the QRS complex is a blend of normal and PVC morphologies, favor a ventricular origin (Fig. 8-35). PVCs usually do not penetrate the SA node and reset its rate, so the pause following a PVC will be longer than ex-

pected. The next normal QRS complex will occur at two cycle lengths after the previous normal QRS complex. The pause is said to be fully compensatory (Fig. 8-33), in contrast to a PAC, which resets the SA node and results in a less than fully compensated pause. A PVC may, however, reset the SA node, so a noncompensatory pause does not totally rule out a ventricular origin.

Unifocal PVCs are commonly seen in otherwise healthy patients.[6] However, multifocal PVCs are associated with a higher risk of degeneration into ventricular tachycardia or fibrillation (Fig. 8-36). A PVC occurring on the peak of the T wave, the vul-

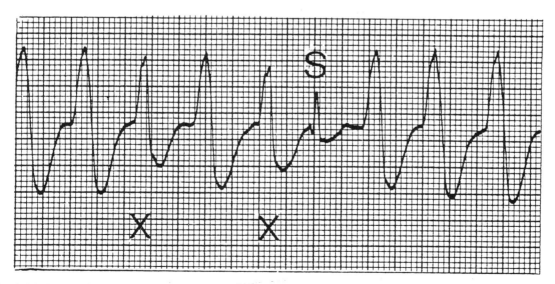

Fig. 8-35. Fusion beats. Ventricular tachycardia is interrupted by two fusion beats (X) with sinus depolarization of the ventricles fusing with the ventricular ectopic activity. Complete capture of the ventricles by the sinus occurs (S). (From Royster and Robertie,[77] with permission.)

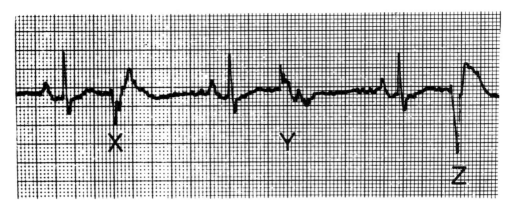

Fig. 8-36. Multifocal PVCs. Note the different morphologies of the three PVCs (X, Y, Z). (From Royster and Robertie,[77] with permission.)

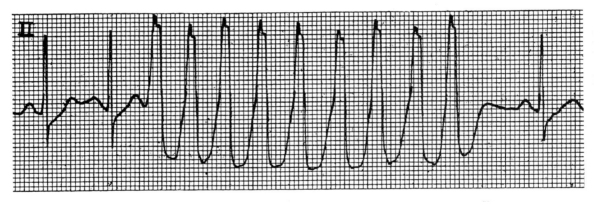

Fig. 8-37. Ventricular tachycardia during sinus rhythm. (From Mangiola and Riotota,[70] with permission.)

TABLE 8-4. Factors in the Electrocardiographic Diagnosis of Ventricular Tachycardia or Supraventricular Tachycardia with Aberration

	VT	SVT with Aberration
AV dissociation	+	−
Fusion beats	+	−
QRS width	>140 ms	<140 ms
QRS morphology		
RBBB	Monophasic, LAD	Triphasic, normal axis
LBBB	Wide R in lead V_1	−
	RAD	−
Onset	PVC	PAC with ↑ QRS
CSM effective	− (<2%)	+ (30%)

Abbreviations: PAC, premature atrial concentration; CSM, carotid sinus massage; LAD, left axis deviation; LBBB, left bundle branch block; RAD, right axis deviation; RBBB, right bundle branch block; SVT, supraventricular tachycardia; PVC, premature ventricular contraction; VT, ventricular tachycardia.

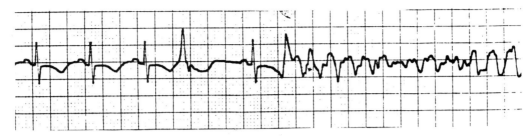

Fig. 8-38. Polymorphic ventricular tachycardia, or torsades de pointes in a patient with prolonged Q-T interval.

nerable period of the ECG, may trigger sustained ventricular tachycardia or fibrillation. In bigeminy, every other beat is a PVC, usually with a fixed coupling interval (Fig. 8-34). This may be from slow reentry or triggered activity. Medical therapy for isolated PVCs remains controversial, but frequent, multiform, or "R on T" beats may trigger sustained ventricular tachycardia or fibrillation, and probably should be suppressed.

Ventricular Tachycardia

Three or more consecutive PVCs occurring at a rate greater than 100 beats/min are defined as ventricular tachycardia (Fig. 8-37). If the rate is less than 100 beats/min, the term accelerated idioventricular rhythm is used. As with PVCs, differentiating ventricular tachycardia from supraventricular tachycardia with aberrancy is often very difficult.[62] Criteria which suggest ventricular tachycardia included wide QRS complex (>0.14 second), left axis deviation (>−60 degrees), fusion beats, certain QRS morphologies, and AV dissociation (Table 8-4). Establishing ventricular tachycardia as the diagnosis is of extreme importance. An AEG or esophageal lead may show evidence of atrioventricular dissociation, establishing the diagnosis of ventricular tachycardia. Immediate treatment, with antiarrhythmic drugs or electrical countershock is almost always indicated.

Polymorphic ventricular tachycardia, also known as torsades de pointes, is associated with prolongation of the Q-T interval on the surface ECG (Fig. 8-38). Acquired prolongation of the Q-T interval is seen with myocardial ischemia, myocarditis, intracranial pathology, hypothermia, and electrolyte abnormalities.[63] A number of drugs, most notably the class I-a antiarrhythmic agents such as procainamide, quinidine, and disopyramide can also cause torsades de pointes.[64] Treatment is aimed at short-

ening the Q-T interval, and includes rapid overdrive pacing, isoproterenol infusion, and intravenous magnesium.[65] In contrast, the congenitally prolonged QT syndromes are treated with beta-adrenergic blockers and/or surgical sympathectomy.[66] Cardiac arrest during anesthesia is a distinct possibility in this syndrome and preoperative institution of beta blockers is critical.[67]

Ventricular Fibrillation

Ventricular fibrillation is chaotic, asynchronous electrical activity of the ventricular myocardium, associated with minimal to no cardiac output. ECG tracings in ventricular fibrillation may show large amplitude (coarse) or low amplitude (fine) fibrillatory activity. Low-amplitude fibrillation may be confused with asystole, depending on the leads used for monitoring. Ventricular fibrillation requires immediate recognition and initiation of cardiopulmonary resuscitation including electrical defibrillation.

Asystole

Asystole is the absence of ventricular electrical activity, also known as cardiac standstill. No ventricular complexes are seen on ECG, although continued atrial activity may be seen. Immediate institution of CPR is required, with atropine, epinephrine, or temporary pacing. Care must be taken when a flat ECG tracing is seen not to assume ECG lead disconnection, and delay the diagnosis of asystole. Presence of an arterial pulse rules out asystole.

REFERENCES

1. Kurtz CM, Bennett JH, Shapiro HH: ECG studies during surgical anesthesia. JAMA 106:434, 1936
2. Vanik PE, Davis HS: Cardiac arrhythmias during halothane anesthesia. Anesth Analg 47:299, 1968

3. Kuner J, Enescu V, Utsu F et al: Cardiac arrhythmias during anesthesia. Dis Chest 52:580, 1967

4. Bertrand CA, Steiner NV, Jameson AG et al: Disturbances of cardiac rhythm during anesthesia and surgery. JAMA 216:1615, 1971

5. Angelini L, Feldman MI, Lufschonowski R et al: Cardiac arrhythmias during and after heart surgery: diagnosis and management. Prog Cardiovasc Dis 16:469, 1974

6. Brodsky M, Wu D, Denes P et al: Arrhythmias documented by 24-hour continuous electrocardiographic monitoring in 50 male medical students without apparent heart disease. Am J Cardiol 39:390, 1977

7. Atlee JL III, Bosnjak ZJ: Mechanisms for cardiac dysrhythmias during anesthesia. Anesthesiology 72:347–74, 1990

8. Wojtczak JA: Basic Cellular Electrophysiology of the Heart. In Thys DM, Kaplan JA (eds): The ECG in Anesthesia and Critical Care. p. 115. Churchill Livingstone, New York, 1987

9. Hoffman BF, Rosen MR: Cellular mechanisms for cardiac arrhythmias. Circ Res 49:1, 1981

10. Gorgels APM, Vos MA, Brugada P et al: In: Brugada P, Wellens HJJ (eds): Cardiac Arrhythmias: Where to Go From Here? p. 147. Futura, New York, 1987

11. Rosen MR: Mechanisms for arrhythmias. Am J Cardiol 61:2A, 1988

12. Manolis AS, Estes NA III: Supraventricular tachycardia. Mechanisms and therapy. Arch Intern Med 147:1706, 1987

13. Akhtar M: Management of ventricular tachyarrhythmias. Part I. JAMA 247:671, 1982

14. Hollifield JW: Thiazide treatment of hypertension: effects of thiazide diuretics on serum potassium, magnesium, and ventricular ectopy. Am J Med 80:8, 1986

15. Denlinger JK, Kaplan JA, Lecky JH, Wollman H: Cardiovascular responses to calcium administered intravenously to man during halothane anesthesia. Anesthesiology 42:390, 1975

16. Royster RL, Johnston WE, Gravlee GP et al: Arrhythmias during venous cannulation prior to pulmonary artery catheter insertion. Anesth Analg 64:1214, 1985

17. Damen J, Bolton D: A prospective analysis of 1400 pulmonary artery catheterizations in patients undergoing cardiac surgery. Acta Anaesthesiol Scand 30:386, 1986

18. Weinberger M: The pharmacology and therapeutic use of theophylline. J Allergy Clin Immunol 73:525, 1984

19. Frommer DA, Kulig KW, Marx JA, Rumack B: Tricyclic antidepressant overdose: a review. JAMA 257:521, 1987

20. Bazaral MG, Norfleet EA: Comparison of CB_5 and V_5 leads for intraoperative electrocardiographic monitoring. Anesth Analg 60:849, 1981

21. Blackburn H, Taylor HL, Okimoto N et al: Standardization of the exercise electrocardiogram: a systematic comparison of chest lead configurations employed for monitoring during exercise. p. 101. In Karvonen MJ, Barry AJ (eds): Physical Activity and the Heart. Charles C Thomas, Springfield, IL, 1967

22. Drew BJ: Bedside electrocardiographic monitoring: state of the art for the 1990s. Heart Lung 20:610, 1991

23. Kates RA, Zaidan JR, Kaplan JA: Esophageal lead for intraoperative electrocardiographic monitoring. Anesth Analg 61:781, 1982

24. Fletcher DR, Saunders RC: Technique of esophageal electrocardiography. p. 1690. In Hurst JW (ed): The Heart. 6th Ed. McGraw-Hill, New York, 1986

25. Katz A, Guetta V, Ovsyshcher IA: Transesophageal electrocardiography using a temporary pacing balloon-tipped electrode in acute cardiac care. Ann Emerg Med 20:961, 1991

26. Rice MJ, Atlee JL III: Electrocardiography: monitoring for arrhythmias. p 53. In Lake CL (ed): Clinical Monitoring. WB Saunders, Philadelphia, 1990

27. Parker EO III: Electrosurgical burn at the site of an esophageal temperature probe. Anesthesiology 61:93, 1984

28. Waldo AL, Henthorn RW, Pluab VJ: Temporary epicardial wire electrodes in the diagnosis and treatment of arrhythmias after open heart surgery. Am J Surg 148:275, 1984

29. Lombness PM: Taking the mystery out of rhythm interpretation: atrial electrograms. Heart Lung 21:415, 1992

30. Waldo AL, Kaiser GA: Electrophysiologic consideration for the cardiac surgical patient. p. 241. In Litwak RS, Jurado RA (eds): Care of the Cardiac Surgical Patient. Appleton-Century-Crofts, East Norwalk, CT, 1982

31. Schultz CK, Woodall CE: Using epicardial pacing electrodes. J Cardiovasc Nurs 3:25, 1989

32. Donovan KD, Power BM, Hockings BE et al: Usefulness of atrial electrocardiograms recorded via central venous catheters in the diagnosis of complex cardiac arrhythmias. Crit Care Med 21:532, 1993

33. Martin JT: Neuroanesthetic adjuncts for surgery in the sitting position. III. Intravascular electrocardiography. Anesth Analg 49:793, 1970

34. Kint PP, Spaa W, van den Berg A et al: Recording the right atrial electrogram through the fluid column of a pulmonary catheter. Crit Care Med 13:982, 1985

35. Vincent JL: New development in pulmonary artery catheterization. Int Care World 3:42, 1986

36. Ehrenwerth J: Electrical safety. p 625. In Barash PG, Cullen BF, Stoelting RK (eds): Clinical Anesthesia. JB Lippincott, Philadelphia, 1989

37. Barker SJ, Tremper KK: Physics applied to anesthesia. In Barash PG, Cullen BF, Stoelting RK (eds): Clinical Anesthesia. JB Lippincott, London, 1989
38. Geddes LA, Tacker WA, Rosborough J et al: The electrical doses for ventricular defibrillation with electrodes applied directly to the heart. J Thorac Cardiovasc Surg 68:593, 1974
39. Watson AB, Wright JS, Loughman J: Electrical thresholds for ventricular fibrillation in man. Med J Aust 1:1179, 1973
40. Becker CM, Malhotra IV, Hedley-Whyte J: The distribution of radiofrequency current and burns. Anesthesiology 38:106, 1973
41. Menon DK, Peden CJ, Hall AS et al: Magnetic resonance for the anesthetist. Part I. Physical principles, applications, safety aspects. Anaesthesia 47:240, 1992
42. Tobin JR, Spurrier EA, Wetzel RC: Anaesthesia for critically ill children during magnetic resonance imaging. Br J Anaesth 69:482, 1992
43. Roth JL, Nugent M, Gray JE et al: Patient monitoring during magnetic resonance imaging. Anesthesiology 62:80, 1985
44. Brown RE, Galford RE: Sinus tachycardia. p. 67. In Galford RE (ed): Problems in Anesthesiology: Approach to Diagnosis. Little, Brown, Boston, 1992
45. Kennedy DJ, Galford RE: Sinus bradycardia. p. 71. In Galford RE (ed): Problems in Anesthesiology: Approach to Diagnosis. Little, Brown, Boston, 1992
46. Zaidan JR: Electrocardiography. p. 587. In Barash PG, Cullen BF, Stoelting RK (eds): Clinical Anesthesia. JB Lippincott, Philadelphia, 1989
47. Singer DH, Ten Eick RE: Aberrancy: electrophysiologic aspects. Am J Cardiol 28:381, 1971
48. Josephson ME, Kastor JA: Supraventricular tachycardia: mechanisms and management. [Review]. Ann Intern Med 87:346, 1977
49. Wu D: Supraventricular tachycardias. JAMA 249:3357, 1983
50. Scarpa WJ: The sick sinus syndrome. Am Heart J 92:648, 1976
51. Shine KI, Kastor JA, Yurchak PM: Multifocal atrial tachycardia: clinical and electrocardiographic features in 32 patients. N Engl J Med 279:344, 1968
52. Levine JL, Michael JR, Guarnieri T: Multifocal atrial tachycardia: a toxic effect of theophylline. Lancet 1:12, 1985
53. Josephson ME, Wellens HJ: Differential diagnosis of supraventricular tachycardia. Cardiol Clin 8:411, 1990
54. Richardson JM: Ventricular preexcitation: practical considerations. Arch Intern Med 143:760, 1983
55. Mandel WJ, Laks MM, Obayashi K et al: The Wolff-Parkinson-White syndrome: pharmacologic effects of procaine amide. Am Heart J 90:744, 1975
56. Platia EV, Michelson EL, Porterfield JK et al: Esmolol versus verapamil in the acute treatment of atrial fibrillation or atrial flutter. Am J Cardiol 63:925, 1989
57. Fenster PE, Comess KA, Marsh R et al: Conversion of atrial fibrillation to sinus rhythm by acute intravenous procainamide infusion. Am Heart J 106:501, 1983
58. Dunn M, Alexander J, de Silva R et al: Antithrombotic therapy in atrial fibrillation. [Review]. Chest 89:68S, 1986
59. Wells JL Jr, MacLean WA, James TN et al: Characterization of atrial flutter: studies in man after open heart surgery using fixed atrial electrodes. Circulation 50:665, 1979
60. Waldo AL, Wells JL Jr, Cooper TB et al: Temporary cardiac pacing: applications and techniques in the treatment of cardiac arrhythmias. [Review]. Prog Cardiovasc Dis 23:451, 1981
61. Platia EV, Waclawski SH, Pluth TA et al: Management of acute-onset atrial fibrillation/flutter: esmolol vs verapamil vs digoxin vs placebo, abstracted. Circulation 76(suppl IV):520, 1987
62. Wellens HJ, Bar FW, Lie KI: The value of the electrocardiogram in the differential diagnosis of a tachycardia with a widened QRS complex. Am J Med 64:27, 1978
63. Galloway PA, Glass PS: Anesthetic implications of prolonged QT interval syndromes. [Review]. Anesth Analg 64:612, 1985
64. Roden DM, Woosley L, Primm PK: Incidence and clinical features of the quinidine-associated long QT syndrome: implications for patient care. Am Heart J 111:1088, 1986
65. Tzivoni D, Banai S, Schuger C et al: Treatment of torsade de pointes with magnesium sulfate. Circulation 77:392, 1988
66. Moss AJ, McDonald J: Unilateral cervicothoracic sympathetic ganglionectomy for the treatment of the long QT interval syndrome. N Engl J Med 285:903, 1971
67. Medak R, Benumof JL: Perioperative management of the prolonged QT interval syndrome. Br J Anaesth 55:361, 1983
68. Royster RL: Causes and consequences of arrhythmias. p. 228. In Benumof JL, Saidman JL (eds): Anesthesia and Perioperative Complications. Mosby Year Book, St. Louis, 1992
69. Stoelting RK: Heart. p. 692. In: Pharmacology and Physiology in Anesthetic Practice. 2nd Ed. JB Lippincott, Philadelphia, 1991
70. Mangiola S, Ritota J: Basic Principles: Cardiac Arrhythmias. JB Lippincott, Philadelphia, 1974
71. Fozzard HA, Arnsdorf MR: Cardiac physiology. p. 24. In Fozzard HA, Haber E, Jennings RB et al (eds):

The Heart and Cardiovascular System. Raven Press, New York, 1986

72. Chung EK: Electrocardiography: Practical Applications with Vectorial Principles. 3rd Ed. Appleton-Century-Crofts, East Norwalk, CT, 1985

73. Kaplan JA, Thys DM: Electrocardiography. In Miller RD (ed): Anesthesia. 3rd Ed. Churchill Livingstone, New York, 1990

74. Zipes DP: Cardiac arrhythmias. p. 176. In Kelley WN (ed): Textbook of Internal Medicine. JB Lippincott, Philadelphia, 1989

75. Conover MB: Understanding Electrocardiography. 6th Ed. Mosby Year Book, St. Louis, 1992

76. Marriott HJL: Practical Electrocardiography. 7th Ed. Williams & Wilkins, Baltimore, 1983

77. Royster RL, Robertie PG: Recognition and treatment of ectopic beats. Anesthesiol Clin North Am 7:315, 1989

Central Venous Pressure Monitoring

9

Charles W. Otto

Over the past quarter-century, central venous cannulation has become a standard part of medical practice and the indications for placement of central venous catheters have expanded rapidly. In the critically ill, measurement of central pressures gives a more accurate assessment of hemodynamic status than clinical evaluation and such measurements prompt changes in therapy.[1] Most discussions of cardiovascular physiology and central pressures focus on pulmonary artery occlusion pressure (PAOP) and left ventricular function because they are the primary determinants of systemic blood flow. Right atrial or central venous pressure (CVP) reflects the preload of the right ventricle. If the function of the right and left ventricles is discordant, a pulmonary artery catheter may be necessary to accurately assess left heart function. However, there are strong theoretical and practical reasons for continuing to measure CVP, whether or not a pulmonary artery catheter is used. There are a significant number of situations in which right ventricular dysfunction is the limiting step in cardiac performance. CVP measurement is invaluable in these circumstances. Conversely, there are also many occasions when right and left ventricular function is consistent, and CVP measurements are as useful as PAOP measurements. Passing a catheter through the right heart is associated with potential complications not found with CVP measurement. As a practical matter, there are times when the urgency of the clinical situation will not allow pulmonary artery catheterization.

This chapter takes the point of view that CVP measurement does provide useful information about cardiovascular status whether or not pulmonary artery occlusion pressures are measured. Throughout this chapter, the terms central venous pressure and right atrial pressure will be used interchangeably. In order to have a pressure gradient for blood flow, there must be a slight pressure difference between the right atrium and the superior vena cava or innominate vein. However, in clinical use, pressure measurement is not always within the right atrium, but the value obtained is treated as right atrial pressure. As with all cardiovascular measurements, a "normal" value and range can be stated (in the right atrium: 3 mmHg with a range of 0 to 7 mmHg). However, the measurement can be interpreted only within the context of overall cardiovascular function and with a thorough understanding of the limitations and possible errors in measurement. Because of the limitations of the technique, *changes* in CVP with changes in patient status or therapeutic intervention are more reliable indicators of hemodynamic function than any single measurement.

CARDIOVASCULAR PHYSIOLOGY

The regulation of cardiac output and its distribution to the tissues is an enormously complex system, even in the normal organism. When derangements such as disease or trauma occur, reflex responses both intrinsic and extrinsic to the cardiovascular system complicate matters even further. Yet, clinicians are frequently required to make therapeutic judgments about the state of the system with less than complete information. To do so with some accuracy requires a thorough understanding

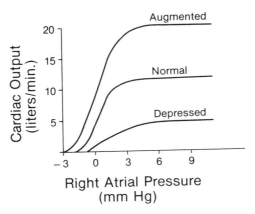

Fig. 9-1. Frank-Starling cardiac function curves.

of basic circulatory physiology and the usual responses to various insults. For a complete review of cardiovascular physiology, the reader is referred to a standard text.[2] In the following sections, we will try to review some essential concepts as they relate to interpreting central venous pressures.

Clinically, measurement of the CVP is used for two purposes: (1) to gain information about cardiac function, and (2) to gain information about the adequacy of vascular volume. It performs this dual function because physiologically the right atrial pressure is the interface between the two major determinants of cardiac output: cardiac function and venous return. Because CVP influences, and is influenced by, both of these physiologic functions, it is an extremely useful measure of car-

diovascular function. For the same reason, it also can be confusing and difficult to interpret.

Right Atrial Pressure and Cardiac Function

The relationship between right atrial pressure and cardiac output is usually expressed by the classic Frank-Starling cardiac function curve (Fig. 9-1). The major determinants of cardiac function are preload, afterload, heart rate, and myocardial contractility. The relationship between preload and cardiac output is expressed in the cardiac function curve where right atrial pressure is a measure of preload. Any factor that increases heart rate or contractility or decreases afterload will cause a greater cardiac output at the same preload (augmented curve in Fig. 9-1). Similarly, a decrease in heart rate or contractility or increase in afterload will result in a lower cardiac output at the same CVP (depressed curve in Fig. 9-1). Some of these factors are summarized in Table 9-1.

Pressure Versus Volume: Variable Compliance Systems

The cardiac function curve uses the right atrial pressure to represent preload. More accurately, preload is the resting myocardial fiber length or, in the intact heart, end-diastolic ventricular volume. Right atrial pressure is used to predict right ventricular end-diastolic volume. Unfortunately, the relationship between pressure and volume is not linear (Fig. 9-2). The ventricles of the heart (as well as many biologic systems) are variable compliance

TABLE 9-1. Factors Influencing Cardiac Output at Constant Right Atrial Pressure

Factors That Increase Cardiac Output	Factors That Decrease Cardiac Output

↑ Heart rate
   Sympathetic stimulation
   β-Adrenergic stimulation
	↓ Heart rate
	   Parasympathetic stimulation
	   β-Adrenergic blockade

↑ Contractility
   Sympathetic stimulation
   β-Adrenergic stimulation
	↓ Contractility
	   Myocardial ischemia
	   Myocardial disease
	   β-Adrenergic blockade

↓ Afterload
   Decreased arteriolar resistance
	↑ Afterload
	   Increased arteriolar resistance
	   Aortic stenosis

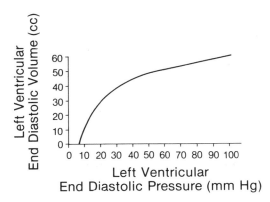

Fig. 9-2. The relationship between left ventricular end-diastolic pressure and left ventricular end-diastolic volume in the dog is an example of a variable compliance system. Compliance is defined as the change in volume divided by the change in pressure ($\Delta V / \Delta P$). A constant compliance system would result in a straight line.

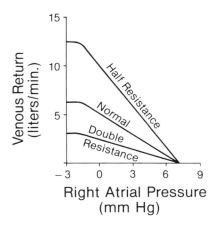

Fig. 9-4. Effect of resistance on venous return.

systems. The ventricles are able to expand to accept a greater volume of blood with very little change in pressure. When the limit of expansion is reached, pressures rises rapidly with little change in volume. Consequently, as diastolic volume increases, cardiac output will increase with little change in right atrial pressure, accounting for the nearly vertical part of the cardiac function curve (Fig. 9-1), until the limits of ventricular expansion are reached. At that point, cardiac output no longer improves, but right atrial pressure increases rapidly.

Just as with the cardiac function curves, the pressure-volume relationship is not constant. Disease states and different physiologic states can change the position and shape of the curve. Consequently, a single measurement of right atrial pressure cannot accurately predict end-diastolic volume, just as it cannot predict the cardiac output. However, determining the compliance (i.e., the change in pressure for a given change in volume) will add valuable information about the system.

Right Atrial Pressure and Venous Return

The relationship between right atrial pressure and venous return is shown in Figure 9-3. Two important concepts are obvious from this graph. Decreasing right atrial pressure below zero causes very little increase in venous return because veins leading into the thorax tend to collapse. Above a right atrial pressure of zero, venous return is linearly related to the difference between mean systemic pressure and right atrial pressure. There are two major determinants of the position of the venous return curve: mean systemic pressure and resistance to venous return. Figure 9-3 demonstrates that changes in mean systemic pressure cause a parallel change in venous return. Changing resistance causes a change in slope of the curve as shown in Figure 9-4. In most clinical situations, changes in mean systemic pressure are much more important than changes in resistance. The major factors influencing venous return through changes in mean systemic pressure and resistance are summarized in Table 9-2.

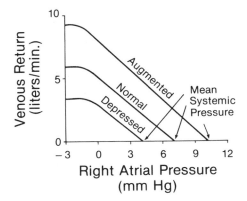

Fig. 9-3. Effect of mean systemic pressure on venous return.

TABLE 9-2. Factors Influencing Venous Return at Constant Right Atrial Pressure

Factors That Increase Venous Return	Factors That Decrease Venous Return

↑ Mean systemic pressure
  ↑ Sympathetic stimulation
  α-Adrenergic stimulation
  ↑ Vascular volume
	↓ Mean systemic pressure
	  ↓ Sympathetic stimulation
	  α-Adrenergic blockade
	  ↓ Vascular volume

↓ Resistance
  Anemia
  Arteriovenous fistulas
  Pregnancy
  Thyrotoxicosis
	↑ Resistance
	  Polycythemia

Venous Return and the Vascular Variable Compliance System

Just as the heart demonstrates variable compliance, the vascular system is able to adjust to changes in volume with minimal changes in pressure. A rapid increase in vascular volume results in a rapid increase in venous return as well as right atrial and mean systemic pressures. Within seconds, circulatory reflexes begin to adjust these pressures and venous return toward normal. In addition, stress relaxation of the vasculature (not dependent on autonomic reflexes) allows further compensation over the ensuing minutes. Similar compensation occurs for decreases in vascular volume. Consequently, a single measurement of right atrial pressure (or even mean systemic pressure, if that were possible) cannot accurately predict vascular volume. However, determining the compliance of the system can provide valuable clues to the status of the vascular volume.

CENTRAL VENOUS PRESSURE MEASUREMENT

Clinical Utilization

From the preceding discussion, it is obvious that CVP is an important determinant of both cardiac output and venous return. It is also obvious that numerous other factors influence the CVP, cardiac output, and venous return. Central venous pressure measurement alone will not allow correct clinical decisions. When the CVP measurement is combined with other clinical observations and other influencing factors are considered, it can be an important adjunct to clinical management.

The most common reasons for CVP measurement are to help determine the state of cardiac function and the state of vascular volume. As can be seen in Table 9-3, a single measurement of the CVP helps somewhat in defining circulatory status but leaves considerable overlap in possible interpretations.

Using Compliance To Improve Interpretation

Rapid changes in vascular volume can help further define the cardiovascular status if the time course of compliance changes are remembered. A rapid infusion of 300 to 500 ml of fluid in a normovolemic adult with good cardiac function will result in a moderate increase in CVP (2 to 4 mmHg) with a return nearly to baseline within 10 to 15 minutes. A minimal initial rise in CVP implies a reduced vascular volume. A large initial rise in CVP implies a heart which is noncompliant or an elevated vascular volume or both. If the CVP returns to baseline rapidly (within 5 minutes), it implies a reduced vascular volume that can accommodate additional volume by rapid changes in vasomotor tone. A slower return toward baseline indicates that stress relaxation is occurring and the vascular volume is closer to normal. A prolonged return to baseline implies that vascular volume is elevated for the current cardiac status. Table 9-4 indicates how a volume challenge can improve the interpretation made on the basis of the CVP alone.

The addition of information about cardiac output can further improve diagnostic accuracy (Table

**TABLE 9-3. Possible Interpretations of a
Single Central Venous Pressure Measurement**

CVP	Cardiac Status	Vascular Volume
Below normal	Depressed	Reduced
	Normal	Reduced
	Hyperdynamic	Reduced
		Normal
Normal	Depressed	Reduced
		Normal
		Elevated
	Normal	Reduced
		Normal
		Elevated
	Hyperdynamic	Normal
		Elevated
Above normal	Depressed	Reduced
		Normal
		Elevated
	Normal	Elevated
	Hyperdynamic	Elevated

9-4). Actual measurement of cardiac output is best, but frequently indirect assessment using clinical signs may be enough to provide the additional data needed. For example, the patient with a low CVP who has a small response to a fluid bolus and moderate return toward baseline could have either a depressed cardiac status with a reduced vascular volume or a hyperdynamic heart with a relatively normal vascular volume. Determining which situation exists in a given patient should not be difficult using clinical signs.

Techniques and Errors

Over the years, a number of techniques have been used to estimate central venous pressure. Inspection of jugular venous pulsations in the neck, comparing the height of pulsations in the neck with the distance above the right atrium, can provide clues to the CVP. Significant hepatojugular reflux (marked increase in the height of jugular venous pulsations during firm pressure over the liver) is particularly indicative of a high CVP. Cannulation and measurement of peripheral venous pressure has also been used, but has many potential errors because valves in the venous system inhibit distal transmission of flow and pressure. These indirect measurements have largely been supplanted by measurement of CVP through catheters placed within the central vessels of the chest.

Calibrated Transducer Versus Water Manometer

Originally, central venous pressures were measured using a column of water in a marked manometer. The CVP is the height of the column in cm of H_2O when the zero point of the column is at the level of the right atrium and the fluid reaches equilibrium when allowed to flow freely into or out of the central venous catheter. Alternatively, CVP is measured using a transducer properly calibrated in mmHg, connected to the central venous catheter, placed at the level of the right atrium and the pressure waveform displayed on an oscilloscope or paper. The difference in units of measurement between these two methods should not be forgotten when switching from one technique to another. The relative density (specific gravity) of mercury to water is 13.6. Thus, a 1-mm column of mercury would have the same weight as a 1.36-cm column of water. At low pressures, these differences are not very great, but at higher pressures they can become significant (Table 9-5).

The main advantage of water manometer measurement is simplicity. The CVP can be measured easily and quickly by connecting widely available disposable plastic tubes to the central venous catheter. The major disadvantages of this system are the inability to analyze the CVP waveform and the relatively slow response of the water column to changes in intrathoracic pressure. The latter can lead to an overestimation of the central venous pressure during mechanical ventilation and, occasionally, an underestimation during spontaneous ventilation (Fig. 9-5). With the widespread use of electronic pressure monitoring for arterial and pulmonary artery pressures, calibrated transducer measurement of CVP has become more common. Because it is generally more accurate and allows observation of the waveform, transducer measurement is preferred when it is available.

The Central Venous Waveform

A typical central venous waveform is shown in Figure 9-5. It consists of three positive deflections labeled the a-, c-, and v-waves as well as two major depressions labeled the x- and y-descents. The a-wave represents the increase in right atrial pressure

TABLE 9-4. Possible Interpretations of Central Venous Pressure Measurement with Volume Challenge

CVP	Initial[a] Increase	Return to Baseline	Cardiac Status	Vascular Volume	Cardiac Output
Below normal	+	Rapid	Normal	Reduced	Low
			Hyperdynamic	Reduced	Low to normal
	+ to ++	Moderate	Depressed	Reduced	Very low
			Hyperdynamic	Normal	High
Normal	+ to ++	Rapid	Normal	Reduced	Low to normal
	++	Moderate	Normal	Normal	Normal
			Hyperdynamic	Normal	High
	++	Slow	Normal	Elevated	High
			Hyperdynamic	Elevated	Very high
	+++	Rapid	Depressed	Reduced	Very low
	+++	Moderate	Depressed	Normal	Low
	+++	Slow	Depressed	Elevated	Low to normal
Above normal	++	Moderate	Normal	Elevated	High
			Hyperdynamic	Elevated	Very high
	+++	Moderate	Depressed	Reduced	Very low
	+++	Slow	Depressed	Normal	Low
			Depressed	Elevated	Low to normal

[a] + = minimal, ++ = moderate, +++ = large.

that occurs during atrial contraction. Originally thought to be related to carotid expansion when observing jugular venous pulsations, the c-wave is more likely caused by a slight elevation of the tricuspid valve into the right atrium during early ventricular contraction. The x-descent corresponds to the period of ventricular ejection and reflects the emptying of blood from the heart. The v-wave is the increase in atrial pressure that occurs as venous return continues while the tricuspid valve is closed. The y-descent is the drop in atrial pressure that occurs when the tricuspid valve opens and blood flows into the right ventricle.

Changes in the typical waveform pattern occur in many pathologic conditions. The a-wave will be absent in atrial fibrillation. In atrioventricular dissociation, frequent cannon a-waves (very large a-waves) will be seen whenever the atrium contracts against a closed tricuspid valve. In cardiac tamponade and constrictive pericarditis, the right atrial, right ventricular diastolic, pulmonary artery occlusion and left ventricular diastolic pressures are elevated and nearly equal to each other. The x- and y-descents are exaggerated and very rapid in constrictive pericarditis, whereas the prominent y-descent is absent is absent in cardiac tamponade.[3] When tricuspid regurgitation is present, the c-wave and x-descent will be replaced by a large positive regurgitant wave. The presence of regurgitant waves can make interpretation of the central venous pressure difficult. By convention, the CVP is usually taken as the mean of the pressure fluctuations in the central venous waveform. A large positive deflection caused by regurgitant flow during right ventricular systole will significantly elevate the mean pressure. However, this pressure does not truly reflect the filling pressure of the right ventricle. In such cases, a better measure of the right ventricular preload is the lower pressure measured between regurgitant waves.

Intrathoracic Pressure

Because the central veins are located inside the thorax, CVP measurements are influenced by changes in intrathoracic pressure. Respiration

TABLE 9-5. Equivalent Pressures with Water Manometer and Calibrated Transducer

cmH$_2$O	mmHg
1	1.36
3	2.2
5	3.7
10	7.4
15	11
20	14.6

causes the CVP to flucuate, decreasing with a spontaneous inspiration and rising with a forced exhalation or with a positive pressure mechanical inspiration (Fig. 9-5). To minimize these effects, CVP measurement should be taken at end exhalation when the muscles of respiration are at rest and intrathoracic pressure is stable at its resting level. Measurements taken at this point in the respiratory cycle will be consistent from breath to breath. When using a water manometer, it has been common practice to disconnect the ventilator for a brief period during CVP measurement. This practice can lead to other errors and is unnecessary when using a calibrated transducer for measurement.

By convention, vascular pressures (CVP, arterial, etc.) are measured relative to atmosphere by opening the transducer system to air to establish the zero baseline. Positive end-expiratory pressure (PEEP) applied to the airway may be partially transmitted to the intrathoracic structures. Therefore, part of the pressure in the central veins measured relative to atmosphere while a patient is receiving PEEP may be due to the airway pressure. This effect rarely is significant if PEEP is less than 7.5 cmH$_2$O. The cardiovascular consequence of an increase in CVP due to airway pressure is to reduce venous return and, thus, cardiac output. The reduction in venous return is easily predicted from the venous return curve (Fig. 9-3). Since most of the vasculature is outside the thorax, an elevation of the CVP relative to atmosphere will reduce the pressure gradient for venous return unless there is a compensatory increase in mean systemic pressure. The effect of PEEP on cardiac output can be more confusing. According to the Frank-Starling curve (Fig. 9-1), if PEEP causes an increase in right atrial pressure, the cardiac output should rise. But the opposite effect is observed. CVP measured relative to atmosphere is a good estimate of preload under many circumstances because intrathoracic pressure remains constant. However, because the heart lies within the thorax, a more accurate measure of preload is the pressure difference across the wall of the heart, intravascular pressure minus intrapleural pressure (transmural pressure). When PEEP is applied, airway pressure is transmitted to all intrathoracic structures and pleural pressure increases more than right atrial pressure so that transmural pressure actually decreases.[4] Consequently, cardiac output is reduced, although the CVP measured relative to atmosphere increases.

Clinically, a reduction in cardiac output and a rise in CVP associated with the application of PEEP could be interpreted as a deterioration in cardiac function. One solution to this problem is to measure the CVP when the PEEP has been removed. However, both practical and theoretical considerations make this approach unadvisable. The beneficial effects of PEEP on gas exchange are lost very quickly when it is removed and may take a prolonged period to recover when PEEP is reapplied. Thus, removing PEEP subjects the patient to the dangers of hypoxemia. If PEEP is causing a significant elevation in CVP and reduction in cardiac output, then removing PEEP will allow an increase in venous return and the cardiovascular status will no longer be the same as when the PEEP is being applied. Therefore, one erroneous measurement is merely being exchanged for another. Although a number of rules of thumb and formulas have been

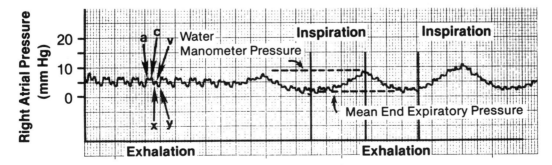

Fig. 9-5. Typical CVP waveform of a patient receiving controlled mechanical ventilation, a-, c-, v-waves and x-, y-descents are indicated (see text). The lowest pressure measured by a water manometer is often the highest pressure seen during the respiratory cycle, whereas the desired pressure is that at the end of exhalation.

proposed, the only accurate method of compensating for the effects of PEEP is to measure transmural pressures. Unfortunately, simple accurate measurement of intrathoracic pressure in the clinical setting is difficult. From a practical standpoint, PEEP does not usually cause a large change in the CVP; and it is best not to remove PEEP for measurements, recognizing that the numbers obtained may be slightly higher than would be found without PEEP.

TECHNIQUES OF CENTRAL VENOUS CANNULATION

General Considerations

Indications

With improvement of techniques leading to increased safety and success in central venous cannulation, the indications for placing catheters in the central circulation have expanded rapidly. The most common indications are listed in Table 9-6.

Venipuncture Techniques

Regardless of the site of insertion, the techniques used for introducing the definitive catheter into the central circulation can be categorized as one of three basic types: catheter-over-the-needle, catheter-through-the-needle, or catheter-over-a-guidewire. In recent years, the last technique has largely superseded the first two.

TABLE 9-6. Common Indications for Central Venous Cannulation

Measurement of central venous pressure
Rapid administration of fluids and blood
Insertion of pulmonary artery catheter
Insertion of transvenous pacemaker
Parenteral alimentation
Temporary single cannula hemodialysis
Long-term chemotherapy
Inability to cannulate peripheral veins for venous
  access
Operations in which venous air embolism is possible
Administration of drugs that cause sclerosis of
  peripheral veins
Frequent blood sampling
Frequent therapeutic plasmapheresis

Catheter-Over-the-Needle

When an over-the-needle catheter is used, the entire assembly of needle and catheter must be of a length sufficient to reach the central circulation. The most common length is 5.5 to 6 inches (12 to 15 cm), which allows the catheter to reach the superior vena cava from the jugular or subclavian veins (Fig. 9-6). The catheter usually is tapered to aid passage through the skin and subcutaneous tissue and fits closely over the needle. Following venipuncture, the needle-catheter assembly is advanced into the vein 3 to 4 mm and the catheter advanced into the vein. The needle is removed and discarded. The most common technical difficulty with this technique is having the needle tip within the vein but the leading edge of the catheter still outside. Consequently, when attempts to pass the catheter are made, it "hangs up" on the vessel wall. This problem can be minimized by ensuring that the distance between the needle bevel and catheter is small (less than ⅛ inch), by ensuring that the entire assembly is well inside the vein before advancing the catheter and by being careful to advance the catheter off the needle and not to withdraw the needle into the catheter before advancing the catheter. An advantage of this technique is that the catheter completely occupies the hole made in the vessel wall, resulting in minimal leakage. Additionally, the entire insertion is accomplished in a single step minimizing the time during which the vein is open to atmosphere and minimizing the risk of air embolism. A disadvantage is that many operators find it unwieldy to manage the long needle-catheter assembly. The tapered catheter tip also may be slightly more prone to perforating vein walls than other catheter types. With this technique, the operator is restricted in the choice of definitive catheter to the single-lumen catheter in the needle-catheter assembly.

Catheter-Through-the-Needle

Catheter-through-the-needle techniques were originally developed for cannulation of arm veins but also have been used for subclavian and, less frequently, internal jugular cannulation. In this technique, a venipuncture is performed with a self-contained device depending on the flashback of blood to indicate entrance into the vein (Fig. 9-7) or with a syringe attached to the needle to aspirate blood upon entrance into the vein. A catheter is

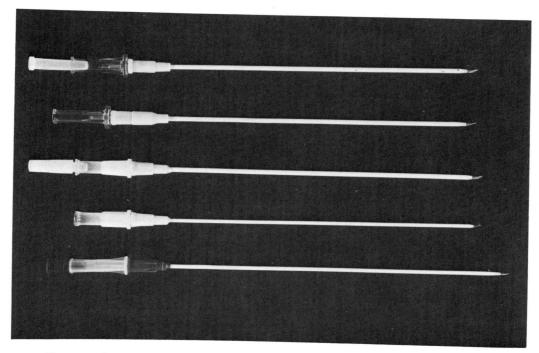

Fig. 9-6. $5^{1}/_{2}$- and 6-inch over-the-needle Teflon catheters of 14 and 16 gauge.

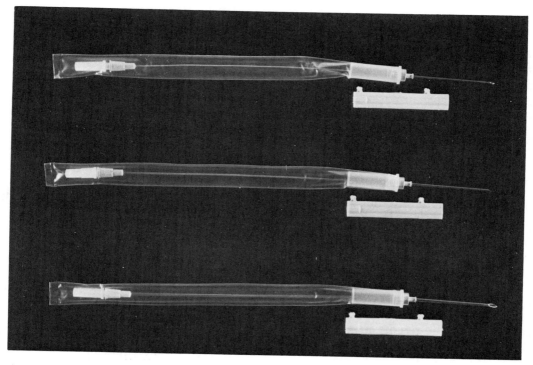

Fig. 9-7. Polyvinyl chloride through-the-needle catheter assemblies. The protective needle sheath is shown just below each needle. *Top:* 19-gauge needle with 22-gauge catheter. *Middle:* 17-gauge needle with 18.5-gauge catheter. *Bottom:* 14-gauge needle with 16-gauge catheter.

then advanced through the needle to its proper position and the needle withdrawn. Since the needle usually cannot be removed past the hub of the catheter, a protective sheath must fix the needle to the catheter to ensure that the catheter is not cut by the sharp edge of the needle. With this technique, it is possible to use a more pliable catheter with a blunt tip because the catheter does not have to pass through subcutaneous tissues.

Disadvantages of this technique include possible leakage around the puncture site because the catheter is smaller than the hole made by the needle and the necessity of making the venipuncture with a very large needle if a large intravenous line is desired (e.g., a 14-gauge needle is necessary to pass a 16-gauge catheter). The major drawback of this technique is the possibility of shearing the catheter on the sharp needle edge and subsequent catheter embolism if attempts are made to withdraw the catheter into the needle during insertion. There is a common variation on this technique that eliminates this danger. The initial venipuncture is performed with an over-the-needle cannula, the needle removed, and the definitive catheter is inserted through the short cannula. Surgical implantation of long-term central venous catheters frequently is performed using this variation and the guidewire and dilator technique. In this way, a very large, breakaway short cannula is placed through which a soft, long-term catheter is inserted. The short cannula then is removed and the wound closed. PICC (peripherally inserted central catheters) inserted via the basilic or cephalic veins utilize this methodology.

Catheter-Over-a-Guidewire

The catheter-over-a-guidewire method has come to dominate vascular access techniques in recent years. Originally described for use in arteriography in 1953[5] by Seldinger, it was adapted in 1974[6] for central venous cannulation through the external jugular vein by Blitt. In the direct Seldinger technique, a needle is inserted into a vessel and an angiographic wire catheter guide is passed through the needle. The needle is removed, and the definitive catheter is passed over the wire. The indirect or modified Seldinger approach uses a short over-the-needle cannula to gain vascular access and the wire is passed through the cannula. This is the preferred technique if manipulation of

wire is anticipated (e.g., external jugular cannulation) because it eliminates the danger of shearing the wire on the sharp edges of the needle. Use of a guidewire allows the initial venipuncture to be accomplished with a small needle or cannula, which is just large enough to accept the wire. This minimizes the danger of trauma to adjacent structures when cannulating deep veins that cannot be directly visualized. The technique also allows a wider selection of definitive catheters because the catheter inserted is not related to the venipuncture technique.

Insertion of relatively rigid, tapered catheters is easiest with this technique. More pliable or blunt catheters can be inserted by using a scalpel to widen the opening in the skin and underlying fascia around the wire. A short, firm, tapered dilator temporarily passed over the wire also helps provide a path through the tissues for the definitive catheter. A dilator is a necessity when inserting a very large cannula, such as a sheath, for use in pulmonary artery catheterization (Fig. 9-8). In such cases, the sheath is fitted over the dilator, and the two are passed over the guidewire and into the vein as a unit. The wire and dilator are removed, leaving the sheath in the vein. The guidewire technique is more elaborate than the other techniques, but it has become the method of choice for most central venous cannulations because it improves safety and success rates and allows selection of the best catheter for the situation.

Choice of Catheter

Intravenous catheters are made of a variety of materials because no single material is ideal for all uses. The most common materials are polyvinyl chloride (PVC), polypropylene, polyethylene, polyurethane, tetrafluoroethylene (Teflon), and Silastic (silicone elastomer or siliconized rubber) (Table 9-7). Most of these materials are relatively chemically inert, having been implant tested. However, leaching of plasticizers, antioxidants, and stabilizing agents from the plastic probably does contribute to the development of phlebitis in smaller veins when the catheters are in place. Silastic catheters are the most chemically inert, with Teflon and polyurethane intermediate in reactivity, and PVC, polypropylene, and polyethylene the most reactive. Thrombogenicity of catheter materials is closely related to chemical inertness but is also related to the

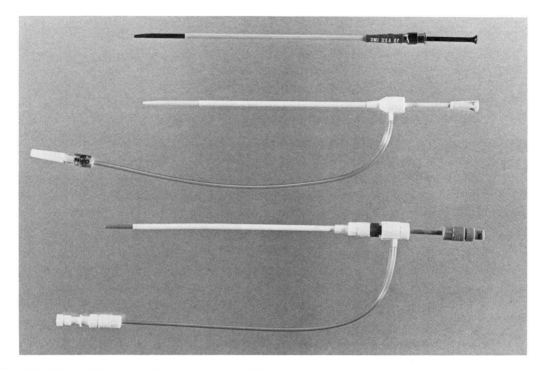

Fig. 9-8. Three dilator-sheath introducer combinations for passage of a pulmonary artery catheter.

smoothness of the catheter surface. Heavy metal salts (barium or bismuth) are added to the plastic to make it radiopaque. These agents increase the thrombogenicity of the catheter by causing the surface to become more irregular. However, radiopacity is important in central venous catheters, since the most commonly used method of determining the position of the catheter tip is by x-ray. Thrombogenicity may be reduced by imbedding the heavy metals within the wall of the catheter or

coating the catheter with a less thrombogenic substance (e.g., polyethylene and PVC can be siliconized). In addition, PVC catheters can be coated with heparin. This is common practice on pulmonary artery catheters and has been shown to decrease thrombus formation on the catheter for at least 48 hours.

Flexibility of a catheter is also related to the catheter material. A catheter that is relatively rigid in its longitudinal dimension helps passage through

TABLE 9-7. Comparison of Central Venous Catheter Materials

Type of Material	Chemical Inertness	Thrombogenicity	Flexibility	Transparent
Polyvinyl chloride	− − −	+ + +	+ +	Yes
Siliconized polyvinyl chloride	−	+ +	+ +	Yes
Polyethylene	− −	+ + +	+ +	Yes
Polypropylene	− −	+ + +	+ +	Yes
Siliconized polypropylene	0	+	+ +	Yes or no
Teflon	−	+	+	No
Silastic	0	0	+ + + +	No
Polyurethane	− −	+	+ + +	No

0 = none, + = minimal, + + moderate, + + + and + + + + large, − less, − − much less, − − − markedly less.

skin and subcutaneous tissues. However, the same rigidity may contribute to the catheter perforating a vessel wall. Teflon is the most rigid of the catheter materials, with PVC, polyethylene, and polypropylene intermediate in stiffness. Polyurethane catheters are significantly softer but retain enough rigidity to enable easy insertion. This combination has led to most multilumen central catheters being made of polyurethane. Silastic catheters are so flexible that they are difficult to manipulate into a vein without a stylet or guidewire, even when there is no drag from skin and subcutaneous tissues.

The choice of a catheter must be made on an individual basis, taking into consideration the primary purpose of the catheter. Long-term intravenous alimentation or chemotherapy probably warrants the most flexible and least reactive material available. Consequently, Silastic catheters would seem to be the best choice, with siliconized polypropylene as an alternative. When rapid central venous access is desired for administration of fluids or blood, a catheter that is easiest to insert is desired. Under such circumstances, the stiffness of Teflon may be helpful, with PVC or polyethylene as alternatives. For general, short-term use, polyurethane catheters provide a good compromise between Teflon and Silastic catheters, although all the materials have proven suitable. Catheters with side holes at the distal end are valuable because they virtually eliminate aspiration difficulties.

Multiple-lumen catheters have become increasingly popular for central venous use. These catheters have two to four lumens with individual connections for infusions and separated openings on the intravascular portion of the catheter (usually at the tip, 2 and 5 cm from the tip) (Fig. 9-9). Lumen size varies with catheter size and number of lumens. Double-lumen catheters as large as two 14-gauge lumens are available in 8-French catheters. The most common multilumen catheter materials are polyurethane and polyethylene. Multiple-lumen catheters are especially useful when multiple drug infusions (that may be incompatible with each other) need to be given centrally.

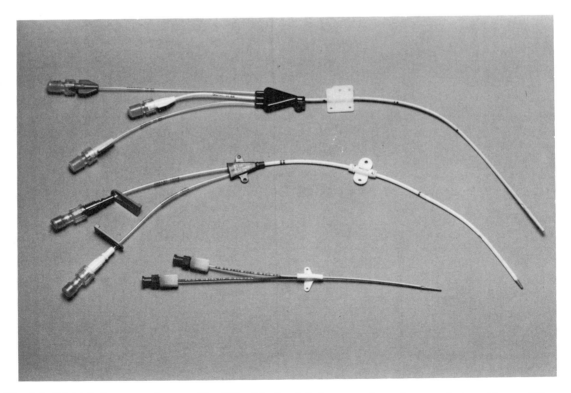

Fig. 9-9. Multiple lumen catheters. *Top:* 7 Fr., 8-inch triple-lumen polyurethane catheter with one 16-gauge and two 18-gauge lumens. *Middle:* 7 Fr., 8-inch double-lumen polyurethane catheter with 14-gauge and 18-gauge lumens. *Bottom:* 5 Fr., 3¹/₄-inch polyethylene double-lumen catheter with two 20-gauge lumens.

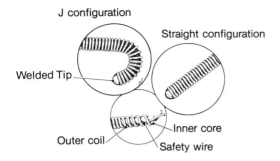

Fig. 9-10. Construction of a flexible angiographic wire catheter guide.

Guidewires

Flexible angiographic wire catheter guides used in the Seldinger techniques of central venous cannulation are available in many sizes, shapes, and lengths. The most common guides consist of an inner core wire with an outer coiled wire (Fig. 9-10). Although the inner core can be movable in relationship to the outer coil, this provides little advantage in central venous cannulation, and the usual wires have the core fixed to the outer coil. To minimize possible vessel damage by the wire, a short length at the end of the wire is made more flexible by tapering the inner core. When using a guidewire, the user should always check that the end of the wire to be inserted is the one with the extra flexibility.

The flexible end of the wire can be made straight or with a permanent curve (J-type configuration) (Figs. 9-11 and 9-12). The straight wires are satisfactory for internal jugular, subclavian, or femoral cannulations. However, the J configuration is necessary to attain a reasonable success rate with external jugular cannulations where the wire and catheter must pass around several sharp bends in the vein.[7] The J configuration also can be used during cannulation of other veins. J-type wires are packaged with a small sheath that is used to temporarily straighten the J to aid insertion of the wire into the needle or cannula. A tapered straightener also can be used as a minidilator. A 3-mm radius of curvature on the J wire has been found optimal for external jugular cannulation in adults and most children.[8] Occasionally, a smaller radius (1.5 or 2.0 mm) may be helpful in very small children, prob-

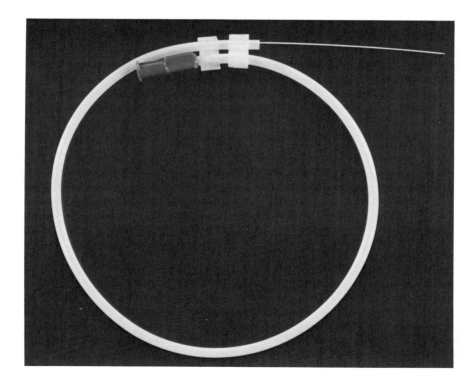

Fig. 9-11. A straight flexible angiographic wire catheter guide in a coiled plastic container.

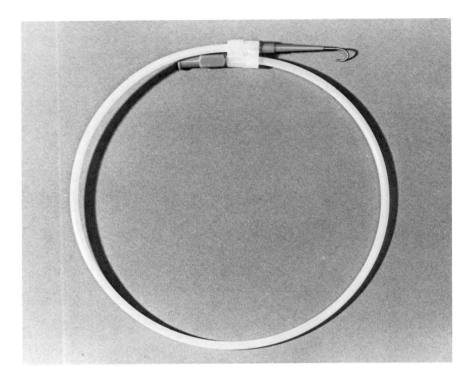

Fig. 9-12. A J-type flexible angiographic wire catheter guide. The tapered sheath is used for straightening the J to aid insertion of the wire into the hub of a cannula. Because of the taper it can also be used to carefully dilate the skin puncture site as an aid in passing the definitive catheter.

ably because of the size of the vessels.[9] Unfortunately, these wires seem to have difficulty maintaining the very small radius of curvature in storage.

Guidewires are sized by the external wire diameter in inches or centimeters. Table 9-8 gives wire sizes that will generally fit through various needles and cannulas. However, the gauge sizing of needles and cannulas also refers to outside diameter. Wall thickness can vary among manufacturers. The wire should always be tested to ensure it will fit through

the introducer selected before venipuncture is begun. The length of the wire should be at least 10 cm longer than the definitive catheter. If a technique is chosen that requires the wire to be fully inserted into the central circulation before the catheter is introduced into the vein (e.g., external jugular), then the wire needs to be twice as long as the definitive catheter plus 5 to 10 cm.

Sterility

Infection is the most common late complication of central venous cannulation. However, infection-free catheters can be maintained for prolonged periods with strict adherence to aseptic protocols.[10,11]

Aseptic Insertion Technique

Prevention of infection begins with an aseptic insertion technique. The individual inserting the catheter should scrub hands and wear a mask, sterile gown, and gloves. Shaving of body hair is not required, but a wide area around the insertion site should be prepared with an antiseptic scrub. Any antiseptic solution used for surgical site preparation is considered suitable. One study found a re-

TABLE 9-8. Relative Sizes of Angiographic Wires, Cannulas, and Needles

Wire Outer Diameter (inches)	Smallest Thin-Wall Needle Through Which Wire Will Fit (Gauge)	Smallest Cannula Through Which Wire Will Fit (Gauge)
0.018 to 0.021	21	22
0.022 to 0.025[a]	19	20
0.028	19	18
0.035	18	16
0.038	18	16

[a] A 0.025-inch or smaller wire will fit through the lumens of most pulmonary artery catheters.

duced incidence of catheter-related local infection (but not bacteremia) when 2% chlorhexadine was used for preinsertion site preparation and postinsertion site care, compared to 10% povidone-iodine or 70% alcohol.[12] The prepped insertion site should be surrounded by a sterile, water-impermeable drape to provide a large work area in order to avoid unintentional contamination of equipment. A number of prepackaged central venous cannulation kits are available that include all the materials needed for sterile insertion except gloves, mask, and gown. These kits can be very helpful in ensuring the availability of all the equipment needed for an efficient, aseptic technique. Of course, there are situations in which the urgency of obtaining intravenous access is extreme and full sterile precautions may be impossible. Under such circumstances, the physician's discretion must be used concerning which precautions to take, with the full realization that every break in technique increases the chance of subsequent infection. Catheters inserted via cutdown are more prone to infection than those inserted percutaneously.

Securing the Catheter

Securing the catheter so that it does not move is an important step in preventing future infection. A catheter that moves in relation to the skin puncture prevents the tissues from closing around it. The primary source of catheter contamination is migration of bacteria from the skin along the insertion tract. With a securely fixed catheter, the closing of the skin and subcutaneous tissues around the catheter provides a natural barrier to this migration. In addition, a catheter that moves within a vein causes mechanical irritation, which leads to thrombophlebitis. For situations in which the risk of infection is high (e.g., insertion sites close to open wounds) or in which prolonged catheterization is anticipated, infection risk can be reduced further by using a subcutaneous tunnel. By moving the skin puncture site several centimeters away from the vein puncture site, advantage is taken of the natural barrier provided by tissues closing around the catheter. A number of techniques have been described that depend on specific equipment.[13,14] In general, the catheter is inserted into the chosen central vein and the free end drawn through a subcutaneous tunnel to the chosen exit site. The original insertion site is then sutured closed over the catheter. A number of the catheters inserted in this manner for long-term use incorporate a synthetic fiber cuff to promote tissue closure and have an exceptionally low rate of catheter-related infections. A similar subcutaneous cuff made of biodegradable collagen and incorporating bactericidal silver is available for use with other central venous catheters. Early studies with these cuffs demonstrated a reduction in local catheter-related infection and showed a trend toward reduced bacteremia, suggesting cost effectiveness.[15,16] More recently, the efficacy of the cuffs for many critically ill patients has been questioned.[17] Bonding of antibiotics to the catheter surface is another method being tested to reduce catheter-related infections with encouraging results. Soaking immediately prior to insertion will bind an anionic antibiotic (e.g., cefazolin) to a cationic surfactant coated polyethelene or PVC catheter.[18] Also available is a polyurethane catheter impregnated with silver sulfadizaine and chlorhexidine.[19]

For catheters that are not tunneled subcutaneously, secure fixation with suture is recommended. In these cases, 2-0 or 3-0 silk or Prolene suture works well and, when affixed to a straight Keith needle, requires no additional instruments for suturing. Monofilament suture is preferable because of decreased surface area. The suture is passed through the skin and a knot tied loosely near the catheter. This ensures that the pressure of tying the catheter firmly will be against the knot rather than the skin. If the skin puncture site is particularly large or gaping, a figure-of-eight or mattress-type suture may be used to close the skin around the catheter. The catheter is secured with a lattice-type maneuver in which the ends of the suture are wrapped in opposite directions around the catheter several times before being tied securely. Some catheters have a groove in the hub or a rubberized catheter clamp around which suture can be tied to aid fixation.

Sterile Dressing

Following insertion and securing of the catheter, a sterile dressing should be applied. There has been considerable controversy for many years over the best type of dressing and antimicrobial preparations to use. The first step in any dressing is to thoroughly clean the insertion site of any blood remaining from the insertion procedure using sterile water or saline. After the site has completely dried, it has been widely recommended that an antimicrobial preparation be applied to the insertion site.[20] Antibacterial ointments containing polymyxin, neomycin, and bacitracin were used for many years but have fallen into disfavor, since fungi and antibiotic-resistant bacteria can proliferate in the preparation.[21,22] Providone-iodine preparations are most widely used today because they have both antibacterial and antifungal activity. However, these preparations have not significantly reduced the incidence of catheter-related infections.[23] All ointments allow a moist atmosphere at the wound edge that prevents the skin from forming a tight seal around the catheter. Current practice is to encourage a clean, dry insertion site by cleansing the site with antimicrobial solutions. Providone-iodine solution is commonly used, although chlorhexadine may provide better protection.[12]

For many years, a tight, occlusive dressing applied over the insertion site was standard practice to prevent outside contamination. However, the dark, moist conditions under such a dressing promote more rapid bacterial and fungal growth. Currently, it is recommended that dressings not be completely occlusive but allow moisture to escape from under the dressing.[24] A simple, effective dressing is a sterile gauze sponge held in place with porous tape. Adhesive, transparent, semipermeable plastic membranes were introduced as dressings in recent years. Early studies suggested they were cost effective because they could be changed much less frequently than standard dressings. However, recent studies are demonstrating that prolonged use of these dressings is associated with increased skin colonization and local catheter infection and, probably, with catheter-related bacteremia.[25,26] If these dressings are used, they probably should be changed at least every 3 to 4 days.

Air Embolism

There is a risk of air embolism whenever a vein is entered, and such risk is exacerbated when dealing with large central veins exposed to negative intrathoracic pressures. Venous air embolism can cause cardiovascular collapse secondary to occlusion of the right ventricular outflow tract. In addition, venous air can reach the arterial circulation through patent atrial or ventricular septal defects or other venoarterial connections with the possi-

bility of stroke, myocardial infarction, bowel infarction, or other arterial compromise. Therefore, precautions are necessary whenever inserting or using central venous lines in order to avoid air embolism. Intravenous tubing should be carefully inspected to ensure it is free of air bubbles.

The danger of air embolism during insertion can be minimized by proper positioning. Placing the insertion site below the level of the right atrium will increase the venous pressure, decreasing the risk of air aspiration. It also has the advantage of distending the vein, which facilitates cannulation.[27] The head-down (Trendelenburg) position is well known for jugular and subclavian insertions. A head-up position provides the same advantages for femoral puncture, as does a tourniquet for arm vein punctures. Any time a needle or cannula is in a vein and the hub is open to the atmosphere, there is a danger of air aspiration. These times should be kept to a minimum by keeping the hub occluded by a syringe or gloved finger. Of particular danger are times when a through-the-needle catheter or guidewire is being inserted, since air may pass around the catheter or wire. These manipulations should be accomplished expeditiously and the introducing needle or cannula removed from the vein as soon as possible.

When a patient is breathing spontaneously, intrathoracic pressure decreases during inspiration. Consequently, air embolism is more likely if the patient takes a deep breath or sighs. Alternatively, a patient receiving mechanical ventilation is at somewhat less risk because intrathoracic pressure is higher and increases during inspiration. When air embolism is of particular concern, it is helpful to have the conscious patient perform a Valsalva maneuver or to have a positive pressure breath given to the ventilated patient at critical points in the procedure.

A less obvious time of danger for air embolism is at the time of removal of a central venous catheter. Particularly if the catheter has been in place for several days, a tract may form around the catheter that does not immediately seal when the line is removed. Consequently, all central lines should be removed with the patient in the recumbent position and firm pressure held over the insertion site to prevent aspiration of air. If there is any question of whether the insertion site has sealed itself, an air-tight pressure dressing should be temporarily applied.

Safely Locating the Vein

Part of a number of techniques for central venous cannulation when the vein cannot be seen involves the use of a small needle (20-gauge or smaller) to locate the vein before cannulation with a larger needle. This is widely recommended for internal jugular cannulation,[28,29] has also been suggested for subclavian punctures,[30] and would seem to have merit for the femoral route as well. Ultrasonography (Site-Rite II, Dymax Corp, Pittsburgh PA) also can help identify anatomic variations in vein location and has been recommended as an adjunct to safe cannulation.[31–34] The rationale for the use of a locator needle is that exploration for the vein with a small needle will cause less damage to adjacent structures should the aim be inaccurate, particularly if an artery is unintentionally punctured. Leaving the needle in place, once the vein has been identified, also provides a guide for venipuncture with a larger needle. Additional protection against unintentional arterial puncture can be gained by briefly attaching the small needle to a transducer and observing the absence of arterial pulsations.[35] Unfortunately, the color of the aspirated blood is not always reliable for detecting arterial puncture, and pulsatile blood flow is not always obvious through a small-gauge needle.

Proper Catheter Position

The ideal location of the tip of the catheter will depend, to some extent, on its purpose. If the catheter is needed for rapid administration of fluids or blood, a location within any large vein is adequate. If a highly accurate measurement of right ventricular filling pressure is needed, then a position in the right atrium may be indicated. The ideal location for a catheter to be used to aspirate potential air emboli during certain surgical procedures is at the superior vena cava-right atrial junction or slightly above.[36]

Extravascular migration of central venous catheters is a serious complication, which may be fatal.[37] Factors contributing to extravascular migration include the debility of the patient, the stiffness and sharpness of the catheter, the anatomic location of the catheter tip, and movement of the catheter tip resulting from patient movement and the dynamic movement of the cardiovascular system. A catheter that is too long should not be cut with scissors or scalpel before insertion because the sharp edges of the catheter tip increase the chances for vessel perforation. Another factor that contributes to catheter erosion is positioning of the catheter tip perpendicular to the vessel wall.[38,39] This is a particular problem with catheters inserted from the left side of the neck. Care must be taken to assure that the catheter is long enough to pass well into the brachiocephalic vein or superior vena cava. Too short a catheter is likely to lie transversely in the brachiocephalic vein with its tip impinging on the lateral wall of the superior vena cava. Erosion at this point is likely to lead to hydromediastinum and hydrothorax.[39] When the tip of the catheter lies below the pericardial reflection, extravascular migration can result in the infusion of intravenous fluids into the pericardial sac. In one series, the resulting cardiac tamponade had an 88 percent mortality.[40] This devastating result most commonly occurs when the catheter erodes through the right atrium or right ventricle, but may also occur with the perforation of intrathoracic venous structures. Any case of unexplained hypotension in a patient with a central venous catheter should suggest the possibility of cardiac tamponade. For most purposes, the ideal position for the catheter tip would seem to be the upper superior vena cava (a compromise between accurate central venous pressures and safety).

The most accurate method of determining the location of the catheter tip is identifying it on chest radiograph. Other methods, such as observing respiratory oscillations, determining the length relative to surface anatomy, and formulas based on anatomy, are only guides to approximate good position.[41] The actual position should be confirmed by radiograph as soon as is feasible after insertion. Radiography, however, can only serve as an estimate of *true* anatomical catheter location (e.g., is the catheter tip in the lower SVC or high right atrium?). A catheter inserted intraoperatively should be accompanied by a chest radiograph immediately postoperatively. If the catheter used is not made of radiopaque material, a useful technique is to fill the catheter with an injectable radiopaque substance (e.g., sodium diatrizoate) before the radiograph.

Long-Term Care

A number of considerations relating to long-term care, such as catheter materials, types of dressing, antimicrobial cleansing, and insertion techniques, have been discussed previously. Most aspects of long-term care focus on minimizing the risk of infection.[42] As with the type of dressing, the frequency with which dressings should be changed is controversial. Recommendations vary from daily[43] to weekly.[44] The consensus would seem to be moving toward less frequent dressing changes for long-term parenteral alimentation lines, which are rarely manipulated. For central lines in critically ill patients, dressing changes every 2 to 4 days seems warranted. Of course, dressings should be changed whenever they become wet. Strict aseptic technique with an established protocol for cleaning and redressing the site should always be used.

As important as the insertion site as a source for contamination of central venous lines is the fluid administration system. Practices that increase the incidence of infection include not having a completely closed system, blood sampling from the lines, the use of stopcocks in the line, injections into the line, and adding drugs to the intravenous fluids outside the pharmacy.[24,45,46] These practices should be avoided assiduously in caring for long-term alimentation lines and minimized whenever possible when caring for other central venous lines. In addition, it is recommended that the entire fluid administration set be changed every 24 hours.[43,46]

Multiple-lumen catheters are useful because they allow multiple separate infusions in a single central venous line. However, the multiple manipulations inherent in the use of these catheters increases the risk of infection. Uncontrolled studies of triple-lumen subclavian catheters reported a three- to fivefold greater incidence of infection than single-lumen catheters when used in a similar patient population.[47,48] The highest risk is encountered when parenteral alimentation is administered through a multiple-lumen catheter. More recent controlled studies have not demonstrated a significant increase in catheter-related infection rates with these catheters.[49]

No consensus exists on the need for changing the central venous catheter. For long-term intravenous alimentation catheters, the incidence of catheter-related sepsis does not seem to be related to the duration of catheterization.[24] Consequently, there seems to be little reason to change these catheters except when there is an indication of sepsis unresponsive to antibiotics. In critically ill patients, the incidence of contaminated central venous lines not used for alimentation appears to

increase significantly after 48 to 72 hours.[50] Significant catheter contamination and catheter-related infections are very low in the first 3 to 4 days after insertion, whether single- or multiple-lumen catheters are used, but increase significantly after that time.[48,51] These findings have led to recommendations that catheters be changed on a routine basis.[50] Catheter changes to new sites or over guidewires in the same site at intervals ranging from every 3 days to every 7 days have been studied. Most studies have demonstrated that changing catheters over guidewires does not reduce the incidence of catheter-related infection, although the ability to do semiquantitative cultures on the removed catheter may improve diagnostic accuracy. Two controlled randomized trials of routine catheter changes demonstrated clearly that the longer a patient had a central line in place, the greater was the risk of a catheter-related infection. However, changing the catheter on a routine basis (every 3 days in one study, every 7 days in the other) did not reduce the incidence of infection.[52,53] Therefore, my current practice in the intensive care unit is to remove central lines as soon as possible and to replace necessary lines only for specific indications, such as malfunction, local inflammation, or sepsis from an unknown source.

Site Selection

A great number of routes and techniques have been described for central venous cannulation, making appropriate selection for the individual patient difficult. The primary considerations should include the experience of the person inserting the catheter, reason for the cannulation, availability of equipment, condition of the patient and ability to withstand the positioning necessary for insertion, and the success rate and complications of the technique. For many techniques, success rates and complications are directly related to the expertise of the operator. Consequently, the experience of the individual inserting the catheter is an extremely important consideration.

For general reference in the following sections, Figure 9-13 is a diagrammatic representation of the relationships of the major venous structures in the neck and thorax, and Figure 9-14 emphasizes the major surface landmarks used in central venous cannulation. There are five major approaches to the central venous circulation: the basilic vein in

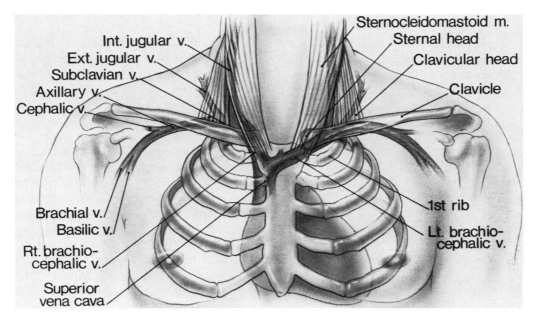

Fig. 9-13. Diagram of the major venous structures of the neck and thorax.

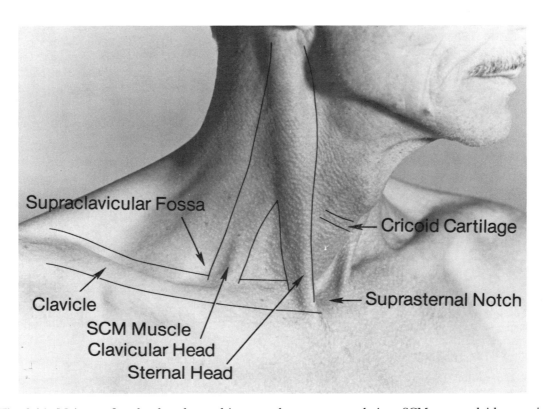

Fig. 9-14. Major surface landmarks used in central venous cannulation. SCM, sternocleidomastoid.

the arm, the external jugular vein, the internal jugular vein, the subclavian vein, and the femoral vein. Table 9-9 describes the author's opinion of how each site would rate relative to the others for several important considerations in selecting a site for cannulation. In the following sections, the advantages, disadvantages, insertion techniques, and complications of each approach will be discussed. A comprehensive discussion of the many insertion variations will not be attempted, but the most common techniques will be discussed with reference to variations.

Basilic Vein Cannulation

Anatomy

Cannulation of the arm veins is one of the oldest techniques for central venous access and also one of the safest. The veins of the forearm empty into the basilic and cephalic systems in the upper arm (Fig. 9-15). The basilic vein passes up the medial aspect of the arm and joins with the deeper brachial vein to form the axillary vein. The cephalic vein passes up the lateral aspect of the arm to the shoulder where it occupies the deltopectoral groove until it plunges to pierce the clavipectoral fascia to enter the axillary vein. The basilic system should be used for percutaneous placement since success rates through the cephalic system are 50 percent or less in most series reported. However, the cephalic system has been used with success for long-term lines when it is approached by cutdown in the deltopectoral groove.

Basic Insertion Technique

The basilic vein is usually approached at the medial side of the antecubital fossa or through the median cubital vein in the middle of the antecubital fossa (Fig. 9-16). The classic technique uses a through-the-needle catheter which is supplied inside a sterile sheath which allows insertion with a "no-touch" technique. Consequently, sterile gown and gloves are not mandatory, but the usual skin preparation should be carried out. PICC insertion protocol usually recommends gown, gloves, and mask. In adults, a 14-gauge needle that allows passage of a 16-gauge catheter is usually used. Smaller sizes are available for use in children. The approximate length of catheter to be inserted should be estimated by laying it out along its route before insertion.

A tourniquet is applied around the upper arm to distend the veins. Venipuncture is performed at a convenient site and when blood returns into the needle indicating the vein has been entered, the catheter is advanced into the vein for a short distance. The tourniquet is released and the catheter is advanced to the predetermined distance. The catheter should be advanced using very little force to avoid perforating the vein. The catheter should never be withdrawn through the needle or the catheter may be severed, resulting in a catheter embolus. If withdrawal is necessary, the catheter and needle should be removed together. If the catheter meets resistance in the axillary region, abduction and external rotation of the arm may facilitate passage, as may ipsilateral flexion and rotation of the neck.

Variations of Insertion Technique

The catheter has a tendency to "hang up" on the venous valves. This problem may sometimes be overcome by using a continuously running intravenous infusion or intermittent boluses from a syringe. Of course, this necessitates breaking the ster-

TABLE 9-9. Relative Rating of Central Venous Access Techniques[s]

	Basilic (Arm Veins)	External Jugular	Internal Jugular	Subclavian	Femoral
Ease of insertion and safety for the inexperienced	1	3	4	5	2
Long-term use	5	3	2	1	4
Success rate	5	4	1	3	2
Complications (technique related)	1	2	3	5	4
Ease of pulmonary artery catheter insertion	5	2	1	3	4

[s]In each category 1 = best, 5 = worst.

ile packaging around the catheter and requires appropriate sterile precautions. Not infrequently the catheter passes up the ipsilateral internal jugular vein. The chance of this occurrence can reportedly be reduced by turning the head toward the side of the venipuncture,[54-56] although not all studies have shown this maneuver to be successful.[57] Another report[58] claimed a high degree of success by using a "soft" catheter passed slowly with the patient in the sitting position, thus allowing gravity to help guide the catheter to its proper position. Greater than 90 percent success has been reported using a J-type angiographic wire catheter guide passed into the central circulation through a short cannula with the definitive catheter passed

over the wire.[59] Some authors[60,61] have advocated cannulation of the proximal basilic or axillary veins in the upper arm or axilla using a combination of direct observation and palpation of the axillary artery for identification. These techniques have not gained widespread use, most likely because they are relatively blind and close to important arteries and nerves.

Success Rate

Peripheral venous cannulation is invariably successful, but obtaining a central position of the catheter is reported in only 60 to 75 percent of patients in most series.[54-56,68,62-67] Use of a long J-type guide

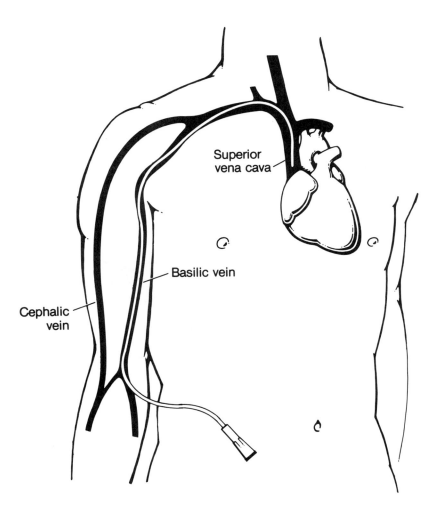

Fig. 9-15. Diagram of central venous cannulation from the arm demonstrating the relationships of the major venous systems in the arm.

wire may improve success.[59] A greater than 90 percent success rate has been claimed for the proximal techniques.[60,61]

Complications

The only significant reported complication with this technique is thrombophlebitis, which occurs in 2 to 10 percent of cases.[62,63,66] Occasional complications include hematoma at the site of puncture (more common with proximal basilic or axillary approaches) and catheter embolism. Catheter-related sepsis and vessel perforation by the catheter are potential complications of all central venous catheters.

Advantages and Disadvantages

Basilic vein cannulation is particularly useful for the inexperienced operator since the technique is simple, the vein is directly visible, and complica-tions of venipuncture are rare. (See Table 9-10). It is also to be recommended for the patient with a bleeding diathesis or for one who is receiving anticoagulants. Certain patients poorly tolerate the Trendelenburg position (because of respiratory distress) or have other relative contraindications to being placed in the head-down position (neurosurgical patients, preeclamptics). In these patients, the antecubital approach provides an alternative to central venous cannulation through neck veins.

External Jugular Vein Cannulation

Anatomy

The external jugular vein is formed by the junction of the posterior division of the posterior facial vein and the posterior auricular vein at the level of the angle of the mandible (Fig. 9-17). It runs obliquely across the body of the sternocleidomas-

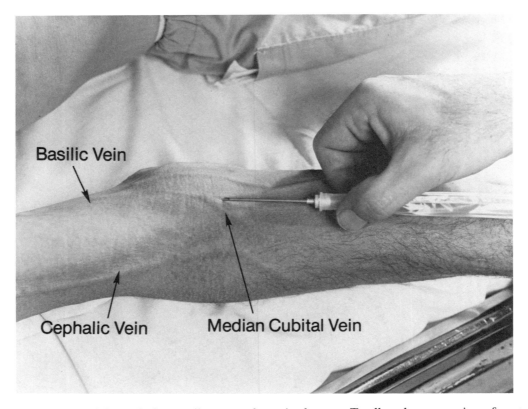

Fig. 9-16. Insertion of through-the-needle type catheter in the arm. To allow demonstration of anatomic relationships, the usual sterile preparation and draping has not been used in this photograph. Appropriate sterile precautions should always be used when inserting central venous catheters.

toid muscle toward the middle of the clavicle where it penetrates the deep fascia of the subclavian triangle and enters the subclavian vein. Although the position of the external jugular vein if quite constant, cannulation is recommended only is it is easily visible or palpable. The vessel is quite thin-walled and movable in the subcutaneous tissues, making cannulation slightly more difficult than most arm veins. However, a minimal amount of practice is necessary to become facile at external jugular cannulation. Two sets of valves, one approximately 4 cm above the clavicle and one at the subclavian junction, plus the acute angle with which the external jugular joins the subclavian vein, can make passage of a catheter into the superior vena cava difficult. However, use of a flexible J-type guidewire markedly improves success.

Basic Insertion Technique

I prefer a modification of the original J-wire technique described by Blitt and colleagues.[6] The patient is placed in the Trendelenburg position with the head turned away from the site of venipuncture. Either the right or left external jugular vein may be used. A wide area of the neck is prepped and draped. The operator should wear gown, mask, and gloves. Local anesthesia is used if the patient is conscious. Venipuncture is performed slightly distal to the midpoint of the vein where it is easily seen (Fig. 9-18). A Valsalva maneuver, sustained positive pressure ventilation, or digital pressure over the vein just above the clavicle may help in distending the vein. Venipuncture is made with a short (2½ inches) over-the-needle cannula attached to a syringe. A 16- or 18-gauge cannula is usually used in adults, and an 18- or 20-

gauge cannula is used in children. Some operators prefer to make a small incision in the skin with a scalpel to minimize the resistance to passage of the needle-cannula assembly.

Venipuncture is made applying intermittent or continuous gentle aspiration on the syringe to identify entry into the vein. Applying large amounts of negative pressure during insertion is discouraged because the vein is easily collapsible and the flash of blood on entry may be missed because of collapse of the vessel walls around the needle point. When free flow of blood is obtained, the cannula is advanced off the needle into the vein. The needle is removed and the syringe reattached to the cannula and aspirated to verify free flow of blood. If free blood return is not obtained, the cannula is slowly withdrawn with intermittent gentle aspiration until free flow returns and the cannula fixed in that position with the nondominant hand.

After this initial cannulation, a J wire with a 3 mm radius of curvature, appropriate to the size cannula being used (Table 9-8) and at least twice as long as the definitive catheter is inserted through the cannula and advanced into the central circulation. To ease introduction of the wire into the hub of the cannula, a plastic sheath is slipped over the tip of the J to straighten it. This should be done before beginning the venipuncture as it may be awkward to accomplish while simultaneously fixing the external jugular cannula in the vein.

When advancing the J wire, it occasionally meets an obstruction and may need to be manipulated. Most success will be found by rotating the wire between the thumb and index finger while simultaneously moving the wire in and out 1 to 2 cm. This

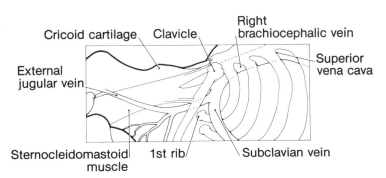

Fig. 9-17. Anatomy of neck and upper thorax emphasizing relationships to the external jugular vein.

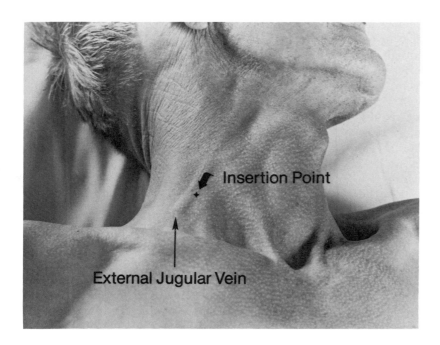

Fig. 9-18. Insertion point for external jugular venipuncture.

method of manipulation is greatly superior to rotating the wire while maintaining constant inward pressure against the obstruction. If an obstruction cannot be passed after multiple attempts, I have had occasional success in passing a smaller diameter wire. Internal rotation of the ipsilateral arm with upward pressure on the scapula may be helpful in difficult wire passages, as the maneuver raises the clavicle, allowing the wire to pass under. Advancing the wire approximately 20 cm will assure passage into the thorax in adults, with shorter lengths necessary for children. Care should be taken not to advance the wire too far because it will easily enter the right ventricle causing arrhythmias and could possibly puncture the ventricular wall.

Once the guidewire is advanced into the chest, the short cannula is removed and the definitive catheter is threaded over the wire using it as a guide. Depending on the type and size of catheter chosen, there may be some resistance to passage through the skin and subcutaneous tissues. A #11 scalpel blade can be used to carefully widen the venipuncture site around the wire. The tapered J-straightener or firm, tapered dilator can also be used to widen the puncture site. Advancing the

catheter with a rotary motion aids passage through the tissues. Care should be taken not to lose grasp of the wire during catheter insertion or the wire may be advanced with the catheter, resulting in a wire embolism. The catheter is inserted 15 to 20 cm on the right side and 20 to 25 cm on the left side. The wire is then removed and a syringe attached to verify free flow of blood from the catheter. An intravenous infusion is attached, the catheter secured in place, and a chest radiograph obtained to confirm catheter position.

TABLE 9-10. Basilic Vein Cannulation

Advantages	Disadvantages
Simplicity	Low success rate
Low complication rate	Successful placement may
Easily visible landmarks	require considerable
May be performed in	time
sitting position if	Difficult route for
patient cannot	pulmonary artery
tolerate head-down	catheter insertion
position (respiratory	
distress, neurosurgical	
patients,	
preeclampsia)	

Variations in Insertion Technique

The original Blitt J-wire technique[6] used a 5½- or 6-inch over-the-needle cannula to perform the venipuncture. Once the cannula is inserted into the vein, the guidewire is passed into the chest and the cannula advanced over the wire. This technique has the advantage of using only the definitive catheter for the entire procedure. However, I prefer the modified technique because performing the venipuncture with the syringe on the end of a 6-inch needle-cannula assembly is cumbersome. Additionally, most long over-the-needle cannulas are made of Teflon and the modified technique allows a wider choice of catheter type.

External jugular vein cannulation can be performed using a pure Seldinger technique of passing the wire through a thin-wall needle used for venipuncture. Generally, this method is not recommended, since the wire frequently has to be manipulated. It is possible to shear the wire with the needle. The wire should not be pulled back through the needle. If more than gentle rotation of the wire while advancing it is needed, the needle should be removed from the vein before additional manipulation is attempted. However, the pure Seldinger technique may be of use in neonates and very small infants where cannulation of the external jugular vein with any size cannula can be difficult.

Percutaneous external jugular cannulation for central venous lines can be performed without use of a J wire with either over-the-needle or through-the-needle catheters.[54,68–72] However, the success of passing a catheter into the central circulation is substantially reduced. Similarly, this route may be approached by a surgical cutdown on the vein.[73] Although reliable central venous pressures have been reported in anesthetized patients from external jugular vein catheters that do not enter the thorax,[74] they should not be relied on with the many alternative techniques available to ensure central placement of a catheter.

Success Rates

Success rates of 75 to 95 percent have been reported in adults using the J-wire technique.[6,75] Approximately 60 percent success rates are reported in children using the J-wire technique.[9] Success rates of 50 to 70 percent are reported in adults without the use of the J wire.[54,71,72]

Complications

Because the external jugular vein is superficial, complications related to insertion are minimal. Local hematoma at the puncture site occasionally occurs. Thrombosis of the vein occurs in 2 to 3 percent of cases.[76] The major complications are those associated with all central venous catheters regardless of site of insertion, that is, perforation of the vessel wall and sepsis. No deaths attributable to external jugular catheterization technique have been reported.

Advantages and Disadvantages

The external jugular approach is preferred under many circumstances. Although the technique is more complicated than the basilic vein approach, it shares many of the same advantages, has a higher success rate, and is usually accessible to the anesthesiologist during an operative procedure. Since the venipuncture is superficial and the vein directly visualized, it can be used safely by an inexperienced operator. It is a safe technique for the patient with a bleeding diathesis or on anticoagulants. It can be used for long-term catheterization and for pulmonary artery catheterization, although the large catheters necessary to accept a pulmonary artery catheter occasionally cannot be successfully passed under the clavicle by this route or the acute angulation as the catheter enters the subclavian vein causes it to kink so that the pulmonary artery catheter will not pass. The disadvantages of the external jugular approach are primarily relative to other approaches that have higher complication rates. Catheters inserted through the neck are more difficult to fix and dress than some other sites and have a tendency to kink when the head is turned. For long-term catheterization, the subclavian vein is the best choice. In the hands of experienced operators, success rates are slightly higher with internal jugular and subclavian approaches. Successful placement of a large cannula for pulmonary artery catheter insertion is higher with the internal jugular vein technique. See Table 9-11.

Internal Jugular Vein Cannulation

Anatomy

The internal jugular vein has become a favorite site for central venous cannulation by anesthesiologists because of its ready accessibility, high success rate, and low incidence of complications. The internal jugular vein begins at the jugular foramen just medial to the mastoid process at the base of the skull and runs directly caudad to pass under the sternal end of the clavicle where it joins the subclavian vein to become the innominate vein (Fig. 9-19). The carotid artery, internal jugular vein, and vagus nerve are all contained within the carotid sheath. At its origin, the vein lies posterior to the carotid then becomes lateral and finally anterolateral to the artery. With the head turned away from the side of anticipated cannulation, the entire course of the vein lies deep to the sternocleidomastoid muscle. Using surface anatomy, the course of the vein is marked by a line drawn from the mastoid process to the medial insertion of the clavicular head of the sternocleidomastoid muscle on the clavicle (Fig. 9-20).

Basic Insertion Technique

Although many approaches to the internal jugular vein have been described,[72] the most widely practiced, and my preference, is a central approach along the axis of the vein with venipuncture occurring several centimeters above the clavicle to minimize risk of puncturing the pleura.[29,77,78] Ultrasonography can be a useful adjuvant to IJV cannulation. The patient is placed in the Trendelenburg position, with the head turned away from the site of venipuncture. Either right or left internal jugular vein may be used, although the right is preferred because of the straight access into the superior vena cava, the presence of the thoracic duct on the left, and performance of the technique is easier for right-handed operators. A wide area of the neck is

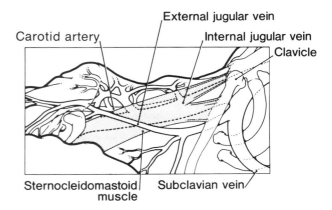

Fig. 9-19. Anatomy of neck and upper thorax emphasizing relationships to internal jugular vein.

prepped and draped. The operator should wear gown, mask, and gloves. Local anesthesia is used if the patient is conscious.

An important landmark is the triangle formed by the sternal and clavicular heads of the sternocleidomastoid muscle and the clavicle (Fig. 9-20). It can be readily identified in nearly all people by placing a finger in the sternal notch and then moving laterally over the sternal head until a depression in the muscle is felt. Tensing the muscle by having the patient raise his head against resistance may help identification. The course of the vein and, therefore, the axis of needle insertion is determined by drawing a line connecting the mastoid process and the medial insertion of the clavicular head of the sternocleidomastoid muscle on the clavicle. This latter point is also the lateral border of the aforementioned triangle. If the triangle cannot be reliably identified, this point can be found at the junction of the medial and middle thirds of the clavicle. Venipuncture is performed along this line with the needle following its course.

Since a line so drawn represents the course of the vein, venipuncture could be performed at any point along the line. However, very high in the neck the carotid artery lies in front of the vein and the cupola of the lung lies low in the neck. Therefore, most operators prefer a puncture site approximately in the middle portion of the neck. I prefer to perform the puncture at the apex of the triangle (which usually falls along the line) to avoid having to pass through the sternocleidomastoid muscle. Occasionally, the triangle is small, with the apex occurring very low in the neck, or the triangle is

TABLE 9-11. External Jugular Vein Cannulation

Advantages	Disadvantages
Low complication rate	Success rates lower
Easily visible landmarks	than internal jugular
High success rate	or subclavian in
Suitable for long-term	hands of experienced
catheterization	operator
Accessible to	Difficult to fix and
anesthesiologist	dress securely
Suitable for pulmonary	Not as reliable for
artery	pulmonary artery
catheterization	catheterization as
	internal jugular

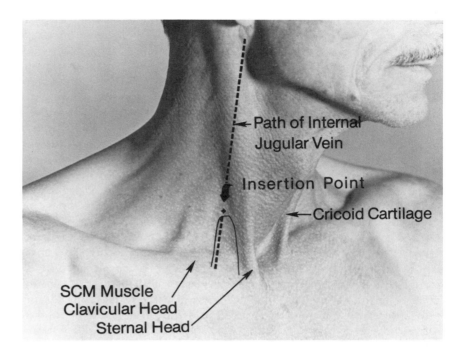

Fig. 9-20. Insertion site for internal jugular venipuncture. See text, SCM, sternocleidomastoid.

difficult to identify. In such cases, the skin puncture site is determined by drawing another line, perpendicular to the first, which intersects with the cricoid cartilage; and venipuncture is performed through the muscle. In most cases, a puncture site determined by this method will lie just above the apex of the triangle (Fig. 9-21).

Before venipuncture, the carotid artery may be palpated to assure it is medial to the intended puncture. However, excessive pressure during venipuncture in attempts to palpate the artery can distort the anatomy, making venipuncture more difficult. Before venipuncture with a larger needle, the internal jugular vein is located with a 22-gauge, 1½-inch needle attached to a syringe. A 23- or 25-gauge needle may be used in children. The needle is inserted from the previously identified entrance point at a 45-degree angle to the skin, caudad, and along the axis of the line from the mastoid to the clavicle. This latter direction is roughly toward the ipsilateral nipple. The angle of insertion should not be too narrow with the skin, or the vein will not be encountered until the needle has passed very low in the neck. Continuous or intermittent gentle aspiration should be applied to the syringe to immediately identify entry into the vein.

The use of the locator needle is important to minimize trauma to adjacent structures should the

vein be missed. Puncture of the carotid artery can usually be identified by the color of the blood and rapidity of blood return when the syringe is removed (although pulsatile flow should not be expected through such a small needle). The vein should be encountered at a depth of ½ to 1½ inches. If blood return is not encountered during insertion, gentle aspiration should be continued during slow needle withdrawal because the needle may have passed completely through the vein. If the vein is not found, changing the direction of the needle slightly lateral or medial should result in success. Once the vein has been located, the sy-

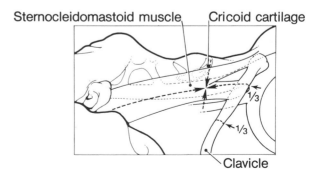

Fig. 9-21. Alternative method for determination of internal jugular venipuncture insertion site.

ringe is removed from the needle and the needle left in place as a guide for insertion of a larger cannula. The needle does represent a potential port for air embolism, but this is minimal in the head-down position.

When the vein has been located, a 16- or 18-gauge, 2½-inch, over-the-needle cannula is inserted immediately adjacent to the locator needle and advanced in the same direction into the internal jugular vein. An 18- or 20-gauge cannula is used in children. It is important to ensure that the tip of the cannula, as well as the tip of the needle, is in the vein. When free flow of blood is obtained, the cannula is advanced into the vein and the needle removed and discarded. The locator needle is removed. A flexible angiographic wire catheter guide of the appropriate size (Table 9-8) is passed through the cannula. Either a straight wire or J wire can be used. After the wire has been inserted 15 to 20 cm, the cannula is removed and the definitive catheter is passed over the wire. Depending on the type and size of catheter chosen, there may be some resistance to passage through the skin and subcutaneous tissues. A #11 scalpel blade can be used to carefully widen the puncture site around the wire. The tapered J-wire straightener or firm, tapered dilator may also be used to widen the puncture site. Advancing the catheter with a rotary motion aids passage through the tissues. Care should be taken to never lose grasp of the wire during catheter insertion or the wire may be advanced with the catheter resulting in a wire embolism. The catheter is inserted 15 to 20 cm on the right side and 20 to 25 cm on the left. The wire is removed and a syringe attached to verify free flow of blood from the catheter. An intravenous infusion is attached, the catheter secured in place, and a chest radiograph obtained to confirm catheter position.

Variations of Insertion Technique

As discussed in the section on external jugular vein cannulation, variations of the guide wire approach just described can be used for internal jugular cannulation. The pure Seldinger technique is of particular value in hypovolemic patients. Cannulation may also be performed without a guide wire with through-the-needle catheters. After locating the vein, venipuncture is performed with the needle attached to a syringe. When free flow of blood is obtained, the syringe is removed and the

definitive catheter passed through the needle into the superior vena cava. The needle is removed from the vein and covered with its protective sheath to avoid shearing the catheter. Similarly, a 5½- or 6-inch over-the-needle catheter can be used for venipuncture with the catheter advanced directly into the vein.

Some operators prefer to remove the locator needle after noting the direction and depth of the vein. This technique removes the hub of the locator needle from the insertion site, making insertion of a larger cannula somewhat easier. The obvious disadvantage is that this technique relies on memory to provide guidance for the larger cannula. Another variation accomplishes the same purpose. Once the entry point has been identified, the locator needle is inserted at a 90-degree angle to the skin at a point approximately 2 cm caudad to the entry point along the line from the mastoid process to the clavicle. When the vein is located, the needle is left in place. Venipuncture is then performed using the over-the-needle cannula inserted at the identified entry point (cephalad to the locator needle) and directed toward the tip of the locator needle, which has been left in the vein. This technique requires a better feeling for the spatial relationships involved in the cannulation. It is recommended only for those who have become comfortable with the basic procedure.

Multiple variations on the landmarks and insertion point have been described.[72] Some authors have described insertion points medial[79] and lateral[70,80,81] to the sternocleidomastoid muscle with good success and low complication rates. Similarly, there are a number of reports of internal jugular cannulation low in the neck with high success and minimal complications.[78,81-83] The internal jugular vein may be approached by surgical cutdown. Clearly, familiarity with a technique breeds success. I prefer the technique described because the basic direction of the needle is along the axis of the vein facilitating smooth cannulation and it is high enough to minimize the danger of pleural puncture.

Success Rates

Most series report a 90 to 98 percent success of venous cannulation and greater than 90 percent of successful cannulations result in the catheter tip resting in the central circulation.[71,75,78,79,81-83]

Complications

It is generally agreed that a high success rate and low complication rate, associated with insertion of percutaneous catheters into veins that cannot be visualized, is directly related to the experience of the operator. Consequently, lack of experience in a technique is a relative contraindication for its use. Experience should be gained under the close supervision of an expert. In experienced hands, the complications associated with internal jugular vein cannulation are infrequent. Carotid artery puncture, the most frequent complication, occurs approximately 2 percent of the time in most series and rarely leads to significant sequelae.[70,76,78–80,83] However, should the carotid artery be unintentionally punctured with a very large cannula, such as a sheath for a pulmonary artery catheter, surgical exploration and repair are advisable. If doubt ever exists as to arterial placement of the locator needle, initial cannula, or Seldinger needle, connection to a transducer will ascertain whether arterial cannulation has transpired, that is, an arterial pressure waveform will be seen.

All other complications occur less than 1 percent of the time. The incidence of pneumothorax in two series using a low approach were 0.2 and 0.3 percent.[78,83] Pneumothorax may also occur rarely with other techniques.[84] Thoracic duct puncture is a concern on the left side and more common with a low technique.[83] Thrombosis of the internal jugular vein is rarely found even after prolonged cannulation,[76] although it has been reported.[70] A single case of superior vena caval thrombosis has also been reported.[85]

Although complications are rare, the physician should be aware that they can occur. Hematomas have caused respiratory obstruction,[86] vocal cord paralysis,[87] Horner's syndrome[88] and cervical nerve damage[89] and may require surgical evacuation.[90] Laceration or puncture of mediastinal structures by errant needles have caused tracheal laceration,[91] endotracheal tube cuff rupture,[92] aortic dissection,[93] pseudoaneurysm of the brachiocephalic artery,[94] aortic catheterization,[95] and fatal hemothorax from laceration of the ascending cervical artery.[96] Perforation of the vessel wall by the catheter has caused hydrothorax,[97,98] hydromediastinum[82,89] and cardiac tamponade.[36] Air embolism may occur during insertion[70] or later if an intravenous port is opened.[100] Ventricular arrhythmias

TABLE 9-12. Internal Jugular Vein Cannulation

Advantages	Disadvantages
High success rate	Requires experience
Low complication rate	Difficult to fix and dress securely
Best for pulmonary artery catheterization	Major complications possible
Suitable for long-term catheterization	
Accessible to anesthesiologist	

may occur during insertion if the wire or catheter enters the right ventricle. Cardiac arrest has been reported with carotid palpation[101] and carotid compression after unintentional puncture.[102] Death has not been reported in any of the large series, but isolated reports of fatalities in association with cannulation of the internal jugular vein do exist.[92,95]

Advantages and Disadvantages

Although internal jugular vein cannulation is not a technique recommended for the inexperienced, it is relatively easy to learn. It has a high success rate and a low rate of complications. (See Table 9-12). It is a useful technique for the anesthesiologist because of the accessibility of the neck. The internal jugular is probably the vein of choice for pulmonary artery catheterization. Internal jugular cannulation is generally not recommended for patients with a bleeding diathesis, although its use in these patients with minimal complications has been reported.[103] The internal jugular vein can be used for long-term catheterization, but catheters inserted through the neck are more difficult to fix and dress than some other sites and have a tendency to kink when the head is turned.

Subclavian Vein Cannulation

Anatomy

The subclavian vein is a continuation of the axillary vein (Fig. 9-13). Beginning at the outer border of the first rib, it inclines up over the first rib then proceeds medially and downward to enter the thorax and join the internal jugular vein behind the sternoclavicular joint to form the brachiocephalic (innominate) vein. If a line is drawn from the junction of the middle and medial thirds of the clavicle posteromedially toward the spine, the following structures are encountered in turn: clavicle, subclavian vein, scalenus anterior muscle, subclavian artery, and dome of the pleura. On the left, the thoracic duct passes over the pleural dome to empty into the angle made by the junction of the subclavian and internal jugular veins. On the right, a similar position is occupied by the smaller right lymphatic trunk. As the vein arches over the first rib, it reaches as high as the upper border of the clavicle just medial to its midpoint. The subclavian vein is anchored by the connective tissue of the surrounding muscles and fascia such that the lumen does not collapse even in marked hypovolemia.

The subclavian vein may be approached from the infraclavicular or supraclavicular routes. First described in 1952,[104] the needle passes between the clavicle and first rib for the infraclavicular subclavian venipuncture. This remains the most popular approach because it is considered safer,[72,77] and because of the greater stability of the catheter on the anterior chest wall. An approach from the supraclavicular fossa above the clavicle was described in 1965.[105] It has gained some popularity because the distance from skin to vein is shorter and the puncture site is more easily accessible to the anesthesiologist during surgery. I prefer the infraclavicular approach because the supraclavicular route offers no advantage over internal jugular cannulation but is associated with more complications. Ultrasonography may facilitate cannulation of the subclavian vein.

Basic Insertion Technique: Infraclavicular

The patient is placed in the Trendelenburg position, arms at sides, with the head turned away from the site of venipuncture. Either right or left subclavian vein may be used, although the right is generally preferred by right-handed operators because of the shorter distance to the superior vena cava and the presence of the thoracic duct on the left. Placing a folded sheet or small pillow under the center of the back may help open the space between the clavicle and first rib and may let the shoulders fall back so that the head of the humerus is out of the way. A wide area of the neck and chest is prepped and draped. The operator should wear gown, gloves, and mask. Local anesthesia is used if the patient is conscious.

The skin puncture site is approximately 1 cm below the midpoint of the clavicle in adults and just below the midpoint of the clavicle in children (Fig. 9-22). In the classic technique, a 14-gauge needle from a through-the-needle catheter assembly is used in adults and a 17-gauge needle is used in children. Although an airtight syringe-needle junction is needed to apply negative pressure during venipuncture, it is important that the syringe can be easily removed from the needle. A sterile clamp to help hold the needle while removing the syringe can be a help. The needle is placed at the insertion site and the index finger of the free hand is placed in the suprasternal notch. The needle is aimed toward the finger and advanced posterior to the clavicle, keeping close to the bone, with the syringe and needle parallel to the coronal plane (i.e., parallel to the bed).

Continuous gentle negative pressure is applied to the syringe as the needle is advanced in order to identify the vein as soon as it is entered. A large needle can remove a core of tissue as it passes through the skin and subcutaneous tissues. Some operators prefer to partially fill the syringe with saline and to inject a small amount once the needle is under the clavicle to clear the needle. In adults the vein should be reached at a depth of 3 to 5 cm. Upon entering the vein, the needle is advanced an additional 1 to 2 mm to ensure that the entire bevel is within the vein. If the venipuncture is performed with the bevel facing anteriorly (up in the supine patient), rotating the needle 180 degrees may aid in passing the catheter.

When free flow of blood is obtained, the syringe is removed and the catheter is advanced through the needle to a depth of 10 to 15 cm on the right and 15 to 20 cm on the left in adults. If the catheter has been advanced beyond the end of the needle but cannot be advanced into position, the catheter should not be withdrawn. Rather, the needle and catheter should be removed together and the venipuncture repeated. Attempting to withdraw the catheter through the needle tip may result in shearing the catheter and catheter embolism. If the vein is not encountered during advancement of the needle, gentle aspiration should be maintained during its withdrawal since it is possible to pass through the vein without encountering the usual flashback of blood. If the vein is not found, the needle should not be redirected until the tip has been withdrawn into the subcutaneous tissues. Laceration of the subclavian artery or pleura may result from movement of the needle beneath the clavicle. When the catheter has been advanced into position, free flow of blood through the catheter is confirmed, and the needle is removed from the skin and covered with its protective sheath. The catheter is secured, an intravenous infusion connected, and a chest radiograph obtained to confirm catheter position and exclude pneumothorax.

Variations of Insertion Technique: Infraclavicular

Most authors prefer a point at the midpoint of the clavicle or slightly lateral as the insertion point.[72,76,77,104,106,107] Although the incidence of complications does not appear significantly different, some authors have suggested that an insertion site at the junction of the medial and middle thirds of the clavicle is safer.[108–111] A more lateral puncture site has also been suggested as being safer.[112] In all these techniques, the direction of the needle is to-

ward the finger in the suprasternal notch with the needle close to the posterior surface of the clavicle and the syringe parallel to the coronal plane.

The Seldinger technique has surpassed in popularity the classic technique of passing the catheter directly through the needle. Most commonly, a large-bore needle is still used for venipuncture, but a wire is passed and the needle removed before a catheter is advanced over the wire. This approach has the advantage of removing the needle entirely from the catheter. Occasional difficulty is encountered in advancing the catheter through the tissues with this technique. The likelihood of difficulty in passing the catheter is increased if smaller gauge needles are used for venipuncture. A vessel dilator can overcome this difficulty, but there is the possibility of vessel perforation by the dilator. Over-the-needle cannulas can be used for subclavian cannulation, 2½ inches for the modified Seldinger technique and 5½ to 6 inches for direct cannulation. However, the latter are unwieldy to manipu-

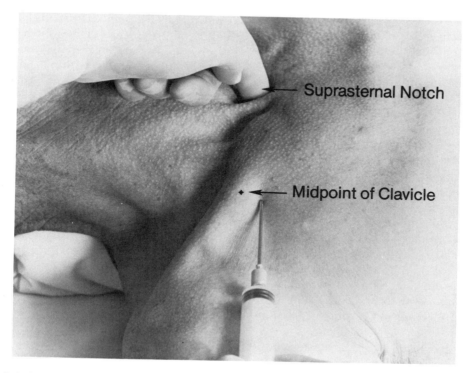

Fig. 9-22. Subclavian venipuncture with the needle from a through-the-needle assembly. To allow demonstration of anatomic relationships, the usual sterile preparation and draping has not been used in this photograph. Appropriate sterile precautions should always be used when inserting central venous catheters.

late and the plastic catheters tend to have more resistance to passage through the fascia and under the clavicle making the "feel" of the procedure less acute. The use of a small-gauge locator needle has not proven to be useful in infraclavicular subclavian cannulation. The flexibility of the small-gauge needle allows it to be easily misdirected from a straight line as it passes under the clavicle.

Basic Insertion Technique: Supraclavicular

The patient is placed in the Trendelenburg position, arms at the sides, with the head turned slightly away from the site of venipuncture. The right side is greatly preferred because there is greater hazard of thoracic duct puncture (on the left) with this approach. A wide area of the neck and chest is prepped and draped. The operator should wear gown, gloves, and mask. Local anesthesia is used if the patient is conscious. Use of the supraclavicular approach has not been described in children.

The skin puncture site is at the lateral border of the clavicular head of the sternocleidomastoid muscle just cephalad to the clavicle (Fig. 9-23). Asking the patient to raise his head against resistance to tense the muscle may help identify this point. Cannulation may be accomplished with a through-the-needle technique, direct long over-the-needle technique, or a pure or modified Seldinger technique using a thin wall needle or short over-the-needle cannula, since only skin and fascia must be pierced. Before venipuncture with a larger needle, the vein is located with a 22-gauge, 1½-inch needle attached to a syringe. The needle is inserted directly in the angle formed by the muscle and clavicle and directed medially at a 45-degree angle to the sagittal plane with the syringe depressed 15 degrees below the coronal plane. Continuous or intermittent gentle aspiration is applied to the syringe as the needle is advanced to immediately identify entry into the vein. The vein is usually encountered only one-half inch under the skin. Probing greater than 1 inch should be unnecessary and is dangerous.

When the vein has been located, the depth and direction of the locator needle are noted and the needle is removed. A 16- or 18-gauge, 2½-inch over-the-needle cannula or 18-gauge, thin-wall needle is inserted in the exact direction and depth of the locator needle. The cannula or needle is advanced into the vein. A flexible wire guide of either the straight or J type is inserted through the cannula or needle, the cannula or needle is removed, and the definitive catheter passed over the wire. Care should be taken to never lose grasp of the wire during catheter insertion to avoid wire embolism. The catheter is inserted 10 to 15 cm on the right and 15 to 20 cm on the left. The wire is removed, free flow of blood from the catheter is confirmed, and an intravenous infusion attached. The catheter is secured and chest radiograph obtained to confirm proper catheter position and to exclude a pneumothorax.

Variations of Insertion Technique: Supraclavicular

The most significant variation on the supraclavicular technique is an approach aimed at puncturing the subclavian vein at its junction with the internal jugular vein.[30] The skin entry point is 2 to 3 cm above the clavicle at the posterior border of the sternocleiodomastoid muscle. The needle is directed medially 35 degrees from the sagittal plane, and the syringe is depressed slightly below the coronal plane. The vein is usually encountered at a depth of 2 to 5 cm. This junctional approach is rarely used because of the increased danger of lymphatic damage and resulting chylothorax. Most other variations use the same entry point as described in the basic technique but use a slightly different needle direction or different catheterization technique.[105,109,113,114]

Success Rates

Most series report an 80 to 95 percent success rate, with greater than 90 percent of successful cannulations resulting in the catheter tip resting in the central circulation with the infraclavicular approach.[109–111,104–107] For the supraclavicular approach, most series report an 85 to 98 percent success rate, with greater than 90 percent of successful cannulations yielding central catheter placement.[30,105,109,113,114]

Complications

As with internal jugular vein cannulation, a high rate of success and low rate of complications during subclavian vein cannulation is directly related to the experience of the operator. Consequently, this technique should be learned under close super-

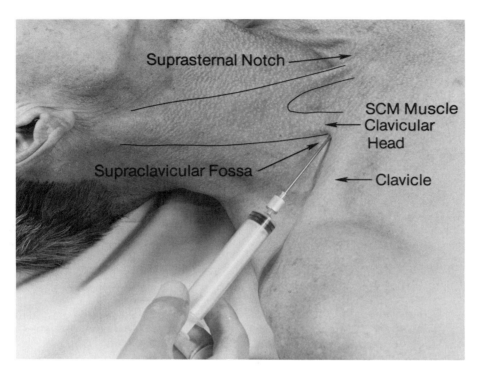

Fig. 9-23. Supraclavicular subclavian venipuncture with a short over-the-needle catheter. To allow demonstration of anatomic relationships, the usual sterile preparation and draping has not been used in this photograph. Appropriate sterile precautions should always be used when inserting central venous catheters. SCM, sternocleidomastoid.

vision. It is uniformly agreed that much caution should be used in infants and children,[106,107,110,118,119] although several authors have reported low complication rates with the infraclavicular approach. A series using the supraclavicular approach has not been reported in children. The complications of most concern are those associated with lacerating adjoining structures during puncture. The incidence of pneumothorax ranges from 0 to 3 percent in reported series with the infraclavicular approach[76,106,109–112,114,116–119] and 0 to 4.7 percent with the supraclavicular approach.[84,105,109,113,114] The overall incidence of pneumothorax appears to be approximately 1 percent, which is high enough to recommend that bilateral attempts at cannulation not be made without an intervening chest radiograph in order to avoid bilateral pneumothorax. A 1 to 2 percent incidence of arterial puncture has been reported in some series,[106,115] and hematomas may occur 1.5 to 3 percent of the time.[110,111,117] Hydrothorax and hemothorax are also reported in a number of series, with incidences ranging from 0.1

to 2 percent.[30,114,119,120] Puncture of the thoracic duct was reported in 0.9 percent of cases with the junctional approach.[30]

Less common complications reported include brachial plexus palsy,[42,120] mediastinal hemorrhage,[42] subclavian vein thrombosis,[30,114,121] arteriovenous fistula,[114] air embolism,[30,114] and catheter embolism.[122,123] This last complication (catheter embolism) of subclavian vein cannulation is important, since through-the-needle catheters are principally used for subclavian cannulation. Subclavian vein stenosis has been reported in nearly 50 percent of a series of patients who had subclavian catheterization for single catheter hemodialysis.[124] None of the patients developed clinically detectable complications and most recanalized the vein. However, such stenosis may lead to upper extremity edema and poor functioning of an arteriovenous fistula subsequently performed on the ipsilateral arm. Whether this complication has clinical significance other than for placement of ipsilateral vascular access is unknown at this time.[125–127]

Advantages and Disadvantages

The major advantage of the infraclavicular subclavian approach is the ability to secure the catheter to the anterior chest wall. In this position, the catheter has minimal movement with changes in body position, dressings stay secure, and the entrance site is away from potential neck wounds, such as tracheostomies. These considerations have dictated that the approach be the site of choice for parenteral alimentation lines. The fact that surrounding tissue connections tend to keep the vein from collapsing has also made it a favorite site for cannulation in the hypovolemic patient. The disadvantages are that it has a higher complication rate than other techniques, is more difficult to master, and is not readily accessible to an anesthesiologist at the head of the table. It is not recommended for patients with a bleeding diathesis or patients receiving anticoagulants. Pulmonary artery catheterization can be accomplished through infraclavicular subclavian vein cannulation. However, the very large cannula introducer may be difficult to pass under the clavicle or it may kink as it does so, making passage of the pulmonary artery catheter through the introducer impossible. (See Table 9-13).

The supraclavicular route to the subclavian vein has little to recommend it. Since the insertion site is in the neck, it has none of the catheter stability advantages of the infraclavicular approach. In many respects, it is similar to internal jugular cannulation but has less well-defined landmarks to direct the operator and a higher complication rate than the internal jugular approach.

TABLE 9-13. Infraclavicular Subclavian Vein Cannulation

Advantages	Disadvantages
High success rate	Requires experience
Best for long-term catheterization	Relatively high complication rate
Suitable for pulmonary artery catheterization	Inaccessible to anesthesiologist
Relatively good success in hypovolemic patient	

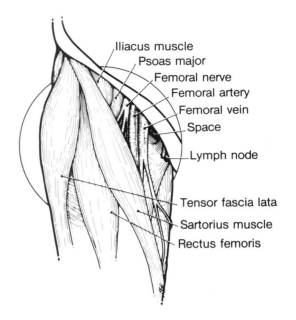

Fig. 9-24. Anatomy of femoral region.

Femoral Vein Cannulation

Anatomy

Venous drainage of the leg consists of a superficial and deep system of veins. The major superficial vein is the great saphenous, which begins in the foot, passes up the medial side of the leg, and empties into the femoral vein just below the inguinal ligament. Cannulation of the great saphenous usually requires surgical exposure. The femoral vein accompanies the femoral artery and becomes the external iliac vein at the inguinal ligament (Fig. 9-24). The femoral vein can be cannulated percutaneously in the femoral triangle just below the inguinal ligament. In the triangle, the major structures from lateral to medial are the femoral nerve, femoral artery, femoral vein, femoral canal (an empty space), and lymph node of Cloquet. In this area, these structures are covered only by the superficial and deep fascia and the arterial pulse can be easily palpated.

Because of the high rate of serious complications (primarily sepsis, thrombosis, and pulmonary embolism) reported in the 1950s, femoral vein cannulation was largely abandoned except when access was urgent or no other site was available. For this reason, much of the literature is decades old. In the mid-1980s, some physicians cautiously began trying the femoral vein for central venous access, especially in small children. The experience has generally been more favorable than previous reports. Consequently, femoral venous cannulation is enjoying a resurgence of interest.

Basic Insertion Technique

The patient is placed in the slightly head-up position and the thigh is abducted and externally rotated. Some operators place a pillow beneath the buttocks to make the groin more prominent. Either right or left femoral vein may be used. A wide area is prepped and draped. The operator should wear a gown, gloves, and mask. Local anesthesia is used if the patient is conscious. The length of catheter to be inserted should be estimated by laying it out along its route before insertion. This length will be approximately 30 to 35 cm in adults. The ideal catheter tip position is just below the diaphragm. A higher position results in the tip being within the heart.

In adults, the skin puncture site is about 1 cm medial to the palpated femoral artery, just below the inguinal ligament. In infants, puncture is made immediately medial to the artery. A small locator needle may be used if desired but is usually not necessary since the only adjacent structure in danger is the artery, which is readily palpated and, thus, avoided. Venipuncture is performed with a 16- or 18-gauge, 2½-inch over-the-needle cannula in adults and an 18- or 20-gauge over-the-needle cannula in infants and children. The direction of aim is slightly medial to the sagittal plane (parallel to the palpated pulse) with the syringe elevated 20 to 30 degrees above the surface of the skin. Continuous or intermittent gentle negative pressure is maintained in a syringe attached to the needle as it is advanced in order to promptly identify the vein as it is entered. The vein should be encountered at a depth of 2 to 4 cm in most adults.

Upon entering the vein, advance the cannula into the vein, remove and discard the needle. An appropriate size guide wire (Table 9-8), either straight or J-type, is advanced through the cannula, the cannula removed, and the definitive catheter advanced over the guide wire. Using a scalpel blade to carefully widen the puncture site around the wire and advancing the catheter with a rotary motion are aids in passing the catheter through the subcutaneous tissues. Care should be taken never to lose grasp of the wire during catheter insertion or a wire embolism may result. The catheter is inserted to its previously determined length and free flow of blood confirmed. The catheter is secured, an intravenous infusion connected, and a radiograph obtained to confirm catheter position.

Variations on Insertion Technique

A direct through-the-needle technique similar to that described for subclavian cannulation was the first technique described.[128] It is quite successful and eliminates the step of passing a guidewire. However, it limits the choice of catheters and results in a needle attached to the catheter. A pure Seldinger technique with a wire passed directly through a thin-wall needle may also be used. Direct over-the-needle cannulation is not feasible if central pressure monitoring is desired because the cannulas are not long enough to reach the central circulation in adults. However, this technique may be used if only large bore intravenous access is needed.

Success Rate

The original series by Duffy[128] reported a 100 percent success rate of cannulation. Recent series have also reported a high rate of success.[128–131] Cannulation should be successful in more than 90 percent of cases in adults and larger children with experienced operators. Success may be less in infants. Ultrasound may be of value in femoral vein cannulation.

Complications

Complications related to insertion are uncommon and minor. Unintentional arterial puncture, hematoma, and local bleeding are most common.[131] The major complications that led to near abandonment of this procedure were related to long term use. Although a few older reports had minimal complications,[131–134] most stressed the dangers of this technique.[76,77,135–138] Deep vein thrombosis or thrombophlebitis occurred in 5 to 50 percent of cases in these series. Pulmonary embolism occurred approximately 2 percent of the time in two series.[76,136] Sepsis was reported in 2 to 20 percent of cases.[76,135,136] Review of the literature by one author yielded an incidence of death of 4 percent

TABLE 9-14. Femoral Vein Cannulation

Advantages	Disadvantages
Simplicity	Inaccessible to
High success rate	anesthesiologist
Low immediate	Difficult to pass pulmonary
complication rate	artery catheter through
Suitable for pulmonary	heart
artery catheterization	Unknown rate of
	thromboembolic
	complications

related to femoral vein catheterization.[76] In contrast, more recent studies in children[129,130,139] and adults[131] have found no higher incidence of catheter-related infections than with other central venous catheter sites. None of these newer studies specifically addressed the issue of deep vein thrombosis, but they noted no clinical evidence of lower extremity edema or pulmonary embolus. However, this remains an issue for further study.

Advantages and Disadvantages

Cannulation of the femoral vein is a relatively simple technique with a high success rate and low incidence of immediate complications. (See Table 9-14). The femoral area is frequently inaccessible to the anesthesiologist during an operative procedure. Although the femoral vein is suitable for pulmonary artery catheterization, it is frequently more difficult to manipulate the catheter through the right heart from the inferior rather than superior vena cava. It is likely that with modern catheter management, the incidence of septic complications from femoral venous catheters is no greater than other central venous sites. Whether thromboembolic complications are similar in frequency and severity as other sites will require further study.

REFERENCES

1. Connors AF Jr, McCaffree DR, Gray BA: Evaluation of right-heart catheterization in the critically ill patient without acute myocardial infarction. N Engl J Med 308:263, 1983
2. Guyton AC, Jones CE, Coleman TG: Circulatory Physiology: Cardiac Output and Its Regulation. 2nd Ed. WB Saunders, Philadelphia, 1973
3. Lake CL: Anesthesia and pericardial disease. Anesth Analg 62:431, 1983
4. Qvist J, Pontoppidan H, Wilson RS et al: Hemodynamic response to mechanical ventilation with PEEP: the effect of hypervolemia. Anesthesiology 42:45, 1975
5. Seldinger SI: Catheter replacement of the needle in percutaneous arteriography. Acta Radiol 39:368, 1953
6. Blitt DE, Wright WA, Petty WC, Webster TA: Central venous catheterization via the external jugular vein: a technique employing the J-wire. JAMA 229:817, 1974.
7. Blitt CD, Carlson GL, Wright WA, Otto CW: J-wire versus straight wire for central venous system cannulation via the external jugular vein. Anesth Analg 61:536, 1982
8. Nordstrom L, Fletcher R: Comparison of two different J-wires for central venous cannulation via the external jugular vein. Anesth Analg 62:365, 1983
9. Humphrey MJ, Blitt CD: Central venous access in children via the external jugular vein. Anesthesiology 57:50, 1982
10. Wilmore DW, Dudrick SJ: Safe long term venous catheterization. Arch Surg 98:256, 1969
11. Faubion WC, Wesley JR, Khalidi N et al: Total parenteral nutrition catheter sepsis: impact of the team approach. J Parenter Enteral Nutr 10:642, 1986
12. Maki DG, Ringer M, Alvarado CJ: Prospective randomised trial of povidone-iodine, alcohol, and chlorhexidine for prevention of infection associated with central venous and arterial catheters. Lancet 338:339, 1991
13. Broviac JW, Cole JJ, Scribner BH: A silicone rubber atrial catheter for prolonged parenteral alimentation. Surg Gynecol Obstet 136:602, 1973
14. Heird WC, Driscoll JM, Schullinger JN et al: Intravenous alimentation in pediatric patients. J Pediatr 80:351, 1972
15. Maki DG, Cobb L, Garman JK et al: An attachable silver-impregnated cuff for the prevention of infection with central venous catheter: a prospective, randomized multicenter trial. Am J Med 85:307, 1988
16. Flowers RH, Schwenzer KJ, Kiple RF et al: Efficacy of an attachable subcutaneous cuff for the prevention of intravascular catheter-related infections. JAMA 261:878, 1989
17. Norwood S, Hajjar G, Jenlins L: The influence of an attachable subcutaneous cuff for preventing triple lumen catheter infections in critically ill surgical and trauma patients. Surg Gynecol Obstet 175:33, 1992
18. Kamal GD, Pfaller MA, Rempe LE, Jebson PJR: Reduced intravascular catheter infection by antibiotic bonding: a prospective, randomized, controlled trial. JAMA 265:2364, 1991

19. Maki DG, Wheeler SJ, Stolz SM, Mermel LA: Clinical trial of a novel antiseptic central venous catheter, abstracted. In: Program and abstracts of the 31st Interscience Conference on Antimicrobial Agents and Chemotherapy (Chicago). Washington, DC. American Society for Microbiology, 1991

20. Ryan JA Jr: Complications of total parenteral nutrition. p. 55. In Fischer JE (ed): Total Parenteral Nutrition. Little, Brown, Boston, 1976

21. Norden CW: Application of antibiotic ointment to the site of venous catheterization: a controlled trial. J Infect Dis 120:611, 1969

22. Zinner SH, Denny-Brown BC, Braun P et al: Risk of infection with intravenous indwelling catheters: effect of application of antibiotic ointment. J Infect Dis 120:616, 1969

23. Maki DG, Band JD: A comparative study of polyantibiotic and iodophor ointments in prevention of vascular catheter-related infection. Am J Med 70:739, 1981

24. Allen JR: The incidence of nosocomial infection in patients receiving total parenteral nutrition. p. 3391. In Johnson IDA (ed): Advances in Parenteral Nutrition. MTP, Lancaster, PA, 1977

25. Hoffmann KK, Weber DJ, Samsa GP, Rutala WA: Transparent polyurethane film as an intravenous catheter dressing: a meta-analysis of the infection risks. JAMA 267:2072, 1992.

26. Richet H, Hubert B, Nitemberg G et al: Prospective multicenter study of vascular-catheter-related complications and risk factors for positive central-catheter culture in intensive care unit patients. J Clin Microbiol 28:2520, 1990

27. Mallory DL, Shawker T, Evans RG et al: Effects of clinical maneuvers on sonographically determined internal jugular vein size during venous cannulation. Crit Care Med 18:1269, 1990

28. Civetta JM, Gabel JC, Gemer M: Internal jugular vein puncture with a margin of safety. Anesthesiology 36:622, 1972

29. Prince SR, Sullivan RL, Hackel A: Percutaneous catheterization of the internal jugular vein in infants and children. Anesthesiology 44:170, 1976

30. Haapaniemi L, Slatis P: Supraclavicular catheterisation of the superior vena cava. Acta Anaesthesiol Scand 18:12, 1974

31. Denys BG, Uretsky BF: Anatomical variations of internal jugular vein location: impact on central venous access. Crit Care Med 19:1516, 1991

32. Troianos CA, Jobes DR, Ellison N: Ultrasound-guided cannulation of the internal jugular vein: a prospective randomized study. Anesth Analg 72:823, 1991

33. Alderson PJ, Burrows FA, Stemp LI, Holtby HM: Use of ultrasound to evaluate internal jugular vein anatomy and to facilitate central venous cannulation in paediatric patients. Br J Anaesth 70:145, 1993

34. Denys BG, Uretsky BF, Reddy PS: Ultrasound-assisted cannulation of the internal jugular vein. Circulation 87:1557, 1993

35. Jobes DR, Schwartz AJ, Greenhow DE et al: Safer jugular vein cannulation: recognition of arterial puncture and preferential use of the external jugular route. Anesthesiology 59:353, 1983

36. Bunegin L, Albin MS, Helsel PE et al: Positioning the right atrial catheter: a model for reappraisal. Anesthesiology 55:343, 1981

37. Duntley P, Siever J, Korwes ML et al: Vascular erosion by central venous catheters: clinical features and outcome. Chest 101:1633, 1992

38. Sheep RE, Guiney WB: Fatal cardiac tamponade: occurrence with other complications after left internal jugular vein catheterization. JAMA 248:1632, 1982

39. Ghani GA, Berry AJ: Right hydrothorax after left external jugular vein catheterization. Anesthesiology 58:93, 1983

40. Greenall MJ, Blewitt RW, McMahon MJ: Cardiac tamponade and central venous catheters. Br Med J 2:595, 1975

41. Peres PW: Positioning central venous catheters: a prospective survey. Anaesth Intens Care 18:536, 1990

42. Kaye W: Catheter- and infusion-related sepsis: the nature of the problem and its prevention. Heart Lung 11:221, 1982

43. Dillon JD Jr, Schaffner W, Van Way CW III, Meng HC: Septicemia and total parenteral nutrition. JAMA 223:1341, 1973

44. Myers RN, Smink RD, Goldstein F: Parenteral hyperalimentation: five year's clinical experience. Am J Gastroenterol 62:313, 1974

45. Goldman DA, Maki DG: Infection control in total parenteral nutrition. JAMA 223:1360, 1973

46. Ryan JA, Abel RM, Abbott WM et al: Catheter complications in total parenteral nutrition. N Engl J Med 290:757, 1974

47. Pemberton LB, Lyman B, Lander V et al: Sepsis from triple- vs single-lumen catheters during total parenteral nutrition in surgical or critically ill patients. Arch Surg 121:591, 1986

48. Yeung C, May J, Hughes R: Infection rate for single lumen v triple lumen subclavian catheters. Infect Control Hosp Epidemiol 9:154, 1988

49. Farkas JC, Liu N, Bleriot JP et al: Single- versus triple-lumen central catheter-related sepsis: a prospective randomized study in a critically ill population. Am J Med 93:277, 1992

50. Maki DG, Goldman DA, Rhame FS: Infection con-

trol in intravenous therapy. Ann Intern Med 79: 867, 1973

51. Miller JJ, Bahman V, Mathru M: Comparison of the sterility of long-term central venous catheterization using single lumen, triple lumen, and pulmonary artery catheters. Crit Care Med 12:634, 1984

52. Eyer S, Brummitt C, Crossley K et al: Catheter-related sepsis: prospective, randomized study of three methods of long-term catheter maintenance. Crit Care Med 18:1073, 1990

53. Cobb DK, High KP, Sawyer RG et al: A controlled trial of scheduled replacement of central venous and pulmonary-artery catheters. N Engl J Med 327: 1062, 1992

54. Dietel M, McIntyre JA: Radiographic confirmation of site of central venous pressure catheters. Can J Surg 14:42, 1971

55. Langston CS: The aberrant central venous catheter and its complications. Radiology 100:55, 1971

56. Burgess GE, Marino RJ, Peuler MJ: Effect of head position in the location of venous catheters inserted via basilic veins. Anesthesiology 46:212, 1977

57. Woods DG, Lumley J, Russell WJ, Jacks RD: The position of central venous catheters inserted through arm veins: a preliminary report. Anaesth Intens Care 2:43, 1974

58. Bridges BB, Carden E, Takacs FA: Introduction of central venous pressure catheters through arm veins with a high success rate. Can Anaesth Soc J 26:128, 1979

59. Smith SL, Albin MS, Ritter RR, Bunegin L: CVP catheter placement from the antecubital veins using a J-wire catheter guide. Anesthesiology 60:238, 1984

60. Spracklen FHN, Niesche F, Lord PW, Beterman EMM: Percutaneous catheterisation of the axillary vein. Cardiovasc Res 1:297, 1967

61. Ayim EN: Percutaneous catheterization of axillary vein and proximal basilic vein. Anaesthesia 32:753, 1977

62. Holt HM: Central venous pressure via peripheral veins. Anesthesiology 28:1093, 1967

63. Johnston AOB, Clark RG: Malpositioning of central venous catheters. Lancet 2:1395, 1972

64. Lumley J, Russell WJ: Insertion of central venous catheters through arm veins. Anaesth Intens Care 3:101, 1975

65. Ng WS, Rosen M: Positioning central venous catheters through the basillic vein: a comparison of catheters. Br J Anaesth 45:1211, 1973

66. Sorenson TIA, Sonne-Holm S: Central venous catheterization through the basillic vein or by infraclavicular puncture. Acta Chir Scand 141:323, 1975

67. Webre DR, Arens JF: Use of cephalic and basilic veins for introduction of central venous catheters. Anesthesiology 38:389, 1971

68. Cockington RA: Silicone elastomer for nasojejunal intubation and central venous cannulation in neonates. Anaesth Intens Care 7:248, 1979

69. Giesy J: External jugular vein access to central venous system. JAMA 219:1216, 1972

70. Jernigan WR, Gardner WC, Mahr MM, Milburn JL: Use of the internal jugular vein for placement of central venous catheter. Surg Gynecol Obstet 120: 520, 1970

71. Malatinsky J, Kadlic M, Majek M, Samel M: Misplacement and loop information of central venous catheters. Acta Anaesthesiol Scand 20:237, 1976

72. Rosen M, Latto IP, Ng S: Handbook of Percutaneous Central Venous Catheterisation. 2nd Ed. WB Saunders, London, 1992

73. Rams JJ, Daicoff GR, Moulder PV: A simple method for central venous pressure measurements. Arch Surg 92:886, 1966

74. Stoelting RK: Evaluation of external jugular venous pressure as a reflection of right atrial pressure. Anesthesiology 38:291, 1973

75. Belani KG, Buckley JJ, Gordon JR, Castenada W: Percutaneous cervical central venous line placement: a comparison of the internal and external jugular vein routes. Anesth Analog 59:40, 1980

76. Burri C, Ahnefeld FW: The Caval Catheter. Springer-Verlag, Berlin, 1978

77. Blitt CD: Catheterization Techniques for Invasive Cardiovascular Monitoring. Charles C Thomas, Springfield, IL, 1981

78. English ICW, Frew RM, Pigott JF, Zaki M: Percutaneous catheterization of the internal jugular vein. Anaesthesia 24:521, 1969

79. Mostert JW, Kenny GM, Murphy GP: Safe placement of central venous catheter into internal jugular veins. Arch Surg 101:431, 1970

80. Brinkman AJ, Costley DO: Internal jugular venipuncture. JAMA 223:182, 1973

81. Hall DMB, Geefhuysen J: Percutaneous catheterization of the internal jugular vein in infants and children. J Pediatr Surg 12:719, 1977

82. Daily PO, Griepp RB, Shumway NE: Percutaneous internal jugular vein cannulation. Arch Surg 101: 534, 1970

83. Rao TLK, Wong AY, Salem MR: A new approach to percutaneous catheterization of the internal jugular vein. Anesthesiology 46:362, 1977

84. Cook TL, Deuker CW: Tension pneumothorax following internal jugular cannulation and general anesthesia. Anesthesiology 45:554, 1976

85. Schuster W, Vennebusch H, Doetsch N, Taube HD: Vena cava superior thrombosis following placement of internal jugular vein catheter. Anaesthetist 27: 546, 1978

86. Knoblanche GE: Respiratory obstruction due to he-

matoma following internal jugular vein cannulation. Anaesth Intens Care 7:286, 1979

87. Butsch JL, Butsch WL, Da Rossa JFT: Bilateral vocal cord paralysis: a complication of percutaneous cannulation of the internal jugular veins. Arch Surg 111:828, 1976

88. Parikh RK: Horner's syndrome: a complication of percutaneous catheterisation of internal jugular vein. Anaesthesia 27:327, 1972

89. Briscoe CE, Bushman JA, McDonald WI: Extensive neurological damage after cannulation of internal jugular vein. Br Med J 1:314, 1974

90. Brown CS, Wallace CT: Chronic hematoma: a complication of percutaneous catheterization of the internal jugular vein. Anesthesiology 45:368, 1976

91. Arnold S, Feathers RS, Gibbs E: Bilateral pneumothoraces and subcutaneous emphysema: a complication of internal jugular venipuncture. Br Med J 1:211, 1973

92. Blitt CD, Wright WA: An unusual complication of percutaneous internal jugular vein cannulation, puncture of an endotracheal tube cuff. Anesthesiology 40:306, 1974

93. McDaniel MM, Grossman M: Aortic dissection complicating percutaneous jugular-vein catheterisation. Anesthesiology 49:213, 1978

94. Shield CF, Richardson JD, Buckley CF, Hagood CO: Pseudoaneurysm of the brachiocephalic arteries: a complication of percutaneous internal jugular vein catheterization. Surgery 78:190, 1975

95. Schwartz AJ: Percutaneous aortic catheterization: a hazard of supraclavicular internal-jugular-vein catheterization. Anesthesiology 46:77, 1977

96. Wisheart JD, Hassan MA, Jackson JW: A complication of percutaneous cannulation of the internal jugular vein. Thorax 27:496, 1972

97. Carvell JE, Pearce DJ: Bilateral hydrothorax following internal jugular vein catheterization. Br J Surg 63:381, 1976

98. Koch MJ: Bilateral "I.V. hydrothorax." N Engl J Med 286:218, 1972

99. Ayalon A, Anner H, Berlatzky Y, Schiller M: A life-threatening complication of the infusion pump. Lancet 1:853, 1978

100. Ross SM, Freeman PS, Farman JV: Air embolism after accidental removal of intravenous catheter. Br Med J 1:987, 1979

101. Sprigge JS, Oakley GDG: Carotid artery palpation during internal jugular cannulation and subsequent ventricular fibrillation. Br J Anaesth 51:807, 1979

102. Ohlgisser M, Kaufman TS, Taitelman V et al: Cardiac arrest following a complication of internal jugular vein cannulation. Anaesthesia 34:1035, 1979

103. Goldfarb G, Lebrec D: Percutaneous cannulation of the internal jugular vein in patients with coagulopathies: an experience based on 1,000 attempts. Anesthesiology 56:321, 1982

104. Aubaniac R: L'injection intraveineuse sousclaviculaire; avantages et technique. Presse Med 60:1456, 1952

105. Yoffa D: Supraclavicular subclavian venipuncture and catheterization. Lancet 2:614, 1965

106. Morgan WW, Harkins GA: Percutaneous introduction of long-term indwelling venous catheters in infants. J Pediatr Surg 7:538, 1972

107. Wilson JN, Grow JB, Demong CV et al: Central venous pressure in optimal blood volume maintenance. Arch Surg 98:256, 1969

108. Borja AR, Hinshaw JR: A safe way to perform infraclavicular subclavian vein catheterization. Surg Gynecol Obstet 130:673, 1970

109. Christensen KH, Nerstrom B, Baden H: Complications of percutaneous catheterisation of the subclavian vein in 129 cases. Acta Chir Scand 133:615, 1967

110. Davidson JT, Ben-Hur N, Nathen H: Subclavian venepuncture. Lancet 2:1139, 1963

111. Mogil RA, Delaurentis DA, Rosemond GP: The infraclavicular venepuncture. Arch Surg 95:320, 1967

112. Tofield JJ: A safer technique of percutaneous catheterisation of the subclavian vein. Surg Gynecol Obstet 128:1069, 1969

113. Freeman J: Subclavian vein catheterization. Med J Aust 2:979, 1968

114. James PM, Myers RT: Central venous pressure monitoring: complications and a new technique. Am Surg 39:75, 1973

115. Blackett RJ, Bakran A, Bradley JA et al: A prospective study of subclavian vein catheters used exclusively for the purpose of intravenous feeding. Br J Surg 65:393, 1976

116. Defalque RJ: The subclavian route: a critical review of the world literature up to 1970. Anaesthetist 21:325, 1972

117. Williams RW, McDonald JC: A prospective study of the dangers of central venous pressure monitoring. Am Surg 37:719, 1971

118. Dudrick SJD, Wilmore DW, Vars HM, Rhodes JE: Can intravenous feeding as the sole means of nutrition support growth in the child and restore weight loss in an adult? Ann Surg 169:974, 1969

119. Groff DB, Ahmed N: Subclavian vein catheterization in the infant. J Pediatr Surg 9:171, 1974

120. Smith BE, Modell JH, Gaub ML, Moya F: Complications of subclavian vein catheterisation. Arch Surg 90:228, 1965

121. Feiler EM, deAlva WE: Infraclavicular percutaneous subclavian vein puncture: a safe technique. Am J Surg 118:906, 1969

122. Longerbeam JK, Vannix R, Wagner W, Joergenson E: Central venous pressure monitoring: a useful guide to fluid therapy during shock and other forms of cardiovascular stress. Am J Surg 110:220, 1965

123. Massumi RA, Ross AM: A traumatic nonsurgical technique for removal of broken catheters from cardiac cavities. N Engl J Med 277:195, 1967

124. Spinowitz BS, Galler M, Golden RA et al: Subclavian vein stenosis as a complication of subclavian catheterization for hemodialysis. Arch Intern Med 147:305, 1987

125. Cimochowski GE et al: Superiority of the internal jugular over subclavian access for temporary dialysis. Nephron 54:154, 1990

126. Wanscher M et al: Thrombosis caused by polyurethane double-lumen subclavian superior vena cava catheters and hemodialysis. Crit Care Med 16:624, 1988

127. Barrett N et al: Subclavian stenosis: a major complication of subclavian dialysis catheter. Nephrol Dialysis Transplant 3:423, 1988

128. Duffy BJ: The clinical use of polyethylene tubing for intravenous therapy. Ann Surg 130:929, 1949

129. Kanter RK, Zimmerman JJ, Strauss RH et al: Central venous catheter insertion by femoral vein: safety and effectiveness for the pediatric patient. Pediatrics 77:842, 1986

130. Newman BM, Jewett TC Jr, Karp MP et al: Percutaneous central venous catheterization in children: first line choice for venous access. J Pediatr Surg 21:685, 1986

131. Williams JF, Seneff MG, Friedman BC et al: Use of femoral venous catheter in critically ill adults: prospective study. Crit Care med 19:550, 1991

132. Hohn AR, Lambert EC: Continuous venous catheterization in children. JAMA 197:658, 1966

133. Ladd M, Schreiner GE: Plastic tubing for intravenous alimentation. JAMA 145:642, 1951

134. Shaw G: Acute renal insufficiency treated by caval infusion of dextrose solutions of high concentration. Lancet 1:15, 1959

135. Bansmer G, Keith D, Tesluk H: Complications following use of indwelling catheters of inferior vena cava. JAMA 167:1606, 1958

136. Bonner CD: Experience with plastic tubing in prolonged intravenous therapy. N Engl J Med 245:97, 1951

137. Lynn KL, Maling TMJ: Case reports: a major pulmonary embolus as a complication of femoral vein catheterisation. Br J Radiol 50:667, 1977

138. Page OC, Stephens JW: Prolonged intravenous alimentation: use of polyethylene tubing in inferior vena cava or common iliac veins. Northwest Med 53:596, 1954

139. Stenzel JP, Green TO, Fuhrman BP et al: Percutaneous femoral venous catheterizations: a prospective study of complications. J Pediatr 114:411, 1989

Pulmonary Artery Catheterization

10

Roberta L. Hines
Paul G. Barash

Since its development more than 20 years ago as a research tool in the study of myocardial infarction, the balloon-tipped pulmonary artery flotation catheter (Swan-Ganz catheter) has become one of the most important and valuable clinical tools for monitoring the critically ill patient. In 1929, Forssmann, a surgical resident, used a mirror to catheterize his own right atrium via the left antecubital vein.[1] Skill in cardiac catheterization increased markedly over the next several decades, until this procedure became commonplace in the cardiac catheterization laboratory. However, the technique required fluoroscopic guidance and was time-consuming, often requiring 20 to 30 minutes for catheter passage. In addition, approximately 30 percent of all attempts at catheter placement were unsuccessful. Fortunately, in 1953, in conjunction with their experiments isolating each lung, Lategola and Rahn[2] developed a catheter with an inflatable balloon at the tip. They reported that the catheter consistently and easily slipped into the pulmonary artery without extensive manipulation. However, no clinical notice was taken of the accomplishment, and it remained for Jeremy Swan, William Ganz, and their colleagues[3,4] to "rediscover" the principle two decades later. "Bedside" monitoring of the critically ill became a reality, since fluoroscopy was no longer needed and rapid passage to the pulmonary artery was easily achieved. As originally designed, the catheter measured pulmonary artery and pulmonary capillary wedge pressures. Subsequently, the catheter has been modified to do the following:

1. Measure cardiac output by thermodilution
2. Allow infusion of drugs
3. Perform angiography
4. Obtain intracavitary electrograms
5. Perform atrial and/or ventricular pacing
6. Calculate lung water
7. Calculate ejection fraction
8. Detect venous air embolism

In short, the pulmonary artery catheter has revolutionized cardiovascular monitoring.[5-14]

CATHETER DESIGN

The standard 7 Fr thermodilution pulmonary artery catheter (PAC) consists of a single catheter, 110 cm in length, containing four lumina.[15] It is constructed of flexible, radiopaque polyvinyl chloride (Fig. 10-1). Beginning at the distal end, 10-cm increments are marked in black on the catheter. At the distal end of the catheter is a latex rubber balloon of 1.5 ml capacity. When inflated, the balloon extends slightly beyond the tip of the catheter, but does not obstruct it. This feature prevents the tip of the catheter from contacting the right ventricular wall during passage and is responsible for the reduced incidence of arrhythmias during insertion. Not only does the balloon reduce the force of contact against the right ventricular wall, but it also acts to float the catheter into the pulmonary artery. Finally, inflation of the balloon allows measurement of the pulmonary capillary wedge pressure. As N_2O can diffuse into the PAC balloon,[16,17] in patients receiving this anesthetic (especially in the pediatric age group), the duration of balloon inflation should be kept to a minimum. In addition, the development of high intraballoon pressure may cause disruption of the pulmonary artery.[18,19] Studies have implicated high peak intraballoon pressures, which are transmitted to the pulmonary artery, as the main etiology of this problem.[18–20] Recently, Ikeda and associates[21] evaluated the pressure-volume relationship of the balloon in four different PACs.[21] In this study, a slower rate of balloon inflation (over 2.5 to 6 seconds) resulted in a lower peak pressure and a lower balloon volume. Therefore, these authors suggest that, to minimize the potential for excessive intraballoon pressure (and secondary increases in volume), air should be injected slowly, preferably over at least 3 seconds. Initial reports suggested that the composition of the PAC balloon (polyvinyl chloride) may also increase the risk for pulmonary artery perforation.[22] As a result, polyurethane has been suggested as an alternative material for balloon manufacture.[23] A potential advantage of the polyurethane balloon is that the material softens at body temperature and does not stiffen over time (a trait of polyvinyl chloride catheters). Although theoretically attractive, the clinical advantages of polyurethane balloons remains to be elucidated. The standard 7 Fr PAC has a relatively low natural frequency (16 to 22 Hz), which is governed mainly by the length of pressure tubing used. This may cause artifacts and introduce errors in interpretation of pulmonary artery and pulmonary capillary wedge pressures.[22,23]

INFORMATION OBTAINED WITH THE PULMONARY ARTERY CATHETER

The marked advance in critical care and intraoperative monitoring brought about by the PAC rests on its ability to provide fundamental hemodynamic information and to provide data necessary for calculation of derived hemodynamic indices. Information provided by the PAC includes (1) right- and left-sided intracardiac pressures, (2) cardiac output by the thermodilution method, and (3) mixed venous blood for gas and chemical analysis. In addition, newer catheters facilitate diagnosis of complex arrhythmias, provide continuous measurement of mixed venous oxygen saturation, and allow for pacing of the atrium and/or ventricle.

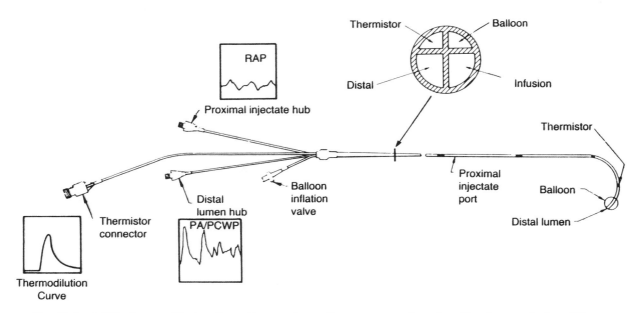

Fig. 10-1. A 7 Fr thermodilution Swan-Ganz catheter. Inset cross section, detailing lumen design. (Courtesy of American Edwards Laboratories.)

Intracardiac Pressure Measurements

Pulmonary capillary wedge pressure is an indirect measurement of left ventricular end-diastolic pressure (Fig. 10-2). Traditionally, left ventricular end-diastolic pressure measurements have been employed to assess left ventricular function. However, a normal left ventricular end-diastolic pressure (6 to 12 mmHg) does not ensure normal ventricular function. Conversely, an abnormal left ventricular end-diastolic pressure (>15 mmHg) cannot directly measure the degree of left ventricular impairment. Left ventricular end-diastolic pressure has also been used to assess preload.

Preload is classically derived from measurement of end-diastolic fiber length (or end-diastolic volume). However, due to logistic problems of routinely obtaining ventricular volume, a pressure measurement has been employed. Depending on the state of ventricular compliance, left ventricular end-diastolic pressure may or may not have a linear relationship to left ventricular end-diastolic volume. In the absence of mitral valve disease, pulmonary capillary wedge pressure approximates left atrial pressure. Therefore, a more clinically available measurement of preload is the pulmonary capillary wedge pressure (normal: 8 to 12 mmHg).

Pulmonary capillary wedge pressure correlates with left ventricular end-diastolic pressure (left atrial pressure) over a wide range of filling pressures (5-25 mmHg).[24-28] Exceptions to this include:

Pulmonary capillary wedge pressure greater than left ventricular end-diastolic pressure
  Mitral stenosis
  Elevated airway pressure (positive end-expiratory pressure [PEEP])
  Left atrial myxoma
  Pulmonary capillary wedge pressure less than left ventricular end-diastolic pressure
  Stiff left ventricle
  Left ventricular end-diastolic pressure >25 mmHg
  Premature closure of mitral valve (aortic insufficiency)

To avoid the potential users associated with PAC balloon inflation, pulmonary artery end-diastolic pressure is frequently used as an estimate of pulmonary capillary wedge pressure.[29-34] In the absence of increased pulmonary vascular resistance (e.g., chronic mitral stenosis, chronic left ventricular failure, pulmonary disease) the gradient between pulmonary artery end-diastolic pressure and pulmonary capillary wedge pressure is approximately 1-4 mmHg.[35-38] Pulmonary artery end-diastolic pressure may be greater than pulmonary capillary wedge pressure in a patient with tachycardia, since diastolic filling time is decreased.[27] The anatomic site of PAC also impacts upon the pulmonary capillary wedge pressure-left atrial pressure relationship. The ideal position for obtaining a pulmonary capillary wedge pressure is in a large branch of pulmonary artery. This will result in a good pulmonary capillary wedge pressure-left atrial pressure correlation. However, wedging in a small artery yields a pulmonary capillary wedge pressure higher than left atrial pressure.[39,40] Occasionally, the transition from pulmonary artery to pulmonary capillary wedge pressure may not be evident by changes in waveform analysis. In these situations

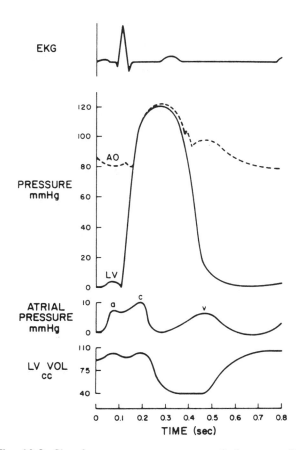

Fig. 10-2. Simultaneous measurement of electrocardiogram, systemic blood pressure (BP), left ventricular pressure (LVP), left atrial pressure (LAP), left ventricular volume (LV).

aspiration of pulmonary capillary blood will confirm PAC location.[41]

A number of additional factors alter the correlation between pulmonary capillary wedge pressure and left atrial pressure, including incorrect catheter placement, transducer related artifacts, eccentric balloon occlusion, non-zone III pulmonary capillary wedge pressure, pulmonary venous occlusive disease, valvular heart disease, pericardial tamponade and altered left ventricular compliance, and the presence of mitral regurgitation (V waves).[42-44] In addition, depending on the state of ventricular compliance, left ventricular end-diastolic pressure may or may not have a linear relationship to left ventricular end-diastolic volume.[45-49] An elegant study by Pichard and colleagues[50] has clearly demonstrated how the left atrial waveforms are affected by compliance changes. They showed that the patient would develop a large v wave without ischemia or mitral regurgitation when the preload was acutely increase; a large cardiac filling volume makes the pulmonary venous and atrial systems noncompliant where a small stroke volume can create a significant v wave. In contrast, if the pulmonary artery opening pressor is low and the pulmonary veins and the atrium are compliant, severe mitral regurgitation may be associated with a normal-sized v wave. This study demonstrated a poor correlation between the severity of mitral regurgitation and the height of the v wave.

Right atrial pressure (normal: 0 to 8 mmHg) obtained from the proximal port of the standard thermodilution catheter, yields valuable information regarding right ventricular performance.[10,51,52] Studies show that right ventricular ischemia has been be detected by continuous monitoring of right atrial pressure and combined with electrocardiography.[53] Right atrial pressure is also critical in the early diagnosis of cardiac tamponade (Fig. 10-3). However, by itself, right atrial pressure has been shown to be a poor predictor of left ventricular filling pressure.[54-56]

To summarize:

LVEDV $\propto$ ventricular compliance $\propto$ LVEDP $\propto$ mitral valve $\propto$ LAP $\propto$ airway pressure $\propto$ PCWP $\propto$ pulmonary vascular resistance

PAEDP $\propto$ right ventricular compliance $\propto$ RVEDP $\propto$ tricuspid valve $\propto$ RAP

When used in combination with a measurement of flow (i.e., cardiac output) the information gained from the pulmonary capillary wedge pressure measurement will be maximized. This is es-

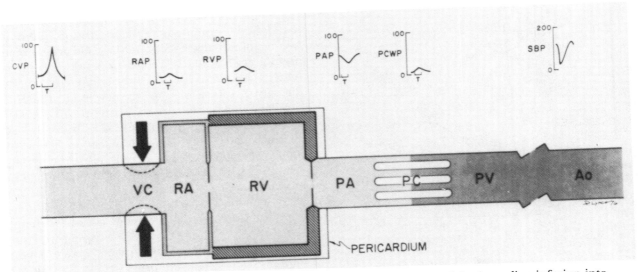

Fig. 10-3. Schematic representation of cardiac tamponade in a canine model using saline infusion into the intact pericardial sac. Due to anatomic relationships of the pericardium, the CVP will give the first indications of tamponade.

pecially applicable when making a diagnosis or instituting a new therapy. For example, a patient may have a reduced blood pressure and decreased pulmonary capillary wedge pressure (e.g., blood pressure 70/50; pulmonary capillary wedge pressure, 4 mmHg). Clinically, this may be interpreted as hypovolemia. This would be true if the patient has a low cardiac output (<3 L/min). However, the patient had the same blood pressure (70/50 mmHg) and pulmonary capillary wedge pressure (4 mmHg) with a high cardiac output state (8 L/min), case septic shock may lead the differential diagnosis list. Therefore, a cardiac output should accompany the measurement of pulmonary capillary wedge pressure determination when any clinically important diagnostic, therapeutic, or prognostic decision is to be made.

Thermodilution Cardiac Output

The ability to obtain accurate, rapid, and repetitive measurements of cardiac output is one of the principal advantages of the pulmonary artery catheter.[57–60] The information gained from serial measurements of cardiac output can be vital in diagnosis, evaluation of therapeutic interventions, and assessing prognosis.[60–63] Estimation of cardiac output from physical diagnosis has been shown to be unreliable,[64–66] and therefore direct measurement is essential.

The thermodilution method of measuring cardiac output was first described in 1954 by Fegler.[67] Subsequent incorporation of a thermistor into the pulmonary artery catheter greatly enhanced the usefulness of the technique in clinical medicine.[1,68,69] An excellent correlation has been reported between thermodilution cardiac output and other techniques, including dye dilution techniques, the Fick method, the Doppler method, and radionuclear and electromagnetic flow meters.[70–81]

Thermodilution cardiac output is a variant of the indicator dilution technique, with "cold" used as the trace indicator. Cooling of the blood is accomplished by the injection of 5 percent dextrose and noting that the change in temperature at the downstream sampling site is proportional to cardiac output.

The thermodilution principle is described by the Stewart-Hamilton equation:

$$Q = \frac{V_I (T_B - T_I) K_1 K_2}{T_B(t)\, dt}$$

where

Q = cardiac output
V_I = injectate volume
T_B = blood temperature
T_I = injectate temperature
K_1 = density factor

$$\frac{(\text{specific heat}) (\text{specific gravity}) \text{injectate}}{(\text{specific heat}) (\text{specific gravity}) \text{blood}}$$

K_2 = a computation constant that includes heat change in transit, dead space of the catheter, and injection rate, and adjusts the units to liters per minute
$T_B(t)\, dt$ = change in blood temperature as a function of time

Solution of this equation is accomplished by the cardiac output computer, which integrates the area under the thermodilution curve and displays a digital readout of cardiac output in liters per minute.[79] Cardiac output is inversely proportional to the area under the curve ($T_B(t)\ dt$).

Volume of Injectate (V_I)

Standard cardiac output measurements are performed with 2.5, 5, or 10 ml of injectate (D_5W). The volume of injectate must be accurately measured as it will affect the total amount of thermal indicator injected. If careful attention is paid to filling syringes, the error introduced by variations in volume is small, amounting to 1 percent. If a separate injectate catheter is used, it should have the same volume as the proximal port of the PAC,[82,83] or the computation constant (K_2) should be changed.

Blood Temperature (T_B)

A stable baseline blood temperature is essential for computing an accurate thermodilution curve. Currently available cardiac output computers utilize a thermistor to measure pulmonary artery temperature. Even so, baseline temperatures can be seen to vary in phase with the respiratory cycle. These variations are small with normal respiration, amounting to 0.01 to 0.02°C, but are accentuated in dyspneic patients or patients being mechanically ventilated. To obviate or minimize the effect of these variations, each injection of the thermal indicator should be performed at the same time in the respiratory cycle.[54]

Injectate Temperature (T_1)

Of equal importance is the accurate measurement of injectate temperature. Temperatures ranging from 0°C to room temperature (19 to 24°C) can be used. However, warm solutions require larger injectate volumes and higher thermistor sensitivities than do iced solutions.[84] The use of iced solutions increases the signal-to-noise ratio by a factor of 2:3. In theory, this may lead to greater reproducibility of results. Commercially, systems are now available for maintaining cold injectate syringes and/or accurately measuring injectate temperature at the proximal port. However, studies using an in vitro model failed to show any difference in accuracy or reproducibility between iced injectate or room temperature injectate. A potential hazard of cold injectate has been recently reported by Nishikawa and Dohi.[85] They observed that a transient bradycardia following injection of 10 ml of iced D_5W (Fig. 10-4).

The time between withdrawal of the injectate and injection should be as short as possible. Significant warming of the iced injectate can occur in handling and during prolonged injection phases. Most computation constants assume injection to have been made in less than 4 seconds. Little warming of room-temperature injectate occurs between filling the syringe and injection. As a result, newer methods, using in-line temperature probes, have been developed that allow for measurement of injectate temperature as the injection proceeds. A 1°C increase in the temperature of the injectate will cause an error of 3 percent in cardiac output. Therefore, to create a smooth thermodilution curve, injection should be made as rapidly and smoothly as possible and at the same point in the respiratory cycle. Most computation constants assume injection to have been made in less than 4 seconds.

Density Factor (K_1)

D_5W and normal saline are the two most commonly used injectates. The choice of solutions *does not* significantly affect the computation of K_1, as both yield nearly identical results (NS/blood K_1 = 1.08, D_5W/blood K_1 = 1.10). Although the specific gravity of blood changes with hematocrit, K_1 shows little variation, decreasing from only slightly 1.13 to 1.07 as hematocrit is significantly changed from 52 to 30 percent.

Computation Constant (K_2)

The computation constant combines several components of the Stewart-Hamilton equation. Calculation is based upon the volume of injectate, temperature change of injectate, and the capacity of the injectate port of the cardiac output catheter.

Correction is required to allow for the warming of injectate as it passes through the intravascular portion of the catheter.[86,87] The magnitude of this change may be appreciated by the fact that a 4°C injectate yields an effective temperature of 12°C at the point of entry into the circulation. It should be noted that each computer manufacturer determines K_2 in a different manner. Therefore, the user should be aware of assumptions made by the manufacturer of their particular cardiac output computer.

Change in Blood Temperature with Time ($T_B(t)\ dt$)

When a bolus of thermal indicator is injected, a time-temperature plot is constructed. The computer then integrates the area under this curve

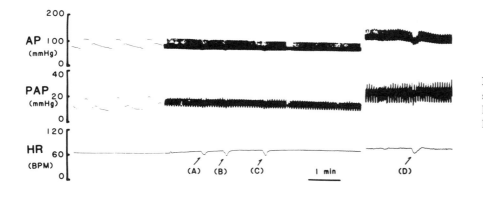

Fig. 10-4. Thermodilution curves showing transient bradycardia following ice injection. (From Mishikawa and Dohi[85] with permission.)

$(T_B(t) \, dt)$. Methods that employ this technique to calculate cardiac output include integrating to a point on the downslope equal to 10 percent of the peak, integrating the entire curve, extrapolating the downslope to zero, or the use of a constant to multiply a certain portion of the curve.[88,89] The thermistor of the PAC is balanced through use of Wheatstone's bridge. As a result, variations in temperature will alter resistance and current flow. To ensure correct calculations, it is important that a smooth thermodilution curve be obtained. Low amplitude curves may be caused by small injectate volumes, a high cardiac output, or inadequate blood:injectate temperature differential. Irregular curves may result from poor mixing, changes in blood pressure or heart rate, or contact between the thermistor and vessel wall.

Other Factors

The location of the thermistor is also important in the determination of an accurate cardiac output. A thermistor located at the catheter tip is likely to impinge upon the vessel wall, giving rise to irregular thermodilution curves. Such curves are characterized by a prolonged upslope, a reduced peak deflection, and an increased downslope. Early models of the thermodilution catheters had the thermistor located in this position and were plagued by this problem. New modifications in PAC design locate the thermistor 4 cm from the catheter tip. By doing this, abnormalities in cardiac output results from contact with the vessel wall have been minimized.[15]

Technique

The clinical determination of cardiac output by the thermodilution method is a simple technique, well suited to the operating room or intensive care unit. However, if accurate, reproducible measurements are to be obtained, careful attention to technique is essential.[43,87] The following is a summary of key features that have been described in detail in previous sections.

1. The correct computation constant (K_2) must be entered into the computer. This may vary with manufacturer and size of catheter, as well as with injectate volume and temperature.
2. The volume of injectate must be accurately measured. For example, an error of 0.5 ml in a 5-ml injection will cause a 10 percent error in the measurement.
3. The time between withdrawal of the sample and injection should be as short as possible, certainly less than 30 seconds if possible. As previously described, a 1°C increase in the temperature of the injectate will cause an error of 3 percent in cardiac output.
4. Each injection should be timed to occur at the same point in the respiratory cycle to assure comparability of measurements.

In summary, to create a smooth thermodilution curve, injection should be made as rapidly and smoothly as possible and at the same point in the respiratory cycle (Table 10-1). Most computation constants assume injection to have been made in less than 4 seconds. To accomplish this, the use of automated injectors may prove helpful[78,90] (Fig. 10-5).

TABLE 10-1. Guidelines for Best Results in Hemodynamic Monitoring

Acquisition of Pressure Data

Completely eliminate any air or blood clots from the system.

Discard catheters or tubes with kinks or bends.

Do not depend on internal calibration alone; use a mercury manometer for external calibration.

Check calibration routinely (3 or 4 times a day) or any time that unexpected pressures are recorded.

Always recheck the zero reference and calibration before measuring pressures.

Measure pressures at end-expiration, regardless of whether the patient is breathing spontaneously or is on mechanical ventilation.

Derive pressures manually off hard copy when tracing artifact is present.

Cardiac Output Measurements

Ensure proper positioning of distal thermistor and right atrial lumen.

Use 5 or 10 ml of cold injectate or 10 ml of room temperature injectate.

Injection should be rapid and smooth, with minimal time wasted between picking up the injectate syringe, turning on the computer switch, and actually injecting the fluid.

Adjust the computer constant according to the type, volume, and temperature of the injectate and the type of catheter used (predetermined constants are available).

Complications

In general, complications of cardiac output measurement are few. The most frequently encountered errors result from inaccurate measurements or misinterpretation of results. Either of these may lead to the initiation of inappropriate therapeutic maneuvers.[20,91] Although there are no published reports documenting the development of septic complications that can be specifically traced to cardiac output determinations, the potential for such contamination does exist.[35,92–95] Inadvertent injection through a catheter containing potent cardiovascular drugs can occur. Fluid overload (2°C to repeated determinations) or hypothermia (if ice injectate is used) are additional possibilities for complications in pediatric patients. As previously stated, bradycardia and atrial fibrillation have been reported following use of iced injectate.[85,86] A new occupational disease has been described as the result of obtaining repetitive cardiac output injections: "Swan-Ganz elbow."[91]

Mixed Venous Oxygen Tension ($P\bar{v}O_2$)

Serial measurements of mixed venous oxygen tension ($P\bar{v}O_2$) can provide valuable diagnostic and prognostic information.[98–103] $P\bar{v}O_2$ is also necessary for the calculation of several important derived respiratory and hemodynamic parameters, such as arteriovenous oxygen content difference [$C(a-v)O_2$], intrapulmonary shunt (Q_s/Q_t), and oxygen consumption (VO_2).[104] Mixed venous carbon dioxide tension is used for calculating carbon dioxide production and respiratory quotient, and can be used for estimating changes in cardiac output. The use of continuous mixed venous oximetry is presently being used to supplement traditional hemodynamic monitoring in critically ill patients.[98,99,105–108]

The technology that measures mixed venous oxygen saturation (by PAC) is based upon the use of reflectance spectrophotometry. Using this technique, the determination of $S\bar{v}O_2$ is based upon the differential capacity of oxyhemoglobin and desaturated hemoglobin to absorb light. Of note, desaturated hemoglobin absorbs more light than saturated (oxy)hemoglobin. When $S\bar{v}O_2$ monitoring was initially developed, the systems transmitted the different wavelengths of light along fiberoptic wires that were incorporated into one of the lumina of the PAC. These fiberoptic components are used to measure hemoglobin oxygen saturation by the process of reflectance spectrophotometry.[109] One of these wavelengths, identified as the *indicator* wavelength is sensitive to changes in oxygen saturation. The second wavelength or *isolestic* wavelength is relatively insensitive to changes in oxygen saturation, but is quite sensitive to potential sources of interference such as temperature, pH, velocity blood flow, and hematocrit. Light from either of these two wavelengths is reflected back along the catheter and then sensed by a photodetector, which is connected to a microprocessor located within the monitor. The microprocessor then computes the ratio of the light reflection from wave-

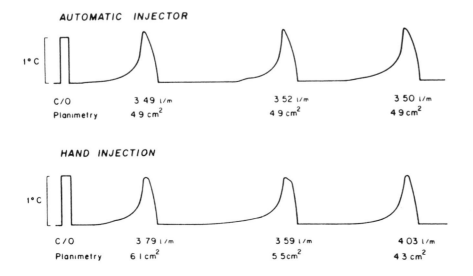

AUTOMATIC INJECTOR

1°C

| C/O | 3 49 l/m | 3 52 l/m | 3 50 l/m |
| Planimetry | 4 9 cm² | 4 9 cm² | 4 9 cm² |

HAND INJECTION

1°C

| C/O | 3 79 l/m | 3 59 l/m | 4 03 l/m |
| Planimetry | 6 1 cm² | 5 5 cm² | 4 3 cm² |

Fig. 10-5. Variability in thermodilution curves obtained by hand injection as compared to those obtained with an automatic injector. (From Dizon et al.,[90] with permission.)

length 1 and wavelength 2 (in an attempt to minimize any effect of the interferences previously described). By doing this, the microprocessor theoretically determines the changes in light intensity due solely to changes in oxygenation. In practice, however, the relationship of light intensity to oxygenation is a nonlinear function. As a result, early prototypes of $S\bar{v}O_2$ monitors often produced at values that only intermittently and or variably correlated with in vitro data that obtained by simultaneously obtained co-oximetry measurements). More recently, a third wavelength was incorporated into the $S\bar{v}O_2$ monitoring system in an attempt to improve the accuracy of this technology. This new modification allows for the nonlinear computation of the relationship between light-intensive and oxygen saturation.[107] Clinical studies comparing their wavelength system in vivo with in vitro (transmission spectrophotometry) technique have demonstrated an excellent correlation between these two techniques (r = .912 to .99).[109,110] Therefore, it appears that the incorporation of this third fiberoptic component has significantly increased the clinical accuracy of $S\bar{v}O_2$ technology. Hecker and colleagues[109] designed a study in patients undergoing cardiac surgery to determine the accuracy of a two-wavelength and the wavelength $S\bar{v}O_2$ system. Their data revealed that the two-wavelength determination varied significantly from co-oximetry values (r = .762) include data from the three-wavelength system did not differ significantly from co-oximetry values (r = .92).

Nelson[111] reported a correlation between $S\bar{v}O_2$ and the oxygen utilization coefficient reflecting the overall balance between oxygen consumption and delivery. Subsequently, decreases in $S\bar{v}O_2$ have been shown to directly correlate with decreases in cardiac output in a variety of clinical settings.[98,104,112–114] When arterial oxygen content and oxygen consumption are held constant, mixed venous oxygen varies directly with cardiac output. Consequently, this value can be used to directly assess the adequacy of cardiac output in relation to tissue oxygen requirements.[98] (Fig. 10-6).

The oxygen tension of venous blood varies according to the location from which the sample is obtained. Due to the large nonmetabolic blood flow (shunt) from the kidneys, blood from the inferior vena cava usually has a higher oxygen tension than superior vena cava blood. The high oxygen extraction ratio of the myocardium results in the low oxygen tension of the coronary sinus. Use of blood from the right atrium for determination of oxygen tension may yield an inaccurate measurement, since streaming is present from the inferior vena cava, superior vena cava, and coronary sinus. Numerous empirical formula have been developed in an attempt to relate right atrial oxygen tension to true mixed venous oxygen tension.[42,115] However, in critically ill patients, measurements of central venous oxygen tension correlate poorly with true mixed venous oxygen tension obtained from the pulmonary artery.[116] It has been shown that mixing of the three streams of venous blood

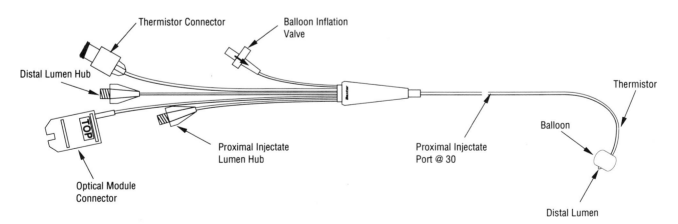

Fig. 10-6. A pulmonary catheter modified to provide continuous mixed venous oximetry measurements. The system allows for determination of cardiac outputs, pressure measurements as well as on line SVO_2. (Courtesy of American Edwards Laboratories.)

occurs in the right ventricle. However, the risk of arrhythmias does not allow a catheter to be placed in the right ventricle. A sample from the superior vena cava is useful when a "true" mixed venous blood cannot be obtained, for example, in children with an intracardiac left-to-right shunt (atrial septal defect).

Mixed venous oxygen tension represents the final balance between total body oxygen supply and demand. The normal Pv_{O_2} is 40 mmHg ($Sv_{O_2} = 75$ percent). Due to regional differences in blood flow, a normal Pv_{O_2} does not necessarily indicate adequate perfusion in each organ system. Factors that reduce Pv_{O_2} include:

Decreased O_2 delivery
Decreased arterial oxygen content (Ca_{O_2})
Decreased arterial O_2 tension
Decreased hemoglobin
Increased tissue requirements
Hypermetabolic states
Fever
Endocrinopathies

An elevated Pv_{O_2} may be seen in patients who have a left-to-right shunt, for example, a ventricular septal defect complicating an acute myocardial infarction.[117,118] Impairment of cellular respiration as seen with sepsis or cyanide poisoning also results in an elevated Pv_{O_2}. The latter is of particular importance to the anesthesiologist. Cyanide ion resulting from sodium nitroprusside administration may poison the cytochrome oxidase system.

Significant errors can result from contamination of mixed venous blood by pulmonary capillary blood. This may occur with distal migration of the catheter to a wedge position or blood withdrawal with the balloon inflated. In these circumstances retrograde flow from pulmonary capillaries is the only possible source of blood. When the catheter tip is positioned more proximally, experimental results have been conflicting. Several studies demonstrate contamination accompanying rapid blood withdrawal, while several investigators could not support this observation.[40,119] Therefore, in light of current evidence, it is recommended that mixed venous blood samples be obtained only from properly positioned catheters and that a slow rate of withdrawal be used. Proponents of the continuous mixed venous saturation monitoring claim it is associated with minimal risk and is cost effective.

Pacing Catheter

A multipurpose pulmonary artery catheter composed of five pacing electrodes is now available. This catheter may be used for atrial, ventricular, or atrioventricular sequential pacing. An additional advantage provided by this catheter is its ability to record an intracardiac electrocardiogram (ECG).[120] In a recent study, the ability of the pacing pulmonary artery catheter to detect endocardial electrical activity during hypothermic cardioplegia arrest.[121] Roth and Zaidan[122] evaluated the pacing Swan-Ganz catheter to detect atrial and ventricular electrical activity was compared with the activity found on the standard ECG. These results demonstrate that the atrial electrodes detected activity that was noted also by visual inspection. However, the ventricular electrodes were detected receiving electrical activity in 7 of 18 patients. Three of these 7 patients did not have simultaneous ECG activity, indicating that, in the usual monitoring circumstance, this ventricular electrical activity would have been untreated. As a result of the ventricular activity seen with the pacing catheter, additional cardioplegia was administered. The authors therefore recommend that when a pacing Swan-Ganz catheter is used for clinical care, it can also be used to monitor myocardial electrical activity during cardioplegia arrest.[122]

The multipurpose PAC that is presently available has five electrodes: two intraventricular electrodes situated 18.5 and 19.5 cm from the distal end and three intra-atrial electrodes situated 28.5, 31.0, and 33.5 cm further from the distal end (Swan-Ganz flow-directing pacing catheter, Model 93-200H-7F, Baxter Healthcare Corp., Irvine, CA). Incorporation of a third intra-atrial electrode enables the proper positioning in hearts of varying chamber sizes. The ability of the catheter to provide successful pacing was evaluated in a series of 30 patients undergoing cardiac surgery.[121] Atrial pacing was possible in 80 percent of patients, ventricular pacing in 93 percent, and atrioventricular sequential pacing in 73 percent.

In addition to the multipurpose PAC, a new modification with an additional right ventricular port placed 19 cm from the catheter tip has been introduced (Pace-port). This additional lumen allows for the introduction of a pacer wire for emergency right ventricular pacing (Fig. 10-7). With the Paceport system, the pacing wire is packaged separately from the PAC. This allows the flexibility of having ventricular pacing compatibility available (i.e., the pacing wire with the additional lumen in the right ventricle) but not having to use the technology unless it becomes indicated. The present Paceport system allows for rapid and accurate placement of the pacing wire into the right ventricle. To ensure the wire is in contact with the right ventricle and to minimize the risk of right ventricular injury, the manufacturer recommends using either an intracavity ECG (looking for injury current, or verifying capture by the pacing wire in the conventional fashion) (Fig. 10-7). A recent modification of the paceport catheter provides an additional right atrial port (in addition to the right ventricular port), which allows for atrioventricular sequential pacing (AV Paceport Catheter Model 93A-991H-7.5F, Baxter Healthcare Corp., Irvine, CA) (Fig. 10-8). Seltzer and associates[123] have reported a high degree of successful placement and atrioventricular pacing ability with this new pace-

port modification. Lumb[124] evaluated the ability of atrioventricular sequelae pacing probes with transluminal atrial and ventricular pacing probes inserted via the PAC; results are obtained using epicardial pacing wires. In this study, there was no statistically significant difference between the electrical currents delivered through either epicardial wires or transluminal pacing probes in the PAC. A subsequent study by Trankina and White[125] revealed a 98 percent rate for atrial capture and a 100 percent rate of ventricular capture using an atrioventricular pacing PAC in 40 cardiac surgical patients. The ability to provide atrial pacing following cardiopulmonary bypass decreased slightly to 95 percent.

Suggested indications for the use of a PAC with pacing capability are as follows[126]:

1. Intermittent third-degree heart block
2. Second-degree heart block (Mobitz II)
3. Left bundle branch block

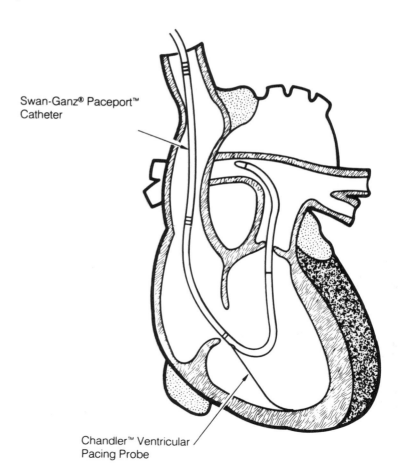

Swan-Ganz® Paceport™ Catheter

Chandler™ Ventricular Pacing Probe

Fig. 10-7. Paceport catheter with a right ventricular port which allows for passage of a ventricular pacing wire (Chandler Ventricular Pacing Probe).

4. Digitalis toxicity
5. Severe bradycardia
6. Need for atrioventricular sequential pacing
7. Need for intracardiac electrocardiogram

Right Ventricular Ejection Fraction

Bing and coworkers[70] pioneered the technology responsible for our present ability to utilize indicator dilution techniques for the determination of ventricular volumes. They developed a method that attempted to estimate the residual end-diastolic blood volume of the right ventricle in normal and diseased human hearts. Following catheterization of the right ventricle and the pulmonary artery with a double-lumen catheter, Evans blue was injected into the right ventricle. The residual volumes were estimated from the slope of photographically recorded dye dilution curves.

Using Bing's original concepts, technological advances in PAC technology have facilitated the measurement of right ventricular ejection fraction (RVEF) and volumes by use of thermodilution techniques.[127] This has occurred as a result of recent advances in the manufacture of thermistors for PACs that have a rapid response time of approximately 50 ms (normal: 300 to 1000 ms). The response time of these catheters is rapid enough to record beat-to-beat temperature variation and thus allow for the calculation of right ventricular ejection fraction (Fig. 10-9). Kay and colleagues[55a] have validated this technique with radionuclear studies both in animal models and in patients after open heart surgery. Subsequently, Jardin and colleagues[26] and Rafferty[128] have also validated this technique using echocardiography.

Using this "rapid-response" catheter (7.5 Fr, Baxter Healthcare, Irvine, CA) and an accompanying computer system (Monarch REF-1, Baxter Healthcare), computation of RVEF is easily accomplished from an experimental decay process of the thermal washout curve.[127] Normal RVEF (thermodilution technique) is approximately 40 percent.

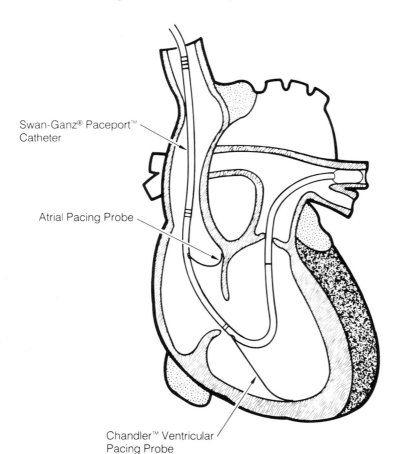

Swan-Ganz® Paceport™ Catheter

Atrial Pacing Probe

Chandler™ Ventricular Pacing Probe

Fig. 10-8. Modification of the original paceport catheter with an additional atrial and ventricular ports which permit passage of pacing wires to allow for atrial, ventricular, or synchronous atrioventricular pacing. (Courtesy of American Edwards Laboratories.)

RVEF, RV stroke volume, RV end-diastolic volume, and RV end-systolic volume may be calculated as follows:

$$RV\ stroke\ volume = \frac{cardiac\ output}{heart\ rate}$$

$$RV\ end\text{-}diastolic\ volume = \frac{RV\ stroke\ volume}{RV\ ejection\ fraction}$$

$$RV\ end\text{-}systolic\ volume = RV\ end\text{-}diastolic\ volume - RV\ stroke\ volume$$

Thus, from the standard **RVEF** catheter the following hemodynamic measurements may be obtained: cardiac output, right ventricular ejection fraction, right atrial pressure, right ventricular pressure, and pulmonary artery and capillary wedge pressure. Hines and Barash[53] have demonstrated the ability to detect right ventricular ischemia by monitoring RVEF and right ventricular end-diastolic pressure in patients with right coronary artery disease. The *newest* modification of the right ventricular ejection fraction system incorporates the measurement of both RVEF and continuous mixed venous oxygen saturation monitoring. Dormann and colleagues[129] evaluated the reproducibility and accuracy of this new system in patients undergoing cardiopulmonary bypass surgery. Catheter-derived mixed venous and arterial oximetry data were compared with simultaneous values using conventional laboratory co-oximetry methods. Their results demonstrated a significant correlation for mixed venous oxygen saturation between catheter-derived and laboratory co-oximetry data ($r^2 = 0.81$; $P < .01$). Their coefficients variation for each set of five repeated measurements for cardiac output was 8 percent, and for computed RVEF, it was 15 percent. The authors conclude that the continuous catheter system provides a reliable method for monitoring both mixed and venous oxygen saturation and RVEF.[129]

However, potential limitations do exist with the use of thermal indicator technique. First, in patients with cardiac arrhythmias such as atrial fibrillation, variations in diastolic filling time may introduce error into the measurement of RVEF. However, since RVEF is computed with 4 to 5 beats, an average RVEF may be obtained. Conversely, a beat-to-beat RVEF can be calculated, so that minimal and maximal RVEF is known. Second, in patients with regurgitant valvular lesions (tricuspid insufficiency), an erroneous RVEF may be seen, since the technique measures forward ejection fraction.[52,127]

The location of the injectate port further influences the accuracy of the cardiac output obtained via the thermodilution technique. Comparison of right atrial and right ventricular ejection sites, both

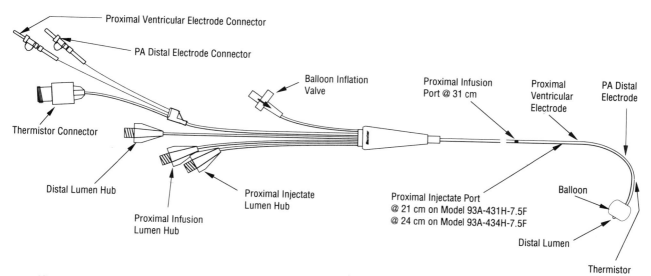

Fig. 10-9. Right ventricular ejection fraction (RVEF) catheter thermister response has been modified to allow for determination of RVEF. Traditional determination of PAD, PCWP, and RAP are also available from this catheter. (Courtesy of American Edward Laboratories.)

in animals and humans, demonstrate that right ventricular injection results in a highly variable and an inaccurate measurement of output when compared to right atrial injection.[55,130] Finally, by increasing the time necessary to equilibrate fully to temperature change present techniques of thermistor mounting may artifactually lower the measurement of RVEF. Despite the limitations, the use of thermodilution technique for measurement of right ventricular function still remains clinically useful.[53,128]

Continuous Cardiac Output Determinations Using Pulmonary Artery Catheter Modification

Recently a method to measure continuous thermodilution cardiac outputs has been developed. Rather than a cold bolus injectate to create a temperature signal, a filament is intermittently heated to provide a very small heat signal.[131] To accomplish this, PACs have been modified such that a 10-cm thermal filament is located within the right ventricle. This filament is coiled over a portion of the PAC that lies in the right atrium and ventricle. The thermometer at the tip of the PAC detects changes in blood temperature, and the heat signal is then analyzed by "stochastic" techniques. Stochastic techniques differ from classical demonstrative techniques in that the statistical properties of the input and output signals are of more interest than the instantaneous values of the signals themselves.[131] Once in place, this thermal filament continually transfers a safe level of heat directly into the blood according to a pseudorandom binary sequence. Any resulting temperature change is then detected downstream in the pulmonary artery and is cross-correlated with an input sequence to produce a thermodilution "washout" curve. This thermodilution curve is presented in millidegrees.[132] The cardiac output is then subsequently computed from a conservative of heat equation using the area under the curve.[131]

With this technique, the average heat infused is usually less than 7.5 W. This temperature was selected so that the catheter surface temperature remains below 44°C, regardless of blood flow conditions. Earlier studies suggest that long-term exposure at this temperature (44°C) has no detrimental effects on red blood cells, the myocardium,[133–135] or other blood components.[136] In prac-

tice, the actual filament surface temperature is continually measured, and the delivered power is either reduced or terminated when the average temperature exceeds 44°C.[132]

The insertion of the PAC is performed by traditional methods allowing for placement of the thermistor in the pulmonary artery outflow tract. Once the correct position of the PAC has been verified (using standard methods such as wave- and/or pressure form analysis), the catheter is connected to the monitor. Once this has been accomplished, the process of continuous cardiac output determination begins. The first cardiac output measurement is computed and displayed within several minutes. The heating sequence is repeated every 30 seconds; the displayed value is based on approximately six determinations and is updated every 30 seconds (137). Thus, the monitor actually provides a time average continuously updated rather than "instantaneous" cardiac output.

This method for measuring cardiac output (i.e., volumetric fluid flow using stochastic techniques) has been evaluated in a laboratory bench model[121] and in sheep.[138] Clinically, Yelderman and associates[132] have studied continuous cardiac output as compared with bolus thermal dilution cardiac outputs in intensive care unit patients. They found an acceptable correlation between thermodilution (cardiac output) and continuous cardiac output measurement ($r = .94$) in this patient population (range: 2.8 to 10.8 per minute). One potential advantage of this system is that it is "user friendly," requiring no calculations and no injection of volume. In addition, it is possible to perform routine bolus cardiac output determination through the same catheter. At present, increased cost is a major factor limiting the clinical application of this technology.

Miyasaka and coworkers[139] have advocated "thermodeprivation" as yet another and different approach for the determination of continuous output. This technique employs the measurement of flow velocity in the pulmonary artery using a continuous arterial thermodeprivation system (KATS) catheter. This catheter is designed such that a continuously heated thermistor is incorporated into the tip of the PAC.[6] The heated thermistor is subsequently cooled by the surrounding blood; the decrease in temperature between the "thermodeprivation" is proportional to the velocity of blood. This system is then calibrated with a simultaneous thermodilution (or injectate, cardiac output) and the velocity signal is subsequently converted into a quantitative flow valve. The caveat here is that a constant blood vessel diameter (the vessel in which the PAC is placed) is assumed by the thermodeprivation method. As a result, variations in pulmonary artery diameter and/or changes in diameter of the pulmonary artery during monitoring (which may be seen with changes in volume status, PEEP, etc.) may prove to be a major limitation to the clinical usefulness of this technology. At present, this methodology has only been studied in an animal model.

Segal and colleagues[140,141] recently evaluated a method for determining instantaneous and continuous cardiac output using a Doppler PAC. This method provides spaced average measurements of blood flow velocity in the pulmonary artery, coupled with continuous measurement of the diameter of the pulmonary artery. In this model quantitative flow is calculated by the use of the instantaneous, spaced average velocity (obtained from the velocity profile) and the instantaneous area (obtained from the vessel diameter). Segal's group compared the results from this Doppler pulmonary artery catheter to measurements made by electromagnetic flow. Their results demonstrated that Doppler catheter-determined flow was highly predictive of electromagnetic flow in both continuous and pulsatile pump models ($r^2 = .89$, $r^2 = .97$, respectively).[134] This catheter system also provides instantaneous diameter measurements and mapping of instantaneous velocity profiles within the main pulmonary artery. Although initial reports were encouraging, this technology failed for economic reasons and is not presently available.[142]

INDICATIONS

As originally reported in 1970, the primary indication for PAC was for hemodynamic assessment of patients following complicated myocardial infarction.[143-145] Since these early reports, the potential benefits of the information gained from the PAC have extended its use to a variety of other clinical areas.[146-149] This expansion is attested to by the fact that an estimated 2 million PACs are sold annually in the United States. However, the debate regarding the appropriate indications for PAC monitoring, which stared over a decade ago, is still ongoing.

The fact that a physician's database is improved by pulmonary artery catheterization is evidenced by several reports documenting the difficulty of correlating physical signs with the severity of myocardial dysfunction.[61,62,65] Connors and colleagues[148] prospectively analyzed 62 consecutive pulmonary artery catheterizations. They found that less than half of a group of clinicians correctly predicted pulmonary capillary wedge pressure or cardiac output, and 48 percent made at least one change in therapy based on data from the PAC.[148] Waller and associates[150] demonstrated that a group of experienced cardiac anesthesiologists and surgeons who were "blinded" to the results of pulmonary artery catheterization during coronary artery bypass surgery, and were unaware of any problem during 65 percent of severe hemodynamic abnormalities. Similarly, Iberti and Fisher[65] showed that a group of physicians was unable to accurately predict hemodynamic data on clinical grounds, 60 percent made at least one change in therapy, and 33 percent changed their diagnosis based on pulmonary artery catheterization data. Recently, Boyd and co-workers[35] studied 528 pulmonary artery catheterizations. In this study, the clinicians caring for these patients reported that the catheter was "felt to be helpful" in the management of 80 percent of these patients.

In an attempt to address the issue of risk versus benefit of PACs, several organizations have published "guidelines" for the appropriate indications for PAC monitoring.[151-154] In 1991, in an attempt to provide practice guidelines for pulmonary artery catheterization, the American Society of Anesthesiologists established a pulmonary artery catheterization task force.[146] The mission of this group was to develop guidelines for the appropriate indications for PAC use. To fulfill its purpose, the task force reviewed a total of 860 clinical trials, controlled observational studies, uncontrolled case reports, and individual case reports. In addition, the task force focused its review on evidence of effectiveness based on clinical outcome. In its report, the task force reported that their survey of the literature demonstrated that PAC data appeared to change therapy in 30 to 60 percent of all cases reviewed. These studies demonstrated no effect on mortality in patients whose therapy was changed (25 percent of adults, 10 percent of children).[12,15] The task force concluded that one of the major deficiencies in these studies is their small sample size, and this may account for lack of change in outcome in these patient groups.

For the purpose of this discussion, the clinical applications of pulmonary artery catheter monitoring will be grouped into the following categories: (1) preoperative assessment, (2) perioperative monitoring (both cardiac and noncardiac surgery, (3) obstetric-gynecological procedures, (4) pediatric patients, and (5) hemodynamic or nonsurgical indications.[155–170].

Preoperative Assessment

The preoperative use of the PAC provides physicians with data that may be used to guide patient therapy. Studies have revealed that this information gained from the PAC would often be undetected by clinical observation alone.[64] Orlando,[114] in a retrospective study of 148 consecutive patients over 65 years of age, who were cleared for surgery by standard clinical assessment, found that preoperative invasive hemodynamic monitoring resulted in 23 percent of patients being classified as having severe cardiopulmonary compromise. As a result, these patients were identified as being at extremely high risk for the planned surgical procedure. All 8 of these patients, who subsequently underwent surgery as originally planned, died. Similarly, Babu and coworkers[168] examined a series of 75 elderly patients (average age: 68) who underwent preoperative PAC placement (168). In this patient population, 40 percent of patients were found to have abnormal left ventricular function (by PAC data), which was not detected by clinical evaluation alone.

In a prospective study of elderly patients with hip fractures ($n = 70$; average age: 72), half of the patients ($n = 35$) were randomized for evaluation either by standard clinical examination combined with central venous pressure placement, or PAC insertion (171). The patients in the PAC group went to surgery only after correction of all hemodynamic abnormalities. Mortality in this group was 2.9 percent as compared to 29 percent in the central venous pressure group.

In an attempt to answer the question of the potential positive effect of preoperative hemodynamic optimization using PAC data on outcome, Berlavk and colleagues[157] prospectively evaluated 89 patients scheduled for peripheral vascular surgery. In this study, patients were randomized into three groups: (1) preoperative optimization in the inten-

sive care unit 12 hours prior to surgery, (2) PAC insertion and hemodynamic manipulation 3 hours prior to surgery, or (3) control group (i.e., arterial line and central venous pressure). Hemodynamic optimization was defined as a pulmonary capillary wedge pressure between 8 and 15 mmHg, a confidence interval > 2.8 L/min/m^2, and an SVR $< 1,100$ dynes/s/cm^{-5}. Patients in groups 1 and 2 were more hemodynamically stable intraoperatively and had a lower incidence of tachycardia, hypotension, and arrhythmias than group 3 patients. In addition, these groups had a lower incidence of postoperative cardiac morbidity and less early graft closure than did the control group ($P < .05$). However, pulmonary artery catheterization 12 hours before surgery did not result in any better outcome than catheterization 3 hours before surgery. In contrast, an observational study was unable to demonstrate any difference in outcome between elderly patients who did not undergo preoperative catheterization and unmatched patients who were admitted to the hospital during the same time period for other diagnosis.[172] The PAC task force of the American Society of Anesthesiologists suggested that, in this study, the similar outcomes may have been due to selection basis.[154]

Perioperative Monitoring

High-Risk General Surgical Patients

The presence of significant cardiac disease (defined as either a recent myocardial infarction or clinical evidence of congestive heart failure) was one of the earliest indications for PAC insertion in noncardiac surgical patients. The presence of clinical CHF has been shown to place patients at an increased risk for postoperative cardiac death following noncardiac surgery.[173–175]

In a report in 1972, Tarhan and associates[13] evaluated patients with a history of recurrent myocardial infarctions who underwent noncardiac surgery. This study revealed a reinfarction rate of 37 percent within the first 3 months following infarction. In this study patients did not receive routine hemodynamic monitoring prior to their procedure.[13] In a later study of 733 patients, Rao and coworkers[176] compared the incidence of reinfarction in noncardiac surgical patients. In this study, PACs and arterial lines were inserted in all patients prior to surgery. Each patient's hemodynamic status was optimized preoperatively using the information obtained from these monitors. Using this technique, Rao's group[176] reported a reinfarction rate (at 3 months) of only 5.8 percent.

Abdominal Aortic Reconstruction

Perhaps the major difficulty with trying to interpret the impact of PAC use in the patient population receiving abdominal aortic reconstruction is the absence of a control group for comparison (i.e., patients who do not receive a PAC). In an early report, utilizing controls, Hesdorffer and colleagues[177] were able to demonstrate a reduction in mortality, perioperative hypertensive events, and renal failure in patients managed using an aggressive fluid loading protocol and a PAC who were undergoing aortic reconstruction. The main problem in this study is that the PAC was only a small part of the overall study design. Several authors have suggested that utilizing pulmonary capillary wedge pressure measurements obtained from the PAC to optimize preoperative volume status may prove beneficial in this patient population.[147,178,179] In a prospective study of 41 patients (18 abdominal aortic aneurysm repairs, 23 other peripheral vascular procedures) who maintained their postoperative pulmonary capillary wedge pressure within 3 mmHg of their best postoperative level, had a decrease in their overall complication rate (14 percent vs 79 percent).[179] However, more recent studies by Joyce and Iaacson[154] reported different results. Using a randomized controlled protocol evaluation of patients undergoing abdominal aortic reconstruction, these authors were unable to show any difference in outcomes between patients monitored by pulmonary artery catheter or central venous pressure.[161,162]

Neurosurgery

The main focus of all studies to date in the area of neurosurgery has been on the ability of PAC to detect air embolism.[180,181] None of the studies has evaluated the impact of PAC use on clinical outcome.

Obstetrics-Gynecology

Once again, the major problems with studies performed using PACs in the obstetrics-gynecology patient population is the lack of historical controls.[155,164-166,182,183] The major focus of PAC utilization has been in patients with severe preeclampsia,[164,165] Spapen and coworkers[182] reported on the potential of PAC monitoring in the early recognition of an amniotic fluid embolus.

Pediatrics

The small number of PACs used in pediatrics and the lack of controlled studies make it difficult to evaluate the effectiveness in the patient population.[118,159,184]

Hemodynamic Disorders

The use of PACs in intensive care units has become widespread both in medical and surgical settings. The data from the medical intensive care units focus primarily on patients with myocardial infarction. Once again, these uncontrolled studies have yielded inconsistent results.[14,142] Opponents of PAC use in this setting argue that patients with an myocardial infarction who were monitored by PAC had a higher in-hospital mortality, longer hospital stay, and shorter short-term survival than patients who did not have a PAC inserted.[185,186] However, it is important to note that the impact of patient pathology on outcome is never addressed in these investigations (i.e., it is not stated whether patients receiving PACs were sicker than in monitored patients.[179]

Data from the surgical intensive care literature supports the ability of data from the PAC studies to aid in diagnosis and to guide therapy.[146,176,177,187,188] However, the major question that still exists is: Does the routine placement of a PAC in selected patients in surgical intensive care units reduce morbidity and mortality? In an attempt to answer this question, Scalea and colleagues[172] studied a group of geriatric blunt trauma patients. They showed that using routine placement of the PAC identified a group of patients in clinically unrecognized shock (46 percent). Shoemaker and colleagues[146] preoperatively randomized high-risk general surgical populations to receive either PAC or central venous pressure placement. For the purpose of this study, patients were randomized into one of two treatment groups: (1) normal values of healthy subjects were used as therapeutic goals or (2) a protocol group in which median values of patients who had survived life-threatening postoperative shock were the therapeutic goals. Controversy still exists about the result of this study (centering around whether the control and protocol group were comparable), which revealed that the PAC protocol group had fewer complications, fewer ICU hospital and ventilator days, and less total cost.

Other recent studies have demonstrated that in patients with sepsis and adult respiratory distress syndrome (ARDS) survival may be improved by therapy guided by the PAC. In a randomized prospective study, Tuchschmidt and associates[189] successfully employed the concept of achieving "supranormal" values in the treatment of 26 septic patients in the ICU. Similarly, Russell and coworkers[142] documented (retrospectively) improved outcome in patients with ARDS who had an elevated cardiac output. There are now several other publications from different institutions validating these higher goals for cardiac output.[146,190] Each of the groups of investigators focused on oxygen delivery and changed the long-established concept that a cardiac index of 2.2 $L \cdot min^{-1} \cdot m^{-2}$ is sufficient in all clinical situations.

Cardiac Surgery

Numerous uncontrolled observational studies have attempted to determine whether PACs change the outcome in cardiac surgical patients[150,191,192] (Table 10-2). Moore and colleagues[192] compared 20 consecutive patients with left main coronary artery stenosis undergoing coronary artery bypass grafting without PAC monitoring to 28 patients undergoing surgery who had a preoperative PAC in-

serted. They demonstrated a decrease in mortality from 20 percent to 3.5 percent and concluded that this improvement was due to the use of vasodilators, inotropic agents, and propanolol. All of these modalities were facilitated by the information obtained using the PAC.

A more recent study by Tuman and coworkers[191] in 1,094 patients undergoing cardiac surgery was unable to demonstrate any positive impact (i.e., a reduction in mortality, cardiac ischemia, or postoperative myocardial infarction) in patients receiving elective or emergent PAC vs central venous pressure placement. The lack of observed differences in outcome may have been due to patient demographics, as assignment to monitoring groups was made solely by the anesthesiologist assigned to the case. Similarly, a randomized controlled study by Pearson and coworkers[193] ($n = 229$) found no difference in death, length of ICU stay, or use of vasopressors between cardiac surgical patients monitored by PAC or central venous pressure. Once again, the anesthesiologist in charge of the case could remove patients from the control (central venous pressure group) and place them into the monitored PAC group at his or her discretion.

INSERTION

Preparation for Insertion

Successful PAC insertion begins with preparation of the site for venipuncture (see Ch. 00 for specific details) and appropriate balancing and calibration of pressure monitoring equipment. Following successful venipuncture (using a classical Seldinger technique),[194] a larger sheath and vessel dilator can then be introduced into the vessel. After placement of the introducer, the dilator is removed, and the larger intravascular sheath remains in place.[195] The PAC can then be inserted into the sheath and threaded into the central circulation. This method may be used whether the internal or external jugular, femoral, or antecubital veins are employed; we use the following check list prior to each insertion[196–199]:

Prior to venous catheterization:

1. Insertion kit available and components checked
2. Pressure monitor balanced and calibrated
3. Transducer and pressure tubing free of air

TABLE 10-2. Recommendations for Pulmonary Artery Catheterization in Patients Undergoing Cardiac Surgery

1. Poor ventricular function
   EF < 0.4, LVEDP > 16 mmHg
   CI < 2 $L \cdot min^{-1} \cdot m^{-2}$
2. Noncompliant ventricle
3. Left main coronary lesion (or ivalent)
4. Aortic stenosis/aortic insufficiency
5. Mitral stenosis/mitral insufficiency
6. Acute ventricular septal defect
7. Acute papillary muscle dysfunction
8. Combined lesions (coronary + valvular)
9. Recent infarct (< 6 months)
10. Intra-aortic balloon counterpulsation
11. Hemodynamic instability

EF, ejection fraction; LVEDP, left ventricular diastolic pressure; CI, cardiac index.

Prior to insertion of PAC:

1. Distal (pulmonary artery pressure) port connected to transducer tubing; all ports free of air and allow infusion of heparinized saline
2. Check to ensure normal balloon inflation
3. A trace is seen in the oscilloscope following manipulation of the catheter.

Insertion Site Selection

A number of venous entry sites are employed for pulmonary artery catheterization. These include internal and external jugular, subclavian, anticubital, and femoral veins (see Ch. 00 for detailed discussion). Ideally, the appropriate site should be easily accessible, a short distance from the right atrium, and be associated with minimal complications. Meticulous attention to detail is essential if complications are to be avoided. There are no short cuts! (See Tables 10-3 and 10-4.)

Based on these goals, most anesthesiologists inserting PACs choose the internal jugular vein approach.[200] Advantages include simplicity,

TABLE 10-3. Guidelines for Safe Insertion of Pulmonary Artery Flow Guided Catheters

1. Balance risk versus benefit.
2. Slowly inflate balloon while continuously monitoring the pulmonary artery waveform.
3. Upon transition from the pulmonary artery to the pulmonary capillary wedge pressure trace, immediately stop inflation.
4. If an overwedge pattern is observed, the balloon should be immediately deflated, and the catheter immediately withdrawn 1–2 cm (Fig. 10-15). The balloon is slowly reinflated and a normal wedge pressure waveform is noted.
5. Minimize duration of pulmonary capillary wedge pressure measurements.
6. If balloon inflates with less than 1.5 ml of gas, the catheter should be withdrawn at least 1–2 cm.
7. Spontaneous tip migration may occur; therefore, continuously monitor the pulmonary artery trace for "spontaneous wedging." If this occurs withdraw the catheter 1–2 cm or until a normal pulmonary artery tracing reappears.
8. Minimize number of pulmonary capillary wedge pressure measurements in patients who are elderly, anticoagulated, or have pulmonary hypertension.
9. If pulmonary artery diastolic pressure is less than 18 mmHg, use pulmonary artery diastolic pressure rather than pulmonary capillary wedge pressure as an index of left ventricular filling pressure.

accessibility of the site during surgery, and a relatively short and direct pathway to the right atrium. Disadvantages include inadvertent carotid artery puncture with hematoma formation or dislodgement of atherosclerotic plaques, nerve injury, and, rarely, pneumothorax.[201–209]

Catheter Insertion

With the introducer sheath in place, the Swan-Ganz catheter is inserted carefully and advanced until the tip lies in a central vein. Approximate distances from various insertion sites are listed in Table 10-5. Intracardiac knotting is a consequence of inserting the PAC too far distally without the appropriate pressure trace being displayed on the monitor.

Location of the tip of the catheter in a central vein can be confirmed by pressure changes related to respiration or coughing. With the catheter in the right atrium, the balloon is inflated with 1.5 ml of air (never more or less), and the catheter slowly advanced. When the right atrium is entered, typical venous A-C and V waves will be noted (right atrial pressure = 0–8 mmHg)[210] (Fig. 10-10). Further advancement of the catheter will produce a dramatic change in the pressure tracing as the tip of the catheter enters the right ventricle. Within one cardiac cycle pressures change from those characteristic of the atrium to a phasic pressure in the range of 25/0–5 mmHg, typical of the right ventricle should be observed. The catheter is then advanced through the right ventricle (as quickly as possible to minimize the potential for arrhythmias until it enters the main pulmonary artery. Location can be verified by an increase in the diastolic pressure 25/12 and a change in the morphology of the waveform. Usually there is no change in the systolic pressure. The catheter is advanced further until it wedges in a branch of the pulmonary artery. At this point, the trace will have the appearance of an atrial pressure pattern with A-C and V wave components transmitted retrograde from the left atrium (pulmonary capillary wedge pressure = 8–12 mmHg).[210] In summary, pulmonary capillary wedge position is verified by (1) a characteristic waveform, (2) a mean pressure lower than the mean pulmonary artery pressure, and (3) the ability to withdraw arterialized blood.

Once the wedge position has been achieved, the balloon is deflated. This should produce a typical

TABLE 10-4. A Comparison of Venous Access Routes

Route	Method of Cannulation	Advantages	Disadvantages
Peripheral external jugular	Percutaneous	Easy to learn Safe Does not interfere with cardiopulmonary resuscitation (CPR)	Valves may hinder catheter or guidewire insertion Stasis, thrombosis, and phlebitis are more common
Antecubital	Percutaneous/cutdown	Easy to learn Safe Preferred route with anticoagulant or thrombolytic therapy, because the site is easily compressible should bleeding occur	Stasis, thrombosis, infection, and venospasm are more common Catheter displacement is frequent
Central internal jugular	Percutaneous	Rapidly accessible Does not interfere with CPR Provides a straight route to the heart Less restrictive to patient movement	Air embolism, carotid artery puncture, tracheal injury may occur Pneumothorax (more common in the left than the right internal jugular vein) Thoracic duct injury (left internal jugular vein only)
Subclavian	Percutaneous	Rapidly accessible Allows free neck and arm movement Easier to keep sterile	Air embolism, more frequent pneumothorax and hemothorax; subclavian artery puncture; injury to nerve bundle may occur
Femoral	Percutaneous	Rapidly accessible Does not interfere with CPR	Sepsis, in situ thrombosis, pulmonary embolism may occur

pulmonary artery pressure tracing.[6] Reinflation of the balloon should reproduce the wedge tracing with 1.5 ml of air. If *less* than 1.5 ml of air results in a wedge trace, the catheter should be withdrawn to the point where 1- to 1.5-ml balloon inflation is associated with a pulmonary capillary wedge pres-

sure. At *no time* should more air be injected into the balloon than is necessary to obtain pulmonary capillary wedge pressure. This will result in distal migration of the catheter. By emphasizing the above technique, pulmonary artery catheterization can be accomplished in expeditious and efficient

TABLE 10-5. Distance to Right Atrium, Pulmonary Artery, and Wedge Position

Vein	Right Atrium (cm)	Right Ventricle (cm)	Pulmonary Artery (cm)
Internal jugular			
Right	20	30	45
Left	25	35	50
Antecubital			
Right	50	65	80
Left	55	70	85
Femoral	40	50	65
Subclavian	10	25	40

Fig. 10-10. Pressure waveforms in relation to catheter position from right atrium to pulmonary capillary wedge position. RA, right atrial pressure; RV, right ventricular pressure; PA, pulmonary artery pressure; PCWP, pulmonary capillary wedging pressure.

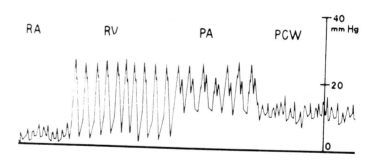

manner (less than 2 minutes in about 90 percent of patients). However, certain disease states such as low output, pulmonary hypertension, and congenital cardiac defects, are commonly associated with difficult catheter insertions. In addition, unrecognized technical difficulties may also result in catheterization failure. Air bubbles in the transducer or tubing may dampen the pressure waves sufficiently to prevent recognition of the waveforms. An improperly set calibration scale can reduce the waveform deflection to such low levels that important pressure changes go unrecognized. Clotting within or at the tip of the catheter can prevent transmission of the characteristic way with the equipment will prevent the complications from interfering with successful catheter passage.

INTERPRETATION OF HEMODYNAMIC DATA

Pressure Measurements

The accurate interpretation of pressure measurements is central to defining the various subsets of patients with abnormal cardiovascular performance. Classically, intravascular pressures have been measured at end exhalation, since no air flow occurs and intrapleural pressure is considered static[211] (Fig. 10-11). In those patients where the point of end exhalation is difficult to discern, direct measurement of respiratory variables (airway pressure, end-tidal CO_2, etc.) may be necessary.[7,212] Numerous reports have documented the effects of airway pressure on the correlation between left atrial pressure and pulmonary capillary wedge pressure.[7,213–216] Spontaneous ventilation and noncompliance lungs *do not* alter the relationship.[7] In contrast, increased airway pressure as seen with positive end expiratory pressure (PEEP), continuous positive airway pressure (CPAP), airway obstruction, PAC tip placement

above the left atrium, hypovolemia, and obesity all serve to increase the gradient between pulmonary capillary wedge pressure and left atrial pressure.[25,27,42,216–220] As a result, controversy exists as to whether PEEP should be temporarily removed in order to accurately measure pulmonary capillary wedge pressure.[44,220] Disadvantages of this technique include a temporary increase in A-aO$_2$ gradient and potential destabilization of the hemodynamic state.[44] Indeed, if a patient is receiving high levels of PEEP (>10 cmH$_2$O), spurious cardiovascular information may be obtained, even with tran-

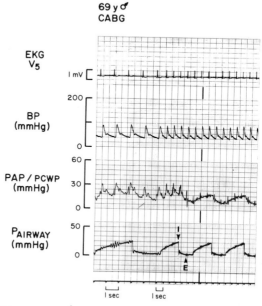

Fig. 10-11. Vascular measurements should be made at end exhalation. This recording of an anesthetized patient receiving positive pressure ventilation shows a significant variation in PCWP during the respiratory cycle. EKG, electrocardiogram; BP, blood pressure; PA, pulmonary artery pressure; AP, airway pressure.

sient removal of PEEP.[33] Errors in interpretation may also occur as a result of transmural pressure gradients across a vessel. Downs[211] has suggested using direct measurement of intrapleural pressure as a means of more accurately assessing this transmural gradient. Finally, the relatively low resonant frequency of currently available clinical monitoring systems (catheter and tubing system) can be another significant cause of artifact.

Analysis of the pressure waveform may also yield information regarding cardiac pump function. Early reports by Kaplan and Wells[221] demonstrated in selected patients, that abnormalities in the A-C wave component of pulmonary capillary wedge pressure may be an early indicator of myocardial ischemia. In addition, acute papillary muscle dysfunction or rupture secondary to ischemia or infarction, respectively, may be detected by the onset of v waves in the pulmonary capillary wedge pressure trace. This may be helpful in selected patients as a specific, if not sensitive, monitor for ischemia. Large v waves may be seen in mitral regurgitation due to a dilated annulus, papillary muscle dysfunction, or ruptured chordae tendineae[222,223] (Fig. 10-12).

Derived Cardiovascular Variables

At present, the anesthesiologist is confronted with a data dilemma. On the one hand, it is possible to obtain extensive physiologic measurements in the critically ill patient. On the other, the volume of data, its organization, and the subsequent calculations necessary for clinical management can be overwhelming. Nowhere is this more obvious than in cardiovascular monitoring. The use of the pulmonary artery thermodilution catheter has facilitated the clinician's ability to perform extensive hemodynamic assessments. Using these data, various circulatory disease states can now be defined in terms of pump failure, hypovolemia, and high/

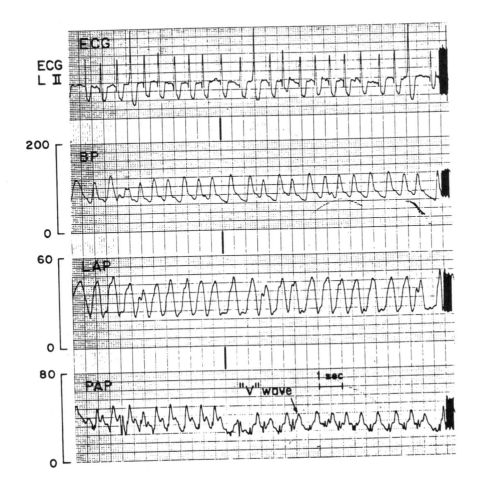

Fig. 10-12. The v waves are shown in the left atrial and pulmonary capillary wedge tracing of a patient with mitral stenosis.

low resistance states. Assessment of cardiac performance using the derived indices of cardiac performance such as: cardiac index, stroke work index, systemic vascular resistance, pulmonary vascular resistance, and the O_2 transport provide the foundation for sound physiologic management of the critically ill patient[166,220,221,224–226,228] (Table 10-6). To accommodate patients of varying body size the use of indexed systemic or pulmonary vascular resistance is often utilized. The sequential and repeated use of these measure provide the opportunity to utilize therapy aimed at treating specific hemodynamic abnormalities.

Cardiac Work

Although some estimation of ventricular function can be obtained by the shape of the ventricular pressure volume loop and its relation to the pressure volume ordinates, the logistical difficulty in obtaining these data limits their clinical utility.[229–231] *Cardiac work* can serve as a more clinically

TABLE 10-6. Hemodynamic Calculations

Cardiac output (CO) L/min = heart rate × stroke volume

Cardiac index (CI) $L \cdot min^{-1} \cdot m^{-2}$ is calculated as follows:

$$CI = \frac{CO}{BSA}$$

Stroke volume (SV) or *stroke volume index* (SVI) overcomes some of the difficulties inherent in the use of CO or CL

$$SV = ml/stroke \frac{CO}{Heart\ rate} \quad or \quad SVI = \frac{CI}{Heart\ rate}$$

SV = End diastolic volume − end systolic volume

Systemic vascular resistance is defined as:

$$SVR\ (RU) = \frac{MBP - RAP}{CO}$$

$$SVRI\ (RU/M^2) = \frac{MBP - RAP}{CI}$$

Pulmonary vascular resistance is:

$$PVR\ (RU) = \frac{PAP - PCWP}{CO}$$

$$PVRI\ (RU/M^2) = \frac{PAP - PCWP}{CI}$$

Measurement of resistance is reported in one of two methods.*
1. Absolute resistance units (ARU) = dynes · s · cm^{-5}
2. Hybrid resistance units (HRU) = RU

To convert HRU to ARU, multiply by 79.9

useful index of cardiac performance. Work is a basic description of the pump function and can be extrapolated from either a pressure volume loop or calculated by use of a formula. The amount of work performed is a function of the load carried and the distance moved (work = force × distance moved). In the operating room or intensive care unit, the most commonly employed formula for calculation of left ventricular stroke work index (LVSWI) is

LVSWI = (Mean BP − Mean PCWP) × SVI × 0.0136

LVSWI = Left ventricular stroke work index (g-m/m^2 per beat)

SVI = Stroke volume index (ml/m^2)

BP = Mean aortic pressure (mmHg)

PCWP = Mean pulmonary capillary wedge pressure (mmHg)

0.0136 = Factor for converting mmHg cm^3 to g-m

Ventricular Function Curve

The ventricular function curve (VFC) defines the relationship between ventricular filling pressure and ventricular stroke work and is a unifying concept to explain the performance characteristics of a given ventricle. The left ventricular function curves possess certain characteristics. Each has a steep ascending limb, which plateaus at higher filling pressures. Since the right ventricle empties into a lower pressure system (pulmonary artery), right ventricular function curves have lower values for stroke work and may *not* possess a plateau. However, with either ventricle, the later the input (end diastolic volume), the greater the output (work) (within the limits of normal contractile performance).

Although more sophisticated indices of cardiac performance have been advocated, the ventricular function curve serves as one of the best clinical means of physiologically describing the performance of the intact heart. This is due, in part, to the fact that both ordinate (LVSWI) and abscissa (LVEDP, LAP, PCWP, etc.) are related qualitatively to the two major symptom complexes of patients with heart disease.

The graphic representation of the ventricular function curve is based upon the work of Ross and Braunwald.[232] They constructed ventricular function curves relating left ventricular filling pressures and left ventricular stroke work index. These curves were derived from data obtained under controlled conditions during cardiac catheterization. From these data they described three classes of ventricular function: normal function, mildly depressed ventricular function, and grossly depressed ventricular function.

Although normal pulmonary capillary wedge pressure is 8 to 12 mmHg, optimal cardiac output in normal patients can usually be achieved with a mean "wedge" pressure between 14 and 18 mmHg. A pulmonary capillary wedge pressure of 18 to 20 mmHg can cause dyspnea, 20 to 30 mmHg transudation of fluid (pulmonary congestion), and 30 to 35 mmHg frank pulmonary edema. However, Packman and Rackow[233] observed that a pulmonary capillary wedge pressure = 12 mg may be optimal in patients with hypovolemic or septic shock. The symptoms and signs of peripheral hypoperfusion appear as cardiac performance (stroke work) deteriorates. Signs of dyspnea appear as the left ventricular filling pressure increases above critical levels. The interpretation of these data provides a useful clinical framework for defining the cardiovascular status of a patient and the response to interventions.

The use of left ventricular stroke work index (LVSWI) rather than cardiac output or stroke volume, has several advantages.

1. Defines the area within a pressure volume loop
2. Includes measurements of both systolic and diastolic performance
3. Contains the major variables that alter cardiac performance (e.g. heart rate, preload, afterload)

An upward shift to the left has been interpreted as an improvement in ventricular performance. A shift downward and to the right has been considered as a deteriorating ventricular performance. In addition to changes in *contractility*, many interventions, including alterations in preload, afterload, heart rate, and ventricular compliance can produce shifts in the ventricular function curve. On this basis, some authorities have held that the use of LVSWI is too global to be informative. However, the directional changes of the ventricular function curve allow qualitative assessment of overall cardiac performance.

In addition to changes in contractility, many interventions can also produce shifts of the ventricular function curve by alterations in preload, afterload, heart rate, and ventricular compliance.

Therefore, stroke volume, stroke work, and other ejection phase measurements cannot be used as direct indices of contractility. Rather, these ejection-phase indices can be useful in assessing directional changes in left ventricular function.

Derived Indices of Respiratory Performance

Derived indices, especially those concerning oxygen delivery, can play an important role in optimizing respiratory evaluation and support of critically ill patients[158,169,227,234] (Table 10-7).

Nowhere is the interplay of respiratory and circulatory function more frequently assessed than in the selection of the optimal level of positive end expiratory pressure (PEEP).[235] Just as there is no one perfect measure of cardiac function, no single parameter will define the optimal level of respiratory performance for all patients. The optimum level of PEEP has been variously defined as follows:

The best PaO_2 does not necessarily infer the optimal level of PEEP. As PaO_2 is increased by higher levels of PEEP, transport of oxygen to the tissues may actually decrease (secondary to decreased cardiac output). Similarly, the lowest $A-aO_2$ gradient may be a function of an improvement in PaO_2 regardless of the effect on cardiac output. A reduction in intrapulmonary shunt to less than 15 percent has been thought to be a therapeutic goal that is consistent with adequate respiratory performance. Other reports emphasize that the best compliance coincides with optimal PEEP. Finally, an optimal level of PEEP has been defined as that which promotes the highest oxygen transport (O_2T) to the peripheral tissues.

COMPLICATIONS

Although the benefits of the PAC are unquestioned, they are not an unmixed blessing. Experience gained with more than a decade of use of the PAC in a wide variety of clinical situations has revealed a large variety of complications which can, and do, occur. These range from minor sequelae of catheter use, without clinical significance, to those with a fatal outcome. As a matter of fact, Alschule has termed "complications of vascular catheters" a new branch of medicine.[236] For an overview, see Table 10-8.

Swan, Ganz, and their colleagues,[3] in their initial

report describing 100 patients, noted only transient premature ventricular contractions, 2 cases of intravascular thrombosis, and 10 cases of balloon failure. The last may have been related to the fact that catheters were reused. Despite numerous case reports that have detailed the occurrence of specific complications resulting from PAC insertion, few large series exist that quantify complication rates. More recent reports have focused on specific complications resulting from PAC insertion (Table 10-9).

For the purpose of this disease, the complications arising from the use of a Swan-Ganz catheter can be usefully grouped in three categories: (1) those associated with venous cannulation, (2) those associated with passing the catheter, and (3) those occurring after the catheter is in place.

Table 10-8 lists the variety of complications, which now numbers over 30, associated with the use of a Swan-Ganz catheter. Most complications are avoidable by meticulous attention to technique.

Venous Cannulation

Arterial Puncture

The complications occurring venous cannulation are, with a few exceptions, the same as those that may occur during insertion of any central venous catheter. The exact frequency of arterial puncture is dependent upon several variables, such as operator skill and experience, site of insertion, and the urgency of the situation. However, it should be noted that arterial puncture has been reported in conjunction with all insertion sites. The carotid artery can be punctured during attempts at cannulating the internal jugular vein.[208,237,238] Shah and coworkers[239] reported a 1.9 percent incidence of carotid artery punctures in more than 6,000 patients receiving PACs. Methods to confirm that the introducer is venous and not arterial in location include pressure waveform analysis, usual comparison with blood in the arterial tubing and blood gas laboratory measurements of P_{IO_2}.[240] Although most arterial punctures result in minimal morbidity, on rare occasions death has been reported.[206,241] Early recognition followed by pressure over the puncture site will lead to immediate cessation of bleeding without further consequence. However, large hematomas can occur, leading to respiratory compromise, arterial compression, or exsanguination. The more serious sequelae are much more likely to occur if the large-bore introducer (sheath) has been inserted into the artery. Arterial perforation in patients who are, or are subsequently to be, heparinized may result in cancellation of sur-

---

TABLE 10-7. Derived Indices of Respiratory Function

Qs/Qt	$=$	$\dfrac{Cc_{O_2} - Ca_{O_2}}{Cc_{O_2} - Cv_{O_2}}$	(normal 7%)
$A - a_{O_2}$	$=$	$PA_{O_2} = Pa_{O_2}$	(normal 9 mmHg if $F_{IO_2} = 0.21$, 34 mmHG if $F_{IO_2} = 1.0$)
V_{O_2}	$=$	$CO\,(a - v_{O_2})$	(normal = 240 ml/min in 70-kg patient)
O_2T	$=$	$CO\,(Ca_{O_2})$	(normal = 1000 ml/min in 70-kg patient)
$A - V_{O_2}$	$=$	$Ca_{O_2} - Cv_{O_2}$	(normal = 4–6 ml/100 ml)

where:

Qs/Qt	$=$	Intrapulmonary shunt
Cc_{O_2}	$=$	Capillary O_2 content (Hgb × 1.39[a]) + [F_{IO_2} × 713) − (Pa$_{O_2}$)] × .0031
Ca_{O_2}	$=$	Arterial O_2 content (Hgb × 1.39 × Sa$_{O_2}$) + (Pa$_{O_2}$ × .0031)
Cv_{O_2}	$=$	Mixed venous O_2 content (Hgb × 1.30 × Sv$_{O_2}$) + (Pv$_{O_2}$ × .0031)
$A - a_{O_2}$	$=$	Alveolar-arterial O_2 gradient
PA_{O_2}	$=$	Alveolar O_2 tension (PB[b] − 47) (F_{IO_2} − PaCO_2)
Pa_{O_2}	$=$	Arterial O_2 tension
V_{O_2}	$=$	Minute O_2 consumption
CO	$=$	Cardiac output
O_2T	$=$	Tissue oxygen transport
$Ca - v_{O_2}$	$=$	Arterio-venous O_2 content difference

[a]Assumes F_{IO_2} .35 (Sa$_{O_2}$ = 100%).
[b]Assumes PB = 760 mmHg.

gical procedures. Another possibility is that athero- sclerotic plaques may be dislodged and embolize to the cerebral circulation. Puncture of the subcla- vian artery may be more insidious. Evidence of bleeding is not readily visible, nor can pressure be easily applied. The first evidence of subclavian ar- tery puncture may be the appearance of a hemo- thorax on chest radiograph.

Presently, insertion techniques are aimed at in- creasing the ease of finding the vein and minimiz- ing the risk of arterial injury. Techniques that re- sult in engorgement of the internal jugular and subclavian veins, such as use of the Trendelenburg position, coughing, the Valsalva maneuver, or the inspiratory phase of mechanical ventilation all con- tribute to a successful cannulation. Similarly, the use of a 20-gauge "finder" needle to preliminary locate the vein will produce a smaller hole in the event of an inadvertent arterial perforation. Once the vein has been located, this small needle can be left in place to serve as a visual guide for insertion of the larger needle. Unfortunately, arterial punc- ture can still occur with the second needle, though much less frequently.[242] The technique described by

TABLE 10-8. Complications (Case Reports) Associated with Pulmonary Artery Catheters

I.	Venous Cannulation
	Air embolization
	Arterial puncture
	Bernard-Horner syndrome
	Hematoma
	Nerve injury
	Phrenic nerve blockade
	Pneumothorax
	Equipment malfunction (Cohen)
II.	Catheter Passage/Removal
	Arrhythmias
	Knotting
	Knotting on papillary muscle
	Pneumoperitoneum
	Separation of introducer from hub
	Bundle branch block
III.	Catheter In Situ
	Aberrant waveform due to balloon rupture
	Bradycardia secondary to thermodilution cardiac output measurement
	Cardiac valve injury
	Catheter fracture
	Deep venous thrombosis
	Endobronchial hemorrhagic
	Endocarditis
	False positive lung imaging
	False positive echocardiography
	Hemoptysis
	Intraoperative transection of a catheter
	Migration of pediatric PA catheters
	PA perforation
	Pulmonary infarction
	Sepsis
	Suturing PA catheter to the heart
	Systolic clicks
	Thrombocytopenia
	Thrombosis caused by starch on PA catheters
	Vertebral arteriovenous fistula
	Pseudoaneurysm
	Errors in cardiac output secondary to catheter malfunction
	Inadvertent passage of catheter into left side of heart
	Hematuria

Civetta and Gabel[187] uses a 20-gauge spinal needle as the "finder" with a 16-gauge over-the-needle catheter threaded on the spinal needle prior to insertion. Schwartz and colleagues[206] have emphasized the important of transducing the intravenous catheter or needle before the wireguide is passed. In their series, a number of patients sustained unrecognized carotid artery puncture with passage of an 8 Fr sheath into the artery. In a subsequent group of patients in whom pressures were transduced, no sheaths were inserted into the carotid artery.

Previous arterial puncture often precludes subsequent use of the vein in the same location. Following the development of a hematoma, attempts at cannulation yield blood from the hematoma that cannot be distinguished from that of venipuncture. If arterial puncture occurs and a hematoma develops, we recommend use of another venous access site when feasible. If the carotid artery is entered prior to cardiac surgery, we recommend postpone-

ment due to heparinization and possible expansion of the hematoma. This may not be possible in urgent or emergent situations. In these cases, the neck is prepped and draped into the surgical field where the hematoma may be observed. Following heparinization, if the hematoma is enlarging, surgical exploration may be necessary prior to cardiopulmonary bypass.

Pneumothorax

Violation of the pleural space during attempts at venous cannulation is a well-recognized complication of both the subclavian and internal jugular vein approaches. The incidence of pneumothorax is dependent upon both operator experience and cannulation site. In patients being mechanically ventilated, a simple pneumothorax may be converted into a tension pneumothorax, resulting in serious respiratory and circulatory compromise. In

TABLE 10-9. Reported Incidence of Adverse Effects

Complication	Reported Incidence (%)
Central Venous Access	
Arterial puncture	1.1–13
Bleeding at cutdown site (children)	5.3
Postoperative neuropathy	0.3–1.1
Pneumothorax	0.3–4.5
Air embolism	0.5
Catheterization	
Minor arrhythmias	4.7–68.9
Severe arrhythmias (ventricular tachycardia or fibrillation)[a]	0.3–62.7
Right bundle branch block[a]	0.1–4.3
Complete heart block (in patients with prior left bundle branch block)	8–8.5
Catheter Residence	
Pulmonary artery rupture[a]	0.1–1.5
Positive catheter tip cultures	1.4–34.8
Catheter related sepsis	0.7–11.4
Thrombophlebitis	6.5
Venous thrombosis	0.5–66.7
Pulmonary infarction[a]	0.1–5.8
Mural thrombus[a]	28–61
Valvular/endocardial vegetations or endocarditis[a]	2.2–100
Deaths (attributed to PA catheter)[a]	0.02–1.5

[a]Complications thought to be more common (or exclusively associated) with PA catheterization than with central venous catheterization.
(From Practice Guidelines for Pulmonary Artery Catheterization,[154] with permission.)

these patients, the insertion of a chest tube is indicated, with more urgency being demanded for a tension pneumothorax. If a chest tube is not immediately available, needle aspiration of the pleural space will relieve symptoms temporarily. If possible, a chest radiograph should be obtained following PAC insertion, not only to confirm catheter position, but to exclude the presence of pneumothorax. However, intraoperatively this is not routinely feasible. Because of differences in solubilities of gases, nitrous oxide will diffuse into any pneumothorax much faster than nitrogen can diffuse out. This can lead to a doubling or tripling of the size of the pneumothorax in a very few minutes leading to the development of cardiovascular compromise. Clinically, unexplained rises in pulmonary capillary wedge pressure and PAD are the earliest signs of pneumothorax.[243] For this reason, attempts at subclavian cannulation are not advised intraoperatively or preoperatively when chest radiographs cannot be obtained on a regular basis. In addition, hemothorax or hemopneumothorax can occur rarely when the subclavian or low internal jugular approach has been used.[92]

Air Embolism

Despite the theoretical likelihood of air embolus occurring with some frequency during venous cannulation (especially through the large bore introducer) very few reports have appeared in the literature documenting its occurrence.[244-246] Fatal air embolism has been reported to occur through smaller bore central venous catheters connected to continuous flush systems.[240] Only three cases of clinically significant embolism have appeared in the literature, which were associated with the insertion of a Swan-Ganz catheter.[245-247] Two of these were in conjunction with an introducer, which had no provision for a self-sealing valve following removal of a Swan-Ganz catheter. The third was detected in a study where Doppler monitors were placed over the right parasternal area specifically to study the occurrence of air embolism.[244] No clinical changes were noted at the time of embolization. Had it not been for the presence of the Doppler, no suspicion of air embolus would have arisen. The utilization of the Trendelenburg position is probably responsible for preventing many air emboli. Nonetheless, air embolus probably occurs more frequently than we are aware, but insufficient

air enters the venous circulation to result in clinical symptoms. A recent report by Moorthy and colleagues[248] illustrates that venous air embolism can also occur during removal of the PAC.

Neurologic Deficit

Nerve injury during percutaneous venous catheterization is rare. Traumatic injury during surgical attempts venous cutdown has been reported.[249] As a result of trauma to the stellate ganglion Horner syndrome has been described during internal jugular catheterization.[250,251] In a series examining neurologic deficits following open heart surgery, 4.1 percent of internal jugular vein catheterization were associated with ipsilateral nerve deficit.[252] A recent report has emphasized the fact that complications of median sternotomy may also result in a similar neurologic presentation as that observed from venous cannulation.[253,254] This makes identifying the precise cause of neurologic deficit difficult. However, when a peripheral neurologic deficit is observed, extensive workup is indicated. Both transient and permanent phrenic nerve injury has been reported with internal jugular and subclavian approaches.[197,254] Brown[238] reported patients in whom an 8 Fr introducer was inserted into the right common carotid artery. Cerebral embolization, rather than prolonged catheterization of the artery, led to a left hemiparesis.

Passage of the Pulmonary Artery Catheter

Arrhythmias

The most common complication during catheter passage is the development of cardiac arrhythmias. Swan and Ganz[255] reported a 13 percent incidence of transient premature ventricular contractions in their original report. Since then, numerous studies have documented an incidence of isolated premature ventricular contractions ranging from 12 to 48 percent.[256-259] Those studies reporting the lower incidence relied on visual observation of an oscilloscopic ECG monitor during insertion, while investigators reporting the higher incidence of this complication (46 and 48 percent relied on continuous ECG tracings for their data collection. As a result, true incidence of premature ventricular contractions is probably closer to the latter. Ventricular tachycardia has been noted in as many as 33 percent of patients.[257] Ventricular fibrillation has been reported as well. The incidence of arrhythmias may be related to time required to float the catheter into the pulmonary artery.[260] In a study by Lopez Seden[50] the presence of a recent right ventricular infarction (RVI) increased incidence of ventricular fibrillation during passage of the PAC (4.2 percent with RVI vs 0.28 percent RVI). In this same study, the incidence of ventricular fibrillation was also higher during PAC insertion in patients suffering from acute myocardial infraction, 1.07 percent vs an 0.85 percent overall rate of ventricular fibrillation.

In a large series of insertions analyzed for new and complex arrhythmias 5 percent of patients sustained a new right bundle branch block.[261] Castellanos and coworkers[262] theorize that damage to the bundle of His may occur during passage of the PAC through the right ventricle, resulting in a right bundle branch block. In the majority of patients, this conduction abnormality has no significance. In one patient, right bundle branch block was seen only during balloon inflation.[263] However, in patients with preexisting left bundle block complete heart block may result with passage of the catheter through the right ventricle chamber.[264] If catheterization is required for these patients, a pacing electrode should be available. Alternatively, transcutaneous pacing could be used in these situations. Using this approach, should complete heart block develop during insertion, the patient can then be transcutaneously paced. The placement of a multipurpose (pacing) Swan-Ganz catheter may be placed in this situation. Parenthetically, the right ventricular section of the pacing catheter shaft is stiffer and may actually predispose to right bundle branch block. Left fascicular or left bundle branch block has also been reported with PAC insertion.

Clinically significant arrhythmias including ventricular tachycardia have also been reported on removal of PAC (63 percent incidence).[265] The mechanism of production of these arrhythmias is the result of mechanical stimulation of the conduction pathways. Theoretically, the design of the catheter balloon prevents the tip of the catheter from contacting the ventricular surface. It was originally believed that this feature would eliminate arrhythmias during insertion. No doubt it has reduced the incidence of serious arrhythmias. Nonetheless, sufficient force is generated when the balloon or free portion of the catheter contacts the ventricular wall to stimulate the conduction system in a high percentage of patients. Production of arrhythmias can

be minimized by passing the catheter rapidly once the right ventricle is reached. Lidocaine, 1 to 1.5 mg/kg intravenously, has been shown to be effective in reducing the occurrence of ventricular arrhythmias.[266] We use lidocaine when previous catheter passage has resulted in hemodynamically significant arrhythmias. However, Salmenpera and colleagues[227] have shown that prophylactic use of lidocaine is ineffective.

In addition to the development of arrhythmias, a recent report by Cohen and Whalen[250] demonstrates that the PAC may lodge in the coronary sinus during insertion. Resistance to passage from the right atrium to the right ventricle, in conjunction with an observation of the systemic pressure trace, should alert the clinician to this possibility. Similarly, Allyn and associates[268] reported in the inadvertent passage of a PAC from the superior vena cava through the left atrium and left ventricle and close observation of acute change in the waveform of the PAC should have altered these authors to a potential change in PAC location.[268] Electrode separation from a multipurpose pacing PAC has been reported. As a result, the manufacturer has made specific recommendations for removal of this type of catheter.

Intracardiac Knotting

Several reports of intracardiac knotting of a pulmonary artery catheter have appeared.[269–275] Most knots probably occur during insertion when coiling in the right atrium or right ventricle can occur.[276] These knots may take the form of free, single, or double knots in the catheter, or more ominously, may incorporate intracardiac structures such as a papillary muscle, chordae tendineae, or the lead from a cardiac pacemaker.[277,278] Knots may be diagnosed from postinsertion radiographs or during attempts to remove the catheter, when resistance to withdrawal occurs.[272,273]

The knot may be withdrawn through the original venotomy site.[279] Most often, it becomes necessary to utilize one of a number of fluoroscopic techniques in the cardiac catheter laboratory in which the knot can be either tightened or untied or the catheter cut.[268,281,282] Occasionally operative intervention becomes necessary.

The suspicion of coiling during insertion should be raised anytime that an undue length of catheter has been inserted without achieving the expected intracardiac pressure tracing. Normal distances from insertion site to right atrium, right ventricle, pulmonary artery and wedge position are shown in Table 10-4. When these reference points are exceeded by about 10 cm without the tip of the catheter reaching the appropriate location, the balloon should be deflated and the catheter withdrawn to the right atrium. If resistance is encountered, all attempts at withdrawal should cease and a chest radiograph should be immediately obtained. Another sign suggestive of coiling is the occurrence of ventricular arrhythmias at a time when pressure tracings indicate the tip is still in the right atrium.

Patients with a transvenous pacemaker in place who also require pulmonary artery monitoring are at risk of having the catheter become entwined around the pacing leads. Insertion of a PAC in such a patient should be performed under fluoroscopy.

Isolated complications occurring during pulmonary artery catheter insertion include torn chordae tendineae, probably caused by multiple attempts at insertion, and withdrawal of the catheter while the balloon was still inflated. Aberrant catheter locations have been reported including the pleural space, the peritoneal cavity, the renal vein, the aorta, and the vertebral artery.[283] Most, if not all, of these complications probably could have been prevented by strict adherence to the previously described insertion techniques (Table 10-3).

The Catheter In Situ

Pulmonary Artery Perforation

Unquestionably the most catastrophic complication that occurs as a result of PAC insertion is pulmonary artery perforation and subsequent hemorrhage.[20,284–304] Reports of this complication were rare for the first 10 years following introduction of the pulmonary artery catheter (only five such reports). Since that time it has become much more commonly reported, and there are now more than 50 reported cases in the English language literature.

Several significant risk factors for the development of PAC perforation have been identified. Advanced age, hypothermia, and pulmonary hypertension place the patient at greater risk for pulmonary artery perforation.[304] Furthermore, females have a higher incidence of perforation. Of 24 patients who had a pulmonary artery perforation, and in whom pulmonary artery pressures

were reported, 22 had pulmonary hypertension. Deviations from standard insertion techniques have been noted in at least 10 of 56 reported cases as well.[304–307,309,310]

The presenting sign of pulmonary artery perforation in most cases is the sudden appearance of hemoptysis. Characteristically, the blood is bright red and may vary in amount from less than 5 ml to massive bleeding.[289,290] Usually this episode of bleeding is related to balloon inflation or catheter manipulation. However, hemoptysis may also be caused by flushing the catheter in the wedge position.[299]

Treatment of PAC perforation is largely supportive in nature. If bleeding is massive, the patient must be intubated. If a double-lumen endotracheal tube is not available, an ordinary single-lumen endotracheal tube should be advanced into the mainstem bronchus of the noninvolved lung, usually the left. If the patient has received heparin, it should be reversed if possible. Massive blood and fluid replacement may be necessary, as well as operative intervention. PEEP has been used, as well, in an attempt to compress the bleeding site.[311–3131] Pulmonary artery perforation has been described as a complication following cardiopulmonary bypass. Rice and associates[314] reported a patient who sustained a pulmonary artery perforation following cardiopulmonary bypass. In these reversals of situations, heparinization with protamine resulted in a resolution of hemorrhage.

Controversy exists about what to do with the PAC once a pulmonary artery perforation is suspected (i.e., do you have the balloon up, put more air in the balloon, or take the PAC out? In these early reports of pulmonary artery perforation Barash and colleagues[22] suggested that pulling the PAC back with the balloon down about 5 to 10 cm was appropriate. They suggested that by doing this one could then inject some contrast media into the PAC to radiographically identify the precise location of the pulmonary artery perforation. This could then be used to guide surgical interventions (i.e., wedge resection vs pneumonectomy) if this becomes necessary.[20] Resnick and coworkers[315] recently reported the ability of angiography to aid in the diagnosis and localization of pulmonary artery perforation.

The common feature of pulmonary artery perforation in most patients is distal location of the tip of the PAC, (although it has been reported with a more central location as well)[316] (Fig. 10-13). When

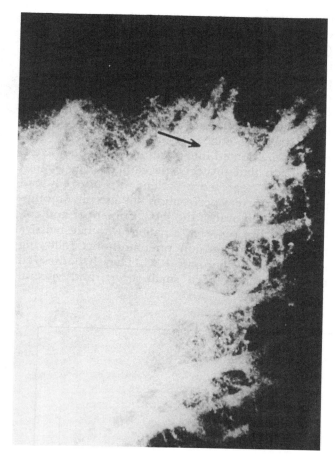

the tip is located too far distally, balloon inflation can distend the vessel wall subjecting it to large transmural pressures.[18] Distal catheter placement can occur as a result of failure to follow currently accepted insertion techniques or in the presence of pulmonary hypertension. The most frequently observed technical error is the use of less than 1.5 ml of air to inflate the balloon during PAC insertion. This allows the tip of the catheter to pass into a smaller, more distal vessels. Subsequent balloon inflation with the full 1.5 ml will then overdistend the vessel increasing the risk for pulmonary artery perforation. The original description of pulmonary artery insertion technique of pulmonary artery perforation by Swan, Ganz, and colleagues suggested advancing the tip of the catheter 1 to 3 cm with the balloon deflated after the initial wedge pressure was obtained. However, this can also lead to distal placement.[317] Pulmonary hypertension may lead to distal placement by distending smaller pulmonary arteries, thus allowing the catheter to wedge in a more distal location. Pulmonary artery hypertension can also lead to degenerative changes in the vessel wall, such as sclerosis and aneurysmal dilatation, which may further predispose the vessel to rupture.

The fact that the catheter tip is in a distal location may be identified by the phenomenon of *overwedging* (Fig. 10-14). Overwedging results from impingement of the tip of the catheter against the vessel wall or herniation of the balloon over the catheter tip.[22] The continuously rising pressure trace seen with this phenomenon results from the high-pressure flush system. Therefore when an overwedge tract is observed the catheter should be withdrawn until a normal wedge tracing is obtained.

Fig. 10-13. Post mortem barium gel studies showing extravasation of gel at the site of pulmonary artery perforation. The distal migration of the catheter presumably occurred with cardiac manipulation during cardiopulmonary bypass. (From Barash et al.,[22] with permission.)

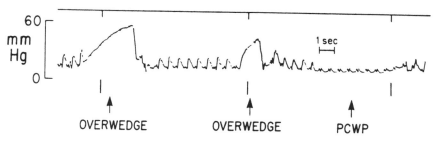

Fig. 10-14. Intraoperative pulmonary artery pressure tracing which demonstrates overwedging patterns observed with balloon inflation. This pattern results from the catheter tip impinging against the vessel wall or balloon herniation over the catheter tip. The pulmonary artery catheter is withdrawn 3 cm and a normal transition from pulmonary artery to pulmonary capillary wedge pressure is obtained. (From Barash et al.,[22] with permission.)

Several mechanisms that may be responsible for pulmonary artery perforation have been described (Fig. 10-15). Inflation of the balloon with a distally located catheter tip can lead to direct tearing of the vessel. Eccentric balloon inflation, as demonstrated by several investigators, can expose the catheter tip and can actually propel it through the arterial wall.[318] This mechanism can be aggravated by the gradient existing with pulmonary hypertension.[22] The tip of the catheter may become lodged in a small vascular branch and may erode or perforate directly. Direct perforation may also occur during insertion. Migration of the catheter tip to more distal location during cardiac surgery has also been postulated as a potential mechanism.[319]

One thing that can clearly reduce the potential for pulmonary artery perforation to minimize the number of balloon inflations. In view of the fact that pulmonary artery diastolic pressure agrees very well with pulmonary capillary wedge pressure (in the absence of pulmonary hypertension), we recommend that the pulmonary artery diastolic pressure be used, whenever possible, as an indirect measurement of left atrial pressure.[22] If this is done, the tip of the catheter can be left in a very proximal location, 4 to 5 cm beyond the pulmonic valve. If a true wedge pressure is required, the catheter can be floated into position through an external sheath that protects the catheter. Farber and associates[289] reported a patient who not only had pulmonary artery perforation but also pneumothorax, upon removal of the PAC. Culpepper and colleagues[285] also reported a patient who had massive hemoptysis and tension pneumothorax following insertion of a fiberoptic PAC. They hypothesized that perforation of a small artery and visceral

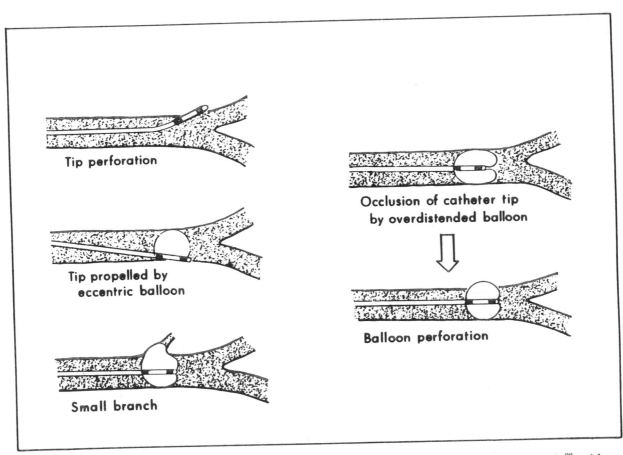

Fig. 10-15. Possible mechanisms of pulmonary artery perforation. (From Barash et al.,[22] with permission.)

pleura occurred following persistent wedging of the catheter. Since these early reports, several authors have demonstrated that the development of hemoptysis in patients with PAC in place should alert the clinician to the possibility of pulmonary artery perforation.[284,312] These authors also suggest that in patients who survive the pulmonary artery rupture (mortality rate of 40 to 70 percent), these patients should undergo further studies aimed at diagnosing a possible catheter induced pseudoaneurysm.[242,303] If such a pseudoaneurysm is found, it must be the obliterated to prevent any further bleeding.[320]

Pulmonary Artery Infarction

Early reports indicated that pulmonary artery infarction also resulted from distal placement of the catheter.[291,321,322] The mechanism responsible for this distal placement has been described in the previous section. The sequelae of pulmonary artery infarction may include deep venous thrombosis with embolization, endothelial damage, or permanent wedging of the catheter tip in a distal pulmonary artery. Clinical states characterized by low cardiac output may further predispose to this complication. Usually the diagnosis or pulmonary infarction is made by chest radiograph.

As with pulmonary artery perforation, prevention is directed at avoiding distal placement of the catheter, avoiding persistent balloon inflation, and use of a continuous high-pressure flush system with heparinized saline.

Thrombosis and Coagulopathies

Several studies have documented the fact that pulmonary artery catheters are thrombogenic. Substantial thrombi (several hundred milligrams) will form on virtually 100 percent of catheter in vivo within 1 to 2 hours of insertion.[205,249,323–325] These thrombi are capable of causing both damped pressure tracings and yielding inaccurately low cardiac output measurements.

Connors and associates[287] performed detailed postmortem examination on 32 consecutive patients brought to autopsy with a PAC in place. Thrombosis or hemorrhage related to PAC was found in 91 percent of patients.[207,287] The incidence of thrombosis was higher after 36 hours of catheterization.

In addition, massive thrombosis of the subclavian

vein[249] and the superior vena cava[326] have been reported. Devitt and colleagues[316] have reported a case where catheter thrombus was apparently stripped off the PAC during removal and embolized across a ventricular sepal defect to the cerebral and coronary circulations.

One hypothesis for the occurrence of pulmonary infarction or emboli, is the development of thrombus on the catheter body. Although no report has directly shown embolization from such thrombi, much circumstantial evidence exists.[321,325–327] In addition to the potential damage to the pulmonary parenchyma, Devitt and coworkers[316] reported embolization across a ventriculoseptal defect, the origin of which was thought to be from the PAC. Early reports by Brunswick and Gionis[328] stated that starch crystals were seen on microscopic examination of the PAC clot. As a result, starch has been advocated in the subsequent manufacture of PAC. In an attempt to reduce thrombotic complications, heparin binding of the catheters is now routine. Heparin bonding prevents thrombosis in a canine model and in humans.[324] However, at present, no published study shows a lower morbidity when heparin-bonded catheters are inserted. Thrombosis has also been reported at insertion sites, such as the internal jugular vein.[329]

At the other end of the spectrum is the possibility of coagulopathies in patients with a PAC. Kim and coworkers originally presented data to show thrombocytopenia related to PAC in a canine model. Richman and coworkers[331] confirmed these data in humans. Although platelet counts were decreased, no patient sustained a bleeding episode on this basis.

Infection

Septic complications of pulmonary artery catheters have been documented by many investigators.[93–95,332,333] While evaluating these studies, it is important to remember that patients with a PAC have other sources of infection present, for example, urinary catheters and intravenous catheters.[94,95] While their occurrence is clearly demonstrated, the incidence and significance of these complications is less well-known. It is difficult to separate colonization, contamination, and infection in published studies. Fortunately, reports of serious sequelae of positive catheter cultures are rare. Elliott and colleagues[304] have provided a useful classification for the study of catheter sepsis. They defined colonization as a positive culture of the catheter tip without evidence of local or systemic infection. Contamination is defined as one of multiple blood cultures yielding a typical non-pathogen and culture of the catheter tip failing to grow any organisms. Infection can be:

1. *Definite*: positive blood and catheter cultures yielding the same organism
2. *Probable*: the same organism cultured from blood and catheter with no other probable source of infection.
3. *Unrelated*: if the same organism had been previously recovered from another source

The reported incidence of catheter related sepsis varies widely from 2 percent[35] to 35 percent.[304] Earlier reports disagreed on the impact of the duration of catheterization on rates of infection. More recent studies by Mermel and Raad[93,334] have provided new evidence for the role of duration of placement as a predictor of PAC-related infections. Mermel and colleagues[93] demonstrated an overall rate of local infection of 22 percent (65 of 29 percent catheters). They further subdivided these PAC-related infections into those that occurred as a result of local infection of the introducer (58/297) or the intravascular portion of the PAC (20/297). In their study only two catheters (0.7 percent) caused bacteremia. About 80 percent of infected catheters (the introducer or the PAC itself) showed concordance with organisms cultures from skin of the insertion site. Of these, 17 percent were the result of a contaminated hub, 18 percent were the result of organisms contaminating the extravascular portion of the catheter beneath the sleeve. The following were identified as increasing the relative risk of pulmonary artery infection: (1) cutaneous colonization of the insertion site with >10^2 colony-forming units (relative risk: 5.5; $P < .001$); (2) insertion into an internal jugular vein (relative risk: 4.3: $P < .001$); and (3) insertion done in the operating room, using less stringent barrier precautions (relative risk: 2.1; $P = .03$). Similarly, Raad and colleagues[334] found that 17 percent (12/71) of PAC in their study produced local infection, and 5.6 percent (4/71) led to septicemia. These episodes of septicemia were directly related to the duration of PAC placement. Catheter-related septicemia occurred at rates of 2 percent and 16 percent, before and after 7 days of catheter placement, re-

spectively. Further analysis from their data (life table analysis) showed that the cumulative risk of developing a catheter infection increased from 9 to 18 percent after *4 days* of placement of the PAC.[325] As a result of the data from those two studies we recommend that PAC should be changed to a new site every 4 to 7 days.

Recently the use of sterile sleeves has been advocated for repositioning the PAC in a sterile fashion.[335–337] However, the precise benefit of these devices in substantially reducing PAC infections remains to be elucidated.

Given the invasive nature of pulmonary artery catheterization the following recommendations are prudent to minimize any infectious complications:

1. Insertion of the catheter should be performed with aseptic technique, including extensive skin preparation.
2. The catheter site should be covered with an antibacterial ointment and a sterile occlusive dressing. This should be repeated daily.
3. Performance of thermodilution cardiac output and changing of infusion sets should be performed as aseptically as possible, and only when necessary.
4. Pulmonary artery catheters should be removed as soon as they are no longer necessary. If the need persists beyond 72 hours, they should probably be replaced with a new one inserted through an entirely new site.

Not only are localized and or systemic infection process of concern but PACs may also be associated with an increased incidence of cardiac valve injury and endocarditis. Smith and coworkers[338,339] reported ruptured chordae tendineae of the tricuspid valve as a result of withdrawing the PAC with the balloon inflated. Isolated case reports of erosion of the pulmonic[277] and tricuspid[278] valves were followed by several series documenting an increased incidence of aseptic endocarditis. In a retrospective analysis, Pace and Horton[340] noted three cases of aseptic endocarditis in 88 catheterized patients compared with 1 in 205 uncatheterized patients. Greene and Cummings[323] found four cases in 24 autopsies. An additional four cases occurred in the 270 noncatheterized patients.[341] Subsequently, they reported that 1 in 493 patients dying prior to the introduction of the PAC developed aseptic endocarditis, while 10 of 483 patients with PAC developed this condition.

Ehrie and colleagues[342] noted that all six burn patients studied developed endocarditis, and Sasaki and colleagues[343] documented a statistically significant increase in the incidence of this complication in 1,105 burn patients following introduction of the PAC. In contrast, Katz and colleagues[159] were unable to find evidence of valvular damage.

LIMITATIONS AND FUTURE DIRECTION

In addition to the complications associated with invasive monitoring a major limitation of pulmonary artery catheters is the assumption that intracardiac pressure measurements (pulmonary capillary wedge pressure) are a good approximation of the volume status of the ventricle. As previously stated, preload can be defined as the force required to stretch the muscle to end-diastolic fiber length. This is clinically translated to measurement of end-diastolic volume. The use of pulmonary capillary wedge pressure to directly or indirectly assess preload assumes a linear relationship between ventricular end-diastolic volume and ventricular end-diastolic pressure. However, alterations in ventricular compliance can affect this pressure-volume relationship (Fig. 10-16). Hansen and associates[344] demonstrated this poor correlation between pulmonary artery pressure and left ventricular end diastolic volume following coronary artery bypass graft surgery. In this study, left ventricular end-diastolic volume was determined using concomitant determinations of ejection fraction, gated blood pool scintigraphy, and stroke volume (determined from thermodilution cardiac output). The authors postulate that an altered ventricular pressure volume relationship may reflect acute changes in ventricular complication in the first few hours following bypass surgery. Reductions in ventricular

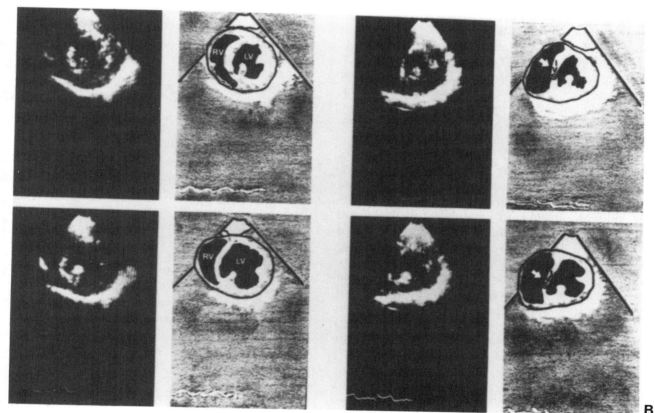

Fig. 10-16. Two-dimensional echocardiograms revealing a leftward shift of the interventricular septum (*arrow*) as increasing levels of PEEP are applied. (**A**) Control period, PEEP = 0 cmH$_2$ (**B**) Obtained at PEEP = 30 cm. (From Jardin et al.,[26] with permission.)

compliance (upward shift to left) can be seen with myocardial ischemia, shock, right ventricular overload and pericardial effusion. Ventricular compliance is increased with vasodilators such as nitroglycerin and sodium nitroprusside.

Calvin and coworkers[345] made simultaneous pressure and volume measurements using radionuclear angiography in patients with sepsis and in another group with acute cardiac illnesses. They found no relationship between left ventricular end-diastolic volume and pulmonary capillary wedge pressure in either group ($r = .58$). The correlation decreased further when PEEP was employed ($r = .30$).[337] Beaupre and colleagues,[91] using two-dimensional echocardiography, reported similar findings in a group of anesthetized patients. They concluded that using pulmonary capillary wedge pressure as a guide to fluid therapy may be misleading. This was further emphasized by Marmana and colleagues[30] who examined the relationship of pulmonary capillary wedge pressure and left atrial pressure in patients undergoing coronary artery bypass surgery. In this study, pulmonary capillary wedge pressure was a poor predictor of left atrial pressure in the early postoperative period. They hypothesized that pulmonary venoconstriction resulting from increased pulmonary extravascular water (due to hemodilution cardiopulmonary bypass) accounted for the difference between left atrial pressure and pulmonary capillary wedge pressure.[30]

Ellis and colleagues[346] also using intraoperative radionuclear monitoring (gated pool) found alterations in ventricular diastolic and systolic performance that were not appreciated by routine hemodynamic monitoring. In patients with a LVEF less than 50 percent undergoing coronary artery bypass operation, a decreased ventricular compliance suggested that this group of patients may require closer observation and increased cardiovascular support in the post-bypass period. On the basis of additional radionuclear data showing a decline in LVEF from 70 to 49 percent, they also concluded that volume loading following cardiopulmonary bypass may be detrimental.

Significant diagnostic errors may result when pulmonary capillary wedge pressure is assumed to be directly related to LVEDV. For example, an elevated pulmonary capillary wedge pressure and a decreased cardiac output can be interpreted as left ventricular failure. However, these hemodynamic findings may also reflect *ventricular interdependence*.[26]

Ventricular interdependence occurs when the interventricular septum encroaches on the left ventricular cavity. This can occur in acute respiratory failure, with high levels of PEEP and so on.[347,348] The differential is made on the basis of knowledge of left ventricular end-diastolic volume. Left ventricular end-diastolic volume is increased in left ventricular failure, while it is decreased when ventricular interdependence is present.

	PCWP	Cardiac Output	LVEDV
LV failure	↑	↓	↑
Ventricular interdependence	↑	↓	↓

Noninvasive assessment of cardiovascular function by radionuclear and echocardiographic methods (particularly the use of perioperative two-dimensional transesophageal echocardiography) offers the anesthesiologist monitoring techniques that overcome these limitations.[266] These techniques will assume greater importance for the clinician in terms of patient care, research, and education. The potential appeal of these methods is a more precise physiologic definition of the patient's cardiac reserve without the risks associated with invasive tests. Just as invasive monitoring with the Swan-Ganz catheter has raised our awareness of cardiovascular physiology, these noninvasive methods offer a unique method of supplementing our knowledge of the cardiovascular system.

Clinically, these modalities, particularly two-dimensional TEE are frequently being utilized in combination with PACs. This combination provides the most and specific methods for cardiac monitoring. In a recent article, Rafferty[128] highlighted the ability of PACs and TEE to complement each in the management of critically ill patients. Pulmonary artery catheterization has transformed the care of critically ill patients.[348] It permits the direct measurement of vital hemodynamic and respiratory parameters and permits rational application of therapeutic modalities. The existence of significant complications, however, mandates care in selecting patients for its use, and in insertion and maintenance of the catheter. The age-old question of risk: benefit of pulmonary artery catheterization continues to be debated. Although precise data are lacking, all of us who rely on the information obtained from PAC are convinced that it has been and will continue to be a vital tool in the management of critically ill patients. It should not be forgotten that it is a tool and that the ultimate monitoring system remains the clinician.

REFERENCES

1. Ganz W, Donoso R, Marcus HS et al: A new technique for measurement of cardiac output by thermodilution in man. Am J Cardiol 27:392, 1971
2. Lategola M, Rahn H: A self-guiding catheter for cardiac and pulmonary arterial catheterization and occlusion. Proc Soc Exp Biol Med 84:667, 1953
3. Swan HJ: The role of hemodynamic monitoring in the management of the critically ill. Crit Care Med 75:83, 1975
4. Swan HJC, Ganz W, Forrester J et al: Catheterization of the heart in man with use of a flow-directed balloon-tipped catheter. N Engl J Med 283:447, 1970
5. Applefeld JJ, Caruthers TE, Reno DJ et al: Assessment of the sterility of long-term cardiac catheterization using thermodilution Swan-Ganz catheter. Chest 74:377, 1978
6. Beique F, Ramsay J: The pulmonary artery catheter: a new look. Semin Anesth, 1993
7. Berryhill RE, Benumof JL: PEEP-induced discrepancy between pulmonary arterial wedge pressure and left atrial pressure: the effects of controlled vs. spontaneous ventilation and compliant vs. noncompliant lungs in the dog. Anesthesiology 51:303, 1979
8. Chun GM, Ellestad MH: Perforation of the pulmonary artery by a Swan-Ganz catheter. N Engl J Med 284:1041, 1971
9. Keefer JR, Barash PG: Pulmonary artery catheterization: a disease of clinical progress? [Editorial]. Chest 84:241, 1983
10. Lopez-Sendon J, Coma-Canella I, Gamallo C: Sensitivity and specificity of hemodynamic criteria in the diagnosis of acute right ventricular infarction. Circulation 64:515, 1981
11. Nehme AE: Swan-Ganz catheter: comparison of insertion techniques. Arch Surg 115:1194, 1980
12. Page DW, Teres D, Hartshorn JW: Fatal hemorrhage from Swan-Ganz catheter. [Letter]. N Engl J Med 291:260, 1974
13. Tarhan S, Moffitt EA, Taylor WF et al: Myocardial infarction after general anesthesia. JAMA 220:1451, 1972
14. Zion MM, Balkin J, Rosenmann D et al: Use of pulmonary artery catheters in patients in the SPRINT Registry. Chest 98:1331, 1990
15. American Edwards Laboratories: Swan-Ganz flow directed thermodilution catheters. Product Information Bulletin 093-4/82
16. Eisenkraft JB, Eger EI: Nitrous oxide and Swan-Ganz catheters. [Letter]. Anesth Analg 61:308, 1982
17. Kaplan R, Abramowitz MD, Epstein BS: Nitrous oxide and air filled balloon-tipped catheters. Anesthesiology 55:71, 1981
18. Hardy JF, Taillefer J: Inflating characteristics of Swan-Ganz catheter balloons: clinical considerations. Anesth Analg 62:363, 1983
19. Hart U, Ward DR, Gillilan R et al: Fatal pulmonary hemorrhage complicating Swan-Ganz catheterization. Surgery, 91:24, 1982
20. Basson MD: Hazards of pulmonary-artery catheterization. [Letter]. N Engl J Med 302:807, 1980
21. Ikeda S, Yagi K, Schweiss JF, Homan SM: In vitro reappraisal of the pulmonary artery catheter balloon volume-pressure relationship: comparison of four different catheters. Can J Anaesth 38:648, 1991
22. Barash PG, Nardi D, Hammond G et al: Catheter-induced pulmonary artery perforation: mechanisms, management, and modifications. J Thor Cardiovasc Surg 82:5, 1981
23. Goldhaber S: Pulmonary embolism thrombolysis: a clarion call for International Collaboration. JACC 2:246, 1992
24. Woods M, Scott RN, Harken AH: Practical considerations for the use of a pulmonary artery thermistor catheter. Surgery 79:469, 1976
25. Hobelmann CF Jr, Smith DE, Vergilio RW et al: Left atrial and pulmonary artery wedge pressure difference with positive end-expiratory pressure. Surg Forum 25:232, 1974
26. Jardin F, Farcot JC, Boisante L et al: Influence of positive end-expiratory pressure on left ventricular performance. New Engl J Med 304:387, 1981
27. Kane PB, Askanazi J, Neville JF Jr et al: Artifacts in the measurement of pulmonary artery wedge pressure. Crit Care Med 6:36, 1978
28. Manjuran RS, Agarwal JB, Roy SB: Relationship of pulmonary artery diastolic and pulmonary artery wedge pressures in mitral stenosis. Am Heart J 89: 207, 1975
29. Moser KM, Spragg RG: Use of the balloon-tipped pulmonary artery catheter in pulmonary disease. Ann Int Med 98:53, 1983
30. Marmana RB, Hiro S, Levitsky S et al: Inaccuracy of pulmonary capillary wedge pressure when compared to left atrial pressure in the early post surgical period. J Thorac Cardiovasc Surg 84:420, 1982
31. Rotman M, Chen JTT, Senngen RP et al: Pulmonary arterial diastolic pressure in acute myocardial infarction. Am J Card 33:362, 1974
32. Robotham JL, Rabson J, Permutt S et al: Left ventricular hemodynamics during respiration. J Appl Physiol 47:1295, 1979

33. Robotham JL, Lixfeld W, Holland L et al: The effects of positive end-expiratory pressure on right and left ventricular performance. Am Rev Respir Dis 121:677, 1980

34. Pichard AD, Diaz R, Marchant E et al: Large V waves in the pulmonary capillary wedge pressure tracing without mitral regurgitation: the influence of the pressure/volume relationship on the V wave size. Clin Cardiol 6:534, 1983

35. Boyd KD, Thomas SJ, Gold J et al: A prospective study of complications of pulmonary artery catheterizations in 500 consecutive patients. Chest 84:245, 1983

36. Bouchard RJ, Gault JH, Ross J Jr: Evaluation of pulmonary arterial end-diastolic pressure as an estimate of left ventricular end-diastolic pressure in patients with normal and abnormal left ventricular performance. Circulation 44:1072, 1971

37. Braunwald E: On the difference between the heart's output and its contractile state. Circulation 43:171, 1971

38. Shah DM, Browner BD, Dutton RE et al: Cardiac output and pulmonary wedge pressure. Arch Surg 112:1161, 1977

39. Sidulka A, Hakim TS: Wedge pressure in large vs. small pulmonary arteries to detect pulmonary venoconstriction. J Appl Physiol 59:1329, 1985

40. Shapiro HM, Smith G, Murray JA et al: Errors in sampling pulmonary arterial blood with a Swan-Ganz catheter. Anesthesiology 40:291, 1974

41. Morris AH, Chapman RH: Wedge pressure confirmation by aspiration of pulmonary capillary blood. Crit Care Med 13:756, 1985

42. Shasby DM, Dauber IM, Pfister S et al: Swan-Ganz catheter location and left atrial pressure determine the accuracy of the wedge pressure when positive end-expiratory pressure is used. Chest 80:666, 1981

43. Teboul JL, Besbes M, Andrivet P et al: A bedside index assessing the reliability of pulmonary artery occlusion pressure measurements ventilation with positive end expiratory pressure. J Crit Care 7:22, 1992

44. Weisman IM, Rinaldo JE, Rogers RM: Positive end expiratory pressures in adult respiratory failure. N Engl J Med 307:1381, 1982

45. Eisenberg PR, Jaffe AS, Schuster DP: Clinical evaluation compared to pulmonary artery catheterization in the hemodynamic assessment of critically ill patients. Crit Care Med 12:549, 1984

46. Dizon CT, Barash PG: The value of monitoring pulmonary artery pressure in clinical practice. Conn Med 41:622, 1977

47. Forrester JS, Diamond G, McHugh TJ et al: Filling pressures in the right and left sides of the heart in acute myocardial infarction. N Engl J Med 285:190, 1971

48. Field J, Shiroff RA, Zelis RF et al: Limitations in the use of the pulmonary capillary wedge pressure. Chest 70:451, 1976

49. Levine HJ, Gaasch WH: Diastolic compliance of the left ventricle. I: Causes of a noncompliant ventricle. Mod Conc Cardiovasc Dis 42:95, 1978

50. Lopez-Sendon J: Right ventricular infarction as a risk factor for ventricular fibrillation during pulmonary artery catheterization using Swan Ganz catheters. Heart J 119:207–290, 1990

51. Hines R, Rafferty T: Right ventricle: toy or tool? in press.

52. Spinale FG, Smith AC, Carabello BA et al: Right ventricular function computed by the thermodilution and ventriculography. J Thorac Cardiovasc Surg 99:141, 1990

53. Hines R, Barash PG: Intraoperative right ventricular dysfunction detected with a right ventricular ejection fraction catheter. J Clin Monitor 2:206, 1986

54. Armengol J, Man GC, Balsys AJ et al: Effects of the respiratory cycle on cardiac output measurements: reproducibility of data enhanced by timing the thermodilution injections in dogs. Crit Care Med 9:852, 1981

55. Bromberger-Barnea B: Mechanical effects of inspiration on heart functions: a review. Fed Proc 40:2172, 1981

55a. Kay H, Afshari M, Barash P et al: Measurement of ejection fraction by thermal dilution techniques. J Surg Rev 34:337, 1983

56. Cengiz M, Crapo RO, Gardner RM: The effect of ventilation on the accuracy of pulmonary artery and wedge pressure measurements. Crit Care Med 11:502, 1983

57. Andreen M: Computerized measurement of cardiac output by thermodilution: methodological aspects. Acta Anaesthesiol Scand 18:297, 1974

58. Kohanna FH, Cunningham JN, Jr, Catinella FP et al: Cardiac output determination after cardiac operation. J Thorac Cardiovasc Surg 82:904, 1981

59. Kressin N, Laravuso RB: Hemodynamic measurements in patients for coronary artery surgery: cath lab vs. operating room. Anesthesiology 59:A6, 1983

60. Shoemaker WC: The efficacy of central venous and pulmonary artery catheters and therapy based upon them in reducing mortality and morbidity. Arch Surg 125:1332, 1990

61. Shaver JA: Hemodynamic monitoring in the critically ill. N Engl J Med 308:277, 1983

62. Shrader LL, McMillen MA, Watson CB, MacArthur JD: Is routine preoperative hemodynamic evaluation of nonagenarians necessary? J Am Geriatr Soc 39:1–5, 1991

63. Starr N, Estafanous FG, Goormastic M, Williams

GW: Operating room monitoring in adult open heart surgery: results of a national survey. Anesthesiology 57:A157, 1982

64. Del Guercio LRM, Cohn JD: Monitoring operative risk in the elderly. JAMA 243:1350, 1980
65. Iberti TJ, Fisher CJ: A prospective study on the use of the pulmonary artery catheter in a medical intensive care unit: its effect on diagnosis and therapy. Crit Care Med 11:238, 1983
66. Waller JL, Zaiden JR, Kaplan JA, Bozeman R: Hemodynamic responses to vascular cannulations before coronary bypass surgery. Anesth Analg 59:563, 1980
67. Fegler G: Measurement of cardiac output in anaesthetized animals by a thermodilution method. Q J Exp Physiol 53:153, 1954
68. Forrester JS, Ganz W, Diamond G et al: Thermodilution cardiac output determination with a single flow-directed catheter. Am Heart J 83:306, 1972
69. Ganz W, Swan HJC: Measurement of blood flow by thermodilution. Am J Cardiol 29:241, 1972
70. Bing R, Heimbecker R, Falholt W: An estimation of the residual volume of blood in the right ventricle and diseased hearts in vivo. Am Heart J 42:483, 1951
71. Bilfinger TV, Lin CY, Anagnostopoulos CE: In vitro determination of accuracy of cardiac output measurements by thermal dilution. J Surg Res 33:409, 1983
72. Branthwaite MA, Bradley RD: Measurement of cardiac output by thermal dilution in man. J Appl Physiol 24:434, 1968
73. Fischer AP, Benis AM, Jurado RA et al: Analysis of errors in measurement of cardiac output by simultaneous dye and thermal dilution in cardiothoracic surgical patients. Cardiovasc Res 12:190, 1978
74. Hendriks FF, Schipperheyn JJ, Quanjer PH: Thermal dilution measurement of cardiac output in dogs using an analog computer. Basic Res Cardiol 73:459, 1978
75. Hoel BL: Some aspects of the clinical use of thermodilution in measuring cardiac output. Scand J Clin Lab Invest 38:383, 1978
76. Jansen JR, Schreuder JJ, Bogaard JM et al: Thermodilution techniques for measurement of cardiac output during artificial ventilation. J Appl Physiol 51:584, 1981
77. Merjavy JP, Hahn JW, Barner HB: Comparison of thermodilution cardiac output and electromagnetic flowmeter. Surg Forum 25:145, 1974
78. Nelson LD, Houtchens BA: Automatic vs manual injections for thermodilution cardiac output determinations. Crit Care Med 10:190, 1982
79. Olsson SB, Wassen R, Varnauskas E et al: A simple analogue computer for cardiac output determination by thermodilution. Cardiovasc Res 6:303, 1972
80. Olsson B, Pool J, Vandermoten P et al: Validity and reproducibility of determination of cardiac output by thermodilution in man. Cardiology 55:136, 1970
81. Sottile FD, Durbin CG, Hoyt JW et al: Evaluation of pulmonary artery oximetry as a predictor of cardiac output. Anesthesiology 57:A127, 1982
82. Maruschak GF, Potter AM, Schauble JF et al: Overestimation of pediatric cardiac output by thermal indicator loss. Circulation 65:380, 1982
83. Mattea EJ, Paruta AN, Worthen LR: Sterility of prefilled syringes for thermal dilution cardiac output measurements. [Letter]. Am J Hosp Pharm 36:1156, 1979
84. Nelson LD, Anderson HB: Patient selection for iced versus room temperature injectate for thermodilution cardiac output determinations. Crit Care Med 13:182, 1985
85. Nishikawa T, Dohi S: Slowing of heart rate during cardiac output measurement by thermodilution. Anesthesiology 57:538, 1982
86. Runciman WB, Ilsley AH, Roberts JG: Thermodilution cardiac output—a systematic error. Anaesth Int Care 9:135, 1981
87. Levine BA, Strinek KR: Cardiac output determination by thermodilution technique: the method of choice in low flow states. Proc Soc Exp Biol Med 167:279, 1981
88. Ross RM: Beside calibration check of pulmonary artery catheters. [Letter]. Chest 79:717, 1981
89. Runciman WB, Ilsley AH, Roberts JG: An evaluation of thermodilution cardiac output measurement using the Swan-Ganz catheter. Anaesth Int Care 9:208, 1981
90. Dizon CT, Gezari WA, Barash PG et al: Hand held thermodilution cardiac output injector. Crit Care Med 5:10, 1977
91. Beaupre PN, Cahalan MK, Kremer PF et al: Does pulmonary artery occlusion pressure adequately reflect left ventricular filling during anesthesia and surgery? Anesthesiology 59:A3, 1983
92. Carlon GC, Howland WS, Kahn RC et al: Unusual complications during pulmonary artery catheterization. Crit Care Med 6:364, 1978
93. Mermel LA, McCormick RD, Springman SR, Maki DG: The pathogenis and epidemiology of catheter related infection with pulmonary artery swan ganz catheters: a prospective study utilizing molecular subtyping. Am J Med 19:3B-197S, 1991
94. Michel L, McMichan JC, Bachy JL: Microbial colonization of indwelling central venous catheters: statistical evaluation of potential contaminating factors. Am J Surg 137:745, 1979
95. Michel L, Marsh HM, McMichan JC et al: Infection of pulmonary artery catheters in critically ill patients. JAMA 245:1032, 1981

96. Todd MM: Atrial fibrillation induced by the right atrial injection of cold fluids during thermodilution cardiac output determination: a case report. Anesthesiology 59:253, 1983

97. Esses G, Feinberg S, Panos T: Swan Ganz elbow. [Letter]. Can Med Assoc J 126:1276, 1982

98. Armstrong RF, St. Andrew D, Cohen SL et al: Continuous monitoring of mixed venous oxygen tension (P$_v$O$_2$) in cardiorespiratory disorders. Lancet 1:632, 1978

99. Armstrong RF, Moxham J, Cohen SL, Vallis CJ: Intravascular mixed venous oxygen tension monitoring. Br J Anaesth 53:89, 1981

100. Kasnitz P, Druger GL, Yorra F et al: Mixed venous oxygen tension and hyperlactatemia. JAMA 236:570, 1976

101. Krauss XH, Verdouw PD, Hugenholtz PG, Nauta J: On-line monitoring of mixed venous oxygen saturation after cardiothoracic surgery. Thorax 30:636, 1975

102. Muir AL, Kirby BJ, King AJ et al: Mixed venous oxygen saturation in relation to cardiac output in myocardial infarction. Br Med J 4:276, 1970

103. Prakash O, Meij SH, van der Borden SG et al: Cardiovascular monitoring with special emphasis on mixed venous oxygen measurements. Acta Anaesthesiol Belg 29:253, 1978

104. Baele PL, McMichan JC, Marsh HM et al: Continuous monitoring of mixed venous oxygen saturation in critically ill patients. Anesth Analg 61:513, 1981

105. Jamieson WRE, Turnbull KW, Larrieu AJ et al: Continuous monitoring of mixed venous oxygen saturation in cardiac surgery. Can J Surg 25:538, 1982

106. Martin WE, Cheung PW, Johnson CC et al: Continuous monitoring of mixed venous oxygen saturation in man. Anesth Analg 52:784, 1973

107. Sperinde JM, Senelly KM: The oximetric opticath system: theory and development. p. 59. In Fahey PJ (ed): Continuous Measurement of Oxygen Saturation in the High Risk Patient: Theory and Practice in Monitoring Mixed Venous Oxygen Saturation. Vol 2. Beach International, San Diego, 1985

108. Waller JL, Kaplan JA, Bauman DI et al: Clinical evaluation of a new fiberoptic catheter oximeter during cardiac surgery. Anesthesiology 61:676, 1982

109. Hecker B, Brown D, Wilson D: A comparison of the pulmonary artery mixed venous oxygen saturation catheters during the changing conditions of cardiac seizure. J Cardiothorac Anesth 3:269, 1989

110. Gettinger A, Glass D: In vivo comparison of two mixed venous oximetrics. Anesthesiology 66:373, 1987

111. Nelson LD: Continuous venous oximetry in surgical patients. Ann Surg 302:329, 1986

112. Norfleet ER, Watson CB: Continuous mixed venous oxygen saturation measurements: a significant advance in hemodynamic monitoring. Clin Monit 1:245, 1985

113. Norwood SH, Nelson LD: Continuous monitoring of mixed venous oxygen saturation in pediatric cardiac surgery. Am Surg 52:114, 1986

114. Orlando R: Continuous mixed venous oximetry in critically ill patients. Arch Surg 121:470, 1986

115. Miller HC, Brown DJ, Miller GAH: Comparison of formulae used to estimate oxygen saturation of mixed venous blood from caval samples. Br Heart J 36:446, 1974

116. Scheinman MM, Brown MA, Rapaport E: Critical assessment of use of central venous oxygen saturation as a mirror of mixed venous oxygen in severely ill cardiac patients. Circulation 40:165, 1989

117. Meister SG, Helfant RH: Rapid bedside differentiation of ruptured interventricular septum from acute mitral insufficiency. N Engl J Med 287:1024, 1972

118. Todres ID, Crone RK, Rogers MC, Shannon DC: San-Ganz catheterization in the critically ill newborn. Crit Care Med 7:330, 1979

119. Mihm F, Feeley TW, Rosenthal M et al: The lack of effect of variable blood withdrawal rates on the measurement of mixed venous oxygen saturation. Chest 78:452, 1980

120. Chatterjee K, Swan HJC, Ganz W et al: Use of a balloon-tipped flotation electrode catheter for cardiac monitoring. Am J Cardiol 35:56, 1975

121. Roth JV: Temporary transmyocardial pacing using epicardial pacing wires and pacing pulmonary artery catheters. J Cardiothorac Vasc Anesth 6:663, 1982

122. Roth JV, Zaidman JR: Use of the pacing pulmonary arterial catheter to detect endocardial electrical activity during hypothermic cardioplegic arrest. J Clin Monit 4:178, 1988

123. Seltzer JL, Mora CT, McNulty SE: Evaluation of ventricular pacing with a new design in pulmonary artery catheter. p. 145. Society of Cardiovascular Anesthesiologists Annual Meeting, 1986

124. Lumb P: Atrioventricular sequential pacing with transluminal atrial and ventricular pacing probes inserted via a pulmonary artery catheter: a preliminary comparison with epicardial wires. J Clin Anesth 1:292, 1989

125. Trankina MF, White R: Perioperative cardiac pacing using an atrioventricular pacing pulmonary artery catheter. J Cardiothorac Anesth 3:154, 1989

126. Zaidan JR: Experience with the pacing pulmonary artery catheter. Anesthesiology 3:S118, 1980

127. Mukherjee R, Spinale FG, VonRecum AF et al: In vitro validation of right ventricular thermodilution

ejection fraction system. Ann Biomed Eng 19:165, 1991

128. Rafferty TD: Transesophageal two dimensional echocardiography in the critically ill: is the Swan-Ganz catheter redundant? Yale J Biol Med 64:375, 1990

129. Dorman BH, Pinale FG, Kratz JM et al: Use of combined right ventricular ejection fraction oximetry catheter system for coronary bypass surgery. Chest 20:1650, 1992

130. Spinale FG, Zellner JL, Mukherjee R et al: Placement consideration for measuring thermodilution right ventricular ejection fractions. Crit Care Med 19:417, 1991

131. Yelderman ML: Continuous measurement of cardiac output with the use of stochastic system identification techniques. J Clin Monit 6:322, 1990

132. Yelderman ML, Ramsey MA, Quinn MD et al: Continuous thermodilution cardiac output measurements in intensive care unit patients. J Cardiothorac Vasc Anesth 6:270, 1992

133. Ham TH, Shen SC, Fleming EM, Castle WB: Studies in destruction of red blood cells. IV. Thermal injury. Blood 3:373, 1948

134. Henriques FC: Studies of thermal injury. V. The predictability and the significance of thermally induced rate processes leading to irreversible epidermal injury. Arch Pathol 43:489, 1947

135. Henriques FC, Moritz AR: Studies of thermal injury. I. The conduction of heat to and through skin and the temperatures attained therein. A theoretical and an experimental investigation. Arch Pathol 43:531, 1947

136. Gillis MF, Smith LG, Bingham DB: Final technical progress report on studies on the effects of additional endogenous heat relating to the artificial heart. National Heart and Lung Institute publication number PH 43-66-1130-5, 1973

137. Yelderman ML, Quinn MD, McKown RC: Thermal safety of a filamented pulmonary artery catheter. J Clin Monit 1994

138. Yelderman ML, Quinn MD, McKown RC: Continuous thermodilution cardiac output measurements in sheep. J Thorac Cardiovasc Surg 1994

139. Miyasaka K, Takata M, Miyasaka K: Flow velocity profile of the pulmonary artery measured by continuous cardiac output monitoring catheter. Can J Anaesth 40:183, 1993

140. Segal J, Pearl RG, Ford AJ Jr et al: Instantaneous and continuous cardiac output obtained with a Doppler pulmonary artery catheter. J Am Coll Cardiol 13:1382, 1989

141. Segal J, Gaudiani V, Nishimura T: Continuous determination of cardiac output using a flow directed Doppler pulmonary artery catheter. J Cardiothorac Vasc Anesth 5:309, 1991

142. Iberti TJ, Silverstein JH: Continuous cardiac output measurements in critically ill patients. J Cardiothorac Vasc Anesth 6:267, 1992

143. Forrester JS, Swan HJC: Acute myocardial infarction: a physiologic basis for therapy. Crit Care Med 2:283, 1974

144. Forrester JS, Diamond G, Chatterjee K et al: Medical therapy of acute myocardial infarction by application of hemodynamic subsets I. N Engl J Med 1356:62, 1976

145. Forrester JS, Diamond GA, Swan HJC: Bedside diagnosis of latent cardiac complications in acutely ill patients. JAMA 222:59, 1972

146. Shoemaker WC, Appel PL, Kram HL: Prospective trial of supranormal values of survivors as therapeutic goals in high risk patients. Chest 94:1176, 1988

147. Russell JA, Ronco JJ, Lockat D et al: Oxygen delivery and consumption and ventricular preload are greater in survivors of the adult respiratory distress syndrome. Am Rev Respir Dis 141:659, 1990

148. Conners AF, Jr, McCaffree DR, Gray BA: Evaluation of right-heart catheterization in the critically ill patient without acute myocardial infarction. N Engl J Med 308:263, 1983

149. Rice CL, Hobelman CF, John DA et al: Central venous pressure or pulmonary capillary wedge pressure as the determinant of fluid replacement in aortic surgery. Surgery 84:437, 1978

150. Waller JL, Johnson SP, Kaplan JA: Usefulness of pulmonary artery catheters during aortocoronary bypass surgery. Anesth Analg 61:221, 1982

151. American College of Physicians/American College of Cardiology/American Heart Association Task Force on Clinical Privileges in Cardiology: Clinical competence in hemodynamic monitoring. J Am Coll Cardiol 15:1460, 1990

152. Technology Subcommittee of the Working Group on Critical Care, Ontario Ministry of Health: Hemodynamic monitoring: a technology assessment. Can Med Assoc J 145:114, 1991

153. European Society of Intensive Care Medicine. Expert Panel: The use of the pulmonary artery catheter. Intens Care Med 17:I-VIII, 1991

154. Practice Guidelines for Pulmonary Artery Catheterization: A Report by the American Society of Anesthesiologists Task Force on Pulmonary Artery Catheterization. Anesthesiology 78:380, 1993

155. Berkowitz RL, Rafferty TD: Invasive hemodynamic monitoring in critically ill pregnant patients: role of Swan-Ganz catheterization. Am J Obstet Gynecol 137:127, 1980

156. Yang SC, P VK: Role of preoperative hemodynamic monitoring in intraoperative fluid management. Am Surg 52:536, 1986

157. Berlauk JF, Abrams JH, Gilmour IJ et al: Preoperative optimization of cardiovascular hemodynamics improves outcome in peripheral vascular surgery: a prospective, randomized clinical trial. Ann Surg 214, 289, 1991

158. Davies MJ, Cronin KD, and Domaingue CM: Pulmonary artery catheterization: an assessment of risks and benefits in 220 surgical patients. Anaesth Intens Care 10:9, 1982

159. Katz RW, Pollack MM, Weibley RE: Pulmonary artery catherization in pediatric intensive care. Adv Pediatr 30:169, 1983

160. Kohanna FH, Cunningham JN Jr: Monitoring of cardiac output by thermodilation after open-heart surgery. J Thorac Cardiovasc Surg 73:451, 1977

161. Isaacson IJ, Lowden JD, Berry AJ et al: The value of pulmonary artery and central venous monitoring in patients undergoing abdominal aortic reconstructive surgery: a comparative study of two selected, randomized groups. J Vasc Surg 12:754, 1990

162. Joyce WP, Provan JL, Ameili FM et al: The role of central hemodynamic monitoring in abdominal aortic surgery: a prospective randomized study. Eur J Vasc Surg 4:633, 1990

163. Katz JD, Cronau LH, Barash PG et al: Pulmonary artery flow-guided catheters in the perioperative period. JAMA 237:2832, 1977

164. Hjertberg R, Belfrage P, Hagnevick K: Hemodynamic measurements with Swan-Ganz catheter in women with severe proteinuric gestational hypertension (preeclampsia). Acta Obstetr Gynecol Scand 70:193, 1991

165. Clark ST, Cotton DB: Clinical indications for pulonary artery catheterization in the patient with severe preeclampsia. Am J Obstet Gynecol 158:453, 1988

166. Cohn JD, Engler PE, Timpawat C et al: Physiologic profiles in circulatory support and management of the critically ill. J.A.C.E.P., 6:479, 1977

167. Benedetti TJ, Cotton DB, Read JC et al: Hemodynamic observations in severe pre-eclampsia with a flow-directed pulmonary artery catheter. Am J Obstet Gynecol 136:465, 1980

168. Babu SC, Sharma PVP, Raciti A, Mayr CH, et al: Monitor-guided responses. Arch Surg 115:1384, 1980

169. Aikawa N, Martyn JA, Burke JF: Pulmonary artery catheterization and thermodilution cardiac output determination in the management of critically burned patients. Am J Surg 136:811, 1978

170. Schrader LL, McMillen MA, Watson CB, MacArthur JD: Is routine preoperative hemodynamic evaluation of nonagenarians necessary? J Am Geriatr Soc 39:1, 1991

171. Schultz RJ, Whitfield GF, Lamura JJ et al: Physiologic monitoring in patients with fractures of the hip. J Trauma 25:309, 1985

172. Scalea TM, Simon H, Duncan AO et al: Geriatric blunt multiple trauma: improved survival with early invasive monitoring. J Trauma 30:129, 1990

173. Goldman L, Caldera DL, Nussbaum SR et al: Multifactorial index of cardiac risk in noncardiac surgical procedures. N Engl J Med 297:845, 1977

174. Larsen SF, Ilesen KH, Jacobsen et al: Prediction of cardiac risk in noncardiac surgery. Eur Heart J 8: 179, 1987

175. Rao TLK, El-Etr AA: Myocardial reinfarction following anesthesia in patients with recent infarction. Anesth Analg 60:271, 1981

176. Rao TL, Jacobs KH, El Etr AA: Reinfarction following anesthesia in patients with myocardial infarction. Anesthesiology 59:499, 1983.

177. Hesdorffer CS, Milne JF, Meyers AM et al: The value of Swan-Ganz catherization and volume loading in preventing renal failure in patients undergoing abdominal aneurysmectomy. Clin Nephrol 28:272, 1987

178. Quinn K, Quebbeman EJ: Pulmonary artery pressure monitoring in the surgical intensive care unit. Arch Surg 116:872, 1981

179. Quintin L, Whalley DG, Wynands JE, Morin JE: The effects of vascular catheterizations upon heart rate and blood pressure before aorto-coronary bypass surgery. Can Anaesth Soc J 28:244, 1981

180. Bedford RF, Marshall WK, Butler A et al: Cardiac catheters for diagnosis and treatment of venous air embolism. J Neurosurg 55:610, 1981

181. Noel TA: Air embolism removal from both pulmonary artery and right atrium during sitting craniotomy using a new catheter: report of a case. Anesthesiology 70:709, 1989

182. Spapen HD, Umbrain V, Brakemans P, Hughens L: Use of the Swan-Ganz catheter in amniotic fluid embolism. [Letter]. Intens Care Med 14:678, 1988

183. Orr JW Jr, Shinglefon HM, Soony ST et al: Hemodynamic parameters following pelvic exenteration. Am J Obstet Gynecol 146:882, 1983

184. Neches WH, Park SC, Lenox CC et al: Pulmonary artery wedge pressure in congenital heart disease. Cathet Cardiovas Diagn 3:11, 1977

185. Gore JM, Sloan K: Use of continuous monitoring of mixed venous saturation in the coronary care unit. Crit Care Med 86:757, 1984

186. Gore J, Goldenberg R, Spodick D et al: A community wide assessment of the use of pulmonary artery catheters in patients with acute myocardial infarction. Chest 92:721, 1987

187. Civetta JM, Gabel JC: Flow directed-pulmonary artery catheterization in surgical patients: indications

and modifications of technic. Ann Surg 176:753, 1972

188. Whittemore AD, Clowes AD, Hechtman HB et al: Aortic aneurysm repair: reduced operative mortality associated with maintenance of optimal cardiac performance. Ann Surg 192:414, 1980

189. Tuchschmidt J, Fried J, Astiz M et al: Elevation of cardiac output and oxygen delivery improves outcome in septic shock. Chest 102:216, 1992

190. Yu M, Levy MM, Smith P et al: Effect of maximizing oxygen delivery on morbidity and mortality rates in critically ill patients: a prospective, randomized controlled study. Crit Care Med 21:830, 1993

191. Tuman KJ, McCarthy RJ, Spless BD et al: Effect of pulmonary artery catherization on outcome in patients undergoing coronary artery surgery. Anesthesiology 70:199, 1989

192. Moore CH, Lombardo TR, Allums JA et al: Left main coronary artery stenosis: hemodynamic monitoring to reduce mortality. Ann Thorac Surg 26:445, 1978

193. Pearson KS, Gomez MN, Moyers JR et al: A cost/benefit analysis of randomized invasive monitoring for patients undergoing cardiac surgery. Anesth Analg 69:336, 1989

194. Seldinger SI: Catheter replacement of the needle in percutaneous arteriography. Acta Radiol 39:368, 1953

195. Barash PG, Dizon CT: An introducer for intraoperative percutaneous insertion of a Swan-Ganz catheter. Anesth Analg 56:444, 1977

196. Brahos GH: Central venous catheterization via the supraclavicular approach. J Trauma 17:872, 1977

197. Dronen S, Thompson B, Nowak R et al: Subclavian vein catheterization during cardiopulmonary resuscitation: a prospective comparison of the supraclavicular and infraclavicular percutaneous approaches. JAMA 247:3227, 1982

198. Pego RF, Luria MH: Left subclavian vein puncture for insertion of Swan-Ganz catheters. Heart and Lung 8:507, 1979

199. DeLange SS, Boscoe MJ, Stanley TH: Percutaneous pulmonary artery catheterization via the arm before anaesthesia: success rate, frequency of complications and arterial pressure and heart rate. Br J Anesth 53:1167, 1981

200. Defalque RJ: Percutaneous catheterization of the internal jugular vein. Anesth Analg 53:116, 1974

201. Ellison N, Jobes DR, Schwartz AJ et al: Cannulation of the internal jugular vein: a cautionary note. Anesthesiology 55:337, 1981

202. Ellison N, Schwartz AJ, Jobes DR et al: Avoidance of carotid artery puncture sequelae during internal jugular cannulation. Anesth Analg 61:181, 1982

203. Ellison N, Jobes DR, Schwartz AJ et al: Cannulation

of the internal jugular vein: another cautionary note. Anesthesiology 57:345, 1982

204. Ellison N, Jobes DR, Schwartz AJ: Internal jugular catheterization. Anaesthesia 37:605, 1982

205. Elinger JH, Bedford RF, Buschi AJ: Do pulmonary artery catheters cause internal jugular vein thrombosis? Anesthesiology 57:A118, 1982

206. Schwartz AJ, Jobes DR, Greenhow DE et al: Carotid artery puncture with internal jugular cannulation. Anesthesiology 51:S160, 1979

207. Conners AF, Castele RJ, Farhat NZ, Tomashefski JF: Complications of right heart catheterization. Chest 88:567, 1985

208. McNabb TG, Green LH, Parker FL: A potentially serious complication with Swan-Ganz catheter placement by the percutaneous internal jugular route. Br J Anaesth 47:895, 1975

209. Birrer RB, Plotz CM: Bernard-Horner syndrome associated with Swan-Ganz catheter. NY State J Med 81:362, 1981

210. Kronberg GM, Quan SF, Schlobohm RM et al: Anatomic locations of the tips of pulmonary-artery catheters in supine patients. Anesthesiology 51:467, 1979

211. Downs JB: A technique for direct measurement of intrapleural pressure. Crit Care Med 4:207, 1976

212. Berryhill RE, Benumof JL, Rauscher A: Pulmonary vascular pressure reading at the end of exhalation. Anesthesiology 49:365, 1978

213. Downs JB, Douglas ME: Assessment of cardiac filling pressure during continuous positive-pressure ventilation. Crit Care Med 8:285, 1980

214. Maran AG: Variables in pulmonary capillary wedge pressure: variation with intrathoracic pressure, graphic and digital recorders. Crit Care Med 8:102, 1980

215. Geer RT: Interpretation of pulmonary-artery wedge pressure when PEEP is used. Anesthesiology 46:383, 1977

216. Benumof JL, Saidman LJ, Arkin DB et al: Where pulmonary arterial catheters go: intrathoracic distribution. Anesthesiology 46:336, 1977

217. Kane PB, Mon RL, Askanazi J et al: Proceedings: the effects of PEEP and left atrial pressure on the correlation between pulmonary artery wedge pressure and left atrial pressure. Br J Anaesth 48:272, 1976

218. Roy R: Pulmonary wedge catheterization during positive end-expiratory pressure ventilation in the dog. Anesthesiology 46:385, 1977

219. Teeple E, Ghia JN: An elevated pulmonary wedge pressure resulting from an upper respiratory obstruction in an obese patient. Anesthesiology 59:66, 1983

220. Vaitkus L: Discontinuing PEEP to measure pulmo-

nary capillary wedge pressures. N Engl J Med 308: 776, 1983

221. Kaplan JA, Wells PH: Early diagnosis of myocardial ischemia using the pulmonary arterial catheter. Anesth analg 60:789, 1981

222. Carlon GC, Kahn RC, Bertoni G et al: Unexpected giant "V" waves during pulmonary artery catheterization. Intens Care Med 5:55, 1979

223. Fuchs RM, Heuser RR, Yin FCP, Brinker JA: Limitations of pulmonary wedge V waves in diagnosing mitral regurgitation. Am J Cardiol 49:849, 1982

224. Cohn JD, Engler PE, Del Guercio LRM: The automated physiologic profile. Crit Care Med 3:51, 1975

225. Boutros AR, Lee C: Value of continuous monitoring of mixed venous blood oxygen saturation in the management of critically ill patient. Crit Care Med 14:130, 1986

226. Sanchez R, WEE M: Perioperative myocardial ischemia: early diagnosis using the pulmonary artery catheter. Cardiothorac Vasc Anesth 5:604, 1991

227. VanRiper DF, Horrow JC, Kutalek SP et al: Mixed venous oximetry during automatic implantable cardioverter defibrillator placement. J Cardiothorac Anesth 4:453, 1990

228. Van Daele ME, Sutherland GR, Mitchell MM et al: Do changes in pulmonary capillary wedge pressure adequately reflect myocardial ischemia during anesthesia? A correlative preoperative hemodynamic, electrocardiographic and transesophageal echocardiographic study. Circulation 81:865, 1990

229. Braunwald E, Ross J Jr, Sonnenblick EH: Mechanisms of Contraction in the Normal and Failing Heart. 2nd Ed. p. 130. Little, Brown, Boston, 1976

230. Scheinman M, Evans GT, Weiss A et al: Relationship between pulmonary artery end-diastolic pressure and left ventricular filling pressure in patients in shock. Circulation 47:317, 1973

231. Sonnenblick EH, Strobeck JE: Current concepts in cardiology: derived indexes of ventricular and myocardial function. N Engl J Med 296:978, 1977

232. Ross J Jr, Braunwald E: The study of left ventricular function in man by increasing resistance to ventricular ejection with angiotensin. Circ 29:739, 1964

233. Packman MI, Rackow EC: Optimal left heart filling pressure during fluid resuscitation of patients with hypovolemic and septic shock. Crit Care Med 11:165, 1983

234. Barash PG: Circulatory strategies in acute respiratory failure. Curr Rev Resp Ther 21:163, 1981

235. Covelli HD, Nessan VJ, Tuttle WK, III: Oxygen derived variables in acute respiratory failure. Crit Care Med 11:646, 1983

236. Alschule M: A new branch of medicine: complications of vascular catheter. Chest 89:242, 1986

237. Matta B, Willatis S: A possible complication with a sheath introducer. Crit Care Med 47:534, 1992

238. Brown CQ: Inadvertent prolonged cannulation of the carotid artery. Anesth Analg 61:150, 1982

239. Shah KB, Rao TLK, Laughlin S, El-Etr AA: A review of pulmonary artery catheterization in 6,245 patients. Anesthesiology 61:271, 1984

240. Landow L: Another problem in differentiating between carotid artery and jugular vein cannulation. Anesthesiology 76:1061, 1992.

241. Krespi YP, Komisar A, Lucente FE: Complications of internal jugular vein catheterization. Arch Otolarynogol 107:310, 1981

242. Dodson T, Quindlen E, Crowell R et al: Vertebral arteriovenous fistulas following insertion of central monitoring catheters. Surgery 87:343, 1980

243. Kenny GN: Effect of haemothorax on pulmonary artery wedge pressure: a case report. Br J Anaesth 51:165, 1979

244. Conahan TJ: Air embolization during percutaneous Swan-Ganz catheter placement. Anesthesiology 50:360, 1979

245. Kopman EA: Preventing air embolism while inserting central catheters. Anesthesiology 57:349, 1982

246. Peters JL, Armstrong, R: Air embolism occurring as a complication of central venous catheterization. Ann Surg 187:375, 1978

247. Doblar DD, Hinkle JC, Fay ML et al: Air embolism associated with pulmonary artery catheter introducer kit. Anesthesiology 56:307, 1982

248. Moorthy SS, Tisinai KA, Speiser BS et al: Cerebral air embolism during removal of a pulmonary artery catheter. Crit Care Med 19:981, 1991

249. Dye LE, Segall PH, Russell RO Jr et al: Deep venous thrombosis of the upper extremity associated with use of the Swan-Ganz catheter. Chest 73:673, 1978

250. Cohen S, Whalen F: Another potential complication of a pulmonary artery catheter insertion. Anesthesiology 75:714, 1991

251. Bradway WR, Gordon R, Ciudice J et al: Thrombosis after pulmonary-artery catheterization via the internal jugular vein. N Engl J Med 306:1486, 1982

252. Lederman R: Peripheral nerve injury after coronary artery bypass surgery. Neurosci Today Cleve Clin Found 4:1, 1981

253. Vander Salm TJ, Cereda JM, Cutler BS: Brachial plexus injury following median sternotomy. Part II. J Thorac Cardiovasc Surg 83:914, 1982

254. Stock MC, Downs JB: Transient phrenic nerve blockade during internal jugular vein cannulation using the anterolateral approach. Anesthesiology 57:230, 1982

255. Swan HJ, Ganz W: Complications with flow-directed balloon-tipped catheters. Ann Intern Med 91:494, 1979

256. Sprung CL, Jacobs LJ, Caralis PV et al: Ventricular arrhythmias during Swan-Ganz catheterization of the critically ill. Chest 79:413, 1981

257. Sprung CL, Pozen RG, Rozanski JJ et al: Advanced ventricular arrhythmias during bedside pulmonary artery catheterization. Am J Med 72:203, 1982

258. Cairns JA, Holder D: Letter: Ventricular fibrillation due to passage of a Swan-Ganz catheter. Am J Cardiol 35:589, 1975

259. Damen J: Ventricular arrhythmias during insertion and removal of pulmonary artery catheters. Chest 88:190, 1985

260. Iberti TJ, Benjamin E, Gruppi L, Rask JM: Ventricular arrhythmias during pulmonary artery catheterization in the intensive care unit: prospective study. Am J Med 78:451, 1985

261. Luck JC, Engel TR: Transient right bundle branch block with Swan-Ganz catheterization. Am Heart J 92:263, 1970

262. Castellanos A, Ramirez AV, Mayorga-Cortes A et al: Left fascicular blocks during right-heart catheterization using the Swan-Ganz catheter. Circulation 64:1271, 1981

263. Strasberg B, Berkowitz CE, Rosen KM: Right bundle branch block reflecting balloon inflation of Swan-Ganz catheter. Chest 81:368, 1982

264. Abernathy WS: Complete heart block caused by the Swan-Ganz catheter. Chest 65:349, 1974

265. Shimm DS, Rigsby L: Ventricular tachycardia associated with removal of a Swan-Ganz catheter. Postgrad Med 67:291, 1980

266. Reitan J, Barash PG: Noninvasive monitoring. In Saidman L, Smith, NT, (eds): Monitoring in Anesthesia. 2nd Ed. Butterworth, London, 1981

267. Salmenpera M, Peltola K, Rosenberg P: Does prophylactic lidocaine control cardiac arrhythmias associated with pulmonary artery catheterization? Anesthesiology 56:212, 1982

268. Allyn J, Lichtenstein A, Koski EG et al: Inadvertent passage of a pulmonary artery catheter from the superior vena cava through the left atrium and left ventricle into the aorta. Anesthesiology 70:1019, 1989

269. Thijs LG, Van-Heukelem HA, Bronsveld W et al: Double intracardiac knotting of a Swan-Ganz catheter. [Letter]. Br J Anaesth 53:672, 1981

270. Trembley N, Taillefer J, Hardy JF: Successful non-surgical extraction of a knotted pulmonary artery catheter trapped in the right ventricle. Can J Anaesth 39:293, 1992

271. Daum S, Schapira M: Intracardiac knot formation in a Swan-Ganz catheter. Anesth Analg 22:862, 1973

272. Dach JL, Galbut DL, Lepage JR: The knotted Swan-Ganz catheter: new solution to a vexing problem. AJR 137:1274, 1981

273. Fibuch EE, Tuohy GF: Intracardiac knotting of a flow-directed balloon-tipped catheter. Anesth Analg 59:217, 1980

274. Graybar GB, Adler E, Smith W, Puyau FA: Knotting of a Swan-Ganz catheter. [Letter]. Chest 84:240, 1983

275. Iberti TJ, Jayagopal SG: Knotting of a Swan-Ganz catheter in pulmonary artery. Chest 83:711, 1983

276. Andreasson S, Appelgren LK: Complication of Swan-Ganz catheter. Crit Care Med 7:256, 1979

277. O'Toole JD, Wurtzbacher JJ, Wearner NE et al: Pulmonary valve injury and insufficiency during pulmonary-artery catheterization. New Engl J Med 301:1167, 1979

278. Boscoe MJ, Delange S: Damage of the tricuspid valve with a Swan-Ganz catheter. Br Med J 283:346, 1981

279. Thomas HA: The knotted Swan-Ganz catheter: a safer solution. [Letter]. Am J Radiol 138:986, 1982

280. McLoud TC, Putman CE: Radiology of the Swan-Ganz catheter and associated pulmonary complications. Radiology 116:19, 1975

281. Block PC: Snaring of a Swan-Ganz catheter. J Thorac Cardiovasc Surg 71:917, 1976

282. Greenfield DH, McMullan GK, Parisi AF et al: Snare retrieval of a catheter fragment with inaccessible ends from the pulmonary artery. Cathet Cardiovasc Diagn 4:87, 1978

283. Kemmots UK: An inadvertent insertion of a Swan Ganz Canter into the intrathecal space. Anesthesiology 62:648, 1985

284. Boncheck LI: Severe endobronchial hemorrhage. Ann Thorac Surg 53:738, 1992

285. Culpepper JA, Setter M, Rinaldo RE: Massive hemoptysis and tension pneumothorax following pulmonary artery catheterization. chest 3:380, 1982

286. Deren MM, Barash PG, Hammond GL et al: Perforation of the pulmonary artery requiring pneumonectomy after the use of a flow-directed Swan-Ganz catheter. Thorax 34:550, 1979

287. Connors JP, Sandza JG, Shaw RC et al: Lobar pulmonary hemorrhage. Arch Surg 115:883, 1980

288. Colvin MP, Savege TM, Lewis CT: Pulmonary damage from a Swan-Ganz catheter. Br J Anaesth 47:1107, 1975

289. Farber DL, Rose DM, Bassell GM et al: Hemoptysis and pneumothorax after a removal of a persistently wedged pulmonary artery catheter. Crit Care Med 9:494, 1981

290. Feng WC, Singh AK, Drew T, Donat W: Swan Ganz catheter induced massive hemoptysis and pulmonary artery false aneurysm. Thorac Surg 50:644, 1990

291. Foote GA, Schabel SI, Hodges M: Pulmonary complications of the flow-directed balloon-tipped catheter. N Engl J Med 209:927, 1974

292. Forman MB, Obel IW: Pulmonary hemorrhage following Swan-Ganz catheterization in a patient without severe pulmonary hypertension. S Afr Med J 58:329, 1980

293. Golden MS et al: Fatal pulmonary hemorrhage complicating use of flow-directed balloon-tipped catheter in a patient receiving anticoagulant therapy. Am J Cardiol 32:365, 1973

294. Hardy JF, Morissett M, Taillefer J, Vauclair R: The pathophysiology of pulmonary artery ruptures by pulmonary artery balloon tipped catheters. Anesthesiology 59:A127, 1983

295. Krantz EM, Viljoen JF: Haemoptysis following insertion of a Swan-Ganz catheter. Br J Anaesth 51:457, 1979

296. Lapin ES, Murray JA: Hemoptysis with flow-directed cardiac catheterization. JAMA 220:1246, 1972

297. Lee ME, Matloff JM, Hackner E: Catheter-induced pulmonary artery hemorrhage [Letter]. J Thorac Cardiovasc Surg 83:796, 1982

298. McDanield DD, Stone JG, Faltas AN et al: Catheter-induced pulmonary artery hemorrhage. Diagnosis and management in cardiac operations. J Thorac Cardiovasc Surg 82:1, 1981

299. Melter R, Kint PP, Simoons M: Hemoptysis after flushing Swan-Ganz catheters in the wedge position. N Engl J Med 304:1171, 1981

300. Ohn KC, Cottrell JE, Turndore H: Hemoptysis from a pulmonary-artery catheter. Anesthesiology 51:485, 1979

301. Pape LA, Haffajee CI, Markis JE et al: Fatal pulmonary hemorrhage after use of the flow-directed balloon-tipped catheter. Ann Intern Med 90:344, 1979

302. Paulson DM, Scott SM, Sethi GK: Pulmonary hemorrhage associated with balloon flotation catheters: a report of a case and review of the literature. J Thorac Cardiovasc Surg 80:453, 1980

303. Rubin SA, Puckett RP: Pulmonary artery-bronchial fistula: a new complication of Swan-Ganz catheterization. Chest 75:515, 1979

304. Elliott CG, Zimmerman GA, Clemmer TP: Complications of pulmonary artery catheterization in the care of critically ill patients. Chest 76:647, 1979

305. Kron IL, Piepgrass W, Carabello B et al: False aneurysm of the pulmonary artery: a complication of pulmonary artery catherization. Ann Thorac Surg 33:629, 1982

306. Lindgren KM, McShane K, Roberts WC: Acute rupture of the pulmonic valve by a balloon tipped catheter producing a musical diastolic murmur. Chest 81:251, 1982

307. Lipp H et al: Intracardiac knotting of a flow-directed balloon catheter. N Engl J Med 284:220, 1971

308. Mayerhofer KE, Billhart RA, Codini MA et al: An aberrant wave form due to rupture of the balloon of the Swanz-Ganz catheter. N Engl J Med 308:594, 1983

309. Moore RA, McNicholas K, Gallagher JD et al: Migration of pediatric pulmonary artery catheters. Anesthesiology 58:102, 1983

310. Kirton O, Varon AJ, Henry R, Civetta JM: Flow directed pulmonary artery catheter induced pseudoaneurysm: Urgent diagnosis and endovascular obliteration. Crit Care 20:1178, 1992

311. Rao TLK, Gorski DW et al: Safety of pulmonary artery catheterization. Anesthesiology 57:A116, 1982

312. Purut CM, Scott SM, Parham JV, Smith PK: Intraoperative management of severe endobronchial hemorrhage. Ann Thorac Surg 51:304, 1991

313. Puri VK, Carlson RW, Bander JJ et al: Complications of vascular catheterization in the critically ill. Crit Care Med 8:495, 1980

314. Rice PL, Piffarre R, El-Etr A et al: Management of endobronchial hemorrhage during cardiopulmonary bypass. J Thorac Cardiovasc Surg 81:800, 1981

315. Resnick JM, Engeler CE, Derauf BJ: Postmortem angiography of catheter induced pulmonary artery perforation. J Forensic Sci 37:1346, 1992

316. Devitt JH, Noble WH, Byrick RJ: A Swan-Ganz catheter related complication in a patient with Eisenmenger's syndrome. Anesthesiology 57:335, 1982

317. Stein JM, Libson A: Pulmonary hemorrhage from pulmonary artery catheterization treated with endobronchial intubation. Anesthesiology 55:698, 1981

318. Gomez-Arnau J, Juan-Montero G, Luengo C et al: Retrograde dissection and rupture of pulmonary artery after catheter use in pulmonary hypertension. Crit Care Med 10:694, 1982

319. Johnson WE, Royster RL, Choplin RH et al: Pulmonary artery catheter migration during cardiac surgery. Anesthesiology 64:258, 1986

320. Yellin LB, Filler JJ, Barnette RE: Nominal hemoptysis heralds pseudoaneurysm induced by a pulmonary artery catheter. Anesthesiology 73:370, 1991

321. Pokora TJ, Boros SJ, Brennom WS, Huseby TL: Fatal neonatal thrombosis associated with a pulmonary arterial catheter. Crit Care Med 9:618, 1981

322. Reinke RT, Higgins CB, Atkin TW: Pulmonary infarction complicating the use of Swan-Ganz catheters. Br J Rad 48:885, 1975

323. Greene JF Jr, Cummings KC: Aseptic thrombotic endocardial vegetations: a complication of indwelling pulmonary artery catheters. JAMA 225:1525, 1973

324. Hoar PF, Wilson RM, Mangano DT et al: Heparin

bonding reduces thrombogenicity of pulmonary-artery catheters. N Engl J Med 305:993, 1981

325. Hoar PF, Stone JG, Wicks AE et al: Thrombogenesis associated with Swan-Ganz catheters. Anesthesiology, 48:445, 1978

326. Snow P: Swan-Ganz catheter and superior vena cava syndrome. [Letter]. JAMA 243:1525, 1980

327. Bennegard I, Curelara B, Gustavsson LE et al: Material thrombogenicity in central venous catheterization. In: Comparison between uncoated and heparin coated, long antebrachial polyethylene catheters. Acta Anaesth Scand 26:112: 1982

328. Brunswick RA, Gionis TA: Starch as a cause of thrombus with Swan-Ganz catheters. [Letter]. Chest 82:131, 1982

329. Chastre J, Cornud F, Bouchama A et al: Thrombosis as a complication of pulmonary-artery catheterization via the internal jugular vein: prospective evaluation by phlebography. N Engl J Med 306:267, 1982

330. Kim YL, Richman KA, Marshall BE: Thrombocytopenia associated with Swan-Ganz catheterization in patients. Anesthesiology 53:262, 1980

331. Richman KA, Kim YL, Marshall BE: Thrombocytopenia and altered platelet kinetics associated with prolonged pulmonary-artery catheterization in the dog. Anesthesiology 53:101, 1980

332. Pinilla JC, Ross DF, Martin T et al: Study of the incidence of intravascular catheter infection and associated septicemia in critically ill patients. Crit Care Med 11:21, 1983

333. Singh S, Nelson N, Acosta I, Check FE: Catheter colonization and bacteremia with pulmonary and arterial catheters. Crit Care Med 10:736, 1982

334. Raad I, Umphrey J, Khan A, Truett LJ, Bodey GP: The duration of placement as a predictor of peripheral and pulmonary arterial catheter infections. J Hosp Infect 23:17, 1993

335. Bessette MC, Quintin L, Whalley DG et al: Swan-Ganz catheter contamination: a protective sleeve for repositioning. Can Anaesth Soc J 28:86, 1981

336. Erceg GW: A sterile cover for repositioning a pulmonary-artery catheter. Anesthesiology, 52:193, 1980

337. Kopman EA, Sandza JG: Manipulation of the pulmonary-artery catheter after placement: maintenance of sterility. Anesthesiology 48:373, 1978

338. Smith WR, Glauser FL, Jemison P: Ruptured chordae of the tricuspid valve: the consequence of flow-directed Swan-Ganz catheterization. Chest 70:790, 1976

339. Smith GB, Willatts SM: A hazard of Swan-Ganz catheterization. Anaesthesia 36:398, 1981

340. Pace NL, Horton W: Indwelling pulmonary artery catheters: their relationships to aseptic thrombotic endocardial vegetations. JAMA 233:893, 1975

341. Greene JF Jr Fitzwater JE, Clemmer TP: Septic endocarditis and indwelling pulmonary artery catheters. JAMA 233:891, 1975

342. Ehrie M, Morgan AP, Moore FD, O'Connor NE: Endocarditis with the indwelling balloon tipped pulmonary artery catheter in burn patients. J Trauma 18:664, 1978

343. Sasaki TM, Panke TW, Dorethy JF et al: The relationship of central venous and pulmonary artery catheter position to acute right-sided endocarditis in severe thermal injury. J Trauma 19:740, 1979

344. Hansen R, Vrquerat C, Matthay M et al: Poor correlation between pulmonary arterial pressure and left ventricular end diastolic volume after coronary artery bypass heart surgery. Anesthesiology 64:764, 1986

345. Calvin JE, Driedger AA, Sibbald WJ: Does the pulmonary capillary wedge pressure predict left ventricular preload in critically ill patients? Crit Care Med 9:437, 1981

346. Ellis RJ, Mangano DT, VanDyke DC: Relationship of wedge pressure to end-diastolic volume in patients undergoing myocardial revascularization. J Thorac Cardiovasc Surg 78:605, 1979

347. King EG: Influence of mechanical ventilation and pulmonary disease on pulmonary artery pressure monitoring. Can Med Assoc J 121:901, 1979

348. Raphael P, Cogbill TH, Dunn EL et al: Routine invasive hemodynamic monitoring does not increase risk of aortic graft infection. Heart Lung 22:121, 1993

Transesophageal Echocardiography

11

Eugenie S. Heitmiller
Joao A. C. Lima
Linda S. Humphrey

Transesophageal echocardiography (TEE) was developed in response to the technical difficulty experienced obtaining images of the heart in certain groups of patients. The location of the esophagus immediately posterior to the heart permits a transducer position that circumvents air, bone, fat, and muscle. Very obese patients or those with extremely muscular chest walls who are often difficult to image with transthoracic echocardiography can be easily studied. In addition, images can be obtained in patients with chronic obstructive pulmonary disease and during mechanical ventilation who would be otherwise difficult or impossible to image due to the air-filled lungs, which produce an impenetrable barrier to ultrasound.

Prior to the development of TEE, epicardial echocardiography had been used in the operating room by both cardiac surgeons[1-4] and anesthesiologists.[5-8] When TEE became available, the potential for intraoperative use and its advantages were immediately apparent. Passage of the probe is simple and painless in the anesthetized patient, access to the chest wall or heart is not required, and surgery need not be delayed to obtain echocardiographic images. These features have led to considerable interest among anesthesiologists in further exploring the potential perioperative applications of TEE.

This chapter reviews the characteristics, instrumentation, and applications of two-dimensional and Doppler echocardiography. It explains the use of TEE as an intraoperative monitor and illustrates

how it can improve patient care and help reduce the incidence of morbidity and mortality.

HISTORY

The first use of an esophageal transducer for imaging is attributed to Frazin who in 1976 placed an M-mode transducer into the esophagus of patients in whom a transthoracic echocardiogram had been unsatisfactory.[9] The potential for intraoperative use was reported in 1980 by Matsumoto and colleagues[10] with a series of 21 cardiac surgery patients who had been successfully monitored by M-mode TEE. Two-dimensional imaging was eventually incorporated into esophageal echocardiography, its use reported by Hisanaga and colleagues.[11] They used a mechanical transducer that rotated at a high speed to produce 180-degree two-dimensional images. The esophagus was protected by housing the mechanism within an oil bag. Development of the phased array transducer was a major step forward for two-dimensional TEE imaging, as awake patients tolerated the motionless transducer more easily. In 1982, Schluter and coworkers[12] reported the use of a miniaturized phased-array transducer housed in a gastroscope. This is the system that is currently in use.

In 1987, color flow imaging was incorporated into the TEE imaging system which enabled the user to obtain information about blood flow in addition to cardiac morphology.[13,14] With the com-

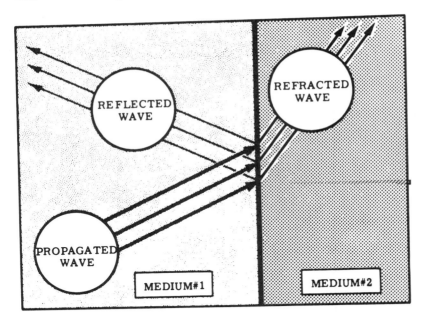

Fig. 11-1. The interface between the two media of differing acoustic impedance causes the ultrasound beam to be both reflected and refracted. (From Feigenbaum,[16] with permission.)

mercial availability of these probes, TEE became increasingly popular. In 1989, Omoto and colleagues[15] reported the development of a biplane TEE probe and in 1991, an omniplane probe became commercially available. These technologic advances have greatly enhanced our understanding of intracardiac and intravascular structure and function.

BASIC ULTRASOUND TECHNIQUES

Two-Dimensional Echocardiography

Echocardiography is the use of high-frequency pulsed ultrasound to create images of the heart and surrounding structures. Ultrasound is defined as sound at a frequency above the audible range (higher than 20,000 Hz), but the ultrasound used in medical imaging has frequencies in the 2 to 7 MHz range.[16]

Acoustic impedance, the product of the density of medium and the velocity of sound in that medium, is the primary characteristic that allows structures to be distinguished by ultrasound.[16] Pulses of ultrasound will traverse tissue until they encounter an interface between two media of differing acoustic impedance (effectively, differing density), such as endocardium and blood. This interface reflects a portion of the ultrasound beam back to the transducer, while the remainder of the beam is refracted

(Fig. 11-1). The intensity of the reflected portion depends on the degree of difference in density at the interface and the angle at which the ultrasound beam encountered the density interface. The clearest images result from interfaces between structures of significantly different density that lie perpendicular to the incident beam. Echoes generated in this fashion are known as specular echoes.

Contrasting with the strong specular echoes are weaker scattered echoes (Fig. 11-2).[16] Scattered echoes are reflections from small, irregular surfaces that tend to disperse the ultrasound in multiple directions. Although some of these reflections return to the transducer, the majority are lost to the system. Along with absorption, scattering results in attenuation or diminution of the ultrasound signal. Attenuation is particularly a problem in those portions of the beam that travel the furthest through tissue, but also depends on the characteristics of the tissue through which the waves are propagated. Less homogeneous tissues produce greater degrees of scattering. Attenuation is extremely high in bone and air, moderate in muscle, and mild in other tissue and blood.

Emission of ultrasound in pulses is necessary to permit determination of depth. Since the speed of sound in soft tissue is more or less constant, the time required for an emitted signal to encounter a structure and return to the transducer is directly related to the distance it traveled. Reconstruction of the spatial orientation of structures is then possible. An added benefit of the pulsed format is that the same transducer element can both send and receive signals.

The quality of the ultimate image depends on many factors, but one of the more important is resolution, the ability to separate adjacent structures. The smallest structure that can be distinguished echocardiographically is one-fourth the wavelength of the ultrasound in size.[16] Higher frequency, shorter wavelength ultrasound therefore provides better resolution than does ultrasound of lower frequency and longer wavelength. Axial resolution, the separation of two objects at different depths, additionally depends on the duration of the ultrasound pulse, whereas lateral, or side-by-side resolution is primarily determined by the width of the ultrasound beam.[17] A 2-MHz transducer has approximately 1 mm axial and 2 to 3 mm lateral resolution.

The same characteristic that makes high-frequency ultrasound desirable for image resolution is also its biggest drawback. The high-frequency beam tends to be reflected by a multitude of small, inconsequential interfaces and thus does not penetrate tissue to a very great distance.[16] Absorption is also greater with high frequency ultrasound, further limiting penetration. Clinically useful ultrasound transducers represent a compromise between these two factors. The average adult is studied with a 2.25 to 3.5 MHz external probe,

whereas infants and small children, with their thinner and less muscular chest walls, often can be studied with transducers of higher frequency and correspondingly superior resolution. Positioning a transducer in the esophagus permits imaging from a location immediately adjacent to the heart, allowing higher frequency transducers to be used than would ordinarily be used to produce transthoracic images in the same patient.[18]

The imaging rate and scan angle also affect the quality of the image. Ultrasound is not a particularly rapid modality compared to other imaging techniques such as x-ray. Obtaining a single line of data requires 0.1 to 0.2 ms, the exact time depending on the depth of the target.[16] Once the maximum depth is set, and allowing for a brief machine lag time, the pulse repetition frequency can be calculated. M-mode echocardiographs generally have pulse repetition rates of approximately 1,000 per second whereas two-dimensional instruments have rates between 3,000 and 5,000 per second.[16] This would seem to suggest that two-dimensional images are of superior quality. In M-mode, however, the pulses continually update information from the single dimension being examined, whereas in two-dimensional echocardiography, the scan lines must be spread out through the scan angle (90 degrees) and the entire two-dimensional image is updated only about 30 times per second. Decreasing the maximum depth of a two-dimensional scan permits an increase in pulse repetition frequency, thereby

SPECULAR ECHOES

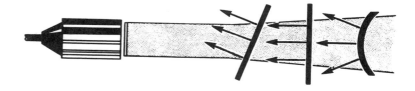

SCATTERED ECHOES

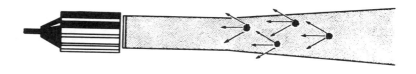

Fig. 11-2. Specular echoes are strong, angle-dependent reflections from relatively large surfaces, while weaker, scattered echoes originate from small, irregular objects. (From Feigenbaum,[16] with permission.)

increasing the number of scan lines per frame enhancing the image. Alternatively, if the angle of a two-dimensional scan is reduced, the same number of lines of information will be closer together, improving image quality. The capacity to vary the depth or narrow the scan angle to examine a small area more closely is incorporated in some echocardiographic equipment. In addition, each echocardiographic frame is composed of two fields, or sweeps of the ultrasound beam through the sector. This effectively doubles the line density and improves the image. Further smoothing results from the tendency of a picture on a television screen to persist, filling in any areas missing from the subsequent frame.

Doppler Echocardiography

Doppler ultrasound is based on a principle described by Christian Johann Doppler, an Austrian physicist. He observed that the color of a star depended on its movement relative to a stationary observer. Similarly, a frequency shift is produced when sound waves are reflected by a moving target. The change in frequency, known as the Doppler shift, is proportional to the velocity of the target. If the angle at which the ultrasound beam encounters the target is known, velocity (*V*) can be calculated from the Doppler equation:

$$V = \frac{\Delta f c}{2} f_0 \times \cos \Theta$$

where Δf is the Doppler frequency shift, f_0 is the fundamental frequency of the emitted ultrasound, c is the velocity of sound in tissue, and Θ is the angle between the beam and the moving object (Fig. 11-3).[19] Since this angle is difficult to determine clinically, most practical applications attempt to align the ultrasound beam in parallel with the moving target (ordinarily red blood cells). This allows the maximal frequency shift to be measured: cos 0 = 1, and the velocity is thus directly proportional to frequency. As the relationship increasingly diverges from parallel, Θ approaches 90 degrees, cos Θ approaches 0, and velocity is underestimated by an increasingly greater amount if the angle is not taken into account. Therefore if the assumption is made that one is parallel to flow, any actual deviation from parallel during data acquisition in-

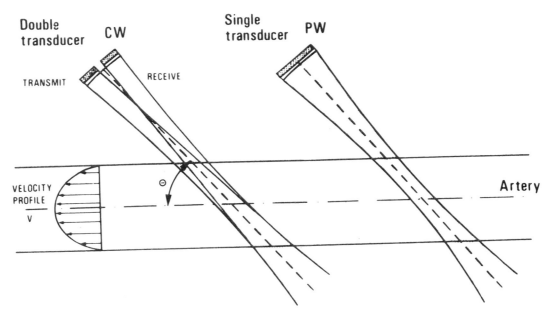

Fig. 11-3. Velocity and direction of blood flow can be determined with a single transducer (pulsed-wave Doppler) or a double transducer (continuous-wave Doppler), the latter containing separate elements to send and receive the Doppler signal, which is emitted continuously. The angle Θ between the velocity vector and the Doppler signal is shown. (From Hatle and Angelsen,[19] with permission.)

troduces potentially significant error. (Practically, deviations of 20 degrees or less introduce an error of only 5 to 10 percent.)

Doppler examination does not reveal morphology, but rather velocity of flow. The combination of Doppler with two-dimensional echocardiography in a duplex transducer allows the techniques to complement each other; two-dimensional echocardiography reveals cardiac structures, whereas Doppler measures the velocity and position of red blood cell flow relative to them. This is achieved as follows: while the cardiac structures are displayed by two-dimensional echocardiography in the usual way, the Doppler beam is emitted either continuously (continuous-wave Doppler) or in pulses (pulsed-wave Doppler). The beam is positioned relative to the two-dimensional image by means of a tracking ball or level, permitting accurate placement of the Doppler signal within the heart or great vessels.

Pulsed-Wave Doppler

In pulsed-wave Doppler echocardiography, a pulse of ultrasound is positioned to interrogate a specific depth and site within the heart, the so-called "sample volume" (Fig. 11-4). The returning signal reflects the velocity and direction of blood flow at that particular point. By moving the sample volume, the pattern of flow at various positions can be mapped out. The results of this interrogation are both audible, as it happens that the frequency shift falls within the audible range, and visually depicted as a real-time spectral display of flow velocity versus time.

The visual display, derived from a fast Fourier transformation of the incoming signal, plots velocity against time, with motion toward the observer displayed above a variable baseline and that away displayed below. Another aspect of the visual display is the distinction between laminar and turbulent flow (Plate 11-1). When laminar flow is sampled, the returning signals are relatively uniform in velocity and direction, because all red blood cells are moving at a uniform velocity at any given moment. The resultant display has a smooth envelope (the outer border of the waveform) with a relatively clear area underlying it. Alternatively, turbulent flow results in a pattern suggestive of the multitude of velocities it contains. This spectrum displays a relatively shaggy curve, with the area below the curve filled in by signals resulting from these many different velocities. This phenomenon is known as spectral broadening.

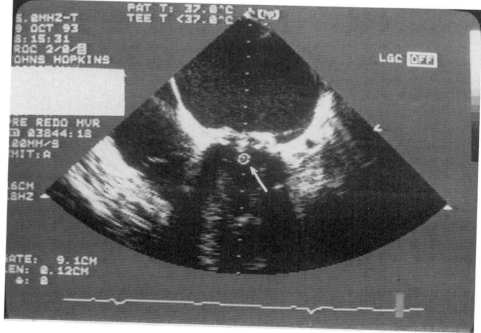

Fig. 11-4. Transesophageal image demonstrating placement of the pulsed Doppler sample volume (*arrow*) just below a prosthetic mitral valve.

The major limitation of pulsed Doppler is its inability to quantify high velocities accurately. When samples frequencies exceed a maximum level (the so-called "Nyquist limit"), the display "wraps around" to the bottom or top so that very high velocities overlie those moving in the opposite direction. This effect is known as aliasing (Fig. 11-5). The maximum velocity that can be detected is related to the transducer's emitted frequency and the maximum range or depth at which the sample volume will be placed. As in echocardiography, range is inversely related to pulse repetition frequency; thus the shorter the range at which the sample volume is placed, the higher the pulse repetition frequency and the higher the velocity that can be measured. This may again represent an advantage of transesophageal ultrasound, which minimizes the distance between the transducer and the heart.[20] *Aliasing* occurs at a lower velocity when simultaneous two-dimensional imaging is occurring because available pulse repetition frequency must be shared. This can be minimized by switching to a lower frequency transducer, which allows more of the ultrasound capability to be applied to Doppler, and by intermittently updating the two-dimensional image while the Doppler signal is being recorded rather than displaying a real-time two-dimensional image. If the peak velocity is only slightly off scale, it sometimes can be measured by lowering the baselines until the entire envelope is visualized.

Continuous-Wave Doppler

Continuous-wave Doppler is employed when the maximum velocity along a range must be known precisely and exceeds the limits of the pulsed format. This method requires two dedicated elements since signals are both sent and received continuously. Flows along the entire length of the beam are sampled, so depth information is no longer available, a situation referred to as range ambiguity; but by eliminating the time consideration required to determine depth, there is no restriction on the velocity that can be measured (Fig. 11-6). Continuous-wave Doppler is used for calculation of valve gradients and area.

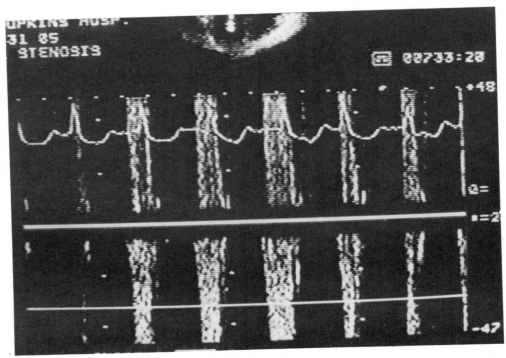

Fig. 11-5. Aliasing occurs when the blood flow velocity exceeds the capacity of the pulsed format; it appears as a "wrap around" of the curve to the top or bottom of the display. In this example, the velocity is so high that one continuous curve is displayed.

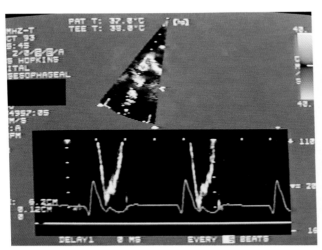

Plate 11-1A.   **Plate 11-1B.**

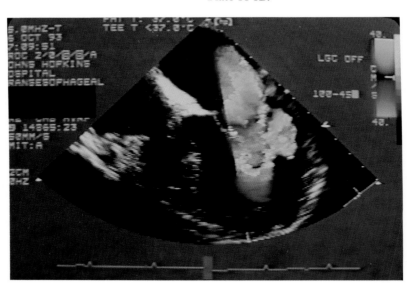

Plate 11-2.

Plate 11-1. The distinction between laminar and turbulent flow. **(A)** Laminar flow across the mitral valve is shown in this transesophageal echocardiography (TEE) study. Laminar flow produces a smooth envelope with a clear space beneath it. **(B)** Turbulent flow across a prosthetic mitral valve produces a curve that is filled to a large extent because of the movement of blood in a disorganized fashion.

Plate 11-2. Color Doppler flow image. In the color scale to the right, red indicates blood moving toward the transducer and blue indicates blood moving away from the transducer. Velocity is represented by the brightness of the color, and high velocity flow is displayed as small echogenic dots.

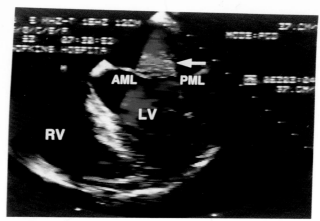

Plate 11-3A.

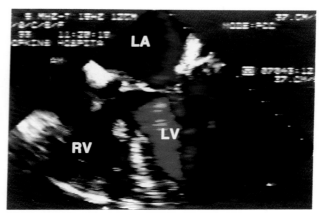

Plate 11-3B.

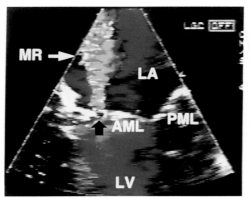

Plate 11-4.

(A) Color Doppler image showing mitral regurgitation seen as a mosaic of color at the arrow (see _1-38_). RV, right ventricle; LV, left ventricle; AML, anterior mitral leaflet; PML, posterior mitral _Color Doppler image of mitral valve after repair. LA, left atrium.

_hole in the anterior leaflet of the mitral valve secondary to endocarditis, resulting in a jet of _itation (MR) in the middle of the leaflet (seen at the black arrow). This was repaired by suturing _n. LA, left atrium; AML, anterior mitral leaflet; PML, posterior mitral leaflet; LV, left ventricle.

The calculation of pressure gradients between two specific chambers of the heart is possible by the application of a modified Bernoulli equation developed by Hatle and associates.[19] The complete Bernoulli equation for fluid flow past an obstruction relates the pressure drop across that obstruction to several parameters including: the density of the fluid (p); the flow velocities before and after the obstruction (V_1, V_2); flow acceleration across the obstruction; and the frictional forces which act to retard blood flow.

$$P_1 - P_2 = \frac{1}{2}\, p(V_2^2 - V_1^2) + p_1 \int^2 (dV/dT)\, ds + R(V)$$

Pressure   Convective   Flow   Frictional
change   acceleration   acceleration   forces

The modified formula is simplified for clinical use by making two principal assumptions: the first, that at the time of maximal velocity flow acceleration is 0, and the second, that in stenotic valves the diameter of the orifice is wide in relation to its length, making the frictional forces negligible. The first term relates to the convective acceleration of flow through the orifice. It can be further simplified if V_1 is normal, that is, less than 1 m/s. If one expresses all velocities and the density of blood in appropriate units, the equation then becomes:

$$P_1 - P_2 \ (\text{mm/Hg}) = 4V_2^2$$

The mean pressure gradient can be calculated by squaring the velocity at each time point and averaging the squared values before multiplying the average by 4.

The calculation of the aortic valve area can be achieved by a different formula called the continuity equation which is based on the formula for instantaneous flow across a distinct obstruction. The rationale behind the derivation of this formula is that the flow (F) through a conduit is a function of the instantaneous velocity (V) of the fluid and the area (A) of the conduit. Thus,

$$F = V \times A$$

If one assumes that all the blood leaving the left

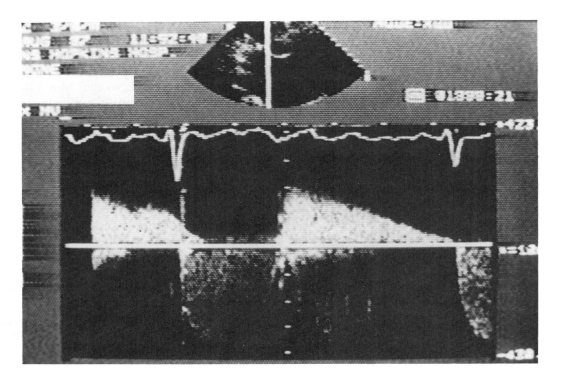

Fig. 11-6. Continuous-wave Doppler recording from a transthoracic apical four-chamber view in a patient with mitral stenosis/regurgitation. Velocities are sampled throughout the length of the cursor. The transmitral flow is toward the transducer and displayed above the baseline, whereas the regurgitant flow is away and displayed below.

ventricle passes through both the left ventricular outflow tract (LVOT) and the aortic valve (AV), then

$$F_{LVOT} = F_{AV}$$

Substituting for the continuity equation,

$$(V \times A)_{LVOT} = (V \times A)_{AV}$$

Rearranging the equation for aortic valve area (A_{AV}),

$$A_{AV} = \frac{(V \times A)_{LVOT}}{V_{AV}}$$

The area of the left ventricular outflow tract (A_{LVOT}) is estimated from the diameter (D) measured immediately below the aortic valve and calculated as: $A = \pi(D/2)^2$. The final equation is thus:

$$A_{AV} = \frac{V_{LVOT}}{V_{AV}} \times \pi\left(\frac{D}{2}\right)^2_{LVOT}$$

Peak velocities are most commonly used in this formula but flow velocity integrals can also be used and may be more stable as estimates of flow over time.

The second important equation in the quantification of valve areas by continuous wave Doppler is the calculation of the pressure half-time. This formula is based on the assumption that the size of a stenotic mitral valve orifice can be estimated from the amount of time it takes the initial pressure gradient to fall to one-half its original value. Although the detailed derivation of this formula is beyond the scope of this text, the velocity at the time the pressure gradient has fallen to half its initial value can be shown to be approximately V_{max} divided by 1.4.[19] The time interval between the time of peak pressure to the time of the pressure half-time $(P_{1/2})$ in milliseconds is then related to 220 ms, which is the time interval corresponding to a valve area of 1 cm^2 across a wide variety of flow values. Thus, the orifice area of a stenotic mitral valve can be estimated by

$$\text{Orifice area} = \frac{220}{P_{1/2}} \text{ (ms)}$$

This formula is extremely useful for estimating valve area and inflow obstruction in cases of significant mitral stenosis or prosthetic valves in the mitral position. The reader is referred to more complete texts for detailed derivation of this formula and discussion of the physical principles behind such derivation.[19]

Finally, a Doppler-based system is theoretically capable of continuous measurement of cardiac output in a relatively non-invasive manner. The problem of assuring parallel alignment of the Doppler beam to blood flow (in the absence of imaging) has been one major obstacle to using Doppler for the clinical determination of cardiac output. Another is that the conversion from velocity to flow requires an accurate measurement of estimate of vessel diameter and the presumption that it will not change appreciably. In addition, laminar flow varies in velocity from the vessel center to the walls.[21] Despite these drawbacks, several instruments that determine cardiac output using an esophageal transducer are used clinically, and reasonable tracking of thermodilution cardiac output has been reported.[22-26]

Color-Flow Doppler Mapping

Color Doppler flow mapping uses a pulsed-wave format with multiple simultaneous sampling gates that map flow by means of color. The magnitude of the velocity is portrayed by color intensity. A scale for comparison is displayed in the corner of the screen (Plate 11-2). Similar scales are available to assess turbulent flow, known as variance, which is displayed as a mosaic of colors. Color-coded Doppler signals are superimposed on a real-time, two-dimensional image, so that blood flow relative to cardiac structures can be appreciated readily.

As in standard pulsed-wave Doppler, *aliasing* can be a problem, appearing as color reversal in areas of high velocity. Color also reverses as flow changes direction, but under this circumstance the change in color is sequential, with a dark area separating the two colors. The dark segment represents flow moving perpendicular to the transducer. Color *aliasing*, on the other hand, appears as a color change in the center of the flow where the velocity is maximal. If the velocity is extremely high, one can see multiple color changes and color mixing. Other dark areas (i.e., not displaying color) contain blood moving at a velocity below the threshold for detection by the color Dopper system.

Since color flow mapping is generally performed along with two-dimensional imaging, the pulse repetition frequency at any depth must be split between the two modes.[27,28] The imaging may or may not continue to be displayed in a 90-degree sector arc, but only about 30 to 52 degrees can be used to detect and display signals for color flow.

Mapping of flow in color can be very useful for localizing maximal forward or regurgitant flow jets, suggesting the appropriate placement of the sample volume or cursor for a standard pulsed or continuous-wave Doppler recording. It can also indicate unsuspected flow patterns resulting from septal defects or valve lesions,[28,29] and has been used to delineate aortic dissections.[29-32] It greatly facilitates Doppler examination by presenting a real-time display of blood flow patterns in the heart, in much the same way as an angiogram.

Contrast

It was discovered during the early development of echocardiography that intravascular injection of a turbulent solution results in a cloud of echoes passing through the cardiac chambers. These microbubbles are easily visualized but do not appear to cause any harm to the patient. Gramiak and colleagues[33] investigated microbubbles resulting from injection of indocyanine, a foamy contrast solution. Less dense but otherwise similar microbubbles are produced by rapid injection of saline or the patient's own blood. Since the contrast effect is lost during passage through the pulmonary bed, they were able to demonstrate intracardiac shunting by appearance of microbubbles on both sides of the interatrial septum. Similarly, aortic regurgitation was documented by supravalvular injection of microbubbles.

Microbubbles have been used extensively for evaluation of valvular function and congenital heart disease.[34] Reid and associates[35] found the technique to be both specific and sensitive for detecting valvular regurgitation during cardiac catheterization. Contrast echo also has been used intraoperatively to assess the adequacy of repair of both valves and congenital defects.[36-40]

The exact nature of the contrast effect is still debated. It appears that actual bubbles of air or water vapor of the micrometer range in size are responsible for the effect, although other explanations such as cavitation or turbulence have also been proposed. The very poor conduction of ultrasound through air makes it a significant reflector of the beam, resulting in high contrast with the surrounding blood (Fig. 11-7). Several studies document the absence of neurologic deficits after the appearance of microbubbles on the left side of the heart, regardless of whether they are intentionally produced by agitation or sonication or whether they appear after cardiac surgery.[39-42] The safety of con-

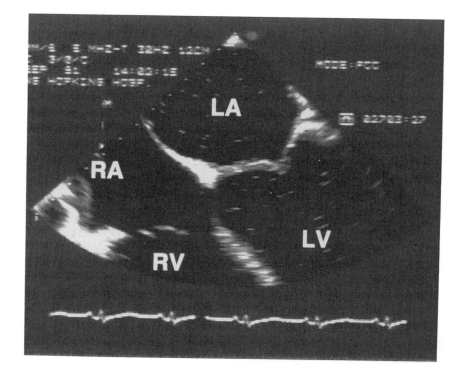

Fig. 11-7. Transesophageal image of the four chamber view showing microbubbles on the left side of the heart, displayed as small echogenic dots. LA, left atrium; LV, left ventricle; RA, right atrium; RV, right ventricle.

trast echocardiography was reviewed by the Committee on Contrast Echocardiography of the American Society of Echocardiography.[41] They surveyed the membership of the Society and reported approximately 51,000 studies with no long-term side effects, although a variety of transient effects were noted. Most likely, the very small size of these bubbles permits them to be readily cleared from the microvasculature.

INSTRUMENTATION

There are two major components to the echocardiographic system: the transmitter and the transducer. The transmitter is a very complex device that controls the pulse repetition frequency and the duration of the emitted ultrasound pulses, processes the returning signals, and displays the resulting image; the transducer physically contacts the patient to emit and receive the ultrasound signals.

Transmitter

The transmitter, known as an echocardiograph, emits the ultrasonic signal and manipulates the reflected signals to generate an image. This signal processing is complex, but in general involves conversion of a radiofrequency signal to a video display. Along the way, the signal is electronically modified and differentiated, then digitized and further modified by the system's microprocessors, enhancing it and transforming it for display on a television screen. Most of this manipulation of preprocessing

is not under user control, but several aspects of signal processing are adjustable. These are described in the following sections.

Gray Scale

Early echocardiograms were recorded simply to locate structures and to observe their motion and thus little variation in brightness was incorporated in the display.[16] This permitted imaging within a relatively narrow dynamic range, that is, the spectrum of signals in decibels that can be detected by the instrument, with those above and below the range discarded. One advantage of this system is the ability to eliminate low-intensity noise. As interest in lower intensity scattered echoes has increased, the capacity to record a range of brightness or gray scale has assumed increasing importance. The dynamic range required to record gray scale is much greater than the capacity of the instrument, a problem resolved by logarithmic compression of the range (Fig. 11-8). Gray scale can be enhanced or accentuated by digital processing.

Gain

The system or master gain control increases the intensity of all returning echoes, bringing more of them into the dynamic range. The time-gain compensation, on the other hand, selectively enhances echoes that are reflected by the deepest structures. Because of the longer distance traveled by these echoes, their attenuation is greater than that of echoes returning from targets closer to the trans-

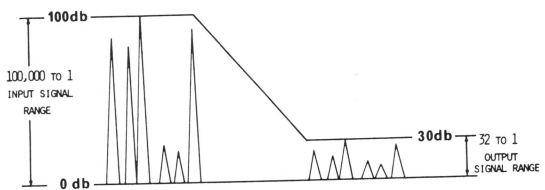

Fig. 11-8. The ability to record gray scale requires a large, dynamic range. In this diagram, 100 dB of ultrasonic information have undergone logarithmic compression to a 30 dB output. (From Feigenbaum,[16] with permission.)

ducer. The time-gain compensation assures that all echoes will be of similar intensity regardless of distance traveled. Time-gain compensation can be adjusted automatically by the instrument, by a single knob, in which case the slope of the compensation is altered, or by a series of levers, allowing the user to modify each level independently.

The price paid for increasing the gain is widening of the returning echoes in all dimensions (Fig. 11-9). In addition to decreasing the resolution, broadening of the image introduces error into calculations that depend on a discrete signal for measurement.

Transducers

The primary component of the transducer is a piezoelectric element, a substance that expands and contracts in the presence of an electric field as the current changes polarity. These expansions and contractions generate the ultrasound waves. The same component senses the returning waves during the pauses between emissions, regenerating an electric signal. Various modulations of this electric signal result in the final displayed image. TEE transducers are miniaturized and affixed to the tip of a gastroscope for esophageal placement (Figs. 11-10 and 11-11).

M-mode echocardiography can be performed with a single crystal and in fact is often recorded simultaneously with two-dimensional echocardiography by using one element of the two-dimensional array.[16] A TEE M-mode scan of the entire heart is obtained by slowly moving between the transducer so that the beam progressively sweeps across the heart at the different imaging levels. (See section on two-dimensional TEE examination for explanation of imaging levels.)

Two-dimensional transducers are somewhat more complicated because of the requirement for steering the echo beam through a sector arc. This was first achieved mechanically, either oscillating or rotating the element(s) to sweep through an angle ranging from 30 to 90 degrees.[16,17] Electronic scanners, which sweep through an arc by varying the time of firing of multiple individual elements, are equally common at present. The elements in an electronic scanner can be arrayed linearly and fired in sequence, but this system requires a large and

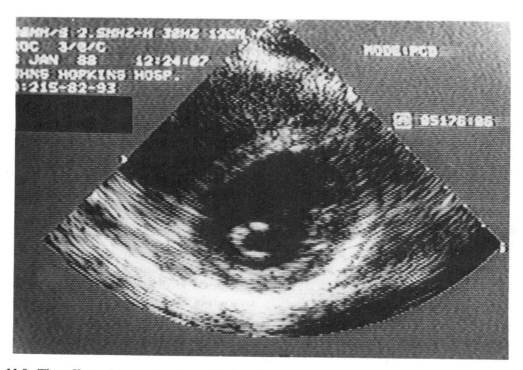

Fig. 11-9. The effect of increasing the gain from low (upper portion) to high (lower portion) is displayed. As the gain increases, the individual echoes widen and resolution is impaired.

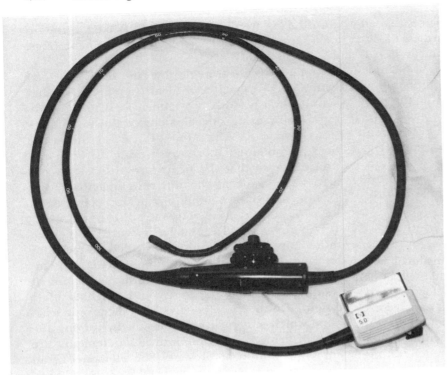

Fig. 11-10. TEE single-plane transducer. The tip is moved by means of the gastroscope control knobs.

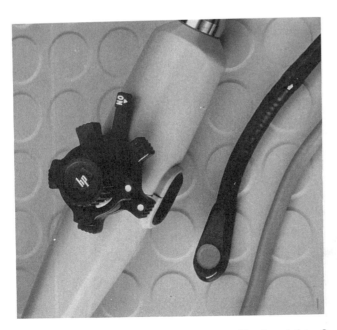

Fig. 11-11. Multiplane TEE transducer. To the right of the control knobs on the handle is a button which controls the rotation of the transducer in the gastroscope tip, enabling 180-degree scan of the heart in each imaging plane.

cumbersome transducer probe and can result in either information gaps or interference between the individual elements.[17] Alternatively, and most commonly, the timing of element discharge is such that a single beam is created by overlap of adjacent small wavefronts from individual crystals (Fig. 11-12).[16,17] This results in a longitudinal waveform comparable to that produced by a single large transducer element. The beam created in this fashion is then steered through the desired sector arc by the individual element firing pattern (Fig. 11-13). The elements of such a transducer are referred to as a phased array.[43]

Timing of element firing can also be used to focus the beam.[16,17] Ultrasound does not travel indefinitely in a straight line; the beam begins to diverge at a distance from the transducer determined by both transducer size and the wavelength of the ultrasound. The point of divergence separates the near field from the far field (Fig. 11-14). Its distance from the transducer can be calculated from the equation

$$1 = \frac{r^2}{\lambda}$$

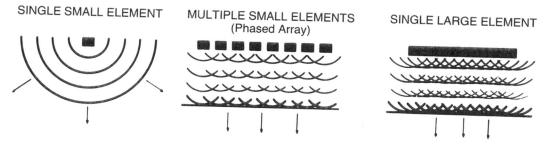

Fig. 11-12. Production of ultrasonic wave fronts. A single small element produces waves that disperse in a circular fashion, whereas both a single large element and multiple small elements produce wavelets that combine, resulting in a single longitudinal wavefront. (From Feigenbaum,[16] with permission.)

where 1 is the length of the near field, r is the radius of the transducer, and λ is the wavelength of the ultrasound.[16,17] Objects are best examined within the near field, where the beam is parallel and narrow. Divergence in the far field can be minimized by further narrowing the beam to a point known as the focal zone, thereby increasing its intensity at the area of interest. Beyond this point it diverges, but from a relatively narrower width. This focusing process can be performed electronically.

The two-dimensional phased-array esophageal probe consists of linearly arranged elements or crystals that fire in a phased manner, resulting in a 90-degree sector arc. The device is housed in a plastic mounting on the anterior face of the tip of a standard gastroscope (Fig. 11-11). The gastroscope controls anteflex and retroflex the tip as well as move it from side to side. In the transgastric view, the tip is anteflexed to improve contact with the mucosa and to obtain an optimal mid-papillary level view of the left ventricle. A locking mechanism, activated by "popping" the control knob inward, permits the tip position to remain fixed. This mechanism should be in the unlocked or free position for insertion or removal of the probe.

The technologic evolution of transducers in the area of TEE has been rapid in the last few years. The newest instruments with full omniplane capability measure 11 mm in shaft diameter and are generally about 100 cm long. However, the tip measures 17 mm by 11 mm and it is flat, containing a mechanism to steer the plane 180 degrees. These transducers enable high resolution imaging of the heart unobstructed by lungs and ribs. The omniplane rotates from the horizontal plane at 0 degrees to the vertical plane at 90 degrees and then to a left/right reversed horizontal plane at 180 degrees. This added omniplane capability allows for

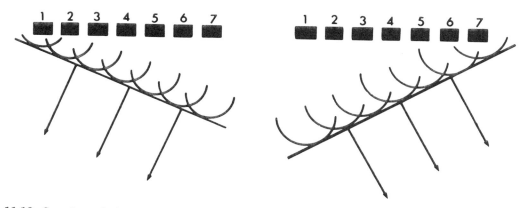

Fig. 11-13. Steering of ultrasonic wave fronts. The ultrasonic wavefront produced from multiple small elements (a linear phased array) can be steered by manipulating the time of firing of the individual elements. (From Feigenbaum,[16] with permission.)

imaging of virtually any structure of the heart in multiple planes. Its only limitation remains the size of its tip, which can be passed without difficulty into the esophagus of most adults, but will occasionally constitute a problem, particularly in elderly and frail individuals. Therefore, the other direction of technologic development has been the miniaturization of transducers which are now available with shafts of 6 mm diameter, tips which do not surpass 7 mm in diameter and with biplane capability. The latter probes are ideal for pediatric examination.

TWO-DIMENSIONAL TRANSESOPHAGEAL ECHOCARDIOGRAPHIC IMAGES

The technique of two-dimensional echocardiography was developed in the late 1960s.[17] Early approaches involved constructing an image from multiple B-mode scan lines. Signals were obtained through several cardiac cycles at points triggered by the electrocardiogram and a non-real-time image was then constructed. Observation of structures in motion was, of course, not possible with this method. Real-time scanning, which allows continuous observation of motion, is performed by rapidly steering the ultrasound beam through the desired angle previously described.

Classically, transthoracic echocardiograms are made from various positions on or around the chest known as "windows." The necessity of imaging through echocardiographic windows results from the very poor transmission of ultrasound through air and bone. Ribs, sternum, and lung tissue all must be avoided to produce a technically satisfactory transthoracic image. As mentioned earlier, the development of TEE was motivated by a desire to circumvent these obstructions.[9] Standard nomenclature has been developed by American Society of Echocardiography to describe the images obtained transthoracically.[44] This nomenclature has

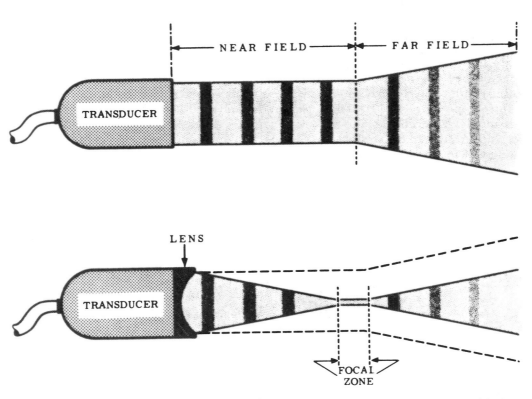

Fig. 11-14. The ultrasound beam remains parallel in the near field but begins to diverge in the far field can be minimized by focusing, accomplished in this instance with an acoustic lens. (From Feigenbaum,[16] with permission.)

been adapted to describe TEE images. The major conventional two-dimensional views fall in one of three planes: basal short axis, four chamber or long axis and transgastric short axis (Fig. 11-15). These planes refer to the manner in which the heart is viewed by the echocardiographic beam. An image inversion switch, incorporated into the echocardiograph, permits displaying the fan with the apex at either the top or the bottom of the monitor. Generally, the image orientation used for TEE is with the transducer (the apex of the fan) at the top of the image. With this orientation, the posterior structure is at the top of the image and the anterior structure at the bottom.

The standard TEE examination starts by inserting the TEE probe into the anesthetized patient by sliding it posteriorly into the hypopharynx. Many users find it helpful to elevate the tongue and larynx anteriorly with a laryngoscope before positioning. The endoscope should slide smoothly into position; no force should be required. The probe is then advanced to about 35 cm inside the esophagus when the aortic root, the superior vena cava and pulmonary artery or right ventricular outflow tract come into view (Fig. 11-16). This upper mediastinum view is used to assess aortic root processes including aortic dissection and aortic root abscesses. Advancing the probe a little further brings the upper portions of the left and right atria into view (Fig. 11-17). The left atrial appendage can be examined at that level by slight anteflexion of the probe with concomitant leftward lateral motion. The left atrial appendage examination is crucial to assess the presence of intra-atrial thrombus. In addition, adjacent to the left atrial appendage and behind a shelf of atrial tissue, the left pulmonary veins can be found and in situations of significant mitral regurgitation, the study of flow in the pulmonary veins is important as an adjunct index of the severity of mitral regurgitation. The right pulmonary veins can also be found by looking in the most medial aspect of the left atrium in the horizontal plane (0 degrees), but are also easily viewed by the multiplane probe by steering the plane to about 100 degrees and looking at the angle formed by the superior vena cava and the left atrium. Again, flow inside the right pulmonary veins can provide information about the severity of mitral regurgitation.

Also seen at this level are the right and left main coronary arteries (Figs. 11-16 and 11-18). The lat-

ter structure can be visualized in its entirety and the bifurcation into the left anterior descending and left circumflex coronary arteries can be seen in many patients. The right coronary artery is found in the majority of patients but it is less clear than the left main coronary artery due to its diameter relative to the resolution of TEE, which is still in the order of 1 to 2 mm.

A cross section of the aortic valve will display three leaflets, distinguishing a trileaflet from a bicuspid aortic valve (Fig. 11-19). Advancing the probe a small distance images the left ventricular outflow tract. The right and noncoronary cusps can be seen at this level, but not the left coronary cusp (Fig. 11-20). It may be hard to obtain a true cross section with the single-plane transducer, but it may be obtained with the multiplane transducer by steering the multiplane transducer to 35 degrees. Further steering of the transducer to 90 degrees will show the aortic root in a longitudinal view which is ideal for the assessment of aortic root abscess and for further assessment of a tissue flap of aortic root dissection. When using the biplane or multiplane transducer in the longitudinal plane (90 degrees), rotating the entire transducer clockwise will bring the superior and inferior vena cava into view, while rotation toward the counterclockwise direction will image the mitral valve and left ventricle. It is important to note that at 90 degrees one generally has a perfect view of the pulmonic valve and pulmonary artery immediately behind the aortic root. The assessment of rare vegetations affecting that valve and the assessment of pulmonic stenosis and infundibular stenosis is easy through this approach.

The mitral valve apparatus is frequently the landmark that most transesophageal echocardiographers seek as they advance the probe down the esophagus. The mitral valve appears with the anterior leaflet to the left and the posterior leaflet to the right if the plane is horizontal (Fig. 11-21). One is able to scan the entire mitral valve by just advancing the transducer 2 or 3 cm further down the esophagus. Alternatively, when using the biplane or multiplane transducer, one can steer the plane from the horizontal position to the vertical position at 90 degrees and observe the anterior leaflet in the center and posterior leaflet on both sides of the mitral annulus (Fig. 11-22). Thus, the mitral valve apparatus can be studied in its entirely by just

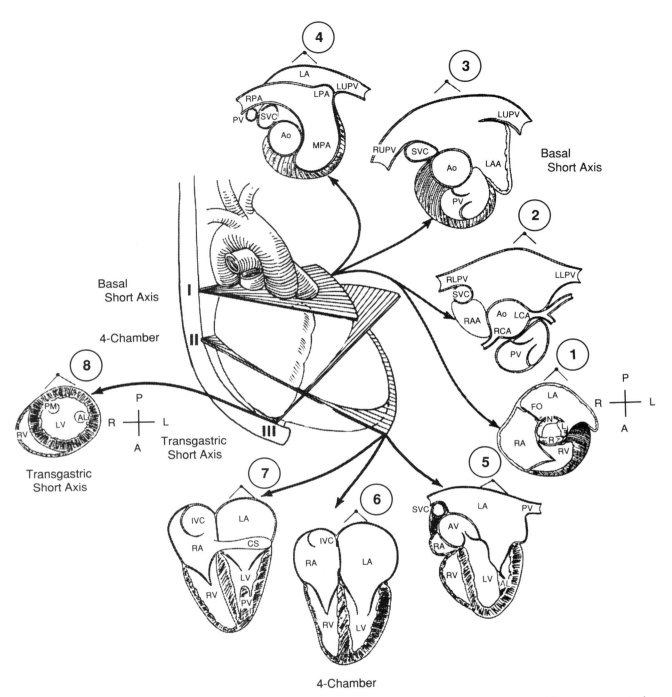

Fig. 11-15. Common horizontal scan planes for TEE studies (*I*) basal short-axis: (*1*) aortic root, (*2*) coronary arteries, (*3*) left atrial appendage, (*4*) pulmonary artery bifurcation. (*II*) Four-chamber (long-axis): (*5*) left ventricular outflow tract, (*6*) four-chamber view, (*7*) coronary sinus. (*III*) Transgastric short-axis: (*8*) ventricular short axis. AL, antero-lateral papillary muscle; AO, aorta; AV, aortic valve; CS, coronary sinus; FO, fossa ovalis; IVC, inferior vena cava; L, left coronary cusp; LA, left atrium; LAA, left atrial appendage; LCA, left coronary artery; LLPV, left lower pulmonary vein; LV, left ventricle; MPA, main pulmonary artery; N, noncoronary cusp; PM, posteromedial papillary muscles; PV, pulmonary valve or pulmonary vein; R, right coronary cusp; RA, right atrium, RAA, right atrial appendage; RCA, right coronary artery; RLPV, right lower pulmonary vein; RPA, right pulmonary artery; RUPV, right upper pulmonary vein; RV, right ventricle; SVC, superior vena cava. Directional axes: A, anterior; L, left; P, posterior; R, right. (From Seward et al.,[263] with permission.)

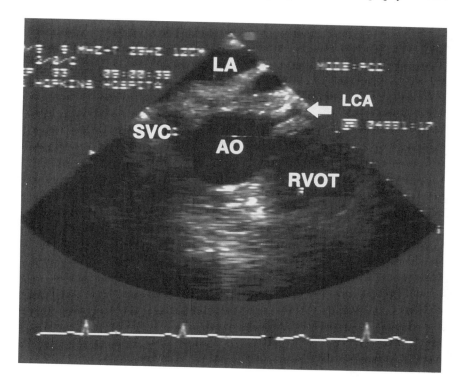

Fig. 11-16. Basal short axis view of the aortic root (AO), superior vena cava (SVC), left atrium (LA), right ventricular outflow tract (RVOT), and left main coronary artery (LCA).

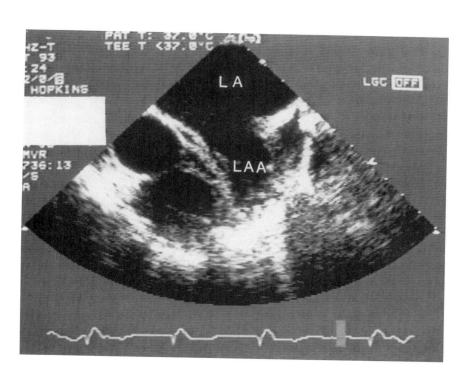

Fig. 11-17. TEE view of the left atrium (LA) and left atrial appendage (LAA).

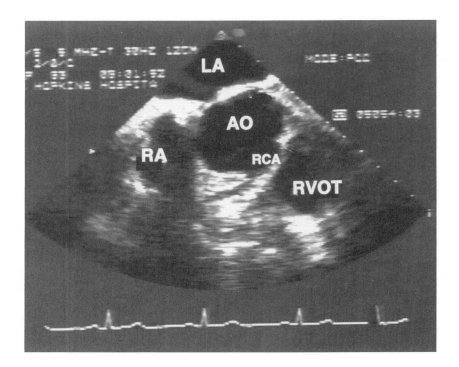

Fig. 11-18. TEE view of the aortic root (AO) at the level of the right coronary artery (RCA). LA, left atrium; RA, right atrium; RVOT, right ventricular outflow tract.

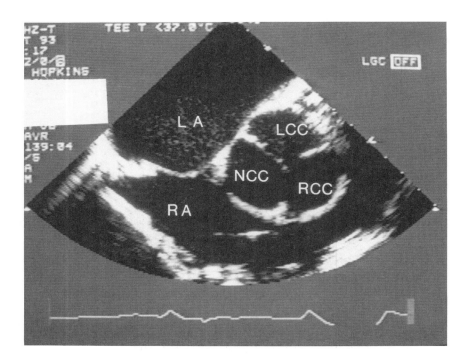

Fig. 11-19. Cross-sectional view of the aortic valve. LA, left atrium; LCC, left coronary cusp; NCC, noncoronary cusp; RCC, right coronary cusp; RA, right atrium.

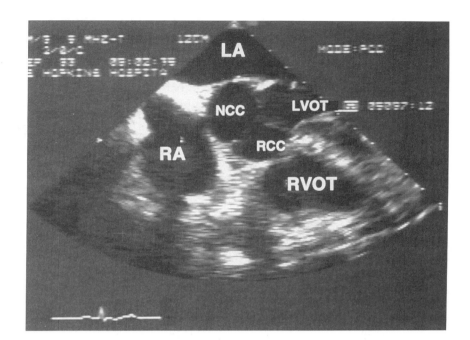

Fig. 11-20. TEE view of the aortic valve at the level of the left ventricular outflow tract (LVOT), also known as the three chamber view. NCC, noncoronary cusp; RCC, right coronary cusp; LA, left atrium; RA, right atrium; RVOT, right ventricular outflow tract.

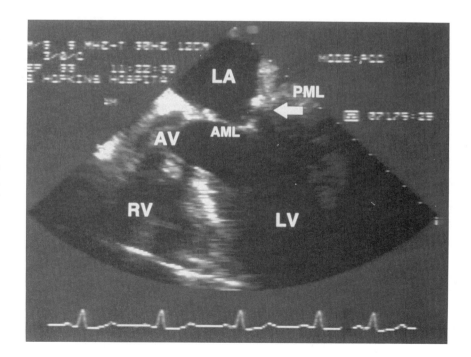

Fig. 11-21. TEE view of the mitral valve. AV, aortic valve; AML, anterior mitral leaflet; LA, left atrium; LV, left ventricle; PML, posterior mitral leaflet; RV, right ventricle.

steering the multiplane transducer or by manually advancing the biplane transducer.

The longitudinal view of the left ventricle is used to assess the size and the relationship between the left ventricle and other cardiac and extracardiac structures (Fig. 11-23). However, because the ultrasound beam is not perpendicular to the left ventricular wall, this view can be misleading in the more refined assessment of left ventricular function. The right ventricle and tricuspid valve can also be seen at this level in the horizontal plane (Fig. 11-24). The relationship of the right ventricle to the left ventricle is generally an important feature in the assessment of its size and function.

The short axis view of the left ventricle is obtained by advancing the transducer into the stomach and flexing the tip upward for better contact with the superior part of the stomach. The inferior wall will be displayed at the top, the septum to the left, the lateral wall to the right and the anterior wall at the bottom of the left ventricular cross section (Fig. 11-25). The left ventricular long axis view

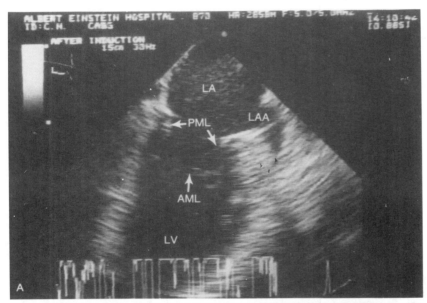

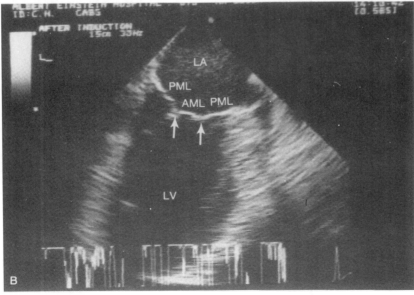

Fig. 11-22. TEE longitudinal view of the mitral valve. **(A)** Mitral valve is open in diastole. **(B)** Mitral valve is closed during systole with the anterior mitral leaflet depicted at the center, just below the mitral annulus. AML, anterior mitral valve leaflet; PML, posterior mitral valve leaflet; LA, left atrium; LV, left ventricle, LAA, left atrial appendage.

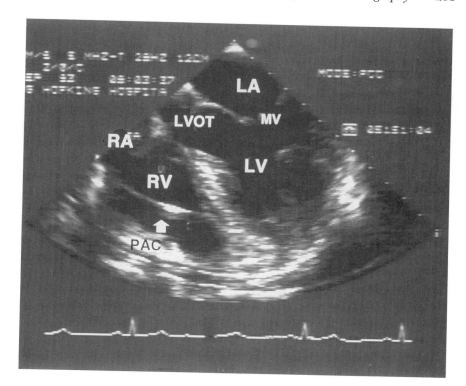

Fig. 11-23. TEE long axis of the left ventricle. LA, left atrium; LV, left ventricle; LVOT, left ventricular outflow tract; MV, mitral valve; PAC, pulmonary artery catheter; RA, right atrium; RV, right ventricle.

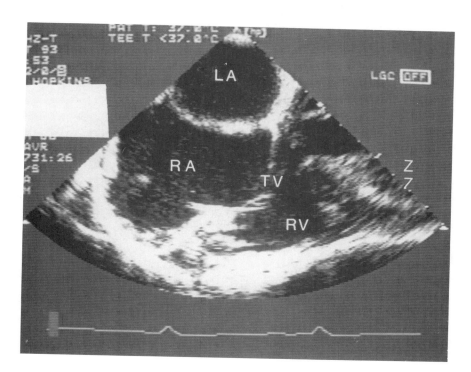

Fig. 11-24. TEE view of the right heart structures. LA, left atrium; RA, right atrium; RV, right ventricle; TV, tricuspid valve.

can be obtained by steering the multiplane transducer from the horizontal position to about 100 to 110 degrees, which will produce an image of the true inferior wall displayed at the top, and the anteroseptal portion of the left ventricle displayed below it. Left ventricular size and function can be assessed in a very precise fashion by the correct utilization of these transgastric views.

The TEE examination also includes viewing the thoracic descending aorta (Fig. 11-26). Obtaining orthogonal views with the biplane transducer or the multiplane transducer is ideal for further assessment of the ascending aorta for atherosclerotic plaques, thrombi, aortic dissection, and other aortic pathologic entities.

INTRAOPERATIVE USES OF TRANSESOPHAGEAL ECHOCARDIOGRAPHY

The indications for using TEE are listed in Table 11-1. It is used as an intraoperative monitor as well as a diagnostic tool in patients undergoing cardiac and non-cardiac surgery.[45] As an intraoperative monitor, it is used to detect air embolism, evaluate signs of myocardial ischemia, determine cardiac preload, and assess ventricular function. As a diagnostic tool, it is used to examine the heart and thoracic aorta for the presence of shunts, masses, and aneurysms. During cardiac surgery it is also used to evaluate the structure and function of native and prosthetic valves and the adequacy of valvular repair. The information obtained from TEE can be invaluable for patient management in the operating room and intensive care unit.

Monitoring for Air Embolism

The extremely intense reflection of ultrasound by air, a characteristic used to great advantage in contrast echocardiography, led investigators to examine the utility of echocardiography as an intraoperative monitor for air. Duff and coworkers[46] were among the first to study the feasibility of using ultrasound to detect intracardiac air. They studied open-chest dogs with epicardial M-mode echocardiography and were able to detect 1 ml of air consistently. False-positive results increased below this level. Furuya and coworkers,[47] using transesophageal M-mode, defined the threshold for air detection as 0.02 ml/kg as a bolus or 0.05 ml/kg/min.

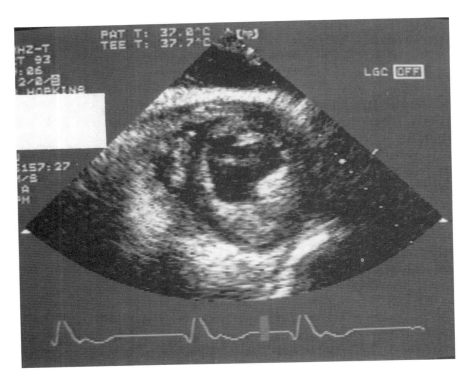

Fig. 11-25. TEE short axis view of the left ventricle.

They were able to detect air in four of five seated neurosurgery patients, often before changes were noted in other parameters, such as pulmonary artery pressure or end-tidal CO_2 concentration. Work by Glenski and colleagues[48] confirmed the sensitivity of TEE in detecting air as compared to other methods but noted the inability to either quantify physiologic changes or determine when air entrainment has ceased. Muzzi and colleagues[49] compared the sensitivity of the precordial Doppler with the TEE Doppler sensor to detect venous air embolism and found TEE Doppler to be more sensitive.

Several studies have demonstrated the usefulness of TEE to detect the presence of a patent foramen ovale and right to left shunting (Fig. 11-27).[50-65] A study comparing TEE with transthoracic echocardiography showed that a patent foramen ovale was found by contrast TEE in 50 of 238 patients compared with 45 patients by color Doppler transthoracic echocardiography.[51] Any condition that increases right atrial pressure in excess of left atrial pressure can result in right to left shunting and paradoxical embolism if a patent foramen ovale is present. Conditions under which this can occur which are pertinent to the operating room include

TABLE 11-1. Common Indications for Transesophageal Echocardiography

Operative	Nonoperative
Intracardiac air or embolism	Inadequate chest wall study
Masses	Low cardiac output
Myoxomas	Tamponade
Thrombus	Acute valve dysfunction
Ventricular function	Vegetations
Wall motion abnormalities (ischemia)	Atrial thrombus
Assess valve structure and function	
Assess shunts and septal repairs	
Aortic aneurysm and dissections	

an increase in right ventricular afterload as air passes through the right side of the heart, or as a result of hemodynamic changes that occur in the seated anesthetized patient, in the mechanically ventilated patient, and in the presence of cardiac tamponade.[59,62-65] Since the incidence of patent foramen ovale is reported to be approximately 25

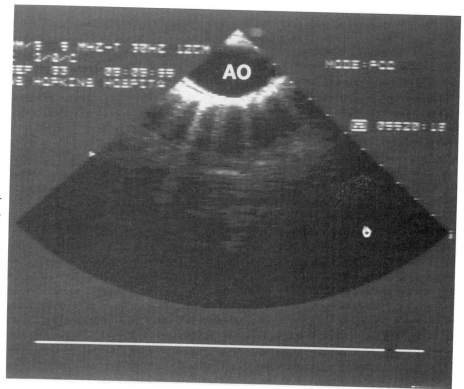

Fig. 11-26. TEE image of the descending thoracic aorta. AO, aorta.

percent by autopsy results[66] as well as by TEE studies,[51,56] using TEE as a preliminary screen could define patients at risk for paradoxical embolism and result in modification of surgical or anesthetic technique.[62] This is particularly important in patients undergoing neurosurgical procedures in the seated position to prevent venous air embolism. If a patent foramen ovale is present, right-to-left shunting at the atrial level is usually demonstrated with contrast echo at 20 cm water peak end-expiratory pressure (PEEP).[56,60,62] The prevalence of a patent foramen ovale has been found to be significantly increased in young adults with otherwise unexplained ischemic stroke.[51]

Persistent air in the left atrium or ventricle after open heart procedures has long been a concern of cardiac surgeons. The use of echocardiography intraoperatively documents the frequency with which microbubbles remain in the left heart after cardiopulmonary bypass.[1,2,42,67,68] Oka et al.[67,68] recommended aggressive maneuvers to eliminate microbubbles detected by echocardiography before discontinuing bypass. One of their patients had air visualized in his coronary arteries coincident with high concentrations of microbubbles, and another required reinstitution of cardiopulmonary bypass

to remove air from the ascending aorta; both patients died in the early postoperative period. On the other hand, microbubbles were detected in most of their noncoronary artery bypass surgery patients at some point after cardiopulmonary bypass with no reported long-term sequelae. In two other series of cardiac patients, Rodigas and colleagues[1] (79 patients) and Topol and colleagues[42] (82 patients) were unable to relate postoperative neurologic events to the presence or density of microbubbles after cardiopulmonary bypass. Topol and associates[42] additionally found that repetitive attempts by the surgeon to eradicate the microbubbles were unsuccessful.

Although it is clear that air is detected readily by TEE, the importance of this capability may depend on the clinical setting. In the case of a seated neurosurgical procedure where a small amount of air may be the forerunner of a sudden large and devastating air embolism, detection of microbubbles by TEE may be crucial. In cardiac surgery, on the other hand, the technique is perhaps overly sensitive, detecting microbubbles which thus far have not been shown to be of any clinical significance. It remains a possibility, however, that more sensitive neuropsychological testing will uncover subtle def-

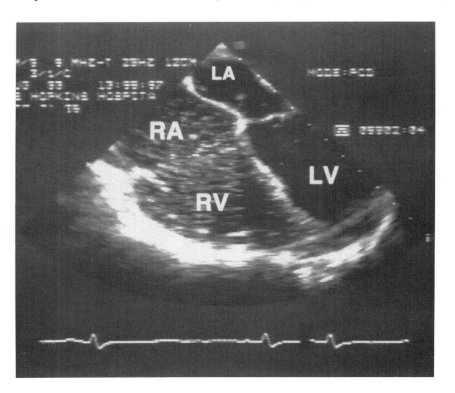

Fig. 11-27. Intracardiac air seen in the right atrium (RA) with a few echogenic bubbles passing across a patent foramen ovale into the left atrium (LA). LV, left ventricle; RV, right ventricle.

icits that could be attributed to the presence of even small amounts of left ventricular microbubbles after open-heart surgery.

Other situations where TEE may be a useful monitor of cardiac embolic phenomenon are during total hip arthroplasty (air and fat embolism)[69] and liver transplantation (air embolism during venoveno bypass).[70]

Monitoring Ventricular Function

Two-dimensional echocardiography is used to determine cardiac function[71,72] by measuring fractional area change, fractional shortening, or by estimating left ventricular volume and ejection fraction. The use of Doppler flow studies to measure cardiac output are currently being investigated.

Fractional Area of Contraction

Left ventricular fractional area change (FAC), also known as area ejection fraction, is the relative change in area of the left ventricular midcavity over

a cardiac cycle and is calculated as follows:

$$FAC = \frac{EDA - ESA}{EDA} \times 100$$

where EDA = end-diastolic area and ESA = end-systolic area (Fig. 11-28). The accuracy of this calculation can be improved by averaging the results from several cardiac cycles, whereas the applicability to global function is enhanced by repeating the calculation at several cross-sectional levels. The areas themselves are obtained by tracing the endocardial borders at end-diastole, synchronous with the R wave of the electrocardiogram, and end-systole, generally defined as the smallest cross sectional area. The tracing can be performed by hand or by a computerized system, for example, light pen. The papillary muscles are excluded from the cavity area by most authors.

The validity of transesophageal FAC measurements was tested by Konstadt and coworkers[73] by comparing them to simultaneous epicardial measurements, previously validated against ventriculo-

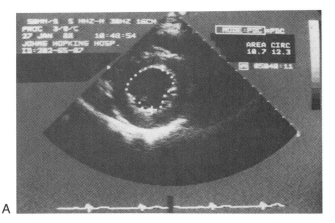

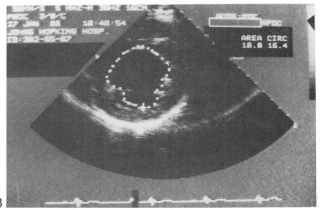

Fig. 11-28. Fractional area change (FAC) is calculated from left ventricular cross-sectional cavity areas at end-systole (**A**) and end-diastole (**B**).

graphic data. End-systolic area, end-diastolic area, and FAC derived by TEE all correlated highly with the respective epicardial measurements. Abel and colleagues[74] confirmed these findings in cardiac surgical patients and concluded that measurements of left ventricular area and FAC intraoperatively obtained by TEE were highly reproducible with minimal interobserver variability, a finding also reported by other groups.[75,76]

It is important to recognize that FAC is approximately 20 percent greater at the apex than at the base in the normal heart. Since absolute area change near the apex is small, the greatest contribution to forward flow comes from the basal region. The contribution of long-axis shortening to ejection fraction is only about 3 to 7 percent,[77] which explains the reasonable correlation obtained when this component is overlooked. Nonetheless, some authors have incorporated a correction factor to account for apical shortening based on visual analysis of apical motion.[3,77] Reproducible cross sections are necessary when serial studies are obtained. It should also be noted that FAC may not be an accurate reflection of ejection fraction in the presence of wall motion abnormalities.

Clinical studies have used FAC measured by TEE to evaluate ventricular function. Reichert and associates[78] studied the prognostic value of biventricular function using FAC assessed by TEE in 60 hypotensive (MAP $\leq$ 65 mmHg) patients after cardiac surgery and found a high mortality rate in patients with biventricular failure, especially right ventricular failure. Ayd and colleagues[79] used FAC to examine the effect of ventricular fibrillation and defibrillation on patients with depressed myocardial function. The results of that study showed that the mean FAC increased significantly while end-diastolic and end-systolic areas decreased significantly, suggesting that the defibrillated heart pumped into a decreased arterial impedance.

If simultaneous left ventricular pressure is available, pressure-area relationships can be plotted. Both systolic and diastolic function can be evaluated in this manner. The slope of the end-systolic pressure-dimension or pressure-area relationship at varied filling pressures (maximum elastance, E_{max}) is felt to be a good load-independent reflection of ventricular contractility.[80] This method of assessing contractility can be applied to the intraoperative investigation of myocardial depression by a variety of anesthetics. A variation of this method is to use systemic arterial pressure and TEE to calculate an end-systolic pressure relationship.[81,82] Similarly, left ventricular relaxation in early diastole[83] and compliance at end-diastole[4] can be assessed from the relationship between pressure and left ventricular cavity area at those time points.

Left Ventricular Volume

Volume of the left ventricle most commonly is obtained from one of the variations on Simpson's rule, which requires an accurate measurement of the long axis of the ventricular cavity. Since this dimension is difficult to obtain with single-plane TEE, most studies have relied on area change to describe left ventricular function.

Several studies document a reasonable correlation between angiographically and echocardiographically derived ejection fraction.[3,77,84–88] Most of these studies were performed transthoracically using orthogonal views, generally felt to improve the accuracy of the measurement[86,87] but difficult to obtain with single plane TEE. Despite the good correlation found for ejection fraction calculations, some,[85,86,89–91] but not all,[88] investigators found that two-dimensional echocardiography consistently underestimated left ventricular volume when compared to ventriculography. This error that influences the measurement of left ventricular volume at both end-diastole and end-systole cancels out when ejection fraction is determined.[77] Volume is thought to be underestimated because the innermost surface of the left ventricle is contoured on the echocardiogram, whereas during ventriculography, contrast material can fill the interstices between trabeculae, leading to endocardial measurement at its outermost point.[90,91]

Folland and colleagues[85] tested a variety of formulas for volume calculation and found a modified Simpson's rule gives the best correlation with angiographic results. Simpson's rule divides the ventricle into serial cross sections that are reconstructed to derive volume. The modified approach uses three equal divisions, modeled as a cylinder, a truncated cone and a cone (Fig. 11-29). Stamm and coworkers[87] concurred that the Simpson's rule model yields the best correlation with ventriculography, but noted that all the requisite measurements may not be obtainable in as many as 50 percent of patients. The lack of an optimal method of calculating left ventricular volume and ejection fraction from two-dimensional echocardiography is apparent from the multitude of variations on this theme that have been reported.[84–89] On the other hand, angiography may not be the best gold standard for volume determination,[60,61] leading to some of the variability in the literature.

Thys and associates[92] used two-dimensional echocardiography in cardiac surgery patients to obtain end-systolic and end-diastolic areas which they used to derive end-systolic and end-diastolic volumes using a modified ellipsoid model. These data were used to compute an echo-derived cardiac index which they found had a good correlation ($r = .80$) with thermodilution cardiac output. Urbanowicz and colleagues[93] compared single plane TEE and scintigraphic estimates of left ventricular end-diastolic volume index and ejection fraction in patients after coronary bypass surgery. A good correlation ($r = .82$) was found between ejection fraction area by TEE and ejection fraction by scintigraphy, but only fair correlation ($r = .74$) between end-diastolic area and left ventricular end-diastolic volume index, which was derived from ejection fraction scintigraphy and cardiac output. Thus, they concluded that a single plane TEE image provided a reasonable estimate of ejection fraction, but not left ventricular end-diastolic index. Martin and colleagues[94] compared left ventricular ejection fraction in dogs measured with reconstructed three dimensional images using a multiplane TEE probe, radionuclide ejection fraction and thermodilution and found a good correlation ($r = .87$) between

them, concluding that the measurements were comparable. This group of investigators then compared single-plane and multiplane TEE with radionuclide derived ejection fraction and found the multiplane probe to be more accurate than the single-plane probe.[95]

Clinical Applicability

Many of the methods of measuring left ventricular function require off-line digitizing of still frames, and they do not lend themselves easily to intraoperative patient care. The TEE technology has now advanced so that beat-to-beat ejection fraction can be calculated on-line and displayed on the echocardiograph monitor. Thus, TEE can be very useful for monitoring global cardiac function during surgery.

With moderate experience, one can acquire sufficient skills to observe major changes in left ventricular function or volume, often at times when invasive hemodynamic measurements are inconclusive. Since preload is better estimated by left ventricular end-diastolic volume than end-diastolic pressure and since changes in compliance can alter the relationship between volume and pressure, left ventricular end-diastolic area may be superior to pulmonary artery occluded (wedge) pressure as a reflection of left ventricular preload.[71,92]

Several investigators have examined the use of Doppler flow studies to measure cardiac output and ventricular filling.[24,25,97–99] Perrino and colleagues[25] and Roewer and colleagues[97] compared thermodilution cardiac output with TEE Doppler derived cardiac output and found very good correlations of $r = .91$ and $r = .95$, respectively. The echo derived cardiac output was obtained by measuring transmitral flow velocity and multiplying the total area under the transmitral Doppler flow velocity display times the cross sectional area of the mitral valve times the heart rate. However, studies by LaMantia and coworkers[98] and Muhuideen and coworkers[24] did not result in such good correlations ($r = .68$ and .24, respectively). Attempts to use pulmonary artery Doppler flow velocities were limited by the ability to adequately visualize the main pulmonary artery.[98] Kuecherer and colleagues[96] showed that pulmonary venous flow measured by TEE pulsed Doppler can be used to estimate mean left atrial pressure.

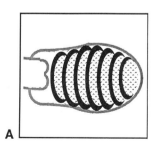
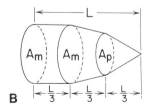

Fig. 11-29. Varying portrayals of Simpson's rule for calculation of left ventricular volume. **(A)** In the original form of Simpson's rule, the ventricle is divided into a series of slices. **(B)** In the modified Simpson's rule, the ventricle is divided into three slices, which can be geometrically modeled as a cylinder, a truncated cone, and a cone. (Figure B modified from Folland et al.,[85] with permission.)

Evaluation of Regional Myocardial Function and Perfusion

Normal Versus Abnormal Motion

The normal ventricular wall thickens during systole with resultant inward motion of the endocardial surface and reduction in ventricular cavity area. The pattern of inward endocardial motion is defined in terms of its vigor, with the terms hypokinesis used to describe segments that move more sluggishly than normal, akinesis to designate segments that neither move nor thicken during systole, and dyskinesis to describe outward or paradoxical systolic motion, often accompanied by thinning. In the clinical setting, endocardial motion is often evaluated qualitatively because normal motion is relatively easily separated from the other three categories.

The evaluation of wall motion abnormalities requires a careful, segment-by-segment visual examination (Fig. 11-30).[16,44,100] The short axis view at the midpapillary muscle is most often used to detect wall motion abnormalities because at this level, areas of myocardium supplied by the three major coronary arteries are represented. The short axis view is divided into segments: anterior, lateral, inferior, and septal. The left anterior descending artery supplies the anterior and anteroseptal wall, the circumflex artery supplies the lateral wall and the right coronary artery supplies the inferior and inferoseptal wall (Fig. 11-31). Of course, wall motion abnormalities may occur at other levels of the ventricle due to disease of more peripheral arterioles. However, the midpapillary muscle level gives the best qualitative impression of ventricular contraction by wall thickening and endocardial motion.

The examination for wall motion abnormalities is aided by several computerized systems. Some equipment allows one to recall earlier scans for simultaneous comparison, so that changes are more readily apparent. Another method allows gating of the image to the electrocardiogram (ECG), so that one may flip back and forth between two time points, such as end-systole and end-diastole, comparing endocardial position without the distraction of the intervening motion. More recently, cine loop technology has become available so that selected images remain in the memory of the echocardiograph computer and can be recalled in a split screen to compare images at different time points.

Various attempts have been made to define endocardial motion more quantitatively and therefore presumably more objectively. The biggest problem is the need to correct for movement of

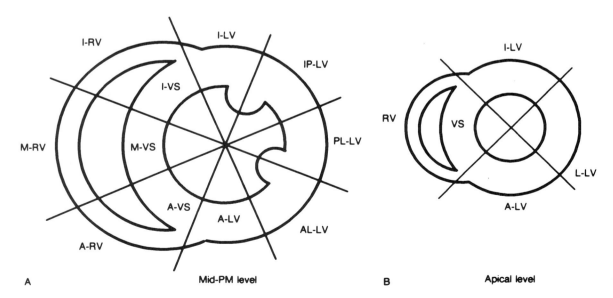

Fig. 11-30. Segmental division of the left ventricle at the midpapillary muscle (PM) level (A) and apical level (B). A, anterior; AL, anterolateral; I, inferior; IP, inferoposterior; LV, left ventricle; M, middle; PL, posterolateral; RV, right ventricle; VS, ventricular septum. (From Hong and Oka,[264] with permission.)

the heart within the thorax when overlaying systolic and diastolic images. Heart motion can be translational, rotational, or both, whereas correction systems fall into two general categories, fixed reference and floating reference. In a fixed reference system, a point either internal or external to the cardiac silhouette is overlaid, and no attempt is made to correct for a change in the position of the heart between systole and diastole. A floating reference system has a reproducible point such as the center of mass determined for both systolic and diastolic images, and these are matched when the images are overlaid (Fig. 11-32). If a radius, such as the left ventricular long axis, or two points, such as the papillary muscles, are used, rather than a single point, rotational correction is also achieved.

The amplitude of motion of various myocardial segments has been shown to vary with the reference system used.[101,102] Parisi and colleagues[103] compared a fixed external reference system to one with a floating reference and found the fixed system to be superior for localizing contraction defects. Schnittger and colleagues[102] evaluated 44 different reference methods in terms of three factors: sensitivity and specificity in separating normal and abnormal hearts, ability to identify abnormal segments as compared to evaluation by an experienced observer, and reproducibility. They found significant differences in measured contraction, both between reference systems and from view to view within one reference system. As a result of their evaluation, they selected optimal systems for each echocardiographic view. For the apical four-chamber and mitral valve short-axis views, this was a floating system with correction for translation only. In the short-axis papillary muscle view, a fixed external method was best, since very little translation or rotation of the heart was seen at this level. The absence of motion was ascribed to the concept that the mid ventricle is the fulcrum around which the other levels move. The papillary view had a narrower band of normal values than the mitral and

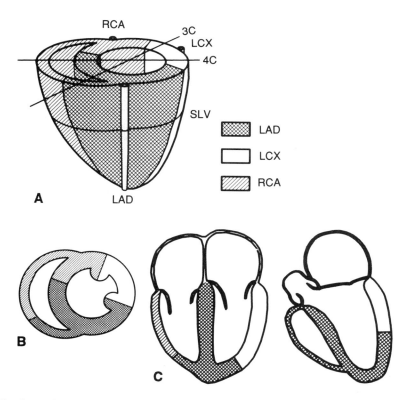

Fig. 11-31. Distribution of the coronary arteries to the ventricles (*top diagram*), in the short axis view (**A**), four-chamber view (**B**), and the three chamber view (**C**). 3C, level of three chamber view; 4C, level of four chamber view; LAD, left anterior descending artery; LCX, left circumflex artery; RCA, right coronary artery; SLV, level of short axis view. (From Hong and Oka,[264] with permission.)

was more sensitive (95 vs 75 percent), although less specific (95 percent vs 100 percent). The apical four-chamber view was the most sensitive (96 percent) but the least specific (69 percent). Reproducibility was good overall, but individual cases showed variation from day to day.

The setting of coronary artery bypass surgery changes some of these relationships. For instance, several investigators have shown significant anteromedial translation of the heart after open heart surgery.[10,104–108] The exaggerated translation leads to apparent abnormal motion of the interventricular septum when the heart is examined from a fixed reference system.[104] This abnormal motion of the interventricular septum commonly seen after cardiopulmonary bypass has been shown not to be caused by removal of restraining forces of the pericardium or anterior mediastinum, but to be directly related to events occurring during cardiopulmonary bypass.[109]

Once the reference system has been selected, wall motion can be quantified by either fractional shortening along multiple radii or fractional area change of wedge-shaped subdivisions of the ventricular cavity. Most investigators have found either no difference between the two or a slight advantage of the area over the radial method.[78,103] Generally, 5- to 30-degree sampling intervals have been recommended, although Schnittger and coworkers[75] found the same sensitivity and specificity up to 45-degree intervals.

Several other problems arise in wall motion anal-

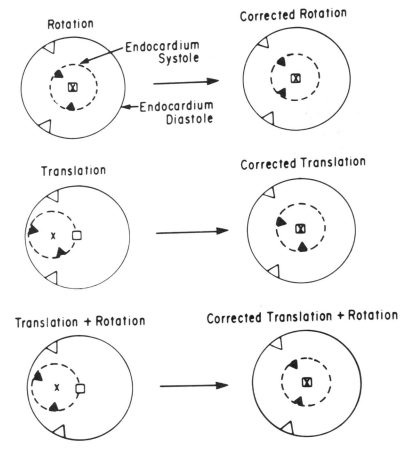

Fig. 11-32. Diagrams of systolic and diastolic endocardial borders as they would appear in a fixed reference system (without correction for translation or rotation of the heart between systole and diastole), left, and after correction for motion by floating axis reference systems, right. (From Clements and de Bruijn,[265] with permission.)

ysis. Under normal conditions, the inward excursion of the endocardium varies a great deal from segment to segment.[76,110] It thus becomes difficult to define hypokinesis as abnormal, when the basis for its definition is merely the movement of adjacent segments or some preconceived notion of what normal motion should be. However, neither akinesis nor dyskinesia is seen in normal ventricles. In addition, temporal heterogeneity of systolic function has been described by Weyman and colleagues.[111] In a group of infarcted segments, maximum outward movement occurred at varying time points during systole. In only 39 percent did the dyskinesia persist to end-systole. The authors concluded that simple measurement of endocardial excursion at two time points (end-systole and end-diastole) may fail to detect important wall motion abnormalities.

To avoid some of the technical difficulties involved in the quantitative assessment of wall motion, some authors have measured systolic wall thickening (SWT).[112–116]

$$SWT\ (\%) = \frac{SWT - DWT}{DWT} \times 100$$

where SWT = end-systolic wall thickness and DWT = end-diastolic wall thickness. Estimates of normal wall thickening in humans range from 0 to 150 percent with means ranging from 20 to 54 percent.[76,113,117] Similar to endocardial motion, heterogeneity has been described both from base to apex and from segment to segment at the same cross sectional level.[76,117] Temporal asynergy of contraction has also been described; that is, some segments reach peak SWT earlier in systole than others.[117] The contraction pattern varies substantially among individuals, but thinning of the ventricular wall during systole is never thought to be a normal event. SWT distinguishes infarcted from noninfarcted tissue better than wall motion.[114]

SWT is generally analyzed off-line using a computerized division of a ventricular cross section into multiple segments (Fig. 11-33).[114,116,117] The use of SWT, rather than wall motion, avoids the problems of translation and rotation and is generally thought to be a more accurate method of assessing regional left ventricular function.[92,114,118] Its major drawback is the need for accurate epicardial as well as endocardial contours,[92] which some investigators have found problematic.[74] Nonetheless, several reports

suggest that SWT measurements in humans are accurate.[113,119] Voci and associates[120] found SWT more reliable and consistent compared with the qualitative assessment of segmental wall motion immediately after coronary bypass surgery. The use of two-dimensional echocardiography for measuring wall thickening has been validated against intramyocardial transmural sonomicrometers.[119]

The epicardium is often hard to adequately visualize, making SWT measurements difficult. As an alternative, observing the movement of the endocardium toward the center of the ventricular cavity during systole can give an assessment of wall motion abnormalities, known as radial shortening.[119] Normal wall contraction is defined as a radial shortening of 30 percent. Mild hypokinesis is associated with radial shortening of 10 to 30 percent and severe hypokinesis with radial shortening of less than 10 percent.

Neither wall motion abnormalities nor decreased wall thickening is 100 percent specific for ischemia. These changes have been seen as well with increased left ventricular wall tension, prior infarction, and focal myocarditis and infiltrative dis-

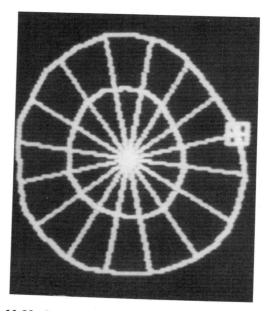

Fig. 11-33. Systolic wall thickening is determined by computerized division of the left ventricular wall into from 8 to 32 separate segments. Wall thickening during systole is then calculated by comparing systolic to diastolic thickness for each segment.

eases.[39,101] Serial observation is critical because acute regional changes are more likely to be indicative of ischemia than chronic or global abnormalities.

Correlation of Regional Function and Perfusion

Since the original observation by Tennant and Wiggers[121] that ligation of a coronary artery would result in immediate and progressively severe wall motion abnormalities in the subtended myocardium, the relationship between perfusion and regional myocardial function has been extensively studied. Investigators primarily have used two approaches to the problem. One compares wall motion or thickening to regional blood flow, assessed by microspheres in the laboratory or by thallium scintigraphy in humans, whereas the other compares regional function to pathologic specimens, correlating the degree of dysfunction with extent of necrosis.

Kerber and colleagues[122] showed a direct relationship between declining perfusion and extent of wall motion abnormalities as assessed by M-mode echocardiography in the dog. These abnormalities persisted after 45 minutes of coronary occlusion and 30 minutes of reperfusion. Similarly, Blumenthal and colleagues[112] demonstrated a linear relationship between regional blood flow and systolic thickening. As with Kerber's animals, in areas of normalized flow the regional thickening remained reduced to 39 percent of control. A biochemical basis was suggested to explain prolonged functional abnormalities in areas of transient ischemia. Finally, Gallagher and colleagues[123] compared wall thickening (measured by sonomicrometry) to transmural flow distribution. They discovered that subendocardial blood flow correlates best with regional thickening. A 45 percent decrease in systolic thickening was seen when flow was reduced only to the inner 25 percent of the left ventricular wall, whereas a 75 percent decrease was seen with reduced flow to the inner 50 percent. Dyskinesia was seen only during transmural ischemia.

Overestimation of both ischemic area and infarct size (based on analysis of regional myocardial function) has been a common finding.[112,118,122,124–127] Various explanations have been proposed for this phenomenon. Since transiently ischemic myocardium can function when abnormally perfused but abnormally functioning segments are always adjacent to ischemic or infarcted tissue, some authors have suggested "partial" or reversible ischemia as the underlying cause.[127] Lima and colleagues[126] however, showed no improvement in function in such regions when local blood flow was significantly enhanced with dipyridamole, making an ischemic basis less likely. Another possibility is that mechanical tethering of the adjacent normal segments to the ischemic ones contributes to their seemingly abnormal function, perhaps as a result of changes in ventricular shape.[112,114,122,126] Force and colleagues[124] analyzed the relative contribution to the overestimate by tethering as opposed to errors introduced as a result of the algorithm used to determine regional function. Tethering was found to cause only about 50 percent of the overestimation. The remainder results from a shift in the center of mass during systole toward the dysfunctional segment as a result of contraction of the normal contralateral wall (Fig. 11-34). Systolic expansion of the dysfunctional segment or hypercontractility of the opposite segment could worsen the overestimate since the abnormal segment would then occupy an even greater percentage of the circumference during systole. The authors concluded that since the function of the uninvolved myocardium is variable, the degree by which infarct size is overestimated is unpredictable.

The ability to detect myocardial infarction in humans using echocardiography has been studied by several groups.[100,127–130] Heger and associates[100] found that asynergy by two-dimensional echocardiography correlated reliably with the site of infarction based on evolving Q waves on the ECG. Horowitz and coworkers[129] studied 80 patients with acute chest pain, obtaining 65 adequate studies. Of 33 patients with clinical evidence of myocardial infarction, 18 of whom had nondiagnostic initial electrocardiograms, 31 had regional wall motion abnormalities on the admission echocardiogram, whereas 27 of 32 patients without infarction had normal wall motion. Of the five patients with false-positive results, three had severe coronary artery disease documented by cardiac catheterization during their hospitalization. Echocardiography proved to be an effective screening tool to select patients who were at high risk for subsequent complications. Additional work by Massie and coworkers[131] supports the finding that asynergy in noninfarcted tissue suggests significant impairment of perfusion.

Intraoperative Monitoring for Ischemia

The major impetus for using echocardiographic monitoring for ischemia in the operating room is the recognition that ischemia will not always be detected by the ECG.[132] This was demonstrated in dogs by Waters and colleagues.[133] Regional mechanical function began to deteriorate when regional coronary flow was decreased to 48 percent of control (simultaneous with the onset of lactate production). In four of six dogs with epicardial ECG recorded, ST-segment changes were not observed until greater reductions in flow were produced. Battler and colleagues[134] further quantified the relationship. Complete coronary occlusion resulted in hypokinesis in 15 seconds and dyskinesis in 1 minute, and ST segments changed on the surface ECG in 30 seconds. During mild partial occlusion, on the other hand, systolic wall thickening decreased by 25 percent but no ECG changes were noted. More severe partial stenosis (25 to 48 percent decrease in wall thickening) produced ECG changes in 4 minutes, significantly later than the onset of functional changes. Ischemia which occurs in the perioperative period is more comparable to that seen during experimental partial stenosis than to total occlusion;[92] in this setting, ECG changes are often not seen or, at best, lag behind regional echocardiographic changes.

Since intraoperative ischemia has been associated with perioperative myocardial infarction, the earliest possible detection and treatment of ischemia should be encouraged.[135] It has been clearly shown that wall motion abnormalities detected by intraoperative TEE are very sensitive markers for myocardial ischemia. Beaupre and colleagues[136] reported intraoperative diagnosis of myocardial infarction despite nonspecific ECG changes in a patient undergoing mitral valve replacement. Smith and colleagues[132] studied 50 patients undergoing either cardiac or major vascular surgery. New wall motion abnormalities developed in 24 patients during surgery, with persistence at the time of skin closure in 8 patients. Only 6 patients had ST-segment changes. Four patients had perioperative infarctions; all had new wall motion abnormalities, but only one had intraoperative ECG evidence of ischemia. Leung and colleagues[137] prospectively studied 50 patients undergoing cardiac surgery using continuous TEE, ECG, and hemodynamic measurements to determine the prognostic importance of wall motion abnormalities pre- and post-cardiopulmonary bypass. Their results showed that

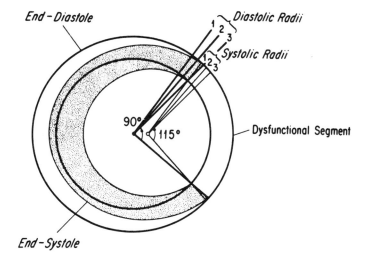

Fig. 11-34. Demonstration of the effect of a shifting center of mass on the apparent size of a dysfunctional myocardial segment. Sixty-four equally spaced radii are generated from both the systolic and the diastolic center of mass, and then compared on the basis of their position. Since the center of mass has shifted between systole and diastole, diastolic radii 1, 2, and 3, which intersect normally contracting myocardium during systole, are matched by the analysis algorithm with systolic radii 1, 2, and 3, which intersect abnormally contracting myocardium. The extent of dysfunction is thereby assessed as 32 percent rather than 25 percent of the left ventricular circumference. (From Force et al.,[124] with permission.)

postcardiopulmonary bypass TEE ischemia was predictive of outcome. Of 18 patients with TEE evidence of ischemia, 6 had adverse outcomes versus none of 32 patients without TEE ischemia. However, some investigators have questioned the value of TEE in predicting adverse outcomes, particularly in patients undergoing noncardiac surgery. London and colleagues[138] continuously monitored 12-lead ECG and TEE in 156 high-risk patients undergoing noncardiac surgery and found that approximately 40 percent of the episodes of TEE ischemia were unaccompanied by clinical events or significant hemodynamic changes and that these episodes were poorly correlated with postoperative cardiac complications.

TEE has been applied to the evaluation of ischemia during various surgical procedures and drug interventions. Topol and coworkers[116] using both systolic wall thickening and visually graded wall motion, showed significant improvement in dysfunctional but noninfarcted myocardial segments immediately after revascularization. Segments demonstrating the most severe dysfunction preoperatively were improved to the greatest extent. The improvement was persistent at the time of postoperative evaluation 1 to 2 weeks later. Abel and coworkers[74] reported approximately equal numbers of segments improving and deteriorating under similar conditions as assessed only by visual wall motion analysis. The effect of thoracic epidural anesthesia combined with general anesthesia on segmental wall motion was assessed using TEE.[139] Segmental wall motion neither worsened nor improved with this anesthetic technique. The effect of varying levels of aortic cross-clamping during surgery for repair of aortic aneurysm was studied by Roizen and colleagues.[140] Most significant effects followed aortic occlusion at the supraceliac level. Left ventricular end-systolic and end-diastolic areas increased significantly, ejection fraction decreased, and wall motion abnormalities were frequently noted. Conventional hemodynamic monitoring, including pulmonary artery pressure measurement, was not sensitive in detecting these changes.

Diagnosis of Shunts

Several studies have described the use of TEE to diagnose the presence of shunts in adults due to septal defects,[141–144] patent ductus arteriosus,[145,146] and fistulas.[147–154] In addition, there are an increasing number of reports on the use of TEE in the evaluation of congenital heart defects in children.[155–161]

When looking for atrial septal defects, the problem of echo "dropout" of the interatrial septum is of particular concern. False-positive diagnoses could be made on the basis of this artifact. The optimal way to avoid such dropout is to image the structure in question perpendicularly. In the case of the atrial septum, TEE is particularly advantageous because the septum is perpendicular to the ultrasound beam from this approach (Fig. 11-35).[143,162] Hanrath and colleagues[162] were able to identify correctly an atrial septal defect in 19 of 20 patients and to diagnose normal atrial septa in 30 of 30 controls. The use of peripheral venous contrast was 100 percent sensitive in confirming the diagnosis. These results were superior to those obtained by transthoracic echocardiography. Mehta and colleagues[163] diagnosed 19 of 19 atrial shunts with TEE in contrast to 16 of 18 shunts with transthoracic echocardiography. Using Doppler color flow mapping the calculated shunt flow volume correlated well ($r = .91$) with that obtained at cardiac catheterization. Morimoto and coworkers[143] had similar results using pulsed and color flow Doppler TEE for diagnosing secundum atrial septal defects.

Diagnosis of Intracardiac Masses

Intracardiac masses that are well visualized by TEE include thrombus (Fig. 11-36),[164–172] myxomas (Fig. 11-37),[39,173–178] and a reported case of intracardiac lymphoma.[179] TEE has been found to be superior to transthoracic echocardiography in identifying left atrial thrombus.[170,180–182] Of 21 patients with mitral stenosis in whom neither transthoracic echocardiography nor cardiac catheterization demonstrated left atrial thrombus, 6 were found to have thrombi in the left atrial appendage by TEE.[170] Of interest, the left atrial appendage was seen in only 4 of 21 transthoracic studies. The presence or absence of thrombus was confirmed at surgery; TEE was 100 percent sensitive and specific in this group of patients for the diagnosis of left atrial thrombus. Likewise, 14 of 29 patients studied by Daniel and associates[171] had left atrial thrombi demonstrated by TEE; none of those thrombi had been detected on transthoracic examination. Cohen and associates[183] used TEE in diagnosing right sided cardiac lesions in 19 patients with indwelling catheters and found TEE to be superior to transthoracic echocardiography. Although intracardiac tumors are generally diagnosed by conventional transthoracic echocardiography, intraoperative echocardiography has proven useful for evaluating the extent of tumor invasion, the adequacy of excision and the competence of the mitral valve and atrial septum before and after tumor removal. TEE has also been used to evaluate pericardial[184] and paracardiac neoplastic masses.[185] An inverted left atrial appendage appearing as a left atrial mass has been reported.[186]

Examination of Native and Prosthetic Valve Structure and Function

Even before TEE became widely available, the significant advantage of immediate and accurate assessment of valvular function after valve repair or replacement was documented with epicardial two-dimensional echocardiography.[37,38,40,187] Eguaras and coworkers[37] demonstrated the high correlation between intraoperative two-dimensional contrast in assessing the presence and severity of valvular regurgitation. Goldman and coworkers[38] reported their experience with intraoperative echocardiography in 263 patients. Of 50 mitral valve repairs for stenosis or regurgitation, 8 were found to be inadequate due to excessive mitral regurgitation af-

ter the repair. These patients underwent immediate mitral valve replacement. Of 120 patients, 9 had residual tricuspid regurgitation after left heart procedures that warranted immediate tricuspid annuloplasty. They concluded that echocardiography permits rapid and accurate assessment of valvular regurgitation after valve repair or replacement and impacts significantly on intraoperative management.

The usefulness of TEE for assessment of valve reconstruction, replacement, and commissurotomy is well known and has become a standard practice at many institutions.[14,39,40,187–200] Drexler and colleagues[188] were one of the first to report on the use of TEE for assessment of valve reconstruction. They reported results similar to Goldman and colleagues[38] using TEE rather than epicardial echocardiography. Schluter and colleagues[20] were among the first to apply TEE pulsed Doppler to the evaluation of mitral regurgitation. They studied 12 patients with and 6 patients without angiographically documented mitral regurgitation from the transesophageal, the parasternal long axis, and the apical positions. In each case, the sample volume was placed in the left atrium just posterior to the valve leaflets. Mitral regurgitation was detected with 100 percent sensitivity by TEE, but with only 58 percent sensitivity by transthoracic examination despite, in some cases, moderately severe regurgitation. In addition to the usual TEE advantage,

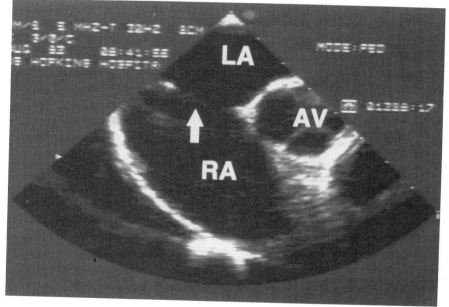

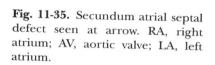

Fig. 11-35. Secundum atrial septal defect seen at arrow. RA, right atrium; AV, aortic valve; LA, left atrium.

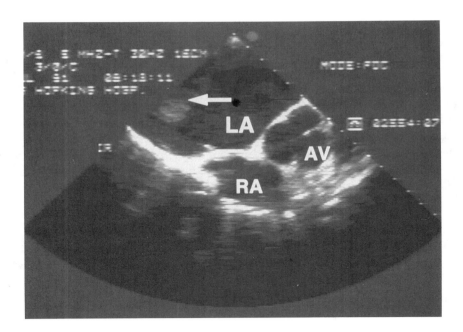

Fig. 11-36. Left atrial thrombus seen at arrow. LA, left atrium; RA, right atrium; AV, aortic valve.

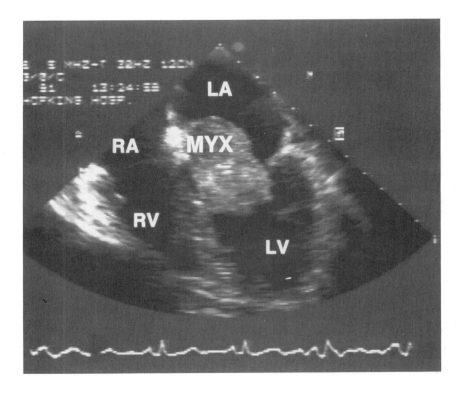

Fig. 11-37. Left atrial myxoma attached to the atrial septum and obstructing the mitral valve. LA, left atrium; RA, right atrium; RV, right ventricle; LV, left ventricle; MYX, myxoma.

namely absence of anatomic interference, they felt the superior results could be explained by the more parallel alignment of the sample volume with blood flow and the higher pulse repetition frequency. The parasternal approach interrogated transmitral flow almost perpendicularly, whereas the apical approach was hindered by the relatively large distance between the transducer and the mitral valve, limiting pulse repetition frequency.

Kenny and colleagues[201] evaluated 21 patients (with Doppler echocardiography) 2 to 14 days after ring annuloplasty for mitral regurgitation, confirming a reduction in regurgitation in most patients. One patient continued to have 4+ regurgitation, was not symptomatically improved, and required subsequent mitral valve replacement. Clearly it would be advantageous to detect such patients intraoperatively to eliminate the need for additional surgery.

The addition of the color flow modality has been of significant benefit. Intraoperative color flow mapping has been shown to correlate well with preoperative angiographic assessment of valvular regurgitation.[198] Doppler echocardiography and color Doppler flow mapping have been touted as permitting immediate intraoperative decision making.[198] In addition, any changes that have developed between the time of preoperative evaluation and surgery will be apparent on the intraoperative Doppler examination.

The main limitation to evaluation of mitral or other valvular regurgitation by Doppler is that the results are at best semiquantitative (as, of course, is angiography). Most studies quantify regurgitation on a 1 to 4+ scale based on extension into the atrium,[198,200–205] yet it is well recognized that a high velocity jet can extend far into the atrium and still represent minor regurgitation in terms of overall volume. Maximal velocity of the regurgitant flow is similarly unhelpful. This problem might be somewhat less significant in the operating room, where regurgitation before and after an intervention is being compared, or when any more than minimal regurgitation is felt to be abnormal, for example after valve replacement. (It should be noted that a small amount of tricuspid and pulmonic regurgitation are seen in a large percentage of normal individuals.)

Another approach, proposed by Helmcke and colleagues,[206] is to express the mitral regurgitant jet area as a fraction of left atrial area. Obtaining valid results by this method requires that the regurgitant jet be examined in three planes to assure that maximal jet area is found. In this series, the ratio of jet area to left atrial area was less than 0.20 in 34 of 36 patients with mild regurgitation, between 0.20 and 0.40 in 17 of 18 patients with moderate regurgitation, and greater than 0.40 in 26 of 28 patients with severe regurgitation by ventriculography. A more recent study reported that the severity of mitral regurgitation is best assessed by measuring the width of the regurgitant jet at its origin.[207]

Generally speaking, patients who are candidates for mitral valve repair have localized pathology (Fig. 11-38; Plate 11-3). Myxomatous degeneration of the mitral valve with localized scalloping of the posterior leaflet, ruptured chordae in the posterior leaflet, ischemic mitral annular dilatation and certain cases of infective endocarditis (Plate 11-4) are ideal for valve repair.[208,209] In most cases of valve repair, the diseased segment of the valve is resected and the valve leaflet is resutured with or without an annuloplasty ring. If the anterior leaflet is primarily involved, surgical repair is technically more difficult and may require mitral valve replacement (Fig. 11-39).

The intraoperative evaluation of the aortic valve by TEE has been reported in multiple studies.[203,204,210,211] The subaortic area is also well visualized with TEE and has been used to diagnose involvement of endocarditis,[205] subaortic stenosis,[212] and subaortic aneurysms.[213] Single-plane TEE Doppler studies of the aortic valve are limited due to the valve position and the direction of blood flow being nearly perpendicular to the ultrasound beam.

Thoracic Aorta Examination

Transesophageal echocardiography has been used to delineate both atherosclerotic and dissecting aneurysms of the thoracic aorta, a site not often well visualized transthoracically.[214–218] Atheromatous plaques (Fig. 11-40) can also be identified.[219–221] TEE has been used for examination of the thoracic aorta for sources of emboli due to thrombus resulting in brain infarct,[222–224] and other major organ involvement.[225–227] During repair of aortic coarctation, TEE was used to diagnose intraaortic thrombus.[228]

In patients with suspected aortic dissection, color flow mapping has proven useful in several ways:

(1) aiding in the initial diagnosis, (2) evaluating communications between true and false lumens, and (3) establishing the presence of aortic valvular regurgitation.[229-231]

Use in the Intensive Care Unit

TEE is being used more and more in the intensive care setting. It has been shown to be a safe and useful monitor and diagnostic tool in critically ill patients.[232,233] Parker and colleagues[234] stated that one-third to one-half of all mechanically ventilated patients cannot be studied transthoracically as a result of poor image quality; those requiring more than 10 cm PEEP have uniformly unsatisfactory transthoracic studies. TEE allows continuous cardiac evaluation in patients treated with up to 15 cm PEEP.[235,236] Koenig and colleagues[237] were able to diagnose one case each of ventricular septal and papillary muscle rupture by TEE after acute myocardial infarction. The sudden onset of cardiogenic shock requiring tracheal intubation and mechanical ventilation had made transthoracic images in this case suboptimal. Postoperative cardiac surgery patients or those with significant thoracic trauma may have bandages that interfere with transthoracic probes.[197]

In both the intensive care unit and the operating room, the cause of hypotension may not always be evident by the hemodynamic measurements from the central venous or pulmonary artery catheters. TEE has been very helpful in determining the cause of hypotension in critically ill patients.[238,239]

ARTIFACTS AND TECHNICAL PROBLEMS

Side Lobes

Side lobes are extraneous beams of ultrasound produced at the edges of the transducer elements.[16,240] These beams are directed away from the main beam, but their reflections are displayed by the echocardiograph as if the reflecting structures were in the line of the main beam. The result is a stray image overlapping the structure being examined by the main beam. If the beam is oscillating, a series of side lobe-generated images will merge together as a curved line (Fig. 11-41). Side lobes are generally weaker than real echoes and are most commonly a problem when they are projected into a relatively echo-free space, such as one of the cardiac chambers. They require a strongly echogenic

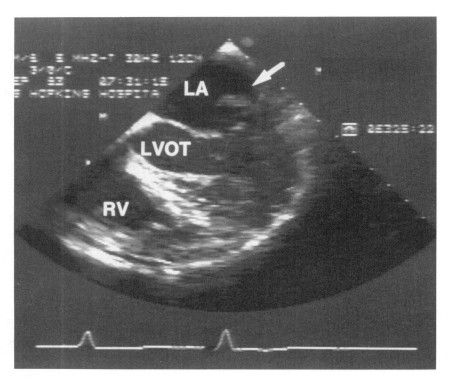

Fig. 11-38. Evaluation of mitral valve before mitral valve repair. Two-dimensional image showing prolapse of posterior mitral valve leaflet (*arrow*) into a dilated left atrium (LA). LVOT, left ventricular outflow tract; RV, right ventricle. See Plate 11-3 for corresponding color Doppler images.

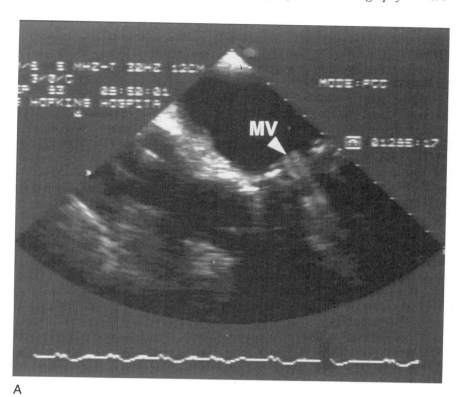

A

Fig. 11-39. Prosthetic (St. Jude) mitral valve in the open (**A**) and closed (**B**) position. LA, left atrium; MV, mitral valve; REV, reverberation from the mitral valve. (See the section *Artifacts and Technical Problems* for explanation of reverberation.)

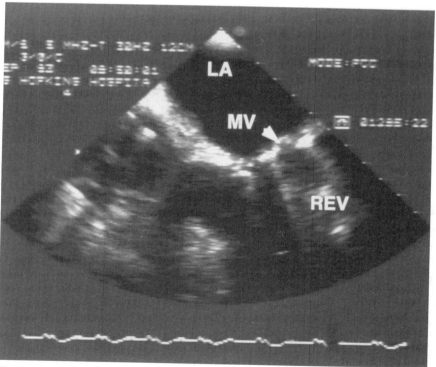

B

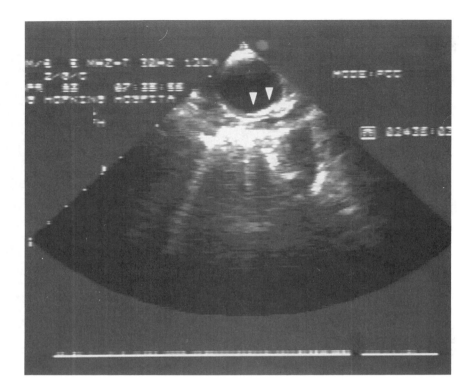

Fig. 11-40. Atheromatous plaque (*arrowheads*) seen in descending thoracic aorta.

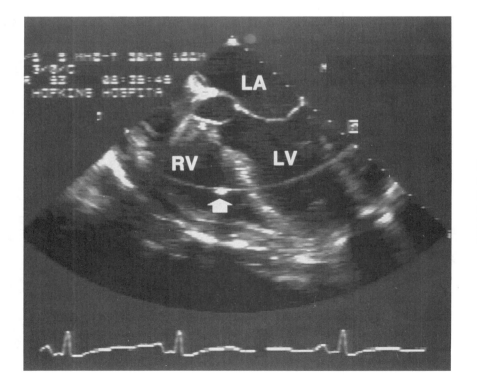

Fig. 11-41. Side-lobe artifact seen as arc-shaped image originating from the strongly echogenic pulmonary artery catheter (*arrow*). RV, right ventricle; LA, left atrium; LV, left ventricle.

structure and are commonly produced by intracardiac catheters (as shown in Fig. 11-41), tissue calcification, or artificial valves. A side lobe artifact across the lumen of the aorta can mimic an aortic intimal flap.[241] Clearly side lobes must be recognized to avoid misinterpreting them as intracardiac masses or structures. Side lobes are primarily a problem of phased array transducers. They can be minimized by decreasing the gain.

Reverberations

Reverberation artifacts are produced when the ultrasound bean is returned into the tissue after its initial reflection back to the transducer.[16] Its subsequent reflection results in an image displayed as a bright tail that originates at a highly echogenic object, such as the mechanical valve shown in Fig. 11-42, and extends toward the side opposite the transducer. Since the echo will have traveled twice as long in being reflected twice, it will be interpreted as having traveled twice as deep as tissues. If the sampling depth of the instrument is less than twice the depth of the structure, the reverberation will "wrap around" to appear at a shallower depth. The reverberation echo is likely to be weaker than the original echo, but its exact position is difficult to predict, as reverberations can originate from numerous structures within the transducer mechanism or chest wall. Reverberations can often be eliminated by changing the transducer angle.

Echo Dropout

Echo dropout is a loss of information in some portion of the echocardiogram (Fig. 11-43). It is typically a problem in two-dimensional echocardiography when imaging the medial and laterals walls of the left ventricle because these structures are encountered in a parallel fashion by the ultrasound beam. In any given frozen frame, though, a certain portion of the echo information will be missing. This problem is partially circumvented by overlapping of individual fields (sweeps of the echo beams) so that each television screen frame represents echoes overlapped from two echocardiographic fields. Similarly, the observer visually compensates in real time for echo dropout, mentally reconstructing a complete image. Dropout creates headaches when still frames are contoured as, for example, in the determination of end-systolic and end-diastolic area. Varying degrees of imagination

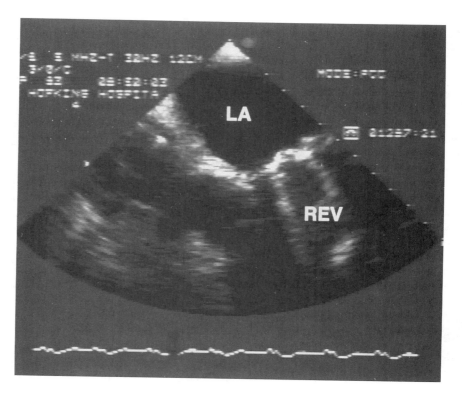

Fig. 11-42. Reverberation artifact seen as multiple reflections from a St. Jude valve in the mitral position. REV, reverberation; LA, left atrium.

are required to cross the gaps created by dropout of the image, and this potential source of error should be borne in mind when quantitative echo data are reviewed.

Gain Artifacts

The gain control should be set to the minimal level that enhances important but weak echoes, such as those of the lateral ventricular walls. Further increases in gain tend to widen the individual echoes, increasing the difference between the leading and trailing edges and decreasing the resolution overall. Gain control tends to be set higher in the operating room because the bright operating room lighting makes it difficult to see images obtained using minimal gain settings. This becomes evident when the TEE study is then viewed in a darkened room. Structures may appear pathologic (e.g., thickened, calcified) due to the high-gain settings, making the study difficult to interpret. The gain setting on the color Doppler imaging must also be set correctly so that flow can be accurately estimated. The gain should be set just below the level where background noise begins to appear.

Interference

Interference is usually considered to be a problem of transthoracic echoes. Unfortunately, use of the transesophageal approach has not totally eliminated interference. Expansion of the lungs occasionally obscures a portion of the cardiac image, either directly by overlapping the heart or indirectly by shifting the mediastinum. Air in the stomach and the presence of a large hiatal hernia can cause loss of contact of the transducer with the esophagus and interfere with the heart images. Similarly, the motion of the heart itself as it beats in the chest can cause a loss of contact with the transducer and result in an image that blinks on and off the screen.

A very strongly reflecting structure, such as an artificial cardiac valve, may screen objects deep to it from the ultrasound beam, a phenomenon known as acoustic shadowing.[16] Acoustic shadowing can occur from sewing rings, struts or the mechanical apparatus of prosthetic valves.

Another type of interference occurs with the use of electrocautery by the surgeon (Fig. 11-44). Several different patterns can be displayed on the echocardiograph monitor screen depending on the type of cautery used. This interference makes two-dimensional imaging difficult and the use of Doppler impossible.

COMPLICATIONS

Large numbers of patients have undergone TEE without problems,[101,242–247] but despite the fact that TEE is overall a ''benign'' procedure, complica-

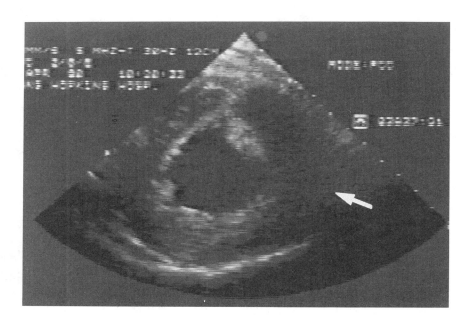

Fig. 11-43. Echo dropout (*arrow*) seen in the short axis view of the left ventricle.

tions have been reported. Studies examining large numbers of patients have reported the risk of major complications ranging from 0.18 to 0.5 percent and the risk of death to be 0.04 percent.[245,247] The main concern is the existence of esophageal pathology which should be elicited from the patient's history. A history of dysphagia, esophageal strictures, esophageal tumors or previous esophageal surgery are usually contraindications to using TEE. One reported fatality associated with TEE was due to a bleeding complication resulting from a malignant lung tumor with esophageal infiltration.[244] A preliminary barium swallow has been recommended in some cases.[39,247] The existence of gastric disease has also been suggested as a possible contraindication because in obtaining a short axis view of the left ventricle, the TEE probe is in the stomach 73 percent of the time and in the cardia 14 percent of the time.[228] A hiatal hernia is not necessarily a contraindication unless it is severe, but it should be noted that due to the patient's anatomy, obtaining an adequate examination may be difficult or impossible.

The potential of the TEE probe to damage the esophagus is illustrated by a case report of a Mallory-Weiss tear occurring secondary to TEE monitoring in a patient who developed a coagulopathy while undergoing cardiac surgery.[249] The patient had a remote history of gastritis, but no known esophageal pathology, and the injury responded to conservative treatment. A study of the effects of prolonged (mean 4.6 hours ± 51 minutes) TEE imaging and probe manipulation in monkeys and dogs showed no significant mucosal or thermal injury on macroscopic and microscopic examination.[250] A similar study by Urbanowicz and colleagues[251] examined the effects of sustained contact and associated surface pressure on the esophagus by a TEE probe in anesthetized dogs and humans. They found that the maximum surface contact pressure between the esophagus and a fully flexed TEE probe is low in dogs and most humans and is not associated with histologic esophageal damage even with long exposure. However, the authors cautioned that potentially dangerous pressure may be generated in some cases in humans and that the TEE probe not be fixed in a flexed position for prolonged periods of time. No difference in the incidence of dysphagia was found between patients who underwent cardiac surgery with TEE monitoring and those who did not.[252]

Inability to flex or extend the neck due to cer-

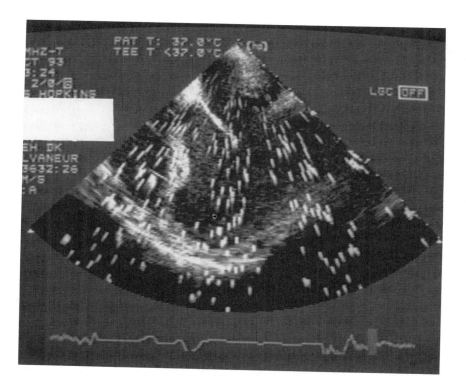

Fig. 11-44. Interference from electrocautery in two-dimensional image of the short axis of the left ventricle.

vical spondylosis or fusion is a potential problem for insertion of the probe[247] and, in addition, the constant pressure of the probe on the posterior pharynx can result in tissue damage. Unilateral vocal cord paralysis (temporary) occurred in several patients studied by Cucchiara and associates,[59] who had undergone seated craniotomies with extreme neck flexion, and had both an endotracheal tube and a single plane TEE probe in place. However, experience with the use of smaller diameter TEE probes has not resulted in vocal cord problems.

Technical complications of intraoperative TEE studies include inability to pass the TEE probe due to operator inexperience or patient anatomy,[244,247] placement of the TEE probe into the trachea[253] and movement of an esophageal stethoscope placed adjacent to the TEE probe. The esophageal stethoscope can be pushed into the stomach due to frictional contact with movement of the TEE probe,[254] so it is usually advised that an esophageal stethoscope *not* be used together with a TEE probe. Buckling of the tip of the TEE probe in the esophagus has been reported, in spite of the fact that the probe was able to be inserted without difficulty and the control knobs were in the release position.[255] In these patients, images could not be easily obtained, manipulation of the probe was difficult, resistance was felt when withdrawal of the probe was attempted and the knob controlling the flexion of the tip of the probe was fixed in the extreme anteflexion position. No symptoms or evidence of injury to the patient was noted in any of the cases.[255]

Cases of bacteremia associated with TEE have been reported by several investigators.[256–258] However, studies which analyzed blood cultures drawn in large groups (100 to 144 patients) of consecutive ambulatory patients (following TEE), showed no increased risk of bacteremia. As a result the authors concluded that it was justified to perform TEE without antibiotics.[259–261] The American Heart Association guidelines do not recommend endocarditis prophylaxis for gastrointestinal endoscopy, with the exception of patients with prosthetic heart valves, a history of endocarditis and surgically constructed shunts and conduits.[262]

In conclusion, we barely have scratched the surface of potential applications of two-dimensional and Doppler echocardiographic techniques to intraoperative events. In particular, use of both echocardiography and Doppler in patients with congenital heart disease could allow intraoperative

monitoring to a degree previously unavailable. Refinement of cardiac output measurements by Doppler, as well as increased acceptance of and familiarity with echocardiographic parameters, could decrease the need for invasive hemodynamic monitoring. Immediate assessment of surgical repairs could become commonplace. Three-dimensional imaging, myocardial textural analysis, and on-line tracking of cavity area are now commercially available. Intraoperative analysis of these exciting techniques remains for future investigators.

REFERENCES

1. Rodigas PC, Meyer FJ, Haasler GB et al: Intraoperative 2-dimensional echocardiography: ejection of microbubbles from the left ventricle after cardiac surgery. Am J Cardiol 50:1130, 1982
2. Spotnitz HM, Malm JR: Two-dimensional ultrasound and cardiac operations. J Thorac Cardiovasc Surg 83:43, 1982
3. Dubroff JM, Clark MB, Wong CYH et al: Left ventricular ejection fraction during cardiac surgery: a two-dimensional echocardiographic study. Circulation 68:95, 1983
4. Spotnitz HM, Bregman D, Bowman FO et al: Effects of open heart surgery on end-diastolic pressure-dimension relations of the human left ventricle. Circulation 59:662, 1979
5. Barash PG, Glanz S, Katz JD et al: Ventricle function in children during halothane anesthesia: an echocardiographic evaluation. Anesthesiology 49:79, 1978
6. Gerson JI, Gianaris CG: Echocardiographic analysis of human left ventricular diastolic volume and cardiac performance during halothane anesthesia. Anesth Analg 58:23, 1979
7. Rathod R, Jacobs HK, Kramer NE et al: Echocardiographic assessment of ventricular performance following induction with two anesthetics. Anesthesiology 49:86, 1978
8. Touze MD, Pinaud M, Rozo L et al: Echocardiography and left ventricular function on recovery from anaesthesia in patients with coronary artery disease. Acta Anaesthesiol Scand 27:149, 1983
9. Frazin L, Talano JV, Stephanides L et al: Esophageal echocardiography. Circulation 54:102, 1976
10. Matsumoto M, Oka Y, Strom J et al: Application of transesophageal echocardiography to continuous intraoperative monitoring of left ventricular performance. Am J Cardiol 46:95, 1980
11. Hisanaga K, Hisanaga A, Nagata K, Ichie Y: Transesophageal cross-sectional echocardiography. Am Heart J 100:605, 1980

12. Schluter M, Langenstein BA, Polster J et al: Transesophageal cross-sectional echocardiography with a phased array transducer system. Technique and initial clinical results. Br Heart J 48:67, 1982

13. Kyo S, Takamoto S, Matsumura M et al: Immediate and early postoperative evaluation of results of cardiac surgery by transesophageal two-dimensional Doppler echocardiography. Circulation 66:386, 1987

14. de Bruijn NP, Clements FM, Kisslo JA: Intraoperative transesophageal color flow mapping: initial experience. Anesth Analg 66:386, 1987

15. Omoto R, Kyo S, Matsumura M et al: Bi-plane color transesophageal Doppler echocardiography (color TEE): its advantages and limitations. Int J Cardiac Imaging 4:57, 1989

16. Feigenbaum H: Echocardiography. 5th Ed. Lea & Febiger, Philadelphia, 1994

17. Talano JV, Gardin JM: Textbook of Two-Dimensional Echocardiography. Grune & Stratton, Orlando, FL, 1983

18. Hisanga K, Hisanga A, Nagata K, Ichie Y: Transesophageal cross-sectional echocardiography. Am Heart J 100:605, 1980

19. Hatle L, Angelson B: Doppler Ultrasound in Cardiology. Lea & Febiger, Philadelphia, 1985

20. Schluter M, Langenstein BA, Hanrath P et al: Assessment of transesophageal pulsed Doppler echocardiography in the detection of mitral regurgitation. Circulation 66:784, 1982

21. Lang-Jensen T, Berning J, Jacobsen E: Stroke volume measured by pulsed ultrasound Doppler and M-mode echocardiography. Acta Anesthesiol Scand 27:454, 1983

22. Gallagher TJ, Banner MJ, Cavallaro DL: Cardiac output measured noninvasively by continuous wave, ultrasonic Doppler compute. Anesth Analg 62:261, 1983

23. Mark JB, Steinbrook RA, Gugino LD et al: Continuous noninvasive monitoring of cardiac output with esophageal Doppler ultrasound during cardiac surgery. Anesth Analg 65:1013, 1986

24. Muhiudeen IA, Kuecherer HF, Lee E et al: Intraoperative estimation of cardiac output by transesophageal pulsed Doppler echocardiography. Anesthesiology 74:9, 1991

25. Perrino AC Jr, Fleming J, LaMantia KR: Transesophageal Doppler cardiac output monitoring: performance during aortic reconstructive surgery. Anes Analg 73:705, 1991

26. Gorscan J III, Diana P, Ball BA et al: Intraoperative determination of cardiac output by transesophageal continuous wave Doppler. Am Heart J 123:171, 1992

27. Hillel Z, Thys D, Ritter S et al: Two-dimensional color flow Doppler echocardiography for the intraoperative monitoring of cardiac shunt flows in patients with congenital heart disease. J Cardiothorac Anesthes 1:42, 1987

28. Sahn DJ: Real-time two-dimensional Doppler echocardiographic flow mapping. Circulation 71:849, 1985

29. Sheikh KH, de Bruijn NP, Rankin JS et al: The utility of transesophageal echocardiography Doppler color flow imaging in patients undergoing cardiac valve surgery. J Am Coll Cardiol 15:363, 1990

30. Iliceto S, Nanda NC, Hsiung MC et al: Assessment of aortic dissection by color Doppler. Circulation 74 (Suppl. II):132, 1986

31. Takamoto S, Kyo S, Adachi H et al: Intraoperative color flow mapping by real-time two-dimensional Doppler echocardiography for evaluation of valvular and congenital heart disease and vascular disease. J Thorac Cardiovasc Surg 90:802, 1985

32. Takamoto S, Kyo S, Matsumura M et al: Total visualization of thoracic dissecting aortic aneurysm by trans-esophageal Doppler color flow mapping. Circulation 74(Suppl. II):132, 1986

33. Gramiak R, Shah PM, Kramer DH: Ultrasound cardiography: contrast studies in anatomy and function. Radiology 92:939, 1969

34. Fraker TD, Harris PJ, Behar VS, Kisslo JA: Detection and exclusion of interatrial shunts by two-dimensional echocardiography and peripheral venous injection. Circulation 59:379, 1979

35. Reid CL, Kawanishi DT, McKay CR et al: Accuracy of evaluation of the presence and severity of aortic and mitral regurgitation by contrast 2-dimensional echocardiography. Am J Cardiol 52:519, 1983

36. Drexler M, Oelert H, Dahm M et al: Assessment of successful valve reconstruction by intraoperative transesophageal echocardiography. Circulation, 74(Suppl. II):390, 1986

37. Eguaras MG, Pasalodos J, Gonzalez V et al: Intraoperative contrast two-dimensional echocardiography. J Thorac Cardiovasc Surg 89:573, 1985

38. Goldman ME, Fuster V, Guarino T, Mindich BP: Intraoperative echocardiography for the evaluation of valvular regurgitation: experience in 263 patients. Circulation 74:I-143, 1986

39. Goldman ME, Mindich BP: Intraoperative two-dimensional echocardiography: new application of an old technique. J Am Coll Cardiol 7:374, 1986

40. Mindich BP, Goldman ME, Fuster V et al: Improved intraoperative evaluation of mitral valve operations utilizing two-dimensional contrast echocardiography. J Thorac Cardiovasc Surg 90:112, 1985

41. Bommer WJ, Shah PM, Allen H et al: The safety of contrast echocardiography: report of the committee on Contrast Echocardiography for the Ameri-

can Society of Echocardiography. J Am Coll Cardiol 3:6, 1984

42. Topol EJ, Humphrey LS, Borkon AM et al: Value of intraoperative left ventricular microbubbles detected by transesophageal two-dimensional echocardiography in predicting neurologic outcome after cardiac operations. Am J Cardiol 56:773, 1985

43. Kisslo J, von Ramm OT, Thurstone FL: Cardiac imaging using a phased array ultrasound system. Circulation 53:262, 1976

44. Henry WL, DeMaria A, Feigenbaum H et al: Report of the American Society of Echocardiography Committee on Nomenclature and Standards: Identification of Myocardial Wall Segments. American Society of Echocardiography, 1982

45. Shantani H, Nakano S, Matsuda H et al: Efficacy of transesophageal echocardiography as a perioperative monitor in patients undergoing cardiovascular surgery: analysis of 149 consecutive studies. J Cardiovasc Surg 31:564, 1990

46. Duff HJ, Buda AJ, Kramer R et al: Detection of entrapped intracardiac air with intraoperative echocardiography. Am J Cardiol 46:255, 1980

47. Furuya H, Suzuki T, Okumura F et al: Detection of air embolism by transesophageal echocardiography. Anesthesiology 58:124, 1983

48. Glenski JA, Cucchiara RF, Michenfelder JD: Transesophageal echocardiography and transcutaneous O_2 and CO_2 monitoring for detection of venous air embolism. Anesthesiology 64:541, 1986

49. Muzzi DA, Lasasso TJ, Black S et al: Comparison of a transesophageal and precordial ultrasonic Doppler sensor in the detection of venous air embolism. Anesth Analg 70:103, 1990

50. Rafferty TD: Intraoperative transesophageal saline-contrast imaging of flow-patent foramen ovale. Anesth Analg 75:475, 1992

51. Hausmann D, Mugge A, Becht I, Daniel WB: Diagnosis of patent foramen ovale by transesophageal echocardiography and association with cerebral and peripheral embolic events. Am J Cardiol 70:668, 1992

52. Chen WJ, Kuan P, Lien WP et al: Detection of patent foramen ovale by contrast transesophageal echocardiography. Chest 101:1515, 1992

53. Siostrzonek P, Lang W, Zangeneh M et al: Significance of left-sided heart disease for the detection of patent foramen ovale by transesophageal contrast echocardiography. J Am Coll Cardiol 19:1192, 1992

54. Siostrzonek P, Zangeneh M, Gossinger H et al: Comparison of transesophageal and transthoracic contrast echocardiography for detection of a patent foramen ovale. Am J Cardiol 68:1247, 1991

55. Goldman AP, Glover MU, Mick W et al: The role of transesophageal echocardiography in the diagnosis and management of patent foramen ovale following aortocoronary bypass graft surgery. Am Heart J 121:1224, 1991

56. Konstadt SN, Louie EK, Black S et al: Intraoperative detection of patent foramen ovale by transesophageal echocardiography. Anesthesiology 74:212, 1991

57. Langholz D, Louie EK, Konstadt SN et al: Transesophageal echocardiographic demonstration of distinct mechanisms for right to left shunting across a patent foramen ovale in the absence of pulmonary hypertension. J Am Coll Cardiol 18:1112, 1991

58. Nagelhout DA, Pearson AC, Labovitz AJ: Diagnosis of paradoxic embolism by transesophageal echocardiography. Am Heart J 121:1552, 1991

59. Cucchiara RF, Nugent M, Seward JB, Messick JM: Air embolism in upright neurosurgical patients: detection and localization by two-dimensional transesophageal echocardiography. Anesthesiology 60:353, 1984

60. Cucchiara RF, Seward JB, Nishimura RA et al: Identification of patent foramen ovale during sitting position craniotomy by transesophageal echocardiography with positive airway pressure. Anesthesiology 63:107, 1985

61. Furuya H, Okumura F: Detection of paradoxical air embolism of transesophageal echocardiography. Anesthesiology 60:374, 1984

62. Black S, Muzzi DA, Nishimura RA, Cucchiara RF: Preoperative and intraoperative echocardiography to detect right-to-left shunt in patients undergoing neurosurgical procedures in the sitting position. Anesthesiology 72:436, 1990

63. Thompson RC, Finck SJ, Leventhal JP et al: Right-to-left shunt across a patent foramen ovale caused by cardiac tamponade: diagnosis by transesophageal echocardiography. Mayo Clin Proc 66:391, 1991

64. Jaffe RA, Pinto FJ, Schnittger I, Brock-Utne JG: Intraoperative ventilator-induced right-to-left shunt. Anesthesiology 75:153, 1991

65. Perkins-Pearson NAK, Marshall WK, Bedford RF: Atrial pressures in the seated position. Implication for paradoxical air embolism. Anesthesiology 57:493, 1982

66. Hagen PT, Scholz DG, Edwards WD: Incidence and size of patent foramen ovale during the first ten decades of life: an autopsy study of 965 normal hearts. Mayo Clin Proc 59:17, 1984

67. Oka Y, Inoue T, Hong Y et al: Retained intracardiac air: transesophageal echocardiography for definition of incidence and monitoring removal by improved techniques. J Thorac Cardiovasc Surg 91:329, 1986

68. Oka Y, Moriwaki KM, Hong Y et al: Detection of air emboli in the left heart by M-mode transesophageal echocardiography following cardiopulmonary bypass. Anesthesiology 63:109, 1985

69. Ereth MH, Weber JG, Abel MD et al: Cemented versus noncemented total hip arthroplasty: embolism, hemodynamics and intrapulmonary shunting. Mayo Clin Proc 67:1066, 1992

70. Prager MC, Gregory GA, Ascher NL, Roberts JP: Massive venous air embolism during orthotopic liver transplantation. Anesthesiology 72:198, 1990

71. Cahalan MK, Muhiudeen IA: Intraoperative TEE: evaluation of left ventricular filling and function, and detection of myocardial ischemia. Am J Cardiol Imaging 4:187, 1990

72. Leung JM, Schiller NB, Mangano DT: Assessment of left ventricular function using two-dimensional transesophageal echocardiography. p 59. In de Bruijn NP, Clements FM (eds): Intraoperative Use of Echocardiography. JB Lippincott, Philadelphia, 1991

73. Konstadt SN, Thys D, Mindich BP et al: Validation of quantitative intraoperative transesophageal echocardiography. Anesthesiology 65:418, 1986

74. Abel MD, Nishimura RA, Callahan MJ et al: Evaluation of intraoperative transesophageal two-dimensional echocardiography. Anesthesiology 66:64, 1987

75. Cahalan MK, Kremer PF, Beaupre PN et al: Consistency and reproducibility of transesophageal two-dimensional echocardiography. Anesth Analg 63:194, 1984

76. Haendchen RV, Wyatt HL, Maurer G et al: Quantitation of regional cardiac function by two-dimensional echocardiography: patterns of contraction in the normal left ventricle. Circulation 67:1234, 1983

77. Quinones MA, Waggoner AD, Reduto LA et al: A new, simplified and accurate method for determining ejection fraction with two-dimensional echocardiography. Circulation 64:744, 1981

78. Reichert CLA, Visser CA, van den Brink RBA et al: Prognostic value of biventricular function in hypotensive patients after cardiac surgery as assessed by transesophageal echocardiography. J Cardiothorac Vasc Anesth 6:429, 1992

79. Ayd J, Bain R, Watkins L et al: Quantitative transesophageal echocardiography during operative automatic internal cardiac defibrillator testing. Society of Cardiovascular Anesthesia 15th Annual Meeting, April 1993

80. Sagawa K: The end-systolic pressure-volume relation of the ventricle: definition, modifications and clinical use. Circulation 63:1223, 1981

81. Mulier JP, Wouters PF, Van Aken H et al: Cardiodynamic effects of propofol in comparison with thiopental: assessment with a transesophageal echocardiographic approach. Anesth Analg 72:28, 1991

82. Dahlgren G, Veintemilla, Settergren G et al: Left ventricular end-systolic pressure estimated from measurements in peripheral artery. J Cardiothorac Vasc Anesth 5:551, 1991

83. Humphrey LS, Topol EJ, Rosenfeld GI et al: Immediate enhancement of left ventricular relaxation by coronary artery bypass grafting: intraoperative assessment. Circulation 77:886, 1988

84. Baran AO, Rogal CJ, Nanda NC: Ejection fraction determination without planimetry by two-dimensional echocardiography: a new method. J Am Coll Cardiol 1:1471, 1983

85. Folland ED, Parisi AF, Moynihan PF et al: Assessment of left ventricular ejection fraction and volumes by real-time, two-dimensional echocardiography: a comparison of cineangiographic and radionuclide techniques. Circulation 60:760, 1979

86. Schiller NB, Acquatella H, Ports TA et al: Left ventricular volume from paired biplane two-dimensional echocardiography. Circulation 60:547, 1979

87. Stamm RB, Carabello BA, Mayers DL, Martin RP: Two-dimensional echocardiographic measurement of left ventricular ejection fraction: prospective analysis of what constitutes an adequate determination. Am Heart J 104:136, 1982

88. Tortoledo FA, Quinones MA, Fernandez GC et al: Quantification of left ventricular volumes by two-dimensional echocardiography: a simplified and accurate approach. Circulation 67:579, 1983

89. Helak JW, Reichek N: Quantitation of human left ventricular mass and volume by two-dimensional echocardiography: in vitro anatomic validation. Circulation 63:1398, 1981

90. Schnittger I, Fitzgerald PJ, Daughters GT et al: Limitations of comparing left ventricular volumes by two-dimensional echocardiography, myocardial markers and cineangiography. Am J Cardiol 50:512, 1982

91. Wyatt HL, Haendchen RV, Meerbaum S, Corday E: Assessment of quantitative methods for 2-dimensional echocardiography. Am J Cardiol 52:396, 1983

92. Urbanowicz JH, Shaaban JM, Cohen NH et al: Comparison of transesophageal echocardiographic and scintigraphic estimates of left ventricular end-diastolic volume index and ejection fraction in patients following coronary artery bypass grafting. Anesthesiology 72:607, 1990

93. Thys DM, Hillel Z, Goldman ME et al: A comparison of hemodynamic indices derived by invasive monitoring and two-dimensional echocardiography. Anesthesiology 67:630, 1987

94. Martin RW, Graham MM, Kao R et al: Measurement

of left ventricular ejection fraction and volumes with three-dimensional reconstructed transesophageal ultrasound scans: comparison to radionuclide and thermal dilution measurements. J Cardiothorac Anesth 3: 260, 1989

95. Nessley ML, Bashein G, Detmer PR et al: Left ventricular ejection fraction: single-plane and multiplanar transesophageal echocardiography versus equilibrium gated-pool scintigraphy. J Cardiothorac Vasc Anesth 5:40, 1991

96. Kuecherer HF, Muhiudeen IA, Kusumoto FM et al: Estimation of mean left atrial pressure from transesophageal pulsed Doppler echocardiography of pulmonary venous flow. Circulation 82:1127, 1990

97. Roewer N, Bednarz F, Dziadka A et al: Intraoperative cardiac output determination from transmitral and pulmonary blood flow measurements using transesophageal pulsed Doppler. J Cardiothorac Anesth 1:418, 1987

98. LaMantia K, Harris S, Mortimore K et al: Transesophageal pulse-wave Doppler assessment of cardiac output. Anesthesiology 69:A1, 1988

99. Nishimura RA, Abel MD, Hatle LK, Tajik AJ: Relation of pulmonary vein to mitral flow velocities by transesophageal Doppler echocardiography: effect of different loading conditions. Circulation 81: 1488, 1990

100. Heger JJ, Weyman AE, Wann LS et al: Cross-sectional echocardiography in acute myocardial infarction: detection and localization of regional ventricular asynergy. Circulation 60:531, 1979

101. Cahalan MK, Litt L, Botvinick EH, Schiller NB: Advances in noninvasive cardiovascular imaging: implications for the anesthesiologist. Anesthesiology 66:356, 1987

102. Schnittger I, Fitzgerald PJ, Gordon EP et al: Computerized quantitative analysis of left ventricular wall motion by two-dimensional echocardiography. Circulation 70:242, 1984

103. Parisi AF, Moynihian PF, Folland ED, Feldman CL: Quantitative detection of regional left ventricular contraction abnormalities by two-dimensional echocardiography. II. Accuracy in coronary artery disease. Circulation 63:761, 1981

104. Force T, Bloomfield P, O'Boyle JE et al: Quantitative two-dimensional echocardiographic analysis of regional wall motion in patients with perioperative myocardial infarction. Circulation 70:233, 1984

105. Force T, Bloomfield P, O'Boyle JE et al: Quantitative two-dimensional echocardiographic analysis of motion and thickening of the interventricular septum after cardiac surgery. Circulation 68:1013, 1983

106. Kerber RE, Litchfield R: Postoperative abnormalities of interventricular septal motion: two-dimen-

sional and M-mode echocardiographic correlations. Am Heart J 104:263, 1982

107. Schnittger I, Keren A, Yock PG et al: Timing of abnormal interventricular septal motion after cardiopulmonary bypass operations. J Thorac Cardiovasc Surg 91:619, 1986

108. Waggoner AD, Shah AA, Schuessler JS et al: Effect of cardiac surgery on ventricular septal motion: assessment by intraoperative echocardiography and cross-sectional two-dimensional echocardiography. Am Heart J 104:1271, 1982

109. Lehmann KG, Lee FA, McKenzie WB et al: Onset of altered interventricular septal motion during cardiac surgery: assessment by continuous intraoperative transesophageal echocardiography. Circulation 82:1325, 1990

110. Klausner SC, Blair TJ, Bulawa WF et al: Quantitative analysis of segmental wall motion throughout systole and diastole in the normal human left ventricle. Circulation 65:580, 1982

111. Weyman AE, Franklin TD, Hogan RD et al: Importance of temporal heterogeneity in assessing the contraction abnormalities associated with acute myocardial ischemia. Circulation 70:102, 1984

112. Blumenthal DS, Becker LC, Bulkley BH et al: Impaired function of salvaged myocardium: two-dimensional echocardiographic quantification of regional wall thickening in the open-chest dog. Circulation 67:225, 1983

113. Feneley MP, Hickie JB: Validity of echocardiographic determination of left ventricular systolic wall thickening. Circulation 70:226, 1984

114. Lieberman AN, Weiss JL, Jugdutt BL et al: Two-dimensional echocardiography and infarct size: relationship of regional wall motion and thickening to the extent of myocardial infarction in the dog. Circulation 63:739, 1981

115. Sasayama S, Franklin D, Ross J et al: Dynamic changes in left ventricular wall thickness and their used in analyzing cardiac function in the conscious dog. Am J Cardiol 38:870, 1976

116. Topol EJ, Weiss JL, Guzman PA et al: Immediate improvement of dysfunctional myocardial segments after coronary revascularization: detection by intraoperative transesophageal echocardiography. J Am Coll Cardiol 4:1123, 1984

117. Pandian NG, Skorton DJ, Collins SM, et al: Heterogeneity of left ventricular segmental wall thickening and excursion in 2-dimensional echocardiograms of normal human subjects. Am J Cardiol 51:1667, 1983

118. Buda AJ, Zotz RJ, Pace DP, Krause LC: Comparison of two-dimensional echocardiographic wall motion and wall thickening abnormalities in relation to the myocardium at risk. Am Heart J 11:587, 1986

119. Pandian NG, Kerber RE: Two-dimensional echocardiography in experimental coronary stenosis. I. Sensitivity and specificity in detecting transient myocardial dyskinesia: comparison with sonomicrometers. Circulation 66:597, 1982

120. Voci P, Bilotta F, Aronson S et al: Echocardiographic analysis of dysfunctional and normal myocardial segments before and immediately after coronary artery bypass graft surgery. Anesth Analg 75: 213, 1992

121. Tennant R, Wiggers C: The effect of coronary occlusion on myocardial contraction. Am J Physiol 112:351, 1935

122. Kerber RE, Marcus ML, Ehrhardt J et al: Correlation between echocardiographically demonstrated segmental dyskinesia and regional myocardial perfusion. Circulation 52:1097, 1975

123. Gallagher DP, Kumada T, Koziol JA et al: Significance of regional wall thickening abnormalities relative to transmural myocardial perfusion in anesthetized dogs. Circulation 62:1266, 1980

124. Force T, Kemper A, Perkins L et al: Overestimation of infarct size by quantitative two-dimensional echocardiography: the role of tethering and analytic procedures. Circulation 73:1360, 1986

125. Homans DC, Asinger R, Elsperger KJ et al: Regional function and perfusion at the lateral border of ischemic myocardium. Circulation 71:1038, 1985

126. Lima JAC, Becker LC, Melin JA et al: Impaired thickening of non ischemic myocardium during acute regional ischemia in the dog. Circulation 71: 1048, 1985

127. Weiss JL, Bulkley BH, Hutchins GM, Mason SJ: Two-dimensional echocardiographic recognition of myocardial injury in man: comparison with postmortem studies. Circulation 63:401, 1981

128. Arvan S, Varat MA: Two-dimensional echocardiography versus surface electrocardiography for the diagnosis of acute non-Q wave myocardial infarction. Am Heart J 110:44, 1985

129. Horowitz RS, Morganroth J, Parrotto C et al: Immediate diagnosis of acute myocardial infarction by two-dimensional echocardiography. Circulation 65: 323, 1982

130. Reeder GS, Seward JB, Tajik AJ: The role of two-dimensional echocardiography in coronary artery disease: a critical appraisal. Mayo Clin Proc 57:247, 1982

131. Massie BM, Botvinick EH, Brundage BH et al: Relationship of regional myocardial perfusion to segmental wall motion: a physiologic basis for understanding the presence and reversibility of asynergy. Circulation 58:1154, 1978

132. Smith JS, Cahalan MK, Benefiel DJ et al: Intraoperative detection of myocardial ischemia in high-risk patients: electrocardiography versus two-dimensional transesophageal echocardiography. Circulation 72:1015, 1985

133. Waters DD, Luz PD, Wyatt HL et al: Early changes in regional and global left ventricular function induced by graded reductions in regional coronary perfusion. Am J Cardiol 39:537, 1977

134. Battler A, Froelicher VF, Gallagher KP et al: Dissociation between regional myocardial dysfunction and ECG changes during ischemia in the conscious dog. Circulation 62:735, 1980

135. Slogoff S, Keats AS: Does perioperative myocardial ischemia lead to postoperative myocardial infarction? Anesthesiology 62:107, 1985

136. Beaupre PN, Kremer PF, Cahalan MK et al: Intraoperative detection of changes in left ventricular segmental wall motion by transesophageal two-dimensional echocardiography. Am Heart J 107:1021, 1984

137. Leung JM, O'Kelly B, Browner WS et al: Prognostic importance of postbypass regional wall-motion abnormalities in patients undergoing coronary artery bypass graft surgery. Anesthesiology 71:16, 1989

138. London MJ, Tubau JF, Wong MG et al: The "natural history" of segmental wall motion abnormalities in patients undergoing noncardiac surgery. Anesthesiology 73:644, 1990

139. Saada M, Catoire P, Bonnet F et al: Effect of thoracic epidural anesthesia combined with general anesthesia on segmental wall motion assessed by transesophageal echocardiography. Anesth Analg 75:329, 1992

140. Roizen MF, Beaupre PN, Alpert RA et al: Monitoring with two-dimensional transesophageal echocardiography. Comparison of myocardial function in patients undergoing supraceliac suprarenal-infraceliac, or infrarenal aortic occlusion. J Vasc Surg 1: 300, 1984

141. Lin SL, Ting CT, Hsu TL et al: Transesophageal echocardiographic detection of atrial septal defect in adults. Am J Card 69:280, 1992

142. Roberson DA, Muhiudeen IA, Silverman NH et al: Intraoperative transesophageal echocardiography of atrioventricular septal defect. J Am Coll Cardiol 18:537, 1991

143. Morimoto K, Matsuzaki M, Tohma Y et al: Diagnosis and quantitative evaluation of secundum-type atrial septal defect by transesophageal Doppler echocardiography. Am J Card 66:85, 1990

144. Shen WK, Khandheria BK: Transesophageal echocardiography: Detection of an acquired left ventricular-right atrial shunt. J Am Soc Echocardiol 4:199, 1991

145. Takenaka K, Sakamoto T, Shiota T et al: Diagnosis of patent ductus arteriosus in adults by biplane

transesophageal color Doppler flow mapping. Am J Cardiol 68:691, 1991

146. Mugge A, Daniel WG, Lichtlen PR: Imaging of patent ductus arteriosus by transesophageal color-coded Doppler echocardiography. J Clin Ultrastruc 19:128, 1991

147. Tsai LM, Chen JH, Teng JK et al: Right coronary artery-to-left ventricle fistula identified by transesophageal echocardiography. Am Heart J 124:1106, 1992

148. Sunaga Y, Taniichi Y, Okubo N et al: Biplane transesophageal echocardiographic study of left coronary artery to right atrium fistula. Am Heart J 123:1058, 1992

149. Varma V, Nanda NC, Soto B et al: Transesophageal echocardiographic demonstration of proximal right coronary artery dissection extending into the aortic root. Am Heart J 123:1055, 1992

150. Liddell NE, Stoddard MF, Prince C et al: Transesophageal echocardiographic diagnosis of complex false aneurysm with aorto-left atrial communication complicating aortic valve and root replacement. Am Heart J 123:543, 1992

151. Kuo CT, Chiang CW, Fang BR et al: Coronary artery fistula: diagnosis by transesophageal two-dimensional and Doppler echocardiography. Am Heart J 123:218, 1992

152. Koh KK: Confirmation of anomalous origin of the right coronary artery from the left sinus of Valsalva by means of transesophageal echocardiography. Am Heart J 122:851, 1992

153. Samdarshi TE, Mahan EF III, Nanda NC et al: Transesophageal echocardiographic assessment of congenital coronary artery to coronary sinus fistulas in adults. Am J Cardiol 68:263, 1991

154. Bansal RC, Graham BM, Jutzy KR et al: Left ventricular outflow tract to left atrial communication infective endocarditis: diagnosis by transesophageal echocardiography and color flow imaging. J Am Coll Cardiol 15:499, 1990

155. Hickey PR: Transesophageal echocardiography in pediatric cardiac surgery. Anesthesiology 77:610, 1992

156. Weintraub R, Shiota T, Elkadi T et al: Transesophageal echocardiography in infants and children with congenital heart disease. Circulation 86:711, 1992

157. Weintraub RG, Sahn DJ: Pediatric transesophageal echocardiography: present and future. Anesthesiology 76:159, 1992

158. Ritter SB: Transesophageal real-time echocardiography in infants and children with congenital heart disease. J Am Coll Cardiol 18:569, 1991

159. Cyran SE, Myers JL, Gleason MM et al: Application of intraoperative transesophageal echocardiog-raphy in infants and small children. J Cardiovasc Surg 32:318, 1991

160. Stumper O, Sutherland GR, Geuskens R et al: Transesophageal echocardiography in evaluation and management after a Fontan procedure. J Am Coll Cardiol 17:1152, 1991

161. Muhiudeen IA, Roberson DA, Silverman NH et al: Intraoperative echocardiography in infants and children with ccongenital cardiac shunt lesions: transesophageal versus epicardial echocardiography. J Am Coll Cardiol 16:1687, 1990

162. Hanrath P, Schluter M, Langenstein BA et al: Detection of ostium secundum atrial septal defects by transesophageal cross-sectional echocardiography. Br Heart J 49:350, 1983

163. Mehta RH, Helmcke F, Nanda NC et al: Transesophageal Doppler color flow mapping assessment of atrial septal defect. J Am Coll Cardiol 16:1010, 1990

164. Cohen GI, Klein AL, Chan KL et al: Transesophageal echocardiographic diagnosis of right-sided cardiac masses in patients with central lines. Am J Cardiol 70:925, 1992

165. Hwang JJ, Kuan P, Lin SC et al: Reappraisal by transesophageal echocardiography of the significance of left atrial thrombi in the prediction of systemic arterial embolization in rheumatic mitral valve disease. Am J Cardiol 70:769, 1992

166. Guindo J, Montagud M, Carreras F et al: Fibrinolytic therapy for superior vena cava and right atrial thrombosis: diagnosis and follow-up with biplane transesophageal echocardiography. Am Heart J 124:510, 1992

167. Kuo CT, Chiang CW, Lee YS et al: Left atrial ball thrombus in nonrheumatic atrial fibrillation diagnosed by transesophageal echocardiography. Am Heart J 123:1394, 1992

168. Pasierski TJ, Alton ME, Van Fossen DB et al: Right atrial mobile thrombus: improved visualization by transesophageal echocardiography. Am Heart J 123:802, 1992

169. Fyfe DA, Kline CH, Sade RM et al: Transesophageal echocardiography detects thrombus formation not identified by transthoracic echocardiography after the Fontan operation. J Am Coll Cardiol 18:1733, 1991

170. Aschenberg W, Schluter M, Kremer P et al: Transesophageal two-dimensional echocardiography for the detection of left atrial appendage thrombus. J Am Coll Cardiol 7:163, 1986

171. Daniel WG, Nikutta P, Schroder E, Nellessen U: Transesophageal echocardiographic detection of left atrial appendage thrombi in patients with unexplained arterial embolism. Circulation 74(Suppl. II):391, 1986

172. Nellessen U, Daniel WG, Matheis G et al: Impending paradoxical embolism from atrial thrombus: correct diagnosis by transesophageal echocardiography and prevention by surgery. J Am Coll Cardiol 5:1002, 1985

173. Gorcsan J III, Blanc MS, Reddy PS et al: Hemodynamic diagnosis of mitral valve obstruction by left atrial myxoma with transesophageal continuous wave Doppler. Am Heart J 124:1106, 1992

174. Aru GM, Cattolica FS, Cardu G et al: A fractured and detached right atrial myxoma: an unusual and threatening condition detected by intraoperative transesophageal echocardiography. J Thorac Cardiovasc Surg 104:215, 1992

175. Samdarshi TE, Mahan EF III, Nanda NC et al: Transesophageal echocardiographic diagnosis of multicentric left ventricular myxomas mimicking a left atrial tumor. J Thorac Cardiovasc Surg 103:471, 1992

176. Fyke FE III: Transesophageal echocardiography and cardiac masses. Mayo Clin Proc 66:1101, 1991

177. Rey M, Tunon J, Compres H et al: Prolapsing right atrial myxoma evaluated by transesophageal echocardiography. Am Heart J 122:875, 1991

178. Mora F, Mindich BP, Guarino T, Goldman ME: Improved surgical approach to cardiac tumors with intraoperative two-dimensional echocardiography. Chest 91:142, 1987

179. Moore JA, DeRan BP, Minor R et al: Transesophageal echocardiographic evaluation of intracardiac lymphoma. Am Heart J 124:514, 1992

180. Mugge A, Daniel WG, Haverich A et al: Diagnosis of noninfective cardiac mass lesions by two-dimensional echocardiography: comparison of the transthoracic and transesophageal approaches. Circulation 83:70, 1991

181. Kronzon I, Tunick PA, Glassman E et al: Transesophageal echocardiography to detect atrial clots in candidates for percutaneous transseptal mitral balloon valvuloplasty. J Am Coll Cardiol 16:1320, 1990

182. Mugge A, Daniel WG, Hausmann D et al: Diagnosis of left atrial appendage thrombi by transesophageal echocardiography: clinical implications and follow-up. Am J Card Imaging 4:173, 1990

183. Cohen GI, Klein AL, Chan KL et al: Transesophageal echocardiographic diagnosis of right-sided cardiac masses in patients with central lines. Am J Cardiol 70:925, 1992

184. Frohwein SC, Karalis DG, McQuillan JM et al: Preoperative detection of pericardial angiosarcoma by transesophageal echocardiography. Am Heart J 122:874, 1991

185. Lestuzzi C, Nicolosi GL, Mimo R: Usefulness of transesophageal echocardiography in evaluation of paracardiac neoplastic masses. Am J Cardiol 15:70:247, 1992

186. Aronson S, Ruo W, Sand M: Inverted left atrial appendage appearing as a left atrial mass with transesophageal echocardiography during cardiac surgery. Anesthesiology 76:1054, 1992

187. Johnson ML, Holmes JH, Spangler RD, Paton BC: Usefulness of echocardiography in patients undergoing mitral valve surgery. J Thoracic Cardiovasc Surg 64:922, 1972

188. Drexler M, Oelert H, Dahm M et al: Assessment of successful valve reconstruction by intraoperative transesophageal echocardiography. Circulation 74:II-390, 1986

189. Freeman WK, Schaff HV, Khandheria BK et al: Intraoperative evaluation of mitral valve regurgitation and repair by transesophageal echocardiography: incidence and significance of systolic anterior motion. J Am Coll Cardiol 20:599, 1992

190. Reichert SL, Visser CA Moulijn AC et al: Intraoperative transesophageal color-coded Doppler echocardiography for evaluation of residual regurgitation after mitral valve repair. J Thorac Cardiovasc Surg 100:756, 1990

191. Wolfe WG, Kisslo J: The utility of transesophageal echocardiography and Doppler color flow imaging in patients undergoing cardiac valve surgery. J Am Coll Cardiol 15:363, 1990

192. Castello R, Lenzen P, Aguirre F et al: Quantitation of mitral regurgitation by transesophageal echocardiography with Doppler color flow mapping: correlation with cardiac catheterization. J Am Coll Cardiol 19:1516, 1992

193. Herrera CJ, Chaudhry FA, DeFrino PF et al: Value and limitation so transesophageal echocardiography in evaluating prosthetic or bioprosthetic valve dysfunction. Am J Cardiol 69:697, 1992

194. Dzavik V, Cohen G, Chan KL: Role of transesophageal echocardiography in the diagnosis and management of prosthetic valve thrombosis. J Am Coll Cardiol 18:1829, 1991

195. Chen YT, Kan MN, Chen JS: Detection of prosthetic mitral valve leak: a comparative study using transesophageal echocardiography, transthoracic echocardiography, and auscultation. J Clin Ultrasound 18:557, 1990

196. Sheikh KH, Bengtson JR, Rankin JS et al: Intraoperative transesophageal Doppler color flow imaging used to guide patient selection and operative treatment of ischemic mitral regurgitation. Circulation 84:594, 1991

197. Kyo S, Takamoto S, Matsumura M et al: Immediate and early postoperative evaluation of results of cardiac surgery by transesophageal two-dimensional Doppler echocardiography. Circulation 76:V-113, 1987

198. Maurer G, Czer LSC, Chauz A et al: Intraoperative Doppler color flow mapping for assessment of valve repair for mitral regurgitation. Am J Cardiol 60: 333, 1987

199. Seward JB, Khandheria BK, Edwards WD et al: Biplanar transesophageal echocardiography: anatomic correlations, image orientation, and clinical applications. Mayo Clin Proc 65:1193, 1990

200. Takamoto S, Kyo S, Adachi H et al: Intraoperative color flow mapping by real-time two-dimensional Doppler echocardiography for evaluation of vulvular and congenital heart disease and vascular disease. J Thorac Cardiovasc Surg 90:802, 1985

201. Kenny J, Cohn L, Shemin R et al: Doppler echocardiographic evaluation of ring mitral valvuloplasty for pure mitral regurgitation. Am J Cardiol 59:341, 1987

202. Abbasi AS, Allen MW, DeCristofaro D, Ungar I: Detection and estimation of the degree of mitral regurgitation by range-gated pulsed Doppler echocardiography. Circulation 61:143, 1980

203. Karalis DG, Chandrasekaran K, Ross JJ et al: Single-place transesophageal echocardiography for assessing function of mechanical or bioprosthetic valves in the aortic valve position. Am J Cardiol 69:1310, 1992

204. Rafferty T, Durkin M, Elefteraides J, O'Connor TZ: Transesophageal echocardiographic evaluation of aortic valve integrity with antegrade crystalloid cardioplegic solution used as an imaging agent. J Thorac Cardiovasc Surg 104:637, 1992

205. Karalis DG, Bansal RC, Hauck AJ et al: Transesophageal echocardiographic recognition of subaortic complications in aortic valve endocarditis: clinical and surgical implications. Circulation 86: 353, 1992

206. Helmcke F, Nanda NC, Hsiung MC et al: Color Doppler assessment of mitral regurgitation with orthogonal planes. Circulation 75:175, 1987

207. Tribouilloy C, Shen WF, Quere JP et al: Assessment of severity of mitral regurgitation by measuring regurgitant jet width as its origin with transesophageal Doppler color flow imaging. Circulation 85: 1237, 1992

208. Cohn LH: Surgery for mitral regurgitation. JAMA 260:2883, 1988

209. Cohn LH, Kowalker W, Bhatia S et al: Comparative morbidity of mitral valve repair versus replacement for mitral regurgitation with and without coronary artery disease. Ann Thorac Surg 45:284, 1988

210. Maurer I, Regensburger D, Bernhard A: Aortic valve reconstruction in Rubinstein-Taybi syndrome: the valuable aid of transesophageal echocardiography. J Cardiovasc Surg 32:327, 1991

211. Rafferty T, Durkin MA, Sittig D et al: Transesophageal color flow Doppler imaging for aortic insufficiency in patients having cardiac operations. J Thorac Cardiovasc Surg 104:521, 1992

212. Essop MR, Skudicky D, Sareli P: Diagnostic value of transesophageal versus transthoracic echocardiography in discrete subaortic stenosis. Am J Cardiol 70:962, 1992

213. Skoularigis J, Deviri E, Wisenbaugh T et al: Role of transesophageal echocardiography in diagnosis of subaortic aneurysm. Am J Cardiol 69:1102, 1992

214. Borner N, Erbel R, Braun B et al: Diagnosis of aortic dissection by transesophageal echocardiography. Am J Cardiol 54:1157, 1984

215. Pfeiffer C, Erbel R, Henkel B, Meyer J: Evaluation of the thoracic aorta by transesophageal echocardiography. Circulation 70:II-293, 1984

216. Adachi H, Takamoto S, Kimura S et al: Early diagnosis and surgical intervention of acute aortic dissection by transesophageal color flow mapping. Circulation 82:IV19, 1990

217. Ballal RS, Nanda NC, Gatewood R et al: Usefulness of transesophageal echocardiography in assessment of aortic dissection. Circulation 84:1903, 1991

218. Chan KL: Usefulness of transesophageal echocardiography in the diagnosis of conditions mimicking aortic dissection. Am Heart J 122:495, 1991

219. Singer RA, Karalis DG, Procacci PM et al: Transesophageal echocardiography for the evaluation of atherosclerosis of the thoracic aorta. AJR 159:285, 1992

220. Matsuzaki M, Ono S, Tomochika Y et al: Advances in transesophageal echocardiography for the evaluation of atherosclerotic lesions in thoracic aorta—the effects of hypertension, hypercholesterolemia, and aging on atherosclerotic lesions. Jap Circ J 56: 592, 1992

221. Katz ES, Tunick PA, Rusinek H et al: Protruding aortic atheromas predict stroke in elderly patients undergoing cardiopulmonary bypass: experience with intraoperative transesophageal echocardiography. J Am Coll Cardiol 20:70, 1992

222. Horowitz DR, Tuhrim S, Budd J et al: Aortic plaque in patients with brain ischemia: diagnosis by transesophageal echocardiography. Neurology 42:1602, 1992

223. Toyoda K, Yasaka M, Nagata S et al: Aortogenic embolic stroke: a transesophageal echocardiographic approach. Stroke 23:1056, 1992

224. Amerenco P, Cohen A, Baudrimont M et al: Transesophageal echocardiographic detection of aortic arch disease in patients with cerebral infarction. Stroke 23:1005, 1992

225. Porembka DT, Johnson DJ, Fowl RJ et al: Descending thoracic aortic thrombus as a cause of multiple system organ failure: diagnosis by transesophageal echocardiography. Crit Care Med 20:1184, 1992

226. Coy KM, Maurer G, Goodman D et al: Transesophageal echocardiographic detection of aortic atheromatosis may provide clues to occult renal dysfunction in the elderly. Am Heart J 123:1684, 1992

227. Tunick PA, Kronzon I: Protruding atherosclerotic plaque in the aortic arch of patients with systemic embolization: a new finding seen by transesophageal echocardiography. Am Heart J 120:658, 1990

228. Thwaites BK, Stamatos JM, Crowl FD et al: Transesophageal echocardiographic diagnosis of intraaortic thrombus during coarctation repair. Anesthesiology 76:638, 1992

229. Illiceto S, Nanda NC, Hsiung MC et al: Assessment of aortic dissection by color Doppler. Circulation 74:II-132, 1986

230. Takamoto S, Kyo Matsumura M et al: Total visualization of thoracic dissecting aortic aneurysm by transesophageal Doppler color flow mapping. Circulation 74:II-134, 1986

231. Troianos CA, Savino JS, Weiss RL: Transesophageal echocardiographic diagnosis of aortic dissection during cardiac surgery. Anesthesiology 75:149, 1991

232. Oh JK, Seward JB, Khanderia BK et al: Transesophageal echocardiography in critically ill patients. Am J Cardiol 66:1492, 1990

233. Pearson AC, Castello R, Labovitz AJ: Safety and utility of transesophageal echocardiography in the critically ill patient. Circulation 83:61, 1991

234. Parker MM, Cunnion RE, Parrillo JE: Echocardiography and nuclear cardiac imaging in the critical care unit. JAMA 254:2935, 1985

235. Hinrichs A, Schluter M, Roewer N et al: Clinical value of transesophageal two-dimensional echocardiography in mechanically ventilated coronary care unit patients. Circulation 68:III-95, 1983

236. Terai C, Uenishi M, Sugimoto H et al: Transesophageal echocardiographic dimensional analysis of four cardiac chambers during positive end-expiratory pressure. Anesthesiology 63:640, 1985

237. Koenig K, Kasper W, Hofmann T et al: Transesophageal echocardiography for diagnosis of rupture of the ventricular septum or left ventricular papillary muscle during acute myocardial infarction. Am J Cardiol 59:362, 1987

238. Glance LG, Keefe DL, Carlon GC: Transesophageal echocardiography for assessing the cause of hypotension. Crit Care Med 19:1213, 1991

239. Reichert CL, Visser CA, Koolen JJ et al: Transesophageal echocardiography in hypotensive patients after cardiac operations: comparison with hemodynamic parameters. J Thorac Cardiovasc Surg 104:321, 1992

240. Bansal RC, Shah PM: Transesophageal echocardiography. Curr Probl Cardiol 15:643, 1990

241. Blanchard DG, Dittrich HC, Mitchell M, McCann HA: Diagnostic pitfalls in transesophageal echocardiography. J Am Soc Echocardiogr 5:525, 1992

242. Schluter M, Hinrichs A, Thier W et al: Transesophageal two-dimensional echocardiography: comparison of ultrasonic and anatomic sections. Am J Cardiol 53:1173, 1984

243. Shively BK, Schiller NB: Transesophageal echocardiography in the intraoperative detection of myocardial ischemia and infarction. Echocardiography 3:433, 1986

244. Daniel WG, Ergel R, Kasper W et al: Safety of transesophageal echocardiography: a multicenter survey of 10,419 examinations. Circulation 83:817, 1991

245. Ofili EO, Rich MW: Safety and usefulness of transesophageal echocardiography in persons aged ≥ 70 years. Am J Cardiol 66:1279, 1990

246. Geibel A, Kasper W, Behroz A et al: Risk of transesophageal echocardiography in awake patients with cardiac diseases. Am J Cardiol 62:337, 1988

247. Chan K, Cohen GI, Sochowdki RA, Baird MG: Complications of transesophageal echocardiography in ambulatory adult patients: analysis of 1500 consecutive examinations. J Am Soc Echocardiogr 4:577, 1991

248. Orihashi K, Hong Y, Sisto DA et al: The anatomical location of the transesophageal echocardiographic transducer during a short-axis view of the left ventricle. J Cardiothorac Anesth 4:726, 1990

249. Dewhirst WE, Stragand JJ, Fleming BM: Mallory-Weiss tear complicating intraoperative transesophageal echocardiography in a patient undergoing aortic valve replacement. Anesthesiology 73:777, 1990

250. O'Shea JP, Southern JF, D'Ambra MN et al: Effects of prolonged transesophageal echocardiographic imaging and probe manipulation on the esophagus: an echocardiographic-pathologic study. J Am Coll Cardiol 17:1426, 1991

251. Urbanowicz JH, Kernoff RS, Oppenheim G et al: Transesophageal echocardiography and its potential for esophageal damage. Anesthesiology 72:40, 1990

252. Messina AG, Paranicas M, Fiamengo et al: Risk of dysphagia after transesophageal echocardiography. Am J Cardiol 67:313, 1991

253. Fagan LF, Weiss R, Castello R, Labovita AJ: Transtracheal placement and imaging with a transesophageal echocardiographic probe. Am J Cardiol 67:909, 1991

254. Humphrey LS: Esophageal stethoscope has complicating transesophageal echocardiography. J Cardiothorac Anesth 2:356, 1988

255. Kronzon I, Cziner DG, Katz ES et al: Buckling of

the tip of the transesophageal echocardiography probe: a potentially dangerous technical malfunction. J Am Soc Echocardiogr 5:176, 1992

256. Foster E, Kusomoto FM, Sobol SM, Schiller NB: Streptococcal endocarditis temporally related to transesophageal echocardiography. J Am Soc Echocardiogr 3:424, 1990

257. Gorge G, Erbel R, Henrichs KJ et al: Positive blood cultures during transesophageal echocardiography. Am J Cardiol 65:1404, 1990

258. Steckelberg JM, Khandheria BK, Anhalt JP et al: Prospective evaluation of the risk of bacteremia associated with transesophageal echocardiography. Circulation 84:177, 1991

259. Nikutta P, Mantey-Stiers F, Becht I et al: Risk of bacteremia induced by transesophageal echocardiography: analysis of 100 consecutive patients. J Am Soc Echocardiogr 5:168, 1992

260. Melendez LJ, Chan KL, Cheung PK et al: Incidence of bacteremia in transesophageal echocardiography: a prospective study of 140 consecutive patients. J Am Coll Cardiol 18:1650, 1991

261. Voller H, Speilberg C, Schroder K et al: Frequency of positive blood cultures during transesophageal echocardiography. Am J Cardiol 68:1538, 1991

262. Dajani AS, Bisno AL, Chung KJ et al: Prevention of bacterial endocarditis. JAMA 264:2919, 1990

263. Seward JB, Khandheria BK, Oh JK et al: Transesophageal echocardiography: technique, anatomic correlations, implementaiton, and clinical applications. Mayo Clin Proc 63:649, 1988

264. Hong Y, Oka Y: Left and right ventricles. p. 70. In Oka Y, Goldiner PL (eds): Transesophageal Echocardiography, JB Lippincott, Philadelphia, 1992.

265. Clements FM, de Bruijn NP: Perioperative evaluation of regional wall motion by transesophageal two-dimensional echocardiography. Anesth Analg 66:249, 1987

Respiratory Monitoring 12

Jeffrey A. Katz
James M. Hynson

The goals of respiratory monitoring are to assess pulmonary oxygen (O_2) and carbon dioxide (CO_2) exchange, and to determine the adequacy and efficiency of respiratory mechanics and ventilatory reserves. The intensity of monitoring ranges from simple clinical observation through various techniques of increasing complexity and invasiveness. Respiratory monitoring has improved significantly during the past decade, based on technologic advances and a better understanding of the pathophysiologic characteristics of respiratory failure. The importance of these changes is demonstrated by the conclusion of the ASA Closed-Claims Analysis that adverse respiratory events could have been prevented with better monitoring.[1,2]

This chapter discusses the respiratory variables monitored in the clinical setting, under the categories of oxygenation, CO_2 elimination, and respiratory mechanics. Clinical considerations governing the selection of these monitors and interpretation of the data are discussed, noting differences between the operating room and critical care settings.

ASSESSING OXYGENATION

Oxygen transport from the environment to body tissues is often described as a cascade (Fig. 12-1), the monitoring of which requires assessing processes at each level of the cascade.[3] Alterations at any level in the transfer process may result in inadequate oxygen delivery.

The whole-body store of oxygen is extremely small—approximately 1,000 ml in the body and 400 ml in the lung during air breathing in the adult.[3] The lung store is augmented when breathing higher oxygen fractions; for example, at an inspired fraction of oxygen (FIO_2) of 1.0, oxygen stores may increase to approximately 3L. Oxygen combined with hemogloblin forms the largest component of the nonpulmonary store; for example, 850 ml while breathing room air, but increasing only to approximately 950 ml with FIO_2 of 1.0. Because the oxygen store is small, changes in uptake or consumption will appear rapidly in the arterial or mixed venous blood. Therefore, blood is an excellent site for sampling the status of the system.

Inspired Oxygen Partial Pressure

Inspired oxygen partial pressure (PIO_2) is determined by barometric pressure (PB) and FIO_2):

$$PIO_2 = FIO_2 \times (PB - 47)$$

where 47 is the vapor pressure exerted by water at 37°C. Intubated patients ventilated with a nonrebreathing system, for example, a critical care ventilator, receive a constant PIO_2 determined by the FIO_2 setting on the ventilator. During ventilation with a partial rebreathing system, PIO_2 will vary slightly during the inspiratory period. In all intubated patients, FIO_2 must be continuously measured using an oxygen analyzer.

Determination of PIO_2 in unintubated patients receiving supplemental oxygen may be difficult due to entrainment of room air. Use of a high-flow system may overcome this problem by exceeding the patient's peak inspiratory flow to maintain a constant FIO_2 throughout the inspiratory phase. High-flow systems usually incorporate a Venturi device with an adjustable valve for controlling the amount of entrained air, permitting the FIO_2 to be varied predictably from room air to that approaching 1.0. As FIO_2 is increased, total flow decreases (because entrained flow decreases). In patients with acute respiratory distress syndrome (ARDS) having high minute ventilation and inspiratory flow, Venturi systems capable of higher flows and higher FIO_2 are required (e.g., the Misty OX, MMCA, Costa Mesa, CA; which provides flows of up to 110 L/min at FIO_2 of 0.7). When the patient's peak inspiratory flow is less than total delivered flow, FIO_2 can be determined from gas samples from the mask; when patient's peak flow demand exceeds delivered flow, the measured FIO_2 exceeds the true inspired value.

PIO_2 cannot be determined easily during use of low-flow systems such as simple face masks or nasal cannulas. However, based on the flow rate and system configuration, PIO_2 can be estimated.[4] For example, with nasal cannulas, at 2 L/min, $FIO_2 \approx$ 0.28, at 4 L/min, $\approx$ 0.36, at 6 L/min, $\approx$ 0.44. With a face mask and a flow rate of 8 L/min, FIO_2 will be $\approx$ 0.6. Finally, a well-fitting face mask with a reservoir bag having a flow of 10 to 15 L/min can provide an FIO_2 of 0.8 or greater. If necessary, PIO_2 can be measured during low-flow oxygen supplementation by sampling gas from a catheter placed in the nasopharynx.[5]

Alveolar Oxygen Partial Pressure

The alveolar partial pressure of oxygen (PAO_2) depends on the combined effects of alveolar ventilation, PIO_2, and uptake of oxygen by pulmonary capillary blood. Failure to replace oxygen removed by pulmonary capillary blood through continued alveolar ventilation will rapidly decrease PAO_2. The "ideal" PAO_2 may be calculated from the alveolar air equation:

$$PAO_2 = PIO_2 - PaCO_2 \left(\frac{PIO_2 - P\bar{E}O_2}{P\bar{E}CO_2} \right)$$

where $PaCO_2$ is the arterial partial pressure of carbon dioxide, $P\bar{E}O_2$ is the mixed-expired O_2 and $P\bar{E}CO_2$ is mixed-expired CO_2. For most clinical applications, a simplified equation for calculating PAO_2 provides an accurate estimate and eliminates the need to collect and measure mixed expired gases:

$$PAO_2 = PIO_2 - PaCO_2 \left(FIO_2 + \frac{1 - FIO_2}{R} \right)$$

where R is the respiratory exchange ratio (quotient) and is assumed to be 0.8.[6]

Alveolar to Arterial Oxygen Partial Pressure Difference

In normal healthy lungs, there is a small alveolar to arterial PO_2 difference ($P(A-a)O_2$) of 15 to 35 mmHg (increasing with age). In disease processes, the effect of right-to-left shunting and/or a low ventilation-to-perfusion ratio (V/Q) adds to this normal gradient. Conceptually, it is useful to consider the $P(A-a)O_2$ as the result of mixing the *content* of oxygen in blood that has perfused normally ventilated alveoli, and the *content* of oxygen in blood that has perfused alveoli that are not ventilated.

Using this two-compartment model, an equation for shunt fraction can be derived as follows: Cardiac output ($\dot{Q}T$) equals the sum of shunt flow ($\dot{Q}s$) and pulmonary capillary blood flow ($\dot{Q}C$).

$$\dot{Q}T = \dot{Q}s + \dot{Q}C$$

The amount of oxygen flowing through any compartment per minute is the product of compart-

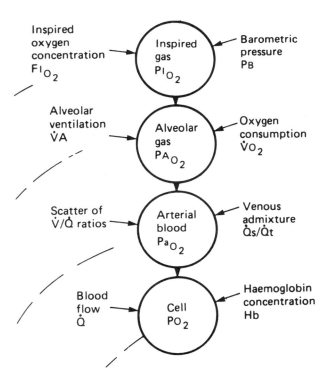

Fig. 12-1. Summary of factors affecting oxygen transport. (From Nunn,[3] with permission.)

ment blood flow and oxygen content. Therefore, the total amount of oxygen flowing through the aorta ($\dot{Q}_T$ · arterial oxygen content [CaO_2]) is the sum of oxygen flowing through the pulmonary capillaries ($\dot{Q}_C$ · pulmonary end-capillary oxygen content [$Cc'O_2$]) and the amount of oxygen flowing through the shunt ($\dot{Q}_S$ · mixed venous oxygen content [$C\bar{v}O_2$]).

$$\dot{Q}_T \cdot CaO_2 = \dot{Q}_C \cdot Cc'O_2 + \dot{Q}_S \cdot C\bar{v}O_2$$

Rearranging these two equations yields the shunt equation:

$$\frac{\dot{Q}_S}{\dot{Q}_T} = \frac{Cc'O_2 - CaO_2}{Cc'O_2 - C\bar{v}O_2}$$

$Cc'O_2$ is derived as follows:

$$Cc'O_2 \text{ (ml/dl)} = PaO_2(0.003)$$

$$+ 1.34$$

$$\times SO_2 \text{ (saturation of hemoglobin)}$$

$$\times Hgb \text{ (g/dl)}$$

Oxygen-combining capacity of hemoglobin is assumed to be 1.34 ml/g and blood oxygen solubility 0.003 ml/dl/mmHg. PaO_2 is calculated from the alveolar air equation as given above.

CaO_2 and $C\bar{v}O_2$ may be calculated from the same capacity and solubility factors as $Cc'O_2$. $C\bar{v}O_2$ measurement from $P\bar{v}O_2$ (mixed venous O_2 partial pressure) may result in substantial variance or errors in calculated $S\bar{v}O_2$ (mixed venous O_2 saturation) due to the shape of the dissociation curve. Finally, in urban populations and persons who are heavy smokers, some hemoglobin-combining capacity may be occupied by carboxyhemoglobin and methemoglobin. A similar problem occurs when methemoglobin has been induced as a side effect of coincidental drug therapy. For these reasons, oxygen content is measured directly; more commonly, oxygen saturation is directly measured using a cooximeter.[7]

For accurate $\dot{Q}_S/\dot{Q}_T$ determination, mixed venous blood (usually from a pulmonary artery catheter) should be sampled. $\dot{Q}_S/\dot{Q}_T$ calculated from an assumed arterial-venous oxygen difference can be grossly inaccurate.

Pulmonary artery catheterization for gas exchange and hemodynamic monitoring is indicated for guiding the management of patients with

a large $P(A-a)O_2$ (e.g., >450 mmHg at an FIO_2 of 1.0) when the etiology is uncertain and complex therapy is being used. A common example is the patient with acute diffuse pulmonary infiltrates, in whom elements of acute lung injury, regional atelectasis, and left heart failure are contributing factors. Therapy aimed at improving myocardial performance should improve pulmonary artery occlusion pressure, $\dot{Q}_T$, and $C(a-\bar{v})O_2$. Changes in the level of ventilatory support [e.g., positive end-expiratory pressure pressure (PEEP)] may improve PaO_2 and decrease $\dot{Q}_S/\dot{Q}_T$ but may adversely affect cardiovascular function.

In evaluating $P(A-a)O_2$ in the critical care setting, certain variables often cause confusion: FIO_2, $\dot{Q}_T$, and the effect of PEEP.

The effect on PaO_2 of increasing FIO_2 depends, in part, on the mechanism causing the increased $P(A-a)O_2$. Figures 12-2 and 12-3 depict the changes

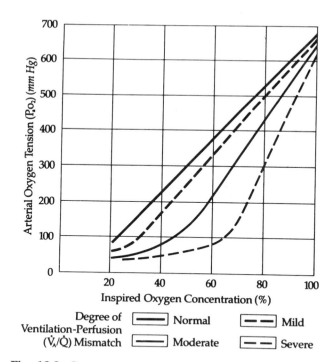

Fig. 12-2. Computer simulation of effect of increasing inspired oxygen concentrations on arterial oxygen tension (PaO_2) for various degrees of V/Q mismatch. In contrast to the negligible effect of FIO_2 on PaO_2 in patients with severe right-to-left shunting, increasing FIO_2 in patients with V/Q mismatch results in a large increase in PaO_2. (From Leatherman and Ingram,[8] with permission.)

in PaO_2 at increasing FIO_2 for conditions of either V/Q scatter or right-to-left shunt.[8] In general, increases in FIO_2 will compensate for V/Q scatter but will not correct hypoxemia due to significant shunting.[9,10]

Changes in $\dot{Q}T$ may also influence PaO_2.[11] Theoretically, a decrease in $\dot{Q}T$, assuming constant oxygen consumption ($\dot{V}O_2$), must result in a decreased $C\bar{v}O_2$:

$$C\bar{v}O_2 = CaO_2 - \frac{\dot{V}O_2}{\dot{Q}T}$$

At a constant $\dot{Q}s/\dot{Q}T$, the lowered $C\bar{v}O_2$ decreases CaO_2 and therefore PaO_2. Frequently, $\dot{Q}s/\dot{Q}T$ varies directly with $\dot{Q}T$, offsetting the anticipated effect.

Increasing end-expiratory pressure has multiple

effects that may alter PaO_2 in opposing directions. These include recruitment of atelectatic or low V/Q lung, redistribution of pulmonary blood flow, and possible decrease in cardiac output. If recruitment is the predominant effect, an increase in PaO_2 may be anticipated.[12] PaO_2 is likely to decrease if pulmonary blood flow is redistributed adversely[13] or if $\dot{Q}T$ and $C\bar{v}O_2$ decrease without an offsetting decrease in $\dot{Q}s/\dot{Q}T$.[11]

Oxygen Transport in the Blood

Oxygen delivery ($\dot{D}O_2$) is the quantity of oxygen transported to the tissues per unit time and is defined as the cardiac output times the arterial oxygen content,

$$\dot{D}O_2 = \dot{Q}T \cdot CaO_2$$

Under normal rest conditions, approximately 1,000 ml of O_2 is delivered to the tissues ($\dot{Q}T$ 5 L/min · CaO_2 20 ml O_2/dl), approximately 250 ml of which is consumed by the body, leaving 75 percent in the mixed venous blood.

$\dot{V}O_2$ is maintained over a wide range of $\dot{D}O_2$ by changes in the O_2 extraction ratio (Fig. 12-4).[14] At a critical lower level of $\dot{D}O_2$, $\dot{V}O_2$ decreases and is linearly dependent on $\dot{D}O_2$. Tissue hypoxia and anaerobic metabolism (i.e., lactic acidosis) occur in this region of delivery-dependent $\dot{V}O_2$. During anesthesia, the critical level of $\dot{D}O_2$ is approximately 330 ml/min/m², or 7 to 8 ml/kg/min[15]; values as low as 5 ml/kg/min have maintained adequate $\dot{V}O_2$.[16]

Experimentally, the critical value of $\dot{D}O_2$ is independent of the etiology of the decrease in $\dot{D}O_2$ (e.g., anemia or hypoxia).[17] During progressive isovolemic anemia, the lower limit of hemoglobin that maintains $\dot{D}O_2$ above the critical level has been estimated to be 4.0 g/dl.[16] However, this value assumes normal cardiovascular function and normal $\dot{V}O_2$.

In many critically ill patients with sepsis and/or respiratory failure, $\dot{V}O_2$ continues to increase as $\dot{D}O_2$ increases above normal levels, making it difficult to determine a critical level of $\dot{D}O_2$ (Fig. 12-4). This relationship is known as "pathologic supply dependency" and may be due to an alteration in oxygen extraction resulting from microcirculatory abnormalities and/or impaired cellular oxygen

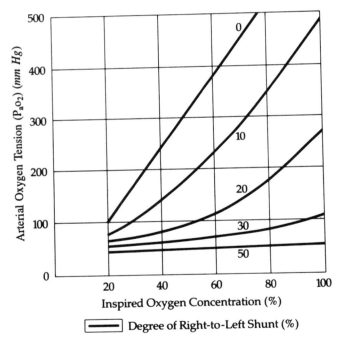

Fig. 12-3. The isoshunt diagram. The arterial concentration of inspired gas is plotted against arterial oxygen tension (PaO_2) for right-to-left shunts ranging from 0 to 50 percent of the cardiac output. The arterial-venous oxygen difference is assumed to be normal (5 ml/100ml), as are the hemoglobin and $PaCO_2$. With right-to-left shunts greater than 30 percent, there is limited increase in PaO_2 with increasing FIO_2. The isoshunt diagram also is useful for adjusting the FIO_2 to obtain a required level of PaO_2 to prevent hypoxemia. (From Leatherman and Ingram,[8] with permission.)

utilization.[18] Maintaining $\dot{D}O_2$ above supranormal levels (e.g., 600 ml/min/m²) may improve survival[19]; decreased blood lactate levels also correlate with improved survival.[19,20]

Monitoring $\dot{D}O_2$ requires measurement of $\dot{Q}T$, most often via a pulmonary artery catheter, and is usually limited to critically ill patients. During anesthesia, oxygen delivery is not routinely monitored but maintained by assuring adequate hemoglobin levels, adequate oxygen saturation (via pulse oximetry), and adequate blood pressure. Refinement of noninvasive techniques for measuring $\dot{Q}T$ (see Chapter 30) may improve clinical monitoring of $\dot{D}O_2$.

Monitoring Cellular Respiration

There is currently no direct method for monitoring the adequacy of cellular respiration. Assumptions of adequacy are based on direct or indirect measures of $\dot{D}O_2$ and indices of vital organ function (e.g., signs of myocardial or cerebral ischemia). Monitoring oxygen partial pressure and metabolite concentrations such as lactic acid in the venous blood from vital organs, might seem a logical method of assessing tissue metabolism. However, regional venous blood is not accessible, and mixed venous blood is less desirable for sampling because it reflects multiple areas of widely varying oxygen consumptions and blood flows. One would prefer to know not only individual organ values but also values from the most vulnerable areas within each organ.

Tissue electrodes (for detection of PCO_2, PO_2, and pH) are available but not clinically applicable. PO_2 varies considerably over short distances within specific tissues because it depends on proximity to the capillaries.

Arterial-Venous Oxygen Content Difference

Arterial-venous oxygen content difference $[C(a-\bar{v})O_2]$ is determined by tissue uptake of O_2 and blood flow. Assuming normal autoregulation, increases in $\dot{V}O_2$ produce metabolites, local acidosis, vasodilation, and a decrease in regional vascular resistance. $\dot{Q}T$ increases and/or peripheral blood flow is redistributed to these more active areas. Typically, this compensation is not complete, resulting in some increases in $C(a-\bar{v})O_2$, (increased extraction). Increased $C(a-\bar{v})O_2$ is manifest as a decrease in mixed venous oxygen saturation ($S\bar{v}O_2$).

Interpretation of $S\bar{v}O_2$ must recognize the influence of several factors, including $\dot{Q}T$, $\dot{V}O_2$, hemoglobin, and SaO_2, through a modified Fick equation:

$$S\bar{v}O_2 \approx SaO_2 - \frac{\dot{V}O_2}{(\dot{Q}T \times Hgb \times 1.34)}$$

$S\bar{v}O_2$ may be abnormally high when peripheral autoregulation is impaired by drugs (vasodilators), sep-

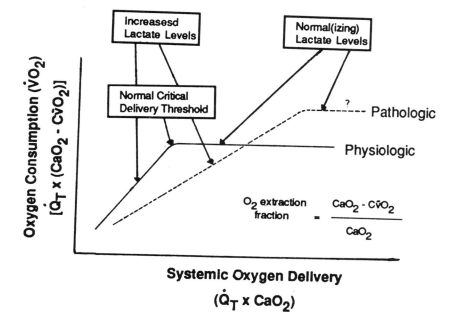

Fig. 12-4. Relationship between oxygen consumption and oxygen delivery in physiologic and pathologic states. The *continuous line* represents normal oxygen extraction and oxygen consumption levels (physiologic relationship). The *dashed line* represents altered oxygen extraction and supranormal oxygen consumption (pathologic relationship associated with sepsis). The oxygen uptake/supply dependency is characterized by increased blood lactate levels. (Modified from Vincent and DeBacker,[14] with permission.)

sis, or diseases such as cirrhosis, and may not accurately reflect the adequacy of tissue oxygen supply.

Mixed venous blood may be intermittently sampled via a pulmonary artery catheter to measure $P\bar{v}O_2$ or $S\bar{v}O_2$; alternatively, $S\bar{v}O_2$ may be measured continuously by reflectance oximetry. To obtain an appropriate mixed venous blood sample, the catheter tip should be in the proximal pulmonary artery and the sample should be drawn slowly to avoid contamination by pulmonary venous blood.[21] An abnormally high $S\bar{v}O_2$ also may indicate that the catheter tip is in a permanently wedged position.

Oxygen Consumption

During anesthesia, $\dot{V}O_2$ decreases by ≈ 15 percent[3] but increases during surgical stimulus and on emergence from anesthesia, especially during shivering.[22] $\dot{V}O_2$ is rarely measured during anesthesia, except for research purposes. Similarly, in critically ill patients, $\dot{V}O_2$ is not often measured, but may provide useful information in guiding hemodynamic (e.g., in determining critical $\dot{D}O_2$ levels) and ventilatory management. Because critically ill patients often have altered metabolism, or simply increased caloric requirements, energy expenditure estimated from $\dot{V}O_2$ and $\dot{V}CO_2$ is helpful in determining nutritional needs.[23]

Methods of Measuring $\dot{V}O_2$

There are three general methods of measuring $\dot{V}O_2$. The *first method* is based on the Fick principle,

$$\dot{V}O_2 = \dot{Q}T \times C(a-\bar{v})O_2$$

and is typically performed in patients with pulmonary artery catheters. $\dot{Q}T$ is measured by thermodilution and oxygen contents by sampling of mixed venous and arterial blood. For accurate determination of oxygen content, saturation must be directly measured by in vitro cooximetry. Inaccuracies are due primarily to errors intrinsic to the $\dot{Q}T$ thermodilution measurement (which can vary by 10 percent or more), and a small and usually negligible error due to exclusion of lung $\dot{V}O_2$.[24]

The *second method* for measuring $\dot{V}O_2$ involves calculating the difference between inspired oxygen volumes ($FIO_2 \times$ the inspired minute ventilation) and expired oxygen volumes ($F\bar{E}O_2$, mixed expired O_2 fraction $\times$ the $\dot{V}E$, expired minute ventilation).

The equation for deriving inspired minute ventilation from a measured expired minute ventilation requires the presence of an insoluble inert gas (usually nitrogen). In steady state, it is assumed that there is no change in inert gas volume during the tidal exchange.

$$\dot{V}O_2 = FIO_2 \times \left[\frac{F\bar{E}N_2 - F\bar{E}O_2}{FIN_2} \right] \times \dot{V}E$$

Gas mixing (for measurement of $F\bar{E}O_2$) can be achieved by passing the expired gas through a baffled box and sampling the gas distally, or by collecting the gas in a container (e.g., Douglas bag). Because the difference between FIO_2 and $F\bar{E}O_2$ will be smaller when FIO_2 is high, the accuracy of this technique at high FIO_2 has been questioned.[25]

Automated $\dot{V}O_2$ monitors based on analysis of inspired and expired gas are fairly accurate up to an FIO_2 of 0.6 (1.4 to 5.7 percent mean relative error) and are usually adequate for clinical application.[26] In unintubated patients, $\dot{V}O_2$ may be measured by the ventilated hood technique, which also uses the expired gas analysis principle.[3]

The *third method* of measuring $\dot{V}O_2$ is based on measurement of volume loss from a closed-circuit breathing system. Volume loss can be determined by measuring loss from a spirometer or by measuring the oxygen inflow required to maintain the volume of the spirometer.[27] This method of $\dot{V}O_2$ measurement requires manipulation of the breathing circuit. However, it is accurate and eliminates the analytic problems associated with high FIO_2. An automated system for use in the operating room or critical care environment is available (VVR Calorimeter, Vital Signs, Totowa, NJ).

ASSESSING CARBON DIOXIDE ELIMINATION

The whole-body store of carbon dioxide in the adult is approximately 100 L or more (of which only 2 to 3 percent is in the blood).[28] In an average-sized, resting, normothermic adult, metabolic CO_2 ($\dot{V}CO_2$) is added to this store at a rate of 200 ml/min, and, in steady state, the same amount is removed by alveolar ventilation. Interpretation of $PaCO_2$ requires recognition of whether the system is in a "steady" or "unsteady" state.

Arterial Carbon Dioxide Partial Pressure

Pa_{CO_2} is *the* measure of the effectiveness of minute ventilation ($\dot{V}E$). Normal $\dot{V}E$ is approximately 80 to 100 ml/kg/min.[29] The volume of gas that enters the respiratory tract in a minute contains two components: alveolar ventilation ($\dot{V}A$), that is, gas that crosses the alveolar capillary membrane, and dead-space ventilation ($\dot{V}D$), that is, gas that is not exchanged in the lungs. The relationship between Pa_{CO_2} and $\dot{V}E$ is such that doubling of ventilation halves the Pa_{CO_2}, and halving ventilation doubles Pa_{CO_2} regardless of the starting point (Fig. 12-5).[30] The factors affecting Pa_{CO_2} are illustrated in the following equation, which assumes no inhalation of CO_2:

$$Pa_{CO_2} = \frac{\dot{V}_{CO_2}(K)}{\dot{V}A}$$

where $\dot{V}_{CO_2}$ = CO_2 production (ml/min); K = 0.863; and $\dot{V}A$ = alveolar ventilation (L/min).

In the unsteady state, due to the time course of intercompartment equilibration, changes in Pa_{CO_2} precede changes in the whole-body CO_2 store (when $\dot{V}A$ changes) or follow such changes (when metabolism changes). After a step change in ventilation, Pa_{CO_2} immediately changes, with half the change occurring approximately 3 to 4 minutes after a step increase in ventilation, and 15 to 20 minutes after a step decrease (Fig. 12-6).[28] Changes in whole-body bicarbonate distribution and, therefore, in pH are related and may be somewhat slower. Arterial blood gas samples intended to reflect whole-body CO_2 production-excretion balance, and other aspects of acid-base balance, should not be drawn for at least 20 minutes after a change in minute ventilation (and preferably longer).

As an indirect measure of Pa_{CO_2}, central or peripheral (superficial) venous blood samples are satisfactory. The normal difference between arterial and mixed venous P_{CO_2} is 6 mmHg. In an inactive limb with no tourniquet, this difference may decrease, particularly when the blood is "arterialized" under conditions of anesthesia.[31]

Minute CO_2 Production ($\dot{V}_{CO_2}$)

During general anesthesia, $\dot{V}_{CO_2}$ decreases to 80 percent of basal levels. However, $\dot{V}_{CO_2}$ may increase during fever, shivering, sepsis, thyroid storm, in-

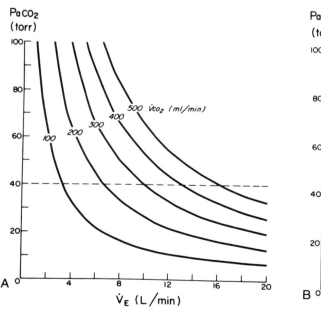

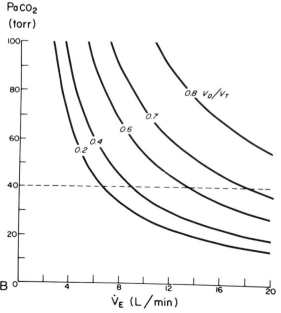

Fig. 12-5. Effects of minute ventilation on Pa_{CO_2}, assuming $P(a - A)_{CO_2} = 0$. **(A)** At various levels of CO_2 production, assuming $V_D/V_T = 0.3$. **(B)** At various levels of V_D/V_T, assuming $\dot{V}_{CO_2} = 250$ ml/min. (From Fairley,[30] with permission.)

creased catecholamine production, seizure activity, hyperalimentation, and malignant hyperthermia. Without a compensatory increase in alveolar ventilation, $PaCO_2$ would increase (Fig. 12-5A).

The rate of CO_2 elimination is the product of the mixed-expired CO_2 fraction ($F\overline{E}CO_2$) and the total volume of all gas expelled over the measurement interval. In clinical practice, a nonreturn valve is connected to the mouthpiece (awake) or endotracheal tube and expired gas is "collected." The system must ensure mixing of early and late expired gas. The $F\overline{E}CO_2$ is then measured, usually by an infrared analyzer (in percent) or by PCO_2 electrode (in mmHg).

Gas mixing (for measurement of $F\overline{E}CO_2$) can be achieved by passing the expired gas through a baffled box (a dry gas meter will suffice) and sampling the gas distally, or by collecting the gas in a container (e.g., Douglas bag).

An inefficient nonreturn valve (i.e., expired gas contaminated by inspired gas) does not influence the accuracy of the value obtained, provided that the diluted value for $F\overline{E}CO_2$ is accurate.

$$\dot{V}CO_2 = \text{measured } \dot{V}E \times F\overline{E}CO_2;$$

$$P\overline{E}CO_2 = F\overline{E}CO_2 (PB - PH_2O \text{ [patient]})$$

Dead Space

The respiratory dead space includes apparatus (if the patient is connected to any form of an external ventilating device), and anatomic and alveolar dead space components.[32] The physiologic dead space is the sum of the anatomic and alveolar dead space and is defined as the component of the tidal volume which does not participate in gas exchange. It is customary to use physiologic dead space ($VD_{physiol}$) in the clinical setting, since respiratory work and required minute ventilation depend, in large part, on the size of the total dead space.

In the healthy, spontaneously breathing person, normal dead space fraction (VD/VT) is approximately 0.3 and is largely related to anatomic dead space (the portion of the tidal volume not in the alveoli). In the clinical setting, VD/VT may increase primarily related to an increase in alveolar dead space (the proportion of tidal volume in nonperfused alveoli). Alveolar dead space increases due to pathologic processes that diminish aerated alveolar volume (e.g., lung cysts) and/or those that inter-

rupt or diminish pulmonary vascular flow (pulmonary embolism, low cardiac output states). In addition, alveolar dead space may increase if lung hyperinflation developed during mechanical ventilation due to differences in regional compliance and ventilation time constants. Indeed, in the terminal phases of acute hypoxemic respiratory failure, VD/VT may increase to values exceeding 0.7, often accounts for the majority of increased $\dot{V}E$, and is a major cause of CO_2 retention.

Exhaled Carbon Dioxide

Capnography analyzes the CO_2 concentration of the exhaled airstream and its principles are described in Chapter 13. This section will discuss the application of exhaled CO_2 monitoring relative to estimating $PaCO_2$ and determining dead space ventilation.

During each exhalation, gases emerge sequentially from the apparatus and anatomic dead space, then the alveoli. The exhaled CO_2 waveform can be examined against time or volume. The CO_2 trace against time is convenient and adequate for

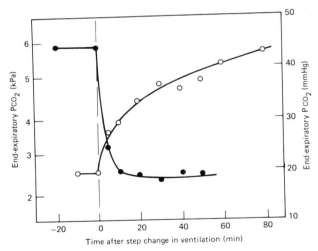

Fig. 12-6. Time course of changes in end-expiratory PCO_2 following step changes in ventilation. The *solid circles* indicate changes in end-expiratory PCO_2, which followed a step change in ventilation from 3.3 to 14 L/min. The *open circles* show the change following a step change in ventilation from 14 to 3.3 L/min. During the decline of PCO_2, half the total change is completed in about 3 minutes. During the increase in PCO_2, half of the change takes approximately 16 minutes. (From Nunn,[28] with permission.)

clinical use and is the method most commonly used by capnographs. However, analysis of the CO_2 against a volume trace gives a better reflection of V̇Q status of the lung and permits calculations of the components of physiologic dead space (Fig. 12-7).[33] When CO_2 is plotted against volume, a correction will be necessary because of the differing time delays of the volume and CO_2 sampling and recording systems.[34]

Whether plotted against time or volume, the CO_2 trace is defined by three phases (Fig. 12-8).[34] Phase I is gas that remains in the anatomic (and apparatus) dead space at the end of the preceding inspiration; phase II is a mixture of dead space and alveolar gas; and phase III reflects the alveolar CO_2 level. If all alveoli were to empty at the same rate (and no additional CO_2 was added from venous blood during expiration), phase III would be "flat" and consist only of a homogeneous mixture of gas from "perfused" and "unperfused" alveoli. The gas in the "perfused" alveoli would equilibrate with its perfusate and be at the same PCO_2 as arterial blood (ignoring any small effect from shunted blood). The gas in the "unperfused" alveoli would be similar to inspired gas and, during exhalation, dilute mixed alveolar (phase III) gas to a level less than arterial. In a normal awake person, this $P(a-ET)CO_2$ (arterial-alveolar gradient) is negligible (Fig. 12-8A); during general anesthesia, and in many patients with respiratory failure and/or

pulmonary embolism (Fig. 12-8C), the $P(a-ET)CO_2$ increases, reflecting the increase in alveolar dead space.[34] For example, during general anesthesia and mechanical ventilation, $P(a-ET)CO_2$ averages 5 mmHg with maximal differences of as much as 15 mmHg.[35,36]

End-tidal CO_2 partial pressure ($PETCO_2$) is a "spot sample" from phase III derived by various methods. Usually, this is the highest value for CO_2 in the respiratory cycle, obtained either by observation of a continuous trace or as an electronically sampled data point. When alveolar emptying is uneven, for example, in pulmonary diseases affecting the airways, there is a greater than normal dispersion of alveolar carbon dioxide partial pressure ($PACO_2$), owing to inhomogeneous V/Q relationships between lung compartments. Compartments with high alveolar ventilation and low $PACO_2$ empty early in expiration and those with low ventilation and high $PACO_2$ empty late in expiration. This asynchronous emptying of the lung compartments results in an increased slope of phase III (Fig. 12-8B). Under these circumstances, $PETCO_2$ may be falsely high (i.e., higher than mean $PACO_2$), reflecting alveoli with the longest time constants, and, in some circumstances, may produce negative values for $P(a-ET)CO_2$.[37] Nevertheless, in most instances, there is sufficient intermixing of alveolar and dead-space gas for the $PETCO_2$ to be considerably less than $PACO_2$. Therefore, the $P(a-ET)CO_2$ depends on both the alveolar dead space and other factors influencing V/Q that affect the slope of phase III. In addition, when phase III has an increasing slope, $PETCO_2$ also depends on the termination of end-expiration, which, during mechanical ventilation, depends on the setting of the inspiration/expiration (I/E) ratio.

Measurement of Dead Space

Anatomic dead space (VD_{anat}) is derived from the Bohr equation, which is derived from the proposition that mixed expired carbon dioxide partial pressure ($P\bar{E}CO_2$) is a mixture of alveolar and dead-space gas. The formula is as follows:

$$VD_{anat} = \frac{PACO_2 - P\bar{E}CO_2}{PACO_2 - PICO_2} \times VT$$

Because a precise definition of $PACO_2$ is difficult, $PETCO_2$ is commonly used. However, if the phase III slope suggests considerable inhomogeneity, an-

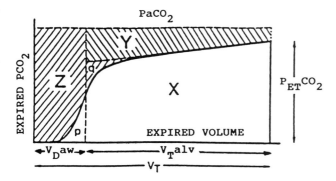

Fig. 12-7. Single-breath test for CO_2 (SBT-CO_2) used to determine physiologic dead space and its subdivisions. Exhaled PCO_2 is plotted against tidal volume (VT). A *dotted horizontal line* representing $PACO_2$ is drawn on the SBT-CO_2 curve. A *vertical dotted line* is constructed (through phase 2) so that the two areas *p* and *q* are equal. Area *Z* represents anatomic dead space, and area *Y* represents alveolar dead space. Physiologic dead space is represented by area *Z* plus area *Y*. (From Shankar et al.,[33] with permission.)

atomic dead space should be calculated by the Fowler method (Fig. 12-7).

Alveolar dead space can be calculated from the CO_2 vs volume trace (Fig. 12-7) or, if the slope of phase III is flat, from the following formula:

$$VD_{alv} = \frac{PaCO_2 - PETCO_2}{PaCO_2 - PICO_2} \times VT$$

If the phase III slope suggests considerable inhomogeneity, calculation of physiologic dead space ($VD_{physiol}$) requires the Enghoff modification of the Bohr equation:

$$VD_{physiol} = \frac{PaCO_2 - P\bar{E}CO_2}{PaCO_2 - PICO_2} \times VT$$

Expired gas volume and $P\bar{E}CO_2$ are derived from a 3-minute gas collection (see discussion of $\dot{V}CO_2$). Respiratory frequency is counted and tidal volume calculated. Note that VD/VT is constant over a wide range of tidal volumes during mechanical ventilation.[38]

When to Measure VD/VT and VCO₂

When the minute volume required to maintain a normal $PaCO_2$ is abnormally large (Fig. 12-5), the cause must be either an unusually large VD/VT or an abnormally high $\dot{V}CO_2$. In most normothermic patients, the assumption can be made that $\dot{V}CO_2$ is near-normal (for each degree centigrade above normal, an increase of 7 percent can be anticipated). Major increases in required minute ventilation usually are due to dead space. (The possibility of rebreathing due to faulty valving must be considered, particularly when the magnitude of cardiopulmonary disorder is not compatible with the data.) In some patients, $\dot{V}CO_2$ can be increased significantly above normal during hyperalimentation with high concentrations of glucose, and with

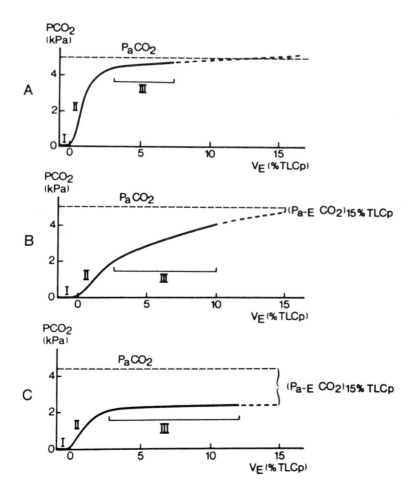

Fig. 12-8. The single-breath test for CO_2 (SBT-CO_2) recording during resting tidal ventilation in (**A**) a healthy subject, (**B**) a patient with obstructive lung disease, and (**C**) a patient with pulmonary embolism. The exhaled PCO_2 is recorded as a continuous trace depicting the three phases, I, II, and III. (From Eriksson et al.,[34] with permission.)

certain topically applied burn dressings (e.g., mafenide acetate cream). Under such conditions, steady-state R (respiratory quotient) values above 1.0 have been measured. If the required degree of minute ventilation generates either unusually high airway pressures or poses difficulties in weaning the patient from mechanical ventilation in the presence of any of the above factors, V_D/V_T and $\dot{V}_{CO_2}$ should be measured to permit identification of the components of the problem and allow appropriate modifications. Direct knowledge of V_D/V_T and $\dot{V}_{CO_2}$ may not be necessary in most clinical circumstances.

ASSESSING RESPIRATORY MECHANICS

Respiratory mechanics encompass an assessment of the mechanical properties of the lung and chest wall, the patient's ability to breathe spontaneously, and the patient's ventilatory reserve or capability. The fundamental indices that characterize the mechanical behavior of the respiratory system are derived from measurements of pressure, volume, and flow. In mechanically ventilated patients, a detailed analysis of respiratory mechanics can be performed readily with simple and commonly available equipment—a pneumotachograph to measure flow, an integrator to measure volume changes from the flow signal, and a transducer to measure pressure at the airway opening. Several commercial ventilators[39] [e.g., Puritan-Bennett 7200a (Puritan-Bennett Corp, Carlsbad, CA); Hamilton Veolar (Hamilton Medical, Reno, NV); Bear 5, (Bear Medical Systems, Riverside, CA)] or stand-alone respiratory monitors[40,41] [e.g., Bicore CP-100, (Bicore, Irvine, CA); Ultima SV (Datex Instruments Corp, Helsinki, Finland)] permit direct measurements of pressure, volume, and flow. When introducing any measurement device into a breathing circuit, consideration must be given to its resistance and mechanical dead space, particularly in patients with poor mechanical reserves.

Measurement of Gas Volumes

The two commonly used methods for measuring gas volumes involve collection devices and flow sensors. Volume changes relative to functional residual capacity (FRC) also can be determined by tracking movements of the chest wall and abdomen (a non-

airway-dependent method), rather than movements of respired gases. Clinical determinations include measurements of tidal volume (V_T), vital capacity (VC), and FRC.

During clinical monitoring, volume values are typically measured at ambient temperature and pressure saturated with water vapor (ATPS). For laboratory testing of pulmonary function, and certainly for research, respiratory volumes generally are expressed at body temperature and pressure saturated with water vapor (BTPS) and require conversion from ATPS. The formula is

$$Vol\ BTPS = Vol\ ATPS$$
$$\times \frac{273 + body\ temp\ °C}{273 + ambient\ temp\ °C}$$
$$\times \frac{P_B - P_{H_2O}\ body\ temp}{P_B - P_{H_2O}\ ambient\ temp},$$

with P_{H_2O} at various temperatures obtainable from standard tables.

Values for $\dot{V}_{O_2}$ and $\dot{V}_{CO_2}$ are always quoted at standard temperature and pressure dry (STPD). The conversion formula is

$$\dot{V}_{O_2}\ (or\ \dot{V}_{CO_2})\ at\ STPD = \dot{V}_{O_2}\ (or\ \dot{V}_{CO_2})\ ATPS$$
$$\times \frac{(P_B - P_{H_2O})0.3592}{(T°C + 273)},$$

using ambient values for T°C and P_{H_2O}.

Collection Devices

A nonreturn valve is placed at the endotracheal tube, and expired gas is collected in a container. This container may be calibrated (e.g., Bennett spirometer bellows, Collins spirometer, wedge spirometer) or its contents ejected (e.g., Douglas bag) into a calibrated device such as a large spirometer or a dry gas meter (see below).

All gas collection techniques are subject to error due to imperfections in valving. If expired tidal or minute volume is to be measured, the valving must *exclude* any contamination by inspired gas or (in an anesthesia circuit) flowmeter output, and must *include* all of each expired tidal volume.

This method of volume measurement is not easily applicable to a rebreathing system or to one that adds gas in excess of the inspired volume. Thus, it is most often used in the critical care setting, where mechanical ventilation systems with nonreturn valves are common, but not in the operating room.

Dry gas meters are housed in metal boxes containing two bellows that fill and empty reciprocally as gas passes through. Each bellows is connected through levers and gears to a common meter display, analogous to that on a commercial gas meter. Thus, a Douglas bag can be emptied through such a device and a reading of the delivered volume obtained, with an accuracy within ±1 percent.[42]

Flow Sensors

Flow sensors are inherently less accurate than collection devices, for reasons that differ with each type. If the sensor is placed between the endotracheal tube and the breathing circuit, errors due to valving inefficiencies are avoided. Placement in other locations in the circuit may incur the same errors associated with collection devices (inspired-expired cross-contamination, added flow augmentation).

Rotor Meters

The measured gas flow of the rotor meter,[43] rotates a vane or rotor on a spindle connected via a geared system to a pointer on a calibrated dial or via electronic integration to a digital display. The gas flow may be directed so that the vane turns when the flow moves in one direction (Wright respirometer) or bidirectionally (Dräger, Ohmeda). These ventilation meters usually include on-off controls and may incorporate timers. Problems include inertia and friction (falsely low readings), collection of moisture and foreign material (falsely low readings), and momentum (overshoot at the end of a high-flow period giving falsely high readings). Most errors occur at low flows. For example, the Ohmeda 5400 and 5410 volume monitors (Ohmeda, Madison, WI) are accurate within 10 percent when tested with ambient air gas at flow rates between 10 and 60 L/min ($\dot{V}E$ 2.4 to 15 L/min).[44] When tested with air saturated with vapor or with a 70 percent N_2O/O_2 gas mixture, both instruments significantly underestimated (20 to 40 percent) the true volume at flow rates less than 12 L/min ($\dot{V}E$ < 3 L/min). Because of impairment by moisture, these instruments are inappropriate for continuous monitoring in the critical care setting but function satisfactorily under other conditions, for example, when incorporated in a circuit that can be switched to bypass the meter.

Pneumotachographs

A low mechanical resistance is placed in the gas flow of the pneumotachograph,[45–47] creating a pressure difference across the resistance that is proportional to flow and electronically transduced. Volume measurement is derived by integration of flow with time. Pneumotachographs can be placed anywhere in the breathing circuit or at the endotracheal tube-circuit interface and are in common use in pulmonary function laboratories and in critical care units. However, pneumotachographs are most accurate over a limited range of flows, becoming inherently nonlinear over a wide range of flows as turbulence increases, resulting in inaccuracy in measurements. Alternatively, their use may require electronic linearizing circuitry that is often unique to each pneumotachograph. The sensitivity and accuracy of the (commonly used) screen type of pneumotachograph are seriously impaired by secretions that decrease the cross-sectional area. If both inspired and exhaled volumes are to be measured, the physical characteristics of the pneumotachograph and its connectors must provide an identical pressure-flow relationship bidirectionally. The pressure difference across the pneumotachograph varies with the viscosity and density of the gas mixture. For example, an error of up to 10 percent may occur in a volume measurement when FIO_2 is changed from 0.21 to 1.0.

Clinically, devices with large dead space (e.g., the Fleisch device) may impose additional ventilatory load during spontaneous breathing. However, commercially available disposable devices incorporating small internal volumes are now available, including the Critikon ring orifice device,[48] the Datex D-lite flow sensor,[41] and the Bicore CP-100.[40] These devices avoid the problems due to collection of moisture, are lightweight, and are streamlined to connect at the endotracheal circuit interface. In addition to flow and volume measurements, the Datex and Bicore monitors also display proximal airway pressure. Manufacturer specifications for the Datex instrument indicate an accuracy of ±6 percent for tidal volumes between 250 and 2,000 ml and $\dot{V}E$ between 2.5 and 40 L/min. Similar levels of accuracy are reported for the Bicore and Critikon monitors.

Ultrasound Flowmeter

The velocity of gas passing between an ultrasound transmitter and receiver influences the received signal of the ultrasound flowmeter. Changes in signal can be calibrated in terms of flow, a principle incorporated in certain pulmonary function and hand-held spirometry devices.

Heated Sensor

A heated element is placed in the (cooler) air flow of the heated sensor. Temperature decreases as flow increases, according to the thermal conductivity of the gas being measured. These sensors readily lose sensitivity when they become coated with foreign material or oxidized. They are not in common use. However, they may serve to indicate the change from inspiration to expiration and vice versa, should this be required (e.g., dynamic compliance measurements, filling pressures at end-expiration).

Thoracic Movement

Changes in thoracicoabdominal dimensions (diameter and circumference) can be measured by plethysmographic techniques and correlated with changes in lung volume during unobstructed respiration.[49] Several types of devices have been developed, but respiratory inductive plethysmography (RIP) is the most commonly used clinically.[50,51]

RIP involves placement of elastic bands about the chest and abdomen. Changes in compartment volume create proportional changes in cross-sectional area of the electrical induction loops. Resulting signal fluctuations track compartmental motion and can be summed to estimate tidal volume changes. RIP allows for the measurement of respiratory frequency, tidal volume, inspiratory time, changes in FRC, and the contributions of the rib cage and abdomen to lung volume changes. Use of RIP will detect discoordinate breathing movements such as asynchrony (a time lag between motion of two compartments) and paradoxical motion (compartments moving in opposite directions). Two types of paradoxical movements may occur, one associated with inward motion of the rib cage during inspiration during airway obstruction, and the other with inward motion of the abdomen during inspiration. Both asynchrony and abdominal paradox are thought to indicate diaphragmatic weakness or fatigue,[52] although these abnormal respiratory motions also may be manifestations of increased respiratory load rather than fatigue per se.[53]

Calibration of Volume Measurement Devices

Volume measurement devices should be calibrated at regular intervals. Rigorous calibration involves either gas displacement by a known volume of water or use of an accurately calibrated spirometer. For calibration of flow-measuring devices, a gas flow may be delivered through highly accurate manufacturer-certified calibration flow meters for a measured time interval. For clinical purposes, a ''supersyringe'' is extremely useful (Fig. 12-9). This is an accurately calibrated giant syringe that has an efficient seal around the plunger. When filled, syringe volume ranges from 500 ml to 3 L, which may be ejected in toto or in mechanically controlled known fractions. The syringe is emptied through the device to be calibrated, and the measured volume noted. If the volume measurement device is flow-sensitive, the speed of emptying the syringe is varied over multiple tests to detect flow-related error.

Lung Volumes

Only a few lung volume divisions are important in clinical monitoring. These include tidal volume (V_T), functional residual capacity (measures of end-expiratory lung volume), and vital capacity (a measure of ventilatory capability).

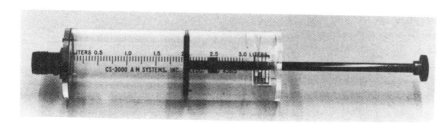

Fig. 12-9. Supersyringe for calibration of volume measurement devices.

Tidal Volume

Measurement of V_T permits calculation of $\dot{V}_E$, a key indicator of work of breathing and an important determinant of Pa_{CO_2}. Shallow V_T (<4 ml/kg) suggests major limitations of respiratory muscle strength or depression of ventilatory drive, and is commonly observed during spontaneous breathing under general anesthesia.

Exhaled V_T can always be assumed to come from the patient's lungs. Ventilation meters should thus be placed on the exhalation side of the breathing circuit or at the endotracheal tube-circuit connection. Although a meter on the inspiratory side offers the advantage of remaining relatively dry (anesthesia circuits), readings from this location (or from a ventilator bellows) cannot be relied upon to provide accurate tidal volume. For example, inspiratory volumes substantially exceeding exhalation volumes on each tidal breath suggest gas leakage in the patient-ventilator system (e.g., from circuit leak, around ET cuff, bronchopleural fistula). The possibility of overestimating V_T also arises when a meter is placed within a breathing circuit (inspiratory or expiratory side) due to continuous cycling of added gases from flow meters.

Gas Compression and Circuit Compliance

The actual V_T delivered (to the patient) may differ from that electronically set on the ventilator or from that apparent by the excursion of the bellows. Discrepancy between set and delivered V_T is a function of several factors, including fresh gas flow, inspiratory time (T_I), circuit volume (including humidifier), distensibility of the breathing circuit, and the ventilator flow generator.[54–56] Under certain conditions, delivered V_T is augmented and in others, decreased.

In anesthesia systems, delivered V_T is augmented by the product of the fresh gas flow and the T_I. (Delivered V_T also might increase in the rare case of a bellows leak.) In contrast, delivered V_T is decreased due to compression of gases and distension of the breathing circuit (ventilator bellows, absorber, and connecting tubing) and the type of flow generator. A typical adult circle circuit with ventilator has a compression volume of 6 to 7 L and a compressibility of 6 to 12 ml/cmH$_2$O.[55] In the operating room, the volume gained by fresh gas flow during inspiration typically is offset by the volume decreased due to compressibility. Therefore, the set

V_T approximates the delivered V_T during conventional mechanical ventilation with peak airway pressures in the 20 to 30 cm H_2O range and a concomitant fresh gas flow of 5 L/min (Fig. 12-10).

Compressibility can critically influence the apparent power of the ventilator. For any V_T setting, ventilator efficiency declines as lung-thorax impedance increases. Figure 12-11 illustrates the decrease in flow with increasing airway pressure for typical anesthesia ventilators and a critical care ventilator.[57] With anesthesia ventilators, inspiratory flow decreases because of compressibility and the type of flow generator used.[56,58] The decreased inspiratory flow that occurs with increasing airway pressure limits the maximum minute ventilation of anesthesia ventilators. In clinical practice, when peak inspiratory pressure is >50 cmH$_2$O and $\dot{V}_E$ exceeds 15 L/min, the commonly used operating room ventilators fail to provide adequate ventilation.[59]

In contrast, critical care type ventilators (e.g., the Siemens 900C or D, Siemens-Elema Ventilators, Schaumberg, IL), maintain near-maximal flow, up to airway pressures of 80 cmH$_2$O (Fig. 12-11). Flow is maintained because the Siemens has minimal compressible volume and a flow generator that is pressure-independent. In the critical care setting, the compressibility ratio generally will be ≤3 ml/cmH$_2$O.[60] Some critical care ventilators can evaluate and compensate for compressibility in their V_T displays. Alternatively, compressibility is compensated by subtracting an estimate of the compressible volume from the total measured exhaled volume, or eliminated from consideration by measuring exhaled V_T at the endotracheal-circuit interface.

Functional Residual Capacity

Functional residual capacity (FRC) is the lung volume at end-expiration and is an index of pulmonary oxygen stores and exchange. In a variety of clinical settings, decreases in FRC have been correlated with impairment of pulmonary oxygen exchange due to an increased venous admixture.[61]

FRC is difficult to measure in the clinical setting, whether in the operating room or the critical care unit. Two methods are commonly used. The first involves measuring end-tidal nitrogen, then washing out this gas by administering a nitrogen-free mixture (e.g., 100 percent oxygen, or a mixture of argon and oxygen).[62] The total quantity of expired nitrogen collected during this washout is used to derive the vol-

$$\text{Delivered} \quad V_T \;=\; V_{SET} \;+\; V_{FGF} \;-\; V_C$$

$$V_{FGF} \;=\; FGF \;\times\; T_I \qquad\qquad V_C \;=\; C \;\times\; PIP$$

$$249\ \text{ml} \;=\; 83\ \text{ml/sec} \times 3\ \text{sec} \qquad 240\ \text{ml} \;=\; 8\ \text{ml/cmH}_2\text{O} \times 30\ \text{cmH}_2\text{O}$$

$$\text{Delivered}\ V_T \;=\; 1000 + 249 - 240 = 1009\ \text{ml}$$

Fig. 12-10. Determinants of delivered tidal volume (VT) during mechanical ventilation. The ventilator is set to deliver a tidal volume of 1,000 ml. The fresh gas flow is 5 L/min. The respiratory rate is 10 breaths per minute with an I:E ratio of 1:1. The compressibility of the anesthesia system is assumed to be 8 ml/cmH$_2$O. During mechanical ventilation, the peak inspiratory pressure is 30 cmH$_2$O. Under these conditions, the delivered tidal volume is slightly larger than that set by the clinician. (From Schwartz and Katz,[57] with permission.)

ume of the lung from which it came. Conversely, an inert gas wash-in technique may be used.[63] The second method involves rebreathing of a gas mixture containing a known quantity of inert "foreign" gas, such as helium. The final diluted concentration of this gas depends proportionately on the lung volume (FRC) and the initial volume of gas in the apparatus.[64] Both of these methods depend on collection and measurement of a gas of extremely low solubility, which, therefore, does not cross the alveolar capillary membrane in any significant quantity.

Vital Capacity

See "Monitoring Respiratory Failure in the Critical Care Unit."

The Use of Airway Pressure To Calculate Compliance and Resistance

Compliance

To expand the lung and chest wall, elastic and flow-resistive opposition must be overcome. The elastic component is defined by static compliance and the flow-resistive component primarily by airway resistance. Figure 12-12 presents a continuous recording of respiratory gas flow, airway pressure, and VT throughout a mechanical ventilation cycle and illustrates the calculations of compliances and total flow resistance of the respiratory system dur-

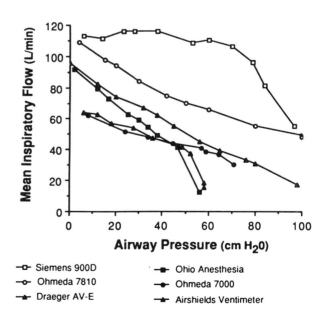

—□— Siemens 900D   —■— Ohio Anesthesia
—○— Ohmeda 7810   —●— Ohmeda 7000
—▲— Draeger AV-E   —▲— Airshields Ventimeter

Fig. 12-11. Effect of increasing airway pressure on mean inspiratory flow for each ventilator/anesthesia machine. The Siemens 900D delivered pressure-independent flow at each airway pressure lower than 80 cmH$_2$O. All other anesthesia ventilators showed decreasing flow with increasing airway pressure. (From Schwartz and Katz,[57] adapted from Marks et al.,[56,58] with permission.)

ing mechanical ventilation.[65] The ventilator incorporates a period of zero flow at end-inspiration. During this period, end-inspiratory airway pressure decreases. The peak airway pressure reflects the pressure generated by both the elastic recoil of the lung-thorax *and* the end-inspiratory flow against

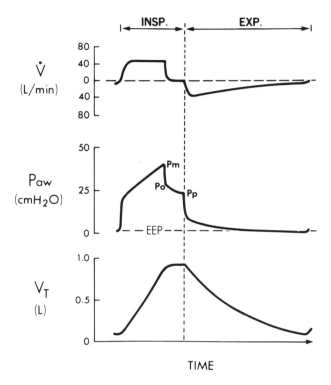

Fig. 12-12. Airflow ($\dot{V}$), airway pressure (Paw), and tidal volume (VT) during mechanical ventilation. Static lung-thorax compliance (VT/[Pp − EEP]): inspiratory plateau pressure (Pp) is measured after 1 to 2 seconds of no flow to allow time for redistribution of VT in accord with time-constant inhomogeneities and viscoelastic properties of the respiratory system (e.g., stress relaxation). End-expiratory pressure (EEP) also is measured at zero flow. Effective dynamic compliance (VT/[Pm − EEP]): inspiratory pressure is measured at its maximum level (Pm). Dynamic compliance (VT/[P0 − EEP]): inspiratory pressure is measured at the instant of zero flow (P0) to eliminate the pressure component resulting from airway resistance. Total flow resistance of the respiratory system, including equipment, is given by two formulas: (Pm − Pp)/($\dot{V}$) or (Pm − P0)/($\dot{V}$). The former identifies the maximum resistance corresponding to a respiratory frequency of zero and the latter, a minimum resistance corresponding to infinite respiratory frequency.

airway resistance. During the period of zero flow, the airway resistance factor is absent and airway pressure decreases. Any unevenness in regional lung expansion, due to variations in regional inflation time constants, tends to redistribute volume. The final, lower end-inspiratory plateau pressure reflects the static lung-thorax compliance (CLT). For clinical measurement purposes, a 1-second period of zero end-inspiratory flow is adequate for redistribution. Patients with severe chronic obstructive pulmonary disease (COPD) might require a longer period of zero flow.

There are three types of compliance: effective (Ceff), dynamic (Cdyn), and static (CLT) (Fig. 12-12). Ceff is derived from measurements made in the ventilator circuit at peak inspiratory pressure, which are commonly obtained from a gauge incorporated in the mechanical ventilator. Ceff therefore includes mechanical resistances in the circuit. Cdyn is derived from measurements made at the airway, usually at the exact moment of initial zero flow. A pneumotachograph or other flow-related trace is necessary to identify this moment.

Ceff is more frequently used in the operating room; both Ceff and CLT are used in the critical care setting. CLT is easily measured in paralyzed or heavily sedated patients. In a paralyzed patient, the lung-thorax can be inflated to a known volume using a "supersyringe"; while the syringe is held steady, airway pressure is measured, providing an excellent measure of CLT.

For the typical adult patient without lung or chest wall pathology, normal CLT is 60 to 100 ml/cmH$_2$O. Values for patients with severe acute hypoxemic respiratory failure are generally <30 ml/cmH$_2$O.[66] Serial CLT measurements have therapeutic and prognostic value in patients with acute respiratory failure (see "Monitoring Respiratory Failure in the Critical Care Unit").

Lung Versus Chest-Wall Compliance

Because airway pressure (during mechanical ventilation) reflects the combined opposing forces of both the lung and the chest wall, separating the components requires knowledge of the pressure difference between the airway and pleural cavity.

Separation of the components usually is accomplished by measuring esophageal pressure via an esophageal balloon. In the clinical setting, this balloon is available as part of a nasogastric tube. The balloon is passed into the stomach, then evacuated and filled with approximately 0.5 ml of air. After the top of the balloon enters the esophagus (negative deflection with spontaneous respiration), it is withdrawn 10 to 15 cm.[67] Appropriate positioning can be confirmed by simultaneously measuring airway and esophageal pressure deflection during respiratory efforts against an occluded airway.[68] Deflection of airway and esophageal pressure should agree within 10 percent. When the balloon is positioned in this manner, changes in esophageal pressure likely reflect changes in pleural pressure accurately, even in the supine position.[69]

Distinguishing the contributions of lung and chest wall distensibility to determine transpulmonary pressure affects lung mechanics and hemodynamics in critically ill patients. The relative compliance of the lung (C_L) and chest wall (C_W) determines the fraction of the airway (alveolar) pressure (Paw) transmitted to the pleural space.[70,71]

$$\Delta Ppl = \Delta Paw \times \frac{C_L}{C_L + C_W}$$

When C_L and C_W are equal, a change in pleural pressure will equal 0.5 of the applied airway pressure. With stiffer lungs, this fraction decreases; with a stiff chest wall, it increases. Thus, for a given airway pressure plateau, conditions associated with decreased C_L will have increased end-inspiratory transpulmonary pressure and conditions associated with decreased C_W, decreased end-inspiratory transpulmonary pressure. The amount of positive end-expiratory pressure (PEEP) transmitted to the pleural space would be similarly affected, and would influence the interpretation of the pulmonary artery occlusion pressure. For most critically ill patients, changes in lung-thorax compliance generally reflect changes in lung rather than chest wall (Fig. 12-13),[72] except in instances of unusually low C_W (e.g., gross obesity, abdominal distension, severe kyphoscoliosis, prone position).

Airway Resistance

The resistance (R) of the airways is defined as the relationship of pressure difference (ΔP) divided by flow ($\dot{V}$), $R = \Delta P / \dot{V}$ and expressed in $cmH_2O/L/s$.[73] Approximately 50 percent of the airway resistance in a normal lung resides above the cricoid cartilage. As the lung expands, the remainder of the resistance decreases as peripheral airway

cross-sectional area increases. Thus, airway resistance is lung-volume-dependent, decreasing with increasing lung volume.

During mechanical ventilation, total flow resistance of the respiratory system, including the endotracheal tube and equipment, is determined by two formulas: $(Pm-Pp)/\dot{V}$ or $(Pm-P0)/\dot{V}$ (Fig. 12-12). The former identifies maximum resistance (Rmax) corresponding to a respiratory frequency of zero, and the latter, a minimum resistance corresponding to infinite respiratory frequency. In clinical practice, Rmax is most commonly measured—the difference between peak and plateau pressures at end-inspiration is divided by the inspiratory flow rate. Ventilators functioning as flow generators (i.e., "square" inspiratory flow wave) are best to obtain the R measurements. Values for Rmax in healthy subjects during anesthesia and mechanical ventilation are approximately 7 $cmH_2O/L/s$.[74] In patients with acute respiratory failure receiving mechanical ventilation, Rmax increases to 12 to 15 $cmH_2O/L/s$ for those with ARDS and to 26 $cmH_2O/L/s$ for COPD patients.[75] These values are important and of potential ther-

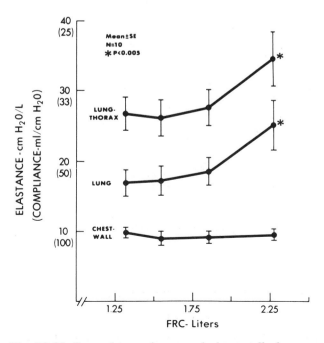

Fig. 12-13. Lung-thorax, lung, and chest wall elastance (compliance) at increments of FRC caused by increasing PEEP. (Data from Katz et al.[72])

apeutic value in evaluating the effectiveness of bronchodilators on the respiratory system.

Resistances should be compared at constant flow rates because pressure across an orifice is logarithmically related to flow, and gross errors can be introduced by flow changes that suggest change in patient resistance. The endotracheal tube also contributes to total flow resistance, increasing it markedly with increasing flow; resistance varies inversely with the size of the tube.[76]

Resistance to expiration also should be considered. While rarely measured, indirect evidence of increased expiratory resistance can be obtained from the auscultation of breath sounds (wheezing or prolonged expiratory phase) and, during mechanical ventilation, by observing the time for airway pressure and flow to return to zero from peak inflation.

RESPIRATORY MONITORING DURING ANESTHESIA

In planning intraoperative monitoring, the patient is carefully evaluated preoperatively to identify problems or clinical factors that may affect pulmonary gas exchange. Appropriate monitoring can be planned, including additional invasive monitoring via arterial and/or pulmonary arterial cannulation where indicated. A partial list of conditions predisposing to perioperative problems includes the following:

1. Conditions suggesting abnormal respiratory mechanics, indicating the need for controlled ventilation intraoperatively and, possibly, in the early postoperative period
2. Conditions likely to cause abnormalities of pulmonary oxygen exchange, such as pulmonary parenchymal or airway disease, obesity, kyphoscoliosis, old age, and congestive heart failure
3. The presence of actual or potential upper airway obstruction
4. Conditions likely to cause or potentiate bronchospasm intraoperatively, such as asthma or bronchitis
5. The presence of abnormal air- or fluid-filled spaces such as air cysts, pneumothorax, lung abscess, or empyema
6. Surgery that will or may encroach on the pleural space, such as thoracotomy, sternotomy, ne-

phrectomy, mediastinoscopy, or cervical rib excision

Routine Monitoring of Respiration

Anesthesia systems contain a number of devices routinely used for intraoperative monitoring of respiratory function. Modern anesthesia systems [e.g., the Ohmeda Modulus Plus system with the 7810 ventilator (Ohmeda, Madison, WI) and the Narkomed 3 with the Dräger AVE ventilator (North American Dräger, Telford, PA)] incorporate monitors of airway pressure, tidal volume, respiratory rate and FIO_2 to alert the anesthesiologist to abnormal intraoperative conditions in either the patient or the system. It is standard practice to measure FIO_2 continuously and, during mechanical ventilation, to record V_T, respiratory frequency, and peak inflation pressure. An audible alarm is sounded for low or high airway pressure and for elevations in circuit pressure persisting longer than 15 seconds. Alarms also sound for apnea, low minute ventilation, low FIO_2, low pressure of the gas supply, power or battery failure, error in ventilator settings, reversal of flow in the circuit, and failure of the ventilator hardware.

Anesthesia systems also incorporate the monitoring of inhalation anesthetics and CO_2 concentration in respiratory gases (see Chapter 13). The combined display of FIO_2, end-tidal CO_2, nitrous oxide concentration, and anesthetic vapor "dosage" (end-tidal concentration) greatly adds to clinical capabilities in respiratory monitoring. "Preoxygenation" can be monitored by observing end-tidal oxygen or, if mass spectometry is used, end-tidal nitrogen, which also facilitates detection of air emboli. The output of a vaporizer unintentionally filled with the wrong anesthetic is immediately detected, as are errors due to vaporizers "full on" instead of "full off." During uptake or elimination of an anesthetic vapor, the alveolar (end-tidal) concentration at which an event occurs (hypotension, hypertension, arrhythmia, patient movement) is recorded.

Pulse oximetry and capnography have become standard monitors. In fact, the pulse oximetry "sentry," which is continuously present at the edge of the desaturation cliff is, to some extent, replacing intermittent but more informative $P(A-a)O_2$ data on pulmonary oxygen exchange.

Clinical applications of capnography during anesthesia include the following:

1. To confirm tracheal intubation.
2. To assess alveolar ventilation and estimate $PaCO_2$ (see earlier comments on $P(a-ET)CO_2$ and VD_{alv}).
3. To detect apnea and/or breathing circuit disconnection.
4. To detect inspired CO_2.
5. To evaluate airway obstruction by assessing distortions of CO_2 waveform (prolonged phase II, steeper phase III).
6. To facilitate respiratory monitoring in the sedated unintubated patient who has received local or regional anesthesia.
   a. Gas is sampled from the nasal cavity using a simple modification of the standard nasal cannula.
   b. One nasal cannula prong is used as a sampling port for exhaled CO_2 measurement, leaving the other for delivering supplemental O_2.
   c. Respiratory frequency and CO_2 waveform are recorded and observed.
   d. Excessive sedation accompanied by mouth breathing, or obstruction, is immediately obvious.
7. As an index of pulmonary embolism (thrombus or gas).

Although the modern generation of anesthesia systems have incorporated redundancy in monitoring and alarm functions, vigilance—including examination of the patient—remains an important defense against the delivery of inadequate ventilation and impaired oxygenation during anesthesia.

Inspection of Respiratory Movement

In the supine position, the rib cage expands during inspiration. The sternum moves anteriorly and the upper rib cage moves anteriorly and cephalad (ribs 1 to 4). These changes are comparable during spontaneous and mechanical ventilation. Anterior abdominal wall movement is consistent during the inspiratory phase of mechanical ventilation, but differs from patient to patient during spontaneous breathing. Exaggerated anterior movement during mechanical ventilation, with minimal recoil, suggests esophageal intubation.

During quiet breathing, there is no clearly visible movement of the alae nasae or accessory neck muscles. During light anesthesia, tightening of the abdominal muscles is observed.

In respiratory obstruction, the power of the diaphragm overcomes chest wall inspiratory muscle force. There is indrawing of the intercostal spaces and the upper chest moves paradoxically: both posteriorly and caudad during inspiration. (The relatively less calcified ribs of small children permit grosser paradoxical movement of this type.) The forceful movement of the diaphragm causes jerky caudad motion of the mediastinum, trachea, and larynx—a "tracheal tug" is observable in the neck. The alae nasae "flare" on inspiration and accessory muscles may contract visibly. The same paradoxical movement of the upper chest occurs as respiratory musculature weakens (e.g., during deep anesthesia or partial myoneural block). The alae nasae may not flare nor neck muscles contract because they weaken before the diaphragm.

Chest Auscultation

During induction of anesthesia, a weighted chest piece may be placed in the suprasternal notch for continuous auscultation of air entry and monitoring for airway obstruction. To detect endobronchial intubation, *air entry* should be monitored by listening in both axillae. Auscultation of the anterior chest can be misleading due to conduction of sounds from one side to the other. In adults, palpation of the endotracheal tube cuff above the suprasternal notch during inflation and deflation will avoid endobronchial intubation. Breath sounds may be auscultated throughout anesthesia, using a weighted chest piece and earpiece, or an esophageal stethoscope if the trachea is intubated. Wheezing during anesthesia is discussed later (see "High Airway Pressure").

Respiratory Function During General Anesthesia

It is widely known that general anesthesia has profound effects upon the respiratory system. In patients with normal pulmonary function, the changes in ventilation, lung mechanics, and gas exchange resulting from general anesthesia are consistent, predictable, and usually non-life-threatening. Knowledge of the expected anesthesia-induced changes in respiratory function is therefore critical to recognizing abnormal respiratory variables that may require clinical action.

Ventilation

All general anesthetics decrease ventilation, depress the ventilatory response to added carbon dioxide (CO_2) and displace the apneic threshold to a higher $PaCO_2$ level.[77] The breathing pattern typically is altered during inhalational anesthesia with volatile anesthetics, resulting in lower V_T and increased breathing frequency, and dose-dependent increases in $PaCO_2$ (Fig. 12-14).[78,79] Because nitrous oxide has minimal effects on $PaCO_2$, its substitution for an equal MAC fraction of volatile anesthetics decreases $PaCO_2$. Narcotics also diminish ventilation with an effect proportional to their analgesic potency. Combinations such as sedatives, narcotics, intravenous and inhalational anesthetics, interact to produce more hypoventilation than when administered alone.

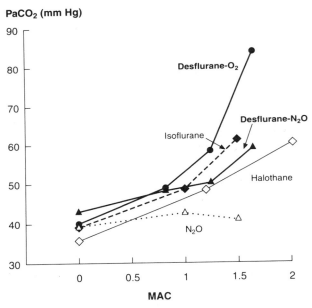

PaCO₂ (mm Hg)

Fig. 12-14. $PaCO_2$ measured in spontaneously breathing volunteers anesthetized with desflurane, enflurane, isoflurane, halothane, or nitrous oxide and oxygen at varying minimum alveolar concentrations. $PaCO_2$ increases in a dose-related manner. The increase found with desflurane and oxygen lies between that found with enflurane and isoflurane. Isoflurane resulted in slightly greater respiratory depression than halothane. Nitrous oxide did not increase $PaCO_2$. For a given MAC-multiple, the combination of 60 percent nitrous oxide and desflurane caused less of an increase in $PaCO_2$ then desflurane alone. (From Eger,[79] with permission.)

During general anesthesia and spontaneous breathing, abdominal respiratory excursion is well-preserved, while rib cage excursion is nearly abolished.[80] This has been interpreted as progressive failure of intercostal muscle function, with preservation of contraction of the diaphragm. Because the major effector of the ventilatory response to added CO_2 is mediated by the intercostal muscles, much of the observed reduced ventilatory response to $PaCO_2$ during anesthesia is impaired intercostal muscle function.[81] The relative loss of the rib cage component during general anesthesia with spontaneous breathing may explain why patients with impediments to abdominal breathing (e.g., obesity), or to diaphragmatic contraction (e.g., COPD), hypoventilate more during anesthesia.[82]

At anesthetizing concentrations (1.0 MAC), inhalation anesthetics suppress the ventilatory response to hypoxemia; the hypoxic ventilatory drive remains attenuated at subanesthetic concentrations (0.1 MAC) that persist into the immediate postoperative period.[83]

Lung Volumes and Mechanics

The shape and motion of the chest wall are affected by general anesthesia, which causes a cephalad shift of the diaphragm and reduces the transverse cross-sectional area of the thorax, thereby decreasing FRC (Fig. 12-15).[84,85] Following induction of general anesthesia in the supine position, FRC immediately decreases by approximately 20 percent; in the obese patient, FRC may decrease below awake supine values by as much as 60 percent.[86] The decrease in FRC occurs independently of whether ventilation is spontaneous or controlled, the duration of anesthesia, the degree of neuromuscular blockade, and the FIO_2.[77] Using computed tomography, several studies have demonstrated dependent-lung crescent-shape densities that appear almost immediately after induction of general anesthesia (Fig. 12-16)[87,88] These densities likely represent atelectasis. Thus, reduced FRC during general anesthesia has major effects on pulmonary function, particularly respiratory mechanics, the distribution of ventilation and perfusion, and gas exchange.

Total respiratory system compliance also decreases, reflecting the decreased FRC.[89] Total compliance depends on multiple factors, including lung volume, surface tension, disease, posture, chest wall mechanics, pulmonary blood volume, and the volume history of the lungs.[90] Shallow V_T breathing further decreases compliance by as much as 30 to 50 percent. This decrease in compliance can be temporarily reversed with maximal inflation or sighs,[91,92] which will increase compliance presumably by recruitment of collapsed alveoli. While periodic hyperinflation improves compliance during small V_T ventilation, it is not necessary when large V_T are used.[93]

Changes in airway resistance during anesthesia are influenced by multiple factors. The increased resistance due to decreased FRC is largely offset by the bronchodilatory effect of most inhalational anesthetics. Although changes in airway resistance due to anesthesia generally are not of significant consequence, other possible causes of increased airway resistance may be serious and life-threatening (see "Increased Airway Pressure").

Pulmonary Gas Exchange

In mechanically ventilated and anesthetized patients in the supine and lateral decubitus positions, the distribution of inspired gas is altered from that in the awake state, while the distribution of regional perfusion does not change significantly.[94] Thus, during anesthesia, and mechanical ventilation, the distribution of V/Q is altered, with some lung regions having low and others high V/Q ratios (Fig. 12-16).

The net effect of these changes in lung volume and distribution of V/Q is to increase the $P(A-a)O_2$ and the V_D/V_T. The average intraoperative PaO_2 is one-half the inspired PO_2, but with wide variation.[77] This is equivalent to an average $\dot{Q}s/\dot{Q}T$ of 0.10 to 0.15. (Acceptable levels of PaO_2 usually are achieved with an FIO_2 of 0.40.)

V_D/V_T increases from 0.3 in awake subjects to approximately 0.4 in anesthetized, mechanically

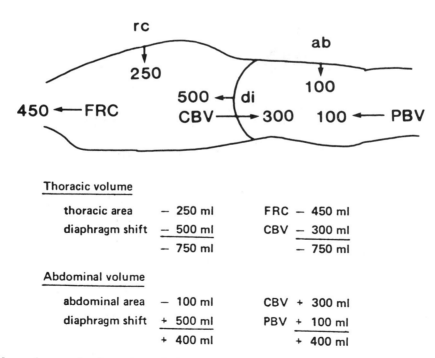

Thoracic volume				
thoracic area	– 250 ml		FRC	– 450 ml
diaphragm shift	– 500 ml		CBV	– 300 ml
	– 750 ml			– 750 ml
Abdominal volume				
abdominal area	– 100 ml		CBV	+ 300 ml
diaphragm shift	+ 500 ml		PBV	+ 100 ml
	+ 400 ml			+ 400 ml

Fig. 12-15. Mean changes in thoracic and abdominal dimensions and in gas and blood volumes after induction of general anesthesia and institution of mechanical ventilation. Volume is expressed in milliliters. FRC, functional residual capacity; CBV, central blood volume; PBV, peripheral blood volume; rc, rib cage; di, diaphragm; ab, abdomen. (From Hedenstierna et al.,[85] with permission.)

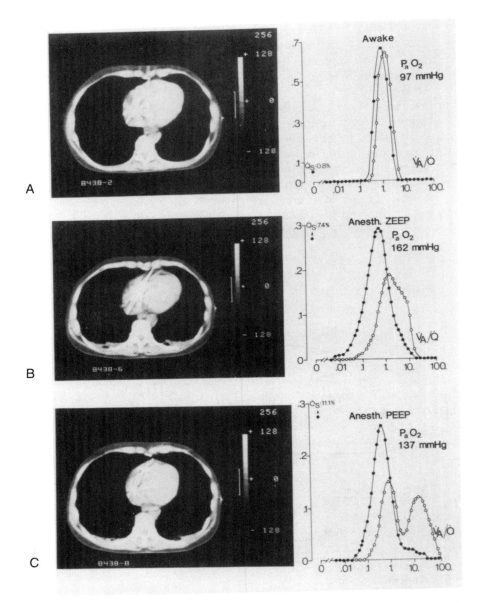

Fig. 12-16. Transverse computed tomography (CT) scans of the chest and VA/Q distribution (○, ventilation; ●, blood flow; L/min) in (**A**) an awake patient, (**B**) during anesthesia with mechanical ventilation, with zero end-expiratory pressure (ZEEP), and (**C**) after the addition of positive end-expiratory pressure (PEEP) of 10 cmH₂O. Note that the CT scan shows no changes in lung tissue and that the unimodal VA/Q distribution shows almost no shunt in the awake state. Also note the appearance of densities in the dependent lung regions and shunt during anesthesia. The addition of PEEP reduces the densities but not the shunt. PEEP also resulted in a distinct high VA/Q region. PaO₂ is presented in each panel. (From Tokics et al.,[88] with permission.)

ventilated subjects.[77] Because anatomic dead space is reduced by endotracheal intubation, alveolar dead space increases due to increased distribution of ventilation to areas of lung having high V/Q ratios.

Abnormal Intraoperative Respiratory Function

Hypoxemia

Hypoxemia may be difficult to recognize clinically, but can be diagnosed reliably by measuring Pa_{O_2} and oxygen saturation of hemoglobin using pulse oximetry. The usual circulatory (e.g., tachycardia and hypertension) and ventilatory (e.g., hyperventilation) responses to hypoxemia may be blunted intraoperatively by anesthetics. Ultimately, severe hypoxemia will lead to sinus bradycardia with widened QRS complexes, progressing rapidly to asystole. In the patient with coincidental heart disease, ventricular arrhythmias, and ventricular fibrillation also may occur.

Dangerous levels of hypoxemia can occur without cyanosis. Cyanosis is related to the amount of desaturated hemoglobin in subcutaneous tissues and is, therefore, dependent on the level of hemoglobin and on skin blood flow rate. Cyanosis can occur without arterial hypoxemia when skin blood flow is low and hemoglobin is high; conversely, hypoxemia can occur without cyanosis when hemoglobin is low and skin blood flow high. Purple or dark-colored freshly shed blood in the operative field should never be ignored, whether the source of bleeding is arterial or venous.

Unrecognized esophageal intubation is a dangerous cause of intraoperative hypoxemia. If the patient is preoxygenated, the store of oxygen in the FRC can permit survival for 10 minutes or more without obvious warning signs. Even experienced anesthesiologists have been misled by clinical tests generally considered reliable in detecting a misplaced endotracheal tube.[95] The only certain signs of tracheal intubation are direct observation of the endotracheal tube inserted in the larynx anterior to the arytenoid cartilages and the maintenance of a near-normal P_{ETCO_2}.[96] Caution must be exercised even with these signs, because visualization of the tube passing through the larynx is not possible in all patients and a correctly placed tube may be withdrawn accidentally. Similarly, several reports

demonstrate that a near-normal P_{ETCO_2} may be detected initially with esophageal intubation when exhaled gas has been forced into the stomach with prior mask ventilation.[97] Differentiating tracheal from esophageal ventilation is then possible because P_{ETCO_2} rapidly diminishes with repeated ventilation of the esophagus.

Intraoperative management of hypoxemia begins with increasing the fresh gas flow to an F_{IO_2} of 1.0, while scanning the anesthesia machine to detect circuit disconnections. Observing chest wall movement, auscultating breath sounds, and examining inspired and end-tidal respiratory gases follows. These sequences should require only a few seconds, and often identify the general problem.

Once decreased F_{IO_2} and hypoventilation have been excluded or corrected as causes of intraoperative hypoxemia, the anesthesiologist should investigate conditions increasing $P_{(A-a)O_2}$. These include endobronchial intubation, massive atelectasis, aspiration into the lung, pulmonary edema, pulmonary emboli, bronchospasm, pneumothorax, intracardiac right-to-left shunting, and conditions decreasing cardiac output and mixed venous oxygen saturation.

Definitive diagnosis is aided by physical findings (e.g., unilateral breath sounds, rales, wheezing, observation of vomitus in the airway, subcutaneous emphysema), respiratory mechanics and hemodynamic measurements, results of a chest radiograph, the response of Pa_{O_2} to an F_{IO_2} of 1.0 and to other therapeutic measures.

Acute lung diseases resulting in increased $P_{(A-a)O_2}$ can be divided into those characterized by decreased FRC and compliance (atelectasis, aspiration, cardiogenic and noncardiogenic pulmonary edema, and pneumonia), or increased FRC and airway resistance (asthma and COPD). Typically, with increased FRC, arterial oxygenation is markedly improved by increasing the F_{IO_2} to 1.0. With decreased FRC, shunting is the primary mechanism of hypoxemia; increasing the F_{IO_2} to 1.0 often fails to improve oxygenation despite ventilation with large V_T (12 to 15 ml/kg). Ventilatory management is thus aimed at increasing FRC (by the application of PEEP) and recruiting collapsed nonventilated lung to decrease intrapulmonary shunting (see ''Monitoring Respiratory Failure in the Critical Care Unit'').

Hypercapnia

Clinical signs of hypercapnia (other than decreased ventilation), such as central nervous system-mediated sympathoadrenal stimulation, respiratory stimulation and peripheral vasodilation, may not be present during anesthesia. Bleeding into the operative site may be increased, intracranial and intraocular pressures increase and, in some cases, arrhythmias may develop. If any of these effects is observed, minute ventilation, $P_{ET}CO_2$ and/or, especially, $PaCO_2$ should be checked. In many instances, ventilation should be increased before results are available. If oxygenation is well maintained, considerable respiratory acidosis can occur without serious harmful effect in normal patients.

The factors affecting $PaCO_2$ ($\dot{V}CO_2$, and $\dot{V}A$) were discussed previously (see "Assessing CO_2 Elimination"). In addition, $PaCO_2$ may increase because of CO_2 inhalation. Intraoperative factors leading or contributing to increased P_ICO_2 include rebreathing of exhaled gases due to a faulty expiratory valve in a circle system, exhaustion of the CO_2 absorber, low fresh gas flow in a nonrebreathing system, and, occasionally, accidental administration of CO_2 in the fresh gas inflow.

To manage hypercapnia due to any of the above factors requires diagnosis of the principal cause and correction.

Abnormal Respiratory Mechanics

During mechanical ventilation, abnormalities in respiratory mechanics may be characterized by conditions resulting in low airway pressure (e.g., endotracheal tube/breathing circuit disconnection) or high airway pressure (i.e., decreased compliance and/or increased resistance). Acute changes in airway pressure-tidal volume relationships often precede detection of changes in oxygenation and other clinical criteria.[98]

Low Airway Pressure

Since pressure equals resistance times flow, the causes of low airway pressure are conditions that decrease flow and/or decrease resistance. Common causes for decreased resistance include complete or partial breathing circuit disconnection, other circuit leaks, excess scavenging system removal of gas from the circuit, accidental extubation, or endotracheal tube malfunction (e.g., cuff deflation, or leak due to a nasogastric tube in the trachea). Conditions decreasing flow include fresh gas flow disconnection, anesthesia machine malfunction, or loss or reduction of pressure in the gas supply.

A comprehensive response algorithm for low pressure in the anesthesia circuit has been described.[99] The low-pressure response algorithm stresses the importance of having the immediate capability for providing manual ventilation (e.g., Ambu-bag) from a gas source separate from the anesthesia machine. This capability is essential to provide adequate ventilation when machine or breathing circuit failures occur that cannot be immediately corrected.

High Airway Pressure

Since most mechanical ventilators used in the operating room deliver a relatively constant tidal volume (constant flow generators), increased peak airway pressure is the most frequent intraoperative sign of conditions associated with decreased compliance or increased flow resistance (Fig. 12-17).[100] Analyzing the difference between peak and plateau airway pressure will distinguish between elastic and flow-resistive abnormalities (Fig. 12-12). If airway resistance is high, and lung-thorax compliance is normal, the difference will be increased. If both peak and plateau pressures are increased, lung-thorax compliance will decrease. However, some anesthesia ventilators do not provide for a period of zero flow at end-inspiration, necessitating clinical assessment for differentiating elastic and flow-resistive conditions. Expiratory flow will decrease (e.g., slow refill of ventilator bellows or reservoir bag) when resistance is high and compliance is normal, and increase during normal resistance and decreased compliance.

When increased peak airway pressure is detected intraoperatively, the conditions outlined in Figure 12-17 must be systematically investigated. In all circumstances, F_IO_2 should be increased to 1.0 until the problem is corrected.

First, equipment-related causes of increased peak airway pressures must be addressed and can be differentiated by examining the level of end-expiratory pressure and expiratory flow before and after disconnecting the endotracheal tube from the breathing circuit. If expiratory obstruction is due to a malfunctioning expiratory valve or mechanical obstruction of the scavenging line, PEEP increases and expiratory flow decreases. Disconnection of the endotracheal tube and circuit will result in vigorous exhalation and deflation of the chest wall. In contrast, when airflow obstruction is in the inspiratory limb or distal to the Y-piece, peak airway pressure increases, but end-expiratory pressure remains unchanged and chest wall deflation is not significant on disconnection. Obstruction of the lumen of the endotracheal tube (due to kinking, an overinflated cuff causing herniation over the tip, severe narrowing of the lumen from secretions, or the bevel of the tube being forced against the lateral tracheal wall) should be explored by passing a suction catheter. Fiberoptic visualization via the tube may define the problem and facilitate correction. If obstruction persists, the tube should be removed and adequate oxygenation and ventilation ensured before laryngoscopy and reintubation.

Increased peak airway pressures due to pathologic conditions should be considered next. Not all wheezing during anesthesia is due to bronchospasm (active bronchoconstriction); most cases are due to other processes that cause airway narrowing without increasing airway smooth muscle tone (passive bronchoconstriction). Conditions causing passive bronchoconstriction are treated by relieving partial airway obstruction and/or increasing lung volume. In some cases, administering 5 to 10 cmH$_2$O PEEP may distinguish wheezing due to passive narrowing of the airway secondary to markedly decreased lung volume, from wheezing due to other causes.

Bronchospasm is treated initially by increasing the depth of anesthesia. Using a potent volatile anesthetic may suffice, since reflex bronchospasm and/or effects of mediators released from sensitized cells may be due to "light" anesthesia.[101] When bronchospasm is severe, increasing the depth of inhalation anesthesia may be difficult, making intravenous drugs a preferable first step. Ketamine appears to be more effective than thiopental in reversing bronchospasm in experimental models.[102]

Bronchodilator therapy is indicated if increasing the depth of anesthesia does not reduce airway resistance and improve ventilation.[103] Use of aerosolized β_2-adrenergic agonists is preferred because high concentrations reach the airways, increasing

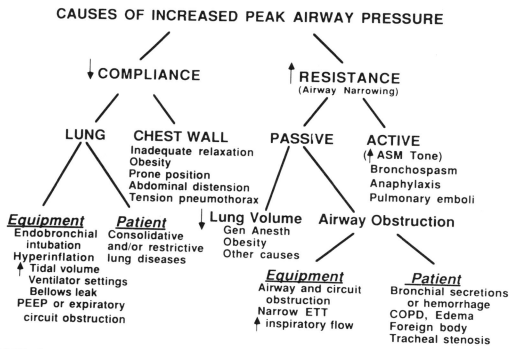

Fig. 12-17. Causes of increased peak airway pressure separated into conditions of decreased compliance and increased flow resistance. (From Katz,[100] with permission.)

the therapeutic effect while possibly reducing systemic toxic effects. When bronchospasm is severe and ventilation minimally effective, systemic β-adrenergic agonists may be required; under these conditions, hydrocortisone (4 mg/kg IV) or its equivalent also should be given.

Because airway resistance is increased markedly, inspiratory flow must be increased to allow for a more prolonged expiratory time (i.e., decreased I:E ratio) to facilitate complete exhalation. In certain cases, complete exhalation may not be achieved, producing dynamic hyperinflation (see "Intrinsic Positive End-Expiratory Pressure").

The clinical presentation of pneumothorax intraoperatively varies from minimal cardiopulmonary dysfunction to acute cardiopulmonary collapse (i.e., tension pneumothorax). The signs of a tension pneumothorax may mimic bronchospasm or other causes of airway obstruction.[104,105] When cardiopulmonary function is stable, a chest radiograph can be obtained for definitive diagnosis. However, in the presence of hemodynamic instability, tension pneumothorax should be emergently treated by placing a 14- or 16-gauge catheter into the second anterior intercostal space in the midclavicular line, or into the fifth intercostal space in the midaxillary line. If the diagnosis is confirmed (observation of gas escaping through the catheter and improvement of hemodynamic function), a tube thoracostomy should be performed; if unconfirmed, the patient should be monitored for development of a pneumothorax secondary to the needle placement.

POSTOPERATIVE MONITORING

Respiratory Muscle Strength After Neuromuscular Blockade

Clinical signs and tests of the degree of reversal of neuromuscular blockade depend on observing, estimating, or measuring the strength of various muscle groups. During recovery from neuromuscular blockade, the diaphragmatic function returns earlier than function of other skeletal muscles, including the upper airway.[106,107] In a study in volunteers comparing the effects of a neuromuscular blocking drug on muscles that protect the airway with effects on respiratory and peripheral muscles, curare was administered in incremental doses up to the elimination of hand-grip strength.[107] At this

degree of neuromuscular blockade, vital capacity was 2.0 L, P_{ETCO_2} was normal and maximum inspiratory pressure (MIP) was −20 cmH$_2$O (Fig. 12-18). However, none of the volunteers could maintain a patent airway without elevation of the mandibles by the investigators. Relief of airway obstruction returned at a MIP level of −39 cmH$_2$O; sustained head lift occurred at a MIP of approximately −50 cmH$_2$O (Fig. 12-19). Thus, the maintenance of a normal ventilatory pattern during quiet tidal breathing through an open airway, while suggestive of a lack of residual weakness, is not a reliable indicator of adequate reversal of neuromuscular blockade.

Further evidence suggesting the return of satisfactory muscular power following myoneural blockade includes the ability to sustain the unsupported head in a flexed position (or to lift the leg) for 5 seconds, or the ability to demonstrate the return of airway function (Fig. 12-19). Other objective tests include demonstrating either a sustained tetanus for 5 seconds or a MIP > −50 cmH$_2$O. When

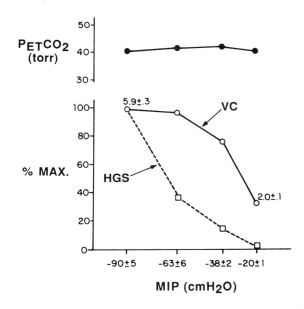

Fig. 12-18. Hand grip strength (HGS), vital capacity (VC), and end-tidal partial pressure of carbon dioxide (P_{ETCO_2}) at three different levels of paralysis with curare measured by maximum inspiratory pressure (MIP). At the lowest level of MIP (−20 cmH$_2$O), HGS is absent, but ventilation is adequate and VC indicates ventilatory reserve. On VC curve, number labels indicate actual values ±SE in liters. (From Pavlin et al.,[107] with permission.)

respiratory muscle strength is in doubt, a conservative approach to withdrawing mechanical support is indicated.

Recovery of Pulmonary Function

Immediate Postoperative Period

Defective pulmonary oxygen exchange is common after all types of surgery and occurs in two phases. The first phase occurs in the immediate postoperative period and is a consequence of general anesthesia and its known effects on respiratory function, including residual central and/or peripheral ventilatory depression, diffusion, and post-*hyperventilation* hypoxia, increased venous admixture, and shivering after anesthesia. In the absence of pre-existing abnormalities in pulmonary function, gas exchange returns to normal within 2 hours following an uncomplicated general anesthetic for a peripheral surgical procedure. During that time, hypoxemia may be difficult to detect by clinical observation because residual anesthetic may still blunt the respiratory distress and tachycardia, which would be obvious in an awake individual.[83] Therefore, if pulse oximetry is not used routinely, oxygen should be given to everyone after general anesthesia.

Site of Surgery

The second phase of impaired oxygenation is attributed to the changes in lung mechanics following operations on the abdomen and thorax.[108] Most often, a restrictive pattern develops, characterized by marked decreases in VC and a smaller, but clinically important, decrease in FRC. After upper abdominal surgery, forced vital capacity (FVC) decreases to 60 percent below preoperative levels and FRC declines by 30 percent (Fig. 12-20).[108] After lower abdominal surgery, FVC and FRC decrease to a lesser extent, that is, by only 30 percent and 10 percent, respectively. Gradually, these deficits improve, returning to preoperative levels within 2 weeks.

After abdominal or thoracic surgery, hypoxemia correlates with decreased FRC and is most severe in the elderly, the obese, and those with preoperative cardiopulmonary disease (conditions that increase the tendency for airway closure).[109] Although the magnitude of hypoxemia is not clinically important in otherwise normal patients, pulse oximetry data will assist in deciding whether supplemental oxygen is necessary when the patient returns to the ward. After thoracic surgery and in other patients with a high probability of a serious degree of gas exchange impairment, minimal additional evaluation (preceding a decision regarding further respiratory management) should include a chest examination, a chest radiograph, and arterial blood gas measurement.

The actual mechanisms of reduced lung volumes and hypoxemia following abdominal and thoracic surgery are not completely known, but spasm and splinting of the abdominal and intercostal muscles,[110] diaphragmatic dysfunction,[111,112] and pain[113] appear to be the primary factors.

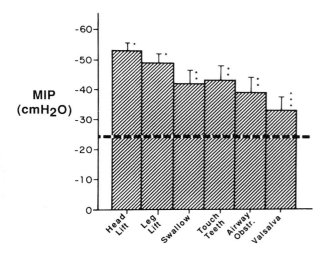

Fig. 12-19. Levels of neuromuscular blockade with curare indicated by maximum inspiratory pressure (MIP ± SE), below which indicated clinical maneuvers could not be accomplished. No maneuvers indicating airway protection could be accomplished by any of the subjects at MIP of −25 cmH$_2$O. *$P < .001$ compared with MIP = −25 cmH$_2$O); **$P < .02$ compared with MIP = −25 cmH$_2$O; ***$P < .05$ compared with MIP = −25 cmH$_2$O. (From Pavlin et al.,[107] with permission.)

Postoperative Analgesia

Systemic narcotics can be administered to provide pain relief nearly equal to that observed with regional therapies, but are associated with greater respiratory depression.[114] In addition, the patient's ventilatory pattern may be altered by elimination of sighs that are essential to maintain normal lung volume. Furthermore, the interaction of sleep and systemically administered morphine following abdominal and peripheral surgery has been shown to produce disturbances in ventilatory patterns (primarily obstructive sleep apnea and paradoxical breathing) that can cause profound oxygen desaturation.[115] These disturbances in breathing patterns and oxygen desaturation are more frequent in the elderly and not observed in a matched group of patients receiving regional analgesia with bupivacaine, even during periods of sleep.[115] Supplemental O_2 may therefore be warranted in high-risk postoperative patients receiving parenteral opioids.

Whether regional techniques improve pulmonary function and reduce pulmonary complications following abdominal and thoracic surgery is unclear: some studies confirm a beneficial effect,[116–119] while others do not.[120,121] Thoracic epidural local anesthesia decreases diaphragmatic dysfunction, increases tidal volume, and decreases respiratory frequency following upper abdominal surgery,[122,123] but epidural opiates do not.[124,125] Even with complete pain relief, both epidural methods only partially restore FVC, minimally improve FRC, and modestly improve oxygenation.[108,113]

Analgesia with both epidural local anesthetics and opioids is comparable. However, the local anesthetics produce undesirable sympathetic blockade, while the opiates impose a risk of delayed respiratory depression. The incidence of the latter in the general surgical population is 0.25 to 0.9 percent,[126] the peak vulnerable period with morphine being 6 to 10 hours after injection. Clinical monitoring should focus on respiratory rate, pattern, and patient sedation (level of consciousness) and should follow a written protocol.[127]

MONITORING RESPIRATORY FAILURE IN THE CRITICAL CARE UNIT

The respiratory variables monitored in the critical care setting are similar to those monitored in patients undergoing anesthesia, with additional attention to the effects of the underlying disease process and the clinical appearance of the patient.

Acute respiratory failure may be classified into two types: hypoxemic and ventilatory.[128] Acute hypoxemic respiratory failure results when disease processes cause airspace filling or collapse (e.g., pulmonary edema, pneumonia, or atelectasis); and acute ventilatory failure results when conditions associated with decreased ventilatory drive, neuromuscular weakness, or increased mechanical load lead to alveolar hypoventilation and hypercapnia.

While patients may exhibit relatively "pure" forms of acute hypoxemic respiratory failure or ventilatory failure, many may exhibit elements of both. For example, patients with severe hypoxemia due to ARDS have decreased respiratory system compliance and increased elastic load which, when combined with increased minute ventilation, may cause respiratory muscle fatigue resulting in ventilatory failure and the need for mechanical ventilatory support. The important clinical aspects of

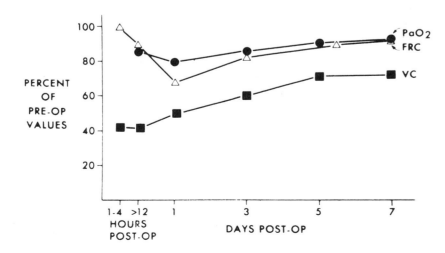

Fig. 12-20. Postoperative vital capacity (VC), functional residual capacity (FRC), and PaO_2 while breathing room air expressed as a percent of preoperative values in patients recovering from upper abdominal surgery (From Craig,[108] with permission.)

monitoring acute hypoxemic and ventilatory failure will be discussed, focusing primarily on the mechanics of breathing.

Acute Hypoxemic Respiratory Failure

Approach to Ventilatory Management

Traditionally, patients with acute hypoxemic respiratory failure receive mechanical ventilatory support with large V_T (12 to 15 ml/kg) and an increased FIO_2. PEEP is applied clinically when satisfactory oxygenation (e.g., $PaO_2 \leq 70$ mmHg with an $FIO_2 > 0.60$) cannot be achieved,[129] but it carries the risks of cardiovascular depression and ventilator-induced lung injury, including pulmonary barotrauma.[130] Most often, PEEP is adjusted according to derived oxygenation variables.[131] A practical approach to applying PEEP is stepwise titration (e.g., in 5 cmH_2O increments from 5 to 20 cmH_2O) evaluating PEEP effects on oxygenation and cardiac function at each increment. Respiratory frequency is adjusted according to $PaCO_2$ and pH measurements, and the I:E ratio is set to prevent dynamic airtrapping.

Recent data indicate that the lungs in patients with ARDS are not homogeneously affected.[132] Pressure/volume relationships in these patients may reflect normal or recruitable lung areas having essentially normal intrinsic properties,[133] which may indicate an abnormally small lung rather than a stiff lung of normal dimensions. These findings have important clinical implications for the ventilatory management of patients with acute hypoxemic respiratory failure.

Ventilator-Induced Lung Injury

Recent evidence suggests that large V_T may propagate and extend pulmonary injury in ARDS. High peak inflation pressure alone can disrupt normal barriers to protein leakage,[134,135] while tidal volume and end-expiratory alveolar pressures[136,137] may influence the shearing forces applied to the alveolar membrane. Repeated opening and closing of susceptible lung tissue also appears to injure alveolar sacs and terminal airways of edematous lung.

An appropriate strategy to avoid ventilator-induced lung injury in patients with ARDS includes the following objectives[138]:

1. To prevent overdistension of alveolar tissues and terminal airways

2. To avoid large tidal volumes
3. To provide enough PEEP to exceed the minimum volume that prevents widespread tidal closure of alveolar units

Under experimental conditions, the safe upper limit of tidal transalveolar pressure (the difference between end-inspiratory alveolar and pleural pressure) should not exceed 30 to 35 cmH_2O (the transalveolar pressure at total capacity of normal lung).[139] Clinically, a transalveolar pressure of 30 to 35 cmH_2O often translates into an end-inspiratory airway plateau pressure of 40 to 50 cmH_2O. In some circumstances, this lung protective strategy requires decreases in tidal volume and/or minute ventilation leading to CO_2 retention.[140,141]

Whenever high-tidal airway pressures are applied, pressure-volume curves of the respiratory system should be analyzed, rather than risk alveolar distension. It is sometimes necessary in severe cases of ARDS to exceed the maximum compliance point to achieve the desired decrease in $P(A-a)O_2$. The end-inspiratory airway plateau pressure must be monitored and, if high (e.g., >40 cmH_2O), decreasing tidal volume at the higher PEEP levels should be considered. Higher plateau pressures may be acceptable with clinical conditions associated with decreased chest wall compliance (i.e., decreased transpulmonary pressure).[142]

Selecting Ventilator Settings from Pressure/Volume Monitoring

Flow-Controlled Volume-Cycled Modes

End-inspiratory and end-expiratory pressure/volume relationships may be used as indices of *optimum pulmonary distension*. Each lung region has its own compliance curve. At low volumes, regional compliance is low. As PEEP is applied and lung volume increases, compliance improves by alveolar recruitment, then declines when lung regions become overdistended.[143] The compliance measurement for the whole lung reflects the status of all regions. An increase in compliance (caused by adding PEEP) usually is associated with an improvement in PaO_2.[144]

Pressure/volume curves also may be used to guide PEEP application. The lowest level of PEEP preventing progressive loss of gas exchanging area should be applied and can be determined as the inflection point on the inflation portion of the pressure/volume curve (Fig. 12-21),[145,146] or as the lowest point of the steepest section of the PEEP vs FRC curve (Fig. 12-22).[147] The lower inflection points tend to emerge during the earliest phases of ARDS and to disappear later in its course. PEEP values in the range of 7 to 15 cmH₂O usually are sufficient

In a study of patients with acute respiratory failure, the increase in FRC per increment of PEEP (end-expiratory compliance) above 8 cmH₂O significantly exceeded that reflected by the end-inspiratory compliance (and demonstrates the inflection point or pressure) (Fig. 12-22).[147] The increase in end-expiratory compliance likely reflects recruitment of nonventilated lung.[147,148] However, with increasing levels of PEEP (to 18 cmH₂O) at constant tidal volume, end-inspiratory compliance

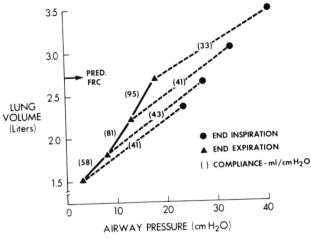

Fig. 12-22. Mean lung-thorax pressure-volume data for 13 patients in acute respiratory failure: measured functional residual capacity (FRC) and end-expiratory pressure, and end-inspiratory lung volume and airway plateau pressures. *Dashed lines* and numbers in parentheses indicate mean lung-thorax compliance at PEEP levels of 3, 8, 13, and 18 cmH₂O. The *solid line* connecting the triangles and numbers in parentheses represents end-expiratory (FRC) compliances. The lung volume achieved by applying PEEP at levels above 8 cmH₂O greatly exceeds that gained by comparable pressures during tidal ventilation. This additional volume (difference between comparable end-expiratory and end-inspiratory pressures) correlated with improvement in arterial oxygenation. (From Katz et al.,[147] with permission.)

decreases and is likely explained by overexpansion at end-inspiration.

The harmful effects of overexpansion at end-inspiration might be avoided by using PEEP to recruit nonventilated lung at end-expiration, while minimizing the end-inspiratory pressure by decreasing tidal volume. Such a strategy was investigated in a group of patients with acute lung injury, and resulted in both improved pressure/volume relationships and improved pulmonary oxygen exchange.[149]

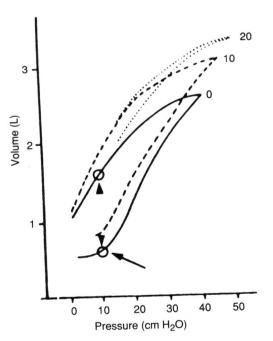

Fig. 12-21. Static pressure-volume curve for a patient with ARDS at 0, 10, and 20 cmH₂O end-expiratory pressure. Without PEEP applied, the pressure-volume curve of the acutely edematous respiratory system often demonstrates marked hysteresis (*arrowheads*) and an inflection point (Pflex) on the inflation limb (*arrow*). At the higher levels of PEEP, Pflex and hysteresis diminish and the pressure-volume curve assumes a monotonic, flattened profile. (From Marini and Truwit,[145] adapted from Benito and Lemaire,[146] with permission.)

Pressure-Controlled Ventilation

Pressure-controlled (PC) ventilation, with or without inverse ratio (IRV, I:E > 1), may be used to effectively control peak, plateau, and mean airway pressures during mechanical ventilation,[150] and to possibly reduce ventilator-induced lung injury. PC with extended inspiration may improve gas exchange by increasing mean airway pressure. Sustained alveolar inflation improves oxygenation and decreases V_D/V_T. The improved CO_2 exchange allows a decreased V_E and peak inspiratory pressure. However, the decreased expiratory time may result in excessive end-expiratory gas trapping (i.e., lung hyperinflation and cardiovascular depression). This may be detected by increased intrinsic PEEP (see "Intrinsic Positive End-Expiratory Pressure") and/or decreased tidal volume.

Because V_T varies inversely with respiratory impedance (decreased compliance, increased resistance), it is necessary to continuously monitor V_T during PC ventilation. At the bedside, the clinician must adjust airway pressure setting, duration of inspiration (e.g., I:E), and respiratory frequency to vary minute ventilation and mean airway pressure. In most cases, it is necessary to suppress breathing efforts with deep sedation and neuromuscular blockade (when appropriate).

Acute Ventilatory Failure

Alveolar hypoventilation arises from an imbalance between the function of the respiratory "pump" (the respiratory muscles, neural connections, and the central nervous system driving center) and the mechanical loads (elastic and resistive opposition) imposed on the system. This section focuses on measurements assessing respiratory muscle function during ventilatory support, the mechanical effects of intrinsic PEEP, assessment of ventilatory capability, and concludes with a discussion of monitoring during weaning from mechanical ventilation.

Monitoring Breathing Effort During Ventilatory Support

Many patients may expend considerable effort during ventilatory support, the magnitude of this effort varying from a small percentage of the normal work-of-breathing to values that greatly exceed the total workload expected in a spontaneously breathing normal subject.[142] While continued respiratory efforts may help to prevent disuse atrophy, a state of chronic respiratory muscle fatigue may result in the presence of limited respiratory reserve.

Several options are available to assess spontaneous respiratory activity during ventilatory support;

in the clinical setting, only clinical assessment and pressure/volume monitoring are commonly used. Respiratory muscle activity also may be assessed by electromyography, but this technique has been used primarily in the laboratory setting.[151]

Clinical Assessment

During spontaneous or ventilator-assisted breathing, clinical assessment includes the patient's spontaneous respiratory rate and associated tidal volume, the use of accessory muscles, abdominal chest wall coordination, and the presence of chest wall retraction.[152] Expiratory muscle contraction may be visualized during expiratory flow obstruction, hyperinflation or high minute ventilation. Patients exhibiting general agitation, rapid, shallow breathing, use of accessory muscles, discoordinate ventilatory patterns including paradoxical breathing, likely are exerting significant respiratory effort to breathe and the workload may be fatiguing.[52] Adjustments to enhance a more appropriate ventilatory pattern such as increasing the synchronized intermittent mandatory ventilation (SIMV) rate, the inspiratory flow rate (in volume-targeted ventilatory modes), and the level of pressure support, or discontinuing a CPAP trial, may be indicated. In some circumstances, patient-ventilator dyssynchrony may be due to excessively high patient ventilatory drive, and may require sedation and neuromuscular blockade (when appropriate).

Pressure-Volume Monitoring

The airway pressure and waveform are very useful for determinating compliance and resistance (see prior discussion), intrinsic PEEP (see later section), and for identifying and quantifying patient effort during ventilatory support.

Patient Workload During Controlled and Assisted Mechanical Ventilation. During positive-pressure mechanical ventilation, the ventilator and the respiratory muscles behave as two pumps in series. If the respiratory muscles are completely relaxed, the ventilator develops all of the pressure required to overcome elastic and flow-resistive opposition of the lung and chest wall to inflate the respiratory system. This is simply the airway pressure (Prs), measured at the airway opening relative to atmospheric pressure; the area subtended by the pressure/volume curve represents the total work of breathing (Fig. 12-23A).[153] When the inspiratory muscles are active, the area contained in the curve represents the work performed by the ventilator, but this is no longer the total work (Fig. 12-23B). The difference between these areas yields the patient's respiratory work on the lungs and chest wall (Fig. 12-23C). Comparison of these curves is valid only if they are generated during constant inspiratory flow, tidal volume, and respiratory frequency.

The area under the transrespiratory pressure-time curve may be evaluated in a similar manner to the pressure-volume curves to yield a pressure-time product of the inspiratory muscles (Fig. 12-24A-C)). The pressure-time product often provides

a better index of the oxygen cost of breathing of the respiratory muscles than the mechanical analysis of work-of-breathing.[154]

In the absence of inspiratory muscle activity, the airway pressure vs time curve is characterized by a smooth rise, with the tracing always concave to the time axis (Fig. 12-24A). Tracings are reproducible from breath to breath. When respiratory muscles become active, the airway pressure vs time curves are not smooth and vary from breath to breath. During controlled mechanical ventilation (CMV), decreases in airway pressure occur after onset of inspiratory flow and reach their nadir near midinspiration, decreasing the airway pressure curve

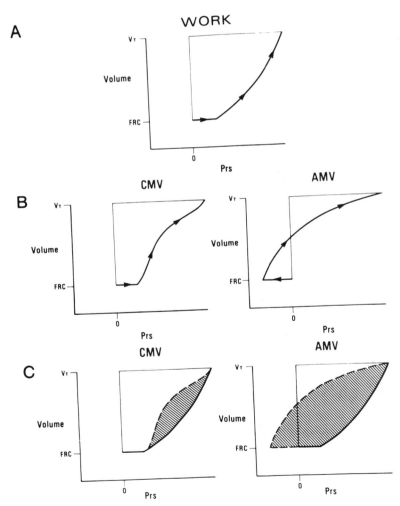

Fig. 12-23. Subtraction of the area subtended by the inflation pressure (Prs)-volume curve in the presence of inspiratory muscle activity (**B**) from that recorded during passive inflation (**A**) yields the work of inspiration performed by the patient (*shaded area,* **C**). (From Ward et al.,[153] with permission.)

(Fig. 12-24B). Increasing the inspiratory flow rate to greater than patient demand (usually >65 L/min) eliminates patient effort during CMV.

During assisted mechanical ventilation (AMV), the respiratory muscles contract to initiate inspiratory flow, decreasing the Prs curve (Fig. 12-24B). The inspiratory muscles continue to contract throughout a large portion of assisted mechanical breaths, resulting in continued decrease in the Prs vs time curve relative to the relaxed state. The patient's component of the total workload may be a large percentage (e.g., 60 percent) of the total inspiratory workload.[153,155] In these circumstances, respiratory muscle strength and ventilatory drive become major determinants of patient work and effort, rather than abnormalities in compliance and resistance.[155]

Other factors influencing patient effort during AMV include ventilator circuits that impose substantial resistance[156] (e.g., excessive trigger threshold, narrow endotracheal tube, bubble-type humidifier) and response time of the ventilator to flow demand.[157] Patient effort also is greatly increased during intrinsic PEEP, which depresses the effective functional triggering sensitivity (see "Intrinsic Positive End-Expiratory Pressure").

Patient Workload During Continuous Positive Airway Pressure. In contrast to mechanical ventilation, evaluating the airway pressure waveform dur-

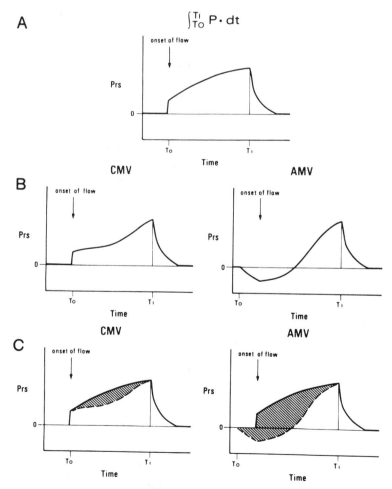

Fig. 12-24. Subtraction of the area subtended by the inflation pressure (Prs)-time curve in the presence of inspiratory muscle activity (**B**) from that recorded during passive inflation (**A**) yields the pressure-time product ($\int P \cdot dt$) of the inspiratory muscles (**C**). (From Ward,[153] with permission.)

ing spontaneous breathing cycles (e.g., CPAP) reflects only the work required by the patient, imposed by the ventilator circuit. To quantify the work of inspiration during CPAP, the esophageal pressure relative to atmospheric pressure must be electronically integrated with V_T to reflect the work done on the lungs, and the work required to overcome the endotracheal tube and ventilatory circuit.[158] Recent instrumentation (Bicore CP-100) has made esophageal pressure monitoring more available, but it is infrequently used in the clinical setting because of remaining technical difficulties.

The application of CPAP may decrease, increase, or produce no change in the patient's work of breathing compared with breathing via T tube (zero end-expiratory pressure) and depends on the patient's lung mechanics and the CPAP delivery system.

Mechanical and ventilatory responses to breathing with CPAP depend on the starting FRC. When FRC is normal, applying CPAP may overdistend alveoli and decrease lung compliance, thereby increasing elastic work and O_2 cost of breathing.[159] Ventilatory responses would include an increase in V_T, respiratory frequency and minute ventilation.

In contrast, when starting FRC is below normal because of processes causing regional atelectasis, applying CPAP normalizes FRC and increases lung compliance. In patients recovering from acute respiratory failure, breathing at optimum CPAP (the level which produced maximum Ceff), compared with breathing via T tube, significantly decreased respiratory frequency while increasing V_T, and was associated with decreased work of breathing.[160]

CPAP delivery systems affect the patient's work of breathing by changes in airway pressure.[161] To the extent and duration that airway pressure decreases below the end-expiratory pressure level, additional inspiratory work performed by the patient will be required. Similarly, during exhalation, increases in airway pressure above the end-expiratory (e.g., nonthreshold PEEP valves) level will lead to additional expiratory work. In the ideal CPAP system, the delivered inspiratory flow should be sufficient (relative to the patient's inspiratory flow) to keep airway pressure close to the end-expiratory level.

CPAP systems fall into two basic categories: continuous-flow and demand-flow. Continuous-flow systems work on the principle of a continuous high flow of pressurized gas, usually in an external circuit from the ventilator. Most mechanical ventilators work via a demand-flow system which may be pressure- or flow-triggered.[162] With some demand-flow systems, airway pressure may decrease further due to poor response time for initiation of gas flow and inability to actively regulate flow to maintain the end-expiratory level.

CPAP systems vary widely in the amount of additional work they impose. Most data suggest that continuous-flow systems are preferable to demand-flow systems because the latter impose additional work.[163] However, the more technologically advanced ventilators, for example, Puritan Bennett 7200 or Siemens 900C, may impose less additional work than a standard continuous-flow device (Fig 12-25).[161] For some demand-flow systems (e.g., Siemens 900B), there is a large but brief decrease in airway pressure (without volume change) due to time delay of inspiratory flow. Although the time delay may not result in increased mechanical work (pressure × volume), the short period of airway obstruction results in additional O_2 consumption for the respiratory muscles[164] and potential patient ventilator dyssynchrony. In such cases, changing to a continuous-flow system would be indicated.

Patient Workload During Pressure-Support Ventilation. Pressure-support ventilation (PSV) is a pressure-targeted, flow-cycled mode of ventilatory support in which each breath is initiated by the patient.[165] PSV is used as a primary mode of ventilatory support and as a method of weaning patients from mechanical ventilation. Because PSV is designed primarily to assist spontaneous breathing, the patient must have an intact respiratory drive.

During inspiration, PSV provides gas flow to the predetermined pressure limit. The pressure level is maintained by a servoloop in the ventilator that continuously adjusts inspiratory flow. The patient regulates the inspiratory flow, the inspiratory time, the expiratory time, and, thus, respiratory frequency and tidal volume with support from the ventilator. Exhalation starts when inspiratory flow to the patient is <25 percent of the maximum flow. Thus, the patient and the ventilator work in synchrony to achieve the total work of each breath.

PSV has been used to compensate for the additional work of breathing due to the endotracheal tube, humidifier, and breathing circuit.[166] For this purpose, low levels of pressure support (5 to 10 cmH_2O) are used. Higher levels (10 to 40 cmH_2O)

also can be used independently or combined with SIMV.

PSV reduces the work of breathing roughly in proportion to the pressure delivered and is associated with an increase in V_T, decrease in respiratory frequency, and esophageal pressure swings (Fig. 12-26).[167] The magnitude of the change in esophageal

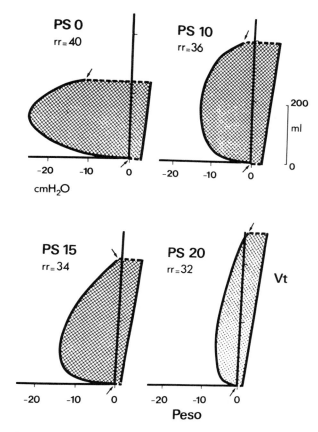

Fig. 12-26. Esophageal pressure plotted against volume for a representative patient from pressure support (PS) 0 to 20 cmH_2O, used to compute the work of breathing. The work per breath is represented by the *hatched area*, subtended by the inspiratory part of the P-V loop on the left and the relaxation curve of the chest wall on the right. *Arrows* indicate beginning and end of inspiration. With increasing levels of PS, tidal volume increases while respiratory frequency and work per breath decrease. (From Brochard et al.,[167] with permission.)

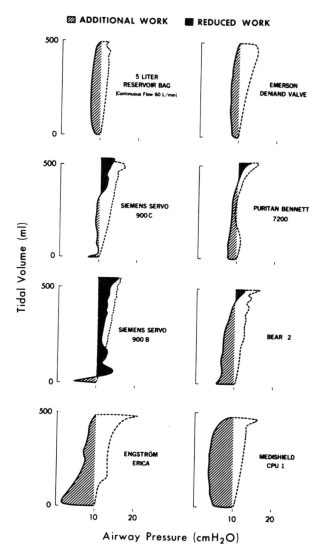

Fig. 12-25. Pressure-volume curves for each CPAP delivery system at 10 cmH_2O end-expiratory pressure at an inspiratory flow of 40 L/min. The airway pressure-volume area below the end-expiratory pressure level reflects the increased patient work of breathing caused by the CPAP delivery system. (From Katz et al.,[161] with permission.)

pressure is proportional to the O_2 cost of breathing and, consequently, the patient's work of breathing.

The level of pressure support may be optimally adjusted to prevent diaphragmatic fatigue in patients recovering from acute respiratory failure. Adjustment can be based on electomyographic criteria and/or reducing the fraction of the inspiratory reserve used to maintain tidal ventilation.[167] The ratio of mean transdiaphragmatic pressure to maximum transdiaphragmatic pressure during inspiration with an occluded glottis (Pdi/Pdi max) is a useful indicator of this fraction. Normal subjects are unable to sustain indefinitely a Pdi/Pdi max in excess of 0.4[168]; a similar relationship was found in COPD patients recovering from acute respiratory failure.[169] Because the application of PSV reduces Pdi, it should be possible to lower this ratio to <0.40 to prevent or minimize diaphragmatic fatigue. Clinically, neither transdiaphragmatic pressure nor diaphragmatic EMG monitoring is routinely performed; fortunately assessing sternocleidomastoid activity (SCM) by palpation may accurately define an optimal level of PSV. At optimum levels of pressure support, SCM has minimal activity.[167] At the bedside, pressure support could be gradually reduced until phasic inspiratory activity of SCM appears to increase; a slightly higher level of pressure support should then be applied, balancing the need to maintain substantial diaphragmatic activity yet avoiding respiratory muscle fatigue.

Intrinsic Positive End-Expiratory Pressure

In lung diseases characterized by increased airway resistance and decreased expiratory flow (e.g., COPD, asthma), and/or in conditions characterized by a short expiratory time (high minute ventilation in patients with acute hypoxemic respiratory failure), expiratory flow continues until interrupted by inspiration producing dynamic hyperinflation of the lungs—often referred to as PEEPi.

In stable patients with COPD, PEEPi levels up to 9 cmH$_2$O have been observed.[170] In COPD patients with acute respiratory failure, the magnitude of PEEPi may be as high as 13 cmH$_2$O during spontaneous breathing,[171] and 22 H$_2$O during mechanical ventilation.[75] In patients with acute respiratory failure, the incidence of PEEPi increased from 39 to 100 percent when mechanical ventilation increased from >10 to >20 L/min. The magnitude of PEEPi varied from 1 to 25 cmH$_2$O, with the majority of patients having 5 to 15 cmH$_2$O.[172]

Implications of PEEPi

High levels of PEEPi have important and often profound hemodynamic and pulmonary consequences. PEEPi has been shown to impair cardiac output, presumably by decreasing venous return secondary to the increased intrathoracic pressure.[173] Additionally, if the effects of PEEPi on transmural filling pressures are not accounted for, measurements of cardiac filling pressures may be seriously overestimated.

Lung hyperinflation from high levels of PEEPi increases the risk of pulmonary barotrauma, increases dead space ventilation, and causes the respiratory muscles to operate on an unfavorable portion of their length-tension curves, functionally decreasing maximal inspiratory pressure. If PEEPi is not accounted for, static compliance will be underestimated.[174]

PEEPi increases patient effort during assisted mechanical ventilation or spontaneous breathing by producing a pressure threshold that must be overcome by the inspiratory muscles.[170] Thus, the onset of inspiratory muscle activity and the commencement of inspiratory flow are not synchronous: inspiratory flow starts only when the pressure within the pleural space (developed by the inspiratory muscles) exceeds PEEPi because alveolar pressure only then becomes subatmospheric. The result is increased O$_2$ consumption by the respiratory muscles and increased requirement for elastic work in response to lung hyperinflation.[171] In patients with high levels of PEEPi (e.g., >10 cmH$_2$O), the inspiratory effort required to trigger the ventilator may be excessive, leading to serious ventilator-patient asynchrony that may require heavy sedation or neuromuscular blockade. Patients with high levels of PEEPi are difficult to wean from mechanical ventilation.

Methods To Measure PEEPi

The presence or level of PEEPi is not detectable by observing the airway pressure manometer (at end-expiration) during mechanical ventilation. The presence of PEEPi is best determined by assessing whether exhalation is still occurring when the next inspiration begins; this can be assessed by chest auscultation and/or by analysis of the pressure-flow relationship during mechanical ventilation. If PEEPi is present, flow continues throughout exhalation, which is abruptly terminated by the next mechanical inflation; in contrast, when PEEPi is absent, the expiratory flow decreases smoothly to zero before the next breath.

During controlled mechanical ventilation, the level of PEEPi can be quantified by measuring the airway pressure at the onset of inspiratory flow or, more commonly, during expiratory port occlusion at end-exhalation (Fig. 12-27).[173,174] (The former technique requires that the airway and flow tracings be synchronized, graphically displayed, and recorded at high speeds). During expiratory port occlusion, distal airway pressure and proximal circuit pressure equilibrate, and PEEPi will be reflected on the ventilator manometer (Fig. 12-28). For accurate measurement, expiratory port occlusion must occur just prior to the next ventilator delivered breath and is easily obtained with the Siemens 900C and Hamilton Veolar ventilators. Activating the expiratory pause button in these ventilators closes the expiratory valve (while inhibiting the next mechanical inspiration) at the end of the set expiratory time. For other ventilators, an external valve is needed to achieve manual occlusion at end-expiration.

In patients breathing spontaneously or during assisted mechanical ventilation, PEEPi can be determined by measuring the esophageal pressure deflection from the start of inspiratory effort to the onset of inspiratory flow.[170] Another approach for measuring PEEPi is to monitor changes in end-expiratory thoracic volume using RIP while adding PEEP or CPAP.[175] The level of end-expiratory pressure at which end-expiratory lung volume begins to increase would correspond to PEEPi.

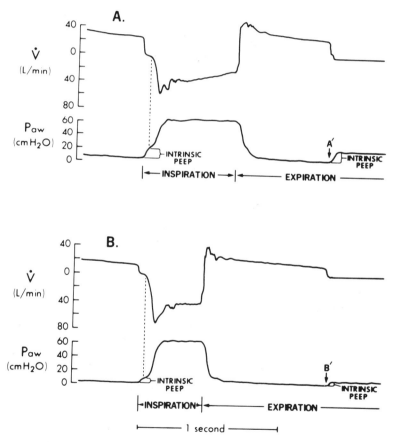

Fig. 12-27. Airway pressure (Paw) and flow ($\dot{V}$) in a patient with acute respiratory failure receiving pressure controlled ventilation. The level of end-expiratory pressure was set at 0 cmH$_2$O. (**A**), Inspiratory time of 50 percent, and (**B**), inspiratory time of 33 percent of the respiratory cycle. The *dashed vertical line* marks the airway pressure at the instant of inspiratory flow. **A'** and **B'** denote the onset of end-expiratory airway occlusion. Two methods of measuring intrinsic PEEP are shown: the airway pressure at onset of inspiratory flow and the airway pressure during airway occlusion at end-expiration. The effect of prolonging expiratory time from 50 to 67 percent of the respiratory cycle is to reduce the level of intrinsic PEEP from 14 to 6 cmH$_2$O. (From Katz,[100] with permission.)

Treatment of PEEPi

Treatment of patients with COPD and acute respiratory failure who have PEEPi should be directed at decreasing flow resistance (e.g., bronchodilation) and reducing respiratory frequency. To the extent that tachynpnea is due to fever and/or airway infection, treatment of these two conditions by conventional methods (e.g., antipyretics, antibiotics, and steroids) should be beneficial.

During mechanical ventilation, reducing respiratory frequency is aimed at prolonging expiratory time (to allow for a more complete exhalation) and can be accomplished by increasing inspiratory flow (decreasing the I:E ratio); in some circumstances a reduction in $\dot{V}E$ is required because of the associated high peak airway pressure with higher inspiratory flows.

A controversial but promising approach to manage PEEPi is the external application of CPAP or PEEP. The application of end-expiratory pressure to a level less than the PEEPi has been shown to diminish the work of breathing in stable patients

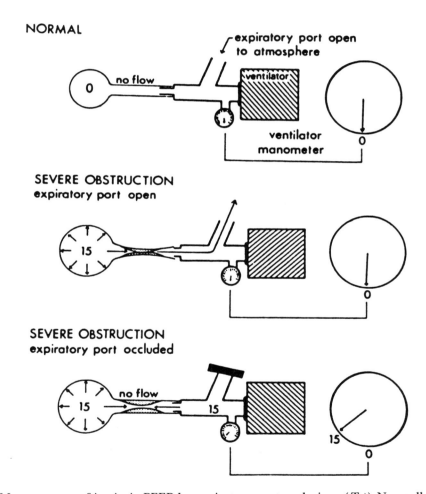

Fig. 12-28. Measurement of intrinsic PEEP by expiratory port occlusion. (*Top*) Normally, alveolar pressure is atmospheric at the end of passive exhalation. (*Middle*) With severe airflow obstruction, alveolar pressure remains elevated (in this example at 15 cmH_2O) and slow flow continues, even at the end of the set exhalation period. The ventilator manometer senses negligible pressure because it is open to atmosphere through large-bore tubing and downstream from the site of flow limitation. (*Bottom*) When gas flow is stopped by occlusion of the expiratory port at the end of the set exhalation period, pressure equilibrates throughout the lung-ventilator system and is displayed on the ventilator manometer. (From Pepe and Marini,[173] with permission.)

with severe COPD and in patient-initiated mechanical breaths.[171,176] During airflow limitation, CPAP or PEEP diminishes the existing airway pressure threshold.[177] The effectiveness of this therapy is assessed by observing reduction in respiratory efforts or by measuring the esophageal deflection with and without PEEP (Fig. 12-29).[178]

To avoid further pulmonary inflation with PEEP application in flow-limited circumstances, end-expiratory lung volume and/or peak inspiratory pressure should remain unchanged until the critical level of PEEPi is exceeded. In contrast, in patients without flow limitations, a progressive increase in lung volume and peak inspiratory pressure should occur starting with the smallest increments in extrinsic PEEP.[179]

Ventilatory Capability

Drive to Breathe

In the clinical setting, ventilatory drive is rarely measured, but indirectly assessed. Drive measures correlate with dyspnea, patient work, minute ventilation and the ability to wean from mechanical ventilation.

Normal drive to breathe in the awake state may be inferred if the patient is alert, follows commands and exhibits an increased respiratory rate ($\dot{V}E$) in response to hypoxemia and hypercapnia. Measurements of $\dot{V}E$ and mean inspiratory flow (VI) correlate well with the output of the respiratory center, but not in the presence of abnormal respiratory mechanics because reduced strength and endurance limit the ability to maintain $\dot{V}E$ in proportion to drive.[180]

Measuring the airway pressure 0.1 seconds ($P_{0.1}$) after initiating an inspiratory effort during airway occlusion provides a measure of drive and, in contrast to VI, $P_{0.1}$ is not affected by abnormal lung mechanics.[180] Clinically, $P_{0.1}$ can be determined during mechanical ventilatory support because most ventilators incorporate a demand valve, which imposes a measurable delay (usually 100 ms) prior to inspiratory flow.[181]

The $P_{0.1}$ in normal subjects is generally less than 2 cmH$_2$O. In addition to impaired respiratory center output causing ventilatory failure, an elevated drive may also signify a problem.[182] High $P_{0.1}$ values (>6 cmH$_2$O) imply high inspiratory muscle activity that may not be sustained for a prolonged period without developing respiratory muscle fatigue.[183] Similarly, $P_{0.1}$ values have been used as a predictor of successful weaning from mechanical ventilation. Two studies have reported $P_{0.1}$ values >6 cmH$_2$O to predict failure of weaning,[183,184] while a third was unable to demonstrate predictive value.[185]

Respiratory Muscle Strength

Two tests are clinically used to assess respiratory muscle strength. These are vital capacity (VC) and maximal inspiratory pressure (MIP). Serial measurements will help determine the progression of weakness and guide the frequency with which measurements should be made. In patients with neuromuscular diseases, such as Guillain-Barre syndrome, tracheal intubation and mechanical venti-

Fig. 12-29. Effect of PEEP on auto-PEEP (intrinsic PEEP). As a positive end-expiratory alveolar pressure (Palv) (*dashed line*), auto-PEEP presents an inspiratory threshold load that must be overcome by inspiratory effort [negative esophageal pressure (Pes) deflection] before external airway pressure (*straight line, upper tracing*) can begin to decrease, triggering an inflation cycle. The addition of PEEP (less than the original auto-PEEP) in a patient with dynamic airway collapse reduces the effective triggering threshold and the work of breathing. (From Marini,[178] with permission.)

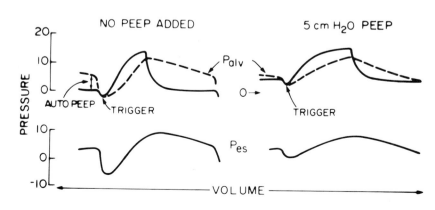

lation should be considered based on abnormal values (e.g., vital capacity < 1 L) that may precede a deterioration in blood gas values.

Vital Capacity. Vital capacity (VC) is a measurement which reflects several components including lung-thorax compliance, volitional effort, and muscle strength. The VC is normally 70 ml/kg and is 10 (or more) times greater than the spontaneous resting tidal volume. Muscle strength must decline to nearly 20 percent of the normal value before significant reductions occur in VC.[186] Despite this limitation, the VC is commonly considered a valuable clinical indicator to assess weaning from mechanical ventilation; values exceeding 10 ml/kg often predict a favorable outcome.[187] However, VC predictive power is rather poor.[188]

In the unintubated patient, VC can be measured using a mouthpiece (and nose clip) and a "spirometer." When a vital capacity is to be measured in an intubated patient, a low-resistance nonreturn value is incorporated at the junction between the endotracheal tube and the breathing circuit. The spirometer is attached to the exhalation port of the nonreturn valve.

Maximal Inspiratory Pressure. The pressure developed at the airway opening during a maximal inspiratory effort against an occluded airway (MIP) is a simple noninvasive test of inspiratory muscle strength.[189] Before measurement of MIP, 100 percent oxygen should be administered. Then, with a tight airway seal by mask or cuffed endotracheal tube, the airway is occluded. Pressure in the closed system is measured, usually by aneroid manometer. The largest negative pressure produced during the next 20 seconds is noted.[190]

In the pulmonary function laboratory, MIP is conventionally measured during inspiratory effort from residual volume, to detect the maximal value resulting from the mechanical advantage of the inspiratory muscles increasing their operating length. When measured in this fashion, MIP is approximately -120 cmH$_2$O. However, in the clinical setting, MIP is measured at FRC, because the latter reflects the pressure available for inspiratory efforts during resting ventilation and should be a better predictor of weaning outcome than MIP measured from residual volume.

In the alert, unmedicated patient (e.g., in the critical care setting when evaluating a patient for withdrawal of mechanical support), the normal value usually is greater than -60 cmH$_2$O. Decreases in MIP may be due to muscle weakness, central nervous system (CNS) depression, hyperinflation or any combination of these factors. An early clinical study of patients recovering from anesthesia suggested that -20 cmH$_2$O was an adequate MIP.[191] Larger values (>-30 cmH$_2$O) may be required for more accurate prediction of successful weaning from mechanical ventilation in the critical care setting,[192] although even these criteria have yielded high rates of false-positive and false-negative results.[188,193,194] The disappointing results may be due, in part, to the fact that MIP measurements do not take into account the demands (e.g., elastic and resistive load) placed on the respiratory system.

Weaning From Mechanical Ventilatory Support

Although many patients receiving mechanical ventilatory support in the critical care unit do not require repetitive measurements or involved plans for discontinuing mechanical ventilatory support, it is desirable to have predictive indices that can be easily measured and widely applied. These indices should help to identify the earliest time that a patient can resume spontaneous unassisted breathing, or possible failure to wean, so that cardiorespiratory distress and/or pulmonary function deterioration may be prevented. Requirements common to all patients to initiate weaning from mechanical ventilation include resolution of a large P(A $-$ a)O$_2$ (e.g., <450 mmHg) or $\dot{Q}$s/$\dot{Q}$t < 0.2, cardiovascular stability, and an adequate drive to breathe.

Much of the clinical literature pertaining to the process of discontinuing mechanical ventilatory support has focused on measurable bedside parameters that, when applied to large series of patients, have some predictive value for successful outcome. Threshold values of these parameters include: MIP > -30 cm H$_2$O[192]; VC > 10 mg/kg[187]; P$_{0.1}$ < -6 cm H$_2$O[183]; V$_T$ > 4 ml/kg[195]; respiratory frequency < 35/min[196]; $\dot{V}$E < 10 L[192]; maximal voluntary ventilation > twice the resting $\dot{V}$E[192]; V$_D$/V$_T$ < 0.6[197]; P(A $-$ aO)$_2$ < 450 mmHg[197]; and C$_{LT}$ > 25 ml/cmH$_2$O[198]. Although these threshold values are useful, they are not fully reliable predictors of weaning outcome.

An alternative approach to discontinuing mechanical ventilatory support integrates the measurement of respiratory muscle strength and of respiratory load. Thus, the load imposed on the respiratory system and the patient's ability to perform the required work of breathing is evaluated.

In the laboratory setting, a mean inspiratory pressure ($\overline{P}_{Imus}$) per breath exceeding 0.4 of the maximum pressure for the respiratory muscles (P_{Imax}) or a pressure time index $[PTI] = (\overline{P}_{Imus}/P_{Imax}) \times (T_I/T_{TOT})$ exceeding 0.15 to 0.18 seconds predicts the inability to sustain spontaneous breathing indefinitely without developing respiratory muscle fatigue.[168] Although these data were collected in normal healthy volunteers, the basic relationship is applicable to the vast majority of mechanically ventilated patients.[169]

In the clinical setting, the PTI has been referred to as the inspiratory effort quotient (IEQ)[199] and can be quantified using

$$IEQ = \frac{(k V_T / C_{eff}) \times (T_I/T_{TOT})}{MIP}$$

where k is considered to be 0.75, and MIP is measured in the standard fashion. The advantage of this equation is that it takes into account some of the major factors that promote respiratory muscle fatigue, specifically, the load to breathe (C_{eff}), the breathing pattern (V_T and T_I/T_{TOT}), and the available inspiratory pressure (MIP). All but the MIP value are easily obtained from the settings during mechanical ventilation. Based on this equation, the MIP should be 2.5 times the pressure predicted from the C_{eff} for the patient to be capable of sustained spontaneous breathing.

This concept was evaluated in a large group of patients being weaned from mechanical ventilation using the CROP (an acronym for compliance, respiratory rate, oxygenation, and pressure) index.[195] This index integrates respiratory load (C_{eff} and respiratory rate), respiratory muscle strength (MIP), and gas exchange (P_{aO_2}/P_{AO_2}). The integrative index equation is

$$CROP = \frac{[C_{eff} \times MIP \times (P_{aO_2}/P_{AO_2})]}{\text{respiratory rate}}$$

Patients with a CROP index of ≥ 18 ml/breath per minute had an 87 percent likehood of successful weaning outcome compared with 55 percent and 61 percent, respectively, for $\dot{V}_E < 10$ L or a MIP of > -30 cmH$_2$O.[195]

One of the best predictors of sustained successful breathing during weaning from mechanical ventilation is the respiratory rate. In general, when the respiratory rate is >35 breaths per minute, reassessment for further mechanical ventilatory support is indicated.[196] The development of hypercapnia and respiratory acidosis in patients who fail to successfully wean from mechanical ventilation is associated with rapid and shallow breathing. A rapid shallow breathing index <105 breaths/min/L [derived by the respiratory frequency divided by the V_T (L)] is a more accurate predictor of weaning success than traditional indices such as $\dot{V}_E$ and MIP, and is slightly more predictive than the CROP index.[195]

SUMMARY

In summary, assessment of pulmonary oxygen and carbon dioxide exchange, and of the adequacy and efficiency of respiratory mechanics and ventilatory reserves are the goals of respiratory monitoring. The last decade has brought technologic advances in monitoring and an increased understanding of the pathophysiologic characteristics of respiratory failure. Our capability to manage and treat respiratory complications as they occur during anesthesia and critical illness is significantly enhanced.

REFERENCES

1. Tinker JH, Dull DL, Caplan RA et al: Role of monitoring devices in prevention of anesthetic mishaps: a closed claim analysis. Anesthesiology 71:541, 1989
2. Caplan RA, Posner K, Ward RW, Cheney FW: Adverse respiratory events in anesthesia: a closed claim analysis. Anesthesiology 72:828, 1990
3. Nunn JF: Oxygen. p. 247. In: Applied Respiratory Physiology. 4th Ed. Butterworth, London, 1993
4. Shapiro BA, Harrison RA, Kacmarek RM, Cane RD: Oxygen therapy. p. 176. In: Clinical Applications of Respiratory Care. 3rd Ed. Year Book Medical Publishers, Chicago, 1985
5. Leigh JM: Variation in performance of oxygen therapy devices. Anaesthesia 25:230, 1970
6. Johnston WE, Vinten-Johansen J, Strickland RA, Bowton DL: Comparison of two formulas to calculate alveolar oxygen tension in canine oleic acid pulmonary edema. Crit Care Med 17:176, 1989
7. Cole PV: Bench analysis of blood gases. p. 33. In Spence AA (ed): Respiratory Monitoring in Intensive Care. Churchill Livingstone, Edinburgh, 1982
8. Leatherman J, Ingram RH: Respiratory failure. In

Rubernstein E, Federman DD (eds): Scientific American Medicine. Scientific American, New York, 1992

9. West JB, Wagner PD: Pulmonary gas exchange. p 361. In West JB (ed): Bioengineering Aspects of the Lung. Marcel Dekker, New York, 1977

10. Benatar SR, Hewlett AM, Nunn JF: The use of iso-shunt lines for control of oxygen therapy. Br J Anaesth 45:711, 1973

11. Cheney FW, Colley PS: The effect of cardiac output on arterial blood oxygenation. Anesthesiology 52:496, 1980

12. Falke KJ, Pontoppidan H, Kumar A et al: Ventilation with end-expiratory pressure in acute lung disease. J Clin Invest 51:2315, 1972

13. Kvetan V, Carlon GC, Howland WS: Acute pulmonary failure in asymmetric lung disease: approach to management. Crit Care Med 10:114, 1982

14. Vincent JL, DeBacker D: Initial management of circulatory shock as prevention of MSOF. Crit Care Clin 5:369, 1989

15. Shibutani K, Komatsu T, Kubal K et al: Critical level of oxygen delivery in anesthetized man. Crit Care Med 11:640, 1983

16. van Woerkens ECSM, Trouwborst A, van Lanschot JJB: Profound hemodilution: what is the critical level of hemodilution at which oxygen delivery-dependent oxygen consumption starts in an anesthetized human? Anesth Analg 75:818, 1992

17. Cain SM: Oxygen delivery and uptake in dogs during anemic and hypoxic hypoxia. J Appl Physiol 42:228, 1977

18. Schumacker PT, Samsel RW: Oxygen delivery and uptake by peripheral tissues: physiology and pathophysiology. Crit Care Clin 5:255, 1989

19. Hayes MA, Yau EHS, Timmins AC et al: Response of critically ill patients to treatment aimed at achieving supranormal oxygen delivery and consumption: relation to outcome. Chest 103:886, 1993

20. Bakker J, Coffernils M, Leon M et al: Blood lactate levels are superior to oxygen-drived variables in predicting outcome in human septic shock. Chest 99:956, 1991

21. Suter PM, Lindauer JM, Fairley HB, Schlobohm RM: Errors in data derived from pulmonary artery blood gas values. Crit Care Med 3:175, 1975

22. Bay J, Nunn JF, Prys-Roberts C: Factors influencing arterial PO_2 during recovery from anesthesia. Br J Anaesth 40:398, 1968

23. Bursztein S: Monitoring of metabolic response in multisystem organ failure. Anesthesiol Clin North Am 6:39, 1988

24. Smithies MN, Royston B, Makita K et al: Comparison of oxygen consumption measurements: indirect calorimetry versus the reversed Fick method. Crit Care Med 19:1401, 1991

25. Westenskow DR, Cutler CA, Wallace WD: Instrumentation for monitoring gas exchange and metabolic rate in critically ill patients. Crit Care Med 12:183, 1984

26. Makita K, Nunn JF, Royston B: Evaluation of metabolic measuring instruments for use in critically ill patients. Crit Care Med 18:638, 1990

27. Nunn JF, Makita K, Royston B: Validation of oxygen consumption measurements during artificial ventilation. J Appl Physiol 67:2129, 1989

28. Nunn JF: Carbon dioxide. p 219. In: Applied Respiratory Physiology. 4th Ed. Butterworth, London, 1993

29. Radford EP: Ventilation standards for use in artificial respiration. J Appl Physiol 7:451, 1955

30. Fairley HB: Management of respiratory failure. In Hershey SG (ed): Refresher Courses in Anesthesiology. Vol 1. JB Lippincott, Philadelphia, 1973

31. France CJ, Eger EI, Bendixen HH: The use of peripheral venous blood for pH and carbon dioxide tension determinations during general anesthesia. Anesthesiology 40:311, 1974

32. Nunn JF: Distribution of pulmonary ventilation and perfusion. p 156. In: Applied Respiratory Physiology. 4th Ed. Butterworth, London, 1993

33. Shankar KB, Moseley H, Kumar AY, Delph Y: Capnometry and anaesthesia. Can J Anaesth 39:617, 1992

34. Eriksson L, Wollmer P, Olsson CG et al: Diagnosis of pulmonary embolism based upon alveolar dead space analysis. Chest 96:357, 1989

35. Nunn JF, Hill DW: Respiratory dead space and arterial to end-tidal CO_2 tension difference in anesthetized man. J Appl Physiol 15:383, 1960

36. Pansard JL, Cholley B, Devilliers C et al: Variation in arterial to end-tidal CO_2 tension differences during anesthesia in the "kidney rest" lateral decubitus position. Anesth Analg 75:506, 1992

37. Fletcher R, Jonson B: Deadspace and the single breath test for carbon dioxide during anaesthesia and artificial ventilation. Br J Anaesth 56:109, 1984

38. Cooper EA: Physiological deadspace in passive ventilation: relationships with tidal volume, frequency, age and minor upsets of respiratory health. Anaesthesia 22:199, 1967

39. Korst RJ, Orlando R, Yeston NS: Validation of respiratory mechanics software in microprocessor-controlled ventilators. Crit Care Med 20:1152, 1992

40. Bicore: Bicore CP-100 pulmonary monitor product literature. Bicore, Irvine, CA, 1991

41. Bardoczky GI, Engelman E, D'Hollander A: Continuous spirometry: an aid to monitoring ventilation during operation. Br J Anaesth 71:747, 1993

42. Adams AP, Vickers MDA, Munore JP, Parker CW: Dry displacement gas meters. Br J Anaesth 39:174, 1967

43. Byles PH: Observations on some continuously-acting spirometers. Br J Anaesth 32:470, 1960

44. Ilsley AH, Hart JD, Withers RT, Roberts JG: Evaluation of five small turbine-type respirometers used in adult anaesthesia. J Clin Monit 9:196, 1993

45. Grenvik A, Hedstrand U: The reliability of pneumotachography in respiratory ventilation, an experimental study. Acta Anaesthesiol Scand 10:157, 1966

46. Kafer ER: Errors in pneumotachography as a result of transducer design and function. Anesthesiology 38:275, 1973

47. Yeh MP, Adams TD, Gardner RM, Yanowitz FG: Effect of O_2, N_2, and CO_2 composition on nonlinearity of Fleisch pneumotachograph characteristics. J Appl Physiol 56:1423, 1984

48. Osborn JJ: A flowmeter for respiratory monitoring. Crit Care Med 6:349, 1978

49. Konno K, Mead J: Measurement of the separate volume changes of rib cage and abdomen during breathing. J Appl Physiol 22:407, 1967

50. Milledge JS, Scott FD: Inductive plethysmography: a new respiratory transducer. J Physiol 267:4, 1979

51. Chadha TS, Watson H, Birch S et al: Validation of respiratory inductive plethysmograph using different calibration procedures. Am Rev Respir Dis 125:644, 1982

52. Cohen CA, Zagelman G, Gross D et al: Clinical manifestations of inspiratory muscle fatigue. Am J Med 73:308, 1982

53. Tobin MJ, Perez W, Guenther SM et al: Does rib cage abdominal paradox signify respiratory muscle fatigue? J Appl Physiol 63:851, 1987

54. Gravenstein N, Banner MJ, McLaughlin G: Tidal volume changes due to the interaction of anesthesia machine and anesthesia ventilator. J Clin Monit 3:187, 1987

55. Coté CJ, Petkau AJ, Ryan JF, Welch JP: Wasted ventilation measured in vitro with eight anesthetic circuits with an without inline humidification. Anesthesiology 59:442, 1983

56. Marks JD, Schapera A, Kraemer RW, Katz JA: Pressure and flow limitations of anesthesia ventilators. Anesthesiology 71:403, 1989

57. Schwartz DE, Katz JA: Mechanical ventilation during general anesthesia. p 529. In Tobin M (ed): Principles and Practice of Mechanical Ventilation. McGraw-Hill, New York, 1994

58. Marks JD, Katz JA, Schapera A, Kraemer RW: Evaluation of a new operating room ventilator: the Ohmeda 7810. Anesthesiology 71:A462, 1989

59. Schapera A, Marks JD, Minagi H et al: Perioperative pulmonary function in acute respiratory failure: effect of ventilator type and anesthetic gas mixture. Anesthesiology 71:396, 1989

60. Bartel LP, Bazik JR, Powner DJ: Compression volume during mechanical ventilation: comparison of ventilators and tubing circuits. Crit Care Med 13:851, 1985

61. Whaba RW: Perioperative functional residual capacity. Can J Anaesth 38:384, 1991.

62. Ozanne GM, Zinn SE, Fairley HB: Measurement of functional residual capacity during mechanical ventilation by simultaneous exchange of two insoluble gases. Anesthesiology 54:413, 1981

63. Larsson A, Linnarsson D, Jonmarker C et al: Measurement of lung volume by sulfur hexafluoride washout during spontaneous and controlled ventilation: further development of a method. Anesthesiology 67:543, 1987

64. Suter PM, Schlobohm RM: Determination of functional residual capacity during mechanical ventilation. Anesthesiology 41:605, 1974

65. Milic-Emili J, Ploysongsang Y: Respiratory mechanics in adult respiratory distress syndrome. Crit Care Clin 2:573, 1986

66. Matamis D, LeMaire F, Harf A et al: Total respiratory pressure volume curves in adult respiratory distress syndrome. Chest 86:58, 1984

67. Macklem PT: Procedures for Standardization Measurements of Lung Mechanics. Bethesda, National Heart Institute, 1974

68. Baydur A, Behrakis PK, Zin WA et al: A simple method for assessing the validity of the esophageal balloon technique. Am Rev Respir Dis 126:788, 1982

69. Milic-Emili J, Mead J, Turner FM: Topography of esophageal pressure as a function of posture in man. J Appl Physiol 19:212, 1964

70. O'Quin R, Marini JJ, Culver BH, Butler J: Transmission of airway pressure to the pleural space during lung edema and chest wall restriction. J Appl Physiol 59:1171, 1985

71. Chapin JC, Downs JB, Douglas ME et al: Lung expansion, airway pressure transmission and positive end-expiratory pressure. Arch Surg 114:1193, 1979

72. Katz JA, Zinn SE, Ozanne GM, Fairley HB: Pulmonary, chest wall and lung-thorax elastances in acute respiratory failure. Chest 80:304, 1981

73. Nunn JF: Non-elastic resistance to gas flow. p 61. In Applied Respiratory Physiology. 4th Ed. Butterworth, London, 1993

74. D'Angelo E, Calderini E, Torri G et al: Respiratory mechanics in anesthetized paralyzed humans: effects of flow, volume, and time. J Appl Physiol 67:2556, 1989

75. Broseghini C, Brandolese R, Poggi R et al: Respi-

ratory mechanics during the first day of mechanical ventilation in patients with pulmonary edema and chronic airway obstruction. Am Rev Respir Dis 138: 355, 1988

76. Wright PE, Marini JJ, Bernard G: In vitro versus in vivo comparison of endotracheal tube airflow resistance. Am Rev Respir Dis 140:10, 1989

77. Nunn JF: Respiratory aspects of anaesthesia. p 384. In: Applied Respiratory Physiology. 4th Ed. Butterworth, London, 1993

78. Fourcade HE, Stevens WC, Larson CP Jr et al: The ventilatory effects of Forane®, a new inhaled anesthetic. Anesthesiology 35:26, 1971

79. Eger EI: Respiratory effects. p 30. In: Desflurane (Suprane): A Compendium and Reference. Healthpress Publishing Group, Rutherford, NJ, 1993

80. Jones JG, Faithfull D, Jordan C et al: Rib cage movement during halothane anaesthesia in man. Br J Anaesth 51:399, 1979

81. Tusiewicz K, Bryan AC, Froese AB: Contributions of changing rib cage-diaphragm interactions to the ventilatory depression of halothane anesthesia. Anesthesiology 47:327, 1977

82. Pietak S, Weenig CS, Hickey RF, Fairley HB: Anesthetic effects on ventilation in patients with chronic obstructive pulmonary disease. Anesthesiology 42: 160, 1975

83. Knill RL, Clement JL: Variable effects of anaesthetics on the ventilatory response to hypoxaemia in man. Can Anaesth Soc J 29:93, 1982

84. Schmid ER, Rehder K: General anesthesia and the chest wall. Anesthesiology 55:668, 1981

85. Hedenstierna G, Strandberg Å, Brismar B et al: Functional residual capacity, thoracoabdominal dimensions, and central blood volume during general anesthesia with muscle paralysis and mechanical ventilation. Anesthesiology 62:247, 1985

86. Don HF, Wahba M, Cuadrado L, Kelkar K: The effects of anesthesia and 100 per cent oxygen on the functional residual capacity of the lungs. Anesthesiology 32:521, 1970

87. Brismar B, Hedenstierna G, Lundquist H et al: Pulmonary densities during anesthesia with muscular relaxation: a proposal of atelectasis. Anesthesiology 62:422, 1985

88. Tokics L, Hedenstierna G, Strandberg Å et al: Lung collapse and gas exchange during general anesthesia: effects of spontaneous breathing, muscle paralysis, and positive end-expiratory pressure. Anesthesiology 66:157, 1987

89. Westbrook PR, Stubbs SE, Sessler AD et al: Effects of anesthesia and muscle paralysis on respiratory mechanics in normal man. J Appl Physiol 34:81, 1973

90. Nunn JF: Elastic forces and lung volumes. p 36. In

Applied Respiratory Physiology. 4th Ed. Butterworth, London, 1993

91. Ferris BG Jr, Pollard DS: Effect of deep and quiet breathing on pulmonary compliance in man. J Clin Invest 39:143, 1960

92. Egbert LD, Laver MB, Bendixen HH: Intermittent deep breaths and compliance during anesthesia in man. Anesthesiology 24:57, 1963

93. Bendixen HH, Hedley-Whyte J, Laver MB: Impaired oxygenation in surgical patients during general anesthesia with controlled ventilation. N Engl J Med 269:991, 1963

94. Rehder K: Anaesthesia and the respiratory system. Can Anaesth Soc J 26:451, 1979

95. Pollard BJ, Junius F: Accidental intubation of the esophagus. Anaesth Intens Care 8:183, 1980

96. Birmingham PK, Cheney FW, Ward RJ: Esophageal intubation: a review of detection techniques. Anesth Analg 65:886, 1986

97. Linko K, Paloheimo M, Tammisto T: Capnography for detection of accidental oesophageal intubation. Acta Anaesthesiol Scand 27:199, 1983

98. Bone RC: Diagnosis of causes for acute respiratory distress by pressure-volume curves. Chest 70:740, 1976

99. Raphael DT, Weller RS, Doran DJ: A response algorithm for the low-pressure alarm condition. Anesth Analg 67:876, 1988

100. Katz JA: Management of intraoperative ventilatory emergencies. p 155. In Barash PG (ed): Refresher Courses in Anesthesiology. Vol 17. JB Lippincott, Philadelphia, 1989

101. Kingston HGG, Hirshman CA: Perioperative management of the patient with asthma. Anesth Analg 63:844, 1984

102. Hirshman CA, Downes H, Farbood A et al: Ketamine block of bronchospasm in experimental canine asthma. Br J Anaesth 51:713, 1979

103. Tobias JD, Hirshman CA: Attenuation of histamine-induced airway constriction by albuterol during halothane anesthesia. Anesthesiology 72:105, 1990

104. Hamilton WK, Moyers J: Pneumothorax during surgery. JAMA 198:187, 1966

105. Gold MI, Joseph SI: Bilateral tension pneumothorax following induction of anesthesia in two patients with chronic obstructive airway disease. Anesthesiology 38:93, 1973

106. Gal TJ, Goldberg SK: Relationship between respiratory muscle strength and vital capacity during partial curarization in awake subjects. Anesthesiology 54:141, 1981

107. Pavlin EG, Holle RH, Schoene RB: Recovery of airway protection compared with ventilation in humans after paralysis with curare. Anesthesiology 70: 381, 1989

108. Craig DB: Postoperative recovery of pulmonary function. Anesth Analg 60:46, 1981

109. Alexander JI, Spence AA, Parikh RK, Stuart B: The role of airway closure in postoperative hypoxemia. Br J Anaesth 45:34, 1973

110. Duggan J, Drummond GB: Activity of lower intercostal and abdominal muscle after upper abdominal surgery. Anesth Analg 66:852, 1987

111. Dureuil B, Cantineau JP, Desmonts JM: Effects of upper or lower abdominal surgery on diaphragmatic function. Br J Anaesth 59:1230, 1987

112. Maeda J, Nakahara K, Ohno K et al: Diaphragm function after pulmonary resection: relationship to postoperative respiratory failure. Am Rev Respir Dis 137:678, 1988

113. Bromage PR, Camporesi E, Chestnut D: Epidural narcotics for postoperative analgesia. Anesth Analg 59:473, 1980

114. Keats AS, Girgis KZ: Respiratory depression associated with the relief of pain by narcotics. Anesth Analg 29:1006, 1968

115. Catley DM, Thornton C, Jordan C et al: Pronounced episodic oxygen desaturation in the postoperative period: its association with ventilatory pattern and analgesic regimen. Anesthesiology 63:20, 1985

116. Rawal N, Sjostrand U, Christoffersson E et al: Comparison of intramuscular and epidural morphine for postoperative analgesia in the grossly obese: influence on postoperative ambulation and pulmonary function. Anesth Anal 63:583, 1984

117. Spence AA, Smith G: Postoperative analgesia and lung function: a comparison of morphine with extradural block. Br J Anaesth 43:144, 1971

118. Cushieri RJ, Morran CG, Howie CJ, McArdle CS: Postoperative pain and pulmonary complications: comparison of three analgesic regimens. Br J Surg 72:495, 1985

119. Hasenbos M, Van Edmond J, Gielen M, Crul JF: Postoperative analgesia by high thoracic epidural versus intramuscular nicomorphine after thoracotomy. Acta Anaesthesiol Scand 31:608, 1987

120. Hjortso NC, Andersen T, Frosig F et al: A controlled study of the effect of epidural analgesia with local anesthetics and morphine on morbidity after abdominal surgery. Acta Anaesthesiol Scand 29:790, 1985

121. Jayr C, Mollie A, Bourgain JL et al: Postoperative pulmonary complications: general anesthesia with postoperative parenteral morphine compared with epidural analgesia. Surgery 104:57, 1988

122. Mankikian B, Cantineau JP, Bertrand M et al: Improvement of diaphragmatic function by a thoracic extradural block after upper abdominal surgery. Anesthesiology 68:379, 1988

123. Pansard JL, Mankikian B, Bertrand M et al: Effects of thoracic extradural block on diaphragmatic electrical activity and contractility after upper abdominal surgery. Anesthesiology 78:63, 1993

124. Clergue F, Montembault C, Despierre O et al: Respiratory effects of intrathecal morphine after upper abdominal surgery. Anesthesiology 61:677, 1984

125. Simonneau G, Vivien A, Sartene R et al: Diaphragm dysfunction induced by upper abdominal surgery. Am Rev Respir Dis 128:899, 1983

126. Gustafsson LL, Schildt B, Jacobsen KJ: Adverse effects of extradural and intrathecal opiates: report of a nationwide survey in Sweden. Br J Anaesth 54:479, 1982

127. Ready LB, Oden R, Chadwick HS et al: Development of an anesthesiology-based postoperative pain management service. Anesthesiology 68:100, 1988

128. Roussos C, Macklem PT: The respiratory muscles. N Engl J Med 307:786, 1982

129. Bolin RW, Pierson DJ: Ventilatory management in acute lung injury. Crit Care Clin 2:585, 1986

130. Eissa N, Ranieri M, Corbeil C et al: The effects of inflation volume on the elastic properties of the total respiratory system and the risk of pulmonary barotrauma in ARDS patients. Intens Care Med 16:S39, 1990

131. Nelson LD, Civetta JM, Hudson-Civetta J: Titrating positive-end-expiratory pressure therapy in patients with early, moderate arterial hypoxemia. Crit Care Med 15:14, 1987

132. Gattinoni L, Pesenti A, Bombino M et al: Relationships between lung computed tomographic density, gas exchange, and PEEP in acute respiratory failure. Anesthesiology 69:824, 1988

133. Gattinoni L, Pesenti A, Avalli L et al: Pressure-volume curve of total respiratory system in acute respiratory failure. Am Rev Respir Dis 136:730, 1987

134. Webb H, Tierney D: Experimental pulmonary edema due to intermittent positive pressure ventilation with high inflation pressures: protection by positive end-expiratory pressure. Am Rev Respir Dis 110:556, 1974

135. Dreyfuss D, Basset G, Soler P, Saumon G: Intermittent positive-pressure hyperventilation with high inflation pressure produces pulmonary microvascular injury in rats. Am Rev Respir Dis 132:880, 1985

136. Dreyfuss D, Soler P, Basset G, Saumon G: High inflation pressure pulmonary edema: respective effects of high airway pressure, high tidal volume, and positive end-expiratory pressure. Am Rev Respir Dis 137:1159, 1988

137. Corbridge TC, Wood LDH, Crawford GP et al: Adverse effects of large tidal volume and low PEEP in

canine acid aspiration. Am Rev Respir Dis 142:311, 1990

138. Marini JJ: New options for the ventilatory management of acute lung injury. New Horizons 1:489, 1993

139. Tsuno K, Prato, Kolobow T: Acute lung injury from mechanical ventilation at moderately high airway pressures. J Appl Physiol 69:956, 1990

140. Darioli R, Perret C: Mechanical controlled hypoventilation in status asthmaticus. Am Rev Respir Dis 129:385, 1984

141. Hickling KG, Henderson SJ, Jackson, R: Low mortality associated with low volume pressure limited ventilation with permissive hypercapnia in severe adult respiratory distress syndrome. Intens Care Med 16:372, 1990

142. Slutsky AS: Mechanical ventilation. Chest 104:1833, 1993

143. Suter PM, Fairley HB, Isenberg MD: Effect of tidal volume and PEEP on compliance during mechanical ventilation. Chest 73:158, 1978

144. Suter PM, Fairley HB, Isenberg MD: Optimum end-expiratory airway pressure in patients with acute pulmonary failure. N Engl J Med 292:284, 1975

145. Marini JJ, Truwit J: Monitoring the respiratory system. p 197. In Hall JB, Schmidt GA, Wood LDH (eds): Principles of Critical Care. McGraw-Hill, New York, 1992.

146. Benito S, Lemaire F: Pulmonary pressure-volume relationships in acute respiratory distress syndrome in adults: role of positive end-expiratory pressure. J Crit Care 5:27, 1990

147. Katz JA, Ozanne GM, Zinn SE, Fairley HB: Time course and mechanisms of lung-volume increase with PEEP in acute pulmonary failure. Anesthesiology 54:9, 1981

148. Ranieri VM, Eissa NT, Corbeil C et al: Effects of positive end-expiratory pressure on alveolar recruitment and gas exchange in patients with the adult respiratory distress syndrome. Am Rev Respir Dis 144:544, 1991

149. Putensen C, Baum M, Hörmann C: Selecting ventilator settings according to variables derived from the quasi-static pressure/volume relationships in patients with acute lung injury. Anesth Analg 77:436, 1993

150. Marcy TW, Marini JJ: Inverse ratio ventilation in ARDS: rationale and implementation. Chest 100:495, 1991

151. Gross D, Grassino A, Ross WRD, Macklem PT: Electromyogram pattern of diaphragmatic fatigue. J Appl Physiol 46:1, 1979

152. MacIntyre NR: Respiratory monitoring without machinery. Respir Care 35:546, 1990

153. Ward ME, Corbeil C, Gibbons W et al: Optimiza-

tion of respiratory muscle relaxation during mechanical ventilation. Anesthesiology 69:29, 1988

154. Field S, Sanci, Grassino A: Respiratory muscle oxygen consumption estimated by diaphragm pressure-time index. J Appl Physiol 57:44, 1984

155. Marini JJ, Rodriguez RM, Lamb V: The inspiratory workload of patient initiated mechanical ventilation. Am Rev Respir Dis 134:902, 1986

156. Dennison FH, Taft AA, Mishoe SC et al: Analysis of resistance to gas flow in nine adult ventilator circuits. Chest 96:1374, 1989

157. Cox D, Niblett DJ: Studies on continuous positive airway pressure breathing systems. Br J Anaesth 56:905, 1984

158. Fleury B, Murciano D, Talamo C et al: Work of breathing in patients with chronic obstructive pulmonary disease in acute respiratory failure. Am Rev Respir Dis 131:822, 1985

159. Roussos CS, Fixley MS, Gross D, Macklem PT: Respiratory muscle fatigue in man at FRC and higher lung volumes. Physiologist 19:345, 1976

160. Katz JA, Marks JD: Inspiratory work with and without continuous positive airway pressure in patients with acute respiratory failure. Anesthesiology 63:598, 1985

161. Katz JA, Kraemer RW, Gjerde GE: Inspiratory work and airway pressure with continuous positive airway pressure delivery systems. Chest 88:519, 1985

162. Banner MJ, Blanch PB, Kirby RR: Imposed work of breathing and methods of triggering a demand-flow, continuous positive airway pressure system. Crit Care Med 21:183, 1993

163. Beydon L, Chasse M, Harf A, Lemaire F: Inspiratory work of breathing during spontaneous ventilation using demand valves and continuous flow systems. Am Rev Respir Dis 138:300, 1988

164. McGregor M, Becklake M: The relationship of oxygen cost of breathing to respiratory mechanical work and respiratory force. J Clin Invest 40:971, 1961

165. MacIntyre NR: Respiratory function during pressure support ventilation. Chest 89:677, 1986

166. Brochard L, Rua F, Lorino H et al: Inspiratory pressure support compensates for the additional work of breathing caused by the endotracheal tube. Anesthesiology 75:739, 1991

167. Brochard L, Harf A, Lorino H, Lemaire F: Inspiratory pressure support prevents diaphragmatic fatigue during weaning from mechanical ventilation. Am Rev Respir Dis 139:513, 1989

168. Roussos CS, Macklem PT: Diaphragmatic fatigue in man. J Appl Physiol 43:189, 1977

169. Pourriat JL, Lamberto CH, Hoang PH et al: Diaphragmatic fatigue and breathing pattern during weaning from mechanical ventilation in COPD patients. Chest 90:703, 1986

170. Haluszka J, Chartrand DA, Grassino AE et al: Intrinsic PEEP and arterial P_{CO_2} in stable patients with chronic obstructive pulmonary disease. Am Rev Respir Dis 141:1194, 1990

171. Petrof BJ, Legare M, Goldberg P et al: Continuous positive airway pressure reduces work of breathing and dyspnea during weaning from mechanical ventilation in severe obstructive pulmonary disease. Am Rev Respir Dis 141:281, 1990

172. Brown DG, Pierson DJ: Auto-PEEP is common in mechanically ventilated patients: a study of incidence, severity, and detection. Respir Care 31:1069, 1986

173. Pepe PE, Marini JJ: Occult positive end-expiratory pressure in mechanically ventilated patients with airflow obstruction: the auto-PEEP effect. Am Rev Respir Dis 126:166, 1982

174. Rossi A, Gottfried SF, Zocchi L et al: Measurement of static compliance of the total respiratory system in patients with acute respiratory failure during mechanical ventilation: the effect of "intrinsic PEEP." Am Rev Respir Dis 131:672, 1985

175. Hoffman RA, Ershowsky P, Krieger BP: Determination of auto-PEEP during spontaneous and controlled ventilation by monitoring changes in end-expiratory thoracic gas volume. Chest 96:613, 1989

176. Smith TC, Marini JJ: Impact of PEEP on lung mechanics and work of breathing in severe airflow obstruction. J Appl Physiol 65:1488, 1988

177. Ranieri V, Giuliani R, Cinnella G et al: Physiologic effects of positive end-expiratory pressure in patients with chronic obstructive pulmonary disease during acute ventilatory failure and controlled mechanical ventilation. Am Rev Respir Dis 147:5, 1993

178. Marini J. Ventilatory management of COPD. p 495. In Cherniack N (ed): Chronic Obstructive Pulmonary Disease. WB Saunders, Philadelphia, 1991

179. Tobin MJ, Lodato RF: PEEP, auto PEEP, and waterfalls. Chest 96:449, 1989

180. Milic-Emili J: Recent advances in clinical assessment of control of breathing. Lung 160:1, 1982

181. Fernandez R, Benito S, Sanchis J: Inspiratory effort and occlusion pressure in triggered mechanical ventilation. Intens Care Med 14:650, 1988

182. Aubier M, Murciano D, Fournier M et al: Central respiratory drive in acute respiratory failure of patients with chronic obstructive pulmonary disease. Am Rev Respir Dis 122:191, 1980

183. Murciano D, Aubier M, Bussi S et al: Comparison of esophageal, tracheal, and mouth occlusion pressure in patients with chronic obstructive pulmonary disease during acute respiratory failure. Am Rev Respir Dis 128:837, 1982

184. Sassoon CSH, Te TT, Mahutte CK, Light RW: Airway occlusion pressure: an important indicator for successful weaning in patients with chronic obstructive pulmonary disease. Am Rev Respir Dis 135:107, 1987

185. Montgomery AB, Holle RHO, Neagley SR et al: Prediction of successful weaning using airway occlusion pressure and hypercapnic challenge. Chest 91:496, 1987

186. Macklem PT: Muscular weakness and respiratory function and fatigue. N Engl J Med 314:775, 1986

187. Feeley TW, Hedley-Whyte J: Weaning from controlled mechanical ventilation and supplemental oxygen. N Engl J Med 292:903, 1975

188. Tahvanainen J, Salmenperä M, Nikki P: Extubation criteria after weaning from intermittent mandatory ventilation and continuous positive airway pressure. Crit Care Med 11:702, 1983

189. Derenne JPH, Macklem PT, Roussos C: State of the art: the respiratory muscles: mechanics, control, and pathophysiology. Am Rev Respir Dis 118:113 (part I); 373 (part II); 581 (part III), 1978

190. Marini, JJ: Smith TC, Lamb V: Estimation of inspiratory muscle strength in mechanically ventilated patients: the measurement of maximal inspiratory pressure. J Crit Care 1:32, 1986

191. Westcott DA, Bendixen HH: Neostigmine as a curare antagonist: a clinical study. Anesthesiology 23:324, 1962

192. Sahn SA, Lakshminarayan S: Bedside criteria for discontinuation of mechanical ventilation. Chest 63:1002, 1973

193. DeHaven CB, Hurst JM, Branson RD: Evaluation of two different extubation criteria: attributes contributing to success. Crit Care Med 14:92, 1986

194. Krieger BP, Ershowsky PF, Becker DA, Gazeroglu HB: Evaluation of conventional criteria for predicting successful weaning from mechanical ventilatory support in elderly patients. Crit Care Med 17:858, 1989

195. Yang KL, Tobin MJ: A prospective study of indexes predicting the outcome of trials of weaning from mechanical ventilation. N Engl J Med 324:1445, 1991

196. Tobin MJ, Perez W, Guenther SM et al: The pattern of breathing during successful and unsuccessful trials of weaning from mechanical ventilation. Am Rev Respir Dis 134:1111, 1986

197. Pontoppidan H, Geffin B, Lowenstein E: Acute respiratory failure in surgical patients. N Engl J Med 287:690 (part I); 743 (part II); 799 (part 3), 1972

198. Tobin MJ: Respiratory monitoring in the intensive care unit. Am Rev Respir Dis 138:1625, 1988

199. Milic-Emili J: Is weaning an art of science? Am Rev Respir Dis 134:1107, 1986

Monitoring Anesthetic and Respiratory Gases

13

James H. Philip
David M. Feinstein
Daniel B. Raemer

During the past fifteen years, many technological developments have facilitated, improved, and encouraged airway gas monitoring. Practical instruments are now available that continuously monitor airway O_2, CO_2, N_2O, volatile anesthetics and sometimes N_2. This chapter presents the various methods used to measure these gases and vapors. The principles of operation are described, as well as the implementations available in commercial devices. Important clinical issues regarding proper use and misuse of these devices are also presented. An indepth discussion of clinical aspects of inhalation anesthetic monitoring is not presented here but can be found elsewhere.[1]

SPECTROSCOPY

Infrared Spectroscopy

Absorption

Many substances, including several of the respiratory and anesthetic gases, absorb infrared energy. Infrared absorption at a particular wavelength is characteristic of a polyatomic molecule's interatomic bond energy, degrees of freedom, and dipole moment.[2,3] Strong infrared absorption occurs when a molecule's atoms rotate or vibrate asymmetrically, resulting in a change in dipole moment. Among the respiratory gases and anesthetics, CO_2, N_2O, H_2O, and the fluorinated hydrocarbons exhibit strong absorption peaks throughout the infrared spectrum; the nonpolar molecules Ar, N_2, and O_2 do not. Figure 13-1 shows the infrared spectrum with gas absorption bands identified.

Measuring the energy absorbed from a single wavelength infrared light beam passing through a gas is termed *nondispersive infrared spectroscopy* (NDIR spectroscopy). The relationship between light energy absorbed and other factors was originally stated by Bouguer, rediscovered by Lambert and refined by Beer.[3] These laws are usually lumped together and termed the Lambert-Beer or Beer-Lambert law, expressed mathematically as

$$A_a = 1 - e^{-aDC} \qquad (13\text{-}1)$$

where A_a is the fraction of incoming energy which is absorbed, a is the absorption coefficient characteristic of the particular gas species, D is the distance the beam travels through the gas, C is the molar gas concentration, and e is the base of natural logarithms. Equation 13-1 can be solved for concentration if the other variables are known. In commercial instruments, the energy fraction absorbed is measured and the path length (D) and absorption coefficient of the gas (a) are known. Thus, concentration is calculated by substituting values into transposed Equation 13-1, as follows:

$$C = \frac{-\ln\,(1 - A_a)}{aD} \qquad (13\text{-}2)$$

There are wavelengths in the infrared region of the spectrum where each of the respiratory and

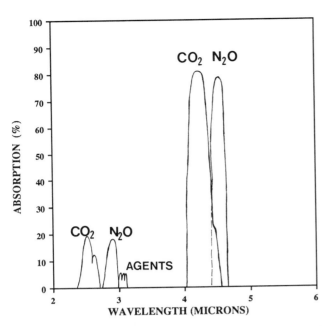

Fig. 13-1. The infrared spectrum for the respiratory and anesthetic gases and agents measurable with clinical devices.

anesthetic gases exhibit unique absorption. Unfortunately, some of these bands are quite near each other (Fig. 13-1). For example, CO_2 absorbs strongly between 4.2 and 4.4 μm, while N_2O absorbs strongly between 4.4 and 4.6 μm. At the 4.4-μm edges of both absorption bands, CO_2 and N_2O overlap slightly. Consequently, practical CO_2 analyzers can exhibit inaccuracy in the presence of high concentrations of N_2O.[4] Many commercial instruments measure N_2O to correct the CO_2 reading for this cross-sensitivity.

A separate phenomenon, termed *collision broadening*, causes additional inaccuracy in an infrared analyzer. Molecules in the gas mixture being analyzed are constantly colliding with each other, exchanging energy with each collision. Depending on the size and dipole moments of the gas molecules, these energy exchanges add energy to or remove it from the gas being measured. As a result, the infrared absorption band is broadened, and the apparent absorption at the measurement wavelength is altered.[5] Notably, O_2 and N_2O cause collision broadening when CO_2 is measured. In a typical nondispersive infrared CO_2 analyzer, this effect will result in inaccuracies of about 0.01 percent CO_2 per percent N_2O and -0.005 percent CO_2 per per-

cent O_2.[5,5a] By measuring or estimating concentrations of interfering gases, CO_2 readings are corrected automatically.

All the anesthetic vapors absorb strongly near 3.6 μm, and many infrared anesthetic analyzers measure at this wavelength. Because the absorption signatures for halothane, enflurane, isoflurane, desflurane, and sevoflurane are indistinct at this wavelength, these analyzers cannot distinguish among the various anesthetics. To achieve agent identification, analysis at multiple wavelengths is performed, and the relative absorptions at the various wavelengths allow identification. Absorption at longer wavelengths—in the range of 9 to 12 μm—also occurs, and some analyzers use these wavelengths.

Infrared Analyzers

Clinical infrared analyzers are available to measure CO_2, N_2O, and the anesthetic vapors halothane, enflurane, isoflurane, desflurane, and sevoflurane. Figure 13-2 shows a block diagram of an infrared analyzer. The nondispersive infrared analyzer consists of five systems: light source, optical path, signal detector, signal processor, and gas sampler.

Light Sources

Light sources that emit particular wavelengths of infrared light (corresponding to specific gases) are not readily available. Consequently, respiratory gas analyzers use sources that emit a range of light wavelengths. Tungsten wires and ceramic resistive materials heated to 1,500 to 4,000 K emit energy in the proper range.

Signal Paths and Compensation

The energy output of infrared light sources tends to vary over time and from device to device. For this reason, optical paths have been designed to compensate for these fluctuations. There are three common designs in commercial use. They are distinguished in their use of single and dual infrared beams and by their use of positive or negative filtering.

Single-Beam Positive Filter. Precision optical band-pass filters mounted on a spinning wheel (40–250 rpm) sequentially interrupt a single infrared beam. The beam retains energy at a narrow band of wavelengths during each interruption. For each gas of interest, a pair of band-pass filters are selected at

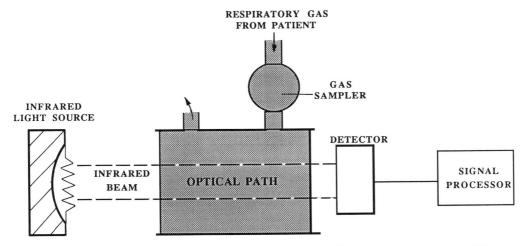

Fig. 13-2. Block diagram of the nondispersive infrared analyzer. The instrument consists of five systems: infrared light source, optical path, detector, signal processor, and gas sampler.

an absorption peak and at a reference wavelength where relatively little absorption occurs. The chopped infrared beam then passes through a cuvette containing the sample gas. The ratio of infrared beam intensity for each pair of filters is proportional to the gas partial pressure and is insensitive to changes in infrared source intensity.

Another single-beam positive filter design uses stationary optical filters instead of a spinning filter wheel. The pairs of filters are mounted close together within the circumference of the infrared beam. A separate infrared detector for each filter is used to measure the infrared intensity. As before, the ratio of intensity at the absorption peak and reference wavelength is used to calculate the partial pressure of each gas in the sample.

Single-Beam Negative Filter Design. In this design, the filters are usually sealed gas-filled cells mounted in a spinning wheel. During each interruption, the infrared beam retains energy at all wavelengths except those absorbed by the gas. For each gas of interest, a cell with a high percentage of that gas and one with a nonabsorbing reference gas are used. The chopped infrared beam then passes through a cuvette containing the sample gas. Analogous to the positive filter design described above, the ratio of infrared beam intensity for each pair of filter cells is proportional to the gas partial pressure and is insensitive to changes in the infrared source intensity.

Dual-Beam Positive Filter Design. The infrared energy from the source is split into two parallel beams. One beam passes through the sample gas, and the other passes through a reference gas. A spinning blade passes through the beams and sequentially interrupts one, the other, and both. The two beams are optically focused to a single point where a band-pass optical filter selected at the absorption peak of the gas of interest is mounted over a single detector. As before, the ratio of the intensity of the sample and reference beams are proportional to the partial pressure of the gas.

Photoacoustic Design. A variation of the single-beam positive filter method is the photoacoustic spectrometer depicted in Figure 13-3. Here the infrared energy is passed through optical filters that select the narrow-wavelength absorption bands. Evenly spaced windows are located circumferentially on a rotating wheel. As the wheel spins, the sample gas is exposed to the pulses of energy at the prescribed wavelength at a frequency depending on the rotation rate of the wheel. The sample gas absorbs the pulsating infrared energy and expands and contracts at those frequencies. The expanding and contracting gas results in sound waves that are detected with a microphone and separated into components by electronic band pass filters. Gases are separated relatively easily because the number of windows on the spinning wheel for each different substance are prime relative to each other. That

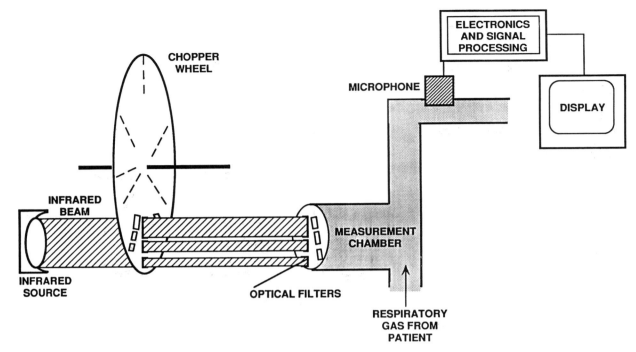

Fig. 13-3. Schematic diagram of a photoacoustic spectrometer. An infrared source emits a beam that passes through a spinning "chopper wheel" having several rows of circumferential slots. The interrupted infrared beams then pass through optical filters that select specific wavelengths of light chosen to be at the absorption peaks of the gases to be measured. Each interrupted infrared light impinges on its respective gas in the measurement chamber causing vibration of the gas as energy is absorbed and released from the molecules. The vibration frequency of each gas is dependent on the spacing of its slots on the chopper wheel. A microphone converts the gas vibration frequencies into a electrical signals that are converted to the gas concentrations for display. (From Raemer,[32] with permission.)

is, their frequencies have no common divisors and thus their frequencies have no common components, even in their harmonic overtones.

Signal Detector

The most commonly used detectors for infrared energy are made of radiation-sensitive solid-state material, usually lead selenide. Over the spectral range of interest, lead selenide changes its electrical conductivity in proportion to the number of impinging infrared photons. Unfortunately, this material also changes its electrical conductivity as a function of temperature, which must be compensated.[3]

Another type of detector, called the *Luft cell,* functions by measuring heat absorbed in a CO_2-filled chamber. An infrared-transparent window serves as one wall of the chamber and a flexible membrane serves as another. Radiation penetrates

the window and heats and expands the CO_2 gas as it is absorbed. The flexible wall of the chamber moves correspondingly against a transducer, which converts the motion to an electrical signal.[6]

Still another detector is the thermopile, consisting of a series of thermocouples or bimetallic thermometers. The thermopile is bonded to an infrared-absorbing substrate, which heats up when struck by radiation. The increase in temperature causes an increase in the electrical voltage produced by the thermopile.[7]

Signal Processor

No matter which detector is chosen, the signal processor converts the measured electrical currents into a signal related to gas partial pressure. First, the ratio of detector currents at various points in the spinning wheel's progress (or from multiple detectors) are computed. Next, scaling corrects for gain and offset errors in the measurement process. Then, filtering is sometimes applied to eliminate electronic noise. Finally, the curvilinear relationship between the absorbed energy and gas concentration (predicted by the Lambert-Beer Law; see equation 13-2) is transformed to a linear relationship. This linearization is usually achieved in a microprocessor programmed with a "look-up" table, which contains the point-by-point conversion from electrical voltage to gas partial pressure. Any cross-sensitivities or known interferences between gases are compensated by the microprocessor after linearization.

Gas Sampler

Respiratory gas monitoring instruments are classified as either mainstream or sidestream, according to how they obtain the gas sample measured. In mainstream instruments, the patient's respiratory gas stream passes through a wide-bore chamber (cuvette) in the airway. There are infrared-transparent (sapphire) windows in two opposing walls of the cuvette. A miniature nondispersive infrared optical system placed over the chamber measures gas partial pressure. To ensure that water vapor does not condense on the windows and obstruct the optical path, the cuvette is heated to slightly above body temperature.

Advantages of the mainstream systems include ease of attachment, simplicity of use, and lack of waste gas to be disposed. Disadvantages include difficulty with face mask use (secondary to size and weight) as well as noise, vibration, and potential for mechanical damage.

Sidestream instruments continuously withdraw a small sample of gas from the airway. Lightweight tubing is attached to the breathing circuit near the airway. A small vacuum pump draws gas from the breathing circuit into the instrument where the sample enters the measurement cuvette. Sample flow rate is usually controlled at a fixed flow between 50 and 300 ml/min. After analysis, gas is expelled through a port and can either be returned to the breathing circuit (and patient) or disposed through the scavenging system.

Sampled gas always contains water vapor from the breathing circuit. Sidestream systems sometimes have difficulty with condensation since fully saturated exhaled gas travels down room-temperature tubing where condensation occurs. Condensed wa-

ter within the sample cuvette can interfere with the transmission of the infrared beam. Water vapor may be eliminated by interposing a length of Naphion tubing, a unique semipermeable polymer that selectively allows water vapor to pass from its interior to the dry exterior.[8]

Sampling systems must be protected from liquid water and body fluids. A mechanical water trap is usually interposed between the patient sample line and the analyzer. Intricate designs prevent gas mixing in this chamber, thus averting slurring of the respiratory waveforms.[9]

One advantage of the sidestream system is that the sample tube does not encumber the breathing circuit. Also, the fragile optical components are housed safely within the instrument. The disadvantages of these systems are a slightly slower response speed, required water trap, and removal of sampled gas from the breathing circuit. If sampled gas is returned to the breathing circuit, heart and breath sounds may be obscured by motor noise.

Raman Spectroscopy

Raman Spectrum

When visible or ultraviolet light strikes gas molecules, energy is absorbed and reemitted. Most energy is reemitted at the same wavelength and direction received in a process called Raleigh scattering. About one millionth (10^{-6}) of the energy absorbed is reemitted at new wavelengths in all directions, including perpendicular to the incident beam in a phenomenon called *Raman scattering*. At room temperature, Raman scattering usually results in reemission at a longer wavelength, producing a so-called "red-shifted" spectrum. The wavelength shift and amount of scattering is proportional to the amount of gas. This is used to discriminate and measure the constituents of the gas mixture. Raman scattering is not limited to polyatomic and polar gases as is infrared absorption. O_2, N_2, H_2O, CO_2, N_2O, halothane, enflurane, isoflurane, desflurane, and sevoflurane all exhibit Raman activity and are measured in the available commercial device (RASCAL II, Ohmeda Medical Products, Louisville, CO).

Principles of Operation

The Raman spectrometer designed for use in clinical anesthesia was introduced in the late

1970s.[10] It consists of a laser light source, measurement chamber, optical detection system, and electronics system (Fig. 13-4).

The light source is an argon laser, which emits a pure beam of ultraviolet light with a wavelength of 488 nm. The laser is air-cooled and fairly rugged. The laser in the first commercial version of this product (RASCAL I) consumed 800 watts and needed replacement every 12 to 18 months. The laser in the current version (RASCAL 2) consumes only 15 watts and is rated to last over 10,000 hours. The manufacturer calculates that this works out to 4.8 years if used 5 days per week, 52 weeks per year.

In the instrument, the sampled gas enters the measurement chamber where the focused ultraviolet laser beam strikes the gas molecules. The measurement chamber is actually the resonator chamber for the laser where the beam may strike the gas molecules many times. Raman-scattered light (at various wavelengths) is detected perpendicular to the laser beam axis by sensitive photomultiplier tubes after passing through narrow-band optical filters.

The electric currents from the detectors are used to compute the gas constituent partial pressures. When Raman scattering wavelengths are close together, several weaker Raman wavelengths are used to discriminate among gases. Computer algorithms are used to extract and compute the correct values.

The accuracy of the Raman spectrometer has been shown to be equal to or better than the mass spectrometer for measuring anesthetic and respiratory gases.[11]

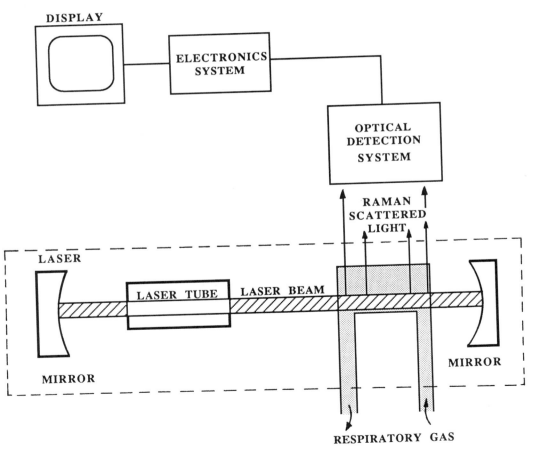

Fig. 13-4. Block diagram of the Raman spectrometer. The instrument consists of a laser system, a measurement chamber, an optical detection system, an electronics system, and a display.

Mass Spectroscopy

Mass and Charge Spectrum

A mass spectrometer measures gas sampled from the breathing circuit. Electrons bombard the gas mixture and ionize gas molecules into fragments of predictable mass and charge. The charged particles are accelerated electrically and deflected magnetically, causing them to be collected and counted at unique locations.

Principles of Operation

There are two types of mass spectrometers: magnetic sector and quadrapole; most mass spectrometers for medical use are the former.

Figure 13-5 shows a block diagram of a magnetic sector mass spectrometer. The measurement chamber is maintained at a pressure of about 10^{-5} mmHg. This low pressure is achieved with a vacuum pump plus an additional device to remove residual ions, either an oil diffusion pump using a jet of oil or noble metal plates (termed simply an ion pump).

An extremely small fraction of the gas sampled from the patient is analyzed in the mass spectrometer. This small quantity of sample gas enters the measurement chamber through a tiny "molecular leak," comprised of either a fine needle valve, a sintered metal filter, a vibrating crystal, or other device. Electrons bombard the gas mixture and ionize gas molecules into fragments of predictable mass and charge. The charged particles are accelerated by an electric field and deflected by a magnetic field to land in ion-specific metal collectors. The heaviest and least charged ions have the shortest trajectories. Each ion produces a tiny electrical current, which is amplified and scaled to represent fractional gas composition. The number and location of the plates determines the gas species the mass spectrometer can measure. The fluorinated volatile anesthetics except desflurane may all be measured at mass 67. The ratio of mass 67 to mass 51 is used to identify the particular agent. Desflurane is measured at mass 101. For dry inspired gas the total count is assumed to represent all gases present.

The composition displayed equals the fractional percentage of counts. Exhaled gas is assumed to have been fully saturated with water vapor (partial pressure of 47 mmHg) at body temperature and to have lost all water vapor before entering the analyzer which has no collector for water. All measured gases are summed to prevailing atmospheric pressure less 47 mmHg. Software in the instrument assesses inspiration and expiration based upon timing of CO_2 (maximally present on expiration).

Clinical mass spectrometers monitor either a single patient (stand-alone) or several patients sequentially (shared or multiplexed). In the stand-alone system, the analysis takes place in the individual operating room and is displayed there.

Shared-systems take two forms. In the first, a

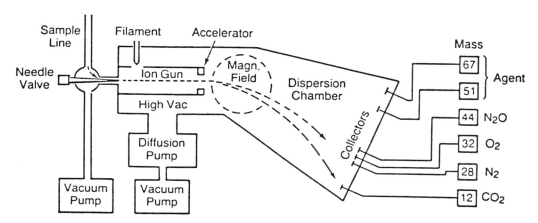

Fig. 13-5. Block diagram of a magnetic sector mass spectrometer. Respiratory gas is sampled and a small fraction is introduced into the high vacuum of the mass spectrometer chamber. The gas is ionized and accelerated in an electric field. The ions are deflected by a magnetic field in the dispersion chamber where they impact appropriately placed fixed metal plate collectors. The ion impacts are counted as a measurement of gas composition.

large vacuum pump draws gas simultaneously from all attached operating rooms through individual lengths of nylon tubing (~50 m) at a rate of about 250 ml/min. A rotary multiplexer valve sequentially directs gas samples to the mass spectrometer through which a second vacuum pump draws the sampled gas for analysis.

In the second method,[12] gas is continuously sampled from all patient locations at 90 ml/min to a waste line; each sample line contains about 20 seconds of inspired and expired gas. Solenoid valves sequentially switch each sample line to the inlet manifold of the mass spectrometer which is maintained at a substantially lower pressure. The gas from the sample line is drawn into the evacuated inlet manifold at twice the original sampling rate and data is displayed at half-speed to recreate the proper gas profile. Less time per patient location is required with this method and there appears to be little waveform degradation.

Up to 31 patients may be connected to a multiplexed system. One and a half to 2 breaths are usu-

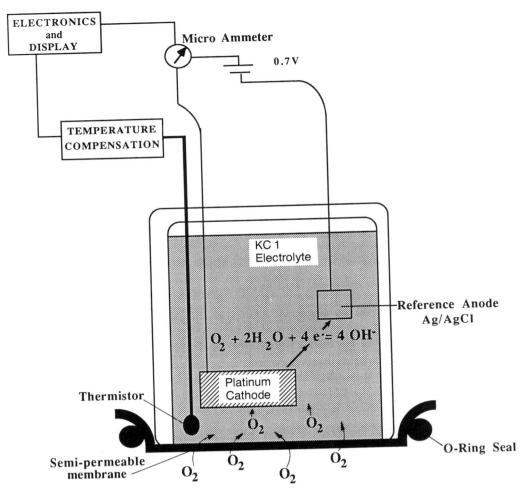

Fig. 13-6. A schematic of a polarographic O_2 sensor. The sensor consists of an O_2-permeable semipermeable membrane, platinum cathode, reference anode, electrolyte, polarizing voltage source (~0.7 V), a microammeter, and electronics and display system. Oxygen molecules diffuse across the semipermeable membrane where they are reduced at the polarized cathode according to equation 13-3. The electric current is proportional to the oxygen pressure at the membrane. Temperature compensation is usually required for accurate measurement.

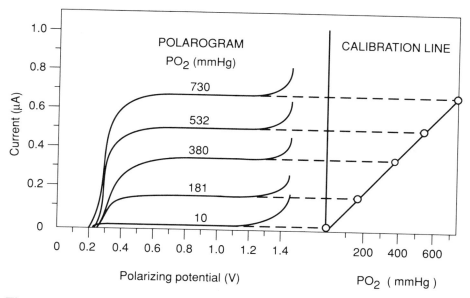

Fig. 13-7. The relationship between polarizing potential and current for different oxygen partial pressures. Within the operational range of polarization potential, the current resulting from oxygen reduction is almost linear with the supply of O_2 molecules at the electrode surface.

ally required to detect a breath and analyze it. In a typical 16-station system with breathing rates of 10 per minute, each patient is monitored every 3 minutes. If 31 patients are ventilated 6 times per minute the sampling interval is 10 minutes.

Since long sample intervals occur with multiplexed systems, continuous infrared CO_2 monitoring at each patient station has been added to each of the two commercial multiplexed mass spectrometer systems: SARACap for the SARA and Lifewatch for the Marquette Advantage system. Each system allows a user to request a STAT measurement that interrupts normal sequencing briefly.

ELECTROCHEMISTRY

Electrochemical Oxygen Sensors

In an electrochemical oxygen sensor, oxygen is chemically reduced in a liquid solution by an electric potential at a metal surface, following the electrochemical reaction:

$$O_2 + 2H_2O + 4e^- = 4OH^-. \qquad (13-3)$$

A fixed number of electrons are consumed for each O_2 molecule reduced, and the electric current produced measures the O_2 in solution. The electric

potential that drives this reaction to the right can be externally applied or can be provided by another chemical reaction within the sensor. The polarographic O_2 sensor uses an externally applied voltage, while the galvanic cell uses an internal chemical reaction.[13]

Both polarographic and galvanic O_2 sensors are available to monitor O_2 concentration in the breathing circuit. Performance of commercial O_2 sensors depends less on sensor technology choice than on ability of the sensor membrane to exclude water.[14]

Polarographic Oxygen Sensors
Principles of Operation

Polarographic O_2 sensors consist of metal electrodes, an electrolyte, a voltage source, an oxygen-permeable semipermeable membrane, and a means to measure electric current (Fig. 13-6). The cathode is made from a noble metal (platinum, gold, or silver) so chosen to reduce the interference from impurity reduction reactions. The anode is made of silver and silver chloride. The electric potential between anode and cathode is usually derived from a battery and controlled to about 0.7 V. At this polarization potential, the current resulting from oxygen reduction is almost linear with the supply of O_2 molecules at the electrode surface (Fig. 13-7). An electrolyte of KOH or KCl is provided as a viscous liquid or gel to transport the electrons between the cathode and anode. A Teflon or polyethylene membrane covers the sensor surface and serves as a diffusion barrier for other molecules, such as halothane, which would otherwise interfere with the sensor. The diffusion of oxygen through the membrane is the major limitation for the supply of O_2 at the cathode and, in turn, determines the current available for the reduction reaction. The diffusion of O_2 through the membrane is a function of the partial pressure of O_2 at its outer surface. Thus, the electric current at the cathode is related to the PO_2 of the gas outside the sensor. The diffusion of O_2 through the membrane is temperature-dependent, and a thermistor is used to compensate for this effect.

Galvanic Oxygen Sensors

Galvanic O_2 sensors are similar to polarographic sensors in that O_2 reduction occurs at the cathode. However, in this sensor the electric potential to reduce the O_2 is provided by an internal chemical reaction rather than an external battery. Usually this reaction is the oxidation of lead. The overall reaction that results between a silver cathode and a lead anode is

$$O_2 + 2Pb + 2OH^- = 2PbO_2H^-. \quad (13\text{-}4)$$

As with polarographic sensors, current used to drive the reaction to the right is related to the PO_2 of the gas outside the membrane.

OTHER TECHNOLOGIES

Paramagnetism

Oxygen possesses two unpaired electrons in its outer shell orbit and thereby exhibits relatively strong paramagnetism. Measurement of oxygen concentration using this property was described by Pauling[15] in 1946. Recently, a practical rapid-response oxygen analyzer for anesthesia has been developed (Instrumentarium Oy, Helsinki, Finland). The patient's respiratory gas and reference air continuously flow through rigid sample lines into a magnetic field produced by an electromagnet. The electromagnet is switched on and off at about 100 Hz. The paramagnetic property of oxygen causes the switched magnetic field to produce a changing pressure in each of the sample lines. The pressure pulsations in the sample lines are detected synchronously with the electromagnet switching and measured differentially, producing a signal related to oxygen partial pressure.

Piezoelectric Adsorption

Cooper and colleagues[16] simultaneously but independently with Engstrom Co. (Stockholm, Sweden) developed an anesthetic agent analyzer using a quartz piezoelectric crystal. The crystal vibrates at a particular frequency when stimulated with an electrical voltage. One surface of the piezoelectric crystal is coated with a lipid substance that reversibly adsorbs anesthetic gas molecules, which increases crystal weight and slows oscillation.

The major difficulty with the piezoelectric analyzer is its sensitivity to water vapor, which is also adsorbed to the coating, resulting in an elevated reading. This problem can be reduced by zero-calibrating the device in a warm humidified atmosphere before any agent is introduced.[17]

CLINICAL CONSIDERATIONS

Barometric Pressure Effects

Most of the gas analysis techniques described measure gas partial pressure.[18] Partial pressure is the force exerted by the actual number of gas molecules per unit volume. This is also the variable that affects the patient's physiology.[19]

Although partial pressure is usually the variable actually measured, historically, gas composition measurements in anesthesia are expressed in percent,[20] usually thought of as *concentration*. For example, most clinical polarographic oxygen analyzers measure PO_2 but display percent O_2 on their meters. A measurement of oxygen in air in Boston (sea level) is $PO_2 = 0.21 \times 760$ mmHg $= 160$ mmHg. In Denver where the atmospheric pressure is 620 mmHg, $PO_2 = 0.21 \times 620$ mmHg $= 130$ mmHg, or 0.82 times that at sea level.

A polarographic oxygen analyzer in Boston measures a 3:2 nitrous oxide:oxygen mixture (40 percent) as 0.4×760 mmHg $= 304$ mmHg and displays a concentration of 40 percent. If the analyzer is brought to Denver *without recalibration*, it will measure a 3:2 mixture as 0.4×620 mmHg $= 248$ mmHg, but will display 33 percent O_2. The diminished reading of 33 percent would correctly reflect the lower partial pressure of oxygen while seeming to contradict the 3:2 composition. Thus, routine practice dictates that the analyzer be recalibrated to read 21 percent in air in Denver. When this is done, a 3:2 nitrous oxide:oxygen mixture is measured to contain 40 percent oxygen. This 40 percent oxygen provides the same oxygen partial pressure as 33 percent O_2 provides at sea level and has the same physiologic effect. Thus, expressing readings in percent can cause significant confusion.

Partial Pressure, Concentration, and Altitude Effects

The problem of measuring partial pressure and displaying concentration arises for other gases and analyzers as well. Inhalation anesthetic potency, for example, is expressed in terms of MAC, minimum alveolar concentration [to achieve anesthetization]. If the words "at sea level" are added to this statement, *or* the word "concentration" is replaced with "partial pressure," the definition is useful at any ambient pressure. Otherwise, MAC varies with barometric pressure. To rectify the situation, we recommend interpreting anesthetic agent analyzer readings as partial pressure, expressed in percent of 1 sea level atmosphere. Then, all applications of the concept of MAC (MAP or MAPP representing minimal alveolar partial pressure or MAT representing minimal alveolar tension) are consistent and useful at any atmospheric pressure. To allow MAC to remain independent of altitude, anesthetic analyzers must be calibrated to read percent of 1 sea level atmosphere.

One exception to gas analyzers measuring partial pressure is the mass spectrometer; it measures fraction gas composition by fixing the sum of all gases measured to 100 percent.[21] This has several implications for clinical monitoring. First, the medical mass spectrometer does not measure water vapor. Inspired gas is assumed to be dry. Hence at sea level, inspired compositions are displayed as fractions of 100 percent. When sampled from the patient, expired gas is saturated with water vapor at body temperature (water vapor pressure = 47 mmHg). At sea level, some mass spectrometers display gas concentrations as fractions of 713 mmHg (760 mmHg − 47 mmHg). Hence total gas composition sums to 94 percent, the remaining 6 percent being water vapor. Other devices sum all gases

to 100 percent or to 713 mmHg, depending on the measurement units selected by the clinician.

Unexpected Gases and the Mass Spectrometer

In a mass spectrometer, if an additional unexpected gas is present, it is neither identified nor measured. This occurs with helium, for example.[22] Thus, although the *actual* concentrations of the measured gases are diluted by the unexpected gas, the measurements do not reflect this, and displayed gas concentrations are greater than the actual composition.

Sometimes, an unexpected gas may be misinterpreted as an expected gas. One notable example is Freon-13, the propellant used in many metered dose inhalers which deliver bronchodilator drugs.[23,23a] When Freon-13 is fractured by the electron beam in the mass spectrometer, the ions produced have the same mass:charge ratio as ions produced by fracturing fluorinated anesthetics. The Advantage system (Marquette Gas Systems, St. Louis, MO) interprets Freon-13 as isoflurane, while the SARA system (PPG Medical Systems, Kansas City, MO) interprets Freon-13 as enflurane. For the Advantage system, 0.8 percent Freon-13 appears as 8 percent isoflurane (J. Philip, unpublished data). In addition to the anesthetic agent reading falsely high, all other gases read slightly low because of the summing feature of the system.

Another notable example of misinterpretation is desflurane reading on a mass spectrometer not modified for its detection. The Advantage system reads a high level of enflurane, which causes an alarm at clinical levels. In addition, summing is incorrect so correct measurement requires an additional collector to be added; this can be performed by the manufacturer. No such modification is available for the SARA system.

STANDARDS FOR RESPIRATORY GAS MONITORING

Monitoring oxygen in the breathing circuit has been used routinely in most developed countries for many years. It is a mandatory requirement under the American Society of Anesthesiologists (ASA) Standards for Basic Intraoperative Monitoring.[24] In many countries, respiratory CO_2 monitoring has become routine and even mandated by law.

The ASA Standard strongly recommends its routine use and requires its use to identify correct placement of every endotracheal tube after intubation. Anesthetic agent monitoring has been recommended by some authors, especially when other than direct-reading vaporizers are used[25] (i.e., Copper Kettle or Vernitrol) or when low-flow techniques are employed. In the Federal Republic of Germany, anesthetic agent monitoring somewhere in the machine or breathing circuit is a legal requirement. Agent identification has been recommended but is not universally available. Because the agents themselves and their ions are similar, correct identification is not easy. Most devices that identify agents do so by making several independent measurements, analyzing the relative readings, and determining the agent present and its partial pressure. Some devices detect and alarm on multiple agents, while others measure each relatively independently.

CLINICAL CAPNOGRAPHY

Technology applied to respiratory gas analysis is illustrated throughout this chapter. Among the gases currently monitored, airway CO_2 measurement is fast becoming a standard of anesthesia care.

CO_2 is usually measured near the proximal end of the endotracheal tube. The temporal curve of CO_2 tension or concentration at the patient's airway is known as the capnogram. It is displayed by an instrument called a capnograph. When only numerical end-tidal P_{CO_2} (P_{ETCO_2}) is displayed, the instrument is a capnometer using the technique called capnometry.

For clinical use in safety monitoring, capnography is preferred over capnometry. The shape of the capnogram reveals much about the integrity of the breathing circuit and the status of the patient's cardiopulmonary system.[26]

Normal Capnogram

The characteristic features of a normal capnogram are shown in Figure 13-8.

At the end of normal inhalation, the CO_2 tension in perfused alveoli is in equilibrium with and equal to that in end-capillary blood while a small volume of gas in unperfused alveoli is in equilibrium with inspired gas, assumed zero. At the airway and down to some point proximal to the alveoli, CO_2 is zero (inspired gas). At the start of exhalation (point A) the airway gas sampled is the CO_2-free anatomic dead space so measured CO_2 remains zero. (segment A-B). As exhalation continues, CO_2-containing gas from the respiratory tree enters the trachea and displaces dead-space gas. CO_2 arrives at the airway and first appears on the capnograph at point B, from which it rises. In the normal capnogram, this rise in CO_2 produces a sharp and smooth upstroke (segment B-C). Then, the minimally changing CO_2 concentration over time produces a nearly horizontal alveolar plateau (segment C-D). Near the end of the exhalation when expiratory flow rate approaches zero, the end tidal CO_2 measured approaches the ventilation-weighted average of ventilated lung units. The highest value is end-tidal CO_2 (point D). End-tidal CO_2 approximates alveolar CO_2. This value is often taken as an estimate of arterial P_{CO_2}, neglecting gas exhaled from nonperfused alveoli which reduce the CO_2 measured.[27] As the patient next inhales, airway CO_2 again falls to zero (point E) unless there is CO_2 in inspired gas.

Capnogram Display

The capnogram may be displayed as a normal wave, low-speed wave, or trend. Some monitors show two or more of these simultaneously. Low-speed wave and trend displays obscure details of individual breaths but highlight evolving events. Each breath should rise to the same end-tidal value and fall to the zero baseline. Alterations of the trend and changes in fine detail of the capnogram wave indicate abnormal patient physiology or a malfunctioning gas delivery system.

Differential Diagnosis of Abnormal Capnograms

Because the essence of pulmonary ventilation and gas exchange is elimination of CO_2 from the lung, the capnogram is the single most reliable and effective monitor for the presence of pulmonary ventilation and gas exchange. The integrity and function of both the patient's cardiopulmonary system and the breathing circuit are reflected by the capnogram,[28] and malfunctions often can be detected by changes in it.[29] The following discussion focuses on major categories of capnographic abnormality and presents a brief discussion of the malfunctions that might lead to them.

Decrease in Partial Pressure of End-Tidal Carbon Dioxide

Sudden Decrease to Near-Zero Concentration

A sudden drop of end-tidal CO_2 (Fig. 13-9) to zero or near-zero usually heralds imminent disaster. The possibility of capnograph malfunction must be considered but never assumed. Critical events that may present this way include esophageal intubation,[30] complete airway disconnection, complete ventilator malfunction, and totally obstructed endotracheal tube.[31] Each of these events results in the sudden disappearance of CO_2 at the patient's airway, and nothing in the capnogram distinguishes one event from another. Only after auscultating the chest and verifying pulmonary ventilation should the possibility of machine malfunction be evaluated. Even patient color and oxygen saturation will remain normal for quite sometime after the cessation of ventilation. Once a patient condition has been ruled out as the source of the flat capnogram, capnograph malfunction and sampling system blockage can be considered. Because potentially fatal airway disasters may occur at any time without warning, continuous capnography during anesthesia is needed to provide early detection of problems to avoid catastrophic events.

Sudden Decrease to Low but Nonzero Concentration

Figure 13-10 demonstrates a fall in $PETCO_2$ to values approaching but not reaching zero, indicating that a full exhalation is no longer being detected at the airway. Exhaled gas may be escaping through a poorly fitting mask. If an endotracheal tube is in place, a loosely fitting tracheal tube, or a leaking or defective endotracheal tube cuff should be considered. Mainstream capnography systems may have a partially displaced transducer producing a similar capnogram.

Examination of the airway pressure may be helpful in diagnosing the etiology of a sudden drop in $PETCO_2$. If the airway pressure is low during mechanical ventilation, there is probably a leak somewhere in the delivery system. If the airway pressure is high during mechanical ventilation, there is

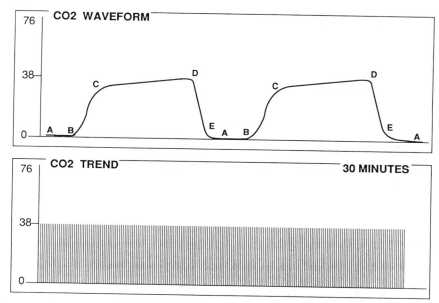

Fig. 13-8. The normal capnogram is shown in the top panel. Exhalation begins at point *A*. Segment *A–B* represents tracheal dead space Segment *B–C* is the early rise in CO_2 concentration as alveolar gas makes its way to the airway. Segment *C–D* is the alveolar plateau. Point *D*, the maximum value in the capnogram, is the end-tidal value of CO_2. Inhalation of CO_2 tree gas begins immediately after point *D* and continues to point *E*. Shown on the bottom panel is the trend display.

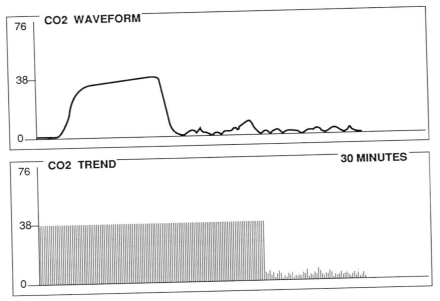

Fig. 13-9. Sudden decrease of $P_{ET}CO_2$ to near-zero values. The trend display demonstrates the sudden occurrence of low $P_{ET}CO_2$ values after a period of normal $P_{ET}CO_2$. The real-time capnogram is disrupted, showing the lack of proper sampling of CO_2 in the airway. Critical events that may present with this pattern include esophageal intubation, complete airway disconnection, ventilator malfunction, and a totally obstructed airway.

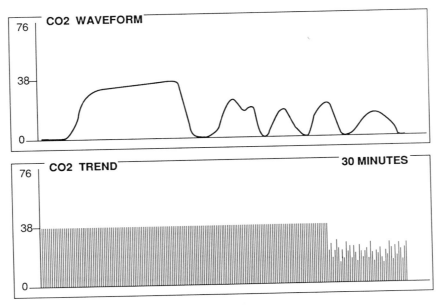

Fig. 13-10. Sudden decrease of $P_{ET}CO_2$ to low, nonzero values. Full exhalation is no longer being detected by the capnograph. A leak in the airway system or poorly fitting anesthesia mask may be the culprit. Note the disappearance of the alveolar plateau on the real-time capnogram and the irregular, nonzero value of $P_{ET}CO_2$ on the trend display.

probably a partial obstruction of the endotracheal tube resulting in lower tidal volumes delivered to the patient, high airway pressure in the circuit, and an obstruction to full emptying of alveolar gas. In this instance, the drop in PETCO$_2$ occurs because the exhalation is not completed before the next mechanical breath starts.

Exponential Decrease

An exponential drop in PETCO$_2$ that occurs within a short time (e.g., a dozen breaths) almost always signals a sudden catastrophic event in the patient's cardiopulmonary system (Fig. 13-11). The cause must be diagnosed and corrected if the patient is to survive. The physiologic basis for this capnogram is an increase in physiologic dead space ventilation or decrease in CO$_2$ returning from tissues to the lungs. Possible causative events include hypotension from blood loss or venae cavae compression, circulatory arrest, and pulmonary embolism by thrombus or air. Immediate diagnosis and treatment is required for all of these conditions. It must be remembered that air embolism can occur whenever the surgical site or an open intravenous site is at a negative circulatory pressure.

The most common noncatastrophic cause of rapid exponential PETCO$_2$ is an increase in ventilation caused by ventilator or fresh gas flow adjustment. However, this benign diagnosis should be entertained only after catastrophic events have been ruled out.

Sustained Low Concentrations

Without Good Plateaus. Occasionally, with no apparent abnormality in the breathing circuit or the patient's cardiopulmonary status, the capnogram shows sustained low PETCO$_2$ values without a good alveolar plateau (Fig. 13-12). The absence of a good alveolar plateau suggests incomplete lung emptying before the next inspiration, or that exhaled gas is diluted with fresh gas during exhalation. The latter can occur with small tidal volumes and high gas sample rate. Several maneuvers are available to differentiate these possibilities.

Incomplete lung emptying may be suggested by adventitial sounds (e.g., wheezing or large airway rhonchi) showing small airway obstruction from bronchospasm or secretions. If rhonchi are present, tracheal suctioning often corrects the partial obstruction and restores full exhalation and the CO$_2$ waveform. Bronchospasm may be treated with

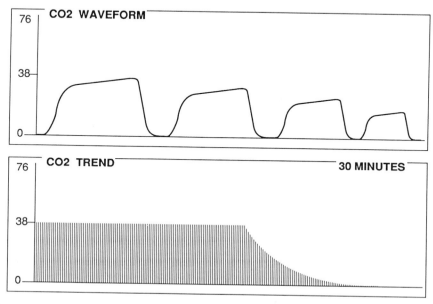

Fig. 13-11. Exponential decrease of PETCO$_2$. This pattern almost always signals a sudden and potentially catastrophic loss of pulmonary perfusion in the patient, such as that caused by a cardiopulmonary arrest or severe pulmonary hypoperfusion or embolism. Note the normal shape of the capnogram in real time but the exponential decay of the PETCO$_2$ on the trend display.

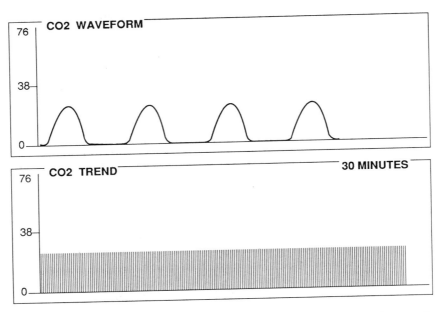

Fig. 13-12. Sustained low PETCO₂ without good plateaus. When this pattern exists on the capnogram, the PETCO₂ does not represent a good estimate of alveolar CO₂ concentration. Often, a gentle squeeze on the patient's chest will produce a full exhalation and the resulting "squeeze PETCO₂" may be used as an estimate of alveolar CO₂.

bronchodilators or halogenated anesthetic vapors. Expiratory obstruction can be caused by a tube kink or obstruction from any cause including a cuff herniating into the lumen. Passing a suction catheter down the endotracheal tube usually confirms or eliminates this possibility. If partial airway obstruction is present, squeezing the patient's chest to force deep exhalation often produces a new, higher plateau, more representative of alveolar CO₂.

After partial airway obstruction is ruled out, excess airway sampling must be considered. When small tidal volumes and large sampling flow rates are employed, sampling during the low or no flow condition at the end of exhalation entrains gas from the inspired limb of the breathing circuit, resulting in a drop-off of end-tidal CO₂. Adding dead space between sampling site and Y-connector usually restores the alveolar plateau. In small newborns, a sample rate of 50 ml/min or less may be required to eliminate this artifact.

With Good Plateaus. In some circumstance of apparently normal ventilation, the capnogram will demonstrate a low PETCO₂ with good alveolar plateau (Fig. 13-13). There may be a large discrepancy between end-tidal CO₂ and arterial PCO₂. This may

indicate capnograph malfunction or miscalibration but is most often associated with a large physiologic dead space in the patient. The anesthetist may check capnograph accuracy by breathing into the gas sampler and ensuring that the reading is between 34 and 46 mmHg. Many conditions are associated with a large arterial to end-tidal CO₂ gradient. Indeed, anesthesia itself tends to increase this gradient to an average of 4 mmHg.[32] Pulmonary disease, pneumonia, and bronchopulmonary dysplasia in children can increase the arterial to alveolar CO₂ gradient. Pulmonary artery hypoperfusion from hypovolemia and high airway pressures (e.g., sitting neurosurgical procedures with dehydration, vasodilators, and hyperventilation) commonly result in wide Pa-PETCO₂ gradients.

Gradually Decreasing Concentration

When the capnogram retains its normal morphology but PETCO₂ (Fig. 13-14) falls slowly over minutes or hours, possible causes include falling body temperature, relative hyperventilation, or decreasing systemic or pulmonary perfusion.

As body temperature falls, so does metabolism and CO₂ production. If ventilation is not de-

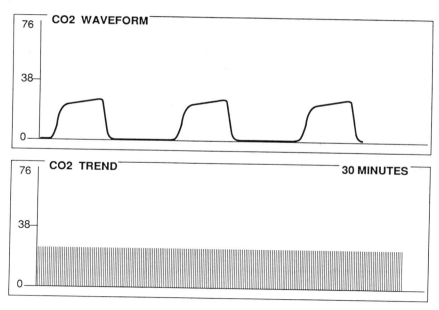

Fig. 13-13. Sustained low P_{ETCO_2} with good alveolar plateaus. This pattern suggests hyperventilation. Other possibilities include a wide $Pa-ACO_2$ in the patient due to excessive physiologic dead space ventilation. The only way to differentiate these two possibilities are to examine the true arterial PCO_2 value.

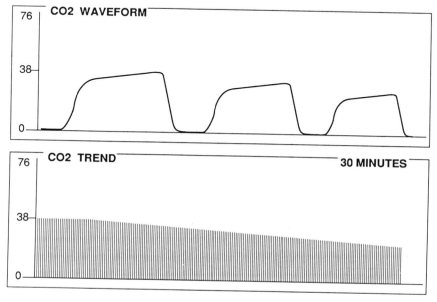

Fig. 13-14. Gradually decreasing P_{ETCO_2}. Possible causes include a falling body temperature, slowly decreasing systemic and pulmonary circulation, or hyperventilation.

creased, alveolar and arterial PCO₂ will fall. A gradual fall in PETCO₂ can arise from growing physiologic dead space from decreased CO₂ return from tissues arising from insufficient cardiac output, secondary to myocardial depression or hypovolemia.

If ventilation is increased by ventilator or fresh gas flow adjustment, PETCO₂ will gradually fall toward a new equilibrium value. This common clinical occurrence is especially obvious when a trend in minute ventilation is temporally aligned with the end-tidal CO₂ trend.

Increase in Partial Pressure of End-Tidal Carbon Dioxide

Gradual Increase in Concentration

A rise in PETCO₂ with unchanged capnogram morphology, (Fig. 13-15) may be associated with decreased minute ventilation, increased CO₂ production, or absorption of insuflating CO₂ during laparoscopy.[33]

Minute ventilation can decrease from many causes including partial airway obstruction, small leaks in the ventilator,[34] or a change in ventilator or fresh gas flow setting. CO₂ production can increase with hyperthermia of any cause, including excessive heating, sepsis, and malignant hyperthermia. When end-tidal CO₂ rises rapidly despite steady state ventilation, malignant hyperthermia must be considered immediately.[35,36]

CO₂ absorption from exogenous sources such as insufflating CO₂ during laparoscopy,[33] may mimic increased endogenous CO₂ production, causing end-tidal CO₂ to rise slowly.

Sudden Increase in Concentration

Sudden, transient increases in PETCO₂ may be caused by any factor that acutely increases the amount of CO₂ reaching the pulmonary circulation. Common causes include intravenous bicarbonate injection and release of a surgical limb tourniquet or aortic cross-clamp.

Sudden Increase in Both the Capnogram Baseline and PETCO₂ Concentration

A sudden rise in the baseline of the capnogram with an approximately equal rise in PETCO₂ value usually indicates some contamination in the sample cell (in the instrument or in the airway, depending on system employed), usually with water, mucus, or dirt. Cleaning the sample cell usually restores proper performance.

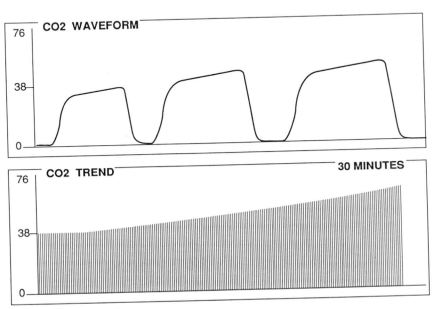

Fig. 13-15. Gradually increasing PETCO₂. This may be associated with a partial airway obstruction, a rising body temperature, or hypoventilation due to a partial leak in the breathing circuit. If the rise is rapid, malignant hyperthermia should be considered.

Gradual Increase in Both the Capnogram Baseline and
PETCO$_2$ *Concentration*

A gradual rise in both baseline and PETCO$_2$ value indicates that previously exhaled CO$_2$ is being re-breathed from the circuit (Fig. 13-16). In this situation, the inspiratory portion of the capnogram fails to reach the zero baseline, and there may actually be a premature rise in CO$_2$ concentration during the inspiratory phase of ventilation; this rise precedes the characteristic sharp upstroke associated with exhalation. The PETCO$_2$ value usually increases until a new equilibrium alveolar CO$_2$ tension is reached, at which time excretion once again equals production.

Some anesthesia circuits, such as the Mapleson D and Jackson-Rees circuits commonly used in pediatric anesthesia, are partial rebreathing circuits by design.[2,27] The user of these circuits should be aware of the characteristic capnogram that results from their use. The exact amount of rebreathing depends on complex interactions among exhaled tidal volume, fresh gas flow, expiratory reservoir volume, APL valve setting, APL valve location, and the expiratory pause time.[37] When using partial rebreathing circuits, these complex interactions make exact prediction of PETCO$_2$ and PaCO$_2$ diffi-

cult or impossible. If there is a good alveolar plateau on the capnogram, PETCO$_2$ value provides a good estimate of alveolar PCO$_2$. Arterial CO$_2$ is then related to alveolar CO$_2$ in the normal manner, either similar or higher, depending on physiologic dead space. Undesired rebreathing in a partial rebreathing circuit can be reduced by increasing fresh gas flow, using larger tidal volumes, and allowing more time for exhalation.

Nonzero inspiratory CO$_2$ in a circle system invariably indicates a circuit malfunction. The most common causes are faulty valves (allowing bidirectional flow), a CO$_2$ absorber bypass circuit enabled, or exhausted CO$_2$ absorbent. Visual inspection of the CO$_2$ cannister, valves and bypass switch (if present), usually identifies these conditions. Occasionally the chemical indicator in soda lime fails to reindicate depletion after the soda lime dries overnight.[38]

Cost Issues

This discussion would not be complete without a brief mention of the costs of using CO$_2$ monitoring techniques. Although each institution establishes its own usage pattern the real expense is ap-

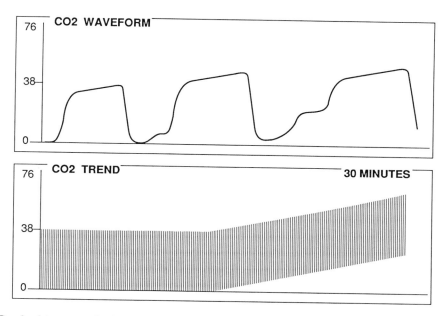

Fig. 13-16. Gradual increase in both the baseline and end-tidal CO$_2$ concentration. This pattern demonstrates that previously exhaled CO$_2$ is being rebreathed from the breathing circuit. The inspired minimum fails to reach the zero baseline, and the PETCO$_2$ steadily rises.

proximately $4 per patient for capnography. This is far less than the cost of an injury.[39]

Summary

Although anesthesia and critical care practice is, for the most part, a safe process, accidents can and do happen, often with devastating results. Capnography provides the clinician with the means for early detection of potential catastrophic events and thus provide the user with sufficient warning to allow early intervention.

HAZARDS OF RESPIRATORY GAS MONITORING

Respiratory gas monitoring has become increasingly common in anesthesia practice. Although this monitoring modality is noninvasive, it is not without hazards. Additional fittings and devices in the breathing circuit can be sources for disconnection, leak, or obstruction.[40] Sampled gas must be disposed of safely. If sampled gas is returned to the breathing circuit, the danger of infectious contamination must be considered. If sampled gas is not returned to the breathing circuit, its loss has further ramifications. In low-flow anesthesia, circuit gas composition becomes difficult to predict (but of course it is measured).[41] Also, circuit volume may decrease, eventually resulting in negative airway pressure[42] and potentially causing harm.[43-45] Negative airway pressure can even occur during cardiopulmonary bypass.[46] Some respiratory gas monitoring systems discontinue sampling when in standby mode, while others merely discontinue analysis while continuing to remove gas from the breathing circuit. As with any monitored variable, incorrect data or misinterpretation can lead to incorrect treatment and potential patient harm.

CLINICAL SUMMARY

Many respiratory gases can now be analyzed and monitored continuously with convenience. Infrared analyzers, mass spectrometers, Raman spectrometers, and electrochemical analyzers reliably measure respiratory and anesthetic gases during anesthesia.

REFERENCES

1. Gravenstein JS: Gas monitoring and pulse oximetry. Butterworth-Heinemann, Boston, 1990
2. Fisher DM: Anesthesia equipment for pediatrics. p. 197. In Gregory GA (ed): Pediatric Anesthesia. 3rd Ed. Churchill Livingstone, New York, 1994
3. Hudson RD Jr: Infrared System Engineering. p. 47. Wiley, New York, 1969
4. Severinghaus JW, Larson CP, Eger EI: Correction factors for infrared carbon dioxide pressure broadening by nitrogen, nitrous oxide, and cyclopropane. Anesthesiology 22:429, 1961
5. Nielsen JR, Thornton V, Dale EB: The absorption laws for gases in the infrared. Rev Modern Phys 16:307, 1944
5a. Raemer DB, Calalang I: Accuracy of end-tidal P_{CO_2} analyzers. J Clin Monit 7(2):195, 1991
6. Luft K: Über eine neue Methode der registrierenden Gasanalyse mit Hilfe der Absorbtion ultratoter Strahlen ohne spektrale Zerlegung. Z Techn Phys 24:97, 1943
7. Cobbold RSC: Transducers for Biomedical Measurement Principles and Applications. p. 91. Wiley, New York, 1974
8. Kertzman J: Paper 73425. p. 121. Instrument Society of America, Analytical Instrumentation Division, 1973
9. Evaluation: carbon dioxide monitors. ECRI Health Dev 15:255, 1986
10. Van Wagenen RA, Westenskow DR, Benner RE et al: Dedicated monitoring of anesthetic and respiratory gases by Raman scattering. J Clin Monit 2:215, 1986
11. Westenskow DR, Smith KW, Coleman DL et al: Clinical evaluation of a Raman scattering multiple gas analyzer for the operating room. Anesthesiology 70:350, 1989
12. Ozane GM, Young WG, Mazzei WJ, Severinghaus JW: Multipatient anesthetic mass spectrometry: rapid analysis of data stored in long catheters. Anesthesiology 55:62, 1981
13. Fatt I: Polarographic Oxygen Sensor: Its Theory of Operation and Its Application in Biology, Medicine, and Technology. p. 1. CRC Press, Boca Raton, FL, 1976
14. Westenskow DR, Jordan WS, Jordan RB, Gillmor ST: Evaluation of oxygen monitors for clinical use. Anesthesiology 53:S382, 1980
15. Pauling L, Wood R, Sturdevant CO: An instrument for determining the partial pressure of oxygen in a gas. Science 103:336, 1946
16. Cooper JB, Edmondson JH, Joseph DM, Newbower RS: Piezoelectric sorption anesthetic sensor. IEEE Trans BME 28:459, 1981
17. Hayes JK, Westenskow DR, Jordan WS: Continuous

monitoring of inspiratory and end-tidal anesthetic vapor using a piezoelectric detector. Anesthesiology 57:A180, 1982

18. James FM, White JF: Anesthetic considerations at moderate altitude. Anesth Analg 63:1097, 1984

19. Kety SS: The physiological and physical factors governing the uptake of anesthetic gases by the body. Anesthesiology 11:517, 1950

20. Eger El, Guadagni NP: Halothane uptake in man at constant alveolar concentration. Anesthesiology 24:299, 1963

21. Sheid P, Slama H, Piper J: Electronic compensation of the effects of water vapor in respiratory mass spectrometry. J Appl Physiol 30:258, 1971

22. Williams EL, Benson DM: Helium-induced errors in clinical mass spectrometry. Anesth Analg 67:83, 1988

23. Gravenstein N, Theisen GJ, Knudsen AK: Misleading mass spectrometer reading caused by an aerosol propellant. Anesthesiology 62:70, 1985

23a. Elliott WR, Raemer DB, Goldman DB, et al: The effects of bronchodilator-inhaler aerosol propellant on respiratory gas monitors. J Clin Monit 7(2):175, 1991

24. American Society of Anesthesiologists: Standards for basic intraoperative monitoring. ASA, Park Ridge, IL, 1994

25. Keenan RL, Boynan CP: Cardiac arrest due to anesthesia: a study of incidence and causes. JAMA 253:2373, 1985

26. Swedlow DB: Capnometry and capnography: an anesthesia disaster warning system. Semin Anesth 5:194, 1986

27. Nightingale DA, Richards CC, Glass A: An evaluation of rebreathing in a modified t-piece system during controlled ventilation in anesthetized children. Br J Anaesth 37:762, 1975

28. Smalhout B, Kalenda Z: An Atlas of Capnography. Vol. 1. Kerckebosch-Zeist, The Netherlands, 1975

29. Smalhout B: A Quick Guide to Capnography and Its Use in Differential Diagnosis. Hewlett-Packard Application Note 78345-90011, Federal Republic of Germany, 1983

30. Linko K, Paloheimo M, Tammisto T: Capnography for detection of accidental oesophageal intubation. Acta Anaesthesiol Scand 27:199, 1983

31. Murray IP, Modell JH: Early detection of endotracheal tube accidents by monitoring carbon dioxide concentration in respiratory gas. Anesthesiology 59:344, 1983

32. Raemer DB: Monitoring Respiratory Function. In Rogers MC, Tinker JH, Covino BG, Longnecker DE (eds): Principles and Practice of Anesthesiology. Mosby–Year Book, St. Louis, 1992.

33. Shulman D, Aronson HB: Capnography in the early diagnosis of carbon dioxide embolism during laparoscopy. Can Anaesth Soc J 31:455, 1984

34. Osborn JJ, Raison JC, Beaumont JO et al: Respiratory causes of "sudden unexplained arrhythmia" in postthoracotomy patients. Surgery 69:24, 1971

35. Baudendistel L, Goudsouzian N, Coté C, Stafford M: End-tidal CO_2 monitoring: its use in the diagnosis and management of malignant hyperthermia. Anaesthesia 39:1000, 1984

36. Triner L, Sherman J: Potential value of expiratory carbon dioxide measurement in patients considered to be susceptible to malignant hyperthermia. Anaesthesiology 55:482, 1981

37. Gravenstein N, Lampotang MS, Beneken JEW: Factors influencing capnography in the Bain circuit. J Clin Monit 1:6, 1985

38. Sato T: New aspects of carbon dioxide absorption in anesthetic circuit. Med J Osaka U 22:173, 1971

39. Philip JH, Raemer DB: Selecting the optimal anesthesia monitoring array. Med Instr 19:122, 1985

40. Cooper JB, Newbower RS, Long CD, McPeek B: Preventable anesthesia mishaps: a study of human factors. Anesthesiology 49:399, 1978

41. Philip JH: GAS MAN: Understanding Anesthesia Uptake and Distribution. Addison-Wesley, Menlo Park, CA, 1984

42. Huffman LM, Riddle RT: Mass spectometer and/or capnograph use during low-flow, closed circuit anesthesia administration. Anesthesiology 66:439, 1987

43. Buda AI, Pinsky MR, Ingels NB et al: Effects of intrathoracic pressure on left ventricular performance. N Engl J Med 301:453, 1979

44. Lee KWT, Downs JJ: Pulmonary edema secondary to laryngospasm in children. Anesthesiology 59:347, 1983

45. Oswalt CE, Gates GA, Holmstrom FMG: Pulmonary edema as a complication of acute airway obstruction. JAMA 238:1833, 1977

46. Mushlin PS, Mark JB, Elliott WR et al: Inadvertent development of subatmospheric airway pressure during cardiopulmonary bypass. Anesthesiology 71:459, 1989

Pulse Oximetry

14

Joyce A. Wahr
Kevin K. Tremper

The introduction of pulse oximetry in the 1980s offered, for the first time, a reliable, noninvasive, easy-to-use means of continuously determining arterial oxygen saturation. Pulse oximetry has been called "arguably the most significant technological advance ever made in monitoring the . . . safety of patients during anesthesia. . .".[1] With a per second consumption of 83 million molecules of oxygen, and virtually no capacity for storage, the average human has only minutes of cell survival following cessation of oxygen delivery. In the operating room and critical care unit, frequent alterations in cardiopulmonary status make it imperative that the patient's oxygenation status be readily monitored. Prior to the advent of pulse oximetry, the only monitor for patient oxygenation was the "trained" eye of the anesthetist observing skin color for cyanosis. Using a primitive oximeter in 1947, Comroe and Botelho[2] concluded that "in the majority of cases, arterial anoxemia is probably unrecognized until the saturation of hemoglobin with oxygen has fallen below 85 percent; in some it is unrecognized even at the 70–75 percent level." Despite identification of a problem, no solution was available until 1983, when Yelderman and New[3] demonstrated that pulse oximetry reliably reports arterial oxygen saturation. Anesthesiologists eagerly embraced the new technology, and in October 1989 the American Society of Anesthesiologists voted to mandate the use of pulse oximetry in all anesthetics after January 1990.

Pulse oximetry is made possible by the combination of two quite simple physical principles. The first is that every substance has a unique absorbance spectra. For example, oxygenated hemoglobin absorbs less red light (600 to 750 nm) and

more infrared light (850 to 1,000 nm) than does deoxygenated hemoglobin (Fig. 14-1). The second principle is that, of all light-absorbing substances in living tissues, only arterial blood is pulsatile. While each of these concepts was recognized decades ago, the juxtaposition of technology from different fields by many researchers was required to bring the pulse oximeter into the everyday world of the anesthesiologist.

TECHNICAL DEVELOPMENT OF THE PULSE OXIMETER

The development of the pulse oximeter really began in the late 1660s, when Isaac Newton[5] came to believe that all the colors demonstrated by a prism actually existed in the beam of light passing through the prism. He thus set the stage for identification of the wavelength spectrum. Nearly 200 years later (1860), Bunson and his colleague Kirchoff[6] developed the first spectroscope and were able to demonstrate that each element in nature has a specific light absorbance "fingerprint." At nearly the same time (1864), Georg Stokes[7] reported that the pigment in blood was the carrier of oxygen. Felix Hoppe-Seyler,[8] a professor of chemistry in Germany, isolated this blood pigment and named it hemoglobin. He further demonstrated that hemoglobin absorbed green and blue light, and that mixing air with hemoglobin altered this absorption. This was the first recognition that oxygenated blood could be differentiated from deoxygenated blood by light absorbance characteristics.

A few years earlier, August Beer,[9] working with the ideas of Heinrich Lambert, had described the

Lambert-Beer law, which states that the transmission of light is a logarithmic function of the density or concentration of the absorbing molecules in the solution. The intensity of the transmitted light is also a function of the pathlength of light through the solution and the absorbance constant for a given absorbing particle at a given wavelength. This law may be written as the equation

$$I_{trans} = I_{in}e^{-D \cdot C \cdot a_1}$$

where I_{trans} = intensity of transmitted light; I_{in} = intensity of incident light; e = natural log base (2.71828); D = distance light is transmitted through the liquid; C = concentration of the solute (hemoglobin), and a_1 = extinction coefficient of the solute, which is a constant for a given solute at a specific light wavelength.

Thus, if a known solute is dissolved in a clear solvent in a cuvette of known dimensions, the solute concentration can be calculated if the incident and transmitted light intensities are measured. Using this principle, Drabkin and Austin[10] were able to measure the saturation of hemoglobin in a cuvette. Laboratory oximeters still use this principle to determine hemoglobin concentration by measuring the intensity of light transmitted through a hemoglobin dispersion produced from lysed red blood cells. For the Lambert-Beer equation to be valid, however, both the solvent and the cuvette must be transparent, the pathlength of the light must be known exactly, and no other absorbers can be present in the solution. Obviously, these requirements could not be fulfilled in clinical application without empirical corrections.

In 1935, Ludwig Nicolai[11] developed an instrument that used blue-green bands of light. With this device, he was able to demonstrate progressive deoxygenation of tissue below a tourniquet. An associate of Nicolai's, Kurt Kramer,[12] developed a slightly different machine, and was able to continuously measure the oxygen saturation of blood moving through the isolated artery of an animal. By substituting red-band light for blue-green, Kramer solved one of the key problems in Nicolai's device, namely, although oxygenated blood absorbs light most intensely in the blue-green bands, these wavelengths are nearly incapable of being transmitted through tissue, while red-band light is transmitted well. Kramer's instrument could transmit light through tissue and determine the saturation of the tissue, but could not isolate blood versus tissue saturation, let alone arterial versus capillary or venous saturation.

JR Squire,[13] working at much the same time as Nicolai and Kramer, was able to develop an instrument capable of measuring blood saturation in the web of the hand. By first compressing the tissue, a bloodless field was obtained and the machine could be "zeroed." Release of compression returned blood to the field, and the change in light absorption was due to absorption by blood (albeit a combination of arterial, venous, and capillary). In 1936, Kramer visited Cambridge and worked with a young American physiologist, Glenn Milli-

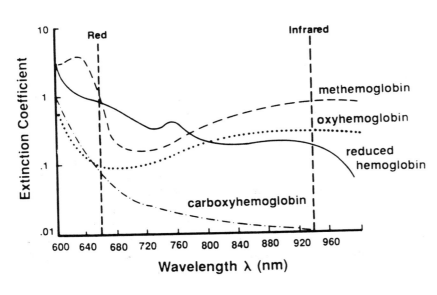

Fig. 14-1. Transmitted light absorbance spectra of four hemoglobin species: oxyhemoglobin, reduced hemoglobin, carboxyhemoglobin, and methemoglobin. (Adapted from Pologe,[4] with permission.)

kan. As World War II became an aerial conflict, Dr. Millikan was approached by the British and asked to develop an oxygen delivery system that would prevent loss of consciousness in aviators at high altitudes. Millikan and John Pappenheimer[14] presented an ear oximeter in 1941 that measured blood saturation using barrier layer photocells and incandescent light with red and green filters. Dr. Millikan gave the name "oximetry" to these measurements of saturation, and his instrument became the first clinically applicable oximeter. The Millikan oximeter was used frequently in research in the years following the end of the war, and was found to agree within ±5 percent with laboratory (Van Slyke) determinations of oxygen saturation.

Earl Wood[15] improved on Millikan's design by adding an inflatable cuff to compress the ear and thus obtain a bloodless reading for the "zero" setting, and improved the infrared filter. He reported on the use of his oximeter in newborns, in infants with congenital heart disease, and in thoracic surgical procedures. By 1950, there were at least 66 publications describing use of the oximeter.[1]

Technical advances over the next decade included defining the absorption characteristics of the two other predominant forms of hemoglobin (carboxyhemoglobin and methemoglobin), improvement in the photoelectric cells, and fiberoptic technology to efficiently deliver the appropriate wavelengths of light to the tissues. Despite these advances, the chief problem remained isolation of arterial blood from venous and capillary blood. The solution to this problem was found serendipitously by a Japanese engineer who was well versed in the status of both oximetry and plethysmography. In 1972, Takuo Aoyagi was working on a photometric means of measuring cardiac output with dye dilution, but was plagued by the pulsatile variation seen due to arterial flow. He noted that the pulsatile components of the absorbances of red and infrared light transmitted through tissue were related to arterial hemoglobin saturation. Application of this principle to oximeters enabled Aoyagi to build an instrument capable of determining the specific saturation of arterial blood and the pulse oximeter was born.[16] Although Aoyagi applied for (in 1974), and was granted (in 1979) the patent in Japan for his discovery, a second Japanese engineer, working at a competing company, was granted patent protection in the United States where the greatest development of oximeters oc-

curred. Aoyagi clearly had an enormous impact on the development of pulse oximetry, yet received little compensation for his discovery. As Severinghaus wrote in his historical review of pulse oximetry, "It is a rare inventor who enjoys financial reward from his or her brilliant insight."[17]

The Aoyagi ear oximeter was marketed by the Nihon Kohden Corporation with little success in the late 1970s. Scott Wilbur, an engineer in Boulder, Colorado, greatly improved the device by developing light-emitting diodes for the light sources, and using photodiodes as detectors.* He also used a small computer to store a complex calibration algorithm based on human volunteer data, which improved accuracy. This oximeter was marketed to pulmonary function laboratories in the early 1980s, but it remained for an anesthesiologist, William New, to recognize the tremendous usefulness of this monitor for the operating and recovery rooms.[3] The Nellcor model N-100 developed and marketed by Dr. New had, by 1985, become almost synonymous with the term "pulse oximeter."

TECHNICAL DESIGN OF CURRENT PULSE OXIMETERS

All currently available pulse oximeters are designed on the principles of light absorbance and pulse detection. They all utilize two wavelengths of light, one in the red band (most commonly 660 nm) and one in the infrared band (most commonly 940 nm). Light-emitting diodes (LED) in the probe transmit light of the appropriate wavelength through the tissue (finger, earlobe, etc.) and the intensity of the transmitted light is measured by a photodetector on the other side. Transmitted light intensities of each wavelength are measured many times each second, and the variation in absorption of light that occurs as the tissue expands and contracts with the pulse of arterial blood is recorded. As arterial blood pulses in the fingertip, the pathlength of light increases slightly. This increase in pathlength and light absorption is due solely to the increased amount of arterial blood (i.e., hemoglobin) in the tissue.

Figure 14-2 schematically illustrates light absorbance in living tissues. The baseline component

---

*Wilber S: Blood constituent measuring device and method. US Patent #4,407,290, April 1, 1981.

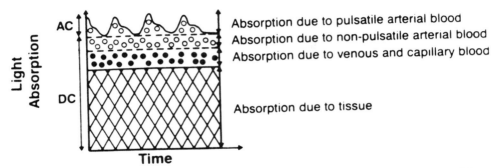

Fig. 14-2. Schematic illustration of light transmission and absorbance through living tissue. Note that the AC signal is due to the pulsatile component of the arterial blood, while the DC signal is composed of the nonpulsatile absorbers in the tissue: nonpulsatile arterial blood, venous and capillary blood, and all other tissues. (Adapted from Ohmeda Pulse Oximetry Model 3700 Service Manual, 1986, p. 22, with permission.)

(analogous to direct current [DC]) represents the absorbance of the tissue bed, including venous blood, capillary blood, and nonpulsatile arterial blood. At the top of the figure is the pulsatile component (alternating current [AC]), which is due to arterial blood. All pulse oximeters assume that the only pulsatile absorbance between the light source and the photodetector is that of arterial blood. The pulse oximeter first determines the AC component of the absorbance at each wavelength and then divides this by the corresponding DC component to obtain a "pulse added" absorbance that is independent of the incident light intensity. It then calculates the ratio of the pulse added absorbances at the two wavelengths, which is empirically related to SaO_2 (arterial oxygen saturation):

$$R = \frac{AC_{660}/DC_{660}}{AC_{940}/DC_{940}}$$

Figure 14-3 is an example of a pulse oximeter calibration curve. These curves are developed by measuring the pulse oximeter absorbance ratios in human volunteers while simultaneously sampling arterial blood for in vitro saturation measurements. Because the calculations are based on alterations due solely to arterial blood, individual variations in skin color, thickness, and composition of tissue (fat versus muscle or bone) should not affect the accuracy of the reported saturation. This fact is reinforced by the finding that SpO_2 (pulse oximeter arterial O_2 saturation) readings are similar whether determined from a finger, a toe, across the bridge of the nose, the earlobe, or other appendage (penis, leg or arm of infant, tongue, etc.). Reflectance

SpO_2 readings such as those obtained from a forehead probe do differ somewhat from transmission SpO_2; reflectance oximetry is discussed separately in a later section.

It should be noted that the pulse oximeter calibration curves do not include specific information

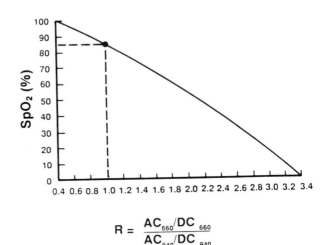

$$R = \frac{AC_{660}/DC_{660}}{AC_{940}/DC_{940}}$$

Fig. 14-3. Example of a pulse oximeter calibration curve. The SaO_2 estimate is determined from the ratio (R) of the pulse-added red absorbance at 660 nm to the pulse-added infrared absorbance at 940 nm. The ratio of red to infrared absorbances varies from approximately 0.4 at 100 percent saturation to 3.4 at 0 percent saturation. The ratio of red to infrared absorbance is 1 at a saturation of approximately 85 percent. This curve can be approximately determined on a theoretical basis, but, for accurate predictions of SpO_2, experimental data are required. (Adapted from Pologe,[4] with permission.)

below a saturation of 70 percent, as safety issues preclude gathering those data in humans. Therefore, calibration curves below 70 percent are based on predictions, not actual data. It should also be noted that an absorbance ratio of 1.0 corresponds to a pulse oximeter saturation of approximately 85 percent.

Although the principles upon which pulse oximetry is based are straightforward, clinical application required a significant engineering effort. The engineering solutions to various clinical problems impact not only on the accuracy and reliability of the instruments, but also define their inherent limitations. The following discussion of these issues is divided into four general areas: dyshemoglobins and dyes, LED center wavelength variability, signal and artifact management, and accuracy and response.

Dyshemoglobins

Adult blood usually contains four species of hemoglobin: oxyhemoglobin (O_2Hb), reduced hemoglobin (Hb), methemoglobin (MetHb), and carboxyhemoglobin (COHb). Laboratory cooximeters measure all four concentrations by utilizing a separate wavelength for each species, and writing a separate Lambert-Beer equation for each. Because pulse oximeters utilize only two wavelengths, they can measure only the ratio of O_2Hb to Hb. In order to understand the impact of this fact on reported saturation, the definition of hemoglobin (or oxygen) saturation must first be discussed. In the rest of this chapter, SaO_2 is used to denote the saturation of arterial blood as determined by laboratory oximetry, and SpO_2 will be used to denote the saturation of arterial blood as determined by pulse oximetry.

Historically, hemoglobin saturation was defined as the oxygen content of blood after it came into equilibrium with room air, expressed as a percentage of oxygen capacity. This definition was developed prior to the clinical availability of supplemental oxygen, so the highest oxygen content of blood came from exposure to room air. By this definition, the two forms of hemoglobin that do not bind oxygen are not included, and this definition is now referred to as "functional hemoglobin saturation" (JW Severinghaus, personal communication):

$$\text{Functional } SaO_2 = \frac{O_2Hb}{O_2Hb + Hb} \times 100\%$$

With the advent of laboratory multiwavelength oximeters that can measure all four species of hemoglobin, fractional saturation has been defined as the ratio of oxyhemoglobin to total hemoglobin:

Fractional SaO_2

$$= \frac{O_2Hb}{O_2Hb + Hb + COHb + MetHb} \times 100\%$$

Referring back to Lambert-Beer's law, absorption (A) can be solved for as follows:

$$A = D_1C_1e_1 + D_2C_2e_2 + D_3C_3e_3 + D_4C_4e_4$$

Each extinction coefficient (e) is a constant for a given wavelength (Fig. 14-1). If COHb and MetHb were not present, their contributions to the absorption of any wavelength of light would be zero and fractional hemoglobin saturation could be determined by a two-wavelength oximeter. Similarly, if two wavelengths existed for which the extinction coefficients for COHb and MetHb were zero, then these absorption terms would again be zero and a two-wavelength oximeter could measure functional saturation. Unfortunately, as shown in Fig. 14-1, the extinction coefficients for COHb and MetHb are not zero in the red and infrared bands, and their presence will contribute to light absorption. Benchtop oximeters utilize four wavelengths, and can therefore precisely determine the percentage of each hemoglobin species present. Being two-wavelength devices, pulse oximeters can deal with only two hemoglobin species. It is not intuitively obvious how a pulse oximeter will behave in the presence of dyshemoglobins, and so each is discussed in turn.

Carboxyhemoglobin

Carboxyhemoglobin, as can be seen in Fig. 14-1, absorbs very little light in the infrared range (940 nm), but absorbs as much light as oxyhemoglobin in the red range (660 nm). This is borne out by the fact that patients with carboxyhemoglobenemia (carbon monoxide poisoning) appear "cherry-red." To the pulse oximeter, therefore, COHb looks like O_2Hb at 660 nm, while at 940 nm COHb is relatively transparent. The Nellcor N100 and Ohmeda Biox III see carboxyhemoglobin as a mixture of approximately 90 percent O_2Hb and 10 percent Hb,[18] thus overestimating the oxygen saturation. Heavy cigarette smokers often have COHb levels of 10 to 15 percent, which may persist up to

8 hours after the last cigarette; the reported SpO$_2$ must be interpreted with caution in these patients.

Patients with carbon monoxide poisoning may have more seriously inaccurate SpO$_2$ readings.[19] In dogs exposed to high levels of carbon monoxide,[18] the pulse oximeter saturation was found to be related to true saturation by the following equation:

$$SpO_2 = \frac{O_2Hb + (0.9)(COHb)}{total\ Hb} \times 100\%$$

In dogs with 70 percent carboxyhemoglobin, the reported pulse oximeter saturation was over 90 percent. Therefore, in any patient at risk for carboxyhemoglobinemia, an arterial sample should be sent for laboratory determination of all hemoglobin species, and the reported SpO$_2$ interpreted in view of these findings.

Methemoglobin

The effects of methemoglobinemia on pulse oximetry are also partially predictable from the extinction curves shown in Fig. 14-1. Methemoglobinemia is seen most commonly as a complication of the use of 20 percent benzocaine sprays and ointments and with the use of dapsone, a sulfonamide derivative used in the treatment of malaria, leprosy, and *Pneumocystis carinii* pneumonia in HIV patients.[20–23] MetHb has nearly the same absorbance as reduced hemoglobin at 660 nm, while it has a greater absorbance than the other hemoglobins at 940 nm. Clinically, methemoglobinemia results in very dark, brownish blood, and in the laboratory, produces a large absorbance signal at both wavelengths. Because MetHb adds significantly to both the numerator and denominator, the absorbance ratio (R) tends toward 1.0, which corresponds to a saturation of 85 percent on the calibration curve. As predicted, dog studies have shown that as MetHb levels increase, SpO$_2$ tends toward 85 percent, and eventually becomes independent of the actual SaO$_2$.[24] In other words, in the presence of high levels of MetHb, SpO$_2$ is erroneously low when SaO$_2$ is above 85 percent, and erroneously high when SaO$_2$ is below 85 percent. The tendency of MetHb to result in a SpO$_2$ of 85 percent regardless of the true SaO$_2$ has been reported in clinical studies as well as dog studies.[20–23] Again, laboratory determination of the concentration of MetHb is useful.

Fetal Hemoglobin

Neonates have a fifth species of hemoglobin, fetal hemoglobin (HbF), which accounts for 50 to 85 percent of the total hemoglobin at birth.[25] HbF differs from adult Hb in the amino acid sequences of two of the four globin subunits. This difference in globin chains has little effect on extinction curves and therefore should not affect pulse oximetry readings.[26,27] HbF does have a small effect on in vitro laboratory oximeters in that O$_2$HbF may be interpreted as consisting partially of COHb.[28]

Dyes

Any substance present in the arterial blood that absorbs light at 660 or 940 nm and which was not present in the same concentration in the volunteers used to generate calibration curves will affect the absorbance ratio and thus the reported SpO$_2$. The detection of intravenous dyes by pulse oximeters should not be surprising because it was this effect that led Aoyagi to the invention of pulse oximetry.

Methylene blue appears to be the dye that affects SpO$_2$ to the greatest degree. Kessler and colleagues[29] first described the effect of methylene blue, citing a case in which this dye had been administered during a transurethral prostate resection, causing a transient, spurious desaturation to 65 percent. Because methylene blue acts to clear MetHb, the picture of a patient with MetHb who has received methylene blue will become confusing. Unfortunately, even laboratory cooximeters will not give a true saturation, for they are affected by methylene blue to the same degree as are pulse oximeters.[30,31] Laboratory oximeter determinations of saturation are affected by methylene blue for up to 48 hours, while pulse oximeters are affected for only a few minutes.[32] No adequate explanation of this difference is available. The most attractive theoretical explanation involves arterial-venous-tissue equilibration, but this theory is not consistent with the observed effect of dyshemoglobins, which alter SpO$_2$ despite being in arterial-venous equilibration.

Scheller and colleagues[33] evaluated the effects of bolus doses of methylene blue, indigo carmine, and indocyanine green in human volunteers. They found that methylene blue caused a spurious fall in SpO$_2$ to approximately 65 percent for 1 to 2 minutes. Indigo carmine produced a very small drop in saturation, while indocyanine green had an intermediate effect (brief decrease, never below 93 percent in the five patients tested). Bilirubin has not been found to affect SpO$_2$, but does affect laboratory determinations of saturation when blood levels pass 20 mg/dl.[27,34]

There is an interesting report that onychomycosis, a superficial fungal infection of the nail, can falsely depress SpO$_2$.[35] The authors report that in five volunteers, the SpO$_2$ determined on unaffected nails was 95 to 98 percent, while the SpO$_2$ on affected nails was 71 to 84 percent. Onychomycosis produces a yellow discoloration of the nail, which may absorb light in either the red or infrared range.

Skin pigment has been reported both to affect and to not affect pulse oximeter readings.[36] In very darkly pigmented individuals the readings may be erroneously high or unobtainable (3 to 5 percent).[37,38] It is not clear whether this is due to inadequate transmission of light or excessive absorption by skin pigment. Certainly, darkly pigmented individuals were not included in the trials from which the calibration curves were generated. Use of the less pigmented nail beds, or use of a buccal probe, may result in appropriate readings.

Many data have been generated concerning nail polish of various colors and brands.[39,40] As might be expected, the interference with pulse oximetry readings depends on the absorption of light in the red or infrared bands by the individual polish colors: blue hues of polish absorb strongly close to 660 nm, while black absorbs in both the red and infrared range. The interference results in spurious decreases in SpO$_2$ of 3 to 5 percent. Clearly, if there is any question of an inappropriate reading, the finger probe can be placed to transmit side to side rather than through the nail with its offending polish, or an ear or nose probe may be used.

Light-Emitting Diode Center Wavelength Variability

The light-emitting diodes used in pulse oximeters are not pure monochromatic light sources. Rather, there is a narrow spectral range over which light is emitted. This range varies not only between manufacturers but also among diodes of the same type from the same manufacturer, with variations of ±15 nm.[4] A shift in the LED center wavelength will change the measured extinction coefficient and thus produce an error in the saturation esti-

mate. This effect will be the greatest for the red wavelength, because the extinction curves have a steeper slope at 660 nm versus 950 nm, and reduced hemoglobin has a steeper extinction curve at 660 nm than does oxyhemoglobin (Fig. 14-1). Therefore, inaccuracy of the probe due to LED wavelength variability will be more significant when the blood is desaturated than when it is well saturated.

Manufacturers use two approaches to correct this problem. The first is to test all diodes, and reject those that are out of their specified wavelength range, e.g., 660 ± 5 nm. This is expensive because of the number of diodes that will be rejected. Alternatively, the pulse oximeter may be programmed to accept several ranges of LED center wavelengths in both the red and infrared band, allowing the device to correct the extinction coefficients internally for different wavelengths. This allows the manufacturer to accept more of the tested diodes, but requires production of a more sophisticated device with a mechanism for identifying the sensor LED wavelengths to the pulse oximeter.[4] Incompletely compensated LED frequency variation will not change the pulse oximeter's ability to trend saturation changes, but will produce probe to probe variability in the absolute measurement of SpO$_2$.

Signal Management and Artifact

Perhaps the most difficult engineering problem in pulse oximeter design is the identification of the "ripple" of arterial blood in a "sea" of electromagnetic artifact. Artifact has three major sources of poor signal-to-noise ratio: ambient light, low perfusion amplitude (low AC/DC signal, too little signal), and motion (large AC/DC signal, too much noise). Two minor sources of artifact (too much noise) are electrocautery and magnetic resonance imaging (MRI).

Ambient Light

The photodiodes used in the sensor as light detectors cannot distinguish one wavelength of light from another. That is, the detector does not know whether the received light originates from the red LED, the infrared LED, or ambient (room) light. This problem is solved by alternating the red and infrared LED light pulses. First, the red LED is pulsed and the photodiode detector generates a current that is a result of red LED plus room light. As the red light is switched off, the infrared LED is switched on, generating a current that is a result of infrared plus room light. Finally, both the red and infrared lights are off, and a current is generated from the room light alone. This process is repeated hundreds of times per second. In this way, the oximeter attempts to eliminate light interference even in a quickly changing background of room light. Nonetheless, interference has been reported both in clinical and laboratory situations involving fluorescent lights,[41] a xenon arc lamp,[42] infrared light,[43] and a fiberoptic cytoscope unit whose stroboscopic effects generated by spinning fan blades near the light source resulted in widely fluctuating SpO_2.[44] Ambient light artifact can most appropriately be minimized using an opaque shield, such as a towel or a foil shield.

Low Perfusion Signal

Determination of pulse saturation is dependent upon detection of a pulse. When a pulse absorbance signal is detected, however small it may be, the oximeter will amplify that signal and estimate the SpO_2 from the ratio of the amplified absorbances. The pulse oximeter can therefore determine arterial saturation even in patients whose pulse amplitude is quite small. Unfortunately, as the pulse signal is amplified, so is the background noise. At the highest amplifications, which may reach one billion times, the oximeter may analyze the noise signal and generate an SpO_2 value from it. Early models would even generate a value from a sheet of paper placed in the probe between the LED and photodiode.[45]

Current models incorporate minimum values for signal-to-noise ratio, and will display either no value or a "low signal strength" message below this value. The minimum signal-to-noise values vary among manufacturers, and while those with lower default levels will report SpO_2 values in a greater percentage of patients, they are more prone to error. Despite these precautions, there are case reports of pulse oximeters displaying pulsatile waveforms, heart rates, and saturation values where none existed. One oximeter maintained readings from a heart transplant donor after the heart had been excised, and another during cardiac arrest (chest open, asystolic heart).[46] There are also reports that pulsations due either to tricuspid regur-

gitation or to an intraaortic balloon pump can interfere with recognition of the true arterial pulse.[47,48] If the saturation has been determined erroneously from background noise, the heart rate displayed will usually be at variance with that determined from the ECG.

It should be clear from the previous discussion that pulse wave amplitude is more critical to determination of SpO_2 than either flow or blood pressure in the monitored appendage. Low pulse wave amplitude results most often during peripheral vasoconstriction due to hypovolemia, hypothermia, or poor cardiac output. Under these circumstances, pulse oximetry may be unobtainable due to low pulse wave amplitude or be unreliable (slow circulation times delaying report of hypoxemia).[49-53] In the critical care setting, extremes of systemic vascular resistance may result in loss of signal or decreased accuracy.[54] In the setting of severe peripheral vasoconstriction, digital nerve blocks have been reported to restore pulse oximetry function.[55] Falconer and colleagues[56] found that pulse pressures less than 11 mmHg increased the inaccuracy of all pulse oximeters when tested in volunteers with SpO_2 values of 80 to 88 percent. Likewise, Severinghaus and Spellman[57] reported that when pulse pressure was normal, average mean pressure at which pulse oximeters failed was approximately 30 mmHg, but diminished pulse wave amplitude resulted in failure of signal detection at higher mean pressures (36 to 47 mmHg). In both of these settings, where SpO_2 was measured in digits with hypotension but not vasoconstriction, saturation values were obtainable despite quite low mean arterial pressures. These findings differ from the misconception that "if the pulse oximeter is working, the blood pressure must be all right."

Indeed, since these devices automatically increase their amplification as the pulse signal decreases, they should be relatively insensitive to decreases in perfusion. Nonetheless, several clinical studies have used the pulse oximeter to assess the adequacy of peripheral perfusion, including use of the device to evaluate perfusion in reimplanted extremities[58] and revascularized bowel,[59,60] as well as to assess the adequacy of collateral circulation.[61,62] As with any plethysmograph, the pulse oximeter will detect a complete loss of peripheral pulse, but it is not a qualitative measure of flow. Lawson and coworkers[63] have shown that correct SpO_2 values and pulse rates can be obtained when flow through the finger is as little as 8.6 percent of baseline, achieved by inflation of a blood pressure cuff to 96 percent of control systolic pressure.[63] This demonstrates the tremendous ability of the pulse oximeter to detect and amplify small pulse signals and thus estimate arterial hemoglobin saturation.

Motion Artifact

Patient motion may be the most difficult artifact to eliminate. This artifact rarely causes difficulties in the operating room, but in the recovery room and intensive care unit it can make the pulse oximeter nearly useless.[64] Shivering is widely held to interfere with saturation estimates,[65] although few clinical data exist. Pulse oximeters have been shown to report accurate values during tonic-clonic seizures[66] and during helicopter transport.[67,68] Still, patient motion has been shown to be the most frequent cause of oximeter failure or spurious desaturation episodes.[69] The body motion generated during cardiopulmonary resuscitation has been shown to generate pulse oximeter saturation values of 85 to 90 percent, despite lack of circulation.[70]

Several approaches have been tried to eliminate the problem of motion artifact, beginning with the signal averaging time. If measurements are averaged over a longer time period, the effect of an intermittent artifact is lessened, but at the expense of a longer response time to acute changes in SaO_2.[71] Many of the pulse oximeters allow the user to select one of several time-averaging modes. In addition, the designer can use sophisticated algorithms to identify and reject spurious signals. These algorithms may assess the AC:DC signal ratio, or they may check the validity of the saturation estimate by calculating its rate of change. For example, if the saturation estimate changes from 95 percent to 50 percent in one-tenth of a second, this sudden change may not be averaged into the displayed SpO_2, or it may be given a lower weighting factor. As stated earlier, these artifact rejection schemes may also affect the accuracy and response time of the pulse oximeter. As with amplified background noise, motion artifact is detected best by observation of the plethysmograph waveform or comparing the heart rate with that determined by ECG.

Electrocautery

Electrocautery can interfere with pulse oximetry by artifactually decreasing SpO_2, or by setting off a false alarm. The cause is ascribed to wide-spectrum radiofrequency emissions picked up directly by the photodiode.[72,73] Careful placement of the electrocautery return plate and pulse oximeter probe may alleviate this problem. Some recent models will report detected electromagnetic interference.

Magnetic Resonance Imaging

Pulse oximetry monitoring of patients in the MRI scanner can be useful, but special care must be taken for peaceful coexistence. Any ferromagnetic materials in or near the scanner as well as the wires in the pulse oximeter cable will interfere with imaging.[74] The MRI scanner itself may cause spurious decreases in SpO_2, again due to wide-spectrum radiofrequency emissions. In addition, there are several case reports of burns developing beneath the probes.[75,76] Few data exist in the literature comparing various oximeter models in this setting, although clinical experience is that accuracy of various models may differ substantially.[65]

Accuracy and Response

There are both technologic and physiologic limitations to the accuracy of a pulse oximeter. The SpO_2 value is only as accurate as the empirical calibration curve programmed into the device, which will be influenced by the volunteers in whom the initial studies were performed (light-skinned vs dark-skinned, grams of hemoglobin present, etc.), the conditions under which arterial saturations were determined (data obtained only above 70 percent saturation), and the accuracy of the in vitro laboratory oximeter used to generate it. The clinician is interested in two measures of accuracy: how closely the device agrees with the accepted gold standard during steady-state conditions, and how closely the device tracks change as it occurs.

Before reviewing pulse oximeter accuracy as reported by clinical studies, statistical interpretation of accuracy data should be discussed. The classic statistical method for comparison of values from two different measurement devices (pulse oximetry versus laboratory oximetry) is a correlation coefficient (r) with a P value, and a linear regression slope and intercept. Unfortunately, the correlation coefficient is not a measure of agreement; it is a measure of association. Because SpO_2 values have been generated from laboratory determinations of saturation, we can expect a very high degree of association, and thus a correlation coefficient that is significant. The *r* value will not tell us, however, to what degree the two oximetry devices agree or what level of confidence we should have in the pulse oximeter.

When trying to determine the accuracy of a new device, what we would really like to know is how well the new device (pulse oximetry) agrees with the "gold standard" (laboratory oximeters) over the range of clinically important values. This involves a "methods comparison" study, as described by Altman and Bland,[77] who recommend calculating the mean difference and standard deviation of the differences between the two methods of measurement. The mean difference is called the *bias*, and the standard deviation of the differences is called the *precision*. The bias will show a systematic overestimation or underestimation of one method relative to the other, while the precision will represent the variability or *random error* of the measurement method. Systematic bias can be corrected using algorithms, while random error cannot be anticipated and thus cannot be corrected. Therefore, it is important for the device of interest to show a good measure of precision (i.e., a low numerical value for standard deviation of the differences).

There have been some 50 published studies of pulse oximetry accuracy and reliability since 1983; comprehensive reviews of these studies exist in the literature[64,65,72] and will not be repeated here. Overall failure rates—patients in whom pulse oximetry readings could not be obtained—range from 2 to 3 percent in the general population, and 7 percent in the sickest patients.[64,65,72,78,79] Most manufacturers claim that their pulse oximeters are accurate to within ±2 percent (SD) from 70 to 100 percent saturation and ±3 percent (SD) from 50 to 70 percent saturation, with no reported accuracy below 50 percent saturation. These numbers imply that, for SaO_2 above 70 percent, approximately 68 percent of the data will fall within ±2 percent of a line of identity, and 95 percent of the data will fall within ±4 percent (±2 SD). The vast majority of the published data support the manufacturers' claim of accuracy; typically bias is between −2 and +3 percent with precisions of 2 to 5 percent for saturations between 70 and 100 percent.[64,65,72,80–82]

Pulse oximetry at saturations below 70 percent is less accurate, both because the calibration curves used to write the individual manufacturers' algorithms do not include experimental data below 70 percent and because clinical studies that test the accuracy below 70 percent are rare. The available clinical data seem to indicate that pulse oximeters will underestimate SaO_2 during rapidly changing conditions. Severinghaus and colleagues[83] tested the accuracy and response of 14 pulse oximeters in volunteers subjected to brief episodes of profound hypoxia (saturations of 40 to 70 percent) and found significant variations between manufacturers in both bias and precision. In all probes tested, precision failed as SaO_2 fell below 70 percent. While clinicians should be aware that reported values below 70 percent may be inaccurate, the average clinician will be less concerned with what the true SaO_2 is than with reinstitution of appropriate oxygenation. Rarely, if ever, will the clinical management change because the true SaO_2 is 60 percent rather than 70 percent! Certainly current pulse oximeters are sufficiently accurate to serve as "desaturation monitors" during routine patient care.

A second measure of device accuracy of importance to the clinician is the response time. That is to say, how closely the monitor tracks events in real time. A glance at the oxygen dissociation curve reveals that the pulse oximeter will continue to report an unchanging saturation of 100 percent while the PaO_2 falls from 500 mmHg to 100 mmHg, and the first note of a change in saturation will occur at a PaO_2 less than 100 mmHg. The time lag between SaO_2 reaching a specific value and the SpO_2 displaying that same value varies, depending on the signal averaging times and circulation time. Due to differences in circulation times and peripheral vasoconstriction, finger probes are consistently slower to report desaturation (or resaturation) than are ear or nose probes. Despite being faster, ear probes still have a substantial response time lag. In various studies of pulse oximeter response times, finger probe response times varied from 20 to 150 seconds, while ear probe response times varied from 10 to 80 seconds.[83–85] Many current pulse oximeters allow the practitioner to alter the signal averaging time or to even request beat-to-beat display.

A brief note should be made of the accuracy of pulse oximetry under conditions of anemia. Studies done in both humans and dogs indicate that SpO_2 will underestimate SaO_2 at low hematocrits. At low saturations (50 percent), mean error is a linear function of hematocrit, with no error seen at normal hematocrit.[86] In dogs, bias and precision were 0.2 ± 7.6 percent at normal hematocrits, and worsened to -5.4 ± 18.8 percent at hematocrits less than 10 percent.[87]

MONITORING APPLICATIONS

The use of pulse oximeters has been described in nearly every setting in the hospital, outpatient and veterinary clinics, and even homes, as shown in Table 14-1. Kelleher reviewed 220 references in a review published in 1989[72]; Severinghaus' follow-up review[65] in 1992 found more than 500 new reports between 1989 and October 1991. Nearly 200 further reports have been published since October 1991. Table 14-1 thus is neither comprehensive nor selective, but is intended as an overview of the wide applicability of this monitor. The reported applications may be divided into monitoring of hypoxemia, hyperoxia, perfusion, and circulation.

Hypoxemia

As early as 1947, oximetry had been recognized to be useful in recognition of intraoperative desaturation events. Yelderman and New's[3] demonstration in 1983 that the Nellcor N-100 correlated well with benchtop oximeters opened the door to large-scale trials of the usefulness of the pulse oximeter in patient care. Far and away the most frequent use for the pulse oximeter is detection of hypoxemia—"the sentry standing at the cliff of desaturation."[64] This application has been studied in the preoperative, intraoperative, and postoperative period, in the catheterization laboratory, in the emergency room, in the labor and delivery room for both the mother and infant, on the general nursing floors, and at home. In every cited instance, the pulse oximeter has uncovered a significant number of previously unrecognized hypoxemic events.

In the first randomized trial of pulse oximetry (in 1988), Coté demonstrated that of 24 hypoxemic events detected by pulse oximetry, only 10 were detected by anesthetists blinded to the oximeter.[90] All observer-detected desaturations involved SpO_2 of less than 73 percent, and nine episodes of desaturation to less than 73 percent were completely missed by the blinded anesthetist. A vast array of studies during preoperative sedation, during anesthesia (including general, regional, or awake-sedated), during postoperative transport to the recovery room, and in the recovery room have similarly shown that pulse oximetry will detect a

significant number of desaturation episodes undetected by trained observers.[83–105]

Despite the overwhelming evidence that pulse oximetry will detect and thereby permit appropriate treatment of desaturation episodes, no study has yet been able to demonstrate a reduction in morbidity or mortality associated with the use of pulse oximetry. The difficulty of demonstrating such a benefit may preclude any such association ever being shown. Foremost, the incidence of morbidity and mortality due to anesthesia alone is extremely difficult to describe accurately, and is itself very low. A recent study of postoperative deaths in Great Britain reported an anesthetic-related mortality of only 1:185,000 (0.005 percent).[173] To show a decrease in mortality due to use of pulse oximetry would require a randomized trial of several million patients. The largest randomized trial done to date is a multicenter Danish study involving 20,802 patients randomly assigned to be monitored with or without pulse oximetry.[78,79] Despite the overwhelming number of patients enrolled, no significant difference between groups in postoperative complications (including death) was found. This was despite the fact that pulse oximetry discovered, and thereby enabled treatment of, a significantly higher number of hypoxemic events than those recognized in patients not monitored. It is not possible to conclude, based on the inadequate sample size of this study, that pulse oximetry does not alter the complication rate. Indeed, the researchers did find a lower incidence of myocardial ischemia in monitored versus nonmonitored patients. Still, due to the low incidence of hypoxemic catastrophes (none occurred in the 20,802 patients with or without pulse oximetry), somewhere in the neighborhood of 10,000 to 70,000 patients would need to be treated with pulse oximetry for one patient to benefit.[174] The cost of pulse oximetry monitoring per patient is approximately $2; "clearly, the benefit of pulse oximetry must be very low."[175]

Should we, then, abandon pulse oximetry? Anesthesia very clearly is safer today than at any time in the past. Eichhorn's classic review of the impact of monitoring standards at Harvard revealed a five-fold decrease in adverse outcomes associated with implementation of those standards.[176] Prior to implementation (1985), the rate of death, central nervous system damage or cardiac arrest was 11/682,000; the rate dropped to 1/319,000 following implementation. Yet this decrease was not statisti-

TABLE 14-1. Overview of Application of the Pulse Oximeter

Indication for Use as Monitor	Author	Ref.
Hypoxemia		
Surgical suite		
Preoperative	Elling and Hanning	88
	Marjot and Valentine	89
Intraoperative		
General anesthesia	Cole et al.	90,91
	Raemer et al.	92
	McKay and Noble	93
	Cooper et al.	94
	Moller et al.	78,79
	Mihm and Halperin	95
Thoracic (one lung anesthesia)	Viitanen et al.	96
	Brodsky et al.	97
Detection of endobronchial intubation	Barker et al.	98
Use during cardiopulmonary bypass	Kurki et al.	99
Congenital heart disease	Stow et al.	100
	Boxer et al.	101
Postoperative	Tyler et al.	102
	Blair et al.	103
	Laycock and McNicol	104
	Smith et al.	105
	Morris et al.	106
	Reeder et al.	107
Critical care units		
Ventilator weaning	Rotello et al.	108
	Withington et al.	109
Surgical intensive care unit	Moore et al.	110
	Bierman et al.	111
Pediatric intensive care unit	Fanconi et al.	112
	Fait et al.	113
Delivery room		
Mother and infant	Pope and Hankins	114
	Minnich et al.	115
	Porter et al.	116
	Deckardt et al.	117
Pain-dependent changes in ventilation of parturient		
Amniotic fluid embolus	Quance	118
Supine hypotensive syndrome	Calvin et al.	119
Fetal monitoring	Johnson et al.	120
	Gardosi et al.	121
Neonates	Durand and Ramanathan	122
	Dimich et al.	123
	Sendak et al.	124
	House et al.	125
Catheterization laboratory	Dodson et al.	126
	Lynn and Bosenberg	127
Magnetic resonance imaging unit	Waggle	74
	Shellock et al.	128
Medical diagnostic units (endoscopy)	Schnapf	129
	O'Connor and Jones	130
	Bell et al.	131
Emergency room		
Prehospital transport	Cydulka et al.	132
	Aughey et al.	133

Table continues

TABLE 14-1. Continued

Indication for Use as Monitor	Author	Ref.
Helicopter transport	Talke et al.	67
	Short et al.	68
Emergency ward	Jones et al.	134
	Yamamoto et al.	135
	Wright	136
Cardiopulmonary resusitation	Narang	137
Ward care		
Supplemental oxygen	King and Simon	138
	Prakash	139
	Jubran and Tabin	140
Ward analgesia-epidural/parenteral narcotics	Choi et al.	141
Outpatient dental units	Anderson and Kafer	142
	Hardeman et al.	143
Sleep disorder study centers	Golding-Wood et al.	144
	Williams et al.	145
Home		
Home oxygen therapy	Adams and Foret	146
	Tiep	147
	Montgomery et al.	148
Sudden infant death syndrome	Poets et al.	149
Veterinary medicine	Jacobson et al.	150
	Schmotzer et al.	151
Hyperoxia		
Premature infants	Cunningham et al.	152
	Dear	153
	Fanconi	154
	Deckardt and Steward	155
	Baeckert et al.	156
	Bossi et al.	157
	Peabody et al.	158
	Hay et al.	159
Perfusion		
Limb ischemia during limb manipulation/ arthroscopy	Ray et al.	160
	Agel and Levy	161
Free flap viability	Lindsay et al.	162
Collateral circulation	Nowak et al.	163
	Rosenberg et al.	164
	Pillow and Herrick	61
Viability of reimplated digits/limbs	Graham et al.	58
Bowel viability	Ferrara et al.	59
	Stolar and Randolph	165
Positioning	Skeehan and Hensley	166
	Hovagim et al.	167
Circulation		
Assessment of central blood volume	Partridge	168
Blood pressure	Wallace et al.	169
	Talke	170
	Chalwa e al.	171
Autonomic dysfunction	Broome and Mason	172

cally significant, again due to the small incidence. In addition to no demonstrated decrease in adverse events due to the use of pulse oximetry, one review of closed claims data showed that adverse events occur despite the use of pulse oximetry.[177] It is highly unlikely that pulse oximetry will ever be demonstrated to significantly decrease the incidence of death associated with anesthesia; it is also highly unlikely that anesthesiologists will ever choose to discontinue the use of such a simple, inexpensive monitor with such theoretically valuable information. It is crucial to recognize, however, that the most vital monitor in the operating and recovery rooms remains a trained, vigilant anesthesiologist/PACU nurse. Severinghaus' quote of Hein is apt: "When technology is master/We shall reach disaster faster."[65] We must not allow the monitors we use make us less vigilant or less intimately involved in the care of our patients.

Hyperoxia

Pulse oximetry has been proposed as a simpler method of monitoring oxygenation to prevent retinopathy of prematurity than transcutaneous oxygen tension.[158] While pulse oximetry is as accurate in neonates and premature infants as it is in adults, it does not provide the requisite information. Although retinopathy is currently believed to be best prevented by maintaining a PaO_2 (i.e., an oxygen tension) of less than 80 to 90 mmHg,[178] in any given infant, it is not predictable what the SpO_2 must be kept below in order to prevent a dangerous PaO_2. In addition, the LED variability between probes is sufficient to report a "safe" SpO_2, while the PaO_2 is, in fact, dangerously high. Prevention of hyperoxia in these infants is best accomplished by a transcutaneous oxygen electrode or frequently determined arterial oxygen tensions, while pulse oximetry plays a peripheral role of monitoring for inadvertent hypoxic episodes.

Perfusion

As noted earlier, pulse oximetry has been used to evaluate reimplanted digits, bowel, and to provide a warning of arterial compression during shoulder manipulation or surgical positioning (see Table 14-1). Even though the flow detected by the pulse oximeter may be extremely low, experimental evidence to date indicates that the presence of a pulsatile signal does appropriately track the viability of the tissue monitored.

Circulation

Pulse oximeters have been used to assess systolic blood pressure, central venous volume, and to assess autonomic dysfunction and pulsus paradoxsis.[171] While of interest, these uses remain ancillary to the primary use—detection of hypoxemia.

COMPLICATIONS

Pulse oximetry is noninvasive and the potential dangers associated with its use are relatively few. Other than false positive (reporting of hypoxia when none exists) and false negative (failure to report hypoxia when present) readings (dealt with in the accuracy section) true complications are rare. There are several reports of severe burns underneath probes used in MRI scanners;[75,76] "suntaning" of digits of neonates when probes were not changed for extended periods of time; burns in neonates,[179,180] burns associated with defective probes[181] or with inappropriate use of one manufacturer's probe with another manufacturer's box,[182] and pressure injury.[183] These complications can be alleviated by checking the digit to which the probe is applied, especially when the probe is used for an extended period of time.

ANTICIPATED ADVANCES: REFLECTANCE OXIMETRY

As discussed earlier, transmission pulse oximeters are usually placed on the most peripheral areas of the body—fingers, toes, ear lobes—which are also the regions most affected by vasoconstriction due to hypovolemia, hypothermia, or infusion of vasoconstrictive drugs. Reflectance pulse oximeters, which determine hemoglobin saturation by means of backscattered light, may be placed on more central body regions such as the forehead or chest. In addition, motion artifact should be less with placement of the sensor on the head or trunk.

The basic principles of light absorption and plethysmography as well as the wavelengths of light used in reflectance oximetry are the same as those for transmission oximetry, with the light emitting diode placed to the side of the photodiode. Like-

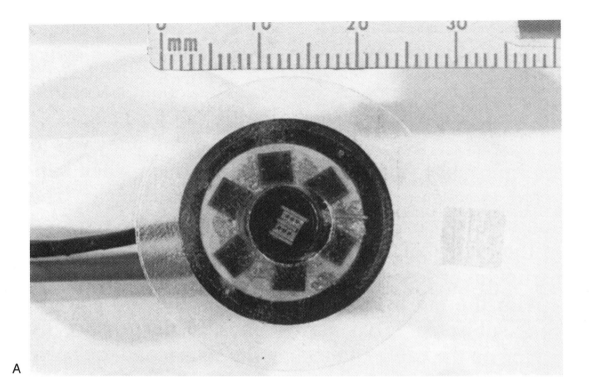

A

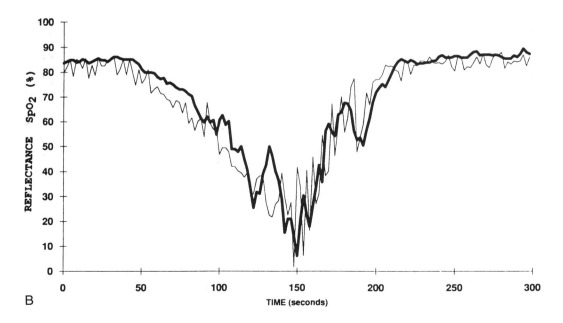

B

Fig. 14-4. (A) Adhesive optical reflectance sensor. The LEDs are the small squares inside the black optical shield in the center of the housing. The large black squares are the photodiodes. **(B)** The response of the adhesive reflectance sensor to a step change in SaO₂. (Adapted from Mendelson and Solomita,[187] with permission.)

wise, the signal-processing method for reflectance oximetry is identical to that used for transmission oximetry. Reflectance oximetry, however, measures backscattered light, while transmission oximetry measure forward-scattered light. Because the backscattered light is order of magnitudes less than forward scattered light, the noise-to-signal ratio is even more problematic, and the pulsatile signal is often weak.[184] In two studies during partial cardiopulmonary bypass, forehead reflectance sensors were compared to transmission probes placed on the earlobe.[185,186] The reflectance probes were shown to be only minimally better than transmission probes both in earlier detection of signal, and in detection of a signal when the transmission probe did not detect a pulse.

Mendelson,[187] who first described reflectance oximetry in 1983, recently described a new reflectance sensor (Fig. 14-4) in which multiple photodetectors surround a central light emitting diode, an arrangement which maximizes the amount of backscattered light detected by the sensor. Although testing of this sensor has been accomplished only in animals to date, the results have been promising.[188] An alternate design has also been described,[184] in which the photodiode is central, surrounded by four of each red and infrared emitting diodes. In this design, the skin is heated to maximize local circulation, and, indeed, the local skin temperature appears to be of "prime importance in the successful operation of the reflectance pulse oximeter."[184] This probe was tested in 18 intensive care unit patients, and appears to be accurate, reliable, and without serious complications (no burns in 5 to 6 hours of continuous operation).

Although reflectance probes may be shown to be slightly more effective in signal detection during low perfusion states, the increased cost (four times the number of diodes) will most likely limit their use. The setting in which reflectance oximetry may offer substantial advantages over transmission oximetry is in monitoring of the fetus during second stage labor, when the only presenting part is the fetal scalp.

SUMMARY

Pulse oximetry is remarkable among monitors in that it involves no calibration, (offers) negligible time lag, and infrequent false negative data . . . requires no routine maintenance, no disposable components, no training and little interpretation while it continuously and noninvasively displays a vital variable.

So wrote Severinghaus and Kelleher[65] in their recent evaluation of pulse oximetry. Despite concerns that this monitor might decrease vigilance and increase anesthetic cost without improving anesthetic outcome, it appears certain that this monitor will continue to play a central role in monitoring of anesthetized patients.

REFERENCES

1. Severinghaus JW, Astrup P: History of blood gas analysis. VI. Oximetry. J Clin Monit 2:270, 1986
2. Comroe JH, Botelho S: The unreliability of cyanosis in the recognition of arterial anoxemia. Am J Med Sci 214:1, 1947
3. Yelderman M, New W: Evaluation of pulse oximetry. Anesthesiology 59:349, 1983
4. Pologe JA: Pulse oximetry: technical aspects of machine design. Int Anesthesiol Clin 25:137, 1987
5. Newton I: Optiks; or a Treatise of the Reflections, Refractions, Inflections and Colours of Light. G. Bull, London, 1672 (reprinted 1931)
6. Kirchkoff GR, Bunsen RWE: Chemische Analyse durch Spectralbeobachtungen. Engleman, Leipzig, 1860
7. Stokes GG: On the reduction and oxygenation of the colouring matter of the blood. London, Edinburgh, Dublin Philos Mag 28:391, 1864
8. Hoppe-Seyler F: Über die chemischen und optischen Eigenschafter des Blutfarbstoffs. Arch Pathol Anat Physiol 29:233, 1864
9. Beer A: Versuch der Absorptions-Verhältnisse des Cordietes für rothes Licht zu bestimmen. Ann Physik Chem 84:37, 1851
10. Drabkin DL, Austin JH: Spectrophotometric studies. V. Technique for analysis of undiluted blood and concentrated hemoglobin solutions. J Biol Chem 157:69, 1945
11. Nicolai L: Uber Sichtbarmachung, Verlauf und chemische Kinetik der Oxyhemoglobinreduktion imlebenden Gewebe, besonders in der menschlichen Haut. Arch Ges Physiol 229:372, 1932
12. Kramer K: Ein Verfahren zur fortlaufenden Messung des Sauerstoffgehaltes im strömenden Blut an uneröffneten Gefassen. Z Biol 96:61, 1935
13. Squire JR: Instrument for measuring quantity of blood and its degree of oxygenation in web of the hand. Clin Sci 4:331, 1940
14. Millikan GA, Pappenheimer JR, Rawson AJ, Hervey

JP: Continuous measurement of oxygen saturation in man. Am J Physiol 133:390, 1941

15. Wood E, Geraci JE: Photoelectric determination of arterial oxygen saturation in man. J Lab Clin Med 34:387, 1949

16. Aoyagi T, Kishi M, Yamaguchi K, Watanabe S: Improvement of the earpiece oximeter. p. 90. [In Japanese]. Abstracts of the 13th Annual Meeting of the Japanese Society of Medical Electronics and Biological Engineering, 1974

17. Severinghaus JW, Honda Y: History of blood gas analysis. VII. Pulse oximetry. J Clin Monit 3:135, 1987

18. Barker SJ, Tremper KK: The effect of carbon monoxide inhalation on pulse oximeter signal detection Anesthesiology 67:599, 1987

19. Vegfors M, Lennmarken C: Carboxyhemoglobinemia and pulse oximetry. Br J Anaesth 66:625, 1991

20. Anderson ST, Hajduczek J, Barder SJ: Benzocaine-induced methemoglobinemia in an adult: accuracy of pulse oximetry with methemoglobinemia. Anesth Analg 67:1099, 1988

21. Watcha MF, Connor MT, Hing AV: Pulse oximetry in methemoglobinemia. Am J Dis Child 143:845, 1989

22. Bardoczky GI, Wathieu M, D'Hollander A: Prilocaine-induced methemoglobinemia evidenced by pulse oximetry. Acta Anaesthesiol Scand 34:162, 1990

23. Trillo RA, Aukburg S: Dapsone-induced methemoglobinemia and pulse oximetry. Anesthesiology 77:594, 1992

24. Barker SJ, Tremper KK, Hyatt J, Zaccari J: Effects of methemoglobinemia on pulse oximetry and mixed venous oximetry. Anesthesiology 70:112, 1989

25. Conley CL: Hereditary persistence of fetal hemoglobin. Blood 21:261, 1962

26. Pologe JA, Raley DM: Effects of fetal hemoglobin on pulse oximetry. J Perinatol 7:324, 1987

27. Anderson JV: The accuracy of pulse oximetry in neonates: effects of fetal hemoglobin and bilirubin. J Perinatol 7:323, 1987

28. Cornelissne PJH, van Woensel CLM, van Del WC, de Jong PA: Correction factors for hemoglobin derivatives in fetal blood as measured with the IL 282 Co-Oximeter. Clin Chem 29:1555, 1983

29. Kessler MR, Eide T, Humayun B, Poppers PJ: Spurious pulse oximeter desaturation with methylene blue unjection. Anesthesiology 65:435, 1986

30. Operator's manual IL 282 Co-Oximeter 79282. Instrumentation Laboratory, Lexington, MA, 1977

31. Eisenkraft JB: Methylene blue and pulse oximetry readings: spriouser and spuriouser! Anesthesiology 68:171, 1988

32. Unger RJ, Scheller MS: More on dyes and pulse oximeters. Anesthesiology 67:149, 1987

33. Scheller MS, Unger RJ, Kelner MJ: Effect of intravenously administered dyes on pulse oximetry readings. Anesthesiology 65:550, 1986

34. Payne JP, Severinghaus JW: Pulse oximetry. Springer-Verlag, Dorchester, UK, 192, 1986

35. Ezri T, Szmuk P: Pulse oximeters and onychomycosis. Anesthesiology 76:153, 1992

36. Gabrielczyk MR, Buist RJ: Pulse oximetry and postoperative hypothermia. Anaesthesia 43:402, 1988

37. Emery JR: Skin pigmentation as an influence on the accuracy of pulse oximetry. J Perinatol 7:329, 1987

38. Ries AL, Prewitt LM, Johnson JJ: Skin color and ear oximetry. Chest 96:287, 1989

39. Rubin AS: Nail polish color can affect pulse oximeter saturation. Anesthesiology 68:825, 1988

40. Coté CJ, Goldstein EA, Fuchsman WH, Hoaglin DJ: The effect of nail polish on pulse oximetry. Anesth Analg 67:683, 1988

41. Hanowell L, Eisele JH, Downs D: Ambient light affects pulse oximeters. Anesthesiology 67:864, 1987

42. Costarino AT, Davis DA, Keon TP: Falsely normal saturation reading with the pulse oximeter. Anesthesiology 67:830, 1987

43. Brooks TD, Paulus DA, Winkel WE: Infrared heat lamps interfere with pulse oximeters. Anesthesiology 61:630, 1984

44. Block FE: Interference in a pulse oximeter from a fiberoptic light source. J Clin Monit 3:210, 1987

45. Wukitsch MW, Tobler D, Pologe J, Petterson M: Pulse oximetry: an analysis of theory, technology and practice. J Clin Monit 4:290, 1988

46. Dawalibi L, Rozario C: Pulse oximetry in pulseless patients. Anaesthesia 46:990, 1991

47. Stewart KG, Rowbottom SJ: Inaccuracy of pulse oximetry in patients with severe tricuspid regurgitation. Anaesthesia 46:668, 1991

48. Smith TC: Intra-aortic balloon pumps and the pulse oximeter. Anesthesia 47:1010, 1992

49. Palve H, Vuori A: Accuracy of three pulse oximeters at low cardiac index and peripheral temperature. Crit Care Med 19:560, 1990

50. Clayton DG, Webb RK, Ralston AC et al: A comparison of the performance of 20 pulse oximeters under conditions of poor perfusion. Anaesthesia 46:3, 1991

51. Langton JA, Lassey D, Hanning CD: Comparison of four pulse oximeters: effects of venous occlusion and cold-induced peripheral vasoconstriction. Br J Anaesth 65:245, 1990

52. Al Khudhairi D, Prabhu R, el Sharkawy M, Burtles R: Evaluation of a pulse oximeter during profound hypothermia: an assessment of the Biox 3700 dur-

ing induction of hypothermia before cardiac surgery in paediatric patients. Int J Clin Monit Comput 7:217, 1990

53. Wilkins CJ, Moores M, Hanning CD: Comparison of pulse oximeters: effects of vasoconstriction and venous engorgement. Br J Anaesth 62:439, 1989

54. Tremper KK, Hufstedler S, Barker SJ, Adams AL: Accuracy of a pulse oximeter in the critically ill adult: effect of temperature and hemodynamics. Anesthesiology 63:A175, 1985

55. Bourke DL, Grayson RF: Digital nerve blocks can restore pulse oximeter signal detection. Anesth Analg 73:815, 1991

56. Falconer RJ, Robinson BJ: Comparison of pulse oximeters: accuracy at low arterial pressure in volunteers. Br J Anaesth 65:552, 1990

57. Severinghaus JW, Spellman MJ Jr: Pulse oximeter failure thresholds in hypotension and ischemia. Anesthesiology 73:532, 1990

58. Graham B, Paulus DA, Caffee HH: Pulse oximetry for vascular monitoring in upper extremity replantation surgery. J Hand Surg 11A:687, 1986

59. Ferrara JJ, Dyess DL, Lasecki M et al: Surface oximetry: a new method to evaluate intestinal perfusion. Am Surg 54:10, 1988.

60. McCleane G, Carragher AM, Bateson PG: Assessment of bowel viability using pulse oximetry. J R Coll Surg Edinb 35:388, 1990

61. Pillow K, Herrick IA: Pulse oximetry compared with Doppler ultrasound for assessment of collateral blood flow to the hand. Anaesthesia 46:388, 1991

62. Glavin RJ, Jones HM: Assessing collateral circulation in the hand: four methods compared. Anaesthesia 44:594, 1989

63. Lawson D, Norley I, Korbon G et al: Blood flow limits and pulse oximeter signal detection. Anesthesiology 67:599, 1987

64. Tremper KK, Barker SJ: Pulse oximetry. Anesthesiology 70:98, 1989

65. Severinghaus JW, Kelleher JF: Recent developments in pulse oximetry. Anesthesiology 76:1018, 1992

66. James MR, Marshall H, Carew-McColl M: Pulse oximetry during apparent tonic-clonic seizures. Lancet 337:394, 1991

67. Talke P, Nichols RJ, Traber DL: Monitoring patients during helicopter flight. J Clin Monit 6:139, 1990

68. Short L, Hecker RB, Middaugh RE, Menk EJ: A comparison of pulse oximeters during helicopter flight. J Emerg Med 7:639, 1989

69. Wilson S: Conscious sedation and pulse oximetry: false alarms. Pediatr Dent 12:223, 1990

70. Moorthy SS, Dierdorf SF, Schmidt SI: Erroneous pulse oximeter data during CPR. Anesth Analg 70:339, 1990

71. Pan PH, James CF: Effects of default alarm limit settings on alarm distribution in telemetric pulse oximetry network in ward setting. Anesthesiology 75:A405, 1991

72. Kelleher JF: Pulse oximetry. J Clin Monit 5:37, 1989

73. Block FE, Detko GJ: Minimizing interference and flase alarms from electrocautery in the Nellcor N-100 pulse oximeter. J Clin Monit 2:203, 1986

74. Waggle WA: Technique for RF isolation of a pulse oximeter in a 1.5-T MR unit. AJNR 10:208, 1989

75. Shellock FG, Slimp GL: Severe burn of the finger caused by using a pulse oximeter during MR imaging. AJR 153:1105, 1989

76. Bashein G, Syrory G: Burns associated with pulse oximetry during magnetic resonance imaging. Anesthesiology 75:382, 1991

77. Bland JM, Altman DG: Statistical methods for assessing agreement between two methods of clinical measurement. Lancet 1:307, 1986

78. Moller JT, Pedersen T, Rasmussen LS et al: Randomized evaluation of pulse oximetry in 20,802 patients: I. Design, demography, pulse oximetry failure rate, and overall complication rate. Anesthesiology 78:436, 1993

79. Moller JT, Johannessen NW, Espersen K et al: Randomized evaluation of pulse oximetry in 20,802 patients: II. Perioperative events and postoperative complications. Anesthesiology 78:445, 1993

80. Hannhart B, Haberer JP, Saunier C, Laxennaire MC: Accuracy and precision of fourteen pulse oximeters. Sur Respir J 4:115, 1991

81. Lebecque P, Shango P, Stijns M et al: Pulse oximetry versus measured arterial oxygen saturation: a comparison of the Nellcor N100 and the Biox III. Pediatr Pulmonol 10:132, 1991

82. Hannhart B, Michalski H, Delorme N et al: Reliability of six pulse oximeters in chronic obstructive pulmonary disease. Chest 99:842, 1991

83. Severinghaus JW, Naifeh KH, Koh SO: Errors in 14 pulse oximeters during profound hypoxia. J Clin Monit 5:72, 1989

84. Young D, Jewkes C, Spittal M et al: Response time of pulse oximeters assessed using acute decompression. Anesth Analg 74:189, 1992

85. Broome IJ, Harris RW, Reilly CS: The response times during anaesthesia of pulse oximeters measuring oxygen saturations during hypoxaemic events. Anaesthesia 47:17, 1992

86. Severinghaus JW, Koh SO: Effect of anemia on pulse oximeter accuracy at low saturation. J Clin Monit 6:85, 1990

87. Lee S, Tremper KK, Barker SJ: Effects of anemia on pulse oximetry and continuous mixed venous hemoglobin saturation monitoring in dogs. Anesthesiology 75:118, 1991

88. Elling A, Hanning CD: Oxygenation during pre-operative transportation. p. 161. In Payne JP, Severinghaus JW (eds): Pulse oximetry. Springer-Verlag, Dorchester, UK, 1986

89. Marjot R, Valentine SJ: Arterial oxygen saturation following premedication for cardiac surgery. Br J Anaesth 64:737, 1990

90. Coté CJ, Goldstein EA, Coté MA et al: A single blind study of pulse oximetry in children. Anesthesiology 68:184, 1988

91. Coté CJ, Rolf N, Liu LM et al: A single-blind study of combined pulse oximetry and capnography in children. Anesthesiology 74:980, 1991

92. Raemer DB, Warren DL, Morris R et al: Hypoxemia during ambulatory gynecologic surgery as evaluated by the pulse oximeter. J Clin Monit 3:244, 1987

93. McKay WPS, Noble WH: Critical incidents detected by pulse oximetry during anaesthesia. Can J Anaesth 35:265, 1988

94. Cooper JB, Cullen DJ, Nemeskal R et al: Effects of information feedback and pulse oximetry on the incidence of anesthesia complications. Anesthesiology 67:686, 1987

95. Mihm FG, Halperin DH: Noninvasive detection of profound arterial desaturations using pulse oximetry device. Anesthesiology 62:85, 1985.

96. Viitanen A, Salmenpera M, Heinonen J: Noninvasive monitoring of oxygenation during one-lung ventilation: a comparison of transcutaneous oxygen tension measurement and pulse oximetry. J Clin Monit 3:90, 1987

97. Brodsky JB, Shulman MS, Swan M, Mark JBD: Pulse oximetry during one-lung ventilation. Anesthesiology 63:212, 1985

98. Barker SJ, Tremper KK, Hyatt J, Heitzmann H: Comparison of three oxygen monitors in detecting endobronchial intubation. J Clin Monit 4:240, 1988

99. Kurki T, Smith NT, Sanford T, Head N: Pulse oximetry and finger blood pressure measurement during open heart surgery. Anesth Analg 67:S123, 1988

100. Stow PJ, Burrows FA, Lerman J, Roy WL: Arterial oxygen saturation following premedication in children with cyanotic congenital heart disease. Can J Anaesth 35:63, 1988

101. Boxer RA, Gottesfeld I, Singh S et al: Noninvasive pulse oximetry in children with cyanotic congenital heart disease. Crit Care Med 15:1062, 1987

102. Tyler IL, Tantisira B, Winter PM, Motoyama EK: Continuous monitoring of arterial oxygen saturation with pulse oximetry during transfer to the recovery room. Anesth Analg 64:1108, 1984

103. Blair I, Holland R, Lau W et al: Oxygen saturation during transfer from operative room to recovery after anaesthesia. Anaesth Inten Care 15:147, 1987

104. Laycock GJ, McNicol LR. Hypoxaemia during re-covery from anaesthesia: an audit of children after general anaesthesia for routine elective surgery. Anaesthesia 43:985, 1988

105. Smith DC, Canning JJ, Crul JF: Pulse oximetry in the recovery room. Anaesthesia 44:345, 1989

106. Morris RW, Buschman A, Warren DL et al: The prevalence of hypoxemia detected by pulse oximetry during recovery from anesthesia. J Clin Monit 4:16, 1988

107. Reeder MK, Goldman MD, Loh L et al: Late post-operative nocturnal dips in oxygen saturation in patients undergoing major abdominal vascular surgery. Anaesthesia 47:110, 1992

108. Rotello LC, Warren J, Jastremski MS, Milewski A: A nurse-directed protocol using pulse oximetry to wean mechanically ventilated patients from toxic oxygen concentrations. Chest 102:1833, 1992

109. Withington DE, Ramsay JG, Saoud AT, Bilodeau J: Weaning from ventilation after cardiopulmonary bypass: evaluation of a non-invasive technique. Can J Anaesth 38:15, 1991

110. Moore FA, Haenel JB, Moore EE, Abernathy CM: Hypoxic events in the surgical intensive care unit. Am J Surg 160:647, 1990

111. Bierman MI, Stein KL, Synder JV: Pulse oximetry in the postoperative care of cardiac surgical patients. Chest 102:1367, 1992

112. Fanconi S, Doherty P, Edmonds JF et al: Pulse oximetry in pediatric intensive care: comparison with measured saturations and transcutaneous oxygen tension. J Pediatr 107:362, 1985

113. Fait CD, Wetzel RC, Dean JM et al: Pulse oximetry in critically ill children. J Clin Monit 1:232, 1985

114. Pope LL, Hankins GDV: Pulse oximetry: application in the labor-and delivery unit of a tertiary care center. J Reprod 36:853, 1991

115. Minnich ME, Brown M, Clark RB et al: Oxygen desaturation in women in labor. J Reprod Med 35:693, 1990

116. Porter KB, O'Brien WF, Kiefert V, Knuppel RA: Evaluation of oxygen desaturation events in singleton pregnancies. J Perinatol 12:103, 1992

117. Deckardt R, Fembacher PM, Schneider KTM, Graeff H: Maternal arterial oxygen saturation during labor and delivery: pain-dependent alterations and effects on the newborn. Obstet Gynecol 70:21, 1987

118. Quance D: Amniotic fluid embolism: detection by pulse oximetry. Anesthesiology 68:951, 1988

119. Calvin S, Jones OW, Knieriem K, Weinstein L: Oxygen saturation in the supine hypotensive syndrome. Obstet Gynecol 71:872, 1988

120. Johnson N, Johnson VA, Bannister J, Lilford RJ: The accuracy of fetal pulse oximetry in the second stage of labour. J Perinatol 19:297, 1991

121. Gardosi JO, Schram CM, Symonds EM: Adaptation of pulse oximetry for fetal monitoring during labour. Lancet 337:1265, 1991

122. Durand M, Ramanathan R: Pulse oximetry for continuous oxygen monitoring in sick newborn infants. J Pediatr 109:1052, 1986

123. Dimich I, Singh PP, Adell A et al: Clinical investigation: evaluation of oxygen saturation monitoring by pulse oximetry in neonates in the delivery system. Can J Anaesth 38:985, 1991

124. Sendak MJ, Harris AP, Donham RT: Use of pulse oximetry to assess arterial oxygen saturation during newborn resuscitation. Crit Care Med 14:739, 1986

125. House JT, Schultheis RR, Gravenstein N: Continuous neonatal evaluation in the delivery room by pulse oximetry. J Clin Monit 3:96, 1987

126. Dodson SR, Hensley FA, Martin DE et al: Continuous oxygen saturation monitoring during cardiac catheterization in adults. Chest 94:28, 1988

127. Lynn AM, Bosenberg A: Pulse oximetry during cardiac catheterization in children with congenital heart disease. J Clin Monit 2:230, 1986

128. Shellock FG, Myers SM, Kimble KJ: Monitoring heart rate and oxygen saturation with a fiber-optic pulse oximeter during MR imaging. AJR 158:663, 1992

129. Schnapf BM: Oxygen desaturation during fiberoptic bronchoscopy in pediatric patients. Chest 99:591, 1991

130. O'Connor KW, Jones S: Oxygen desaturation is common and clinically underappreciated during elective endoscopic procedures. Gastrointest Endosc 36(Suppl.):S2-S4, 1990

131. Bell GD, McCloy RF, Charlton JE et al: Recommendations for standards of sedation and patient monitoring during gastrointestinal endoscopy. Gut 32:823, 1991

132. Cydulka RK, Shade B, Emerman CL et al: Prehospital pulse oximetry: useful or misused? Ann Emerg Med 21:675, 1992

133. Aughey K, Hess D, Eitel D et al: An evaluation of pulse oximetry in prehospital care. Ann Emerg Med 20:887, 1991

134. Jones J, Heiselman D, Cannon L, Gradisek R: Continuous emergency department monitoring of arterial saturation in adult patients with respiratory distress. Ann Emerg Med 17:463, 1988

135. Yamamoto LG, Wiebe RA, Anaya C et al: Pulse oximetry and peak flow as indicators of wheezing severity in children and the improvement following bronchodilator treatments. Am J Emerg Med 10:519, 1992

136. Wright SW: Conscious sedation in the emergency department: the value of capnography and pulse oximetry. Ann Emerg Med 21:551, 1992

137. Narang VPS: Utility of the pulse oximeter during cardiopulmonary resuscitation. Anesthesiology 65:239, 1986.

138. King T, Simon RH: Pulse oximetry for tapering supplemental oxygen in hospitalized patients: evaluation of a protocol. Chest 92:713, 1987

139. Prakash O: Oximetry in the weaning of the ventilator patient. p 119. In Payne JP, Severinghaus JW (eds): Pulse oximetry. Springer-Verlag, Dorchester, UK, 1986

140. Jubran A, Tobin MJ: Reliability of pulse oximetry in titrating supplemental oxygen therapy in ventilatory-dependent patients. Chest 97:1420, 1990

141. Choi HJ, Little MS, Fujita RA et al: Pulse oximetry for monitoring during ward analgesia: epidural morphine versus parenteral narcotics, abstracted. Anesthesiology 65:A371, 1986

142. Anderson JA, Kafer ER: Evaluation of the accuracy of four pulse oximeters during outpatient dental anesthesia, abstracted. Anesth Analg 67:S2, 1988

143. Hardeman JH, Sabol SR, Goldwasser MS: Incidence of hypoxemia in the postanesthetic recovery room inpatients having undergone intravenous sedation for outpatient oral surgery. J Oral Maxillofac Surg 48:942, 1990

144. Golding-Wood DG, Brockbank MJ et al: Assessment of chronic snorers. J R Soc Med 83:363, 1990

145. Williams AJ, Yu G, Santiago S, Stein M: Screening for sleep apnea using pulse oximetry and a clinical score. Chest 100:631, 1991

146. Adams LP, Foret MD: Monitoring oxygen saturation levels in patients undergoing long-term home oxygen therapy using a portable oximeter. p 179. In Payne JP, Severinghaus JW (eds): Pulse oximetry. Springer-Verlag, Dorchester, UK, 1986

147. Tiep BL: Long-term home oxygen therapy. Clin Chest Med 11:505, 1990

148. Montgomery M, Wiebicke W, Bibi H et al: Home measurement of oxygen saturation during sleep in patients with cystic fibrosis. Pediatr Pulmonol 7:29, 1989

149. Poets CF, Samuels MP, Noyes JP et al: Home monitoring of transcutaneous oxygen tension in the early detection of hypoxaemia in infants and young children. Arch Dis Child 66:676, 1991

150. Jacobson JD, Miller MW, Matthews NS et al: Evaluation of accuracy of pulse oximeter in dogs. Am J Vet Res 53:537, 1992

151. Schmotzer WB, Riebold TW, Rowe KE, Scott EA: Steady-state response characteristics of a pulse oximeter on equine intestine. Am J Vet Res 52:619, 1991

152. Cunningham MD, Shook LA, Tomazic T: Clinical experience with pulse oximetry in managing oxygen therapy in neonatal intensive care. J. Perinatol 7:333, 1987

153. Dear PRF: Monitoring oxygen in the newborn: saturation or partial pressure. Arch Dis Child 62:879, 1987

154. Fanconi S: Pulse oximetry and transcutaneous oxygen tension for detection of hypoxemia in critically ill infants and children. Adv Exp Med Biol 220:159, 1987

155. Deckardt R, Steward DJ: Noninvasive arterial hemoglobin saturation versus transcutaneous oxygen tension monitoring in the preterm infant. Crit Care Med 12:935, 1984

156. Baeckert P, Bucher HU, Fallenstein F et al: Is pulse oximetry reliable in detecting hyperoxemia in the neonate? Adv Exp Med Biol 220:165, 1987

157. Bossi E, Meister B, Pfenninger J: Comparison between transcutaneous PO_2 and pulse oximetry for monitoring O_2 treatment in neonates. Adv Exp Med Biol 220:171, 1987

158. Peabody JL, Jennis MS, Emergy JR: Pulse oximetry: an alternative to transcutaneous PO_2 in sick newborns. Adv Exp Med Biol 220:145, 1987

159. Hay WW, Brockway J, Eyzaguirre M: Application of the Ohmeda Biox 3700 pulse oximeter to neonatal oxygen monitoring. Adv Exp Med Biol 220:151, 1987

160. Ray SA, Ivory JP, Beavis JP: Use of pulse oximetry during manipulation of supracondylar fractures of the humerus. Injury 22:103, 1991

161. Agel J, Levy IM: The use of a pulse oximeter for the monitoring of digital pulse during shoulder arthroscopy. Arthroscopy 4:124, 1988

162. Lindsey LA, Watson JD, Quaba AA: Pulse oximetry in postoperative monitoring of free muscle flaps. Br J Plast Surg 44:27, 1991

163. Nowak GS, Moorthy SS, McNiece WL: Use of pulse oximetry for assessment of collateral arterial flow. Anesthesiology 64:527, 1986

164. Rosenberg B, Rosenberg M, Birkhan J: Allen's test performed by the pulse oximeter. Anaesthesia 43:515, 1988

165. Stolar CJH, Randolph JG: Evaluation of ischemic bowel viability with a fluorescent technique. J Pediatr Surg 13:221, 1978

166. Skeehan TM, Hensley FA Jr: Axillary artery compression and the prone position. Anesth Analg 65:518, 1986

167. Hovagim AR, Backus WW, Manecke G et al: Pulse oximetry and patient positioning: a report of eight cases. Anesthesiology 71:454, 1989.

168. Partridge BL: Use of pulse oximetry as a noninvasive indicator of intravascular volume status. J Clin Minit 3:263, 1987

169. Wallace CT, Baker JD, Alpert CC et al: Comparison of blood pressure measurement by Doppler and by pulse oximetry techniques. Anesth Analg 66:1018, 1987

170. Talke PO: Measurement of systolic blood pressure using pulse oximetry during helicopter flight. Crit Care Med 19:934, 1991

171. Chalwa Rajiv, Kumarvel V et al: Can pulse oximetry be used to measure systolic blood pressure? Anesth Analg 74:196, 1992

172. Broome IJ, Mason RA: Identification of autonomic dysfunction with a pulse oximeter. Anaesthesia 43:833, 1988

173. Lunn JN, Devlin HR: Lessons from the confidential inquiry into postoperative deaths in three NHS regions. Lancet 2:1384, 1987

174. Duncan PG, Cohen MM: Pulse oximetry and capnography in anaesthetic practice: an epidemiological appraisal. Can J Anaesth 38:619, 1991

175. Orkin FK, Cohen MM, Duncan PG: The quest for meaningful outcomes. Anesthesiology 78:417, 1993

176. Eichhorn JH: Prevention of intraoperative anesthesia accidents and related severe injury through safety monitoring. Anesthesiology 7:572, 1989

177. Cheney FW: The ASA closed claims study after the pulse oximeter: a preliminary look. ASA Newslett 54:10, 1990

178. Zierler S: Causes of retinopathy of prematurity: an epidemiologic perspective. Birth Defects 24:23, 1988

179. Pettersen B, Kongsgaard U, Aune H: Skin injury in an infant with pulse oximetry. Br J Anaesth 69:204, 1992

180. Sobel DB. Burning of a neonate due to a pulse oximeter: arterial saturation monitoring. Pediatrics 89:154, 1992

181. Sloan TB. Finger injury by an oxygen saturation probe. Anesthesiology 8:936, 1988

182. Murphy KG, Secunda JA, Rockoff MA: Severe burns from a pulse oximeter. Anesthesiology 73:350, 1990

183. Rubin MM, Ford HC, Sadoff RS: Digital injury from a pulse oximeter probe. J Oral Maxillofac Surg 49:301, 1991

184. Takatani S, Davies C, Sakakibara N et al: Experimental and clinical evaluation of a noninvasive reflectance pulse oximeter sensor. J Clin Monit 8:257, 1992

185. Palve H: Comparison of reflection and transmission pulse oximetry after open-heart surgery. Crit Care Med 20:48, 1992

186. Palve H: Reflection and transmission pulse oximetry during compromised peripheral perfusion. J Clin Monit 8:12, 1992

187. Mendelson Y, Solomita MV: The feasibility of spectrophotometric measurements of arterial oxygen saturation from the fetal scalp utilizing noninvasive skin-reflectance pulse oximetry. Biomed Instrum Technol 26:215, 1992

Blood Gas Monitoring *15*

Jeffery S. Vender
Hugh C. Gilbert

Monitoring arterial and venous blood gases has become an essential aspect of anesthesia and critical care. Blood gas determinations play an important role in diagnosing potentially life-threatening derangements in acid-base balance, oxygenation, and ventilation. Since the mid-1960s, serial blood gas determinations have assumed a central role in evaluating cardiopulmonary homeostasis and monitoring the effectiveness of treatment regimens designed for the restoration of cardiopulmonary homeostasis. This chapter reviews the technologic evolution of modern blood gas analysis and the clinical application of monitoring hydrogen ion content (pH), blood oxygen tension (PO_2), and carbon dioxide tension (PCO_2).

Prior to the development of the modern acid-base laboratory (defined as integrated equipment for measuring "blood gases") monitoring of cardiopulmonary homeostasis was difficult. Volumetric and manometric determinations of the "gas" contents of blood were the only laboratory methods available until the early 1960s when electrode systems were designed to replace these cumbersome and difficult physical methods.

One example of such a methodology based on the principles of physical chemistry is the Van Slyke technique. This laboratory procedure employs an acid-saponin-ferricyanide solution that hemolyzes the red blood cells, liberates oxygen (O_2), carbon dioxide (CO_2), and converts all hemoglobin (Hb) to methemoglobin. The CO_2 is absorbed by sodium hydroxide and the O_2 by sodium hydrosulfite.[1] With each absorption the change in the volume of gas liberated is recorded and the partial pressure of the respective gases calculated. The time and skill required for accurate gas analysis using

this approach restricts its utility to research laboratories.

Automation of "blood gas" measurements occurred as a result of the development of three specific electrodes; the glass pH electrode (Sanz Electrode),[2] the PCO_2 electrode (Severinghuas[3]), and the PO_2 electrode (Clark)[4]

ELECTRODE METHODOLOGY

pH-Specific Electrode

Since the 1960s the most common system employed for measuring arterial blood gases has utilized specialized electrochemical sensors. Understanding how electrodes are used to measure pH and PCO_2 requires a basic knowledge of electricity, ionization potentials, and the chemical reaction which occurs when a metal is placed into a solution containing its salts. The following is a condensed description of the physical principles of electrodes which enable them to perform as electrochemical sensors. A more detailed description is available elsewhere.[5]

All sources of electrical current are capable of creating a separation of positive and negative charges at their terminals. It is the attraction between these charges which results in current flow. The strength of the electrical "pump" which drives the current defines the electromotive force (EMF). Electric current is measured in coulombs (C) per second. The work required to "pump" the electricity can also be measured. In this discussion, current will be defined by the term ampere (1 mA = .001 C/s) and the strength of the EMF is defined by the voltage. Thus a circuit requiring 100 J/C (a joule is a unit of work), would have an EMF of 100. Likewise, a 6-V battery has the potential to do 6 J of work when it pumps a coulomb every second. When electrons or ions are "pumped" through a material under the action of an EMF, the material becomes heated permitting the passage of electrons or ions. Ohm's law describes the restriction of current from an EMF where amperes = volts/resistence. Resistence is measured in ohms where 1 ohm = 1 V/A.

Consider the reaction resulting when metal ions go into solution leaving electrons on their surface. A potential difference between the metal surface and the solution creates a small EMF. The resulting EMF can be measured when two such "half-cells" are interconnected. This technology is incorporated into the pH-specific electrode. The pH-specific electrode quantifies pH by measuring the potential difference between two solutions of differing pH's, which are separated by a thin glass membrane. The pH-selective glass contains oxides of silicone, lithium, and calcium. Hydrogen ions in the unknown solution displace the metal cations from the glass matrix creating an EMF when connected to another "half-cell," the reference electrode. The reference electrode usually consists of mercury beads suspended in mercurous chloride (Hg_2Cl_2 or Calomel). A saturated KCl solution surrounds the reference electrode thereby completing the electrolytic circuit.

An electrolytic circuit ensures uniformity in junction potentials and permits miniaturization. pH electrodes are designed to respond to a change in an EMF of a system where the only variable is the EMF generated at the surface of the glass electrode. The EMF of the glass electrode can be calculated using a modification of the Nernst equation:

$$V = RT/F \log (H + sample/H + known),$$

where R and F are constants and T refers to the absolute temperature. At 37°C, a properly functioning pH electrode system will register a 61.5 mV change for each pH unit difference between a known buffer solution containing the silver/silver chloride metal pair and the unknown blood sample.[6] Figure 15-1A characterizes the components of a pH electrode system. The limits of accuracy of pH-selective glass electrodes is ±0.02 pH units.[7] Modern blood gas analyzers control the temperature of the glass and the reference electrodes at 37 ± 0.1°C.

Carbon Dioxide Electrode

The carbon dioxide electrode (P_{CO_2} electrode) uses the same technology as the pH electrode to measure the partial pressure of CO_2 in a blood sample. CO_2 electrodes have the following modifications[3]:

1. A CO_2 permeable membrane separates the sample, e.g., Teflon
2. A buffer solution of $NaHCO_3$ and NaCl resides on the sample side of a glass pH electrode.

Figure 15-1B depicts the components of a typical Severinghaus electrode. This drawing demonstrates how the electrochemical sensor can be designed to fit into a sample chamber containing a blood sample.

Teflon permits only uncharged molecules to pass through it. Dissolved CO_2 from the blood sample diffuses into the bicarbonate electrolyte solution and equilibrates. Therefore, the pH of the bicarbonate solution changes in proportion to the partial pressure of the CO_2 that drives membrane transport. In the electrolyte buffer, the following chemical reaction occurs:

$$H_2O + CO_2 \rightarrow H_2CO_2 \rightarrow H^+ + HCO_3^-.$$

Using the Henderson-Hasselbalch equation the relationship between pH and P_{CO_2} can be defined:

$$\frac{pH = pK_a + \log (HCO_3^-)}{P_{CO_2} \times solubility\ coefficient\ (CO_2).}$$

In a properly functioning pH electrode system, the electrode potential (EP) = E_0 + 61.5 × pH sample. Therefore, if a linear relationship between P_{CO_2} and pH is assumed:

$$EP = E_0\ (P_{CO_2} = 40)\ -61.5\ (\log P_{CO_2} - \log 40).$$

The Clark Electrode (P_{O_2})

The P_{O_2} electrode system measures the partial pressure of oxygen in the blood sample and is often referred to as a Clark electrode.[4] The oxygen electrode is based upon the oxidation-reduction reaction of dissolved oxygen and water, where

$$O_2 + 4\ electrons\ (e^-) \rightarrow 2O^{2-} \quad (platinum\ cathode)$$

$$2O^{2-} + 2H_2O \rightarrow 4\ OH^-$$

This reaction takes place at a platinum cathode. The electrons are produced when a silver wire is

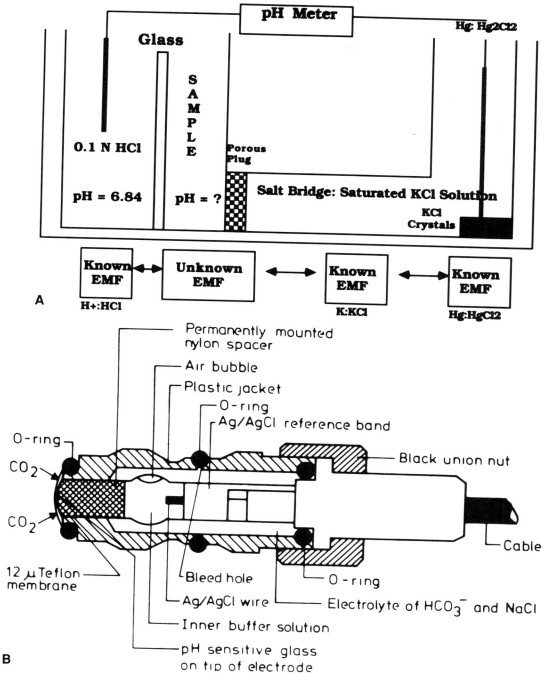

A

Known EMF ⟷ Unknown EMF ⟷ Known EMF ⟷ Known EMF
H+:HCl   K:KCl   Hg:HgCl2

B

Permanently mounted nylon spacer
Air bubble
Plastic jacket
O-ring
Ag/AgCl reference band
Black union nut
O-ring
CO2
CO2
Cable
12 μ Teflon membrane
Bleed hole
O-ring
Ag/AgCl wire
Electrolyte of HCO_3^- and NaCl
Inner buffer solution
pH sensitive glass on tip of electrode

Fig. 15-1. **(A)** The components of a pH electrode. The variables of the system are temperature and pH of the sample. The electrochemical sensor measures the change in electromotive force (EMF), which is proportional to the difference in pH between the sample and the known buffer solution, labeled pH = 6.84. The actual voltage change results from an ion exchange at the surface of the glass. If both buffer and sample contain the same concentration of H^+, then the potential difference across the glass is zero. The equation that characterizes the voltage difference across a glass pH electrode is $E = E_0 + 61.5 \times pH$ (sample), where E_0 = standard potential in millivolts. The theoretical electrode sensitivity at 37°C equals 61.5. **(B)** The components of a P_{CO_2} electrode in common usage for the last several decades. The electrode's specificity depends upon the integrity of the Teflon membrane, which is freely permeable to CO_2. The electrode snaps into a measuring chamber located in the wet section of a blood gas analyzer. (*Figure continues.*)

placed in a potassium chloride solution. Silver chloride is produced at the anode resulting in a constant flow of electrons. Dr. Clark incorporated both the platinum cathode and the reference electrode within a oxygen permeable membrane isolating the electrodes from the influence of plasma proteins. If a constant polarizing voltage (~630 mV) is applied there will always be an excess of electrons available at the platinum cathode to react with oxygen that diffuses across the oxygen permeable membrane. Unlike the pH and PCO_2 electrode systems, the O_2 electrode is polarized at a constant voltage. Under these circumstances the electrode current (I) is dependent on the reduction of oxygen at the platinum cathode:

$$I = S \times PO_2 + I_0$$

where S is the sensitivity and I_0 is the current in the electrode when $PO_2 = 0$. Figure 15-1C depicts the characteristics of a typical Clark electrode.

THE AUTOMATED BLOOD-GAS MACHINE

During the last twenty years, the most significant advance in *in vitro* blood gas analysis has been due to the miniaturization and automation of micro-

processor controlled instruments that simplify the process of blood gas measurements. The components of a blood gas machine often include

1. A gas mixer which produces calibrating gases containing known partial pressures of O_2 and CO_2.
2. A measurement section which contains valves, tubing, pumps, and heaters that transport the sample under controlled conditions to the electrode bank where the measurements are made.
3. A rinsing section containing the maintenance solutions and transport tubing that refreshes the electrode bank following each measurement.
4. An electronics section that monitors the other components, controls the movement of gases and liquids, initiates calibrations, performs diagnostic testing, and prints a report of results of analysis and status of the instrument functions.

Figure 15-2 represents a schematic drawing of the measurement section of the ABL4 acid base laboratory (Radiometer Copenhagen, Copenhagen, Denmark). This instrument is representative of instruments in common use today. When functioning properly, automated blood gas analyzers self-calibrate using a two-point (high and low) check.

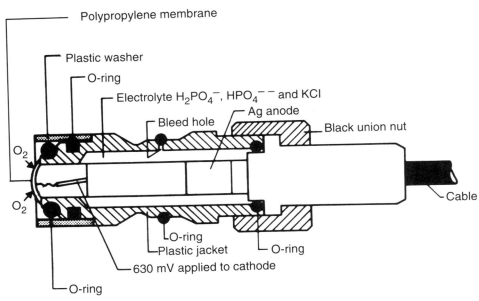

Fig. 15-1. (*Continued*). (**C**) The components of a PO_2 electrode. A polypropylene membrane permits oxygen to equilibrate from the sample chamber and react with water at the platinum cathode. The greater the concentration of oxygen in the electrolyte solution in the electrode, the greater the current measured. (Figs. B and C from Radiometer America Inc., Westlake, Ohio, with permission.)

The exact values of the calibration solutions are calculated electronically using the barometric pressure (BP), and the gas percentages. The ABL4 contains two bubble towers where the premixed gases are heated, humidified and equilibrated with standard solutions of bicarbonate and phosphate buffers. When the barometric pressure and the percentage of CO_2 in the gas mixtures is known, the pH of the solutions can be calculated. The PCO_2 is calculated using the formula:

$$\frac{PCO_2 = \text{barometric pressure} - P_{H_2O}}{100 \times CO_2\%.}$$

The PO_2 electrode is zeroed electronically and than calibrated using a gas mixture of air containing 5.61 percent CO_2. The PO_2 is calculated to establish a single standard PCO_2 using the above gas equation where

$$\frac{PO_2 = \text{barometric pressure} - CO_2\%}{100 \times 20.93\% \text{ (air)}.}$$

Modern blood gas analyzers (BGAs) have the capability of initiating calibration sequences automatically at preprogrammed intervals. The exact values for the calibration (theoretical values) of the standard solutions are then compared to the measured values. On startup, BGAs perform a complete diagnostic check and calibration. During continued usage, it is essential to monitor the performance of the electrode bank. Electrode drift is constantly monitored by comparing the difference between the values measured in the current calibrating sequence to the calculated values.

Normal Values for pH, $PaCO_2$ and PaO_2

Normal values are determined by performing a great many measurements in a representative population and determining the range of values that would include 95 percent (2 standard deviations) of the sampled population.[8] Table 15-1 lists the normal values (healthy volunteers) for pH and PCO_2

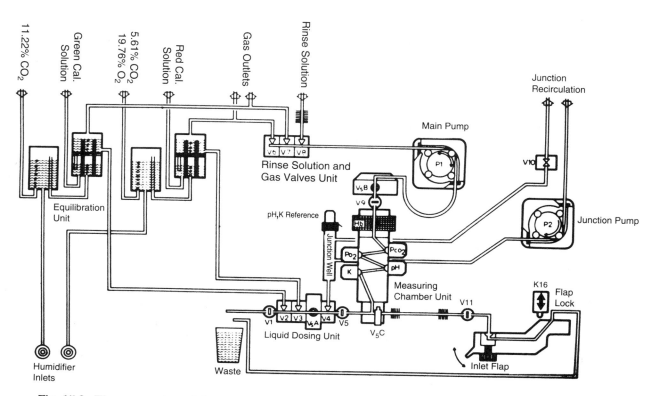

Fig. 15-2. The wet section of the ABL4 Blood Gas Analyzer—the transport system utilized in early blood gas analyzers. New systems eliminate operator contact with medical waste, reduce the sample size, automate diagnostics, and simplify operations.

that are universally accepted for arterial blood samples.

The normal value for PaO$_2$ in healthy adults breathing 21 percent oxygen (air) at sea level is 97 mmHg.[9] Since many factors influence the PaO$_2$, it is necessary to establish the lowest clinically acceptable value of PO$_2$ for various patient populations. Hypoxemia has been defined as an arterial PO$_2$ less than 80 mmHg at sea level in an adult breathing 21 per cent oxygen.[6] Table 15-2 lists the clinically acceptable arterial oxygen tensions based on age.

Clinicians often must decide when to institute measures to augment respiratory function based on the assessment of arterial blood gas measurements. Seriously ill patients often have acid-base, ventilatory, and/or abnormalities of oxygenation which necessitate accurate and frequent arterial blood gas monitoring. Errors in sampling, transport, or analysis may effect the accuracy of the measurements thereby misguiding therapy. The technique used to obtain samples can further interfere with the accuracy of the measurement.

Blood gas samples must be obtained under strict anaerobic conditions, be placed on ice and held at 0°C until analyzed. Blood sampling technique has also been found to influence the reliability of blood gas measurements, particularly the PO$_2$.[10] The presence of air bubbles can cause significant errors in PO$_2$ determinations.[11] Contamination within room air raises the PO$_2$ and lowers the PCO$_2$. The effect of room air contamination (PO$_2$ ~ 150, PCO$_2$ ~ 0) depends upon the physiologic conditions present at the time of sampling and oxygen delivery. Likewise, a properly iced sample reduces the possibility for errors based on the influence of the metabolically active white blood cells in the sample. Kelman and Nunn[12] found a significant effect when blood samples remained at body temperature. Blood gas samples are stable at room temperature for approximately 10 minutes. Thereafter, the samples should be placed in ice until measurement is performed. In addition, spontaneous changes in

TABLE 15-2. Acceptable Arterial Oxygen Tensions

Age	Sea Level Breathing Air (mmHg)
Newborn	40–70
Child	> 90 (expected to be 97)
20–60 y	>80 (expected to be 97)
60 y	> 80 (expected to be 97)
70 y	> 70
80 y	> 60
90 y	> 50
Hypoxemia for an Adult or Child is 80 mmHg or less	

(Modified from Shapiro et al.,[44] with permission.)

oxygen consumption, cardiac output, and systemic distribution of blood flow have been implicated as factors that may influence the variability of arterial blood gas values.[13]

The only suitable anticoagulant for blood gas sampling is neutral, isotonic sodium or lithium heparin. The heparin anticoagulant serves the following three purposes: (1) it prevents the clotting of the sample during transport and analysis, (2) it forms a liquid seal between the plunger and the syringe barrel preventing gas exchange between ambient air and the sample, and (3) it fills the dead space in the needle and syringe hub. Preservatives such as EDTA, citrate or oxalate affect of pH measurements as well. An appropriate amount of heparin is necessary to wet the surfaces of the sampling syringe and fills the dead space of the syringe and needle (0.05 to 0.1 ml per ml of blood sample).[14,15] However, an excessive volume of heparin can decrease the estimate of PCO$_2$ and air pressure introduced into the heparin vial and may also affect estimates of PO$_2$.[16]

CALCULATED PARAMETERS

The values for bicarbonate, standard bicarbonate, and base excess are calculated using equations based on the Henderson-Hasselbalch equation. Calculated parameters were formulated to identify the metabolic (e.g., fixed or related to renal function components) from the respiratory component (e.g., labile or related to PCO$_2$). The two most utilized of these parameters are actual bicarbonate, [HCO$_3^-$]p, and the base excess (BE). The actual bicarbonate represents the concentration of hydrogen carbonate in the plasma. If the pH and PCO$_2$

TABLE 15-1. Laboratory Normal Ranges for PaCO$_2$ and PaH

	Mean	1 SD	2 SD
PaCO$_2$	40 (mmHg)	38–42	35–45
PaH	7.40	7.38–7.42	7.35–7.45

are known, than the $[HCO_3^-]p$ can be calculated using the Henderson-Hasselbalch equation. The actual base excess is the difference in concentration of strong base in whole blood when the blood is titrated with strong acid (base excess) or base (base-deficient) to pH = 7.40 at PCO_2 of 40 mmHg at 37°C. Automated blood gas machines use an empirical formula that describes the Siggard-Andersen nomogram.[17] The $[HCO_3^-]p$ and BE are important components of the clinical interpretation of blood gas measurements.

STANDARDIZATION: AUDITING CONTROL

Legally blood gas laboratories are required to enroll in proficiency testing. Under the auspices of The Health Care Financing Administration (HCFA) and the Clinical Laboratories Improvement Act (CLIA) of 1988, blood gas laboratories (defined as BGAs and the technical support staff that maintain and perform the analysis) must enroll in an accredited proficiency testing program to ensure that measurements of pH and blood gases are accurate.[18] One such program is operated by the American Thoracic Society (ATS). The ATS Blood Gas Survey uses a fluorocarbon-containing emulsion manufactured by Instrumentation Laboratory (Artificial Blood Control, Lexington, MA). Samples are sent to all participating laboratories and the results from these laboratories are than compared. An instrument report is generated for each laboratory and a rating is assigned based on the statistical analysis of the ranges of values submitted by the participants. HCFA defines an acceptable performance for the analysis of a single analyte in one of the test ampules as:

TABLE 15-3. Temperature Effect on Normal Blood Values

	°C	°F	pH	PCO_2	PO_2
Hypothermia	25	77	7.58	24	37
	30	86	7.50	30	51
	35	95	7.43	37	70
	36	97	7.41	38	75
Euthermia	37	99	7.40	40	80
Hyperthermia	38	100	7.39	42	85
	39	102	7.37	45	97

(Modified from Shapiro et al.,[44] with permission.)

PO_2: target value ± SD
PCO_2: target value ± 5 mmHg or ± 8%
pH: target value ± 0.04

Proficiency testing also documents the bias of blood gas instruments and their operators. These testing programs ensure clinicians that the ABG measurements have an accuracy and precision that warrants clinical decisions, since inter- and intrainstrument variability is expected to be present.[19]

TEMPERATURE CORRECTION

Blood gas analysis is carried out at 37°C. Variations in temperature influence gas solubility, ion dissociation, and the off-loading of oxygen from hemoglobin. As a general guideline, oxygen and carbon dioxide tensions decrease and pH increases when temperature falls below 37°C.[20] Table 15-3 lists the pH and gas tensions of CO_2 and O_2 as a function of temperature.

Temperature correction is of clinical importance in patients whose temperatures are outside the range of 35° to 39°C, such as patients undergoing cardiopulmonary bypass.[21] Formulas for temperature correction of PCO_2, pH, and PO_2 have been devised that permit conversion of the values measured at 37°C.[22] The clinical importance of temperature correction is still debated.[23] Hypothermic patients are expected to have normal acid-base balance following rewarming to 37°C.[24] During hypothermia and cardiopulmonary bypass, blood gases may be measured and reported at 37°C or the ABG analysis may be measured at 37°C, and then nomograms for temperature correction are used to report the values at the patient's temperature.

Clinicians who use uncorrected ABGs subscribe to the concept of alpha stat interpretation of ABGs. Alpha refers to histidine's alpha-imidazole locus on hemoglobin, which plays a central role in blood's protein buffer system.[25] In vitro studies demonstrate that the pH of amphibian blood and aqueous solutions containing carbonic acid, bicarbonate, and imidazole behave similarly when temperature is lowered. Observations in poikilothermic animals demonstrate that blood pH is not maintained during hypothermia. On the other hand, hibernating animals can maintain normal pH by increasing the carbon dioxide content of their blood as core temperature falls. The strategy whereby temperature

TABLE 15-4. Primary Blood Gas Classifications

Class	$PaCO_2$	pH	$[HCO_3^-]p$	BE
Ventilatory				
Acute ventilatory failure	↑	↓	N	N
Chronic ventilatory failure	↑	N	↑	↑
Acute alveolar hyperventilation	↓	↑	N	N
Chronic alveolar hyperventilation	↓	N	↓	↓
Acid-Base				
Uncompensated acidosis	N	↓	↓	↓
Uncompensated alkalosis	N	↑	↑	↑
Partially compensated acidosis	↓	↓	↓	↓
Partially compensated alkalosis	↑	↑	↑	↑
Compensated acidosis or alkalosis	↑ Or ↓	N	↑ Or ↓⁻	↑ Or ↓

(Adapted from Shapiro et al.,[44] with permission.)

correction is utilized is based on the premise that hypothermic humans behave as hibernating mammals has been termed pH stat. In order to maintain the pH of hypothermic blood at or near 7.4, carbon dioxide is added to the oxygenator. Animal studies indicate that pH stat management may cause alkalemia when hypothermic animals are administered sodium bicarbonate to correct the "normalized pH" and during rewarming.[26] pH stat management may depress myocardial contractility. Proponents of pH stat management believe that cerebral perfusion is best maintained during hypothermia using this approach.

Changes in temperature affect both the solubility of oxygen as well as the affinity of hemoglobin for oxygen. Alterations in blood temperature will influence the oxygen tension but do not change the *measured* oxygen content. In response to a decreasing temperature, hemoglobin increases its affinity for oxygen (leftward shift of the oxyhemaglobin dissociation curve) resulting in a decrease in the oxygen tension. Conversely, with an elevation in temperature, the affinity for oxygen decreases and oxygen is off-loaded, resulting in an increase in oxygen tension. The influence of temperature on blood PO_2 of an arterial blood sample may reach a threshold for *clinical* significance, for example, PO_2 of 51 mmHg at 30°C is equivalent to a 90 mmHg at 37°C. Therefore, monitoring of oxygenation is best evaluated with the 37°C values, since the tem-

perature at the time of sampling is rarely known. Furthermore, temperature-corrected values may be confused with uncorrected values.[27]

INTERPRETATION OF BLOOD GAS MEASUREMENTS

All blood gas measurements will fall within one of nine primary classifications. Four of the classifications reflect ventilatory derangements and five reflect acid-base. Table 15-4 summarizes the changes in $PaCO_2$, pH, $[HCO_3^-]p$, and BE that are expected for each of the seven primary classifications.

The process of blood gas interpretation begins by evaluating the measured values of $PaCO_2$ and pH and the calculated values of $[HCO_3^-]p$ and BE. The arterial PCO_2 reflects the balance of CO_2 production and the adequacy of alveolar ventilation (VA). CO_2 production may change in critically ill patients. Table 15-5 lists factors that may account for abnormal CO_2 production.

The proportion of expired ventilation (VE) that does not participate in gas exchange is called deadspace ventilation (VD). Changes in VD can influence $PaCO_2$. Circumstances increasing VD require a commensurate increase in total VE in order to maintain adequate alveolar ventilation (VA) since VE = VD + VA.

TABLE 15-5. Abnormal CO$_2$ Production:
Etiologies

Derangement	Magnitude of Change
Hyperthermia	10% increase/°C
Shivering, rigor, seizures	~ 300–400% increase
The stress response	Variable
Sepsis	Variable
Total parenteral nutrition	200–800% increase

Table 15-6 lists clinical conditions that may be associated with increases in V$_D$. Following increases in V$_D$, a compensatory increase in V$_E$ can maintain a normal V$_A$. The Pa$_{CO_2}$ indicates the adequacy of alveolar ventilation. A Pa$_{CO_2}$ less than 30 mmHg defines the presence of alveolar hyperventilation. When the Pa$_{CO_2}$ is between 30 and 50 mmHg, alveolar ventilation is acceptable. A Pa$_{CO_2}$ greater than 50 mmHg defines the presence of alveolar hypoventilation. These liberal ranges are clinically useful for monitoring critically ill patients who may have dynamic changes in cardiopulmonary homeostasis. Classic textbook ranges are as follows:

	Pa$_{CO_2}$
Hyperventilation	>35 mmHg
Normal alveolar ventilation	35–45 mmHg
Hypoventilation	>45 mmHg

The integration of the values for P$_{CO_2}$, pH, and [HCO$_3^-$]p in an arterial blood sample determines whether the acid-base abnormality is partially or completely compensated. Humans maintain the pH of extracellular fluids through the use of buffering systems. Buffers protect cell systems from rapidly changing hydrogen ion concentrations. Buffers represent weak acids, which reversibly bind with H$^+$ as indicated in the equation

$$H^+ + B^+ \rightarrow HB.$$

TABLE 15-6. Factors That Increase Dead-Space
Ventilation

Acute decreases in cardiac output
Acute pulmonary embolus
Acute pulmonary hypertension
Acute lung injury
Positive pressure ventilation

Each of these conditions results in an acute increases in the ratio of ventilation to perfusion. When the proportion of ventilation favors nongravity-dependent lung the proportion of high V/Q units increases and in turn reduces V$_A$.

When a buffer accepts H$^+$ (HB state) that H$^+$ does not contribute to the acidity of blood and is not measured by the pH electrode during blood gas analysis. The dissociation constant (pKa) represents the pH value at which an acid (HB) is 50 percent dissociated. The ability of a buffer to accept a H$^+$ is determined by the relationship of the blood pH and the pKa of the buffer pair. For any buffering system the pKa represents the pH at which maximum buffering capacity occurs. Table 15-7 lists the buffers which are important in maintaining the arterial pH at 7.35 to 7.45. Note that the effectiveness of the blood buffers increases when acidemia is present.

About 90 percent of the carbon dioxide produced as the consequence of normal cellular respiration is transported to the lung by two buffer pairs, the CO$_2$:HCO$_3^-$ and hemoglobin:Hb-carbamino. The interaction of these two systems is demonstrated in Figure 15-3.

Hb is the most effective protein buffer contained in blood. Each reduced Hb molecule can "trap" 38 hydrogen ions and transport them to the lung for removal. The buffering capability of hemoglobin is directly linked to its chemical environment. Reduced Hb is a stronger acid than oxygenated Hb. Bohr demonstrated the phenomenon whereby the addition of CO$_2$ to blood (acidosis) enhances transport of CO$_2$. Haldane found that adding O$_2$ to blood enhances the release of CO$_2$. These effects work in concert to maximize the efficiency of Hb as a respiratory pigment. Figure 15-3 depicts the chemical events which permits Hb to transport H$^+$ from the tissues. At the lung, the events are reversed so that CO$_2$ can be transferred to the alveolus.

ASSESSMENT OF ARTERIAL OXYGENATION

The clinical assessment of a patient's oxygenation status begins with an evaluation of the arterial blood. Modern blood gas machines measure the

TABLE 15–7. Blood Buffers

Buffer	pK_a
Hemoglobin	6.8
H$_2$PO$_4$	6.8
H$_2$CO$_3$	6.1
Other Proteins	Variable

PO_2 and have the capability of estimating the Hb saturation and Hb concentration in the sample. The last two values are essential in calculating the oxygen content which defines the milliliters of oxygen contained in 100 ml of blood. If the Hb concentration and PO_2 are measured, the arterial oxygen content can be estimated using the following calculation:

Oxygen content (vol%) =

$$(1.34 \times \%HbO_2) + (Po_2 \times 0.003).$$

If the oxygen saturation is not measured by cooximetry or pulse oximetry, it can be determined from a measured PO_2 and a "normalized" oxyhemoglobin dissociation curve which plots %Hb saturation against PO_2. The formula for oxygen content focuses attention on the three factors

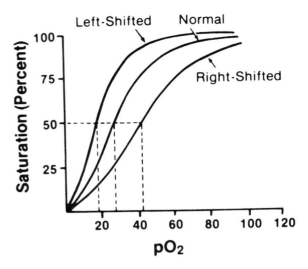

Fig. 15-4. The oxyhemoglobin dissociation curve. The relationship between arterial saturation and hemoglobin and oxygen tension is represented by the sigmoid-shaped dissociation curve. When the curve is left-shifted, the hemoglobin molecule binds oxygen more tightly. The position of the oxyhemoglobin dissociation curve is represented by the p50 that identifies the oxygen tension at which hemoglobin is half-saturated.

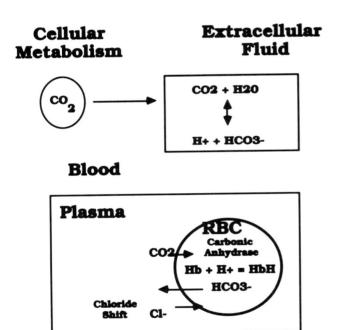

Fig. 15-3. Hemoglobin and the chloride shift. Hemoglobin and bicarbonate are the most important buffers in blood. CO_2 is freely diffusable between plasma and red blood cells. The carbonic anhydrase contained in red blood cells promotes the production of intracellular carbonic acid. The carbonic acid dissociates and the H^+ attaches to reduced hemoglobin. Bicarbonate exchanges with chloride following the hydrogen ion trapping by hemoglobin. At the pulmonary capillary, the process reverses to permit the removal of the H^+ as bicarbonate and H^+ combine to form CO_2.

that determine the quantity of oxygen available for cellular transport:

1. Hemoglobin oxygen affinity
2. Hemoglobin saturation
3. The quantity of oxygen dissolved in blood

While Hb has a strong affinity for oxygen, a shift in the oxyhemoglobin dissociation curve will change the characteristics of oxygen offloading. Figure 15-4 depicts the normal oxyhemoglobin dissociation curve and changes anticipated by shifting the curve. Leftward shifts increase Hb affinity for oxygen reducing oxygen availability at the tissue capillary. Factors affecting the oxyhemoglobin dissociation curve are listed in Table 15-8. The position of the oxyhemoglobin dissociation curve is defined by the p50. The p50 is the PO_2 at which Hb is 50 percent saturated. The p50 measurements are not part of the routine blood gas analysis. Human blood has a p50 of 26.5 mmHg when measured at 37°C, PCO_2 = 40 mmHg, and pH = 7.40.[28]

Hypoxemia defines the clinical significance of an absolute reduction in arterial oxygen tension. The PaO_2 measurement is central to defining the degree of hypoxemia and determining the effective-

TABLE 15-8. Factors Affecting Hb Affinity For Oxygen

Left Shift: Increased Affinity	Right Shift: Decreased Affinity
Alkalosis	Acidosis
Hypocarbia	Hypercarbia
Decreases in temperature	Increases in temperature
Decreases in 2,3-DPG	Increases in 2,3-DPG
Hypophophatemia	
Carbon monoxide	
Sepsis	
(Banked blood)	

ness of therapeutic interventions addressing oxygenation deficits. Blood gas analysis of arterial and pulmonary arterial blood (mixed venous blood gas) are necessary to quantify oxygen delivery, oxygen extraction, and the intrapulmonary shunt fraction.

NEWER TECHNOLOGIES FOR BLOOD GAS MONITORING AND ANALYSIS

Since the 1970s, there has been great interest in exploring techniques which may assist in monitoring cardiopulmonary variables. Methodologies have been utilized to monitor oxygenation, ventilation, and or oxygen delivery. Pulse oximeters and capnographs have become part of the standard regimen for intraoperative monitoring and are increasingly being utilized in monitoring critically ill patients in other intensive care settings. Likewise, devices (see appropriate chapters on these devices) for monitoring transcutaneous or transconjunctional oxygen and carbon dioxide have been designed, studied and have attracted proponents. These technologies are discussed elsewhere.

The trend of the "technologic imperative" of the last several decades has been to develop *clinical analyzers* that served patients by providing historical measurements. Testing required sampling, transport to the laboratory, measurement and reporting. Analyzers were located in laboratories far away from patient care areas. Laboratory analyzers often required sophisticated support to ensure that the systems for analysis were available and trustworthy. Today, there has been great interest in developing "user friendly" analyzers and which measure val-

ues of interest accuratelty and rapidly. Advances in computer design, electronics, biochemistry, and fiberoptics have expanded the potential for point of care devices, making it possible to perform sophisticated analysis far from hospital laboratories.

CONTINUOUS INTRAARTERIAL BLOOD GAS MONITORING (CIABG)

The previous discussion identifies the rationale for blood gas analysis during surgery and the care of critically ill patients. However, the intermittant determination of blood gas analysis does not permit identification of acid-base derragements *as they occur*. Methodology that provides continuous or nearly continuous monitoring of blood gases is desirable. The potential benefits of continuous blood gas monitoring include the following:

1. Prospective identification of clinical derangements.
2. Elimination of the interval between blood gas analysis and the clinical interpretation.
3. Reduction of therapeutic decision time.
4. Introduction of alarms and trending at the bedside.
5. Reduction in the risks of blood contamination to both patient and staff.
6. Reduction in the blood losses attendant to frequent blood sampling.

The suggested design criteria for blood gas biosensors has been previously published.[29] Table 15-9 lists the features that must be engineered into the ideal in vivo blood gas biosensors. Today continuous in vivo blood gas monitoring is clinically available.[30] Table 15-10 lists the methodology, technique, and distinguishing features for technologies

TABLE 15-9. Intravascular Biosensors: Design Requirements

Size: Fit into 20-gauge arterial cannula
Function: Permit continuous arterial pressure monitoring during operation; Measure pH, P_{CO_2}, P_{O_2}, and temperature
Accuracy: Comparable to in vitro methodologies with minimal drift; minimal effect by blood flow
Rapid response time: 90% <2 minutes
Biocompatible and nonthrombogenic
Function automatically with trending and alarms
Economical to operate

TABLE 15-10. In Vivo Blood Gas Technology

Methodology	Technique	Issues
Semipermeable membranes	Gas chromatograph Mass spectrometry	Slow response High failure rate High drift rate No pH measurement
Field-effect transistors (gated by chemicals enxymes, or ions)	Ion-selective pH- and P_{CO_2}-selective P_{O_2} measurement	Thrombus formation Protein adsorption High drift rate Not yet possible
Electrochemical accuracy	Minature Clark electrode	High drift rate Large size Single parameter
Fiberoptic	Optical sensors	All parameters Fast response Small size

that have been adapted to in vivo continuous blood gas monitoring.

Fluorescent optical techniques (for the measurement of continuous blood gas monitoring) have received the most comprehensive and commercial study.[31] Optical sensors function on an interaction between an analyte for example, O_2, CO_2, and a chemical dye to produce a detectable signal. The light passed down a fiberoptic conduit will be affected by the amount of analyte being measured in the presence of the chemical dye. Two types of fiberoptic systems exist: fluorescence or absorbance. Fluorescent sensors are based on a change in wavelength produced by the analyte, while absorbance

sensors measure changes in the light intensity produced by the presence of the analyte measured (Fig. 15-5). A detailed discussion of this technology is beyond the scope of this chapter.[32-34]

The most intriguing advantage of the *in vivo* CIABG technology is the benefit of real-time continuous operation. Therefore, these instruments represent the first proactive blood gas monitoring technology. The advantages of fiberoptic continuous in vivo arterial blood gas monitoring (CIABG) are listed in Table 15-11.

Several manufacturers have ongoing clinical programs for CIABG clinical studies designed to test accuracy, precision, clinical utility, and stability of

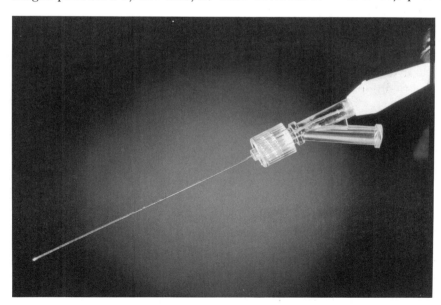

Fig. 15-5. Intravascular blood gas sensor—a fiberoptic sensor that measures arterial pH, P_{CO_2}, P_{O_2}, and blood temperature when inserted through a 20-gauge arterial cannula. Intravascular sensors permit clinicians to trend all measured and calculated blood gas parameters. The fiberoptic sensor is nonthromogenic and allows for arterial pressure monitoring and blood sampling through the arterial cannula. (Photograph courtesy of Puritan-Bennett Corporation, Carlsbad, CA.)

this new technology. Early clinical results are quite encouraging.[35-38]

EXTRACORPOREAL IN-LINE BLOOD GAS MONITORING

An alternative design for bedside monitoring is the development of in-line devices that measure arterial blood gases intermittantly. These systems place microsensors in line with the arterial catheter thereby eliminating the need for arterial sampling and transport for analysis. The proposed benefit of extracorporeal blood gas monitoring is similar to CIABG monitoring.

A rapid on-demand gas monitor incorporating fluorescent sensors placed in line with the arterial catheter is presently undergoing multicenter clinical trials (CDI System 2000, CDI-3M Healthcare, Irvine, CA). This system has a sampling chamber, which requires drawing blood from the arterial catheter when analysis is to be performed. No blood is removed from the patient and there is no interruption in the sterile blood-irrigation fluid interface. The performance of this monitoring system appears to match that of a laboratory instrument.[39]

On demand, ex vivo monitoring systems can incorporate additional biosensors which permit assessment of blood glucose and electrolytes at a push of a button. ABGs may be measured by miniaturized electodes similar to those used in laboratory analysis. Ion specific sensors for Na^+, K^+, Ca^{2+} can be incorporated on the sensor interface. Enzymatic electrodes are available to measure glucose and lactate. A conductance electrode has been designed to measure hematocrit. Clinical evaluation of these devices is presently on-going.[40]

TABLE 15-11. Advantages of CIAGB Monitoring

Technical advantages:
  Electrical isolation
  Immune to electromagnetic noise
  Seamless operation
Physiologic advantages:
  Reduced blood sampling
  Reduced blood losses
  Reduced blood handling
  Real-time data
  Dynamic response time

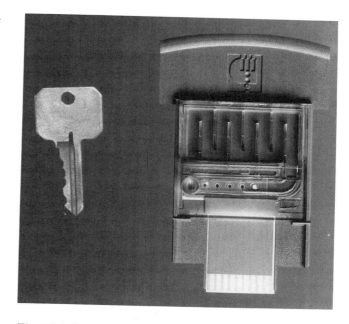

Fig. 15-6. Miniaturized electrochemical sensors used for blood gas analysis. The cartridge represents a single-use, disposable electrode system that attaches to a portable, battery-operated device, which permits assessment of arterial blood gases at a point of care. (Photograph courtesy of Datex Corporation, Minneapolis, MN.)

POINT-OF-CARE ANALYSIS

Bedside testing has been popularized as a more efficient means of obtaining test results.[41] Point-of-care systems represent the attempt by instrument makers to miniaturize laboratory devices to make them portable and simple to operate at "point-of-care." Point-of-care monitoring can be in line and dedicated to a single patient or it can be transportable to any point-of-care for measurements on several patients. The systems currently under study, utilize electrochemical sensors which require periodic verification of accuracy and precision by in vitro testing of the equipment against standard solutions.[42,43] Disposable cartridges containing the biosensors have been designed to simplify startup and quality control (Fig. 15-6). Point-of-Care systems utilizing single patient test cartridges have been designed to provide analysis of ABGs and or electrolytes. Alternatively, systems exists incorporating multitest, disposable cartridges. These systems appear to be promising alternatives to "Stat" laboratories so long as their costs and reliability are validated by clinical study.

REFERENCES

1. Van Slyke DD, Neill JM: The determination of gases in blood and other solutions by vacuum extraction and manometric measurement. J Biol Chem 61:523, 1924

2. Sanz MC: Ultramicro methods and standardization of equipment. Clini Chem 3:406, 1957

3. Severinghaus JW, Bradley AF: Electrodes for blood PO_2 and PCO_2 determination. J Appl Physiol 13:515, 1958

4. Clark LC Jr: Monitor and control of blood and tissue oxygen tensions. Trans Am Soc Artific Intern Organs 2:41, 1956

5. Severinghaus JF, Bradley AF: Electrodes for blood PO_2 and PCO_2 determination. J Appl Physiol 13:515, 1958

6. Shapiro BA, Harrison RA, Walton JR: Clinical application of blood gases. 3rd Ed. Yearbook Medical Publishers, Chicago, 1982

7. Semple SJG: Observed pH differences of blood and plasma with different bridge solutions. J Appl Physiol 16:576, 1967

8. Oldham PD: Measurement in medicine: the interpretation of numerical data. English Universities Press, London, 1968

9. Severinghaus JW: Blood gas concentrations. In Fenn WO, Rahn H (eds): The Handbook of Physiology, Section 3: Respiration, Vol. II. American Physiological Society. Williams & Wilkins, Baltimore, 1964

10. Ladegaard-Pedersen HJ: Accuracy and reproducibility of arterial blood-gas and pH measurements. Acta Anaesth Scand (Suppl.) 67:63, 1978

11. Madiedo G, Sciacca R, Hause L: Air bubbles and temperature effect on blod gas analysis. J Clin Pathol 33:864, 1980

12. Kelman GR, Nunn JF: Nomograpms for correction of blood po2, pCO_2, pH and base excess for time and temperature. J Appl Physiol 21:1484, 1966

13. Thorson SH, Marini JJ, Pierson DJ, Hudson LD: Variability of arterial blood gas values in stable patients in the ICU. Chest 84:14, 1983

14. Hamilton HB, Crockett AJ, Apers JH: Arterial blood gas analysis; potential errors due to the addition of heparin. Anesth Intens Care 6:251, 1978

15. Petty TL: The simplicity and safety of arterial puncture. JAMA 195:181, 1966

16. Bageant RA: Variations in arterial blood gas measurements due to sampling techniques. Respir Care 20:565, 1975

17. Sigaard-Anderson O: Blood acid-base alignment nomogram. Scand Clin Lab Invest 15:211, 1963

18. Clinical Laboratory Improvement Amendments of 1988: Final Rule. Fed Reg 57:7001, February 28, 1992

19. Delaney CJ, Leary ET, Raisys VA, Kenny MA: Proficiency testing of blood-gas quality control. Clin Chem 22:1675, 1976

20. Burnett RW, Noonan DC: Calculations and correction factors used in determination of blood pH and blood gases. Clin Chem 20:1499, 1974

21. Walton JR, Shapiro BA: Value and application of temperature compensated blood gas data. Respir Care 25:260, 1980

22. Andritsch RF, Mauravchick S, Gold MI: Temperature correction of arterial blood gas parameters: a comparative review of methodology. Anesthesiology 55:311, 1981

23. Ream AK, Reitz BA, Silverberg G: Temperature correction of PCO_2 and pH in estimating acid base: an example of the emperor's new clothes? Anesthesiology 56:41, 1982

24. Blayo MC, LeCompte Y, Pocidalo JJ: Control of acid-base status during hypothermia in man. Respir Physiol 42:287, 1980

25. Reeves RB: An imidazole alphastat hypothesis of vertebrate acid-base regulation: tissue carbon dioxide and body temperature in bull frogs. Resp Phys 14:219, 1972

26. Becker H, Vinten-Johansen J, Buckberg GD et al: Myocardial damage caused by keeping pH 7.40 during deep systemic hypothermia. J Thorac Cardiovasc Surg 82:810, 1981

27. Shapiro BA, Peruzzi WT: Arterial blood gas monitoring. Contemp Manage Crit Care I:20, 1993

28. Finch C, Lenfant C: Oxygen transport in man. N Engl J Med 286:407, 1972

29. Mahutte CK: On-line blood gas monitoring. Contemp Manag Crit Care 1:28, 1993

30. Shapiro BA, Cane RD, Chomka C et al: Preliminary evaluation of an inter-arterial blood gas system in dogs and humans. Crit Care Med 17:455, 1987

31. Shapiro BA, Cane RD: Progress in the development of a flourescent intravascular blood gas system in man. J Clin Monit 7:212, 1991

32. Yafuso M, Arick SA, Hansmann D et al: Optical pH measurements in blood. Proc SPIE 1067:37, 1989

33. Regnault WF, Picciolo GL: Review of medical biosensors and associated material problems. J Biomed Mater Res Appl Biomater 21:163, 1987

34. Gehrich JL, Lubbers DW, Opitz N et al: Optical fluorescence and its application to an intravascular blood gas monitoring system. IEEE Trans Biomed Eng 33:117, 1986

35. Depoix JP, Desmonts JM, Camus H et al: Evaluation of a continuous blood gas monitor during open heart surgery. Anesthesiology 79:A563, 1993

36. Vender JS, Gilbert HC, O'Connor BS, Alexander JC: Validation of continuous intra-arterial blood gas monitoring in coronary artery patients. Anesthesiology 79:A564, 1993

37. Haller M. Kilgewr E, Briegel J et al: Continuous intra-Arterial monitoring in patients with severe respiratory failure. Anesthesiology 79:A566, 1993

38. Zimmerman JL, Dellinger RP: Initial evaluation of a new intraarterial blood gas system in humans. Crit Care Med 21:495, 1993

39. Shapiro BA, Mahutte CK, Cane RD, Gilmour IJ: Clinical performance of a blood gas monitor: a prospective, multicenter trial. Crit Care Med 21:487, 1993

40. Wong DK, Jordon WS: Microprocessor-based near real time bedside blood chemistry monitor. Int J Clin Monit Comput 9:95, 1992

41. Chernow B: The bedside laboratory: a critical step forward in ICU care. Chest 97:183, 1990

42. Vender JS, Gilbert HC et al: Validation of a new point of care arterial blood gas analyzer, (abstracted). Crit Care Med (in press)

43. Salem M, Chernow B, Burke R et al: Bedside diagnostic blood testing. JAMA 266:382, 1991

44. Shapiro BA, Harrison RA, Walton JR: Clinical Application of Blood Gases. 3rd Ed. Yearbook Medical Publisher, Chicago, 1982

The Electroencephalogram and Evoked Potential Monitoring

16

Betty L. Grundy

The nervous system is affected more profoundly by anesthetics than any other system of the body, and the methods used for monitoring the nervous system during anesthesia are in a period of rapid development. Clinical signs of anesthetic depth are less reliable with today's agents and techniques than with older agents such as ether, chloroform, and cyclopropane. With the widespread use of neuromuscular blocking agents, even the simplest sign of anesthetic depth—movement in response to stimulation—is lost. Unsuspected awareness during anesthesia, often associated with considerable psychic and physical pain,[1,2] is not uncommon. At the same time, the anesthetic state itself limits our ability to monitor parts of the nervous system that may be at risk during complex neurosurgical, orthopedic, or cardiovascular operations. In the critical care unit, the patient's altered state of consciousness often hampers clinical neurologic assessment just when information is most needed to guide treatment or predict outcome.

Electrophysiologic monitoring of the nervous system[3–6] allows noninvasive assessment of the functional integrity of neural structures when clinical neurologic assessment is severely limited or impossible because of anesthesia or other altered states of consciousness. Both the electroencephalogram and evoked potentials are currently used to monitor patients at risk for neurologic injury in the operating room and in the critical care unit. In attempting to predict the position that electrophysiologic monitoring of the nervous system may ultimately come to occupy in anesthesiology and critical care medicine, we should perhaps recall the history of other monitoring techniques now in common use. For example, Harvey Cushing was told, after his initial study of blood pressure monitoring during anesthesia, that one should not monitor the blood pressure during anesthesia because it was clearly too variable to be of any significance.[7,8]

The electroencephalogram (EEG) reflects the spontaneous ongoing electrical activity of the brain. Evoked potentials (EP) are electrophysiologic responses to sensory, electrical, or magnetic stimulation.[9,10] When recorded noninvasively in humans, these electrical potentials are of such low amplitude that special methods of signal processing are needed to separate the EP signal from the background EEG activity and other electrophysiologic "noise."[11] Although other methods of signal processing have been employed, EP are most often made apparent by using a computer to sum or average responses to multiple stimuli. With the increasing availability of improved computer hardware and software, both EEG and EP monitoring enjoy progressively wider application in the acute care setting.

This chapter introduces the practicing anesthesiologist to the present state of the art in electrophysiologic monitoring of the nervous system in the operating room and critical care unit. Basic concepts of EEG and EP recording and applications of these techniques in diagnostic neurology are described. A section on methods includes discussions of signal acquisition, processing, and display; safety considerations; quality control; and measurement and interpretation of waveforms. The bulk of the chapter is devoted to contemporary applications, many of which remain controversial.

RATIONALE FOR ELECTROPHYSIOLOGIC MONITORING

The electroencephalogram and evoked potentials serve four main purposes in the operating room and critical care unit[3,4]: monitoring of the functional integrity of neural structures that may be at risk; identification of specific neural structures; monitoring the effects of anesthetic agents and other drugs that affect the nervous system; and diagnosis and monitoring of various pathophysiologic conditions that can alter neurologic function in critically ill patients. A major advantage of these techniques is that the EEG and EP are noninvasive and monitor actual neurologic function, which persists to some extent even when the patient is unconscious. Therefore the step of relating intracranial pressure, mean arterial pressure, cerebral perfusion pressure, or cerebral blood flow to neuronal function at a given value is not necessary. Many factors that interfere with neurologic function, such as hypoxia, hypercarbia, and ischemia, may be reflected at once as EEG or EP changes.

Electrophysiologic monitoring of the nervous system may be useful in the operating room or critical care unit when four conditions are met.[3] First, a structure amenable to monitoring is at risk or requires identification. Second, equipment and personnel are present to record and interpret waveforms. Third, appropriate sites are available for stimulation and recording. Finally, if the monitoring is to be of more than academic interest, there should be some possibility of intervention to improve function in the event that deterioration is detected. For example, EEG can be monitored during carotid endarterectomy, somatosensory EP during operations on the spine or spinal cord, auditory EP during operative procedures in the cerebellopontine angle, and multimodality EP in victims of head injury. Because of the devastating nature of the neurologic injuries that can occur in these situations, considerable effort seems warranted to reduce the possibility of permanent damage to the brain or spinal cord.

In contrast, cost-effectiveness considerations at the present state of the art argue against routine use of these methods to monitor depth of anesthesia. Clinical signs of anesthetic depth and information obtained from monitors of cardiovascular function serve well in most instances. As techniques are simplified and methods of display and interpretation are improved, electrophysiologic assessment of anesthetic depth may become more useful. EEG or EP may eventually give some warning of unsuspected awareness during light anesthesia, especially when movement is abolished by pharmacologic blockade of the neuromuscular junction and cardiovascular responses to stimulation are modified by vasoactive drugs.

In considering the methods used to monitor patients in the operating room and critical care unit, some distinction must be made between diagnosis and prediction on the one hand and monitoring with titrated care on the other. In the acute situation we are less interested in identifying those parameters absolutely predictive of neurologic injury than in identifying undesirable trends as early as possible. We intervene early to optimize function and minimize the possibility of permanent injury. Just as we strive to maintain arterial blood pressure within limits that seem safe for a particular patient, we attempt to maintain electroencephalographic and evoked potential parameters within limits that seem clinically acceptable under specific circumstances. The primary goal is to avoid *any* serious neurologic injury rather than to minimize the frequency of reasonable interventions.

NEUROPHYSIOLOGIC BASIS OF THE ELECTROENCEPHALOGRAM AND EVOKED POTENTIALS

To understand and interpret EEG and EP data, the anesthesiologist needs an understanding of the mechanisms and origins of waveform generation, the types of electrical potentials involved, and the mechanisms responsible for variations in frequency and amplitude.

Genesis of the Electroencephalogram

The EEG signals recorded from the scalp reflect the graded summations of excitatory and inhibitory postsynaptic potentials generated by cortical neurons.[12] The pyramidal cells, found in layers II,

III, and V of the cerebral cortex, have long dendritic trees oriented perpendicularly to the cortical surface. These are the only cells so situated as to produce the dipole fields recorded from the scalp.

Classification and Characterization of Evoked Potentials

The terminology used to describe EP is confusing, and the literature contains many terms and abbreviations that appear to be unrelated or conflicting. This chapter employs primarily those terms and abbreviations recommended in the Guidelines on Evoked Potential Studies[13] adopted by the American Electroencephalographic Society in 1983 and revised in 1991. Table 16-1 shows a number of commonly used abbreviations.

Sensory EP can be classified according to four characteristics: the mode of sensory stimulation; the poststimulus latency of a peak, trough, or complex in the elicited waveform; the distance separating the neural generator of the EP from the recording electrode; and the neural structures in which EP are thought to arise (Table 16-2). Motor EP can be used not only to monitor the effects of neuromuscular blocking agents used during anesthesia[14] but also to assess the function of descending motor pathways in the spinal cord.[15] Neither of these techniques has yet found such widespread use as sensory EP.

Modes of Sensory Stimulation

Sensory EP are commonly elicited by somatosensory, auditory, or visual stimulation. Trigeminal, tooth pulp, and olfactory stimulation have also been employed. The mode of stimulation chosen for a particular patient depends on the part of the nervous system that requires assessment. Of the various sensory EP described, this chapter considers only those elicited by somatosensory, auditory, visual, and trigeminal stimulation. Motor EP are also discussed.

Poststimulus Latencies

The poststimulus latency of a peak or complex in the EP waveform is the time after stimulation at which this peak or complex occurs. Poststimulus latencies are measured in milliseconds and loosely subdivided into short (less than 40 ms), intermediate (40 to 120 ms), and long (120 to 500 ms).

These divisions are somewhat arbitrary, and no general agreement has been reached as to the precise values separating these groupings. Nevertheless, because some clinically important characteristics of EP are related to poststimulus latency, these divisions are useful.

Short-latency EP arise closer to the site of sensory stimulation than do EP of intermediate and long latency. Relatively few synapses have been crossed in the transmission of these impulses, and the effects of anesthetic agents and other drugs on these EP are minimal. When recorded from scalp electrodes, short-latency EP are of lower amplitude than the spontaneous background EEG. Thus, large numbers of individual responses must be averaged to demonstrate the electrophysiologic activity related to sensory stimulation. As a rule, the poststimulus latencies and waveform configurations of short-latency EP are less variable within and among subjects than are EP of intermediate and long poststimulus latency. The short-latency EP elicited by auditory and somatosensory stimulation can be effectively used for intraoperative monitoring. Much less is known of short-latency visual EP, and no monitoring applications for these EP have yet been described. This area invites further investigation.

Sensory EP of intermediate poststimulus latency arise in the cerebral cortex and include those components sometimes referred to as the "primary specific complex." These EP are thought of as fairly well localized to specific sensory areas of the cortex. They are altered by anesthetic agents and other drugs as well as by such physiologic factors as hyperventilation. With appropriate anesthetic management, these EP can be successfully monitored in the operating room. They are particularly valuable when the related areas of cerebral cortex may be at risk from either regional or systemic insults. Both somatosensory and visual EP of intermediate latency are used to monitor patients in the operating room and the critical care unit. The intermediate-latency auditory EP have, to date, found less wide application. Early data were confused by the presence of a myogenic potential often seen at the poststimulus latencies of interest. The myogenic potential would not be a problem in the presence of neuromuscular blockade.[16] The auditory EP of intermediate latency deserve reevaluation as monitors of cortical function in the operating

TABLE 16-1. Abbreviations Used in Clinical Electrophysiology

General and miscellaneous terms

CCT	Central conduction time (ms)
CNV	Contingent negative variation, a steady potential shift seen during expectancy, as after a conditional stimulus prior to the stimulus associated with an expected reward
CV	Conduction velocity (m/s)
EEG[a]	Electroencephalogram or electroencephalograph; usually refers to spontaneous rather than evoked activity
EMG[a]	Electromyogram
EP[a]	Evoked potentials, or sensory evoked potentials; may also refer, especially in illustrations, to Erb's point
MEP	Motor evoked potentials
SEP[a]	Somatosensory evoked potentials; has also been used to refer to sensory evoked potentials; also known as SER: somatosensory evoked responses
TEP	Trigeminal evoked potentials
TPEP	Tooth pulp evoked potentials

Auditory system

AEP	Auditory evoked potentials
AP[a]	Auditory nerve compound action potential; may also refer nonspecifically to any action potential
BAEP	Brainstem auditory evoked potentials
	Also known as
	ABR: auditory brain stem responses
	BSEP: brainstem auditory evoked potentials
	BSER: brainstem auditory evoked responses
	BAER: brainstem auditory evoked responses
CM[a]	Cochlear microphonic, a cochlear receptor potential
ECochG[a]	Electrocochleogram, including the cochlear microphonic, the summating potential, and the auditory nerve compound action potential
ERA	Evoked response audiometry
MLR	Middle-latency response
SAEP[a]	Short-latency auditory evoked potentials, including the electrocochleogram and brainstem auditory evoked potentials
SP[a]	Summating potential, a cochlear receptor potential

Somatosensory system

CPN-SEP[a]	Somatosensory evoked potentials elicited by stimulation of the common peroneal nerve
MN-SEP[a]	Somatosensory evoked potentials elicited by stimulation of the median nerve at the wrist
PTN-SEP[a]	Somatosensory evoked potentials elicited by stimulation of the posterior tibial nerve
SCEP	Somatosensory cortical evoked potentials
SEP[a]	Somatosensory evoked potentials, or sensory evoked potentials
	Also known as SER: somatosensory evoked responses
SSEP[a]	Short-latency somatosensory evoked potentials; has also been used to refer to somatosensory evoked potentials
SpEP	Spinal evoked potentials

Visual system

EOG	Electrooculogram
ERG[a]	Electroretinogram
FEP[a]	Flash evoked potentials (visual)
LED	Light-emitting diodes
PREP	Pattern-reversal evoked potentials (visual)
PREP (FF)[a]	Visual evoked potentials produced by full-field pattern-reversal stimulation
PREP (HF)[a]	Visual evoked potentials produced by hemifield pattern-reversal stimulation
S-VEP	Steady-state visual evoked potentials
T-VEP	Transient visual evoked potentials
	Also known as VEP: visual evoked potentials
VEP[a]	Visual evoked potentials
	Also known as VER: visual evoked responses

[a]Abbreviation recommended by the American Electroencephalographic Society.

TABLE 16-2. Classifications of Evoked Potentials

Mode of stimulation (for intraoperative EP
    monitoring)
    Somatosensory: electrical current
    Auditory: clicks or tones, delivered by ear-insert
       transducers
    Visual: flash, delivered by light-emitting diodes
       mounted on opaque goggles over closed eyes
    Trigeminal: electrical current
    Motor: electrical current or magnetic transients
Poststimulus latency
    Short (<10 to <40 ms after stimulus)
    Intermediate (~20 to 120 ms)
    Long (~120 to 500 ms)
Distance from neural generator to recording electrode
    Near-field evoked potentials
    Far-field evoked potentials
Purported neural generators
    Cerebral cortex
    Subcortical structures of the brain
    Spinal cord
    Cranial nerve, peripheral nerve, or nerve plexus
    Sensory receptor

room and critical care unit. They offer some promise in monitoring depth of anesthesia.[17]

Sensory EP of long poststimulus latency (event-related potentials) are thought to arise in the association areas of the cerebral cortex. They are essentially abolished by general anesthesia and are markedly affected by factors such as attention, expectancy, drowsiness, and emotional state.[18] Long-latency EP have not been made useful for intraoperative or critical care monitoring. The late EP may yet be of interest to the anesthesiologist, however. The so-called "cognitive evoked potentials" elicited by the unusual signals in a train of repetitive stimuli (e.g., high-pitched tones randomly interspersed in a series of lower pitched tones) are altered in dementia.[19] Furthermore, a large positive wave, occurring approximately 300 ms after a painful stimulus, may come near to representing a physiologic manifestation of pain.[20] These long-latency or "late" EP may prove useful as investigational tools in anesthesiology.

Distances Separating Neural Generators from Recording Electrodes

Evoked potentials may be generally divided into near-field and far-field. In near-field recordings, each electrode detects primarily that activity within a radius of approximately 2 to 2.5 cm. Far-field EP arise in structures farther away from the electrode. Because signal strength decreases as the distance between the neural generator and the electrode increases, far-field EP are of low amplitude and cannot be seen in the unprocessed spontaneous background EEG activity. Some of the clinically important differences between near-field and far-field EP are shown in Table 16-3. Near-field EP recorded from scalp electrodes originate in the cerebral cortex. Far-field EP seen in scalp recordings may arise in sensory receptors, peripheral or cranial nerves, nerve plexus, spinal cord, or subcortical structures of the brain. These far-field EP reach the scalp by volume conduction, which, compared to neural transmission, is virtually instantaneous. Thus, far-field EP are of short poststimulus latency. They are relatively insensitive to the effects of anesthetics. Both auditory and somatosensory far-field EP are clinically useful. Less is known of far-field visual EP.

Short-latency EP are near-field when the recording electrodes are placed in close physical proximity to the neural generators. Short-latency near-field EP include the electroretinogram[21] recorded

TABLE 16-3. Comparisons of Near-Field and Far-Field Evoked Potentials[a]

	Far-Field EP	Near-Field EP
Distance separating neural generator from recording electrode	Inches or feet	Within 2–3 cm
Amplitude	<1 µV	1–50 µV
Number of responses averaged	1000–8000	64–256
Rate of stimulation	4–15 Hz	0.9–5 Hz

[a]In scalp recordings, brainstem auditory evoked potentials and subcortical short-latency somatosensory evoked potentials are far-field evoked potentials. Intermediate-latency potentials elicited by somatosensory, auditory, or visual stimulation are cortical in origin and are near-field evoked potentials. Potentials that are far-field evoked potentials when recorded from the scalp may be near-field evoked potentials when recorded from invasive electrodes placed near the neural generators. For example, potentials arising in the spinal cord and recorded from the scalp are far-field evoked potentials. The same impulses recorded from epidural electrodes within the spinal canal are near-field evoked potentials even though they are short-latency potentials.

from electrodes placed in the conjunctival sac, subcortical brain EP recorded from stereotactically placed depth electrodes, electrodes placed with the surgical field during craniotomy, spinal EP recorded from electrodes placed within the spinal canal; and brachial plexus EP recorded from Erb's point.

Neural Structures of Signal Origin

Sensory EP that can be recorded noninvasively may originate in sensory receptor, peripheral nerve, nerve plexus, nerve root, spinal cord, subcortical structures of the brain, or cerebral cortex. Potentials thought to arise from each of these sites have been used to monitor patients in the operating room or critical care unit. Not all purported neural generators have been definitely proved; but clinically useful postulates have been developed using information gained from studies in animals, clinical pathologic studies in humans, mathematical modeling of electrical fields, and correlations between electrical or magnetic activity, magnetic resonance images, and radiologic studies of metabolic activation with magnetic resonance spectroscopy (MRS), positron emission tomography (PET), or single photon emission computerized tomography (SPECT). In selecting the most appropriate monitoring for a particular patient, care must be taken to consider the neural structures at risk and to monitor those EP most likely to be affected by the events of interest in the acute situation.

METHODS AND TECHNIQUES

Electrophysiologic monitoring is feasible in the operating room or critical care unit only when reliable equipment and well-trained personnel are available. Much can be done to increase the efficiency and reliability of monitoring by close communication among those who will care for a patient in the acute situation. Such mundane considerations as placement of equipment in the operating room, availability of sites for application of stimulating devices and recording electrodes, and time requirements become important. With a well-trained team and detailed planning, satisfactory monitoring can be done in most operating suites. The situation is somewhat less complex in the critical care unit, but in some older units the electrical noise level may be so high that recording of EP is virtually impossible.

The American Electroencephalographic Society published Guidelines for Intraoperative Monitoring of Sensory Evoked Potentials in 1987, and these have recently been republished.[22] Careful attention is needed not only to the technical details of signal acquisition and processing but also to the monitoring and constraint of multiple factors that can affect EP in the acute care setting.[3,4]

Signal Acquisition

Because the neurophysiologic signals to be recorded are so small, and because both the operating room and the critical care unit present electrically hostile recording environments, meticulous attention to the technical details of signal acquisition is essential. Compare the usual standardization mark on the electrocardiogram, 1 mV, to the standardization marks on EEG or EP records, which range from 50 μV for standard EEG recording to a few microvolts or a few hundred nanovolts for EP.

All electrodes are placed according to the International 10-20 System[23] (Fig. 16-1). Studies in cadavers and magnetic resonance imaging have shown reproducible placement of electrodes over particular portions of the cerebral cortex using this method. Useful monitoring requires that electrodes be positioned where events of interest are expected to occur. Monitoring of regional activity requires multiple electrodes. Precise localization of electrodes is more important for near-field cortical EP than for far-field EP recorded from the scalp.[24]

The particular combination of electrodes being examined at any one time is referred to as a montage. The neurologic literature refers to three types of montages. The bipolar montage is made up of sequential connections of channels along anteroposterior or transverse rows of electrodes. Each channel is connected to a pair of active electrodes and thus measures the potential difference between them. In the common reference or monopolar montage each channel records between one active scalp electrode and an "indifferent" electrode that may be located on the chin or neck but is most often linked ears. These references are not truly indifferent. When each channel records between an active electrode and a common average reference obtained by joining all the scalp electrodes to a common point through high resistors of equal value, the montage is called an average reference montage. This is not optimal for identifying focal changes. The diagnostic EEG most often uses 16 to 32 channels and optimal EEG monitoring in the operating room uses 8 to 16. Nevertheless, fewer channels are often used due to constraints on equipment, time, and personnel. EP monitoring can be done satisfactorily with two channels for brainstem auditory EP, four for somatosensory EP.

Cup or disk electrodes are ideal for recording. Freshly chlorided silver-silver chloride electrodes are best. Subdermal needle electrodes should be made of precious metals, usually platinum, and preferably should be used only for sensory stimulation or to place an electrode within the sterile surgical field. The recording characteristics of these small needle electrodes are less desirable than those of disk or cup electrodes, primarily because of the very small surface area available for recording and the tendency toward polarization.[11] Electrodes should be attached with collodion.

Small pieces of gauze impregnated with collodion can be placed on top of the electrodes to make them even more secure. The cup or disk electrodes are filled with salt gel and may be sealed with collodion or plastic tape to prevent drying. Strain is relieved by taping all electrode wires to the skin. Electrodes placed in this manner can remain physically and electrically stable for 24 hours or longer.

The anesthesiologist working alone has little chance of placing a full set of electrodes (23 or more) with collodion. Simple 2-channel EEG monitoring can be done in this setting, however. Although less information is gleaned than with additional electrodes and channels, two symmetrical bipolar channels can be used to reflect gross asymmetries of EEG activity. This is better than no monitoring at all during carotid endarterectomy or cardiopulmonary bypass. The electrode requirements can be somewhat relaxed for this type of recording, and subdermal or adhesive electrocardiographic

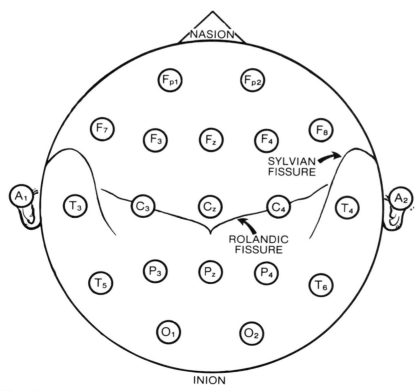

Fig. 16-1. Positions for EEG electrodes according to the International 10-20 System. Reference points are the nasion and the inion. Odd numbers are used for the left side, even numbers for the right side, and z for the midline. Initial letters represent anatomic areas: F, frontal; C, central; T, temporal; P, parietal; O, occipital; A, ear.

electrodes can be used so long as impedances are no greater than 5,000 to 6,000 Ω and are matched. Many anesthesiologists monitoring intraoperative EEG now use standard, adhesive electrocardiographic (ECG) electrodes. Although these electrodes can only be applied to glabrous or shaved areas of skin, they are uniformly available, inexpensive, and provide excellent electrical contact once the site has been prepared. Skin preparation is essential for either cup or adhesive electrodes and consists of removing surface oils and the upper layers of the stratum corneum, wherein most of the resistance to electric current passage resides. Preparation need not be burdensome and takes no more than 15 seconds per site. An efficient means to accomplish this is with OMNI-Prep (D.O. Weaver Co., Denver, CO) rubbed vigorously into the skin. Electrodes difficult to access intraoperatively may be additionally secured with tincture of benzoin, collodion, or adhesive tape.

Interelectrode impedances must be measured before initial recording, at intervals during the procedure (particularly when unexpected changes are seen), and at the termination of recording. For recording EP, impedances should be maintained at or below 3,000 Ω, and matched; impedances up to 6,000 Ω may be acceptable for EEG recording. In any case, impedances between electrodes must be closely matched; mismatches can introduce serious artifacts.

Great care should be taken to position electrodes and wires securely and as far as possible from known sources of artifact, whether mechanical or electrical. Physical disturbance of electrodes and wires can be minimized by twisting the electrode wires together and taping them to the operating table or to the neurosurgical head holder. The electrode wires should not be allowed to cross ventilator tubings, intravenous infusion or pressure monitoring lines, or other devices, such as suction tubings or stethoscopes, that will be frequently moved. Recording electrodes, electrode wires, and cables should be kept away from the cables connected to the sensory stimulators; and cables should not be near power cords leading to either the EP machine or other electrical devices.

Electroencephalographic Signal Processing, Display, and Measurements

For both EEG and EP recording, the signal is initially magnified (by about 100,000) and filtered to minimize unwanted frequencies. Analog filtering is needed whether or not subsequent digital filtering is planned. Most commercial EEG monitors designed for intraoperative use contain filters that limit signals outside the range of 0.5 to 30 Hz. Many also have 50/60 Hz "notch" filters to reduce power line noise that escapes the amplifier. Some monitors have adjustable filters that allow further restriction of the signals they pass, but these adjustments should be used sparingly because they may attenuate legitimate EEG signals. For example, a filter set to attenuate frequencies below 5 Hz (i.e., to reduce motion artifact) would be inappropriate during a high-dose narcotic anesthetic because most of the EEG signal is itself below 5 Hz.

Classical diagnostic EEG is typically recorded as a plot of voltage against time on a paper strip chart using from 8 to 32 channels (Fig. 16-2). Most commonly, the sensitivity is set so that 50 μV causes the pen to deflect 7 or 10 mm, and 30 mm on the horizontal axis represents 1 second. Both parameters are variable, between and within recording sessions, so calibration values must be noted on each record. If the EEG is being used to detect the presence or absence of electrocerebral activity in cases of suspected brain death, it is necessary to calibrate using a 2 μV calibration signal.[25] EEG signals recorded from the scalp are normally in the range of 10 to 200 μV, with peak voltages of approximately 1,000 μV during seizure activity. As considerable variability in the signal may be seen in the operating room, variable calibration is also needed here and must be documented.

Interpretation of the electroencephalographic record involves pattern recognition and quantification.[26] Rudimentary quantification is done by measuring frequency and amplitude either manually or with a computer. Pattern recognition is more complex and involves evaluation of the morphology, spatial and temporal distribution, and reactivity of the waveforms. EEG records contain three basic kinds of activity: continuous and often rhythmical, transient, and the background activity on which the continuous and transient waves are superimposed. EEG frequencies are nominally divided as follows:

Delta: <4 Hz
Theta: 4 to <8 Hz
Alpha: 8 to 13 Hz
Beta: >13 Hz

Amplitude is measured peak-to-peak and expressed in microvolts.

True cerebral electrical activity must be differentiated from electrical or mechanical interference and from extracerebral potentials arising from the patient. Sources of these biopotentials include eye movements, muscle tension, movements of the head and neck, respiration, and the electrical potentials generated by the heart. If an electrode is placed near an artery, a waveform occurring simultaneously with arterial pulsation may be seen. Roller-pump artifact is sometimes seen during cardiopulmonary bypass, particularly from an electrode on a free earlobe. Moving the electrode will often eliminate pulsatile artifact. Artifacts due to muscle movement and to the ECG are not so easily eliminated, but simultaneous recording of the ECG and an electromyogram (EMG) of the muscles involved can aid the clinician in differentiating these from true cerebral activity.

Several microcomputer-based monitors have been designed to facilitate integration of EEG monitoring into the operating room routine. These monitors provide semiquantitative measurement of the EEG and a high degree of data compression. Some information is lost with all the available methods, and it is very important to examine unprocessed EEG to detect artifact, at least at intervals.

Commercially available EEG processors all have amplifiers and filters; they differ in their algorithms, or the methods by which they process the data. All convert the analog EEG voltages into digital numbers, usually at a rate from 100 to 200 per second per channel, and group this sampled data into "epochs," usually 2 to 4 seconds in length, for analysis. As greater computational power becomes readily accessible at the bedside, more complex methods of waveform analysis are incorporated into clinical monitors.

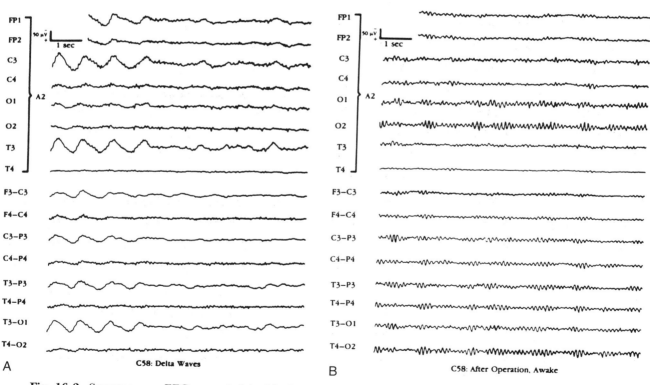

Fig. 16-2. Spontaneous EEG recorded in 16 channels during and after general anesthesia for carotid endarterectomy. **A:** Delta waves and attenuation of fast activity during test occlusion of the left carotid artery. Because of these changes a shunt was inserted. **B:** Normal EEG after successful endarterectomy. Note the normal alpha rhythm, most prominent in posterior channels. The first eight channels use the left ear electrode as "grid two." The low amplitude of the T4 channel is due to the close proximity of the temporal electrode (T4) to the ear electrode (A2) rather than to any pathology. (From Grundy,[320] with permission.)

Details of the methods used for signal analysis are beyond the scope of this chapter, but a brief summary of types of technology used for EEG signal processing may be helpful. Clinical use of these methods has generally paralleled the availability of computers sufficiently powerful to reliably perform the computations required on-line in the acute care setting. The best performance in pattern recognition, however, remains the well-trained human observer.

Computationally simplest is *processing in the time domain*—basically making measurements of amplitude (height of the waveform in the plot of voltage against time) and frequency (by counting baseline- or zero-crossings). (See Figure 16-3.) Data compression is achieved by summing or averaging data over time, or by displaying representation of only a proportion of the individually measured waveforms in a display. Suppressing a proportion of the data in an epoch loses less information than averaging and is used in one form of aperiodic analysis (Fig. 16-4). Aperiodic methods of analysis are in general better at preserving information on varying patterns within an epoch, such as seizure activity, burst suppression, or artifact, than are methods that assume that the EEG signal is stochastic (random). The raw (unprocessed) EEG gives more information in each of these three cases than does processed EEG.

Somewhat more computationally intensive is *power spectral analysis*, which converts the raw EEG from the time domain to the frequency domain.

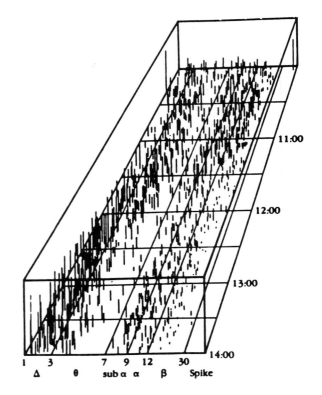

Fig. 16-4. Aperiodic analysis was used to generate this display of EEG during enflurane anesthesia, light to deep. Two channels can be displayed side by side. Time (24-hour clock) is shown at the right of the figure. (From Grundy,[320] with permission.)

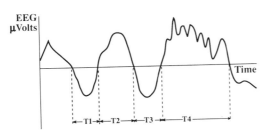

Fig. 16-3. EEG analysis in the time domain. The zero-crossing approach becomes inaccurate when the EEG waveform consist of combinations of different frequency and amplitude wavelets, as usually occurs in nature. For example, here the algorithm does not detect the small fast waves superimposed on the larger slow waves. A contemporary version of aperiodic analysis analyzes the fast and slow components separately, then combines them for display. See Figure 16-4.

This method transforms the raw EEG voltage into a histogram of power (essentially μV^2) versus frequency (Fig. 16-5). This histogram is called a spectrum and is analogous to a light-ray spectrum created by passage through a prism. Sequential spectral histograms are then smoothed and stacked to form a display pattern showing changes over time. Currently popular spectral displays are the compressed spectral array (Fig. 16-6) and the density-modulated spectral array (Fig. 16-7). These spectral arrays are available on several commercially produced monitors. The origin of the plot shifts vertically with time, producing a three-dimensional graph which is plotted with the z axis (power) shown as hills and valleys (compressed spectral array) or by variations in the darkness at each frequency in an epoch (density-modulated spectral array). In the compressed spectral array, "hills" appear at frequencies making a large contribution to the EEG, and "valleys" at frequencies that contain less power. The clinician should choose the method with which he or she is most comfortable. For acute decision making, many clinicians prefer to switch to the unprocessed analog EEG.

Several numerical descriptors of the EEG have evolved. Some, like the zero-crossing frequency or the burst-suppression ratio are derived from the time domain; others, such as the median power frequency or the spectral edge frequency, are based on the spectral array. All of these quantitative descriptors reduce the EEG to a single number with the obvious loss of much of the information contained within. Although none of these is optimal in extracting the maximal relevant information from the EEG, they may provide a useful level of abstraction. Most anesthesiologists are more comfortable comparing numbers than patterns, and these numbers permit simple quantitative comparisons. Three spectral descriptors have been frequently cited in the anesthesia literature: the peak power frequency, the median power frequency, and the spectral edge frequency (Fig. 16-8). The median power frequency bisects the power spectrum and has been correlated with serum concentrations of various narcotics and of methohexital.[27,28] The spectral edge frequency is the high-frequency "edge" of the spectrum, showing the frequency below which a particular percentage of power (usually 95 percent) is found. The spectral edge frequency

has been described as useful in detection of cerebral ischemia[29] and in correlating with clinical criteria of anesthetic depth.[30] It is most helpful when acute changes are fairly dramatic. (See Figure 16-6.)

So-called "brain mapping" (Fig. 16-9) sounds intuitively appealing but is fraught with potential problems. Most important, it is based on power spectral analysis. It may include artifact. For example, eye blinks are plotted as delta activity. This may be suspected by its exclusively frontal location, but true frontal delta activity might then be missed. Motion artifact is often included and may appear anywhere. Both these problems may be reduced by examining the raw EEG. Another pitfall is the use of interpolation to add information to the display that does not truly exist in the acquired signals. Even with electrode densities on the order of that provided by the International 10-20 System, interpolation can increase errors almost without limit.[31] Even at its best, EEG brain mapping produces less accurate localization than does magnetoencephalography.[32] Detection of magnetic fields produced by the brain is more expensive, however, and is not amenable to use in the acute care setting. Finally, we do not at present have sufficient experience to know exactly what to map in the operating room or critical care unit. Dozens of maps, according to frequencies, amplitudes, and combinations

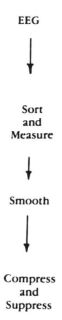

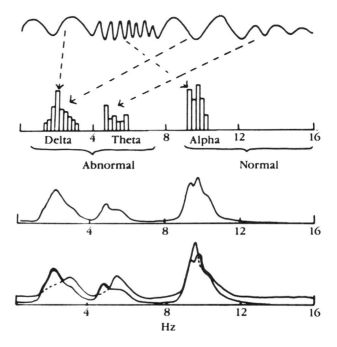

Fig. 16-5. Signal processing for the compressed spectral array (CSA), as popularized by Bickford. (From Bickford,[321] with permission.)

thereof, can be generated from a single 2- or 4-second epoch of EEG. The level of potential information overload is unmanageable in the acute care setting. A great deal more clinical experience is required to solve this problem.

A serious limitation of spectral analysis is its assumption that the component frequencies are independent and do not interact. The brain, however, like most biologic systems is nonlinear.[33] A recently introduced monitor uses a method that addresses the nonlinearity of the EEG: bispectral analysis.[34] The method is not new,[35] but was previ-

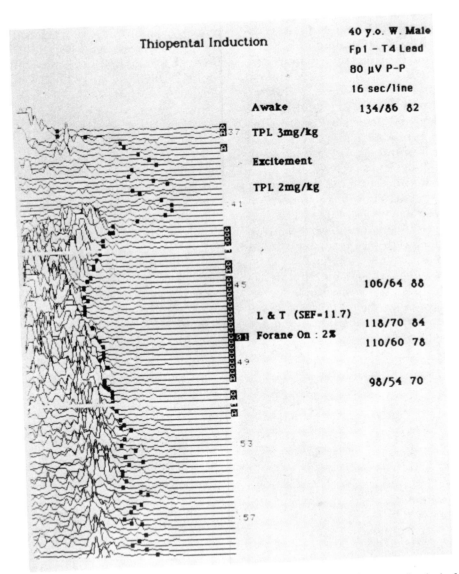

Fig. 16-6. A single-channel compressed spectral array display (CSA) during anesthetic induction. This CSA display contains frequency data from 0.5 to 30 Hz, and each spectral line represents data averaged over a 16-second epoch. In this case, while the patient is awake (*top*), the CSA shows predominantly delta frequencies, probably a result of eye-blink artifact. With the administration of thiopental, the low-frequency activity is replaced by diffuse high-frequency (beta) activity. A second dose of thiopental deepens the anesthesia, and the EEG slows with the spectral edge frequency (*black rectangle*) declining from 24 to 10 Hz.

ously beyond the computational capability of bedside monitors. It detects coherence between any two components in the spectral analysis (biocoherence) and to this extent can show the nonlinear characteristics of the EEG. Reports of bispectral analysis of EEG appeared more than 20 years ago,[36,37] but the literature on intraoperative applications is still limited.[38–41] Only reports of extensive clinical experience as related to other EEG methods and patient outcomes will clarify the eventual position of this promising technology.

The EEG is actually chaotic rather than periodic or quasi-periodic.[42] It manifests "deterministic chaos," which means that the dynamics of the signal are sensitively dependent on initial conditions. As with weather systems, which also exhibit deterministic chaos, epochs arbitrarily chosen initially (as all our sampling must be) may be so widely separated that components appear to be independent and unpredictable, even though they are closely related initially. Thus, both the weather and the EEG are deterministic chaotic processes, which should not be mistaken for truly random patterns (simple noise).

Computational requirements for analyses of chaotic systems are far greater than those for spectral analysis, and no commercially available monitors employing such methods are currently available. A number of reports appear in the current engineering literature, however.[33,42,43] Analyses of deterministic chaos of the EEG may well replace spectral analysis early in the twenty-first century.

Stimulation for Evoked Potential Monitoring

Recording EP requires stimulation to evoke responses. Technical and safety aspects of this stimulation, whether motor or sensory, require consideration. In the operating room and the critical care unit, methods of sensory stimulation differ somewhat from those used in the diagnostic laboratory. Special consideration must be given to factors of patient safety; accessibility to the patient for the surgeon, anesthesiologist, and electrophysiologist; and the inability of anesthetized or comatose patients either to cooperate actively with the testing procedure or to warn of impending iatrogenic injury. Comfort, greater with magnetic than with electrical stimulation, is not a factor during general anesthesia.

Somatosensory Stimulation

Somatosensory stimulation is most often a brief electrical current[44] delivered to a sensory or mixed nerve via paired electrodes traditionally placed approximately 3 cm apart with the cathode proximal

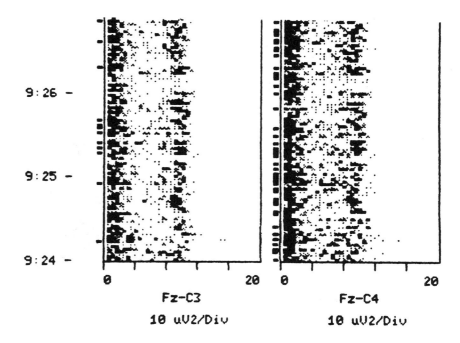

Fig. 16-7. A two-channel density spectral display. (From Grundy,[320] with permission.)

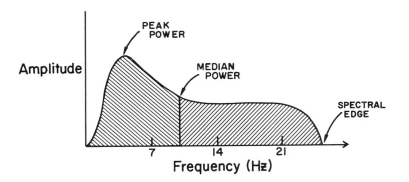

Fig. 16-8. Quantitative spectral frequency parameters are defined by the EEG spectrum. The peak power frequency is that frequency at which the highest power (or amplitude) exists. The median power frequency is that frequency at which half the spectral power is above and half is below, and the spectral edge frequency is that frequency which is the high-frequency "limit" or edge of the spectrum.

to prevent anodal block. In the diagnostic laboratory, the surface electrodes are commonly mounted on a rigid bar so that some pressure may be exerted to increase the proximity of the stimulating electrodes to the nerve. Hand-held ball stimulators are also used, and ring electrodes can be applied to the fingers.[45] Subdermal platinum electrodes or disposable adhesive electrodes such as those used for monitoring the ECG, are preferable to bar electrodes during anesthesia and operation; continuous pressure on the skin during anesthesia might produce ischemic damage. This is a particular risk during induced hypotension. Furthermore, a slight physical displacement of the elec-

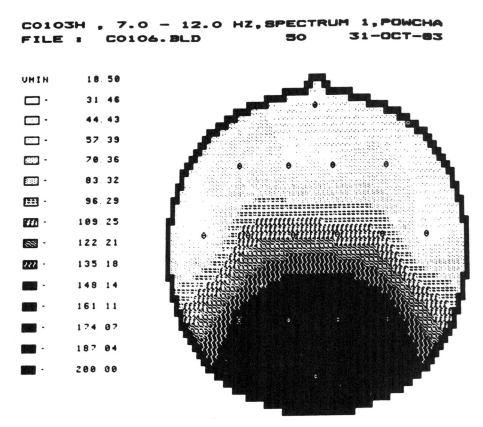

Fig. 16-9. EEG map representing power distribution within the alpha band of a subject during rest with eyes closed. The scale on the left side marks absolute power in μV^2. (From Pfurtscheller et al.,[322] with permission.)

trode, increasing the distance from the electrode to the nerve, might alter or obliterate the somatosensory EP because of inadequate stimulation. The visible motor twitch which confirms adequate simulation of a mixed nerve in the diagnostic laboratory can rarely be used to confirm continuous adequate stimulation intraoperatively. Pharmacologic blockade of the neuromuscular junction is frequently employed to provide muscle relaxation during general anesthesia, and the extremities may not be accessible to continuous observation once the patient is positioned for operation and sterile surgical drapes are in place. The small surface area of the subdermal (needle) electrode is not a problem for somatosensory stimulation if constant-current stimulators are used. The duty cycle of these electrodes is very short, approximately 250 μs one to five times per second, and the constant-current stimulators automatically compensate for impedance changes related to any electrode polarization. Disposable adhesive ECG electrodes are a good alternative and may be preferable except when positioning of the patient might compress the adhesive electrode and its connector, posing a risk of ischemic injury.

Somatosensory EP can also be elicited by magnetic stimulation of sensory or mixed nerves[46,47] or by stimulation of muscle.[48] The main advantages are greater comfort for the alert patient and greater ease in noninvasive stimulation of proximal nerves and plexi—both factors rarely of interest in the operating room. Relative disadvantages are important intraoperatively: (1) the large size of the magnetic stimulator can make for awkward positioning in the operating room; (2) the area stimulated is more diffuse and less exactly reproducible over time during continuous monitoring; (3) the possibility of propelling ferromagnetic objects within the field of stimulation is ever present; (4) EP at the brachial plexus and for the cortical N20-P25 complex (after stimulation of the median nerve at the wrist), the complexes most important in clinical monitoring, are less distinct and of lower amplitude than with electrical stimulation. No reports have appeared advocating this technique during surgery, but it may prove useful in a few special situations or in the critical care unit. The somatosensory EP produced by magnetic stimulation of muscle appear to be fairly specific in quantifying the function of muscle afferents.[48] Effects of anesthesia on these responses are unknown.

Somatosensory EP can also be elicited using a laser heat stimulus[20] or mechanical devices that touch or tap the skin.[49] A single filtered response evoked by a laser heat stimulus of sufficient intensity to produce a second-degree burn, a large-amplitude positive potential occurring approximately 300 ms after stimulation, may be a true physiologic manifestation of pain.[20] Laser and mechanical stimulation are primarily investigational tools at the present time.

Auditory Stimulation

Auditory stimulation is most commonly produced by clicks or tones. For monitoring, broadband filtered clicks are used to minimize effects of the high-frequency hearing loss so common in the elderly. In the diagnostic laboratory these signals are presented through stereo headphones. In the operating room, ear-insert transducers are usually employed to avoid the surgical field. However auditory stimuli are delivered, care must be taken that the pathway for sound transmission is not compromised by compression of the ear canals when headphones are too tight or by compression of either soft ear inserts or the pliable extension tubings commonly used to connect the transducers to ear pieces. Compression at any of these sites can alter or abolish the auditory EP by compromising the transmission of sound to the tympanic membrane. Ear-insert transducers that snap onto rigid or semirigid ear molds minimize this technical difficulty. Transducers should be calibrated at regular intervals. Audiology laboratories can provide this service.

In the diagnostic laboratory, shielded headphones inhibit detection of a sound delivered to one ear by the opposite ear. Broad band or "white" noise is nevertheless often delivered to the contralateral ear only (not to the ear being stimulated) to further prevent such an eventuality. This "masking" of the contralateral ear is vital in the operating room, as the sound delivered by ear-insert transducers is easily heard by the opposite ear.

Visual Stimulation

In the diagnostic laboratory, visual EP are most often elicited by reversal of a checkerboard pattern on a television screen. Other patterns have also been used. A normal pattern-reversal EP is shown in Figure 16-10. The edges in the patterns are particularly important for stimulating specific retinal receptors. Flash EP are less sharply defined than pattern-reversal EP (Fig. 16-11). In anesthetized or comatose patients, flash stimulation is accomplished by using light-emitting diodes mounted in opaque goggles positioned over the patient's closed eyelids (Fig. 16-12). Bland ointment is placed in the eyes, and clear plastic tape is used to keep the eyelids closed under the visual stimulator. Visual EP can be more reliably recorded if mydriatic eyedrops are used to dilate the pupil, but pharmacologic mydriasis may hamper subsequent clinical neurologic assessment.

Some investigators use light-emitting diodes mounted in scleral contact lenses for visual stimulation (M. Mahla, unpublished data). This seems justified when a large scleral lens of methyl methacrylate is used to protect the globe of the eye during major craniofacial operations. The contact lens and the eye are then in full view throughout the procedure. Some anesthesiologists, however, are concerned about placing a foreign body in the eye

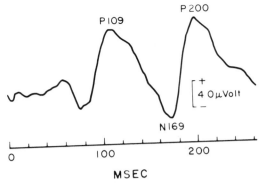

Fig. 16-11. Normal flash evoked potential. This visual EP was recorded from the left occiput to the right ear during flash stimulation of both eyes. Peaks are labeled *P* for positive and *N* for negative, with numbers indicating poststimulus latency. (From Grundy,[320] with permission.)

for long periods during anesthesia when the eye cannot be observed directly but might be subject to pressure or other manipulation, as during neurosurgical operations in the anterior cranial fossa or other procedures near the eye. The danger of keeping the eye open or opening it repeatedly during anesthesia in attempts to perform pattern stimulation of the retina would seem to pose unacceptable dangers of damage to the cornea from drying or trauma. Thus, only flash stimulation can be used for monitoring during anesthesia and operation. Even a pattern shown over closed eyelids is perceived through the lids as a flash.

Trigeminal Stimulation

These potentials, like somatosensory EP, are elicited by electrical current. Electrodes are placed on the face, gingiva, or teeth. Potentials elicited by stimulation of the tooth pulp are of experimental interest because they represent a relatively pure pain stimulus.

Motor Stimulation

Motor activity can be elicited by stimulating at virtually any level of the motor system, from cortex to peripheral nerve. At most sites, however, the stimuli are not specific to the motor system but affect sensory structures and pathways as well. This is no problem when evoked movements or muscle potentials are recorded. It has, however, produced confusion and misleading results when only nerve

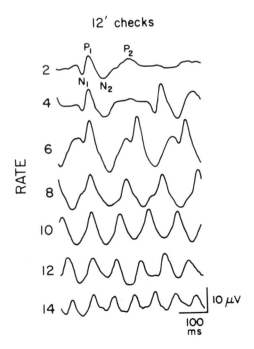

Fig. 16-10. Pattern reversal visual EP elicited by 12-minute checks at different alternation rates. Alternation rate per second is shown to the left of the records. Note the change from transient to steady-state visual EP at 8 alternations per second. (From Sokol,[323] with permission.)

action potentials or spinal cord EP were recorded. The latter may be motor EP; but, except when stimulation is of the motor cortex only, they may be antidromically conducted activity in sensory pathways or nerves. Uninterrupted sensory pathways extend from neck to toe, with no synaptic interruptions. As there is no uninterrupted sensory pathway to carry such antidromic impulses after cortical stimulation, cortically elicited potentials in spinal cord or nerve can be safely assumed to travel in motor pathways.

Stimulation of peripheral nerves is done just as that for somatosensory EP, except that the cathode should be distal rather than proximal to prevent anodal block. Intraoperative monitoring of cranial or peripheral nerves or spinal motor roots is commonly done with monopolar exploratory stimulation in the operative field by the surgeon. Inadvertent mechanical stimulation of the facial nerve by the surgical drill produces electromyographic activity which can provide audible feedback to the surgeon. Stimulation of the spinal cord with subdural or epidural electrodes, or with needles placed near the cord in interspinous ligaments or intervertebral disks, clearly activates both motor and sensory pathways.

Direct electrical stimulation of the motor cortex is done either during open craniotomy or by implanted electrodes placed for electrophysiologic studies prior to epilepsy surgery. With the anode directly on the pia, current levels of 0.25 to a few mA are sufficient. Pulses of 0.3 ms duration are routinely applied at 50 to 60 Hz for 5 to 15 seconds. Short episodes of such stimulation have not been associated with adverse effects in patients.

Repetitive cortical stimulation in animals, when sufficient to elicit afterdischarges, can produce an epileptic focus, which continues to fire after stimulation is stopped, a phenomenon known as *kindling*. Current density is the factor associated with injury due to excessive stimulation; this is minimized by using lower currents and larger electrodes. No reports have appeared of kindling due to direct cortical stimulation in the clinical setting. Seizures can be produced in epileptics, however.

Transcranial stimulation of the motor cortex can be used to evoke motor potentials. More experience has been gathered with electrical than with magnetic stimulators. Levy and colleagues[50] used a 3 × 5.5 cm plate attached to the scalp over the motor cortex as the anode, a curved 4-cm disk on the hard palate in the mouth as the cathode. Calculated current densities at the cortical surface were near those previously described for direct cortical stimulation. With stimulation rates of 17 to 28 Hz, and biphasic pulses of about 20 mA and duration 50 μs to 10 ms (usually 750 μs to 1 ms), EP

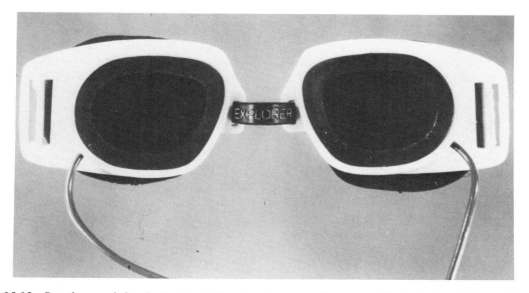

Fig. 16-12. Goggles used for flash stimulation in the operating room. Technical problems with this stimulator are discussed in the text.

could be recorded directly from the spinal cord when 250 to 500 (up to 4,000) responses were averaged. Production of movement required greater stimulation, and currents above about 15 mA were painful in awake volunteers. For intraoperative monitoring Levy used 20 to 40 mA currents several milliseconds in duration at repetition rates of 5 to 25 Hz. Lower current levels can be used with multiple cathodal plates or with a headband placed around the base of the skull. Levy's technique produced hypertension and tachycardia in some patients; these could usually be minimized by reducing the rate and duration of stimulation. No seizure activity was seen. Single shocks of 500 to 700 V and 1,000 mA have been used to demonstrate slowed conduction in patients with multiple sclerosis; no apparent adverse effects were produced.[51]

Transcranial magnetic stimulation[52] is appealing because there is no need to apply scalp electrodes and less pain is produced than with electrical stimulation. The stimulation is less well localized than electrical stimulation, however, and possible explosive propulsion of ferromagnetic objects must be avoided. Further, discharge of the stimulators is noisy, and at least some models may produce hearing loss in both patient and physician.[53,54]

Commonly used magnetic stimulators are limited to rates of approximately 0.3 to 1 Hz.[55] A commercially available magnetic stimulator capable of rates up to 60 Hz was recently evaluated and may be more dangerous.[56] Nine normal volunteers were tested with four 10-second trains of stimuli at each of six locations. Each subject was studied at a single frequency ranging from 1 to 25 Hz, and at the maximum output of the stimulator. In all five subjects stimulated at 5 Hz or higher, movements evoked by stimulation over the motor cortex increased in amplitude and complexity with each train. One subject, a 35-year-old woman, had a seizure after the third train of 10-Hz stimuli, having had a total 30 seconds of stimulation. The seizure began locally and spread, with a secondarily generalized convulsion lasting 57 seconds. It was followed by postictal confusion for 20 minutes and flaccid paralysis of the right side of the body, which resolved over 35 minutes. This subject's only potential risk factors were in the family history: uncomplicated febrile convulsions in a sister and a daughter and a drug-induced convulsion (drug not specified) in another sister.

Three of the nine subjects in this experiment had decreased hearing just after the stimulation,

which had resolved 4 hours later. All these decrements in hearing occurred after a total of only 240 seconds of stimulation. It is probable that intraoperative elimination of the protective middle ear acoustic reflex by muscle relaxants would magnify the effects of magnetic stimulation on hearing.[57]

In 10 other subjects described in the same report, rapid transcranial magnetic stimulation was applied over the motor cortex of the dominant hemisphere at frequencies of 1 to 25 Hz, beginning at each subject's motor threshold and progressing in 10 percent increments to the maximum output of the stimulator. Maximum stimulus intensity ranged from 140 to 220 percent of threshold intensity in different subjects. In this experiment, each train of stimulation caused the spread of cortical excitation in *all* subjects. Evidence of this excitatory spread resolved within five minutes after the end of the stimulus train. The number of pulses required to produce excitatory spread decreased as stimulus frequency and intensity increased. See Figure 16-13.

When transcortical magnetic stimulation is used to evoke descending motor potentials, it also activates excitatory intracortical axon collaterals to neighboring pyramidal cells[58] and to inhibitory neurons which then project to the same pyramidal cells.[59] Normally, these connections balance each other and there is no horizontal spread of excitation. At higher frequencies, however, temporal summation of excitatory postsynaptic potentials outstrips that of inhibitory potentials because conduction is faster in the myelinated monosynaptic excitatory collaterals. The imbalance in excitatory and inhibitory corticocortical connections after prolonged (10-second) trains of rapid transcranial magnetic stimulation may produce such widespread horizontal activation of the cortex that reentering self-generating activity may produce a seizure, even in subjects without predisposing factors.

The authors of this important report[56] propose that all investigators using rapid transcranial magnetic stimulation at rates of 1 Hz or faster wear earplugs; that precautions be taken to prevent burns from metal electrodes that can be overheated by magnetic pulses[60]; that subjects be informed of the possibility of seizures, particularly if there is a family history of seizures; and, as EEG afterdischarges are not sufficiently reliable to predict a risk of seizure induction, that clinical (motor) evidence of spreading cortical excitation should be considered the earliest sign of epileptogenic activity. Parameters derived from the data in this report can be used as a guide. For example, according to these data (Fig. 16-13), rapid transcranial magnetic stimulation at 25 Hz and 200 percent of threshold can be safely applied for a total of *only four impulses.*

How all this relates to safety of transcranial magnetic stimulation intraoperatively is far from clear. Much additional work is needed. For the present it seems that electrical stimulation, though more cumbersome than magnetic, may be both more precise and less dangerous.

Several workers have sought methods for enhancing motor EP. Either partial voluntary contraction of the muscle affected by motor stimulation[15] or a conditioning sensory stimulus given just prior to motor stimulation[61] can produce a marked facilitation of the next motor EP. Only the latter method would normally be available intraoperatively. A recent proposal for short trains (five pulses) of very rapid electrical stimulation of the exposed cortex (300 to 500 Hz) to facilitate motor EP recording during anesthesia[62] would seem to deserve further testing.

Evoked Potential Signal Processing, Display, and Measurement

Although processing of EP is similar in many respects to EEG processing, several essential differences exist. First, EP are precisely time-locked to a triggering stimulus. Second, far-field EP are lower in voltage than the near-field EEG, so that greater amplification is necessary. Far-field EP recorded from the scalp are smaller than the background EEG and must be extracted from this "noise."

Even though some cortical activity related to sensory stimulation can be observed in the unprocessed electroencephalogram, special techniques are required to demonstrate EP reliably. Most EP recording at present is based on averaging of multiple individual responses precisely time-locked to repeated stimuli.[11] This process extracts the electrophysiologic signals evoked by stimulation from the "noise" of background activity and artifact, much of which is chaotic or random. The signal-to-noise ratio increases according to the square root of the number of repetitions. Many other methods of signal processing have been developed,[63] but none are in common clinical use at present. Reports can be found in contemporary literature on engineering and clinical neurophysiology.

Currently, all systems display EP as plots of voltage against time, in the time domain. Other displays may be available, but they are not clinically important today. Measurements of displayed waveforms are made by using electronic cursors, with amplitude and latency reported quantitatively and precisely. Desirable capabilities of EP equipment include secure electronic storage of data and provision for printing at least intermittent paper records. It is very helpful to be able to designate, store,

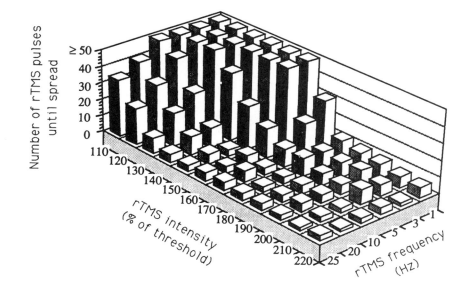

Fig. 16-13. Diagram showing the intensity, frequency, and number of transcranial magnetic stimulation pulses required to produce excitatory spread in normal volunteers. (From Pascuel-Leone,[56] with permission.)

and display a reference waveform from baseline or later episodes for immediate comparisons with current data.

No agreement exists regarding the polarity of displayed EP waveforms, even within the anesthesia literature. Usage is perpetuated in each laboratory by the ability of investigators and clinicians to perform gestalt pattern recognition, using the polarity convention to which they are accustomed. Thus, each representation of EP waveforms must include a designation of polarity. In this chapter, grid-one-positive peaks are up.

The confusion about polarity is compounded by the fact that waveform polarity is reversed by reversing the inputs of an electrode pair. For example, the brainstem auditory EP waveform shown in Figure 16-14 was recorded with the vertex electrode (CZ) in "grid 1" of the input box, the ipsilateral ear electrode (Ai) plugged into "grid 2," and the polarity convention showing positive up. This representation may be described as "vertex-positive up." The waveform would have precisely the same appearance if it were described as "ear-negative up," with the ear electrode plugged into "grid 1," the vertex electrode plugged into "grid 2," and the polarity convention "negative up." Multiple display factors can hinder comparison of

waveforms. Electrode montage, voltage calibration, time calibration, stimulus onset, and polarity convention should always be shown.

Characterization of EP waveforms depends on both qualitative and quantitative methods. First, the overall configuration and reproducibility of waveforms, as shown by superimposition of replicated records, are examined. Then measurements are made of the poststimulus latencies and amplitudes of individual peaks or troughs. These peaks and troughs must be identified using the gestalt pattern recognition skills of a trained observer. Automatic measurement of the minimum or maximum amplitude in a given time window, or even the calculated rates of change in slope, cannot be relied on to identify these peaks or troughs. Pathologic conditions, drug effects, and reversible physiologic alterations can alter poststimulus latencies dramatically, so that any identification of peaks based solely on time-window criteria is likely to be deceptive. The human brain recognizes patterns more accurately than any computer programs so far devised, and peaks must be identified by a trained observer before definitive measurements are taken.

Once the points of interest in the waveform are identified using qualitative techniques, quantitative methods are used to describe the waveform more precisely. Accurate measurements are made by using movable cursors on an oscilloscope screen to select points for quantitative measurement by the computer. Poststimulus latencies are measured in milliseconds after stimulus onset. Amplitudes are measured as microvolts: from peak to peak, from an average zero baseline before stimulus, from the zero point at the onset of the recording, or from a designated point in the waveform. Each method of amplitude measurement has advantages and disadvantages, and no general agreement exists at present as to the most appropriate method.

Secondary measurements may be derived from the absolute values for amplitudes and poststimulus latencies. Interpeak latencies and ratios between the amplitudes of different peaks are clinically useful. Central conduction times are calculated by subtracting the latencies of early subcortical peaks from the latencies of later peaks that arise in the midbrain or cerebral cortex. Central conduction times are particularly useful for distinguishing those EP alterations due to brain dysfunction from EP changes related to failure of sensory input, ab-

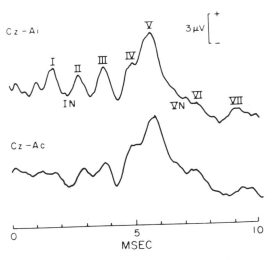

Fig. 16-14. Normal brainstem auditory evoked potential. *CZ-Ai*, vertex to ipsilateral ear; *CZ-Ac*, vertex to contralateral ear. Peaks in the upper waveform are labeled to show the customary designations. The purported generators are shown in Table 16-5. (From Grundy et al.,[249] with permission.)

normalities of sensory receptors, or normal differences among subjects such as the differences in height that affect absolute latencies of somatosensory EP.

Conduction velocities can be calculated for peripheral nerve, spinal cord, or central structures, using interpeak latencies and measured or estimated distances between the known or purported generators of these peaks. Similarly, the time intervals between peaks of ascending or descending volleys recorded from sets of electrodes separated by known distances can be used to calculate the conduction velocities in peripheral nerves or spinal cord.

Other methods of analyzing EP signals can be used. For the EP represented as a plot of voltage against time in the traditional way, one can measure centroids for particular peaks or component wave areas.[64] If the EP activity is represented in the frequency domain rather than in the time domain, power spectra can be described.[65] Significance probability mapping,[66] noise estimation,[67] correlation analysis,[68] and parametric modeling[69] have also been used. Stepwise discriminant analysis has been employed both to detect and to compare EP.[70]

The optimal methods for display and measurement of EP data in the operating room and critical care unit have not yet been fully defined. Stacked plots of sequentially recorded waveforms with multiple channels arranged side by side and events marked in the margins, coupled with trend plots of quantitative measurements (or derived measurements such as central conduction times or conduction velocities), may well be best at present.

Steady-state EP, elicited by a regular train of stimuli, can be measured in terms of amplitude and phase angle.[71] The phase angle describes the relationship between the constant train of stimuli and the resulting train of responses. Measurements of steady-state EP, quantitatively characterized by only two numerical values that can be updated every few seconds, may offer important advantages for intraoperative monitoring. This possibility awaits clinical evaluation.

The 40-Hz response is a steady-state EP elicited by a train of auditory stimuli delivered at a rate of about 40 Hz with a constant interstimulus interval. The amplitude of the response, which approximates a sine wave after the first few stimuli, is much greater with stimulation near this frequency than at higher or lower frequencies, probably because of overlapping components of the middle-latency auditory response. The 40-Hz response is thought to arise in the auditory cortex and/or the thalamus or rostral reticular formation. It has been considered as an index of the depth of anesthesia, but observations of the effects of isoflurane on the feline 40-Hz response show little difference between responses recorded at 0.3 MAC and those obtained at 1.0 MAC.[72]

Electrical Safety

All monitoring equipment to be taken into the operating room or critical care unit must meet the generally accepted standards of safety for the electrically susceptible patient. Leakage current to the patient should be less than 10 μA, and leakage current to the instrument case must be less than 100 μA. When recording directly from neural structures in the operating room, some investigators insert semiconductor switches that automatically disconnect the patient from the machine when current exceeds 10 μA. Others consider this additional precaution unnecessary and find that the switches add noise to the recorded electrophysiologic signals.

All line-powered electrical devices attached to the patient must be connected to an appropriate isolated power source. Provision must be made for dissipation of static electricity. Extension cords should not be employed. Broken or frayed wires should not be used. Monitoring systems should be engineered to minimize the risks of injury to personnel and patients when bulky equipment must be moved in close quarters. All components should be secured to an appropriate rack, and the equipment must be protected from fluids, blood, and overheating.

Some manufacturers are well aware of the requirements for monitoring the electrically susceptible patient. Others, and some in-house technical personnel assembling systems from hardware components, may not have these factors in mind. The anesthesiologist should be sure that all the relevant safety principles are observed.

Quality Control

Spontaneous EEG activity should be monitored at least at intervals during EEG processing or recording of EP, and data acquisition should be suspended when the signal is noisy. Most of the commercially available EEG and EP monitors have options for automatic artifact rejection, but this is usually based only on amplitude criteria. Much of the artifact observed in the spontaneous EEG tracing does not meet the amplitude criteria for rejection. For example, signals generated by the unipolar electrosurgical machine are rejected automatically, but signals from the bipolar coagulator are much smaller and are not automatically excluded. Other low-voltage artifacts may be related to small movements of electrode wires or cables. These movements may be produced by suction tubings within the operative field that lie across electrode wires under the surgical drapes, or by movements of the surgeon and his or her assistants. Electrocardiographic leads crossing the EEG wires are another source of low-voltage artifact that is not automatically eliminated.

EEG or EP should be recorded before induction of anesthesia, when they can be correlated with preoperative neurologic assessment, and continually thereafter until the patient leaves the operating room. Preoperative recording is particularly important when neurologic deficits exist before surgery and baseline waveforms may be abnormal. In most cases, it should be possible to continue monitoring until the patient can be awakened for at least rudimentary clinical neurologic assessment.

Use of pseudorandom interstimulus intervals helps to eliminate contamination of EP waveforms by rhythmic EEG activity in the frequency range of interest. When this kind of contamination is suspected, an average should be recorded with no sensory stimulation. Averaged background EEG activity may sometimes appear distressingly similar to the waveforms obtained after sensory stimulation.

The technologist recording EP should tabulate as closely as possible the pharmacologic, physiologic, and other variables that affect EP in the operating room and critical care unit. Accurate tabulation is greatly facilitated by the use of procedure-specific protocols with coded key strokes for variables and events of interest. Such programs are currently available.

Representative waveforms should be printed or plotted in the operating room or critical care unit immediately after they are recorded. Waveforms electromagnetically stored on disk or tape may occasionally be lost. Excessive time is required to recall these waveforms from the storage medium for on-line comparison to signals recorded subse-

quently. Selected quantitative measurements of EP should be made and automatically logged when EP are recorded.

Whenever possible, EP thought not to be at risk from the operative procedure should be recorded at intervals to help distinguish regional from systemic causes of intraoperative EP alteration. For example, during operations on the thoracic or lumbar spine, somatosensory EP should be recorded not only during stimulation of the posterior tibial nerve at the ankle, but also during stimulation of the median nerve at the wrist. This will help to distinguish the changes produced by operative manipulation from those related to the effects of anesthetics or to innocuous alterations in systemic physiology. In addition, dangerous systemic deterioration can be promptly detected.

Stimulation and recording parameters used should not be indiscriminately altered during monitoring. Alterations in these parameters can in themselves change EP,[73,74] confusing interpretation. Filters are set to admit frequencies of interest but eliminate as much noise as possible. Excessive filtering can, in the process of making waveforms more pleasing to the eye, distort waveforms or even eliminate the information of greatest interest. The rate at which the analog signal is sampled for conversion to digital format must be more than twice the highest frequency admitted by the analog filters.[11] This is to prevent distortion of the waveforms by a process known as *aliasing*. Currently available equipment can enhance quality control by automating appropriate steps in data acquisition and documentation.

Anesthetic Management for Electrophysiologic Monitoring

Several factors must be considered in selecting an anesthetic regimen for the patient who needs intraoperative EEG or EP monitoring. The pathophysiologic conditions or contemplated risks that provide the indication for neurologic monitoring may place other constraints on anesthetic management. For example, the patient with a spinal cord tumor and partial loss of cord function needs not only intraoperative monitoring of cord function but also, and even more critically, vigilant maintenance of spinal cord perfusion and oxygenation.

The anesthesiologist has at hand a variety of pharmacologic agents and physiologic manipulations that must be combined in the best possible way to provide safety and comfort for the patient, optimal operating conditions so that the contemplated procedure can be accomplished with minimal trauma, and reliable monitoring of those body systems at risk during the procedure. No single anesthetic regimen can be prescribed for all patients who require intraoperative monitoring of EEG or EP, but some guidelines for use in clinical decision-making are available. The patient's best interest is served by a closely coordinated team approach to overall optimization of care.

A special consideration in many patients who need intraoperative electrophysiologic monitoring is the need for early awakening after operation to facilitate clinical neurologic assessment. Agents that may needlessly delay either emergence from anesthesia or rapid recovery of mental alertness in the early postoperative period are avoided.

Premedication with agents of relatively short duration of action, such as meperidine and hydroxyzine, if otherwise appropriate, can facilitate the recording of preanesthetic baseline EP by reducing apprehension and the associated muscle activity. Balanced anesthesia, including moderate dosages of a narcotic, is often appropriate. Intravenous agents should be given as constant infusions to avoid the effects of intermittent bolus injections on EEG or EP. Relaxation is provided with neuromuscular blocking agents, and cardiovascular responses to stimulation are controlled with vasoactive drugs rather than deep anesthesia. Deep general anesthesia with inhaled or injected agents seriously hampers monitoring of cortical or motor EP evoked by transcranial cortical stimulation.

The use of halogenated anesthetic agents when EP of cortical origin are to be monitored is controversial. When they are used, isoflurane at concentrations below 0.5 MAC, combined with narcotics, is probably best. The volatile agents decrease amplitudes and increase latencies of cortical EP, sometimes obliterating them at deeper levels of anesthesia.[75–78] Nitrous oxide also decreases amplitudes of cortical EP,[79,80] but this agent has virtually no effect on poststimulus latencies. The effects of halogenated anesthetics and of nitrous oxide seem to be additive.[80] These agents do affect EP of subcortical origin, but their effect on the short-latency EP is not so great that it interferes with monitoring.[81,82] When neuromuscular blockade must be allowed to dissipate so that the surgeon can identify motor nerves by stimulating them directly and observing the muscle twitches that result, halogenated agents may be specifically indicated to assure immobility of the patient. Use of partial neuromuscular blockade when motor nerves or motor EP are being monitored is controversial and may sometimes produce misleading results.

Injectable agents that can alter EP, such as sedatives,[83,84] narcotics,[85] and intravenous anesthetics,[86–91] should not be given by bolus injection during critical operative or physiologic manipulations. Accurate interpretation of changes in the EP may be difficult or impossible when alterations might be related either to the surgical procedure or to the predictably reversible effects of drugs. For example, the surgeon might be misled into abandoning resection of a difficult spinal cord tumor or removing Harrington rod instrumentation from a scoliotic spine because of EP changes that were actually related to the effects of anesthetics. Conversely, a bolus of etomidate (which increases somatosensory EP amplitudes) could conceivably mask an important EP change, so that injury might not be detected.[86,87]

The anesthesiologist can make a valuable contribution to patient safety by monitoring and constraining physiologic variables that affect EEG or EP, such as the patient's body temperature,[92–94] arterial blood pressure, and tensions of arterial blood gases.[95–97] When deliberate physiologic manipulations, such as induced hypothermia or hypotension, are used to facilitate the surgical procedure or to minimize the risk of neurologic damage, the state of the patient should be changed as expeditiously as safely possible, and a new relatively constant physiologic status should be established. Waveforms recorded during the new steady state can then be used for comparison with those recorded subsequently under similar physiologic conditions but during critical operative manipulations.

In summary, the anesthesiologist makes three important contributions to the success of electrophysiologic monitoring even when he or she is not directly involved in the monitoring itself. First, the anesthetic is planned to provide for continuous monitoring of neurologic function, with early awakening after the completion of the surgical procedure to facilitate at least a rudimentary clinical neurologic assessment. Second, anesthetic agents and techniques that will hamper the projected electrophysiologic monitoring are avoided. Third, the anesthesiologist, as far as possible, maintains the patient in a relatively constant pharmacologic and physiologic state so that changes in EEG or EP can be attributed with greater reliability to the surgeon's manipulations. Clearly, the anesthesiologist must make many pharmacologic and physiologic interventions that can alter electrophysiologic waveforms. Close communication must be maintained not only with the surgeon but also with monitoring personnel.

ELECTROPHYSIOLOGY IN DIAGNOSTIC NEUROLOGY

The last several years have seen a decline in the use of diagnostic EEG for diagnoses other than epilepsy or sleep disorders. At the same time there has been a virtual explosion in the use of EP in clinical neurology.[98–101] Visual and auditory EP are used to assess sensory function in infants,[102] in patients who are mentally handicapped or otherwise unable to cooperate, and in patients suspected of hysteria or malingering.[103] These tests are also used in conjunction with behavioral testing to more specifically delineate disorders of hearing and vision. Nerve conduction studies are used to assess peripheral neuropathy and to measure responses to treatment.[104] Use of either EEG or EP to detect mass lesions in the central nervous system becomes progressively less important with the ascendency of neuroradiologic diagnostic techniques.

The most widespread use of EP measurement in the neurologist's office is undoubtedly in the diagnosis of multiple sclerosis.[98,105] EP are often abnormal even before clinical signs of neurologic dysfunction become apparent. Thus, EP studies are particularly important in making the differential diagnosis between multiple sclerosis and other disorders when a single pathway is abnormal clinically. The presence of isolated lesions at multiple sites is an important diagnostic characteristic of multiple sclerosis. For example, if a patient with weakness and ataxia also has abnormal visual EP, the likelihood that a diagnosis of multiple sclerosis may be correct is greatly increased.

Electroencephalogram

The most important application of EEG in diagnostic neurology is in the diagnosis and management of epilepsy. No other method can be used to definitively diagnose this disorder. When medical therapy is less than satisfactory and surgical treatment is contemplated, intensive monitoring of EEG with simultaneous video is vital to identification and localization of the epileptic focus. Correlations between magnetic resonance images and EEG[106] or magnetoelectroencephalography[107] provide identification of epileptic foci with a high degree of reliability. Both preoperative and intraoperative corticography, discussed below, play key roles in the surgical treatment of epilepsy.

Somatosensory Evoked Potentials

In clinical practice, somatosensory EP are most often elicited by electrical stimulation of mixed nerves,[9,10] particularly the median nerve at the wrist, the posterior tibial nerve at the ankle, or the peroneal nerve at the popliteal fossa or just below the knee. As these are mixed nerves, and muscle contraction is usually produced, the initial activation of these sensory pathways is followed by activation of the muscle and tendon afferent pathways. The information transmitted is therefore complex, with input reaching central structures at different times. Somatosensory EP in response to stimulation of sensory nerves are less robust but can be reproducible. Somatosensory EP (Fig. 16-15) are transmitted by peripheral nerves, plexi, nerve roots, the dorsal columns of the spinal cord, and the lemniscal pathways to the thalamus and the primary sensory cortex. The ascending volley can be recorded from any of several sites along this pathway. Purported neural generators of the early peaks are listed in Table 16-4. Conduction velocities in peripheral nerves are determined by recording nerve action potentials that arise in nerve trunks and in the brachial or lumbar plexus. These early EP are also important for confirming adequate sensory input when function at higher levels is to be evaluated. Impulses arising in the spinal cord are recorded from electrodes placed over the spines of lumbar, thoracic, and lower cervical vertebrae.

A negative potential recorded from the skin overlying the second cervical vertebra approximately 14 ms after stimulation of the median nerve at the wrist is thought to arise in the dorsal column nuclei. A negative wave seen over the specific sensory cortex contralateral to the site of the stimulation occurs approximately 20 ms after stimulation of the median nerve at the wrist and seems to be the first cortical event of the somatosensory EP. Some observers think this wave, called N20, originates in either the thalamus or the thalamocortical radiations. The letter designates negative polarity and the number indicates the nominal poststimulus latency of 20 ms.[108] All observers agree that a preceding positive wave seen 13 to 17 ms after stimulation and distributed widely over the scalp is subcortical in origin. This early positivity is not well seen in frontally referenced recordings. When a noncephalic reference such as the knee, hand, or shoulder is used, the early positive activity as well as the even earlier potentials originating in the brachial plexus or spinal cord can be recorded from the scalp. A close correlation exists between cortical activation and regional cerebral blood flow during somatosensory stimulation.[109]

Because of the greater distances that must be traversed, somatosensory EP elicited by stimulation of

TABLE 16-4. Purported Generators of Short-Latency Somatosensory Evoked Potentials[a]

Peak	Generator
N9	Brachial plexus
N11	Spinal roots or dorsal columns
N13, 14	Spinal cord gray matter or dorsal columns
N14, 15	Brain stem and/or thalamus
N20	Primary somatosensory cortex

[a]Stimulation: median nerve; recording: clavicle, mastoid process, 2nd cervical vertebra, primary somatosensory cortical area; reference electrode: FZ or noncephalic. (Early positive waves are obscured in frontally referenced recordings.) N, negative peak. See text for references.

the posterior tibial nerve at the ankle have greater poststimulus latencies than do somatosensory EP elicited by stimulation of the median nerve at the wrist. The initial cortical positivity occurs approximately 25 ms after the stimulation of the median nerve at the wrist but 35 to 40 ms after stimulation of the posterior tibial nerve at the ankle. Poststimulus latencies of somatosensory EP are directly related to patient height.

Pathologic change at any point along the conducting pathway from the site of stimulation to the specific somatosensory cortex can affect somatosensory EP. Localization of a lesion is often possible if early peaks are present and stable, but later peaks are absent or abnormal.

Auditory Evoked Potentials

After far-field recording of brainstem auditory EP[110] was introduced in 1970, this testing largely replaced testing of the nonspecific and more variable intermediate-latency auditory EP (often called middle latency response) in both clinical neurology and audiology. A normal brainstem auditory EP is shown in Figure 16-14. Generators of specific peaks in the brainstem auditory EP waveform have been proposed (see Table 16-5).

Brainstem auditory EP may be useful in diagnosing multiple sclerosis if the patient has a clinically demonstrable lesion elsewhere in the nervous system and a second isolated neurologic abnormality can be demonstrated on brainstem auditory EP testing.[105] In addition, brainstem auditory EP are useful for localizing vascular or mass lesions involving the auditory pathway.[111] These short-latency potentials show characteristic changes with transtentorial herniation.[112] Either unilateral lesions of the

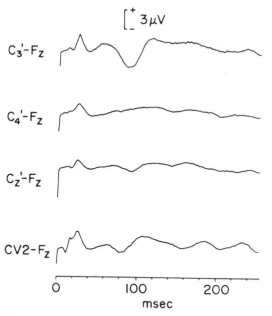

Fig. 16-15. Normal somatosensory evoked potentials recorded simultaneously from the scalp and neck following stimulation of the right median nerve at the wrist. The patient was anesthetized with nitrous oxide, thiopental, and fentanyl. The stimulus rate was 0.9 Hz. Both cortical and subcortical peaks are apparent, and the same recording montage can be used during stimulation at anyone of four stimulus sites: right or left median nerve, right or left posterior tibial or peroneal nerve. (From Grundy,[3] with permission.)

brainstem auditory pathway or lesions that compromise the crossed auditory projections can produce asymmetries of bilaterally recorded brainstem auditory EP.[105,113,114]

Visual Evoked Potentials

Both the electroretinogram (ERG)[115] and the cortical visual EP elicited by pattern reversal stimulation have been well characterized and are clinically useful.[116] Subcortical visual EP[117,118] have yet to receive widespread attention. Cortical visual EP vary according to the type of stimulation, the part of the retina stimulated, degree of pupillary dilation, and the patient's attention level.[21,116] They may be useful in distinguishing among various causes of visual loss,[118] and they are quite sensitive to the subclinical demyelination seen in early multiple sclerosis.[119,120] In addition, visual EP show characteristic changes in coma, hydrocephalus,[121] and some forms of epilepsy.[21] Flash EP (Fig. 16-11) are less well defined and less reproducible than pattern reversal EP.

Trigeminal Evoked Potentials

The function of the trigeminal nerve can be tested by recording from the scalp the potentials elicited by electrical stimulation of the face, gums, or tooth pulp[122,123] (Fig. 16-16). These potentials may be abnormal in trigeminal neuralgia.[124,125] Preoperative recordings of trigeminal EP may help to predict therapeutic results in patients with classic trigeminal neuralgia who undergo microvascular decompression of the fifth cranial nerve or percutaneous retrogasserian glycerol rhizotomy.[122,126]

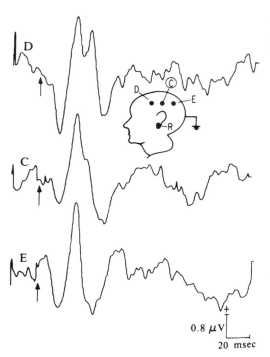

Fig. 16-16. Trigeminal evoked potentials to electrical stimulation of the gingiva above the first maxillary bicuspid at four times threshold. Stimulus rate was 0.9 Hz, duration 200 µs; 128 responses were averaged. Filters were 3 to 3,000 Hz, sweep time 205 ms. (From Bennett et al.,[122] with permission.)

Motor Evoked Potentials

Motor EP are used to measure the latency relaxation as well as the excitability and contractility of muscle in patients with muscle disorders.[15] These potentials have also been used to measure conduction velocity in the pyramidal tract[127,128] and to detect neuropathy in the nerves supplying the external sphincter ani.[129] Except for conduction studies in peripheral and cranial motor nerves, these methods have not achieved widespread popularity; but motor EP elicited by electrical or magnetic stimulation have been described in a number of clinical reports.

Recordings of motor EP after percutaneous electrical stimulation in the cervical region can be used as a rapid noninvasive method for quantitative electrophysiologic evaluation of damage to the brachial plexus.[130] Motor EP have been used to diagnose a spinal cord lesion following epidural anesthesia.[131] After minor cerebral ischemia of the lacunar type,

TABLE 16-5. Purported Generators of Brain stem Auditory Evoked Potentials[a]

Peak	Generator
I	Acoustic nerve
II	Intracranial acoustic nerve and/or cochlear nucleus (medulla)
III	Superior olive (pons)
IV	Lateral lemniscus (pons)
V	Inferior colliculus (midbrain)
VI	Medial geniculate (thalamus)
VII	Thalamocortical radiations

[a]Listed peaks are positive at the vertex. See text for references.

motor EP are altered more frequently than somatosensory EP.[128] Transcortically elicited motor EP in patients with hyperreflexia, spasticity, and weakness often show increased thresholds and/or prolonged central conduction times.[132]

A study of motor EP produced by transcranial magnetic stimulation in five normal subjects showed random variability in responses, perhaps due to spontaneous fluctuations in levels of corticospinal and segmental motoneuron excitability.[133] In patients with hemiplegia due to stroke or those with motor neuron disease, transcranial magnetic stimulation revealed many fewer abnormalities than did electrical stimulation.[134] It was postulated that magnetic stimulation repetitively discharges pyramidal cells and, by temporal summation, produces more powerful excitatory potentials at the lower motoneuron synapse. The role of motor EP in diagnostic neurology is not yet clearly defined.

Cost Effectiveness of Diagnostic Electrophysiology

General consensus exists that EEG is highly cost effective in epileptology and sleep studies but not in the diagnosis of structural abnormalities. Controversy has arisen regarding the appropriateness of much of the EP testing performed in clinical neurology. At least a few nationally prominent neurologists who are experienced in the field believe that much current diagnostic EP testing is superfluous and represents a needless expense.[135] They hold that neuroradiologic procedures and clinical assessment will answer most of the questions posed when EP tests are performed. These workers recognize the possibility that multiple sclerosis can be diagnosed at an earlier stage using EP testing in conjunction with clinical neurologic examination than using clinical assessment alone. However, they question the value of earlier diagnosis when no treatment is available for the disorder.

Perhaps most other neurologists would disagree. In some instances, EP may be important for distinguishing disorders amenable to treatment from those that are not. For example, EP may help to distinguish the dementia related to Alzheimer's disease from dementia of ischemic origin, and some dementia due to ischemia is amenable to either medical or surgical therapy. EP may also be important for evaluating responses to therapy.

One great advantage of electrophysiologic testing is its noninvasive nature. EP recordings are more expensive than clinical neurologic assessments alone, assuming that a thorough neurologic assessment will be performed in any case, but they are both safer and less expensive than many of the neuroradiologic procedures currently used. Furthermore, electrophysiologic testing can be performed at frequent intervals and in a variety of settings. The most important neurologic applications of EP testing in the future may be in assessing acute responses to therapy and in monitoring anesthetized or comatose patients who are at risk for serious neurologic injury.

INTERPRETATION OF ELECTROENCEPHALOGRAM AND EVOKED POTENTIALS

Once the hurdles of data acquisition and processing are cleared, the clinician faces the challenge of interpretation.

In the Diagnostic Laboratory

Although interpretation of EEG and EP in the operating room differ somewhat from interpretation in the diagnostic laboratory, the underlying principles are similar. The anesthesiologist should be acquainted with the principles of interpretation used by the clinical neurologist in diagnostic testing.

Electroencephalogram

Diagnostic EEG interpretation consists of complex pattern recognition and depends on extensive clinical experience. Despite a volume of research on quantitative EEG analysis and brain mapping, no consensus exists on how quantitative EEG should be used in the care of the individual patient. Application of quantitative methods requires substantial expertise in EEG interpretation. These methods should be viewed as adjunctive to traditional EEG testing.[136,137]

Evoked Potentials

Interpretation of diagnostic EP depends on recognition of reproducible characteristic patterns in the waveforms and comparison of quantitative measurements to measurements of EP recorded from a population of normal subjects. Guidelines have been developed by a committee of the American Electroencephalographic Society.[13] Normal subjects should have no personal or family history of neurologic disease or disease in the system being studied and should meet other specified conditions. Furthermore, each control group should contain an equal number of age-matched male and female subjects. The distribution of normal values in a particular group should be examined to determine its approximation to a gaussian distribution, and if significant deviations from normality such as skewness, kurtosis, or both are seen, the observed data should be transformed to obtain a more nearly gaussian curve. Once a normal distribution is obtained, the mean and standard deviation are calculated for each measurement. In subsequent diagnostic testing, clinically observed values exceeding 2, 2.5, or 3 standard deviations of the mean from the normal group are interpreted as abnormal.

Tolerance limits may be employed to give a quantitative appreciation of the statistical significance of the abnormality. for example, a laboratory may elect to choose as its normal limit for a given EP measurement the 98 percent tolerance limits for 95 percent of the normal population. This implies a 98 percent chance that 95 percent of the normal population will fall within the specified limits. As latencies and conduction times are regarded as abnormal when they are excessively long, and amplitudes are called abnormal when they are excessively small, one-tailed tolerance limits are used. A laboratory may decrease the proportion of false-positive results by adopting more stringent normal limits, but this choice is associated with the penalty of increasing the proportion of false-negative interpretations. Conversely, when more liberal limits of normal are chosen, false-positive reports will be increased and false-negative reports decreased.

Once normal limits are determined within a laboratory, each EP can be classified as normal, abnormal, or technically inadequate. According to the guidelines published by the American Electroencephalographic Society, it is acceptable for a new laboratory to use the normative data published by another center, providing two requirements are met. First, the conditions of stimulation, recording, and so on must be either identical to or fully compatible with those of the reference laboratory. Second, the new laboratory should study at least 20 normal subjects spanning the age range of the patients that will be examined there, and it should be determined that a specific proportion of these subjects, for example, 95 or 99 percent, are within the limits derived from the reference laboratory's data.

In the Acute Care Setting

Interpretation of EEG data in the operating room or critical care unit poses difficulties not usually encountered in the diagnostic laboratory. The goals of recording EEG or EP in the acutely changing clinical situation differ from the goal of distinguishing normality from abnormality in diagnostic neurology. Meaningful interpretation of EP in the operating room or critical care unit requires a global assessment of all that is happening to a patient physiologically, pharmacologically, and pathophysiologically. Only in this way can the most likely causes of EEG or EP alterations be determined and the information gained from electrophysiologic monitoring made useful in clinical decision-making.

In the operating room, waveforms recorded before induction of anesthesia are correlated with the patient's clinical neurologic status and serve as control measurements for that patient. Continuous electrophysiologic monitoring is then performed to detect departures from the preoperative baseline status.

In the critical care unit, monitoring is often required when baseline data are not available. This presents little difficulty when waveforms are within normal limits, but when waveforms are abnormal or absent, particular care must be taken to ensure technical adequacy of monitoring. For example, the absence of brainstem auditory EP in a comatose patient might be due to technical difficulty with the ear stimulator, deafness due to a middle ear or inner ear problem, or neurologic abnormality of either the eighth cranial nerve or the brainstem auditory pathways. In such a case, recording of a normal electrocochleogram would rule out the peripheral causes of deafness and localize the abnormality to the eighth nerve or brainstem. Similarly, the ERG provides evidence of effective visual stimulation, and recording of an electrical complex generated by the brachial plexus confirms both adequate somatosensory stimulation and the functional integrity of the peripheral nerve trunk. Documentation of sensory input is particularly important when EP are recorded as part of an electrophysiologic evaluation of brain death.[138–140]

Electroencephalogram

EEG interpretation in the operating room or critical care unit again depends on pattern recognition of the unprocessed EEG, but the range of patterns requiring recognition is narrower than for diagnostic EEG. The most important EEG patterns in the operating room and critical care unit are artifacts, changes from the individual patient's baseline records, slowing, loss of amplitude, burst suppression, seizure activity, and new asymmetries. Interpretation is impossible without relating changes to clinical events of interest; the interpreter should be in the operating room and must be well informed about clinical events and their implications for the EEG.

Evoked Potentials

A number of potentially confusing variations other than injury to neural structures can alter the EP recorded in the acute care setting. These may be considered in three main categories: technical difficulties, drug effects, and physiologic alterations. Whenever a sudden unexpected EP change occurs in the operating room or critical care unit, the operator's initial step should be to rule out some technical problem as the source of change. Once technical difficulties have been ruled out, one assesses the possibility that changes are related to drug administration or benign physiologic changes. If EP changes are seen with induced hypotension or hemodilution, neurologic function may be at risk. Physiologic homeostasis should be restored to reduce the possibility of permanent injury.

Criteria for Abnormality

The clinician is now faced with another pattern-recognition task: integrating all the information available in a given situation and assessing it in light of data gleaned not only from personal professional experiences but also from the general body of medical knowledge in the field. The physician recognizes the patterns that emerge and uses them to reach the most appropriate decision for a given patient in a particular situation. Electrophysiologic waveforms that would be definitely abnormal in the diagnostic laboratory may be completely normal during anesthesia. Furthermore, intraoperative monitoring of EEG or EP can be valuable even when the preoperative waveforms are clearly abnormal, provided the waveforms are sufficiently reproducible to allow tracking of function.

In light of these considerations, we have categorized intraoperative EP findings[81] as follows:

Category I: Minimal change (presumably due to anesthesia and temperature changes only)

Category II: Transient latency increase, with return toward normal before the end of anesthesia

Category III: Obliteration of the evoked potential, with return toward normal before the end of anesthesia

Category IV: Evoked potential obliteration, with no recovery before the end of anesthesia

Category V: Study abandoned because of technical problems

Category VI: Absent evoked potential preoperatively and intraoperatively, with associated preoperative neurologic deficit

Available data do not allow precise quantitative delineation of the acceptable tolerance limits for intraoperative variability of EEG or EP. One should note that definitions of the acceptable limits for intraoperative variability of arterial blood pressure and heart rate are similarly lacking. The clinician can nevertheless use these monitoring modalities to advantage, continually trying to optimize intraoperative function in hopes of avoiding postoperative disability. Modeling the performance of a single experienced observer, we derived a quantitative criterion for warning of intraoperative alterations in brainstem auditory EP: an increase in the post-stimulus latency of wave V exceeding 0.07 ms/min between successive measurements or a cumulative increase 1.5 ms from baseline. This criterion held up fairly well in clinical testing.[81]

Cranial and peripheral nerves are more resistant to the effects of ischemia and hypoxia than are more proximal neural structures. The cauda equina is more sensitive to these insults than the peripheral nerve, the lumbar cord more sensitive than the cauda equina, the thoracic cord more sensitive than the lumbar, and the cervical cord more sensitive than the thoracic. Similarly, the brainstem is more sensitive to hypoxia and ischemia than the spinal cord but less sensitive than the cerebral cortex.[96,141] It follows that the EP changes due to compression of a cranial or peripheral nerve may remain reversible for a longer time than EP changes due to ischemia of the spinal cord or brain. In practice this seems to be true. Brainstem auditory EP changes associated with positioning or with retraction of the eighth cranial nerve may be readily reversible even after relatively long periods of obliteration.[142] This has led some electrophysiologists to wait for virtual loss of brainstem auditory EP before warning the surgeon, particularly when the most likely compromise of the auditory pathway is at the level of the auditory nerve.[143] Others advocate warning the surgeon when brainstem auditory EP amplitude falls by 50 percent because it is not possible to predict whether the waveform will reappear intraoperatively after it is lost.[144]

Greenberg and his coworkers[145,146] presented a multimodality system of grading sensory EP recorded from patients with head injuries that categorized the abnormal EP by grouping them as follows: grade 1: mildly abnormal; grade 2: moderately abnormal; grade 3: severely abnormal; grade 4: absent. This classification, though crude, was useful in predicting the outcome of severe head injury.

Possibilities for totally automated interpretation of electrophysiologic data in the acute care setting seem remote. The pattern recognition skills of the trained observer still far exceed those that can be automated. An experienced physician must perform the final interpretation of electrophysiologic data, considering the totality of all that is happening to the patient pharmacologically, physiologically, and pathophysiologically. The clinician uses this information not for prescribing automatic decisions but rather as an aid to clinical decision-making.

ELECTROENCEPHALOGRAPHIC AND EVOKED POTENTIAL APPLICATIONS IN THE OPERATING ROOM

Intraoperative monitoring of EEG and EP is now part of the usual standard of care for numerous operations in many medical centers and community hospitals. Carotid endarterectomy is probably the most frequent indication for intraoperative EEG monitoring and risk of injury to the spinal cord the most frequent clinical indication for EP monitoring. Other indications are also important. Many anesthesiologists have familiarized themselves with these techniques, and technical personnel with appropriate training are becoming more widely available. Many observers believe that the anesthesiologist is the most appropriate physician to oversee EEG or EP monitoring in the operating room, as the surgeon may need to concentrate on the operation and the neurologist may not be able to spend long hours away from other areas of responsibility. An obvious exception is during corticography for epilepsy surgery, when the epileptologist routinely comes to the operation room for interpretation and to assist with surgical decision-making.

Many reports of EEG and EP monitoring speak in terms of "false positive" and "false negative" results and of the sensitivity and specificity of monitoring methods. Selecting the most appropriate threshold for acting on monitoring data inevitably requires value judgments. When the purpose of monitoring is to prevent a neurologic injury that may be severe and permanent, and when risks of projected interventions are relatively low, sensitivity becomes more important than specificity. That is, numerous false positive results are much more acceptable than even one false negative result that ends in tragedy for the individual patient. Specificity may be more important in the diagnostic setting.

A practical caveat relates to individual practice patterns of surgeons and anesthesiologists. If these clinicians are unwilling or unable to change management of the individual patient on the basis of monitoring data, the monitoring is unlikely to benefit that patient.

Carotid Endarterectomy

Immense controversy surrounds many aspects of carotid endarterectomy.[147] Only recently have large clinical trials demonstrated the value of this procedure in patients with neurologic symptoms and high degrees of stenosis.[148-154] Electrophysiologic monitoring during carotid endarterectomy will be discussed in some detail to illustrate the diversity of techniques, results, and opinions surrounding practical application of these techniques.

Not all clinicians agree that intraoperative monitoring of brain function is worthwhile. Much of the controversy surrounding monitoring of the brain during carotid endarterectomy stems from the misconception that placement of an intraluminal shunt is the only available intraoperative intervention in the event of deteriorating function. Some practitioners limit monitoring to the period of time surrounding carotid occlusion. Others feel no need to monitor the brain at all if they use a shunt routinely. These practices are based on erroneous assumptions.

In actual fact, most perioperative strokes related to carotid endarterectomy are embolic in nature,[155] and use of a shunt may itself increase the possibility of artery-to-artery embolism.[156] Nevertheless, there are clearly a few patients with cerebral blood flow so low during carotid occlusion that failure to use a shunt will result in a very high risk of neurologic deficit. Furthermore, many observers fail to recognize the possibility of intervention to prevent or minimize brain injury in the event of embolism. Many episodes of deteriorating brain function during carotid occlusion can be resolved by methods short of shunting, most often by raising arterial blood pressure. Problems can certainly occur either before or after carotid occlusion[155,157]; if monitoring has been suspended, these will not be detected. When a shunt is used, it may become occluded. Even when deterioration is due to embolism, changes may be transient. For example, small platelet thrombi may break up within several hours. In such cases, optimization of oxygen delivery by manipulation of arterial pressure, blood volume, hematocrit, and so on, can limit or prevent permanent injury. Ischemia due to more substantial embolism may be reduced by immediate intravascular thrombolysis.

Carotid endarterectomy performed in alert patients under regional anesthesia provides an opportunity to observe the precise time of onset of neurologic deficits and thereby deduce the probable cause of each deficit.[155,158] Good evidence supports the presumption that the onset of the neurologic deficit occurs when the insult occurs.[159,160] In a series of 359 patients having carotid endarterectomy under cervical plexus block, 14 (4 percent) had neurologic deterioration during test occlusion of the carotid artery and had shunts inserted.[155] Of the 345 patients having the operation without shunting, 15 had deficits resolving within 24 hours (4.3 percent) and 6 had deficits lasting longer than 24 hours. Only one patient had a deficit that could be attributed to cerebral hypoperfusion during carotid occlusion. Of the 21 deficits, 20 were thromboembolic, reperfusion phenomena, or related to arterial hypotension.

In analyzing conflicting reports, it is essential to remember that levels of cerebral blood flow associated with irreversible brain injury are far lower than the levels at which brain electrical activity stops.[161,162] Once electrical activity is affected, it is not possible to determine whether cells are dying or are merely in the "ischemic penumbra." As most EEG changes during carotid occlusion resolve promptly after insertion of a shunt, many surgeons prefer to use selective shunting based on some kind of brain monitoring.[159,163] In attempting to reduce the rate of brain injury to as near zero as possible, these surgeons inevitably use shunts in some patients who would do well without them. They choose to tolerate a relatively high rate of "false positive" monitoring results in striving to eliminate "false negatives."

Much of the debate about brain monitoring during carotid endarterectomy dwells only on whether a shunt should be used, ignoring other factors that may lead to stroke in this high-risk population. Best results are achieved when monitoring is continuous. Continuous monitoring can be achieved either by doing the procedure under regional anesthesia and keeping the patient alert for clinical neurologic assessment or by instituting electrophysiologic monitoring before induction of general anesthesia and monitoring without interruption until the patient is sufficiently awake for clinical evaluation.

Numerous monitoring methods have been tried during carotid endarterectomy. These can be compared to the two methods with which greatest satisfactory experience has accumulated: (1) clinical neurologic assessment of the alert patient and (2) 16-channel analog EEG continuously monitored by a knowledgeable observer. Each method has advantages and disadvantages, but both are effective.

Clinical evaluation requires minimal sedation so that the patient is indeed alert. Most patients tolerate this well so long as they are comfortably positioned, regional anesthesia is adequate, and both surgeon and anesthesiologist transmit a feeling of confidence that this management is fully acceptable and appropriate. This method avoids the costs and complexities of electrophysiologic monitoring. In patients who need shunts, all observers are readily convinced of the need for action by the complete loss of responsiveness that typically occurs within seconds of test occlusion of the carotid artery. Possible disadvantages of this technique include concerns that the patient may become uncomfortable or restless during the procedure, the need to avoid sedation (which might obscure neurologic assessment), the possible duration of the operation, fear that the patient may move during critical stages of the operation, and concerns about access to the airway should complications arise. The typical abrupt loss of responsiveness upon test occlusion is often seen before dramatic EEG change is apparent. Minimal deficits not amenable to clinical assessment intraoperatively may be associated with small asymmetries in EEG that are apparent only with quantitative methods.[164]

Most surgeons today prefer general anesthesia for this procedure. Clinical evaluation of cerebral function then becomes essentially unavailable. Perhaps the largest series of carotid endarterectomies monitored by 16-channel EEG is that at the Mayo Clinic,[159] now encompassing more than 4,000 cases. To date, no serious new neurologic deficits have occurred in patients whose EEG showed no persistent intraoperative deterioration (F. Sharbrough, personal communication, 1994). This series is often quoted by advocates of using EEG monitoring to determine the need for a shunt.

Advocates of performing carotid endarterectomy under general anesthesia without monitoring and without shunting often refer to the work of the group at the University Hospital in London, Ontario.[165] In a series of 176 operations, clinicians used EEG monitoring but never inserted a shunt. Of 55 patients with intraoperative EEG changes, 5 (9 percent) awoke postoperatively with related neurologic deficits. Two of these were severe and permanent. EEG changes were considered to be major (attenuation of 8 to 15 Hz activity to minimal or nil and/or a twofold or greater increase in delta activity at 1 Hz or less) in 22 cases, and both of the severe and permanent injuries occurred in this group. In contrast, none of the 121 patients with no intraoperative EEG changes awoke with new deficits. In the two patients with intraoperative strokes, major EEG changes occurred within 12 and 20 seconds, respectively. One patient had marked attenuation and marked delta activity; the other had marked attenuation and mild delta activity. The delta activity resolved in one patient even though no shunt was used. Augmentation of delta activity reflects a less severe reduction in the blood flow than does attenuation of all EEG activity.[166] The amplitude attenuation did not resolve in either of these cases. Thus, 2 of 22 patients with major EEG changes, again 9 percent, had intraoperative strokes, compared to none of 121 without EEG changes. It is not unreasonable to assume that insertion of a shunt in the only patients who suffered major neurologic injury may have improved the outcomes for these two individuals.

Although this report closes with the suggestion that preoperative data may be more valuable than intraoperative EEG monitoring in predicting postoperative neurologic deficits, and this paper is often cited as support for the concept that EEG monitoring has no value during carotid endarterectomy, interventions other than shunting were made in this series on the basis of intraoperative EEG changes. The report states that the surgeon who performed all the operations in this series had the "policy of performing the operation himself when an EEG change is observed instead of supervising the resident's performance."[165] When an EEG change occurred, clamp time was 16 to 56 minutes, averaging 32.6 minutes. When no EEG change occurred, clamp time was 22 to 60 minutes and averaged 37.9 minutes. It may be reasonable to assume that efforts were made to increase arterial blood pressure when EEG changes occurred, but these data are not provided. When at least one intervention was routinely made (senior surgeon vs resident performing the endarterectomy) it is no longer possible to state that the intraoperative monitoring made no difference in outcome. True "blinding" of surgeon and anesthesiologist to the EEG findings would give a clearer picture, but such a study may no longer be possible.

Continuous intraoperative monitoring of the 16-channel EEG by a skilled observer is equipment- and personnel-intensive. A number of clinicians use either a limited number of EEG channels or processed EEG, as described above, during carotid endarterectomy. When major EEG changes occur, as in most cases when patients need a shunt, the change can be seen in only two or four symmetrical channels placed over watershed areas of the middle cerebral arteries. Most focal changes in the EEG (seen in only a few channels) that are not associated with clamping of the carotid artery are related to asymmetrical effects of anesthesia on a preexisting focal abnormality.[159] About 1 percent of these, however, are followed by neurologic deficits in the immediate postoperative period.[166] Such focal deficits are not detected by monitoring only two or four channels. In a series of 103 operations monitored with 2-channel compressed spectral array and observation of the raw EEG in the same two channels, monitoring indicated ischemia on test occlusion of the carotid in 14 patients and bypass shunts were inserted.[167] Six postoperative neurologic deficits occurred, and in five of these the monitoring indicated a late ischemic event when it was no longer possible to insert a shunt. In the sixth patient with a new deficit, the EEG monitoring never indicated ischemia. This may have been a limitation of the minimal number of channels monitored. Aperiodic analysis of 2-channel EEG in 70 patients having carotid endarterectomy under cervical plexus block was less reliable than clinical neurologic assessment.[168]

Assuming the same signals, does processed EEG add valuable information not available in the analog EEG? This is controversial. The answer obviously depends on the quality of the data, skill in interpreting both the processed and analog signals, the specific algorithms used in processing the signals, and the pattern recognition skills of the observer present during the operation. At least two reports suggest that it may.[164,169] By contrast, two careful investigations found that neither the 4-channel density modulated spectral array[170] nor a group of 18 spectral descriptors[171] adequately substituted for the neurologist's interpretation of the 16-channel analog record. A comparison of two measurements derived from spectral analysis of the 2-channel EEG showed that EEG power changes were more sensitive indicators of intraoperative cerebral ischemia than variations in the spectral edge frequency.[172] Not surprisingly, surgeons who did not allow EEG data to influence the surgical procedure were unimpressed with the value of intraoperative EEG monitoring.[173]

The cortical areas perfused by the middle cerebral artery are the most vulnerable during and after carotid endarterectomy. This is the artery most frequently embolized in the perioperative period, and its watershed areas are the most at risk during cerebral hypoperfusion due to carotid occlusion. Because the primary cortical response to stimulation of the median nerve at the wrist arises in the area at risk, a number of investigators have monitored somatosensory EP during carotid endarterectomy.[174–176] Somatosensory EP monitoring during 38 operations was used to determine whether a shunt was needed.[177] Of 10 patients under general anesthesia, 3 had marked somatosen-

sory EP changes that were reversed by shunt insertion. In 28 patients under cervical plexus block, only 1 showed somatosensory EP change within 1 minute of test occlusion and had a shunt inserted. Both EEG[178] and somatosensory EP[179] have been successfully used to detect otherwise unsuspected shunt occlusion during carotid endarterectomy.

There is no general consensus on criteria for abnormality of either EEG or somatosensory EP. This helps to explain apparent discrepancies among series regarding the sensitivity and specificity of these two methods. For example, in one series of 193 carotid endarterectomies under general anesthesia, every patient with early postoperative neurologic morbidity had an increase in central conduction time of more than 20 percent from the anesthetic baseline control.[180] Prolongation of central conduction time was 100 percent sensitive and 89 percent specific for early postoperative neurologic morbidity. In contrast, using the criterion of amplitude reduction exceeding 50 percent, the sensitivity was 86 percent and specificity 96 percent. For loss of the cortical response, sensitivity was 71 percent and specificity 99 percent. As false-positive results are far more acceptable than false-negative results (occurrence of undetected brain injury), most clinicians would prefer a criterion with sensitivity as close to 100 percent as possible.

In a series of 400 carotid endarterectomies, complete loss of somatosensory EP amplitudes was seen during 17 procedures.[181] Of 7 patients without a bypass shunt, 5 had neurologic deficits after surgery, while 3 of 10 patients who had shunts inserted had postoperative neurologic deficits. Thus, patients who lost somatosensory EP during carotid occlusion had a much greater incidence of postoperative neurologic deficit when no shunt was used. A report of 675 carotid endarterectomies monitored with somatosensory EP gave a diagnostic sensitivity in predicting neurologic outcome of 60 percent with a specificity of 100 percent.[182] Four of 586 patients with no somatosensory EP change had immediate postoperative neurologic deficits. Reversible somatosensory EP abnormalities were seen in 83 cases, mainly during carotid clamping. All 6 patients with irreversible somatosensory EP changes awoke with new deficits. A more sensitive criterion of somatosensory EP change would have given greater sensitivity with less specificity—a desirable tradeoff for the clinician wishing to completely avoid permanent neurologic injury.

Three studies directly comparing somatosensory EP and EEG monitoring during carotid endarterectomy under general anesthesia reached differing conclusions. One concluded that conventional EEG and somatosensory EP monitoring had similar sensitivity and specificity.[183] In this series, however, somatosensory EP were monitored only before, during, and for 15 minutes after carotid occlusion rather than continuously from before induction of the anesthesia until the patient awakened. Further, no shunt was used in any patient regardless of any EEG or somatosensory EP changes. In the two other reports of such comparison, selective shunting was used. In a series of 53 cases, 23 patients had EEG evidence of ischemia during carotid occlusion.[184] Of these 23 patients, 10 had an increased somatosensory EP latency of 0.1 ms or greater, and 1 of these 23 had a decrease in somatosensory EP amplitude of 50 percent or greater. This report concludes that somatosensory EP monitoring is less sensitive for detecting cerebral ischemia than 16-channel EEG recording. The third report compared EEG and somatosensory EP changes during 151 carotid endarterectomies in which 120 cases had no change in either EEG or somatosensory EP upon carotid occlusion. A shunt was used only in the 16 patients who showed severely depressed EEG and cortical somatosensory EP. When somatosensory EP were less affected, no shunt was used. No new neurologic deficits occurred in the 15 patients with less severely affected somatosensory EP, while one occurred in a patient who had no change in either EEG or somatosensory EP and two occurred in patients who had shunts inserted because of EEG changes accompanied by severe somatosensory EP abnormalities.[185]

In summary, many methods of brain monitoring during carotid endarterectomy have been tried. The two "gold standards" are clinical assessment of the alert patient operated upon under regional anesthesia and 16-channel analog EEG interpreted by an experienced observer and monitored from before induction of anesthesia until the patient is sufficiently awake for clinical neurologic assessment postoperatively. In settings where neither of these techniques is available, somatosensory EP monitoring or 2- or 4-channel EEG monitoring can provide useful information to guide intraoperative management.

Cardiac Surgery

Management of the patient during cardiopulmonary bypass and monitoring of the brain during cardiac surgery are no less controversial than management and monitoring during carotid endarterectomy. Several methods have been used to monitor the brain during cardiac surgery, and results differed in ways that might be expected. The quality control in many of these studies was less than ideal, and only a very few studies emphasized actions on the basis of data obtained by electrophysiologic monitoring rather than attempts to predict outcome. As in other situations, if no action will be taken on the basis of the data, the monitoring is not useful for that particular patient.

An early report of EEG monitoring in 75 patients described visual analysis of the EEG supplemented by power spectral analysis, peak power frequency computation, and average EEG amplitude integration.[186] Of the 75 patients, 15 had significant episodes of hypotension during cardiopulmonary bypass, and all showed associated bilateral EEG slowing or loss of amplitude; 7 patients whose EEG changes were transient had no postoperative neurologic deficits; 8 patients who had EEG disturbances beginning at the time of hypotensive episodes during cardiopulmonary bypass developed postoperative neurologic deficits: their EEG abnormalities persisted postoperatively and correlated with the nature and evolution of the deficits. A 1984 report describes a comparison of visual versus processed EEG analysis in 25 patients during cardiac surgery, with visual analysis only in an additional 5 patients.[187] Burst-suppression activity was seen in 26 percent of the patients during cardiopulmonary bypass, and processing by spectral analysis destroys this characteristic pattern. The report concludes that univariate descriptors of the processed EEG appear inadequate to describe the behavior of EEG during anesthesia in a large percentage of patients.

Despite the above considerations, a more recent report describes 2-channel EEG recordings made from 78 patients during cardiopulmonary bypass and analyzed by descriptors of the Fourier power spectrum.[188] The quality control was obviously less than optimal during data acquisition, complete data being of acceptable quality for only 58 patients. The authors concluded that, under the conditions studied, except for gross loss of signal, the

EEG had little value for predicting brain injury. It seems not unlikely, however, that with more EEG channels, improved quality control in signal acquisition, on-line feedback to the surgeon, anesthesiologist, and perfusionist, and visual analysis in addition to signal processing, a different conclusion might have been reached. Even a gross loss of signal, if detected and acted upon by the team in the operating room, may be valuable during such procedures.

EEG monitoring has been used to detect burst-suppression after administration of thiopental as a measure to protect the brain before aortic declamping.[189] The EEG has also been used to determine safe levels of hypothermia for circulatory arrest during cardiovascular procedures such as replacement of the ascending aorta or aortic arch.[190] This would appear to be particularly valuable in light of the extreme variability in temperatures recorded from different sites during the induction of hypothermia prior to circulatory arrest.

Multimodality EP were monitored in 16 adults during cardiopulmonary bypass and moderate hypothermia.[92] Hypothermia progressively increased the latencies of all the major components in all modalities. This effect was more profound on later components of the EP. Visual EP always disappeared below 25°C, while short-latency somatosensory EP and brainstem auditory EP were always recordable at this temperature. Intraoperative somatosensory EP elicited by stimulation of the median or ulnar nerve at the wrist have been used to predict peripheral nerve injury during cardiac surgery with self-retaining sternal retractors.[191] Somatosensory EP changes were seen in 21 patients. In 16 of these, the changes resolved intraoperatively, but in 5 they persisted throughout the procedure. None of the patients in whom the waveforms reverted toward baseline but all of the five patients in whom the SEP change did not resolve had neurologic deficits postoperatively. Again, this report emphasized prediction rather than intervention to prevent deficits. Many informal anecdotal reports from other clinicians indicate that adjustment of retractors is usually followed by recovery of somatosensory EP and no postoperative deficit.

Two reports give much more optimistic assessment of electrophysiologic monitoring during cardiac surgery than described above. One of these states that intraoperative interventions based on quantitative EEG decreased postoperative neuropsychological dysfunction from 44 percent without intervention to 5 percent with intervention.[192] In the other, a quantitative criterion was developed to provide feedback to the operating team: focal increases in relative low-frequency power (1.5 to 3.5 Hz) lasting longer than 5 minutes and greater than 3 standard deviations from the anesthetic baseline control established in the individual patient.[193] In an initial 38 cases, this descriptor was used to predict a crude evaluation of neuropsychological outcome. It gave a 68 percent false-positive rate but only an 8 percent false-negative rate. Of 48 intraoperative quantitative EEG episodes, 19 were associated with pump perfusion pressures below 50 mm of mercury. In an additional 48 patients, this quantitative EEG descriptor was used in an attempt to prevent postoperative deterioration in neuropsychological outcome: 31 episodes of quantitative EEG abnormality were detected and these ischemic events resolved after prompt elevation of perfusion pressure. The rate of postoperative disorientation fell from 29 percent in the first group, without interventions, to 4 percent in the second group, with interventions.

Both anesthesia and the hypothermia often used during cardiopulmonary bypass affect the electrical activity of the brain, and these two factors may interact. For example, in patients having deep hypothermia under ether anesthesia, without cardiopulmonary bypass, EEG isoelectricity developed at an average esophageal temperature of 27.2°C, while EEG activity persisted throughout procedures done with morphine anesthesia and cardiopulmonary bypass, even at the lowest esophageal temperature of 22.3°C.[194] Thus, it is difficult to compare EEG recordings during hypothermia when different anesthetics are used.

Evoked Potentials in Spinal Surgery

Since the introduction of somatosensory EP monitoring for scoliosis surgery in 1977,[195] its use to monitor spinal cord function during these procedures has become relatively widespread. Neurologic deficits occur in less than 1 percent of Harrington rod instrumentation cases, but injury is far more common with sublaminar wiring techniques such as placement of Luque rods. Although somatosensory EP travel primarily in the posterior columns of the spinal cord, and greatest concern exists about motor rather than sensory function, in all well-documented cases to date with technically adequate recording and continuous monitoring, acute injury to the cord has been detected by changes in somatosensory EP lasting for at least 15 to 30 minutes and usually longer.

A 1991 report described experience with 1,168 consecutive cases[196]: 119 patients had decreases of somatosensory EP amplitude greater than 50 percent, and 32 of these had clinically detectable neurologic changes postoperatively. In 35 cases, somatosensory EP amplitude was rapidly restored either spontaneously or by repositioning of the recording electrode with no postoperative neurologic change. In 52 patients, persistent and significant somatosensory EP changes were seen but were not followed by neurologic sequelae. None of the cases with falls in somatosensory EP amplitude of less than 50 percent had neurologic problems postoperatively. Factors identified in this series as associated with increased risk of postoperative neurologic deficit included neuromuscular scoliosis, the use of sublaminar wires, the magnitude of somatosensory EP decrement, and limited or absent intraoperative recovery of somatosensory EP amplitude.

A sizable number of smaller series and clinical case reports have appeared, some of these perhaps shedding light on methods that can be used to facilitate recovery of somatosensory EP amplitude and latency. Presumably, interventions leading to prompt recovery of somatosensory EP amplitude may have had a positive impact on the outcomes of the individual patients (Fig. 16-17). Interventions that have been described include adjustment of spinal instrumentation, reversal of induced hypotension, decreasing the amount of surgical correction of the deformity, and removing bone grafts.[195,197–199] If changes are seen in somatosensory EP, most surgical and anesthetic teams perform an immediate wake-up test. If no somatosensory EP changes are detected, however, many teams omit wake-up tests during operations for scoliosis.

It is important in monitoring spinal cord function to stimulate each lower extremity separately. Simultaneous bilateral stimulation can lead to false-negative results.[200] Injury to one side of the cord can obliterate somatosensory EP elicited by stimulation of the lower extremity on that side, while those potentials following stimulation of the extremity on the uninjured side are unchanged.[201]

Somatosensory EP have proved useful in neurosurgical procedures within the spinal canal. They provide valuable information during operations to relieve intractable pain by placing deliberate lesions in the dorsal route entry zone of the cord.[202] Monopolar recordings from the dorsal route entry zone of the cord after peripheral nerve stimulation are used at multiple levels for segmental localization and to monitor the state of the afferent pathway and the dorsal horn. Intraoperative loss of somatosensory EP during resection of a large arteriovenous malformation from the posterior aspect of the cord (Fig. 16-18) was associated with loss of spinal cord function in the postoperative period.[203]

The spinal cord EP has also been monitored intraoperatively. It has a relatively large amplitude that is fairly stable in the presence of anesthetics and related drugs.[204] The stimulus is delivered to the spinal cord either above or below that section of the cord at risk intraoperatively, and recording is in the opposite position. Experience with spinal cord EP is still less than the collective experience with somatosensory EP monitoring.

In a report of 6 extramedullary and 14 intramedullary spinal cord tumors, the cord was stimulated from an epidural electrode caudal to the level of the tumor and spinal cord EP were recorded from an epidural electrode rostral to the tumor.[205] An increase in the amplitude of the recorded potential was seen after removal of the tumor in four extramedullary and three intramedullary cases. Five of the six patients who had decreased amplitude of this potential after removal of the tumor went on to develop postoperative motor deficits. Unfortunately, however, four patients developed postoperative neurologic deficits despite stable spinal cord EP intraoperatively. One patient had changes in the EP amplitude but no postoperative deficit. Two of the four false results that occurred in patients with intramedullary tumors had postoperative symptoms consistent with unilateral damage to the spinal cord. The authors concluded that, despite the reproducible waveforms of the spinal cord EP, the sensitivity of this monitoring method for patients having spinal cord tumors resected was unsatisfactory.

The introduction of motor EP monitoring to the clinical environment engendered considerable excitement. An initial report of motor EP monitoring in 98 cases indicated that responses to stimulation of the motor cortex, which were recorded from the spinal cord, changed so little in amplitude and latency with injury conditions that their use was compromised.[206] Recordings from peripheral nerve and muscle gave much more helpful data. The so-called *neurogenic motor evoked potential* recorded from a peripheral nerve after rostral stimulation of the cord

at first seemed attractive because it could be used in the presence of muscle relaxants and was thought to represent the function of motor pathways.[207] Subsequent studies in animals demonstrated that the sciatic nerve response to spinal

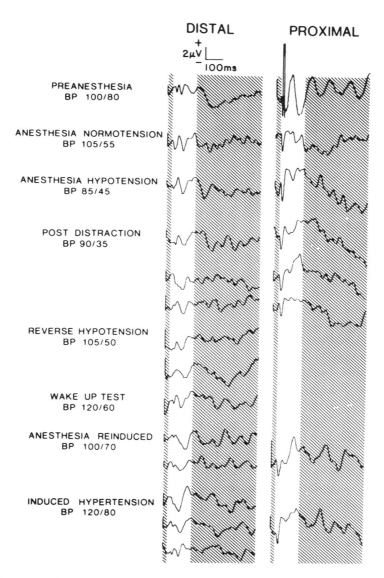

Fig. 16-17. SEP changes related to manipulation of arterial blood pressure during spinal fusion for scoliosis. Unshaded areas highlight the primary specific cortical responses. After induction of anesthesia, responses evoked by stimulation of the median nerve (initial *V*-shaped peak in unshaded area, in column labeled "proximal") are stable. By contrast, the *W*-shaped complex elicited by stimulation of the posterior tibial nerve (in the column labeled "distal") deteriorated markedly with mild-to-moderate hypotension and returned toward normal when blood pressure was raised. The wake-up test was normal, and instrumentation was kept in place. The patient remained neurologically intact. (From Grundy et al.,[198] with permission.)

cord stimulation was not traveling through ventral nerve roots as had been assumed, but was actually conducted antidromically through sensory fibers in dorsal routes. The sciatic nerve response to spinal cord stimulation was abolished by dorsal column transection.[208]

Recording from muscle, however, does ensure that the signals are being carried by motor pathways. In 30 patients who had spine fusion and Cotrel-Dubousset instrumentation, the compound muscle action potential was recorded from the lower limb after stimulation of the upper spinal cord.[209] In three of these patients, the derotation maneuver altered the compound muscle action potential, but not the po-

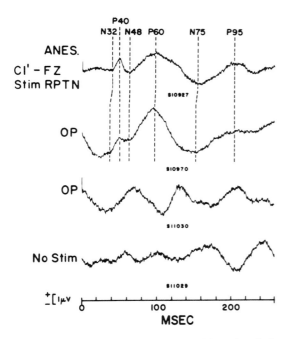

Fig. 16-18. Somatosensory EP elicited by stimulation of the right posterior tibial nerve in a patient with an arteriovenous malformation of the spinal cord. The first waveform, abnormal but reproducible, was recorded before opening the dura. The second, recorded 3 hours later, showed increasing loss of definition of the initial cortical positivity (P40). The third waveform, recorded after 5 hours of intradural operation, was not distinguishable from an average recorded without stimulation. The artifact seen in the last two tracings probably stems from spontaneous EEG rhythms. Artifact of this kind is now eliminated by using pseudorandom interstimulus intervals. Potentials evoked by stimulation of the median nerve (not shown) remained stable throughout. This patient was paraplegic postoperatively. (From Grundy et al.,[203] with permission.)

tential recorded from the caudal epidural space after the same stimulation of the upper spinal cord. The authors concluded that the compound muscle action potential and the spinal somatosensory EP are mediated through independent pathways in the anterior and posterior cord, respectively.

Noninvasive monitoring of motor EP elicited by transcranial stimulation of the motor cortex remains controversial. Numerous attempts to provide adequate anesthesia without abolishing these potentials have shown that best results can be obtained with intravenous anesthesia and nitrous oxide in concentrations no greater than 50 to 60 percent.[210-212]

Evoked Potentials During Aortic Surgery

Paraplegia is a tragic complication of operations on the aorta, rare after operations on the abdominal aorta but common after operations for large, complex thoracoabdominal abnormalities. In patients at highest risk, it may be seen in up to 40 percent. Many attempts have been made to reduce the incidence of spinal cord injury during these procedures by monitoring somatosensory, motor, or spinal cord EP. This area remains controversial.

The anterior two-thirds of the spinal cord are perfused by the anterior spinal artery, which traverses the length of the anterior aspect of the cord. Blood reaches this artery via branches of the vertebral arteries and by numerous other tributaries, including branches of the thyrocervical trunk and numerous radicular branches from the thoracic and lumbar aorta. One radicular branch is usually dominant, the great medullary artery or the artery of Adamkowitz, and arises as a left intercostal branch between T9 and L2 in most patients. Two posterior spinal arteries supply the posterior one-third of the cord, deriving their flow from the vertebral arteries. Occlusion of the anterior spinal artery causes infarction of the anterior part of the cord, which presents with paraparesis or paralysis, loss of pain and temperature sensation, and some decrease in the appreciation of touch. When the posterior spinal arteries remain intact, somatosensory EP are normal after a transient initial loss from which they seem to recover in 1 to 7 days. Transient somatosensory EP alterations intraoperatively may be followed by this syndrome. Estimates of the value of somatosensory EP monitoring during aortic surgery seem directly related to the use of immediate intervention to improve signals should they deteriorate and to continual somatosensory EP monitoring throughout the operation.

The impact of distal aortic perfusion and somatosensory EP monitoring on the postoperative incidence of paraplegia was examined in a series of 198 patients.[213] Patients were not randomized to operation with or without these techniques; the patients who did not have distal aortic perfusion and somatosensory EP monitoring were those in whom, for one reason or another, these could not be adequately obtained. No statistical difference was found between the two groups. False-negative somatosensory EP were seen in 13 percent and false-positive in 67 percent of the patients. Several factors in the study design in addition to the lack of randomization may help to explain these results. First, all patients who were paraplegic or paraparetic were included in the analysis, regardless of the time of onset of the neurologic insult. Of the 20 deficits seen, 11 were delayed from 12 hours to 21 days after the initial postoperative examination. In the postoperative period, 9 patients died, and 6 of these had delayed onset of neurologic injury 24 hours to 21 days after surgery. In these 9 cases cord dysfunction progressed to complete paraplegia before death.

A second confusing factor in this report arises from the fact that patients were not monitored until completion of the operation. If EP were unchanged, monitoring was usually discontinued 30 minutes after aortic reconstruction. If abnormal, recordings were variably continued up to 2 hours. Thus, in the three patients with immediate neurologic complications despite lack of intraoperative somatosensory EP change, it is quite possible that somatosensory EP may have deteriorated, perhaps during an episode of hypotension, between cessation of monitoring and awakening from anesthesia. Immediate postoperative neurologic complications were seen in 3 of 53 patients with no somatosensory EP change, in 1 of 11 patients showing change with return within 30 minutes, in 1 of 10 patients who had change with inconsistent return, and in 3 of 25 patients showing change with no return. There was an association between the level of somatosensory EP change and final neurologic outcome. Neurologic complications developed in 13 percent of patients with no somatosensory EP change, compared to 32 percent of those who had change with no recovery.

It also appears that in this study the same interventions were attempted in all patients, regardless of somatosensory EP data. Interestingly, in 12 patients the somatosensory EP was normal during aortic reconstruction but changed after restoration of flow. An immediate deficit occurred in one of these patients and delayed deficits occurred in three others.

A more recent report from this same group summarizes experience with 1,509 patients who had thoracoabdominal aortic operations by a single surgeon between 1960 and 1991.[214] In this series, 234 patients (16 percent) had paraplegia or paraparesis. Significant predictors of these complications were total aortic clamp time, extent of aorta repaired, aortic rupture, patient age, proximal aortic aneurysm, and history of renal dysfunction. Although the more recent patients in this series had better survival rates, little headway was made in reducing the incidence of paraplegia. Spinal cord injury of late onset was related to postoperative complications, particularly respiratory failure and hypotension. In the patients who developed paraplegia or paraparesis hours or days after surgery, the most commonly associated factor was thought to be decreased oxygenation of the spinal cord, related to either hypotension or respiratory failure.

Another report from the same group described variables predictive of outcome in 832 patients who had repairs of the descending thoracic aorta.[215] Factors associated with paraplegia or paraparesis were the extent of the repair (proximal versus entire), clamp time, postoperative gastrointestinal hemorrhage, and renal complications. The use of atriofemoral bypass eliminated the risk associated with duration of aortic occlusion time in the logistic regression model. The authors concluded that the two most important factors associated with postoperative paraplegia or paraparesis were the degree and duration of ischemia to the spinal cord and failure to successfully reimplant critical intercostal arteries that supply the cord.

Several other groups have had better results with use of EP during smaller series of operations on the thoracic and thoracoabdominal aorta than that described above. In one series of 19 patients who required cross-clamping of the descending thoracic aorta, temporary axillofemoral shunt was used in 10 patients and partial cardiopulmonary bypass in 9 patients.[216] Ischemic somatosensory EP changes were seen in five patients. Two patients, whose spinal cord perfusion pressures were 32 and 35 mmHg, had complete loss of somatosensory EP and developed paraplegia. In the other three patients, the mean distal aortic pressure was increased and/or cerebrospinal fluid was withdrawn to increase the spinal cord perfusion pressure to more than 40 mmHg when ischemic somatosensory EP changes occurred. In two of these, somatosensory EP gradually recovered with the increased perfusion pressure. The third patient underwent reimplantation of intercostal arteries because the ischemic somatosensory EP changes did not revert. All three patients recovered without any neurologic deficit. In the 14 patients without ischemic somatosensory EP changes, spinal cord perfusion pressure was kept at more than 40 mmHg during aortic cross-clamping.

In another series, 33 patients undergoing operations on the descending thoracic or thoracoabdominal aorta were monitored to evaluate causes and effects of spinal cord ischemia as manifested by changes in somatosensory EP.[217] Distal aortic perfusion pressure was maintained at greater than 60 mmHg by either shunt or bypass techniques in 17 patients. In these cases, somatosensory EP were stable, and patients were normal neurologically after surgery regardless of the duration of cross-clamping of the thoracic aorta (range: 23 to 105 minutes). In 16 other patients, cross-clamp times ranged from 16 to 124 minutes and somatosensory EP loss was associated with lack of distal perfusion, inadequate maintenance of distal perfusion pressure despite shunt or bypass, or interruption of intercostal arteries. The incidence of paraplegia in the entire group was 15.1 percent and was limited to only those patients in whom loss of somatosensory EP occurred. Loss of somatosensory EP for more than 30 minutes was followed by a 71 percent incidence of paraplegia. In contrast, when the somatosensory EP loss was either avoided or limited in duration to less than 30 minutes, there was no spinal cord injury.

Another group reported on 6 patients having operations on the descending thoracic aorta and 10 having operations on the abdominal aorta who were monitored with somatosensory EP recorded from subdermal electrodes over the third lumbar vertebra (spinogram) and on the scalp.[218] Stimulation was of one or both posterior tibial nerves at the ankle or peroneal nerves over the head of the fibula. The patients having operations on the tho-

racic aorta had aortic occlusions 32 to 69 minutes in duration. All six patients showed a progressive reduction in amplitude and prolongation in latency of cortical somatosensory EP, beginning within a few minutes of aortic occlusion, and these were lost after 18 to 20 minutes. In five of the six patients, EP recovered within 16 to 20 minutes after their disappearance whether or not the aorta was still occluded. At the end of surgery these somatosensory EP always regained their preclamp amplitudes and had a change in peak latency of 0 to 4 ms. The spinogram was essentially unmodified. Similar somatosensory EP changes were seen during occlusion of the abdominal aorta, and this was attributed to ischemia of the nerves in the legs. The single patient in this series who had paraplegia postoperatively had an aortic occlusion time of 69 minutes and an absence of cortical SEP for 73 minutes (from 20 minutes after aortic occlusion to 24 minutes after unclamping). When the somatosensory EP could again be recorded, the initial cortical positivity showed a latency increase of 11.2 ms with respect to preclamp values. This did not resolve during the remainder of the operation.

These observations suggest the importance of recording from both spinal and cortical sites. The changes seen in the patients with occlusion of the abdominal aorta or the femoral artery suggest that the early loss of lumbar potentials is related to a conduction disturbance in the ischemic peripheral nerve rather than to any problem at the level of the spinal cord. The cortical potential, which persisted while the lumbar potential disappeared, was probably due to the arrival of a desynchronized afferent volley from a partially ischemic peripheral nerve. Support was given to this assumption by monitoring somatosensory EP elicited by stimulation of the right peroneal nerve during an operation that required occlusion (38 minutes) of the right femoral artery alone. No aortic clamp was placed. The lumbar spinogram was obliterated immediately after arterial occlusion, while the cortical somatosensory EP was always present and showed a latency increase of 4 ms.

In a series of 150 consecutive patients undergoing thoracoabdominal aortic replacement from 1980 to 1991, a multimodality prospective perioperative protocol was initiated to reduce the risk of spinal cord injury.[219] This included complete intercostal reimplantation whenever possible, cerebrospinal fluid drainage, maintenance of proximal hypertension during cross-clamping, moderate hypothermia, high-dose barbiturates, and avoidance of hyperglycemia. Mannitol, steroids, and calcium channel blockers were used to minimize reperfusion injury. About 97 percent of the patients lived long enough for evaluation of postoperative spinal cord function. In the preprotocol group of 108 patients, 6 were paraplegic (6 percent), whereas none of the 42 patients in the protocol group had spinal cord injury.

A more recent report from the same group describes results with a further developed protocol.[220] In 23 patients with aortic repair from the proximal descending thoracic aortic to the upper abdominal aorta or from the proximal descending thoracic aorta to below the renal arteries (Crawford types I and II) three methods were combined in an attempt to minimize the incidence of paraplegia and kidney failure. Atriofemoral bypass was used with local cooling of the intercostal and visceral arteries and segmental resection of the aneurysm. The segmental resection allowed perfusion of the spinal cord and abdominal viscera while the proximal anastomosis was completed and as each pair of intercostal arteries was reimplanted. Attempts were made to reimplant all pairs of intercostal arteries from T8 to L2. Each segment of the aorta was perfused with cold crystalloid solution before implantation. Thus, no segment of the aorta was exposed to warm ischemia for more than 30 minutes. With the left-sided atriofemoral bypass, systemic temperatures could be maintained between 35 and 37°C despite the local hypothermia. Of the 23 patients, 7 had dissection or rupture associated with the aneurysm and underwent emergency operations. One of these seven patients was paraplegic postoperatively, giving a 4.3 percent rate of paraplegia in these high-risk patients.

In spinal cord ischemia induced in rabbits, normothermic animals had a high incidence of paraplegia.[221] After 20 minutes of ischemia, 40 percent were paraplegic, 75 percent after 40 minutes, and 100 percent after 60 minutes. In a comparison group of animals the epidural space around the lumbar segments was continually perfused with cold (5°C) isotonic saline through two communicating spinal canal openings. The animals with epidural cooling by this technique had full neurologic recovery even after 60 minutes of ischemia. This technique would seem to deserve clinical exploration.

Both motor EP and spinal cord EP elicited by direct stimulation of the spinal cord were monitored in 27 dogs subjected to 60 minutes of cross-clamping of the proximal descending aorta with (*n* = 18) or without (*n* = 9) cerebrospinal fluid drainage.[222] Somatosensory EP were more sensitive indicators of postoperative paraplegia than were motor EP. Motor EP elicited by direct electrical stimulation of the motor cortex and recorded over the lumbar spinal cord were lost in 9 of 20 dogs with ischemic cord injury and were not lost in any of the 7 dogs that were neurologically normal. Somatosensory EP elicited by stimulation of the sciatic nerve and recorded over the thoracic spinal cord were lost in 19 of 20 paraplegic or paraparetic dogs but also in 3 of 7 normal dogs. After reperfusion, motor EP returned in all the neurologically injured dogs that had lost the potentials, and these recovered motor EP were still present at 24 hours. Thus, loss of somatosensory EP had a high sensitivity (95 percent) but low specificity (67 percent) because of peripheral nerve ischemia. A loss of motor EP recorded from the spinal cord was highly specific (100 percent) but had such a low sensitivity (46 percent) that the motor EP was not a reliable predictor of neurologic injury. Further, return of motor EP after reperfusion did not correlate with functional recovery. Many clinicians would consider the relatively high rate of false-positive somatosensory EP recordings to be perfectly acceptable in this situation, as opposed to the high rate of false-negative results (undetected injury) with motor EP. With distal aortic perfusion (partial cardiopulmonary bypass or bypass shunt) ischemia of the peripheral nerve should be reduced or eliminated and the rate of false-positive somatosensory EP changes considerably reduced.

In 21 patients having operations for thoracic or thoracoabdominal aortic aneurysms, spinal cord EP were elicited by direct stimulation of the cord.[223] Thirteen patients who had only minor alterations of the evoked complex during test occlusion for 15 to 20 minutes were operated on without reimplantation of intercostal vessels. Two patients had sudden cardiac arrests, with complete disappearance of the spinal EP. In another patient, the spinal EP was lost immediately after incision of the aneurysm, presumably due to distal aortic hypoperfusion. This patient suffered prolonged distal hypotension and postoperatively had flaccid paraplegia. Another patient has been described, however, who had paraparesis postoperatively despite well-maintained spinal EP throughout aortic cross-clamping.[224]

Of 22 patients who had somatosensory EP monitoring during operations for coarctation, 10 had somatosensory EP changes.[225] Absence of somatosensory EP for 30 minutes in one patient was followed by paraplegia. Somatosensory EP obliteration for 14 minutes in another patient was associated with transient parerethesias in the lower extremities postoperatively. In a third patient, somatosensory EP were lost abruptly and reproducibly upon test occlusion of the aorta. Because of these changes, a subclavian-aortic bypass was done rather than resection of the coarctation. After full restoration of flow, somatosensory EP recovered, and the patient had no neurologic injury.

In comparing somatosensory, spinal, and motor EP, the somatosensory EP is most sensitive to spinal cord insult during operations on the thoracic and thoracoabdominal aorta. Spinal and motor EP have given disappointing results. Progress made in recent years by a few groups with aggressive protocols and intensive monitoring offers hope for reduction in the incidence of spinal cord injury after aortic surgery.

Evoked Potential and Nerve Conduction Studies in Peripheral Nerve Surgery

Many surgeons consider EP and nerve conduction studies indispensable during operations on peripheral nerves or plexi.[5,226] The early treatment of closed peripheral nerve injuries is conservative. Surgical exploration is usually delayed. If there is no clinical or electrophysiologic evidence of returning function within 2 to 3 months, the area of injury is explored. Often a fusiform swelling is found in the injured area called *neuroma-in-continuity*. Its appearance does not reveal the nature of the internal pathology. The lesion may be reversible with a variable loss of distal function due to such factors as electrolyte imbalance, ischemia of the nerve, and acute or chronic compressive or shearing forces. This type of injury, called neurapraxia, generally improves within days or weeks of injury without surgical intervention. In this case, the only electrical dysfunction is at the site of injury. Stimulation of the nerve distal to the injury produces a muscle contraction. Nerve action potentials can be generated above and below the injury but cannot cross the dysfunctional part of the axon.

A second possibility is that both axons and myelin are interrupted but the surrounding connective tissue elements are preserved (axonotmesis). As the axon grows about 1 mm per day, at 2 months after injury growth will have passed the neuroma-in-continuity. Muscle reinnervation, however, has usually not occurred. Therefore, nerve stimulation will not produce muscle contraction. It is important that the surgeon not resect the neuroma-in-continuity in this situation. The natural process of reinnervation within uninterrupted connecting structures is far more efficient and effective than transection and suturing. An axonotmetic lesion can be detected by recording nerve action potentials across the lesion. Stimulation and recording with electrodes placed just above and below the lesion often produces potentials of sufficient amplitude to be seen without averaging.

When axons, myelin, and the surrounding connective tissue are disrupted (neurotmesis), there is no natural pathway for regeneration of the nerve. This type of lesion can also be detected by recording nerve action potentials. No conduction will be seen across the neuroma, and no muscle contraction will be seen with stimulation either proximal or distal to the area of injury. Although complete transection of the nerve is one form of neurotmesis, the same lesion may exist within a neuroma-in-continuity. No functional recovery can be expected without resection of the lesion and reanastomosis of the nerve either directly or with a graft.

In a series of 171 patients with brachial plexus injuries, 63 of 282 injured nerve elements were spared because nerve action potentials could be detected.[227] After neurolysis, 57 plexus elements recovered function without resection of the nerve segment. On the basis of the electrophysiologic testing, 121 nerve elements were resected, and pathologic examination confirmed neurotmesis in all cases. Somatosensory and spinal cord EP have also been used to detect electrophysiologic continuity during surgical exploration after traumatic brachial plexus injuries.[228]

Corticography for Seizure Surgery or Cortical Mapping

Corticography to precisely localize the somatosensory and motor cortex is vital during certain operations near the sensorimotor strip of the cortex.[229] EP are recorded from several electrodes placed directly on the surface of the cortex in the area of interest, and a phase reversal of the somatosensory EP elicited by stimulation of the median nerve at the wrist is seen as the central sulcus is crossed. Recording from multiple pairs of electrodes on nearby areas of the cortex is necessary to confirm precisely the location of the rolandic fissure. Knowing exactly which area of the cortex to avoid in attempting to prevent postoperative motor deficits, the surgeon can appropriately judge the extent of resection or choose to accept remaining pathology.

The motor cortex can also be precisely identified by electrical stimulation of the cortex and recording of the spinal cord direct (D) response. Magnetic stimulators are not sufficiently localized for this purpose and would probably give misleading results on a regular basis. The corticospinal direct response to stimulation of the motor cortex is resistant to anesthesia and unaffected by muscle relaxants.[230]

Electrocorticography is indispensable for assisting the surgeon in determining the extent of resection when epileptogenic foci are removed as treatment for medically refractory seizure disorders.[231,232] Intraoperative EEG changes during corpus callosotomy are not helpful in predicting the postoperative effect of the surgery.[233]

Intracranial Operations for Aneurysms and Arteriovenous Malformations

Simultaneous monitoring of EP and spontaneous EEG is valuable during intracranial vascular neurosurgical procedures.[234] The combination of monitoring techniques is particularly helpful when adjuncts such as high-dose barbiturate anesthesia or hypothermia may be employed. In these situations, the EEG can be used to confirm burst-suppression, but short-latency EP can still be recorded. Cortical EP are sensitive to local ischemia. In baboons, somatosensory EP elicited by stimulation of the median nerve begin to deteriorate at flows of 15 ml/100 g per minute.[235] Flows between 10 and 15 ml/100 g per minute produce electrical failure but permit maintenance of cellular metabolism.[236] EP may provide warning of ischemia before irreversible damage occurs.[237]

Cortical ischemia during intracranial operations for aneurysms or arteriovenous malformations may be due to intended or unintended arterial hypotension, surgical retractors, deliberate or accidental arterial occlusion, or arterial spasm. EP over both cortices may be altered if arterial hypotension is marked. A trial of deliberate hypotension before placement of brain retractors has been suggested to determine whether somatosensory EP are affected.[174] Pressures below those that affect the EP can then be avoided. Lower levels of cerebral blood flow may be tolerated during anesthesia with agents such as barbiturates or isoflurane, which themselves can depress electrical activity of the brain at clinically useful concentrations.

Central conduction time of the somatosensory EP (the time separating the peak that arises at the second cervical vertebrae from that representing the initial cortical activity) can be an important indicator during operations for aneurysm, as can reduction in amplitude or loss of the cortical response. Such changes have been used as guides for repositioning imperfectly placed aneurysm clips, manipulating arterial blood pressure, and timing of temporary vascular occlusion.[238,239] See Figure 16-19. Postoperative neurologic deficits are less likely when flow can be reestablished within 10 to 12 minutes after loss of the EP.[240,241] Best results are obtained during operations for aneurysms of the middle cerebral artery[239,242] or internal carotid artery.[241] Deficits in areas not monitored by EP, such as aphasia, may not be detected.[238] Similarly, injury to areas adjacent to but not included in the monitored pathway will not be detected unless the ischemia is so severe as to extend into areas that are within the monitored pathway.

Perhaps the most important example of undetected injury in unmonitored pathways is that of the aneurysm at the basilar tip. In a series of 16 patients, 10 were monitored with brainstem auditory and somatosensory EP, 4 with brainstem auditory EP only, and 2 with somatosensory EP only.[242] In 14 patients, no EP changes that were considered significant were detected: 1 patient had transient brainstem auditory EP changes with retraction of the auditory nerve and pons, and another had progressive attenuation and transient loss of somatosensory EP during a period of intermittent basilar artery occlusion. Of the 16 patients, 4 had new ischemic brainstem deficits immediately after surgery that were not predicted by the intraoperative EP monitoring. The ischemic injuries involved relatively small anatomic areas outside the monitored pathways. Unpredictable motor deficits were particularly likely in patients with aneurysms at the basilar bifurcation, which is the most common location of aneurysms in the posterior circulation. In this case, motor tracts are much closer than sensory pathways to the area in question and may become ischemic while sensory pathways are spared and somatosensory EP unchanged. In some cases, however, ischemic changes are sufficiently extensive to involve the somatosensory pathways and somatosensory EP can then be used to guide intraoperative management, probably improving outcome in some patients. An occasional late change in somatosensory EP may indicate a need for additional intervention.[243]

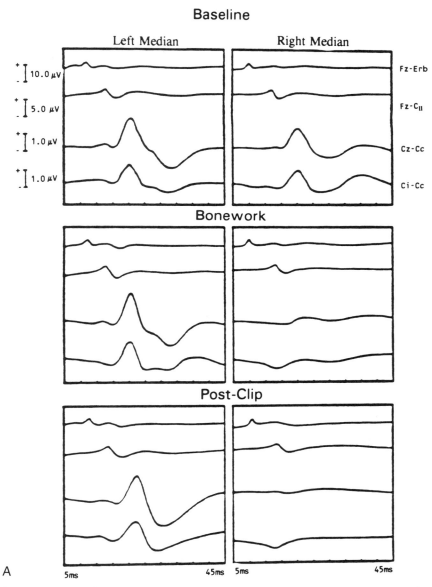

Fig. 16-19. Somatosensory EP recorded during operations for aneurysms of the middle cerebral artery. **(A)** Irreversible loss of cortical somatosensory EP, followed by a major new neurologic deficit. (*Figure continues.*)

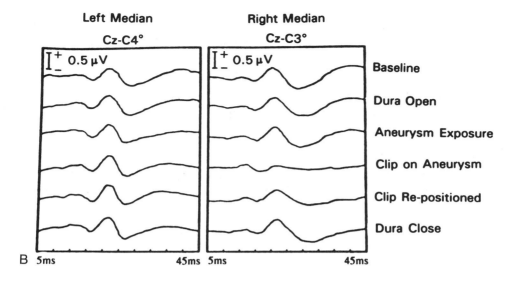

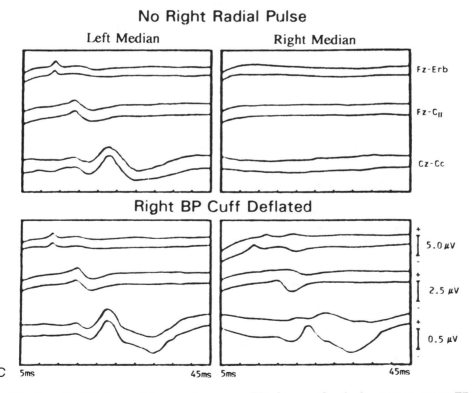

Fig. 16-19 (*Continued*). **(B)** Reversible somatosensory EP change. Cortical somatosensory EP deteriorated after clip was applied, recovered after clip was repositioned. The patient had no new neurologic deficit postoperatively. **(C)** Loss of all EP following stimulation of the right median nerve. Peripheral nerve was ischemic due to an otherwise undetected constant inflation of an automatic blood pressure cuff. EP showed progressive recovery after deflation of cuff. No new neurologic deficit occurred. (From Friedman et al.,[239] with permission.)

Cranial Nerve Monitoring During Posterior Fossa or Cranial Base Surgery

Monitoring of the facial nerve by visual observation of evoked muscle activity has long enjoyed virtually universal acceptance. Monopolar exploratory stimulation in the surgical field is used to identify branches of this motor nerve. In recent years, visual or palpatory monitoring has been to some extent replaced, particularly during neurosurgical procedures, by electrical recording of compound muscle action potentials from muscles around the eye, lip, and chin.[244] A useful supplement to this technique rapidly gaining acceptance is audible monitoring of the electromyographic activity inadvertently elicited by surgical instruments, which can rapidly alert the surgeon to facial nerve fascicles being stimulated by surgical instruments.[245–247] This technique was used during partial neuromuscular blockade in 10 surgical patients,[248] 6 of whom showed marked decreases in the compound muscle action potentials and had severe facial nerve injury postoperatively. Could some of these injuries have been prevented if no neuromuscular blocking agents had been present to interfere with monitoring? Many anesthesiologists prefer that no muscle relaxants be used during monitoring of the facial nerve.

Brainstem auditory EP are often monitored during operations in the posterior fossa. Intraoperative brainstem auditory EP changes were reported to the surgeon and the anesthesiologist in 37 of 54 operations in the cerebellopontine angle.[81] This series used an increase in wave-5 latency of 1.5 ms as a criterion of abnormality. In 22 patients, brainstem auditory EP changes were related to retraction of the cerebellum or brainstem, and changes progressed to virtual obliteration in 6 of these. (See Figure 16-20.) The combination of hypocarbia and relative hypotension was associated with brainstem auditory EP changes as well (Fig. 16-21). In 6 of the 54 cases, brainstem auditory EP were obliterated upon positioning for retromastoid craniectomy. The acoustic nerve was deliberately sacrificed

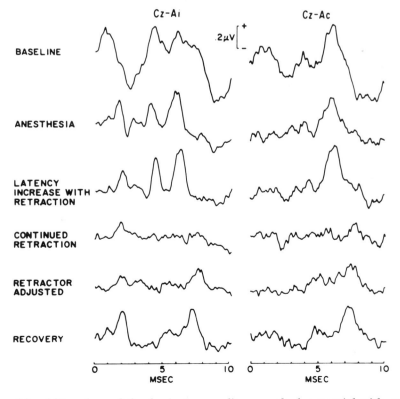

Fig. 16-20. Reversible obliteration of the brainstem auditory evoked potential with retraction of the eighth cranial nerve. (From Grundy et al.,[249] with permission.)

in two of these cases, but in the others brainstem auditory EP substantially recovered when the head was returned to a neutral position at the end of the procedure, and hearing was preserved. (See Figure 16-22.) Of the 37 patients in this series who had brainstem auditory EP changes reported intraoperatively, 32 recovered waveforms well toward baseline in the operating room. Hearing was diminished preoperatively in the other 5 patients and brainstem auditory EP recorded before the induction of anesthesia were abnormal but reproducible. All 5 patients with irreversible brainstem auditory EP loss intraoperatively were deaf in the affected ear postoperatively. Thus, the presence or absence of brainstem auditory EP at the conclusion of an-

esthesia correctly predicted the presence or absence of hearing postoperatively in all 54 cases.

Before the introduction of brainstem auditory EP monitoring during microvascular decompression of the cranial nerves,[81,249] ipsilateral hearing loss was reported in 1 to 4 percent of patients having decompression of the fifth nerve for trigeminal neuralgia[250] and partial hearing loss occurred in as many as 20 percent of these cases.[251] Because of the proximity of the facial and auditory nerves, the risk was greater during decompression of the seventh nerve for treatment of hemifacial spasm.[250] In a subsequent series of 21 patients undergoing microvascular decompression of cranial nerves, increases in the latencies of brainstem auditory EP peaks 1,

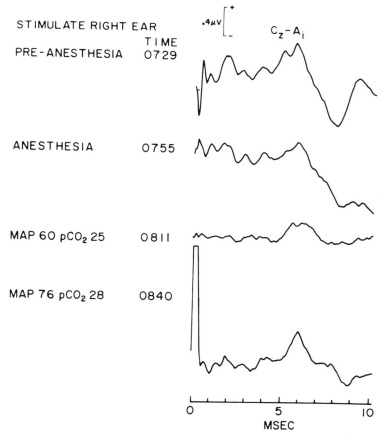

Fig. 16-21. Changes in brainstem auditory evoked potentials associated with hypocarbia and modest hypotension in a patient undergoing microvascular decompression of the eighth cranial nerve for Menière's disease. These changes, seen before skin incision, were partially reversed by reducing minute ventilation to increase the $PaCO_2$, while infusing albumen to raise the arterial blood pressure. MAP, mean arterial blood pressure. (From Grundy et al.,[81] with permission.)

3, and 5 were predictable. The surgeon was warned only for obliteration of brainstem auditory EP, which occurred in four cases.[143] It may be appropriate to withhold warnings to the surgeon until the brainstem auditory EP is lost when compression of the cranial nerve is the primary risk. By contrast, the brainstem is far more sensitive to ischemia and hypoxia than are the cranial nerves; earlier warning should be given when the brainstem or its perfusion is primarily at risk. Insults to the brainstem that do not include the auditory pathways will not be reflected in brainstem auditory EP until secondary changes affect these pathways.[242]

Several reports describe attempts to preserve hearing by monitoring brainstem auditory EP during acoustic neuroma removal.[252–256] Simultaneous recording of the cochlear microphonic, electrocochleogram, and brainstem auditory EP permitted definition of three patterns of loss.[255] Loss of all the evoked auditory components, including the cochlear microphonic, suggested vascular compromise, which may have been due to coagulation of small labyrinthine arteries. Loss of all brainstem auditory EP components, with preservation of the cochlear microphonic, suggested trauma to the cochlear nerve. Loss of brainstem auditory EP wave 5 with preservation of wave 1 was followed by good postoperative hearing. This may have been related to known interactions between potent inhalational

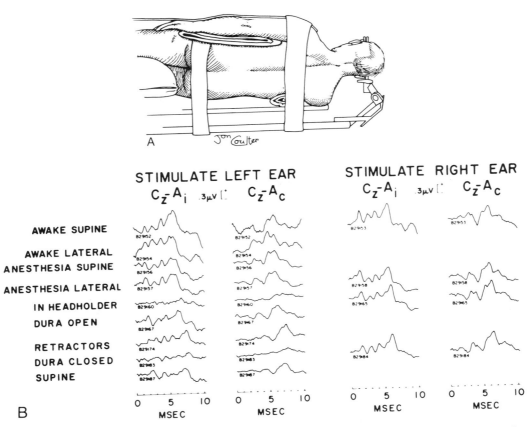

Fig. 16-22. Evoked potential changes produced by positioning for retromastoid craniectomy. **(A)** Lateral decubitus position for retromastoid craniectomy. The neck is stretched slightly and flexed, and the head is rotated 10 to 20 degrees to the ipsilateral side. **(B)** Brainstem auditory EP changes occurred not with the lateral decubitus position but with stretching and flexion of the neck. The waveform alterations partially resolved when the dura mater was opened, were exacerbated on closing of the cervical fascia, and improved dramatically when the head and neck were returned to a neutral position. (From Grundy et al.,[142] with permission.)

anesthetics, the rate of rapid stimulation used in this study, and desynchrony of the brainstem auditory EP caused by surgical manipulation of the tumor.

Brainstem auditory EP were monitored in another series of 31 operations in the posterior fossa for various diagnoses.[144] A postoperative decrease in hearing was associated with either a reduction in amplitude of waves 1 to 5 or loss of one of the waves. Transient loss of a peak followed by recovery did not portend a loss of hearing. Intraoperative appearance of a wave not seen in preoperative recordings was a good prognostic sign.

During resection of acoustic neuromas, 90 patients who had brainstem auditory EP monitored were compared with 90 historical controls matched for tumor size and preoperative hearing.[256] In those with tumors less than 2 cm in size, monitoring was associated with a greater likelihood that hearing would be preserved and also indicated a greater chance that preserved hearing would be useful. Overall, there was a good correlation between intraoperative brainstem auditory EP changes and postoperative hearing.

Less work has been done with monitoring other cranial nerves intraoperatively, although extensive monitoring of multiple cranial nerves has been reported.[257] The optic nerve can be monitored by recording visual EP or action potentials from the optic nerve.[258] The third, fourth, and sixth cranial nerves can be monitored by recording EMG from the respective extraocular muscles.[257] Short-latency trigeminal EP can be used to monitor the integrity of the extra-axial trigeminal nerve but not the central trigeminal circuitry.[123,259] In 10 of 17 patients monitored during operations in the posterior fossa, changes in brainstem trigeminal EP were identified with cerebellar retraction and with tumor dissection from the brainstem.[260] In 7 of these 10 patients, adjustment of cerebellar retractors or changing the surgical approach produced partial or complete return of the waveform. In most of these 17 cases, the brainstem trigeminal EP at the conclusion of surgery correlated with the immediate surgical outcome.

In summary, extensive monitoring of cranial nerves can be performed during operations in the posterior cranial fossa or during skull base surgery. The most widely accepted techniques are monitoring of the facial nerve and the brainstem auditory

EP. Less experience has accumulated with intraoperative monitoring of other cranial nerves.

Other Intraoperative Applications

EP monitoring has been used in attempts to prevent injury to sciatic nerve during total hip arthroplasty.[261] Visual EP elicited by flash stimulation have been monitored during operations on the pituitary gland or in the anterior cranial fossa[3,258] (Fig. 16-23). Flash-elicited visual EP are not specific for visual acuity, and they may predict changes in visual fields more accurately than changes in visual acuity.[262] For these reasons and because of problems with stimulation as described above, intraoperative visual EP monitoring has not found wide acceptance.[263]

EEG of the fetus and neonate have been used to help evaluate the neonatal effects of maternal general or regional anesthesia.[264] These techniques remain experimental.[265,266]

EEG changes have been documented during fulminant porcine malignant hyperpyrexia. After treatment with dantrolene, EEG total power and median frequency improved before significant changes were seen in mean arterial blood pressure,

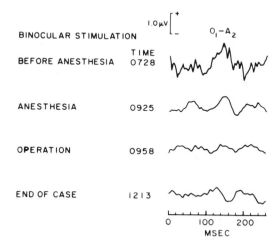

Fig. 16-23. Visual evoked potentials recorded during transsphenoidal resection of a pituitary tumor. The muscle artifact seen before anesthesia is abolished by anesthesia and muscle relaxation. Transient deterioration during the procedure is followed by return of the waveform with a shorter (more normal) latency of the "P100" peak than preoperatively. This improvement was associated with improved visual fields on postoperative testing. (From Grundy et al.,[4] with permission.)

arterial partial pressures of O_2 or CO_2, or plasma potassium concentrations.[267] It seems likely that this will remain a laboratory tool rather than a widely accepted clinical monitor in this situation.

Hypovolemic hypotension led to progressive increases in latency and decreases in amplitude and conduction velocity of both somatosensory and spinal motor EP when mean arterial pressure fell to less than 30 mmHg in anesthetized cats.[268] With immediate blood transfusion, activity at the cortical and spinal levels resumed within 30 minutes of reinfusion but did not reach baseline latency and amplitude values within 1 hour. Spinal somatosensory EP were more resistant to hypotension than either cortical somatosensory or spinal motor EP. When 15 minutes elapsed between loss of responses and transfusion, cortical somatosensory EP and spinal motor EP did not reappear within 1 hour after reinfusion. No return of any signals occurred if 30 minutes elapsed between loss of EP and blood reinfusion.

EVOKED POTENTIAL MONITORING IN NEURORADIOLOGY

An important and currently underused technique is monitoring of EP during diagnostic and therapeutic radiologic interventions. This monitoring can be valuable during such procedures such as local intra-arterial thrombolytic therapy, embolization and occlusion of arteries supplying the brain, percutaneous transluminal angioplasty, and intra-arterial application of drugs. The radiologist can use acute changes in EP waveforms to help evaluate the safety or risk of the next step during a procedure.[269] Important new information can be gained in identifying functional territories of single or multiple feeding vessels and in understanding hemodynamics. The adequacy of collateral circulation can be determined when occlusive procedures are contemplated.

ELECTROENCEPHALOGRAM DURING ELECTROCONVULSIVE THERAPY

The EEG is now frequently used to monitor the characteristics of electroconvulsive therapy. A comparison of the EEG characteristics of four forms of electroconvulsive therapy known to differ in effi-

cacy determined that seizure duration was not a useful marker of therapeutic efficacy. Other features of the EEG may be more useful markers of adequate treatment.[270] Specific features of the ictal and immediate postictal EEG varied significantly with stimulus intensity and electrode placement. Low-dose right unilateral therapy differed from more effective forms of electroconvulsive therapy in having the longest polyspike phase duration and the smallest likelihood of postictal EEG suppression. By contrast, high-dose bilateral electroconvulsive therapy, which has particularly rapid antidepressant effects, produced the highest amplitude peak-and-slow-wave complexes in both hemispheres.

ELECTROENCEPHALOGRAM AND EVOKED POTENTIALS FOR DETERMINING THE DEPTH OF ANESTHESIA

Numerous electrophysiologic methods have been used in attempts to monitor depth of anesthesia and to detect unsuspected awareness during anesthesia. Although correlations between depth of anesthesia with specific drugs and various parameters derived from EEG or EP monitoring have been described, none of the suggested analyses are universally applicable. There is no clear evidence to suggest that, in a large population of patients, these methods are more effective than simple clinical assessment. The polypharmacy currently practiced in the operating room and differing effects of different agents multiply the complexities of electrophysiologic methods for monitoring depth of anesthesia. Contributions have nevertheless been made to our understanding of the pharmacodynamics of anesthetics, particularly with single agents.[271,272] Perhaps most promising of the modalities suggested for this purpose is the middle latency auditory evoked potential.[273-276] This seems most useful during anesthesia with potent inhaled agents or intravenous barbiturates or propofol. Clear dose-response relationships could not be identified with opioids,[85] benzodiazepines,[84] or ketamine.[89] The auditory steady-state response has also been suggested as a monitor of anesthetic depth,[277] but in animal studies this response has been shown to plateau at a level of anesthesia not associated with unconsciousness in humans.[278]

In summary, intraoperative monitoring of EEG

and EP has numerous applications, a number of which are widespread clinical use. In many cases, monitoring to identify structures or pathways or to avert serious neurologic injury seems cost effective. In contrast, use of these techniques solely to identify depth of anesthesia is probably not warranted at present.

ELECTROENCEPHALOGRAM AND EVOKED POTENTIALS IN THE CRITICAL CARE UNIT

Among the inviting applications for EEG and EP monitoring in the critical care unit are monitoring and management of such conditions as status epilepticus, embolic or drug-induced coma, traumatic brain injury, acute cerebrovascular disease such as stroke or hypertensive encephalopathy, and spinal cord injury. Efforts have been made to predict outcomes of severe brain insults using electrophysiologic monitoring, and these techniques play a secondary role in diagnosing brain death.

The great majority of EEG and EP recording in the critical care unit has been done in attempts to predict outcome rather than to detect acute deterioration so that timely intervention might prevent or minimize lasting damage. Only when these techniques are applied on a continual or continuous basis and used to help manage treatments will their full promise be realized.

Predicting Outcome

In posttraumatic coma, EEG patterns reflect the degree of rostrocaudal deterioration. An unfavorable prognosis is indicated by the loss of sleeplike activity, alternating patterns, and reactivity.[279] In a series of 370 comatose patients, however, the sleep spindles that were seen in 5.7 percent of the cases were unrelated to prognosis.[280] Serial recordings assist interpretation, as does knowledge of the underlying clinical picture. Serial brainstem auditory EP recordings in 30 severely head-injured patients showed that all patients who recovered had normal brainstem auditory EP throughout the clinical course, while those who were severely disabled and vegetative showed at least transient brainstem auditory EP abnormalities.[281]

Patterns of EP change in head-injured patients differ according to the supratentorial or brainstem site of the primary injury. Of 85 patients comatose after injury, only in those with supratentorial lesions were nearly normal central conduction times and amplitudes of somatosensory EP correlated with good outcomes.[282] As the central conduction times increased and amplitudes decreased, outcomes were worse. When the primary injury was in the brainstem, however, prolonged central conduction times could also be seen in patients who made good recoveries; and normal central conduction times were sometimes seen in patients with severe disability or death as outcomes. In the latter case, cortical somatosensory EP were often absent on one side. Brainstem auditory transmission times were also correlated with outcome status. Brainstem auditory EP did not differ between patients with primary and secondary brainstem lesions. Patients with absent somatosensory EP bilaterally and bilaterally absent brainstem auditory EP (not related to traumatic or preexisting hearing disorders) all died or were severely disabled. Most of the patients who died or survived with severe disabilities had abnormal somatosensory and brainstem auditory EP.

In a series of patients with Glasgow coma scale scores of 7 or less, brainstem auditory and visual EP were reliable predictors of unfavorable but not of favorable outcomes, while somatosensory EP reliably predicted both favorable and unfavorable outcomes.[283] In this series, EP measurements were better predictors of outcome than were motor findings, intracranial pressure measurements, or pupillary light reaction. In 17 children with mild to moderately severe closed head injuries, abnormalities of the P300 peak of long-latency somatosensory EP were correlated with long-term deficits in school performance.[284]

Simultaneous monitoring of brainstem auditory EP and intracranial pressure in 53 comatose patients showed that acute rises in intracranial pressure to levels greater than 40 mmHg were not always followed by changes in brainstem auditory EP.[285] Stable brainstem auditory EP in the presence of these intracranial pressure rises were associated with a high probability of survival, while prolongation of central latency of brainstem auditory EP in response to intracranial pressure elevations was almost always followed by brain death.

Development of EEG grading scales for 75 patients with anoxic encephalopathies permitted prediction of survival or death in 90 percent.[286] In 50 consecutive comatose patients studied within 8 hours after cardiopulmonary resuscitation, 30 had no cortical somatosensory EP.[287] None of these patients recovered cognition. Of 20 patients with cortical somatosensory EP present, 5 recovered. In another series of 40 patients who were comatose at least 6 hours following cardiac arrest and resuscitation, all had preserved brainstem function. However, 65 percent died without awakening.[288] Cortical somatosensory EP were absent in 19 of these 26, and marked deterioration of the EEG was seen in 11. Of the 14 patients who awakened, 5 recovered completely while 9 had varying degrees of motor or cognitive impairment. Somatosensory EP and EEG findings did not distinguish between these latter outcomes.[288]

Highly accurate prediction was obtained by recording intermediate-latency somatosensory EP to median nerve stimulation in 66 patients resuscitated from cardiac arrest but still unconscious and mechanically ventilated.[289] In this group of patients, predictive ability was 100 percent. In all 17 patients with favorable outcomes, the N70 peak was detected between 74 and 116 ms. By contrast, the N70 peak in 49 patients with poor outcomes was either absent ($n = 35$) or delayed to a latency between 121 and 171 ms ($n = 14$). This report highlights the importance of recording later cortical activity rather than only the initial cortical positivity. Most intraoperative somatosensory EP monitoring, and probably most such recording done in the acute care environment, never examines this activity. A reexamination of current practice in this area is indicated.

Somatosensory and visual EP were recorded in 57 asphyxiated term infants during the first 3 days of life, again during the first week, and at follow-up visits.[290] After 18 to 24 months, 34 infants were normal, 12 had severe neurologic sequelae, and 11 had died. Normal somatosensory EP virtually guaranteed normal outcome (sensitivity 96 percent, negative predictive power 97 percent). Visual EP were 100 percent specific and had a positive predictive power of 100 percent. In these patients, abnormal visual EP guaranteed abnormal outcome. Somatosensory and visual EP together were better predictors than either alone. In infants with an ultrasound diagnosis of cystic leukomalacia, however, little additional information regarding prognosis was provided by median nerve somatosensory EP recordings.[291]

Somatosensory EP were recorded in 19 patients in an attempt to predict progress in rehabilitation following strokes that damaged the dominant hemisphere.[292] The seven patients with no cortical potentials had the worst outcomes, but the existence of cortical potentials in the remaining patients did not give a precise prediction of their progress in rehabilitation.

Motor and somatosensory EP were recorded in 60 patients with traumatic coma and 35 with nontraumatic coma.[293] Somatosensory EP were better predictors of outcomes than the motor EP. All patients with bilaterally preserved somatosensory EP and central conduction times less than or equal to 6.5 ms survived; all with bilaterally absent cortical responses died. In contrast, 31 percent of patients with traumatic coma and 39 percent of those with nontraumatic coma had bilaterally preserved electromyographic responses to transcranial stimulation but died. Only the bilateral absence of motor EP was an unerring unfavorable prognostic sign. In another 22 patients with coma of diverse etiology, motor EP were significantly related to outcomes and appeared to be more accurate prognostic indicators than the Glasgow coma scale.[127] One of six patients with bilaterally absent motor EP, however, had a good recovery. The combined use of somatosensory and motor EP improved outcome prediction in this series. Grading of coma by using combined brainstem auditory and brainstem trigeminal EP in 45 comatose patients showed no significant difference between the accuracy of outcome predictions provided by combined clinical data and those predictions provided by neurophysiologic data.[294] The combination of clinical and neurophysiologic data, however, markedly increased both the accuracy and the confidence of outcome prediction.

Monitoring and Intervention

As technology advances and logistics become simpler, we can hope that some of the methods used in these predictive studies will be more widely applied for monitoring to detect deterioration early so that interventions can be made to improve outcomes.

Electroencephalography and Evoked Potentials in Metabolic or Drug-Induced Coma

Several investigators have drawn attention to changes produced in EEG and EP by drugs used for sedation in the critical care unit.[295–299] Of particular interest is a report of transient drug-induced abolition of brainstem auditory EP in a comatose patient treated with combined high doses of lidocaine and thiopental, which were sufficient to produce long-lasting periods of burst-suppression but not an isoelectric EEG.[297] The brainstem auditory EP returned to normal after the drugs were discontinued. Except for this case, changes in EEG and EP produced by sedation in the critical care unit parallel those already known with the same drugs in the operating room.

EEG recording is more sensitive than computed tomography (CT) in detecting the extent of brain pathology in eclamptic women. CT of the cerebrum was compared with EEG findings in 32 women with eclampsia.[300] Approximately 45 percent of the women had CT abnormalities, while 90 percent had EEG abnormalities. Burst-suppression patterns were recorded from four women.

The frequency and degree of EEG abnormalities declined after institution of extracorporeal membrane oxygenation in 145 neonates with reversible respiratory failure.[301] Of 11 infants with electrographic seizures during extracorporeal membrane oxygenation, seven either died or were developmentally handicapped. This was a significantly greater rate of adverse outcomes than in infants without EEG seizure activity. Cannulation of the right common carotid artery in these patients did not result in lateralized abnormalities of cerebroelectrical activity.

Encephalographic Management of Status Epilepticus

EEG recording in comatose patients may reveal that the alteration in consciousness is due to continual epileptic activity (without motor manifestations) that has not been previously suspected.[302] A predictable pattern of progressive EEG changes is seen during untreated generalized status epilepticus.[303] A sequence of five patterns has been described: discreet electrographic seizures, waxing and waning, continuous, continuous with flat periods, and periodic epileptiform discharges on a relatively flat background. A patient actively having seizures or comatose who shows any of these EEG patterns should be considered to be in generalized status epilepticus and should be treated aggressively to stop all clinical and electrical seizure activity in order to prevent further neurologic injury. Refractory status epilepticus has been successfully treated by surgical removal of a lesion documented to be the focus of seizure onset.[304]

Of 33 patients with status epilepticus but no focal neurologic findings, 30 percent had abnormal somatosensory EP on combined conventional and rapid-stimulation recording. Somatosensory EP abnormalities in this population were significantly correlated with poor outcomes.[305] Seizures are relatively common in the previously healthy young infant with an acute critical illness. Prompt recognition and treatment may influence outcome in the patient with a potentially reversible encephalopathy.[306]

Electroencephalography and Evoked Potentials in Traumatic Brain Injury

EEG and/or EP monitoring has been found useful in the acute management of patients with head injuries.[307,145,146,308-310] A comparison of intracranial pressure measurements to steady-state EP showed that the steady-state visual EP changed within seconds of surgical and/or medical decompression of increased intracranial pressure.[310]

Electroencephalogram and Evoked Potentials in Cerebrovascular Disease

In patients with subarachnoid hemorrhage, both EEG and EP have been used to predict the clinical onset of cerebral ischemia and angiographic vasospasm.[311-313] EEG was recorded in 151 patients on the first day and the fifth day after subarachnoid hemorrhage from ruptured aneurysms.[313] Of the 46 patients with normal EEG on day 1, 72 percent developed neither further electrical ischemic features nor delayed angiographic vasospasm. Of the 78 patients with bilateral bursts of slow waves, however, 97 percent developed EEG signs of ischemia and angiographic vasospasm a few days later. On day 5, 107 patients had focal or asymmetrical bilateral delta waves. Angiographic vasospasm was seen in 96 percent of these, and the extent of the electrical abnormality was related to the degree of arterial narrowing.

Evoked Potentials in Spinal Cord Injury

Most patients with spinal cord injuries do not lose consciousness and can describe their symptoms. Electrophysiologic evaluation of the spinal cord is particularly valuable, however, when patients cannot cooperate for clinical neurologic assessment, as in head injury or intoxication. These techniques may also be useful in neonates, infants, and children. They are of particular interest during manipulations such as traction to reduce displaced spinal fractures.

An extensive review of correlations of outcomes with somatosensory EP findings analyzed reports of several clinical series.[314] A clinical system for automated recording of somatosensory EP at 30-minute intervals was used during nonoperative treatment of acute spinal cord injuries in five patients. Monitoring was continued for 3 to 7 days. Only one of the five patients had abnormal somatosensory EP, and none of the patients had changes during the monitoring period.[315] Localization of sensory levels, particularly helpful in traumatic quadriplegia, can be accomplished by using segmental sensory stimulation. Fluctuations in the level of spinal cord dysfunction can thus be identified.[316]

Several investigators have used somatosensory EP recordings after spinal cord injury in attempts to predict neurologic outcomes. Although signals were not transmitted past complete cord lesions, ultimate outcomes could not be predicted with absolute certainty on the basis of somatosensory EP recorded soon after injury. Normal somatosensory EP recordings after acute spinal cord injury, however, are associated with a very high probability of recovery. In a few cases, function has recovered after complete absence of somatosensory EP.

A 20-ms train of percutaneous electrical stimulation applied to the plantar surface was used to condition muscle responses evoked in the tibialis anterior by transcranial magnetic stimulation of the motor cortex.[317] The interval between conditioning and the motor stimulus was 15 to 60 ms. This technique was used to unmask preserved corticospinal innervation in some spinal cord injury patients with absent motor EP. Four subjects with clinically complete spinal cord injury had no response to either cortical stimulation or combined subliminal percutaneous electrical stimulation and cortical stimulation. Another four subjects did show muscle responses time-locked to percutaneous electrical stimulation when the conditioning subliminal stimulation was given 15 to 40 ms prior to the cortical stimulation. Three of these patients had clinically incomplete lesions and one had a clinically complete injury. In three of the four subjects showing preserved electrophysiologic cortico-

spinal activity, motor EP were absent following cortical stimulation without the preceding conditioning stimulus. Use of such a conditioning stimulus may uncover preserved corticospinal innervation in some patients with spinal cord injury who do not have motor EP activity without conditioning stimulation.

Electroencephalography and Evoked Potentials in Determination of Brain Death

The most recently revised guidelines for EEG recording in suspected brain death were published in 1994 by the American Electroencephalographic Society.[25] Rigorous technical standards must be met. Sources of artifact must be controlled to the extent possible and otherwise meticulously documented. No clinician, however, should depend on electroencephalography alone for making a conclusive diagnosis of brain death. Clinical assessment is far more important and documentation of the absence of brain perfusion is more conclusive. Brainstem auditory and somatosensory EP have also been recorded in brain death. Although these techniques provide an objective electrophysiologic assessment of brainstem function, they are of no value for determination of brain death when used in isolation.[138,140]

CURRENT LIMITATIONS

The reliability of intraoperative electrophysiologic monitoring and of EEG and EP recording in the critical care unit varies to some extent among the reported series. Several inaccurate predictions have been described. Some erroneous results may be explained by technical difficulties, lapses in quality control, and lack of experience. The extent to which a degree of unreliability may be inherent in the methodology cannot yet be determined.

The collective clinical experience with EP monitoring in the operating room and critical care unit is still somewhat limited, with the result that the available clinical data base is relatively small. Furthermore, quantitative characterization of EP waveforms is not yet fully developed. Acceptable tolerance limits for degree and duration of EP alteration in the operating room and critical care unit have not been defined. One can no more expect absolute tolerance limits for variability in EP, however, than one could expect similar absolute tolerance limits for changes in temperature, heart rate, and arterial blood pressure. Continuous evaluation and titrated care are the appropriate goals for monitoring in the acute clinical situation.

Most of the current limitations of intraoperative and critical care unit EEG and EP monitoring are amenable to solution. Techniques are still somewhat cumbersome, equipment and personnel expensive, and interpretation sometimes difficult. With adequate attention to quality control, monitoring and constraint of potentially confounding variables, and formal and informal training in electrophysiologic monitoring, these limitations can be overcome. As equipment and techniques improve, the barriers to successful application of these techniques will continue to diminish.

COSTS VERSUS BENEFITS

Equipment for monitoring EEG and EP may cost $20,000 to $90,000 or more. The full attention of a highly trained operator may be required for several hours, and a physician must be available for interpretation while acute changes are occurring. Thus, monitoring of EEG and EP in the operating room or critical care unit is expensive. Charges for intraoperative monitoring of EP in various regions of the country range from approximately $300 to $1,500 per case. Can this expenditure be justified as cost-effective in the face of pressures to restrain the increasing costs of health care? Decisions about the allocation of scarce resources are difficult. Few guidelines are available. One court, however, ruled that the omission of monitoring may be negligent whenever the incidence of untoward events that could be prevented by monitoring multiplied by the anticipated cost of a single such event is greater than the cost of monitoring.[318] Application of this general guideline is not simple, however. There are difficulties in estimating the incidence of neurologic complications in the operating room and critical care unit, the costs of these complications, and the reliability with which monitoring may be able to help prevent them. On the basis of estimates that are probably quite conservative, we might assume that paraplegia occurs in 0.3 percent of those patients who undergo spine fusion (without sublaminar wiring) for scoliosis.[319] We might further assume, very conservatively, that one case of paraplegia costs $300,000. According to the Learned Hand rule, spinal cord function should be monitored during this operation if reliable monitoring can be provided for less than $900. Greater risk or greater cost of injury would, according to this guideline, justify even greater expenditures. Diminished reliability of monitoring or a decreased possibility of preserving function through the use of monitoring would decrease the allowable cost of monitoring. Cost-benefit studies would, of course, require consideration of the relative costs, risks, and benefits of an alternative test such as intraoperative awakening to test voluntary motor function.

EXPECTATIONS

Monitoring of EEG and EP in the operating room and critical care unit offers real promise as a useful means for reducing the incidence of neurologic injury. It seems likely that electrophysiologic monitoring of the nervous system will be available in the operating rooms and intensive care units of most medical centers where large numbers of complex neurosurgical, orthopedic, and cardiovascular operations are performed. Quality control will continue to require meticulous attention, and the application of electrodes will require care and skill. Many steps in monitoring that must now be done manually will be automated. Once electrodes are in place, signal acquisition, checking, and processing will proceed according to programs in microprocessor-based instruments. Potentially confounding variables will be automatically monitored, and new "baseline" waveforms will be automatically recorded whenever a new steady state, either pharmacologically or physiologically, is established.

As clinical experience with well-documented clinical cases grows, the interpretation of EEG and EP changes in the operating room and critical care unit will be based on statistical probabilities that particular patterns of EP change, quantitatively described, will be associated with untoward neurologic sequelae. Once the patterns of interest are defined and acceptable tolerance limits are determined, automatic alarm functions can be generated. Each waveform measurement, or each set of amplitude and phase measurements for steady-state EP, will be classified by the computer as acceptable, not acceptable, or technically inadequate. Still, absolute tolerance limits for EP change are expected to remain elusive. Decision-making in the operating room will continue to depend on clinical judgment, but more precise information will be made available to the clinician who makes these judgments. The costs of EP monitoring are expected to diminish as personnel requirements diminish and automated devices are manufactured in quantity.

In conclusion, it seems that EP monitoring in the acute care setting as performed today resembles in many respects the intraoperative monitoring of the electrocardiogram a generation ago. The techniques are cumbersome. Quality control is difficult. Equipment is bulky, delicate, and expensive. We know that loss of the waveform is ominous, but we lack quantitative criteria for more subtle changes. Those teams of anesthesiologists, surgeons, and intensivists willing to take the necessary precautions for successful monitoring today will be rewarded by information that facilitates management of patients at risk for neurologic injury. By reporting their carefully documented experiences, these practitioners will contribute not only to new developments in signal acquisition and analysis but also to better understanding of the clinical importance of EEG and EP changes seen in the operating room and critical care unit.

ACKNOWLEDGMENT

This work was supported in part by the Department of Anesthesiology at the University of Florida and by the Medical Research Service of the Veterans Administration.

REFERENCES

1. Anonymous: On being aware. Br J Anaesth 51:711, 1979
2. Blacher RS: On awakening paralyzed during surgery: a syndrome of traumatic neurosis. JAMA 234:67, 1975
3. Grundy BL: Monitoring of sensory evoked potentials during neurosurgical operations: methods and applications. Neurosurgery 11:556, 1982
4. Grundy BL: Intraoperative monitoring of sensory-evoked potentials. Anesthesiology 58:72, 1983
5. Friedman WA, Theisen GJ, Grundy BL: Electrophysiologic monitoring of the nervous system. p. 231. In Stoelting RK, Barash PG, Gallagher TJ (eds): Advances in Anesthesia. Year Book Medical Publishers, Chicago, 1988
6. Grundy BL, Villani RM et al: Evoked Potentials: Intraoperative and ICU Monitoring. p. 1. Springer-Verlag, New York, 1988
7. Beecher HK: The first anesthesia records (Codman, Cushing). Surg Gynecol Obstet 71:689, 1940
8. Bendixen HH: A forword: the tasks of the anesthesiologist. p. xi. In Saidman LJ, Smith NT (eds): Monitoring in Anesthesia. Butterworth, Boston, 1983
9. Chiappa KH, Ropper AH: Evoked potentials in clinical medicine: Part I. N Engl J Med 306:1140, 1982
10. Chiappa KH, Ropper AH: Evoked potentials in clinical medicine: Part 2. N Engl J Med 306:1205, 1982
11. Cooper R, Osselton JW, Shaw JC: EEG Technology. Butterworth, London, 1980
12. Speckmann E-J, Elger CE: Introduction to the neurophysiological basis of the EEG and DC potentials. p. 15. In Niedermeyer E, Lopes Da Silva F (eds): Electroencephalography: Basic Principles, Clinical Applications, and Related Fields. Williams & Wilkins, Baltimore, 1993
13. American Electroencephalographic Society: Guidelines on evoked potentials. J Clin Neurophysiol 11:40, 1994
14. Lee C, Katz RL, Lee AS, Glaser B: A new instrument for continuous recording of the evoked compound electromyogram in the clinical setting. Anesth Analg 56:260, 1977
15. Merton PA, Hill DK, Morton HB, Marsden CD: Scope of a technique for electrical stimulation of human brain, spinal cord, and muscle. Lancet 2:597, 1982
16. Harker LA, Hosick E, Voots RJ, Mendel MI: Influence of succinylcholine on middle component auditory evoked potentials. Arch Otolaryngol 103:133, 1977
17. Schwender D, Kaiser A, Klasing S et al: Midlatency auditory evoked potentials and explicit and implicit memory in patients undergoing cardiac surgery. Anesthesiology 80:493, 1994
18. Velasco M, Velasco F, Olvera A: Effect of task relevance and selective attention on components of cortical and subcortical evoked potentials in man. Electroencephalogr Clin Neurophysiol 48:377, 1980
19. Polich J: P300 in clinical applications: meaning, method, and measurement. Am J EEG Technol 31:201, 1991
20. Carmon A, Mor J, Goldberg J: Evoked cerebral responses to noxious thermal stimuli in humans. Exp Brain Res 25:103, 1976
21. Celesia GG: Visual evoked potentials and electroretinograms. p. 911. In Niedermeyer E, Lopes Da

Silva F (eds): Electroencephalography: Basic Principles, Clinical Applications, and Related Fields. Williams & Wilkins, Baltimore, 1993

22. American Electroencephalographic Society: Guidelines for intraoperative monitoring of sensory evoked potentials. J Clin Neurophysiol 11:77, 1994

23. Jasper HH: The ten-twenty electrode system of the International Federation. Electroencephalogr Clin Neurophysiol 10:371, 1958

24. Goff GD, Matsumiya Y, Allison T, Goff WR: The scalp topography of human somatosensory and auditory evoked potentials. Electroencephalogr Clin Neurophysiol 42:57, 1977

25. American Electroencephalographic Society: Minimum technical standards for EEG recording in suspected cerebral death. J Clin Neurophysiol 11:10, 1994

26. Lopes da Silva F: EEG analysis: theory and practice. p. 1097. In Niedermeyer E, Lopes Da Silva F (eds): Electroencephalography: Basic Principles, Clinical Applications, and Related Fields. Williams & Wilkins, Baltimore, 1993

27. Schwilden H, Stoeckel H: Effective therapeutic infusions produced by closed-loop feedback control of methohexital administration during total intravenous anesthesia with fentanyl. Anesthesiology 73: 225, 1990

28. Schwilden H, Schuttler J, Stoeckel H: Closed-loop feedback control of methohexital anesthesia by quantitative EEG analysis in humans. Anesthesiology 67:341, 1987

29. Rampil I, Correll JW, Rosenbaum SH et al: Computerized electroencephalogram monitoring and carotid artery shunting. Neurosurgery 13:276, 1983

30. Sidi A, Halimi P, Cotev S: Estimating anesthetic depth by electroencephalography during anesthetic induction and intubation in patients undergoing cardiac surgery. J Clin Anesth 2:101, 1990

31. Deleon MG: Electrical source analysis by brain mapping techniques. Physiol Meas 14:A95, 1993

32. Schuler P, Vieth J, Schnabel M, Frey M: Advantages of magnetoencephalography (AC and DC) in focal and generalized brain activity. Psychiatry Res 29: 377, 1989

33. Pradhan N, Dutt DN: A nonlinear perspective in understanding the neurodynamics of EEG. Comput Biol Med 23:425, 1993

34. Nakamura M: Waveform estimation from noisy signals with variable signal delay using bispectrum averaging. IEEE Trans Biomed Eng 40:118, 1993

35. Hasselman K, Munk W, MacDonald G: Bispectra of ocean waves. p. 125. In Rosenblatt M (ed): Time Series Analysis. Wiley, New York, 1963

36. Barnett TP, Johnson LC, Naitoh P et al: Bispectrum analysis of EEG signals during waking and sleeping. Science 172:401, 1971

37. Dumermuth G, Huber PJ, Lkeiner B, Gasser T: Analysis of the interrelations between frequency bands of the EEG by means of the bispectrum: a preliminary study. Electroencephalogr Clin Neurophysiol 31:137, 1971

38. Kearse LA Jr, Manburg P, DeBros F, Chamoun N, Saini V: Bispectral analysis of the electroencephalogram during induction of anesthesia may predict hemodynamic responses to laryngoscopy and intubation. Electroencephalogr Clin Neurophysiol 90:194–200, 1994

39. Sebel PS, Bowles S, Saini V, Chamoun N: Accuracy of EEG in predicting movement at incision during isoflurane or propofol anesthesia. Anesthesiology 75:A446, 1991

40. Lien CA, Berman M, Saini V et al: The accuracy of the EEG in predicting hemodynamic changes with incision during isoflurane anesthesia. Anesth Analg 74:S187, 1992

41. Vernon J, Bowles S, Sebel PS, Chamoun N: EEG bispectrum predicts movement at incision during isoflurane or propofol anesthesia. Anesthesiology 77:A502, 1992

42. Fell J, Roschke J, Beckmann P: Deterministic chaos and the 1st positive lyapunov exponent: a nonlinear analysis of the human electroencephalogram during sleep. Biol Cybern 69:139, 1993

43. Law SK, Nunez PL, Wijesinghe RS: High-resolution EEG using spline generated surface laplacians on spherical and ellipsoidal surfaces. IEEE Trans Biomed Eng 40:145, 1993

44. Burke D, Skuse NF, Lethlean AK: Cutaneous and muscle afferent components of the cerebral potential evoked by electrical stimulation of human peripheral nerves. Electroencephalogr Clin Neurophysiol 51:579, 1980

45. Aminoff MJ, Eisen A: Somatosensory evoked potentials. p. 571. In Aminoff MJ (ed): Electrodiagnosis in Clinical Neurology. Churchill Livingstone, New York, 1992

46. Zarola F, Rossini PM: Nerve, spinal cord and brain somatosensory evoked responses: a comparative study during electrical and magnetic peripheral nerve stimulation. Electroencephalogr Clin Neurophysiol 80:372, 1991

47. Kunesch E, Knecht S, Classen J et al: Somatosensory evoked potentials (seps) elicited by magnetic nerve stimulation. Electroencephalogr Clin Neurophysiol 88:459, 1993

48. Yu Z, Starr A: Magnetic stimulation of muscle evokes cerebral potentials. Muscle Nerve 14:721, 1991

49. Pratt H, Starr A: Mechanically and electrically evoked somatosensory potentials in humans: scalp and neck distributions of short-latency compo-

nents. Electroencephalogr Clin Neurophysiol 51: 138, 1981

50. Levy WJ, York DH, McCaffrey M, Tanzer F: Motor evoked potentials from transcranial stimulation of the motor cortex in humans. Neurosurgery 15:287, 1984

51. Cowan JM, Rothwell JC, Dick JP et al: Abnormalities in central motor pathway conduction in multiple sclerosis. Lancet 2:304, 1984

52. Barker AT, Freeston IL, Jalinous R, Jarratt JA: Magnetic stimulation of the human brain and peripheral nervous system: an introduction and the results of an initial clinical evaluation. Neurosurgery 20:100, 1987

53. Counter SA, Borg E, Lofqvist L, Brismar T: Hearing loss from the acoustic artifact of the coil used in extracranial magnetic stimulation. Neurology 40: 1159, 1990

54. Counter SA, Borg E, Lofqvist L: Acoustic trauma in extracranial magnetic brain stimulation. Electroencephalogr Clin Neurophysiol 78:173, 1991

55. Burgess RC: Technical review: magnetic stimulators. J Clin Neurophysiol 8:121, 1991

56. Pascual-Leone A, Houser CM, Reese K et al: Safety of rapid-rate transcranial magnetic stimulation in normal volunteers. Electroencephalogr Clin Neurophysiol 89:120, 1993

57. Counter SA, Borg E: Acoustic middle ear muscle reflex protection against magnetic coil impulse noise. Acta Otolaryngol (Stockh) 113:483, 1993

58. DeFelipe J, Conley M, Jones EG: Long-range focal collateralization of axons arising from cortico-cortical cells in monkey sensory-motor cortex. J Neurosci 6:3749, 1986

59. Stefanis C, Jasper H: Recurrent collateral inhibition in pyramidal tract neurons. J Neurophysiol 27:855, 1964

60. Roth BJ, Pascual-Leone A, Cohen LG, Hallett M: The heating of metal electrodes during rapid rate transcranial magnetic stimulation: a possible safety hazard. Electroencephalogr Clin Neurophysiol 85: 116, 1992

61. Kasai T, Hayes KC, Wolfe DL, Allatt RD: Afferent conditioning of motor evoked potentials following transcranial magnetic stimulation of motor cortex in normal subjects. Electroencephalogr Clin Neurophysiol 85:95, 1992

62. Taniguchi M, Cedzich C, Schramm J: Modification of cortical stimulation for motor evoked potentials under general anesthesia: technical description. Neurosurgery 32:219, 1993

63. Grundy BL: Sensory-evoked potentials. p. 375. In Boulton AA, Baker GB, Boisvert DPJ (eds): Neuromethods-8. Humana Press, Clifton, NJ, 1988

64. Anthony PF, Durrett R, Pulec JL, Hartstone JL: A new parameter in brain stem evoked response: component wave areas. Laryngoscope 89:1569, 1979

65. Boston JR: Spectra of auditory brainstem responses and spontaneous EEG. IEEE Trans Biomed Eng 28: 334, 1981

66. Duffy FH, Bartels PH, Burchfiel JL: Significance probability mapping: an aid in the topographic analysis of brain electrical activity. Electroencephalogr Clin Neurophysiol 51:455, 1981

67. Wong PK, Bickford RG: Brain stem auditory evoked potentials: the use of noise estimate. Electroencephalogr Clin Neurophysiol 50:25, 1980

68. Keller I, Madler C, Schwender D, Poppel E: Analysis of oscillatory components in perioperative AEP-recordings: a nonparametric procedure for frequency measurement. Clin Electroencephalogr 21:88, 1990

69. Cerutti S, Chiarenza G, Liberati D et al: A parametric method of identification of single-trial event-related potentials in the brain. IEEE Trans Biomed Eng 35:701, 1988

70. Donchin E, Herning RI: A simulation study of the efficacy of stepwise discriminant analysis in the detection and comparison of event related potentials. Electroencephalogr Clin Neurophysiol 38:51, 1975

71. Tang Y, Norcia AM: Improved processing of the steady-state evoked potential. Electroencephalogr Clin Neurophysiol 88:323, 1993

72. Grundy BL, Castenholz RH, Erdmann K et al: Effects of isoflurane dose and stimulus rate on feline BAEPs (abstracted). Electroencephalogr Clin Neurophysiol 72:18P, 1989

73. Lesser RP, Koehle R, Lueders H: Effect of stimulus intensity on short-latency SEPs. Electroencephalogr Clin Neurophysiol 47:377, 1979

74. Stockard JE, Stockard JJ, Westmoreland BF, Corfits JL: Brainstem auditory-evoked responses: normal variation as a function of stimulus and subject characteristics. Arch Neurol 36:823, 1979

75. Peterson DO, Drummond JC, Todd MM: Effects of halothane, enflurane, isoflurane, and nitrous oxide on somatosensory evoked potentials in humans. Anesthesiology 65:35, 1986

76. Salzman SK, Bechman AL, Marks HG et al: Effects of halothane on intraoperative scalp-recorded somatosensory evoked potentials to posterior tibial nerve stimulation in man. Electroencephalogr Clin Neurophysiol 65:36, 1986

77. Samra SK, Vanderzant CW, Domer PA, Sackellares JC: Differential effects of isoflurane on human median nerve SEPs. Anesthesiology 66:29, 1987

78. Sebel PS, Erwin CW, Neville WK: Effects of halothane and enflurane on far and near field somatosensory evoked potentials. Br J Anaesth 59:1492, 1987

79. Sebel PS, Flynn PJ, Ingram DA: Effect of nitrous oxide on visual, auditory and somatosensory evoked potentials. Br J Anaesth 56:1403, 1984

80. McPherson RW, Mahla M, Johnson R, Traystman RJ: Effects of enflurane, isoflurane, and nitrous oxide on somatosensory evoked potentials during fentanyl anesthesia. Anesthesiology 62:626, 1985

81. Grundy BL, Jannetta PJ, Procopio PT et al: Intraoperative monitoring of brain-stem auditory evoked potentials. J Neurosurg 57:674, 1982

82. Sebel PS, Ingram DA, Flynn PJ et al: Evoked potentials during isoflurane anaesthesia. Br J Anaesth 58:580, 1986

83. Sloan TB, Fugina ML, Toleikis JR: Effects of midazolam on median nerve somatosensory evoked potentials. Br J Anaesth 64:590, 1990

84. Schwender D, Klasing S, Madler C et al: Effects of benzodiazepines on mid-latency auditory evoked potentials. Can J Anaesth 40:1148, 1993

85. Schwender D, Rimkus T, Haessler R et al: Effects of increasing doses of alfentanil, fentanyl and morphine on mid-latency auditory evoked potentials. Br J Anaesth 71:622, 1993

86. McPherson RW, Sell B, Traystman RJ: Effects of thiopental, fentanyl, and etomidate on upper extremity somatosensory evoked potentials in humans. Anesthesiology 65:584, 1986

87. Sloan TB, Ronai AK, Toleikis JR, Koht A: Improvement of intraoperative somatosensory evoked potentials by etomidate. Anesth Analg 67:582, 1988

88. Kalkman CJ, Drummond JC, Ribberink AA et al: Effects of propofol, etomidate, midazolam, and fentanyl on motor evoked responses to transcranial electrical or magnetic stimulation in humans. Anesthesiology 76:502, 1992

89. Schwender D, Klasing S, Madler C et al: Mid-latency auditory evoked potentials during ketamine anaesthesia in humans. Br J Anaesth 71:629, 1993

90. Taniguchi M, Nadstawek J, Langenbach U et al: Effects of four intravenous anesthetic agents on motor evoked potentials elicited by magnetic transcranial stimulation. Neurosurgery 33:407, 1993

91. Scheepstra GL, de Lange JJ, Booij LH, Ros HH: Median nerve evoked potentials during propofol anaesthesia. Br J Anaesth 62:92, 1989

92. Markand ON, Warren CH, Moorthy SS et al: Monitoring of multimodality evoked potentials during open heart surgery under hypothermia. Electroencephalogr Clin Neurophysiol 59:432, 1984

93. Short LH, Peterson RE, Mongan PD: Physiologic and anesthetic alterations on spinal-sciatic evoked responses in swine. Anesth Analg 76:259, 1993

94. Panjwani GD, Mustafa MKY, Muhailan A et al: Effect of hyperthermia on somatosensory evoked potentials in the anaesthetized rat. Electroencephalogr Clin Neurophysiol 80:384, 1991

95. Haghighi SS, Keller BP, Oro JJ, Gibbs SR: Motor-evoked potential changes during hypoxic hypoxia. Surg Neurol 39:399, 1993

96. Haghighi SS, Oro JJ, Gibbs SR, McFadden M: Effect of graded hypoxia on cortical and spinal somatosensory evoked potentials. Surg Neurol 37:350, 1992

97. Kalkman CJ, Boezeman EH, Ribberink AA et al: Influence of changes in arterial carbon dioxide tension on the electroencephalogram and posterior tibial nerve somatosensory cortical evoked potentials during alfentanil/nitrous oxide anesthesia. Anesthesiology 75:68, 1991

98. Michels R, Wessel K, Klohn S, Kompf D: Long-latency reflexes, somatosensory evoked potentials and transcranial magnetic stimulation: relation of the three methods in multiple sclerosis. Electroencephalogr Clin Neurophysiol 89:235, 1993

99. Ragazzoni A, Amantini A, Lombardi M et al: Electric and CO_2 laser SEPs in a patient with asymptomatic syringomyelia. Electroencephalogr Clin Neurophysiol 88:335, 1993

100. Huttunen J, Homberg V, Lange HW: Precentral and postcentral somatosensory evoked potentials in huntington's disease—effects of stimulus repetition rate. J Neurol Sci 116:119, 1993

101. Murrison AW: The contribution of neurophysiologic techniques to the investigation of diving-related illness. Undersea Hyperbar Med 20:347, 1993

102. Hume AL, Cant BR: Diagnosis of hearing loss in infancy by electric response audiometry. Arch Otolaryngol 103:416, 1977

103. Jellinek DA, Bradford R, Bailey I, Symon L: The role of motor evoked potentials in the management of hysterical paraplegia: case report. Paraplegia 30:300, 1992

104. Ziegler D, Muhlen H, Dannehl K, Gries FA: Tibial nerve somatosensory evoked potentials at various stages of peripheral neuropathy in insulin dependent diabetic patients. J Neurol Neurosurg Psychiatry 56:58, 1993

105. Chiappa KH: Pattern shift visual, brainstem auditory, and short-latency somatosensory evoked potentials in multiple sclerosis. Neurology 30:110, 1980

106. Williamson PD, French JA, Thadani VM et al: Characteristics of medial temporal lobe epilepsy: 2. Interictal and ictal scalp electroencephalography, neuropsychological testing, neuroimaging, surgical results, and pathology. Ann Neurol 34:781, 1993

107. Stefan H, Abrahamfuchs K, Schneider S et al: Multichannel magnetoelectroencephalography recordings of interictal and ictal activity. Physiol Meas 14:A109, 1993

108. Donchin E, Callaway F, Cooper R: Publication criteria for studies of evoked potentials (EP) in man. p. 1. In Desmedt JE (ed): Attention, Voluntary Contraction and Event-Related Cerebral Potentials. S. Karger, Basel, 1977

109. Lindauer U, Villringer A, Dirnagl U: Characterization of CBF response to somatosensory stimulation—model and influence of anesthetics. Am J Physiol 264:H1223, 1993

110. Jewett DL, Romano MN, Williston JS: Human auditory evoked potentials: possible brain stem components detected on the scalp. Science 167:1517, 1970

111. Nagao S, Roccaforte P, Moody RA: Acute intracranial hypertension and auditory brain-stem responses. Part 3: the effects of posterior fossa mass lesions on brain-stem function. J Neurosurg 52:351, 1980

112. Nagao S, Roccaforte P, Moody RA: Acute intracranial hypertension and auditory brain-stem responses. Part 2: the effects of brain-stem movement on the auditory brain-stem responses due to transtentorial herniation. J Neurosurg 51:846, 1979

113. Celesia GG, Brigell M: Auditory evoked potentials. p. 937. In Niedermeyer E, Lopes Da Silva F (eds): Electroencephalography: Basic Principles, Clinical Applications, and Related Fields. Williams & Wilkins, Baltimore, 1993

114. Stockard JJ, Pope-Stockard JE, Sharbrough FW: Brainstem auditory evoked potentials in neurology: methodology, interpretation, and clinical application. p. 503. In Aminoff MJ (ed): Electrodiagnosis in Clinical Neurology. Churchill Livingstone, New York, 1992

115. Armington JC: Electroretinography, Electrodiagnosis in Clinical Neurology. p. 433. In Aminoff MJ (ed): Churchill Livingstone, New York, 1992

116. Celesia GG: Visual evoked potentials in clinical neurology. p. 467. In Aminoff MJ (ed): Electrodiagnosis in Clinical Neurology. New York, Churchill Livingstone, 1992

117. Sanarelli L, Rossini PM, Rizzo P, et al: Short-latency sinusoidal wavelets to bright flashed stimuli: studies with corneal lens, nasopharyngeal, retrobulbar and scalp recordings. Eur Neurol 29:306, 1989

118. Celesia GG, Bushnell D, Toleikis SC, Brigell MG: Cortical blindness and residual vision: is the second visual system in humans capable of more than rudimentary visual perception? Neurology 41:862, 1991

119. van Dijk JG, Jennekens-Schinkel A, Caekebeke JF et al: What is the validity of an abnormal evoked or event-related potential in MS? Auditory and visual evoked and event-related potentials in multiple sclerosis patients and normal subjects. J Neurol Sci 109:11, 1992

120. Papakostopoulos D, Fotiou F, Hart JC, Banerji NK: The electroretinogram in multiple sclerosis and demyelinating optic neuritis. Electroencephalogr Clin Neurophysiol 74:1, 1989

121. Taylor MJ, McCulloch DL: Visual evoked potentials in infants and children. J Clin Neurophysiol 9:357, 1992

122. Bennett MH, Jannetta PJ: Trigeminal evoked potentials in humans. Electroencephalogr Clin Neurophysiol 48:517, 1980

123. Stechison MT, Kralick FJ: The trigeminal evoked potential. 1. Long-latency responses in awake or anesthetized subjects. Neurosurgery 33:633, 1993

124. Cruccu G, Leandri M, Feliciani M, Manfredi M: Idiopathic and symptomatic trigeminal pain. J Neurol Neurosurg Psychiatry 53:1034, 1990

125. Leandri M, Parodi CI, Favale E: Early trigeminal evoked potentials in tumours of the base of the skull and trigeminal neuralgia. Electroencephalogr Clin Neurophysiol 71:114, 1988

126. Bennett MH, Lunsford LD: Percutaneous retrogasserian glycerol rhizotomy for tic douloureux: part 2. Results and implications of trigeminal evoked potential studies. Neurosurgery 14:431, 1984

127. Facco E, Baratto F, Munari M et al: Sensorimotor central conduction time in comatose patients. Electroencephalogr Clin Neurophysiol 80:469, 1991

128. Abbruzzese G, Morena M, Dall'Agata D et al: Motor evoked potentials (MEPs) in lacunar syndromes. Electroencephalogr Clin Neurophysiol 18:202, 1991

129. Wright AL, Williams NS, Gibson JS et al: Electrically evoked activity in the human external anal sphincter. Br J Surg 72:38, 1985

130. Abbruzzese G, Morena M, Caponnetto C et al: Motor evoked potentials following cervical electrical stimulation in brachial plexus lesions. J Neurol 241:63, 1993

131. Sawaya R: Spinal cord lesion after epidural anesthesia diagnosed by motor evoked potentials. Muscle Nerve 16:883, 1993

132. Caramia MD, Cicinelli P, Paradiso C et al: Excitability changes of muscular responses to magnetic brain stimulation in patients with central motor disorders. Electroencephalogr Clin Neurophysiol 81:243, 1991

133. Kiers L, Cros D, Chiappa KH, Fang J: Variability of motor potentials evoked by transcranial magnetic stimulation. Electroencephalogr Clin Neurophysiol 89:415, 1993

134. Berardelli A, Inghilleri M, Cruccu G et al: Electrical and magnetic transcranial stimulation in patients with corticospinal damage due to stroke or motor neurone disease. Electroencephalogr Clin Neurophysiol 81:389, 1991

135. Eisen A, Cracco RQ: Overuse of evoked potentials: caution. Neurology 33:618, 1983

136. Nuwer MR: Quantitative EEG: I. Techniques and problems of frequency analysis and topographic mapping. J Clin Neurophysiol 5:1, 1988

137. Nuwer MR: Quantitative EEG: II. Frequency analysis and topographic mapping in clinical settings. J Clin Neurophysiol 5:45, 1988

138. Machado C, Valdes P, Garciatigera J et al: Brainstem auditory evoked potentials and brain death. Electroencephalogr Clin Neurophysiol 80:392, 1991

139. Chancellor AM, Frith RW, Shaw NA: Somatosensory evoked potentials following severe head injury: loss of the thalamic potential with brain death. J Neurol Sci 87:255, 1988

140. Buchner H, Ferbert A, Hacke W: Serial recording of median nerve stimulated subcortical somatosensory evoked potentials (SEPs) in developing brain death. Electroencephalogr Clin Neurophysiol 69:14, 1988

141. Cracco RQ, Evans B: Spinal evoked potential in the cat: effects of asphyxia, strychnine, cord section and compression. Electroencephalogr Clin Neurophysiol 44:187, 1978

142. Grundy BL, Procopio PT, Jannetta PJ et al: Evoked potential changes produced by positioning for retromastoid craniectomy. Neurosurgery 10:766, 1982

143. Friedman WA, Kaplan BJ, Gravenstein D, Rhoton AL Jr: Intraoperative brain-stem auditory evoked potentials during posterior fossa microvascular decompression. J Neurosurg 62:552, 1985

144. Schramm J, Mokrusch T, Fahlbusch R, Hochstetter A: Detailed analysis of intraoperative changes monitoring brain stem acoustic evoked potentials. Neurosurgery 22:694, 1988

145. Greenberg RP, Mayer DJ, Becker DP, Miller JD: Evaluation of brain function in severe human head trauma with multimodality evoked potentials: Part 1. Evoked brain-injury potentials, methods, and analysis. J Neurosurg 47:150, 1977

146. Greenberg RP, Becker DP, Miller JD, Mayer DJ: Evaluation of brain function in severe human head trauma with multimodality evoked potentials: Part 2. Localization of brain dysfunction and correlation with posttraumatic neurological conditions. J Neurosurg 47:163, 1977

147. Grundy BL, Heros R: Ischemic cerebrovascular disease. p. 1. In Matjasko J, Katz J (eds): Clinical Controversies in Neuroanesthesia and Neurosurgery. Grune & Stratton, Orlando, 1986

148. European Carotid Surgery Trialists' Collaborative Group: MRC European carotid surgery trial: interim results for symptomatic patients with severe (70–99%) or with mild (0–29%) carotid stenosis. Lancet 337:1235, 1991

149. North American Symptomatic Carotid Endarterectomy Trial (NASCET) Steering Committee: North American symptomatic carotid endarterectomy trial: methods, patient characteristics, and progress. Stroke 22:711, 1991

150. Wiebers DO: Results of a randomized controlled trial of carotid endarterectomy for asymptomatic carotid stenosis. Mayo Clin Proc 67:513, 1992

151. Barnett HJM, Barnes RW, Clagett GP et al: Symptomatic carotid artery stenosis: a solvable problem—North American symptomatic carotid endarterectomy trial. Stroke 23:1048, 1992

152. Taylor DW: Beneficial effect of carotid endarterectomy in symptomatic patients with high-grade carotid stenosis. N Engl J Med 325:445, 1991

153. Mayberg MR, Wilson SE, Yatsu F et al: Carotid endarterectomy and prevention of cerebral ischemia in symptomatic carotid stenosis. JAMA 266:3289, 1991

154. Easton JD, Wilterdink JL: Carotid endarterectomy: trials and tribulations. Ann Neurol 35:5, 1994

155. Steed DL, Peitzman AB, Grundy BL, Webster MW: Causes of stroke in carotid endarterectomy. Surgery 92:634, 1982

156. Halsey JH Jr, The International Transcranial Doppler Collaborators: Risks and benefits of shunting in carotid endarterectomy. Stroke 23:1583, 1992

157. Grundy BL, Webster MW, Richey ET, Karanjia PN: EEG changes during carotid endarterectomy: drug effect and embolism. Br J Anaesth 57:445, 1985

158. Peitzman AB, Webster MW, Loubeau JM et al: Carotid endarterectomy under regional (conductive) anesthesia. Ann Surg 196:59, 1982

159. Sundt TM, Sharbrough FW, Piepgrass DG: Correlation of cerebral blood flow and electroencephalographic changes during carotid endarterectomy: with results of surgery and hemodynamics of cerebral ischemia. Mayo Clin Proc 56:533, 1981

160. Stanford JR, Lubow M, Vasko JS: Prevention of stroke by carotid endarterectomy. Surgery 83:259, 1978

161. Symon L, Lassen NA, Astrup J, Branston NM: Thresholds of ischaemia in brain cortex. Adv Exp Med Biol 94:775, 1977

162. Astrup J, Symon L, Branston NM, Lassen NA: Cortical evoked potential and extracellular K^+ and H^+ at critical levels of brain ischemia. Stroke 8:51, 1977

163. Chiappa KH, Burke SR, Young RR: Results of electroencephalographic monitoring during 367 carotid endarterectomies: use of a dedicated microcomputer. Stroke 10:381, 1979

164. Grundy BL, Sanderson AC, Webster WW et al: Hemiparesis following carotid endarterectomy: comparison of monitoring methods. Anesthesiology 55:462, 1981

165. Blume WT, Ferguson GG, McNeill DK: Significance of EEG changes at carotid endarterectomy. Stroke 17:891, 1986

166. Blume WT, Sharbrough FW: EEG monitoring during carotid endarterectomy and open heart surgery. p. 747. In Niedermeyer E, Lopes Da Silva F (eds): Electroencephalography Basic Principles, Clinical Applications, and Related Fields. Williams & Wilkins, Baltimore, 1993

167. Tempelhoff R, Modica PA, Grubb RL Jr et al: Selective shunting during carotid endarterectomy based on two-channel computerized electroencephalographic/compressed spectral array analysis. Neurosurgery 24:339, 1989

168. Silbert BS, Koumoundouros E, Davies MJ, Cronin KD: Comparison of the processed electroencephalogram and awake neurological assessment during carotid endarterectomy. Anaesth Intensive Care 17:298, 1989

169. Ahn SS, Jordan SE, Nuwer MR et al: Computed electroencephalographic topographic brain mapping. A new and accurate monitor of cerebral circulation and function for patients having carotid endarterectomy. J Vasc Surg 8:247, 1988

170. Kearse LA, Martin D, McPeck K. Lopezbresnahan M: Computer-derived density spectral array in detection of mild analog electroencephalographic ischemic pattern changes during carotid endarterectomy. J Neurosurg 78:884, 1993

171. Young WL, Moberg RS, Ornstein E et al: Electroencephalographic monitoring for ischemia during carotid endarterectomy: visual versus computer analysis. J Clin Monit 4:78, 1988

172. Hanowell LH, Soriano S, Bennett HL: EEG power changes are more sensitive than spectral edge frequency variation for detection of cerebral ischemia during carotid artery surgery: a prospective assessment of processed EEG monitoring. J Cardiothorac Vasc Anesth 6:292, 1992

173. van Alphen HA, Polman CH: The value of continuous intra-operative EEG monitoring during carotid endarterectomy. Acta Neurochir (Wien) 91:95, 1988

174. Hargadine JR: Intraoperative monitoring of sensory evoked potentials. p. 92. In Rand RW (ed): Microneurosurgery. CV Mosby, St. Louis, 1985

175. Hargadine JR, Snyder E: Brain stem and somatosensory evoked potentials: application in the operating room and intensive care unit. Bull Los Angeles Neurol Soc 47:62, 1982

176. Moorthy SS, Markand ON, Dilley RS et al: Somatosensory-evoked responses during carotid endarterectomy. Anesth Analg 61:879, 1982

177. Markand ON, Dilley RS, Moorthy SS, Warren C Jr: Monitoring of somatosensory evoked responses during carotid endarterectomy. Arch Neurol 41:375, 1984

178. Artru AA, Strandness DE Jr: Delayed carotid shunt occlusion detected by electroencephalographic monitoring. J Clin Monit 5:119, 1989

179. Sasaki T, Takeda R, Ogasawara T et al: [Monitoring of somatosensory evoked potentials during extracranial revascularization]. Neurol Med Chir (Tokyo) 29:280, 1989

180. Russ W, Thiel A, Moosdorf R, Hempelmann G: [Somatosensory evoked potentials in obliterating interventions of the carotid bifurcation]. Klin Wochenschr 66 (Suppl.): 14:35, 1988

181. Schweiger H, Kamp HD, Dinkel M: Somatosensory-evoked potentials during carotid artery surgery: experience in 400 operations. Surgery 109:602, 1991

182. Horsch S, De Vleeschauwer P, Ktenidis K: Intraoperative assessment of cerebral ischemia during carotid surgery. J Cardiovasc Surg 31:599, 1990

183. Lam AM, Manninen PH, Ferguson GG, Nantau W: Monitoring electrophysiologic function during carotid endarterectomy: a comparison of somatosensory evoked potentials and conventional electroencephalogram. Anesthesiology 75:15, 1991

184. Kearse LA Jr, Brown EN, McPeck K: Somatosensory evoked potentials sensitivity relative to electroencephalography for cerebral ischemia during carotid endarterectomy. Stroke 23:498, 1992

185. Fava E, Bortolani E, Ducati A, Schieppati M: Role of SEP in identifying patients requiring temporary shunt during carotid endarterectomy. Electroencephalogr Clin Neurophysiol 84:426, 1992

186. Stockard JJ, Bickford RG, Myers RR et al: Hypotension-induced changes in cerebral function during cardiac surgery. Stroke 5:730, 1974

187. Levy WJ: Intraoperative EEG patterns: implications for EEG monitoring. Anesthesiology 60:430, 1984

188. Bashein G, Nessly ML, Bledsoe SW et al: Electroencephalography during surgery with cardiopulmonary bypass and hypothermia. Anesthesiology 76:878, 1992

189. Metz S, Slogoff S: Thiopental sodium by single bolus dose compared to infusion for cerebral protection during cardiopulmonary bypass. J Clin Anesth 2:226, 1990

190. Coselli JS, Crawford ES, Beall AC Jr, et al: Determination of brain temperatures for safe circulatory arrest during cardiovascular operation. Ann Thorac Surg 45:638, 1988

191. Hickey C, Gugino LD, Aglio LS et al: Intraoperative somatosensory evoked potential monitoring predicts peripheral nerve injury during cardiac surgery. Anesthesiology 78:29, 1993

192. Arom KV, Cohen DE, Strobl FT: Effect of intraoperative intervention on neurological outcome

based on electroencephalographic monitoring during cardiopulmonary bypass. Ann Thorac Surg 48: 476, 1989

193. Edmonds HL, Griffiths LK, Vanderlaken J et al: Quantitative electroencephalographic monitoring during myocardial revascularization predicts postoperative disorientation and improves outcome. J Thorac Cardiovasc Surg 103:555, 1992

194. Andoh T, Ka K, Suzuki H, Okutsu Y: [Power spectral analysis of EEG during simple deep hypothermia under ether anesthesia]. Masui 38:765, 1989

195. Nash CL Jr, Lorig RA, Schatzinger LA, Brown RH: Spinal cord monitoring during operative treatment of the spine. Clin Orthop 126:100, 1977

196. Forbes HJ, Allen PW, Waller CS et al: Spinal cord monitoring in scoliosis surgery: experience with 1168 cases. J Bone Joint Surg [Br] 73:487, 1991

197. Wilber RG, Thompson G, Shaffer JW et al: Postoperative neurological deficits in segmental spinal instrumentation: a study spinal cord monitoring. J Bone Joint Surg 66:1178, 1984

198. Grundy BL, Nash CL Jr, Brown RH: Arterial pressure manipulation alters spinal cord function during correction of scoliosis. Anesthesiology 54:249, 1981

199. Grundy BL, Nash CL Jr, Brown RH: Deliberate hypotension for spinal fusion: prospective randomized study with evoked potential monitoring. Can Anaesth Soc J 29:452, 1982

200. Molale M: False negative intraoperative somatosensory evoked potentials with simultaneous bilateral stimulation. Clin Electroencephalogr 17:6, 1986

201. Friedman WA, Richards R: Somatosensory evoked potential monitoring accurately predicts hemispinal cord damage: a case report. Neurosurgery 22:140, 1988

202. Nashold BS Jr, Ovelmen-Levitt J, Sharpe R, Higgins AC: Intraoperative evoked potentials recorded in man directly from dorsal roots and spinal cord. J Neurosurg 62:680, 1985

203. Grundy BL, Nelson PB, Doyle E, Procopio PT: Intraoperative loss of somatosensory-evoked potentials predicts loss of spinal cord function. Anesthesiology 57:321, 1982

204. Tamaki T, Tsuji H, Inoué S, Kobayashi H: The prevention of iatrogenic spinal cord injury utilizing the evoked spinal cord potential. Int Orthop 4:313, 1981

205. Koyanagi I, Iwasaki Y, Isu T et al: Spinal cord evoked potential monitoring after spinal cord stimulation during surgery of spinal cord tumors. Neurosurgery 33:451, 1993

206. Levy WJ Jr: Clinical experience with motor and cerebellar evoked potential monitoring. Neurosurgery 20:169–182, 1987

207. Owen JH, Bridwell KH, Grubb R et al: The clinical application of neurogenic motor evoked potentials to monitor spinal cord function during surgery. Spine 16:S385, 1991

208. Su CF, Haghighi SS, Oro JJ, Gaines RW: "Backfiring" in spinal cord monitoring. High thoracic spinal cord stimulation evokes sciatic response by antidromic sensory pathway conduction, not motor tract conduction. Spine 17:504, 1992

209. Machida M, Weinstein SL, Yamada T et al: Dissociation of muscle action potentials and spinal somatosensory evoked potentials after ischemic damage of spinal cord. Spine 13:1119, 1988

210. Zentner J: Noninvasive motor evoked potential monitoring during neurosurgical operations on the spinal cord. Neurosurgery 24:709, 1989

211. Jellinek D, Jewkes D, Symon L: Noninvasive intraoperative monitoring of motor evoked potentials under propofol anesthesia: effects of spinal surgery on the amplitude and latency of motor evoked potentials. Neurosurgery 29:551, 1991

212. Jellinek D, Platt M, Jewkes D, Symon L: Effects of nitrous oxide on motor evoked potentials recorded from skeletal muscle in patients under total anesthesia with intravenously administered propofol. Neurosurgery 29:558, 1991

213. Crawford ES, Mizrahi EM, Hess KR et al: The impact of distal aortic perfusion and somatosensory evoked potential monitoring on prevention of paraplegia after aortic aneurysm operation. J Thorac Cardiovasc Surg 95:357, 1988

214. Svensson LG, Crawford ES, Hess KR et al: Experience with 1509 patients undergoing thoracoabdominal aortic operations. J Vasc Surg 17:357–370, 1993

215. Svensson LG, Crawford ES, Hess KR et al: Variables predictive of outcome in 832 patients undergoing repairs of the descending thoracic aorta. Chest 104: 1248, 1993

216. Maeda S, Miyamoto T, Murata H, Yamashita K: Prevention of spinal cord ischemia by monitoring spinal cord perfusion pressure and somatosensory evoked potentials. J Cardiovasc Surg 30:565, 1989

217. Cunningham JN Jr, Laschinger JC, Spencer FC: Monitoring of somatosensory evoked potentials during surgical procedures on the thoracoabdominal aorta: IV. Clinical observations and results. J Thorac Cardiovasc Surg 94:275, 1987

218. Fava E, Bortolani EM, Ducati A, Ruberti U: Evaluation of spinal cord function by means of lower limb somatosensory evoked potentials in reparative aortic surgery. J Cardiovasc Surg 29:421, 1988

219. Hollier LH, Money SR, Naslund TC et al: Risk of spinal cord dysfunction in patients undergoing thoracoabdominal aortic replacement. Am J Surg 164:210, 1992

220. Fehrenbacher JW, McCready RA, Hormuth DA et al: One-stage segmental resection of extensive thoracoabdominal aneurysms with left-sided heart bypass. J Vasc Surg 18:366, 1993

221. Vanicky I, Marsala M, Galik J, Marsala J: Epidural perfusion cooling protection against protracted spinal cord ischemia in rabbits. J Neurosurg 79:736, 1993

222. Elmore JR, Gloviczki P, Harper CM et al: Failure of motor evoked potentials to predict neurologic outcome in experimental thoracic aortic occlusion. J Vasc Surg 14:131, 1991

223. Okamoto Y, Murakami M, Nakagawa T et al: Intraoperative spinal cord monitoring during surgery for aortic aneurysm: application of spinal cord evoked potential. Electroencephalogr Clin Neurophysiol 84:315, 1992

224. Ihaya A, Morioka K, Noguchi H et al: [A case report of descending thoracic aortic aneurysm associated with anterior spinal artery syndrome despite no marked ESP changes]. Kyobu Geka 43:843, 1990

225. Kaplan BJ, Friedman WA, Alexander JA, Hampson SR: Somatosensory evoked potential monitoring of spinal cord ischemia during aortic operations. Neurosurgery 19:82, 1986

226. Kaplan BJ, Gravenstein D, Friedman WA: Intraoperative electrophysiology in treatment of peripheral nerve injuries. J Florida Med Assoc 71:400, 1984

227. Kline DG, Judice DJ: Operative management of selected brachial plexus lesions. J Neurosurg 58:631, 1983

228. Murase T, Kawai H, Masatomi T et al: Evoked spinal cord potentials for diagnosis during brachial plexus surgery. J Bone Joint Surg [Br] 75:775, 1993

229. Allison T: Localization of sensorimotor cortex in neurosurgery by recording of somatosensory evoked potentials. Yale J Biol Med 60:143, 1987

230. Katayama Y, Tsubokawa T, Maejima S et al: Corticospinal direct response in humans: identification of the motor cortex during intracranial surgery under general anaesthesia. J Neurol Neurosurg Psychiatry 51:50, 1988

231. Tsai ML, Chatrian GE, Pauri F et al: Electrocorticography in patients with medically intractable temporal lobe seizures: 1. Quantification of epileptiform discharges prior to resective surgery. Electroencephalogr Clin Neurophysiol 87:10, 1993

232. Tsai ML, Chatrian GE, Holubkov AL et al: Electrocorticography in patients with medically intractable temporal lobe seizures: 2. Quantification of epileptiform discharges following successive stages of resective surgery. Electroencephalogr Clin Neurophysiol 87:25–37, 1993

233. Fiol ME, Gates JR, Mireles R et al: Value of intra-

operative EEG changes during corpus callosotomy in predicting surgical results. Epilepsia 34:74, 1993

234. Drummond JC, Todd MM, Schubert A, Sang H: Effect of the acute administration of high dose pentobarbital on human brain stem auditory and median nerve somatosensory evoked responses. Neurosurgery 20:830, 1987

235. Hargadine JR, Branston NM, Symon L: Central conduction time in primate brain ischemia: a study in baboons. Stroke 6:637, 1980

236. Branston NM, Strong AJ, Symon L: Extracellular potassium activity, evoked potential and tissue blood flow: relationships during progressive ischaemia in baboon cerebral cortex. J Neurol Sci 32:305, 1977

237. Strong AJ, Goodhardt MJ, Branston NM, Symon L: A comparison of the effects of ischaemia on tissue flow, electrical activity and extracellular potassium ion concentration in cerebral cortex of baboons. Biochem Soc Trans 5:158, 1977

238. Friedman WA, Kaplan BL, Day AL et al: Evoked potential monitoring during aneurysm operation: observations after fifty cases. Neurosurgery 20:678, 1987

239. Friedman WA, Chadwick GM, Verhoeven FJ et al: Monitoring of somatosensory evoked potentials during surgery for middle cerebral artery aneurysms. Neurosurgery 29:83, 1991

240. Symon L, Momma F, Murota T: Assessment of reversible cerebral ischaemia in man: intraoperative monitoring of the somatosensory evoked response. Acta Neurochir Suppl (Wien) 42:3, 1988

241. Mizoi K, Yoshimoto T, Piepgras DG, Schramm J: Permissible temporary occlusion time in aneurysm surgery as evaluated by evoked potential monitoring. Neurosurgery 33:434, 1993

242. Little JR, Lesser RP, Luders H: Electrophysiological monitoring during basilar aneurysm operation. Neurosurgery 20:421, 1987

243. Ishikawa T, Kamiyama H, Tada M et al: Giant internal carotid aneurysm at the cavernous portion with abrupt disappearance of N20 100 minutes after carotid occlusion: case report. Neurol Med Chir (Tokyo) 30:417, 1990

244. Delgado TE, Buchheit WA, Rosenholtz HR, Chrissian S: Intraoperative monitoring of facial muscle evoked responses obtained by intracranial stimulation of the facial nerve: a more accurate technique for facial nerve dissection. Neurosurgery 4:418, 1979

245. Harner SG, Daube JR, Ebersold MJ: Electrophysiologic monitoring of facial nerve during temporal bone surgery. Laryngoscope 96:65, 1986

246. Harner SG, Daube JR, Ebersold MJ, Beatty CW: Improved preservation of facial nerve function with

use of electrical monitoring during removal of acoustic neuromas. Mayo Clin Proc 62:92, 1987

247. Harner SG, Daube JR, Beatty CW, Ebersold MJ: Intraoperative monitoring of the facial nerve. Laryngoscope 98:209, 1988

248. Lennon RL, Hosking MP, Daube JR, Welna JO: Effect of partial neuromuscular blockade on intraoperative electromyography in patients undergoing resection of acoustic neuromas. Anesth Analg 75: 729, 1992

249. Grundy BL, Lina A, Procopio PT, Jannetta PJ: Reversible evoked potential changes with retraction of the eighth cranial nerve. Anesth Analg 60:835–838, 1981

250. Jannetta PJ: Neurovascular compression in cranial nerve and systemic disease. Ann Surg 192:518, 1980

251. van Loveren H, Tew JM, Keller JT, Nurre MA: A 10-year experience in the treatment of trigeminal neuralgia. Neurosurgery 57:757, 1982

252. Hardy RW Jr, Kinney SE, Lueders H, Lesser RP: Preservation of cochlear nerve function with the aid of brain stem auditory evoked potentials. Neurosurgery 11:16, 1982

253. Ojemann RG, Levine RA, Montgomery WM, McGaffigan P: Use of intraoperative auditory evoked potentials to preserve hearing in unilateral acoustic neuroma removal. J Neurosurg 61:938, 1984

254. Glasscock ME, Hays JW, Minor LB et al: Preservation of hearing in surgery for acoustic neuromas. J Neurosurg 78:864, 1993

255. Levine RA, Montgomery WW, Ojemann RG, McGaffigan PM: Monitoring auditory evoked potentials during acoustic neuroma surgery. Ann Otol Rhinol Laryngol 93:116, 1984

256. Harper CM, Harner SG, Slavit DH et al: Effect of BAEP monitoring on hearing preservation during acoustic neuroma resection. Neurology 42:1551, 1992

257. Sekhar LN, Moller AR: Operative management of tumors involving the cavernous sinus. J Neurosurg 64:879, 1986

258. Harding GF, Bland JD, Smith VH: Visual evoked potential monitoring of optic nerve function during surgery. J Neurol Neurosurg Psychiatry 53:890, 1990

259. Stechison MT: The trigeminal evoked potential. 2. Intraoperative recording of short-latency responses. Neurosurgery 33:639, 1993

260. Soustiel JF, Hafner H, Chistyakov AV et al: Monitoring of brain-stem trigeminal evoked potentials: clinical applications in posterior fossa surgery. Electroencephalogr Clin Neurophysiol 88:255, 1993

261. Schoenfeldt R, Groce R, Laurenzi B: Motor system monitoring during joint replacement operations. Neurosurgery 20:197, 1987

262. Cedzich C, Schramm J: Monitoring of flash visual evoked potentials during neurosurgical operations. Int Anesthesiol Clin 28:165, 1990

263. Cedzich C, Schramm J, Mengedoht CF, Fahlbusch R: Factors that limit the use of flash visual evoked potentials for surgical monitoring. Electroencephalogr Clin Neurophysiol 71:142, 1988

264. Rosen MG, Scibetta JJ, Devroude PJ: The use of fetal EEG in the study of obstetric anesthesia. Clin Anesth 10:103, 1974

265. Modena G, Angiolillo M, Bertelli R, Bini M: EEG activity in newborns delivered from mothers with and without full anesthesia. Electroencephalogr Clin Neurophysiol 27:701, 1969

266. Hollmen AI, Eskelinen P, Tolonen U et al: Effects of anaesthesia for caesarean section on the computerized EEG of the neonate. Eur J Anaesthesiol 2:39, 1985

267. Kochs E, Hoffman WE, Esch JSA: Improvement of brain electrical activity during treatment of porcine malignant hyperthermia with dantrolene. Br J Anaesth 71:881, 1993

268. Haghighi SS, Oro JJ: Effects of hypovolemic hypotensive shock on somatosensory and motor evoked potentials. Neurosurgery 24:246, 1989

269. Hacke W, Hundgen R, Zeumer H et al: [Monitoring of therapeutic neuroradiologic examination and therapeutic procedures using evoked potentials]. EEG EMG 16:93, 1985

270. Nobler MS, Sackeim HA, Solomou M et al: EEG manifestations during ECT: effects of electrode placement and stimulus intensity. Biol Psychiatry 34:321, 1993

271. Buhrer M, Maitre PO, Hung OR et al: Thiopental pharmacodynamics: 1. Defining the pseudo-steady-state serum concentration-EEG effect relationship. Anesthesiology 77:226, 1992

272. Hung OR, Varvel JR, Shafer SL, Stanski DR: Thiopental pharmacodynamics: 2. Quantitation of clinical and electroencephalographic depth of anesthesia. Anesthesiology 77:237, 1992

273. Newton DE, Thornton C, Creagh-Barry P, Dore CJ: Early cortical auditory evoked response in anaesthesia: comparison of the effects of nitrous oxide and isoflurane. Br J Anaesth 62:61, 1989

274. Chassard D, Joubaud A, Colson A et al: Auditory evoked potentials during propofol anaesthesia in man. Br J Anaesth 62:522, 1989

275. Munglani R, Andrade J, Sapsford DJ et al: A measure of consciousness and memory during isoflurane administration: the coherent frequency. Br J Anaesth 71:633, 1993

276. Sebel PS, Heneghan CP, Ingram DA: Evoked responses—a neurophysiological indicator of depth of anaesthesia? Br J Anaesth 57:841, 1985

277. Plourde G, Boylan JF: The auditory steady state response during sufentanil anaesthesia. Br J Anaesth 66:683, 1991

278. Castenholz RH, Grundy BL, Bauman AW et al: Effect of increasing doses of isoflurane on the feline 40-Hz response (abstracted). Electroencephalogr Clin Neurophysiol 72:18P, 1989.

279. Rumpl E: [Electro-neurological correlations in early stages of posttraumatic comatose states. I. The EEG at different stages of acute traumatic secondary midbrain and bulbar brain syndrome (author's transl)]. EEG EMG 10:148, 1979

280. Hansotia P, Gottschalk P, Green P, Zais D: Spindle coma: incidence, clinicopathologic correlates, and prognostic value. Neurology 31:83, 1981

281. Facco E, Munari M, Casartelli Liviero M et al: Serial recordings of auditory brainstem responses in severe head injury: relationship between test timing and prognostic power. Intensive Care Med 14:422, 1988

282. Rumpl E, Prugger M, Gerstenbrand F et al: Central somatosensory conduction time and acoustic brain-stem transmission time in post-traumatic coma. J Clin Neurophysiol 5:237, 1988

283. Anderson DC, Bundlie S, Rockswold GL: Multimodality evoked potentials in closed head trauma. Arch Neurol 41:369, 1984

284. Ruijs MBM, Keyser A, Gabreels FJM, Notermans SLH: Somatosensory evoked potentials and cognitive sequelae in children with closed head-injury. Neuropediatrics 24:307, 1993

285. Garcia-Larrea L, Artru F, Bertrand O et al: The combined monitoring of brain stem auditory evoked potentials and intracranial pressure in coma: a study of 57 patients. J Neurol Neurosurg Psychiatry 55:792, 1992

286. Uldry PA, Despland PA, Regli F: [Modifications in and prognostic value of the EEG in anoxic encephalopathy: 75 cases]. Schweiz Med Wochenschr 121:1453, 1991

287. Brunko E, Zegers de Beyl D: Prognostic value of early cortical somatosensory evoked potentials after resuscitation from cardiac arrest. Electroencephalogr Clin Neurophysiol 66:15, 1987

288. Rothstein TL, Thomas EM, Sumi SM: Predicting outcome in hypoxic-ischemic coma: a prospective clinical and electrophysiologic study. Electroencephalogr Clin Neurophysiol 79:101, 1991

289. Madl C, Grimm G, Kramer L et al: Early prediction of individual outcome after cardiopulmonary resuscitation. Lancet 341:855, 1993

290. Taylor MJ, Murphy WJ, Whyte HE: Prognostic reliability of somatosensory and visual evoked potentials of asphyxiated term infants. Dev Med Child Neurol 34:507, 1992

291. Pierrat V, Eken P, Duquennoy C et al: Prognostic value of early somatosensory evoked potentials in neonates with cystic leukomalacia. Dev Med Child Neurol 35:683, 1993

292. Keren O, Ring H, Solzi P et al: Upper limb somatosensory evoked potentials as a predictor of rehabilitation progress in dominant hemisphere stroke patients. Stroke 24:1789, 1993

293. Zentner J, Ebner A: [Somatosensory and motor evoked potentials in the prognostic assessment of traumatic and non-traumatic comatose patients]. EEG EMG 19:267, 1988

294. Soustiel JF, Hafner H, Guilburd JN et al: A physiological coma scale: grading of coma by combined use of brain-stem trigeminal and auditory evoked potentials and the Glasgow Coma Scale. Electroencephalogr Clin Neurophysiol 87:277, 1993

295. Lehmkuhl P, Lips U, Pichlmayr I: [EEG parameters in the monitoring of ventilated intensive care patients under various sedation methods]. Anasth Intensivther Notfallmed 20:6, 1985

296. Herkes GK, Wszolek ZK, Westmoreland BF, Klass DW: Effects of midazolam on electroencephalograms of seriously ill patients. Mayo Clin Proc 67:334, 1992

297. Garcia-Larrea L, Artru F, Bertrand O et al: Transient drug-induced abolition of BAEPs in coma. Neurology 38:1487, 1988

298. Freye E, Neruda B, Falke K: [EEG power spectra and evoked potentials during alfentanil/midazolam analgesia-sedation in intensive care patients]. Anasthesiol Intesivmed Notfallmed Schmerzther 26:384, 1991

299. Sneyd JR, Wang DY, Edwards D et al: Effect of physiotherapy on the auditory evoked response of paralysed, sedated patients in the intensive care unit. Br J Anaesth 68:349, 1992

300. Moodley J, Bobat SM, Hoffman M, Bill PLA: Electroencephalogram and computerised cerebral tomography findings in eclampsia. Br J Obstet Gynaecol 100:984, 1993

301. Streletz LJ, Bej MD, Graziani LJ et al: Utility of serial EEGs in neonates during extracorporeal membrane oxygenation. Pediatr Neurol 8:190, 1992

302. Brenner RP: The electroencephalogram in altered states of consciousness. Neurol Clin 3:615, 1985

303. Treiman DM: Generalized convulsive status epilepticus in the adult. Epilepsia 34:S2, 1993

304. Gorman DG, Shields WD, Shewmon DA et al: Neurosurgical treatment of refractory status epilepticus. Epilepsia 33:546, 1992

305. Sgro JA, Jaitly R, Delorenzo RJ: Conventional and rapid stimulation evoked potential changes in patients with status epilepticus. Epilepsy Res 15:149, 1993

306. Tasker RC, Boyd SG, Harden A et al: The clinical significance of seizures in critically ill young infants requiring intensive care. Neuropediatrics 22:129, 1991

307. Mackey-Hargadine JR, Hall JW III: Sensory evoked responses in head injury. Central Nervous System Trauma 2:187, 1985

308. Stone JL, Ghaly RF, Hughes, JR: Evoked potentials in head injury and states of increased intracranial pressure. J Clin Neurophysiol 5:135, 1988

309. Stone JL, Ghaly RF, Hughes JR: Electroencephalography in acute head injury. J Clin Neurophysiol 5:125, 1988

310. Zaaroor M, Pratt M, Feinsod M, Schacham SE: Real-time monitoring of visual evoked potentials. Isr J Med Sci 29:17, 1993

311. Wang AD, Cone J, Symon L, Costa da Silva IE: SEP monitoring during the management of aneurysmal subarachonid hemorrhage. J Neurosurg 60:264, 1984

312. Symon L, Hargadine JR, Zawirski M, Branston NM: Central conduction time as an index of ischaemia in subarachnoid hemorrhage. Adv Exp Med Biol 44:95, 1977

313. Rivierez M, Landau-Ferey J, Grob R et al: Value of electroencephalogram in prediction and diagnosis of vasospasm after intracranial aneurysm rupture. Acta Neurochir (Wien) 110:17–23, 1991

314. Grundy BL, Friedman W: Electrophysiological evaluation of the patient with acute spinal cord injury. Crit Care Clin 3:519, 1987

315. Larson SJ, Walsh PR, Ackmann JJ, Sances A Jr: Neurophysiological aids in diagnosis evaluation and prognosis. J Am Paraplegia Soc 7:66, 1984

316. Louis AA, Gupta P, Perkash I: Localization of sensory levels in traumatic quadriplegia by segmental somatosensory evoked potentials. Electroencephalogr Clin Neurophysiol 62:313, 1985

317. Hayes KC, Allatt RD, Wolfe DL et al: Reinforcement of subliminal flexion reflexes by transcranial magnetic stimulation of motor cortex in subjects with spinal cord injury. Electroencephalogr Clin Neurophysiol 85:102, 1992

318. Schwartz WB, Komesar NK: Doctors, damages and deterrence: an economic view of medical malpractice. N Engl J Med 298:1282, 1978

319. MacEwen GD, Bunnell WP, Sviram K: Acute neurologic complications in the treatment of scoliosis: a report of the Scoliosis Research Society. J Bone Joint Surg 57A:404, 1975

320. Grundy BL: Electrophysiologic monitoring: electroencephalography and evoked potentials. p. 30. In Newfield P, Cottrell JE (eds): Neuroanesthesia: Handbook of Clinical and Physiologic Essentials. Little, Brown, Boston, 1991

321. Bickford RG: Computer analysis of background activity. p. 215. In Remond A (ed): EEG Informatics: A Didactic Review of Methods and Applications of EEG Data Processing. Elsevier, Amsterdam, 1977

322. Pfurtscheller G, Ladurner G, Maresch H, Vollmer R: Brain electrical activity mapping in normal and ischemic brain. Prog Brain Res 62:287, 1984

323. Sokol S: Visual evoked potentials. p. 441. In Aminoff MJ (ed): Electrodiagnosis in Clinical Neurology. 2nd Ed. Churchill Livingstone, New York, 1986

Monitoring Anesthetic Depth

17

Stuart R. Hameroff
J. Scott Polson
Richard C. Watt

Monitoring anesthetic depth is essential to prevent patients' perception of pain, awareness, and recall; to judge autonomic status and prevent untoward effects of excessively light or deep anesthesia; to minimize stress and its manifestations; and to facilitate prompt emergence when indicated. Technologic advances are not significant in assessment of anesthetic depth, which still rests on clinically relevant signs. These signs, variable among different anesthetics and in the presence of other drugs, correlate imperfectly with anesthetic depth. Despite these limitations, we often have no other means to assess anesthetic depth. The vagaries of correlation between clinical signs and anesthetic depth, as well as the lack of developments in monitoring anesthetic depth, stem partially from our incomplete understanding of the brain activities most closely linked to perception, awareness, and consciousness. This chapter reviews the question of what consciousness is, clinical correlates of anesthetic depth, awareness and recall under anesthesia, some new monitoring technologies, and theoretical models of brain and anesthetic mechanisms.

WHAT IS CONSCIOUSNESS?

Brains of adequately anesthetized patients are commonly quite active: EEG, evoked potentials, respiratory and autonomic drives, and other brain functions persist. Thus, as we monitor depth of anesthesia we are measuring largely the absence of consciousness, an entity whose nature remains a huge mystery and perhaps the last great frontier in modern science. Recently, consciousness has been approached on more than grounds of philosophy and religion and metaphors of information technology. This is evidenced by a general willingness to discuss consciousness, numerous books that deal head-on with the subject, and participation in the question from a broad range of disciplines. For example, within psychology the concept of consciousness has returned to prominence after a long period of neglect during the behaviorist era. Current approaches to the psychology of consciousness[1] have emphasized natural science and cognitive psychology viewpoints, and have included studies of relationships between the brain and consciousness, daydreaming, sleep, dreams, psychedelic drug states, meditation, and hypnosis. A particularly vigorous area of research involves studies of dissociations between aware and unaware processes following focal and diffuse brain damage.[2] Phenomena of particular interest in this area include so-called "blindsight" in patients with blindness secondary to occipital cortex damage (but who have "subconscious" perception via preoccipital visual pathways), unawareness of hemiplegia, and the preservation of "implicit" aspects of memory in patients with amnesia or dementia.

In neurophysiology, electrical recordings of neuronal activity related to conscious events demonstrate coherent (40 to 70 Hz) firing among widely distributed neurons[3] and behavior analogous to chaotic attractors.[4] Other disciplines approaching consciousness include neuroscience, computer science (e.g., neural networks, artificial intelligence, and artificial life), physics/mathematics (e.g., quantum theory, self-organization, coherent/emergent phenomena, chaos), medicine (e.g., neurology, psychiatry), pharmacology, philosophy, and religion. Anesthesiology is poised to contribute immensely to the understanding of consciousness.

Approaches to consciousness form a spectrum that considers consciousness (on one extreme) as, purely and simply, the sum total of brain activities. This *reductionist* view is best exemplified by Dennett[5] who purports that consciousness may be reduced to an algorithm. On the other end of the spectrum is a dualistic view that considers the brain and mind as distinct, separate entities and consciousness as ineffable and existing in a separate reality.[6] Between these extremes lies ample evidence for views that contend consciousness has a distinct quality, which emerges from neural processes based on natural science.

A self-organized brain function, consciousness has evolved to be the mind's observer/controller. Numerous authors have described consciousness as a collective phenomenon that emerges from a hierarchy of lower level brain processes. One such hierarchical scheme (AC Scott, personal communication, 1993) is depicted in Table 17-1. This hierarchy may be extended in both directions: higher levels could include cultures and societies, lower levels could include subatomic particles. How these levels interact, and how and where consciousness emerges remain unclear. Haken[7] has mathematically described hierarchical systems with emergent properties whose levels are nonlinearly coupled ("synergetically") by "order parameters." In synergetic hierarchies, the emergent property (in this case consciousness) is extremely sensitive to inhibition at lower levels. Thus anesthetics, acting by weak, physical forces at the level of the hydrophobic space within biomolecules (proteins, membranes), have profound effects on consciousness.

In the human brain, certain areas have been suggested as likely foci for consciousness. These include parts of the thalamus, which direct attention to different regions of the brain,[8] the reticular activating system which regulates wakefulness, the superior colliculus, which integrates sensory information,[9] and widespread areas of the cortex.

Aspects of consciousness, in all likelihood, are distributed throughout wide areas of the brain. Crick and Koch[3] have proposed that consciousness is a function of widely distributed neurons, which coherently oscillate (40 to 70 Hz) in conjunction with a given mental state. What binds these regions together into a "unitary" sense of *self* is enigmatic and a rationale for quantum coherence.[10] In quantum coherence, spatially separated particles share identical states over time. Penrose[11,12] has proposed a biomolecular—perhaps cytoskeletal—role for quantum coherence, and for an extended quantum theory in human consciousness.

The property of consciousness appears to have emerged at some point in evolution. Presumably occurring initially as a "helpless spectator" epi-

TABLE 17-1. Hierarchy of Brain Organization

Consciousness
  Perceptions
  Feelings
  Mood
Phase sequence (serial thought)
Brain regions
  Homunculi
  Centers
  Nuclei
Parallel assemblies of parallel assemblies of neurons
Parallel assemblies of neurons
Multiplex neurons
Nerve impulses
  Synaptic transmission
  Dendritic processing
Neuronal regions
  Axons-dendrites-synapses
Biomolecular assemblies
  Mitochondria-nucleus-cytoskeleton
Biomolecules
  Proteins
  Membranes
  Nucleic acids
Biomolecular regions
  Hydrophobic space
  Hydrophilic space
Biomolecular components
  Phospholipids-amino acids
Calcium ion flux
Organized water
Biochemical energy
  Adenosine triphosphate
  Guanosine triphosphate
  Phosphorylation
Atomic elements
Quantum events

(After Scott, personal communication).

phenomenon, consciousness assumed control of its biologic environment.[13] The emergence of consciousness (during evolution and during development of each human being) may be likened to new properties of materials that can develop from microscopic, even quantum level, events. For example, the distinct properties of superconductivity and supermagnetism emerge from materials as their individual atoms reach a high level of coherence. In these cases, coherence is due to lowering temperature to near absolute zero to reduce thermal oscillations. Consequently, at a certain degree of coherence, totally new properties of superconductivity or supermagnetism emerge. Similarly, consciousness may emerge from a critical level of coherence of quantum level events in hydrophobic pockets of proteins (e.g., membrane proteins, arrays such as the cytoskeleton, etc.) in neurons throughout the brain.

The question may then be asked, "is consciousness a property of protoplasm in general?" For example, do single-cell organisms, such as paramecia, contain consciousness? If not, at what point in the evolutionary hierarchy does consciousness emerge? This may be a somewhat arbitrary distinction, but the important feature is that the fabric of consciousness is present within all eucaryotic cells—the essence being perhaps quantum coherence of proteins and associated water and ions. This then can provide a bottom level substrate in the dimensional hierarchy from whose highest level consciousness emerges.

The reductionist view that consciousness is "nothing more than" the activities of the brain's neurons[5] is mirrored in the realm of anesthesiology. Kissin[14] has described anesthesia as "component therapy," providing a spectrum of pharmacologic actions: analgesia, anxiolysis, amnesia, unconsciousness, muscle relaxation, and suppression of somatic motor, cardiovascular, and hormonal responses. Kissin further remarks that because of such component therapy, "the very meaning of the depth of anesthesia disappears." To the contrary, studying anesthetic depth and mechanisms may help to understand consciousness as a unique property that emerges from lower hierarchical levels.

HISTORY OF "DEPTH OF ANESTHESIA"

In 1847 Plomley[15] made the first attempt to define anesthetic depth. He described three stages of ether anesthesia, progressing from "half-intoxica-

tion" to "extreme pleasure" and finally to "profound intoxication and insensibility." Attainment of this third stage, he felt, was necessary for surgery. Plomley's classification was essentially subjective.

Later that same year, John Snow[16] described "five degrees of narcotism" for ether anesthesia. His classification was an improvement over Plomley in that it relied on objective observation of physical signs. These signs included conjunctival reflex, breathing pattern, eye movement, and inhibition of intercostal muscles.

In 1937, Guedel[17] published his classic description of the clinical signs of ether anesthesia. He used somatic muscle tone, respiratory pattern, and ocular movement to define four "stages" of anesthesia. These stages progressed from "analgesia" to "delirium" to "surgical anesthesia," which was subdivided into four "planes." The fourth and final stage was "respiratory paralysis." In 1954, Artusio[18] expanded on Guedel's description and further characterized amnesia as a component of anesthetic depth.[19] Other schemes were devised based on EEG,[20] jaw and forearm relaxation,[21] and "nothria."[22] These are all depicted in Figure 17-1.

These early classifications had significant practical utility for the administration of the first inhalational anesthetics. However, all that changed with the introduction in the 1930s of thiopentone. This agent made it possible to progress from a fully awake state to stage four in a matter of 30 seconds, thus effectively obliterating nearly all the previously described signs of increasing depth of anesthesia.

When curare was introduced in 1942, and controlled ventilation became the norm, use of respiratory pattern and muscle tone as depth indicators was also lost. The anesthesiologist came to rely on signs of autonomic nervous system activity to judge whether the patient was adequately anesthetized. Not surprisingly, it was around this time that reports of intraoperative patient awareness first began to appear in the literature.

Shortly thereafter, the concept that anesthesia consisted of various components was introduced. These components included hypnosis, amnesia, paralysis, analgesia, and attenuation of the stress response. Specific drugs would provide these various components necessary for "general anesthesia." While this component theory helped define what anesthesia is, it also helped to define the problem of monitoring anesthetic depth. Because, while determining degree of paralysis is relatively easy, determining intraoperative degree of amnesia and hypnosis (i.e., unconsciousness) has, thus far, proven impossible.

CLINICAL SIGNS OF ANESTHETIC DEPTH

For lack of a more precise method, assessment of depth of anesthesia has relied on monitoring clinical signs. These signs have included skeletal muscle activity (spontaneous movement or increased tone), aberrations in respiration (sighing, breath holding, bronchospasm or change in respiratory pattern), and evidence of increased autonomic activity (hypertension, tachycardia, and diaphoresis). Unfortunately, all of these signs can be attenuated or eliminated by the various drugs patients may be taking preoperatively (beta blockers,

vasodilators), or by adjuvant drugs given by the anesthesiologist (beta blockers, vasodilators, muscle relaxants, or anticholinergics). Be that as it may, a brief discussion of these various signs will be undertaken.

Thus far, the most widely recognized correlation between clinical signs and anesthetic depth is based on the concept of minimum alveolar concentration (MAC), as described by Eger and colleagues.[19] MAC is defined as that concentration of an inhalation anesthetic that will prevent 50 percent of patients from responding to a painful stimulus with ''gross purposeful movement.'' Equilibrated end-tidal anesthetic concentration in the alveoli is assumed to indicate anesthetic concentration in the brain.

While the original work done with the MAC concept involved the clinical sign of skeletal muscle movement, other researchers defined MAC for other clinical signs. Stoelting and colleagues[23] de-

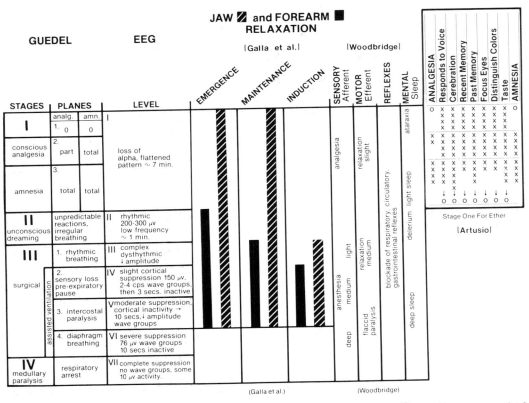

Fig. 17-1. Levels of anesthetic depth displayed on a common axis. Guedel's[17] (1937) stages and planes serve as a standard. Courtin's[20] (1950) EEG levels, Galla's[21] (1958) jaw and forearm relaxation, Woodbridge's[22] (1957) classification of ''nothria,'' and Artusio's[18] stage one for ether are represented.

scribed "MAC awake" as the minimum alveolar concentration of an inhalation anesthetic that would allow patients to open their eyes in response to command. Yakaitis and coworkers[24] described MAC EI as the end-tidal concentration of halothane or enflurane necessary to prevent 50 percent of patients from moving in response to endotracheal intubation. Finally, Roizen and coworkers[25] described MAC BAR (blockade of autonomic response) as the end-tidal concentration of halothane or enflurane needed to prevent an increase in sympathetic tone in response to skin incision in 50 percent of the patients studied. Sympathetic tone was assumed to have increased if the clinical signs of increased blood pressure or heart rate occurred coincident with skin incision. Concentration of plasma norepinephrine was also measured in this study.

Several studies have been done looking at how anesthetic depth affects an array of clinical signs. Cullen and colleagues[26] studied the effects of halothane and isoflurane, both with and without nitrous oxide, on several clinical signs. These and other investigators[27] found that respiratory signs (changes in tidal volume and rate) are least affected by autonomic activity and may be the best index of anesthetic depth in the patient spontaneously breathing a volatile anesthetic. A sustained increase in minute ventilation in response to surgical stimulation may indicate light anesthesia when using halothane. However, this did not hold true for isoflurane, where even at deep levels of anesthesia, minute ventilation increased in response to surgical stimulation.[28,29]

Cullen's study[26] also showed that blood pressure varied predictably with halothane and isoflurane dose during the first hour of anesthesia. However, after 5 hours of halothane, both with and without nitrous oxide, blood pressure remained constant despite increases in anesthetic concentration. The authors attributed their findings to increased sympathetic activity with prolonged halothane anesthesia. Eye signs were not useful indicators of anesthetic depth for halothane or isoflurane. Cullen concluded that it is difficult to characterize useful clinical signs of anesthetic depth for one agent, let alone for inhalation anesthetics in general.

While the correlation between inhalation anesthetic concentration and clinical signs (i.e., MAC) has been fairly well investigated and found to be less than perfect, no such clinical "scale" presently even exists for intravenous anesthetics—at least none that is in widespread use. This is because there is no way to easily obtain continuous plasma levels of the fixed agents which would be analogous to MAC for the inhalation anesthetics. Therefore the ability to use clinical signs as an indicator of intravenous anesthetic depth is even more limited.

Nonetheless, a few general observations can be made. Usually, sighing, breath-holding and irregular breathing are signs of light anesthesia. Heart rate alone is a poor guide to anesthetic depth, as several drugs both suppress or augment heart rate. Arrhythmias, such as bigeminy, often occur during light anesthesia. However, when anesthesia is too deep, more malignant arrhythmias may be induced. Tachycardia, in the absence of any other cause, should suggest light anesthesia.

With regard to anesthetic-induced muscle relaxation, intravenous induction agents and volatile anesthetics cause a dose-related reduction in muscle tone, eventually leading to respiratory paralysis. Ketamine and opioids do not share this depressant effect. In fact, opioids in large doses cause an increase in muscle tone, which can result in chest wall rigidity. Again, with the use of neuromuscular blocking drugs, these signs are obliterated.

Both diaphoresis and lacrimation may occur during light anesthesia with both volatile and intravenous agents. However, excessive sweating has been observed in the presence of adequate anesthesia.[30] Drugs that modify autonomic response may also affect these signs. Under thiopental anesthesia (induction), the presence of a lid reflex is thought to indicate insufficient anesthesia.

The discussion and data presented suggest that, even in a carefully controlled experimental situation, clinical signs offer a rough estimate at best of anesthetic depth. In the typical operative setting, with its myriad of uncontrolled variables, clinical signs become an even weaker gauge of anesthetic depth. Certainly, there is room in anesthesia for a more sensitive "depthometer."

AWARENESS AND MEMORY

General anesthesia is often thought of as consisting of several components: motionlessness, control of autonomic response or hemodynamic stability, absence of pain or analgesia, absence of recall or amnesia, and a fifth more nebulous component variously referred to as lack of awareness, unconsciousness, hypnosis, or sleep. The patient who consents to general anesthesia has implicitly contracted for all these components and usually does not expect to experience intraoperative awareness or postoperative recall. Intraoperative awareness has been associated with both hypertensive crisis[31] and a syndrome of posttraumatic neurosis.[32] Stress-induced perioperative myocardial infarction has also been claimed as a consequence of awareness.[33]

While preventing intraoperative awareness and recall are clearly desirable objectives, doing so in every instance may not be so easily accomplished. An editorial in *Trends in Neuroscience*[34] concluded that it is not possible to reliably determine whether a given anesthetized patient is conscious during surgery and warned that, contrary to popular belief, intraoperative pain and fear cannot always be detected by changes in heart rate or blood pressure. Jones[35] states in an editorial in the *British Medical Journal* that we should assume any anesthetized patient is capable of retaining verbal and other high-level inputs into long-term memory. This position is further supported by an editorial in *Lancet*,[36] which states that evidence has been accumulating for 25 years suggesting that auditory stimuli are registered in the cortex even during surgical anesthesia. This author suggests that active measures (earplugs and headphones) be taken to prevent every anesthetized patient from hearing conversation during surgery, as it is unlikely that unconscious auditory perception can be prevented by pharmacologic means alone.

Definitions and Models

Clearly, awareness is not synonymous with recall as some authors have implied. Consider the patient premedicated with a benzodiazepine who watches as the intravenous catheter is placed but postoperatively has absolutely no recall of the event. Or

consider the patient under general anesthesia who does not respond hemodynamically or otherwise to incision, but who then obeys the instruction to "raise your index finger if you can hear me." Postoperatively, the patient has no recall of the event.[37] Furthermore, a different patient, under identical circumstances, may fail to respond to the intraoperative instruction but clearly recall the event postoperatively.[38] Therefore, it is probably best to consider awareness and recall as two related, but distinct, phenomena.

Awareness has been defined as consciousness, wakefulness, cognition of ongoing events, or the ability to monitor the present situation and environment. Recall or memory has been subdivided in various ways. Several authors describe two distinct types of memory. *Explicit memory* entails conscious, deliberate recollection of events. A patient stating post-CABG that he/she remembers the noise of the sternotomy saw would be displaying explicit memory. The patient knows he/she knows (remembers) something. The term "recall," as used by most anesthesiologists, is probably most synonymous with explicit memory.

Implicit memory does not require conscious recognition. It manifests itself by changes in task performance or behavior that are attributable to past (intraoperative) events.[39] The patient who develops a new, unexplained disdain for the surgeon postoperatively may be manifesting implicit memory of an insulting comment made by the surgeon about the patient while the patient was "asleep." The patient does not recall the comment, but it has unconsciously affected his/her behavior. The patient doesn't know he/she knows (remembers) something, but he does. Experimental and clinical data indicate that these types of memory are separate and dissociable from each other.

Other authors describe memory in different terms. For example Cherkin and Harroun[40] define a two-story theory of memory (Fig. 17-2). They pos-

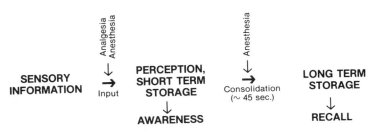

Fig. 17-2. Model of awareness and recall modified from Cherkin and Harroun[40] (1971). Painful or other sensory input may reach perception and awareness but be blocked prior to long-term storage. Thus, awareness does not necessarily result in recall.

tulate that information is first perceived and stored in an unstable, dynamic form. This short-term memory lasts only a few seconds and has a limited capacity, containing only what the person is currently thinking or perceiving. This short-term memory may constitute awareness. Information in this form may then be consolidated into a stable physical memory trace in the brain and become long-term memory. This information could later be retrieved (i.e., recall). The development of the long-term memory trace may depend on the initial significance of the incoming information. Thus threatening or derogatory remarks that are perceived and enter short-term memory are more likely to be consolidated into long-term memory.

Amnesia (lack of recall) would then result from blockade of memory assimilation at any point from initial input to consolidation as long-term memory. Narcotic effects might predominate at the input stage, whereas volatile anesthetics, barbiturates, and benzodiazepines might act at the consolidation stage. Although this model lacks biochemical correlates, it is conceptually useful because it suggests that, clinically, memory consolidation takes a finite amount of time (about 45 seconds). Thus, specific incidents of awareness, if detected quickly, might be prevented from entering long-term memory by promptly increasing anesthetic depth.

Incidence

Various prospective and retrospective studies have attempted to determine the incidence of awareness and recall during anesthesia.[41–44] Most studies cite the incidence around 1 to 2 percent. These studies used various anesthetic techniques and, just as importantly, various methods to determine recall. Petersen and Johansen[45] reported a surprisingly low incidence of recall of 0.1 percent in 5,926 patients. However, only patients who spontaneously reported intraoperative awareness were counted as having experienced recall. Utting[46] determined explicit recall by postoperatively asking specific questions regarding recall. In a series of 500 patients who received only 70 percent nitrous oxide for maintenance of anesthesia, the reported incidence of recall was 2 percent.

Patients may not report recall unless specifically asked, due to fear of not being believed or fear of ridicule. Therefore Brice and associates[47] suggest that all postoperative interviews include the follow-

ing three questions: What is the last thing you remember before going to sleep for your operation? What is the first thing you remember after your operation? Do you remember anything in between?

Determining the true incidence of intraoperative awareness and recall may be further confounded by the notion that recall can occur to different degrees. Patients may recall "dreams" associated with their surgery as opposed to recalling actual intraoperative events.[47] Some of these dreams can be distressing to the patient. "Dreams" are apparently recalled much more frequently than actual events. Utting,[46] in a series of 500 patients under nitrous oxide anesthesia, reported a 7 percent incidence of intraoperative dreaming, felt by the patients to be their worst perioperative experience. This was in contrast to a 2 percent incidence of recall of specific intraoperative events. Utting has suggested that there could be a continuum, with deep anesthesia resulting in complete amnesia, lighter anesthesia resulting in "dream" recall, and still lighter anesthesia resulting in recall of actual events. Wilson and colleagues[44] reported a 1 percent incidence of awareness during surgery, 2 percent incidence of dreaming, and an 8 percent incidence of "hallucinations" associated with surgery in 490 patients. These authors found no correlation between the incidence of mental aberration and anesthetic agent, sex of the patient, or length of surgery.

While there is still debate on the actual incidence and nature of awareness and recall, it is generally agreed that these unwanted events occur more frequently during specific types of surgery. Significantly higher incidences of recall have been reported during obstetrics[38,48] (7 to 28 percent), major trauma[49] (11 to 43 percent), cardiopulmonary bypass[58] (up to 23 percent), and bronchoscopy[51] (8 percent).

Specific Anesthetic Agents and Memory

Nitrous oxide's effect on memory has been fairly well characterized. The drug's ability to impair memory appears dose-dependent as indicated by Crawford's studies.[48] Using 67 percent nitrous oxide in obstetric cases, he found an incidence of recall of 2.5 to 4 percent. This increased substantially to as much as 25 percent when the concentration was reduced to 50 percent.

The memory effects of the volatile agents have

also been extensively studied. Cook and coworkers[52] examined the memory effects of three concentrations of halothane and enflurane and found both drugs produced dose-related impairment in digit span (longest sequence of digits that can be repeated without error, thought to indicate short-term memory), and two pyschomotor tests. Work by Newton and colleagues[53] showed a marked impairment in memory function as the concentration of isoflurane was increased from 0.1 to 0.4 MAC in healthy volunteers. This suggests a steep dose response curve as is seen with nitrous oxide.

Kihlstrom and coworkers[54] showed that patients under isoflurane anesthesia demonstrated no explicit memory as measured by tests of free recall and recognition. However, a majority of these same patients displayed implicit memory for the same material, as evidenced by a priming effect on a postoperative word-association test. They concluded that implicit and explicit memory were dissociable under isoflurane anesthesia.

While there has been no exact determination of "MAC remember," it is assumed that the concentration of volatile anesthetic needed for amnesia is less than that needed for analgesia because patients may briefly move and supposedly feel pain during surgery, but not have any recall of the event.[55] Nonetheless, occasional reports of recall in well-anesthetized patients suggest "MAC remember" may be variable (Table 17-2).

At least one case of awareness without recall during total intravenous anesthesia with propofol has been reported.[56] Without any change in hemodynamic measurements, this patient spontaneously opened her eyes, responded to instructions not to move and indicated that she felt fine. Anesthesia was deepened with a bolus of propofol. Postoperatively, despite specific questioning, she had no recall of the event.

Studies of thiopental's effect on memory have shown mixed results. Dundee and Pandit[57] suggest that neither thiopental (6 mg/kg) nor methohexital alone have significant amnesic effects. However, Osborn and colleagues[58] provided evidence that a continuous infusion of 0.3 percent thiopental significantly impaired learning and retention.

Benzodiazepines clearly interfere with the acquisition of new information but seem not to impair retrieval of information acquired before drug administration (retrograde amnesia). It is also known that benzodiazepines have profound effects on explicit memory; however, their effects on implicit memory have not been well documented.[59] Ghoneim[60] has recently reviewed the amnestic properties of benzodiazepines.

Causes of Intraoperative Awareness and Recall

Scott[61] proposes that a distinction exists between awareness secondary to "insufficient anesthesia" and awareness during apparent "surgical anesthesia."

The former situation is most often caused by equipment failure as illustrated by Winterbottom's[62] patient who was mistakenly "anesthetized" with pure oxygen and obviously remembered the unfortunate event. Intentional light anesthesia often results in recall and thus could be considered "insufficient." This most often occurs during cesarean section, and surgery for major trauma in a hemodynamically unstable patient.

In contrast, awareness during apparently adequate anesthesia does not involve problems with the administration of the anesthetic. Why some patients experience recall, whereas the vast majority do not remains unknown. Certainly, it seems reasonable to expect a variable amnestic response to anesthetics with some patients being more "resistant."[55] Perhaps a tolerance to the amnestic effects can be induced by chronic alcohol[63] or sedative abuse. This tolerance may even be iatrogenic as suggested by the patient who received two high-dose fentanyl-oxygen anesthetics 1 week apart and had significant recall only during the second anesthetic.[64]

Obesity has been suggested, but never proven, as a cause of increased awareness and recall.[55]

TECHNOLOGY IN ANESTHETIC DEPTH ASSESSMENT

Despite difficulties in defining anesthetic depth and measuring aspects of consciousness (or unconsciousness), a variety of devices and technologic approaches have been developed and used experimentally and clinically. In most cases, devices measure a single physiologic variable, which, along with appropriate signal processing is purported to be an index of general anesthetic depth. While such single-parameter approaches are appealing in their simplicity, it seems unlikely that a successful depthometer will be developed without a combined variable approach.

A review of anesthetic depth assessment literature exemplifies the need for an integrated multiparametric approach. Some of the approaches (and derived variables) are sensitive for light anesthetic ranges and others are sensitive at deep anesthetic ranges. Some are plagued with interference during certain surgical techniques and some are useful only when used with particular anesthetic techniques. No device or technology has yet been developed which by itself provides a foolproof anesthetic ''depthometer.'' However, many of the techniques show promise under specific conditions. A successful depthometer may someday be developed using a combination of techniques and physiologic variables in conjunction with appropriate pattern recognition technology such as rule based expert systems or artificial neural networks.

Spontaneous Electroencephalography

Since the brain is the target organ of general anesthetic effects it is not surprising that the electroencephalograph (EEG) has been the focus of most research aimed at developing anesthetic depth assessment technology. The EEG is a complex waveform resembling noise in the 0.5 to 100 Hz range. General anesthetic effects on the EEG correspond roughly to the changes seen during natural sleep. With increasing depth of anesthesia there is an increasing ablation of high frequency content (EEG slowing) and an increase in amplitude progressing toward burst suppression (bursts of activity interspersed with isoelectric waveform) (Fig. 17-3). At extremely high doses the EEG becomes flatline. Unfortunately, the foregoing generalization of anesthetic effects on the EEG is fraught with exceptions, ambiguities, and paradoxical effects. Hypothermic and hypoxic conditions

can mimic increasing depth of anesthesia. Anesthetic effects on EEG frequency content are generally nonlinear, sometimes causing an increase in high-frequency content at light levels and a decrease in high-frequency content at deeper levels. Profound interpatient differences in EEG response to anesthetics contribute to ambiguous and sometimes contradictory research study results.

For instance, it is generally assumed that surgical stimulation reduces anesthetic depth. Therefore, one would expect to see the EEG exhibit apparent lightening of anesthesia during intense surgical stimulation. However, a recent study of EEG activity during steady-state isoflurane-nitrous oxide anesthesia revealed that surgical stimulation resulted in EEG slowing, as if depth of anesthesia had increased![65]

Interpreting changes in the complex EEG waveform is a difficult task, and much research has been devoted to extracting features or derived variables from this waveform for characterizing anesthetic effects on the EEG. Derived variables such as spectral edge frequency (the frequency below which 95 percent of the power in an EEG epoch resides) have been shown to correlate with depth of anesthesia under specific circumstances.[66] EEG-derived variables have also been correlated with plasma concentrations of anesthetics.[67-70] One of the difficulties with such studies is choosing measurable benchmarks of anesthetic depth (as opposed to dosing levels). Many endpoints have been used experimentally at light anesthetic levels such as loss of lid response, loss of response to verbal commands, and lack of movement in response to noxious stimulus.[71-73] However, at deeper levels of anesthesia there are no reliable measurable endpoints of anesthetic depth that can be related to awareness or lack thereof. In fact, as previously mentioned, even during deep anesthesia auditory information can be assimilated by patients.[37] Therefore, even though specific EEG-derived variables correlate with changing anesthetic concentrations, such correlations may not be meaningful with regard to anesthetic depth. Most EEG-derived variables have been developed from spectral (frequency domain) features.[74-76] Table 17-3 includes a list of some common EEG-derived variables and their definitions. The EEG has also been studied in the context of chaos theory, yielding a correlation between anesthetic depth and dimensionality (a measure of complexity) of the EEG waveform.[77] Dimensional-

TABLE 17-2. Patients' Responses to Halothane

	Ratio to MAC
$MAC_{remember}$	0.4 to 1.5?
MAC_{awake}	0.6
MAC	1.0
MAC_{EI}	1.33
MAC_{BAR}	1.45

MAC, minimum alveolar concentration.

ity calculations are computer-intensive mathematical computations that can only be performed off-line, rendering this technique unsuitable as a clinical depthometer.[77–79] Recent studies using bispectral analysis of the EEG (a technique that quantifies interfrequency phase coupling) have also yielded interesting results, showing in some cases a correlation between movement/no movement and a bispectral index.[80–83] Recent studies in rats have shown that anesthetic-induced unresponsiveness to noxious stimuli does not depend on cortical or forebrain structures.[84,85] Assuming the EEG is primarily a cortical process, it is not surprising that correlations between EEG and depth of anesthesia have remained contradictory.

Spontaneous Electromyogram

Spontaneous EMG activity is present even in motionless patients as the background activity required to maintain muscle tone, and this electrical activity tends to decrease as general anesthesia increases. Although the spontaneous EMG is largely ablated by muscle relaxants, certain muscles (notably the frontalis) are relatively immune to neuromuscular blockade and may therefore preferentially reflect general anesthetic levels. Just as facial grimacing and movement are used as clinical signs of inadequate anesthesia, more subtle changes in spontaneous EMG can be measured which are unaccompanied by observable motion or facial

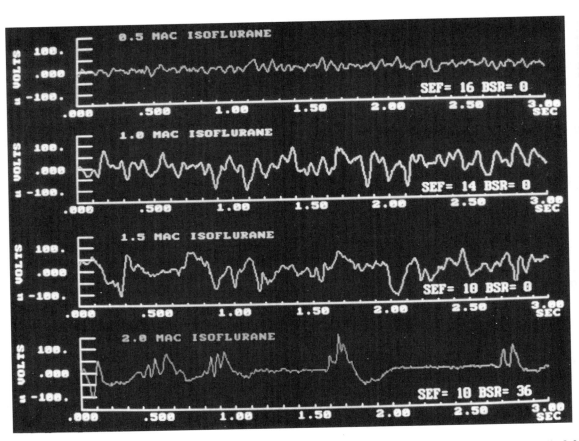

Fig. 17-3. Sample epochs of EEG are shown for isoflurane at four anesthetic levels; 0.5, 1.0, 1.5, 2.0 MAC. Spectral edge frequency (SEF) is an EEG-derived variable defined as that frequency below which 95 percent of the power in a given EEG epoch resides. SEF (shown in the lower right-hand corner of each waveform) is seen to decrease with increasing anesthetic level. Burst suppression ratio (BSR) (also shown to the lower right of each waveform sample) is an EEG-derived variable defined as the percentage of time in an EEG sample that the waveform is isoelectric. BSR is suitable for characterizing EEG waveforms exhibiting burst suppression activity.

changes.[86,87] Several investigations of spontaneous frontalis EMG (facilitated by the introduction of a special-purpose device: DATEX Anesthesia and Brain Activity Monitor: Datex Medical Instrumentation, Inc Tewksbury, MA) yielded inconsistent results.[88–90] Although impending arousal is often forecast by a precipitous rise in frontalis EMG activity, the phenomenon is not consistent enough to be reliable. To gain maximum benefit from monitoring spontaneous EMG, the anesthetic technique must include fine control over neuromuscular blockade with consistent dosing and avoidance of heavy blockade (which would ablate spontaneous activity even in the frontalis).

Evoked Electroencephalographic Responses

Various modalities of central nervous system stimulation (visual, auditory, and somatosensory) cause small fluctuations in cortical electrical potentials which are usually indistinguishable from the background EEG. If the stimulus is presented repeatedly and the background EEG activity is averaged out, then the specific evoked potential can be recorded. Evoked responses are themselves complex waveforms that are usually characterized in terms of latency and amplitude. Most general anesthetics have been shown to produce a dose-related reduction in amplitude and an increase in the latency of evoked responses.[30] Recently, auditory evoked responses have proven useful in the measurement of higher frequency oscillations in the cortex, which are apparently linked to awareness. Oscillations at the upper frequency range of spontaneous EEG (30 to 70 Hz), which are "coherent" (correlated in firing) over wide regions of cortex appear to be related to cognition. Thus "conscious" events may involve coherent activity of distributed neurons. How those neurons may be "bound" together to provide a unity of consciousness is unknown.[3,34,91–94] These auditory steady-state responses have been correlated to level of consciousness during anesthesia and may be useful as a tool for monitoring depth of anesthesia.[95,96]

Esophageal Contractility

Esophageal contractility received some attention as a potential measure of anesthetic depth. With the introduction of a device specifically designed to monitor lower esophageal contractility (American Antec) both spontaneous activity and evoked contractions were reported to correlate with anesthetic level.[97–99] A subsequent study designed to assess the relationship between lower esophageal contractility, EEG spectral edge frequency, and autonomic responsiveness during general anesthesia reported that neither esophageal contractility nor spectral edge frequency could predict whether patients manifested a hypertensive response to surgical stimulation.[99] In summary, while spontaneous and evoked activity in the lower esophagus appeared to correlate with impending arousal on occasion, the phenomenon is not consistent enough to provide a reliable anesthetic depthometer. The American Antec device is no longer available in the United States.

Heart Rate Variability

Heart rate variability (HRV) is a phenomenon that has been studied under a variety of clinical conditions but not extensively investigated during anesthesia. The dominant component of heart rate variability is the respiratory effect. Other cyclical changes in heart rate appear to reflect the balance between sympathetic and parasympathetic reflexes.[101] HRV may therefore provide a measure of

TABLE 17-3. Selected Common EEG-Derived Variables and Their Definitions

Variable	Description
RMS amplitude	EEG amplitude averaged over a sample EEG epoch
Delta power	Average power in the 0–4 Hz range for a sample EEG epoch
Beta power	Average power in the 4–8 Hz range for a sample EEG epoch
Alpha power	Average power in the 8–13 Hz range for a sample EEG epoch
Beta power	Average power in the 13–25 Hz range for a sample EEG epoch
Spectral edge frequency	The frequency below which 95% of the power in a given EEG sample epoch resides
Zero crossing frequency	A simple measure of average frequency content in a sample EEG epoch

autonomic reflex activity and as such may be useful as an anesthetic depthometer. Dose-related decreases in several frequency components of HRV have been characterized during isoflurane anesthesia.[102] Recent studies have confirmed a similar correlation during sevoflurane general anesthesia.[103] Further study is required to determine how consistent HRV effects are among all general anesthetics and how sensitive the technique may be over the clinical dosing range.

Other Physiologic Variables

Preliminary studies have suggested that several other physiologic variables may be useful in assessing anesthetic depth. An interesting correlation between isoflurane concentration and pupillary light reflex has been shown in humans.[104,105] This study was conducted with a small hand-held device typically used for assessing narcotization in emergency rooms. Results have not been extended to include other anesthetics and anesthetic conditions. The electroretinogram (ERG) is a diagnostic tool used in ophthalmology that measures retinal response to photic stimulation. The effects of methoxyflurane, halothane, and enflurane on the ERG were studied in rabbits, revealing a dose-dependent change in latency over the clinically useful range.[106] The swallowing reflex in felines can be provoked by electrical stimulation of the superior laryngeal nerve and thus quantified. Simultaneous activity in the hypoglossal nerve and phrenic nerve can be measured and has been correlated with depth of halothane anesthesia.[107,108] These and other variables warrant further investigation for their potential in contributing to anesthetic depth assessment. Ultimately a combination of many physiologic variables may provide a reliable anesthetic depth assessment tool in conjunction with appropriate pattern recognition tools. Unfortunately, it is difficult to do high-quality investigations of even single variables (especially in humans) for depth of anesthesia studies. Investigating a dozen such variables simultaneously (each requiring its own special purpose device) is fraught with methodological challenges and protocols, which are extremely difficult to implement.

Future Technologies: Automatic Control of Anesthetic Depth

Computer-controlled administration of halothane has been performed using spectral edge frequency (SEF) and mean arterial pressure.[109] Other experimental models of closed-loop control have been successfully implemented in animal anesthesia using a variety of single physiologic variables, including mean arterial blood pressure, spectral edge frequency, and other EEG-derived variables.[110] Recently, sophisticated computer technologies such as fuzzy logic and artificial neural networks have been applied to anesthetic depth control.[111] Artificial neural networks have been used to successfully classify EEG patterns at distinct anesthetic levels and depth of sedation.[73,112–117] Such techniques may improve the accuracy of the EEG, providing a more useful tool in the assessment of anesthetic depth. A progressive step beyond single-variable input systems has shown that a combination of neurologic EEG-derived variables and cardiovascular/hemodynamic-derived variables were far superior in predicting anesthetic depth than any of the variables used separately.[118] While these results are intriguing, closed-loop automation of anesthetic delivery may face considerable opposition from practicing anesthesiologists even if such systems performed flawlessly.

THEORETICAL MODELS OF BRAIN AND ANESTHETIC MECHANISMS

We can monitor anesthetic depth by empirical correlation with clinical signs, but anesthetic depth and anesthesia remain enigmatic due mainly to our lack of understanding of levels of brain function contributing to consciousness. Studies and models of anesthetic action may illuminate these cognitive functions and contribute to an understanding of anesthesia and anesthetic depth.

Anatomic sites of anesthetic action may vary among different anesthetics and may be altered at different concentrations of given anesthetics.[119] Multisynaptic pathways are thought to be more sensitive to effects of anesthetics, and important anesthetic effects in the reticular-activating system, cerebral cortex, and thalamus, as well as spinal cord (particularly in relation to muscle relaxation) have been shown. Within individual neurons or neuronal groups, synapses appear most sensitive to clinically relevant concentrations of anesthetics.[8] Higher concentrations of anesthetics than those required to produce general anesthesia can cause conduction block (as seen with local anesthetics), inhibit axoplasmic transport and enzymatic function, deactivate and depolymerize cytoskeletal proteins,[120] and have other effects. The means by which anesthetic molecules inhibit synaptic and other functions at clinically relevant concentrations remain unclear. Possible mediators include synaptic membrane ion channels, neurotransmitter-releasing mechanisms, postsynaptic receptors and surrounding membranes, retrograde signaling mechanisms, G proteins and other "second messengers," hydrophobic connections of cytoskeletal networks,[121] or combinations of these effects.

Clinically relevant anesthetic concentrations apparently inhibit the conformational responsiveness of functional neural proteins.[122] Thus an ion channel or receptor that changes its conformation in response to a stimulus such as voltage change or binding of a neurotransmitter is prevented from doing so by the presence of anesthetic molecules. Because of the excellent correlation between potency of anesthetic molecules and their solubility in a lipid medium, the molecular site of action of anesthetics is thought to be hydrophobic regions with solubility comparable to a lipid environment.[119] This implies that the anesthetic molecules tend to reside in the interior of a lipid membrane, and within hydrophobic, "lipid-like" regions of proteins. Thus, by weak physical attractions such as van der Waals forces, anesthetic molecules are thought to inhibit conformational responsiveness of membrane proteins, either extrinsically from the lipid phase or (more likely) intrinsically from within hydrophobic regions of proteins. This leads to the question of the role of hydrophobic regions in governing conformational states of proteins. Several lines of evidence point to coordinated conformational oscillations of proteins (in nanosecond/picosecond time scale) by electronic dipole oscillations within protein hydrophobic regions.[123-125] Theoretical models including Fröhlich coherent oscillations[126] and Davydov solitons[127] describe nonlinear couplings of electronic and protein mechanical states, which may be the link sensitive to anesthetics.[128]

While these effects may account for anesthetic inhibition of neural processes, do they explain the "selective" ablation of consciousness? Several authors[129] have linked quantum effects (probabilistic rather than precise deterministic behaviors, nonlocality, quantum coherence, etc.) to consciousness. "Perhaps our minds are qualities rooted in some strange and wonderful features of those phys-ical laws which actually govern the world we inhabit," states Penrose,[12] who suggests that quantum coherence can explain the "unitary" nature of consciousness.[10] Anesthetic inhibition of quantum events (e.g., electronic dipole oscillations coupled to neural protein conformational states, quantum coherence in hydrophobic space) may account for reversible ablation of consciousness. Although speculative, these notions suggest that future modes of anesthetic monitoring may rely on some method of observation of nanosecond oscillations or quantum coherence of brain proteins. Further, such direct monitoring may enable decoding and transfer of molecular cognition to an alternative "computer-like" medium. The "science fiction-like" possibilities and implications of such a merger of mind and technology are reviewed in a book[130] that includes speculation on the future role of anesthesiologists in caring for artificial consciousness.

CONCLUSIONS

Assessment of anesthetic depth requires assimilation and interpretation of multiple indices and confounding variables. Accordingly, technologic advances that have modernized cardiovascular monitoring have yet to make significant inroads in monitoring anesthetic depth. Perhaps capable artificial intelligence computer systems, including fuzzy logic and neural networks, will emerge to integrate and refine the ever-increasing barrage of monitoring sensors. Even then, clinical signs developed 50 years ago for ether anesthesia will be useful, though imperfectly correlated with newer anesthetics and techniques. Presently, excessively light or deep levels of anesthesia remain potential problems that demand clinical acumen and await future developments in our understanding of brain and anesthetic mechanisms and related technologies.

REFERENCES

1. Farthing GW: The Pyschology of Consciousness. Prentice Hall, Englewood Cliffs, NJ, 1992
2. Milner AD, Rugg MD: The Neuropsychology of Consciousness. Academic Press, San Diego, CA, 1992
3. Crick F, Koch C: Towards a neurobiological theory

of consciousness. Seminars in the Neurosciences 2: 263, 1990

4. Freeman WJ: Simulation of chaotic EEG patterns with a dynamic model of the olfactory system. Biol Cybern 56:139, 1987

5. Dennett D: Consciousness Explained. Little Brown, New York, 1991

6. Popper, KR, Eccles JC: The Self and Its Brain. Springer-Verlag, New York, 1977

7. Haken H: Synergetics. Springer-Verlag, Berlin, 1977

8. Angel A: Central neuronal pathways and the process of anaesthesia. Br J Anaesth 71:148, 1993

9. Strehler BL: Where is the self?: a neuroanatomical theory of consciousness. Synapse 7:44, 1991

10. Marshall IN: Consciousness and Bose-Einstein condensates. New Ideas in Psychology 7:73, 1989

11. Penrose R: Shadows of the Mind. Oxford University Press, Oxford, 1994

12. Penrose R: The Emperor's New Mind. Oxford University Press, Oxford, 1989

13. Jaynes J: The Origin of Consciousness and Breakdown of the Bicameral Mind. Alan Layne, Penguin Books, London, 1976

14. Kissin, I: General anesthetic action: an obsolete notion? Anesth Analg 76:215, 1993

15. Plomley F: Operations upon the eye. [Letter]. Lancet 1:134, 1847

16. Snow J: On the Inhalation of the Vapour of Ether in Surgical Operations. London, 1847.

17. Guedel AE: Inhalational Anesthesia: A Fundamental Guide. Macmillan, New York, 1937

18. Artusio JF Jr: Di-ethyl ether analgesia: a detailed description of the first stage of ether anesthesia in man. J Pharmacol Exp Ther 111:343, 1954

19. Eger EI II, Saidman LJ, Brandstater B: Minimum alveolar anesthetic concentration: a standard of anesthetic potency. Anesthesiology 26:756, 1965

20. Courtin RF, Bickford RG, Faulconer A Jr: The classification and significance of electroencephalographic patterns produced by nitrous oxide-ether anesthesia during surgical operations. Mayo Clin Proc 25:197, 1950

21. Galla SJ, Rocco AG, Vandam LD: Evaluation of the traditional signs and stages of anesthesia: an electroencephalographic and clinical study. Anesthesiology 19:328, 1958

22. Woodbridge PD: Changing concepts concerning depth of anesthesia. Anesthesiology 18:536, 1957

23. Stoelting RK, Longnecker DE, Eger EI II: Minimum alveolar concentration in man on awakening from methoxyflurane, halothane, ether and fluoxene anesthesia: MAC awake. Anesthesiology 33:5, 1970

24. Yakaitis RW, Blitt CD, Angiulo JP: End tidal enflurane concentration for endotracheal intubation. Anesthesiology 50:59, 1979

25. Roizen MF, Horrigan RW, Frazer BM: Anesthetic doses blocking adrenergic (stress) and cardiovascular responses to incision—MAC BAR. Anesthesiology 54:390, 1981

26. Cullen DJ, Eger EI II, Stevens WC et al: Clinical signs of anesthesia. Anesthesiology 36:21, 1972

27. Royston D, Snowdon SL: Comparison of respiratory characteristics during enflurane and halothane anaesthesia. Br J Anaesth 53:357, 1981

28. Eger EI II, Dolan WM, Stevens WC et al: Surgical stimulation antagonizes the respiratory depression produced by Forane. Anesthesiology 36:544, 1972

29. Fourcade HE, Stevens WC, Larson CP Jr et al: The ventilatory effects of Forane, a new inhaled anesthetic. Anesthesiology 35:26, 1971

30. Sebel PS: Evaluation of anaesthetic depth. Br J Hosp Med 38:116, 1987

31. Mark JB, Greenberg LM: Intraoperative awareness and hypertensive crisis during high-dose fentanyl diazepam-oxygen anesthesia. Anesth Analg 62:698, 1983

32. Blacher RS: On awakening paralysed during surgery, a syndrome of traumatic neurosis. JAMA 234:67, 1975

33. Anonymous: The depth of anaesthesia. [Editorial]. Lancet 2:553–554, 1986.

34. Kulli J, Koch C: Does anesthesia cause loss of consciousness? Trends Neurosci 14:6, 1991

35. Jones JG, Konieczko K: Hearing and memory in anaesthetised patients. [Editorial]. Br Med J 292:1291, 1986

36. Anonymous: Advertising during anesthesia. [Editorial]. Lancet 2:1019, 1986

37. Tunstall ME: Detecting wakefulness during general anaesthetic for caesarean section. Br Med J 1:1321, 1977

38. Bogod DG, Orton JK, Yau HM, Oh TE: Detecting awareness during general anaesthetic caesarean section. Anaesthesia 45:279, 1990

39. Cork RC, Kihlstrom JF, Schacter DL: Absence of explicit or implicit memory in patients anesthetized with sufentanil/nitrous oxide. Anesthesiology 76:892, 1992

40. Cherkin A, Harroun P: Anesthesia and memory process. Anesthesiology 34:469, 1971

41. Abouleish E, Taylor FH: Effect of morphine-diazepam on signs of anesthesia, awareness and dreams of patients under N_2O for cesarean section. Anesth Analg 55:702, 1976

42. Hutchinson R: Awareness during surgery: a study of its incidence. Br J Anaesth 33:463, 1961

43. Wilson J, Turner DJ: Awareness during caesarean section under general anesthesia. Br Med J 1:280, 1969

44. Wilson SL, Vaughan RW, Stephen CR: Awareness,

dreams and hallucinations associated with general anesthesia. Anesth Analg 54:609, 1975

45. Pederson T, Johansen SH: Serious morbidity attributable to anaesthesia. Anaesthesia 44:504, 1989

46. Utting JE: Awareness. p. 171. In Rosen M, Lunn JN (eds): Clinical Aspects of Consciousness, Awareness and Pain in General Anesthesia. Butterworths, London, 1987

47. Brice DD, Hetherington RR, Utting JE: A simple study of awareness and dreaming during anesthesia. Br J Anaesth 42:535, 1970

48. Crawford JS: Awareness during operative obstetrics under general anaesthesia. Br J Anaesth 43:179, 1971

49. Bogetz MS, Katz JA: Recall of surgery for major trauma. Anesthesiology 61:6, 1984

50. Goldmann L, Shah MV, Helden MW: Memory of cardiac anesthesia. Anaesthesia 42:596, 1987

51. Moore JK, Seymour AH: Awareness during bronchoscopy. Ann R Coll Surg Engl 69:45, 1987

52. Cook TL, Smith M, Starkweather JA, Eger EI II: Effects of subanesthetic concentrations of enflurane and halothane on human behavior. Anesth Analg 57:434, 1978

53. Newton DEF, Thornton C, Konieczko K et al: Levels of consciousness in volunteers breathing sub-MAC concentrations of isoflurane. Br J Anaesth 65:609, 1990

54. Kihlstrom JF, Schacter DL, Cork RC et al: Implicit and explicit memory following surgical anesthesia. Psychol Sci 1:303, 1990

55. Ghoneim MM, Block RJ: Learning and consciousness during general anesthesia. Anesthesiology 76:279, 1992

56. Rupreht J: Awareness with amnesia during total intravenous anaesthesia with propofol. Anaesthesia 44:1005, 1989

57. Dundee JW, Pandit SK: Studies on drug induced amnesia with intravenous anaesthetics in man. Br J Clin Pract 26:164, 1972

58. Osborn AG, Bunker JP, Cooper LM et al: Effects of thiopental sedation on learning and memory. Biol Psychol 23:179, 1986

59. Curran HV: Tranquilizing memories: a review of the effects of benzodiazepines on human memory. Biol Pyschol 23:179, 1986

60. Ghoneim MM, Mewaldt SP: Benzodiazepines and human memory: a review. Anesthesiology 72:926, 1990

61. Scott DL: Awareness during general anesthesia. Can Anaesth Soc J 19:173, 1972

62. Winterbottom EH: Insufficient anaesthesia. BR Med J 1:247, 1950

63. Tammisto T, Tigerstedt I: The need for halothane supplementation of N_2O-O_2 relaxant anesthesia in chronic alcoholics. Acta Anaesthesiol Scand 21:17, 1977

64. Mummaneni N, Rao TKL, Montoya A: Awareness and recall with high dose fentanyl-oxygen anesthesia. Anesth Analg 59:948, 1980

65. Kochs E, Bischoff P: Intraoperative topographical electroencephalographic monitoring during steady-state isoflurane-N_2O anesthesia: effect of surgical stimulation. J Clin Monit 9:123, 1993

66. Rampil IJ, Sasse FJ, Smith NT et al: Spectral edge frequency: a new correlate of anesthetic depth. Anesthesiology 53:S12, 1980

67. Bührer M, Maitre PO, Hung OR et al: Thiopental pharmacodynamics. Anesthesiology 77:226, 1992

68. Hudson RJ, Stanski DR, Saidman LJ, Meathe E: A model for studying depth of anesthesia and acute tolerance to thiopental. Anesthesiology 59:301, 1983

69. Hung OR, Varvel JR, Shafer SL, Stanski DR: Thiopental pharmacodynamics: II. Quantitation of clinical and electroencephalographic depth of anesthesia. Anesthesiology 77(2):237, 1992

70. Scott JC, Ponganis KV, Stanski DR: EEG quantitation of narcotic effect: the comparative pharmacodynamics of fentanyl and alfentanil. Anesthesiology 62:234, 1985

71. Borgeat A, Dessibourg C, Popovic V et al: Propofol and spontaneous movements: an EEG study. Anesthesiology 74:24, 1991

72. Levy WJ: Power spectrum correlates of changes in consciousness during anesthetic induction with enflurane. Anesthesiology 64:688, 1986

73. Veselis RA, Reinsel R, Alagesan R et al: The EEG as a monitor of midazolam amnesia: changes in power and topography as a function of amnesic state. Anesthesiology 74:866, 1991

74. Berezowskyj JL, McEwen JA, Anderson GB, Jenkins LC: A study of anesthesia depth by power spectral analysis of the electroencephalogram (EEG). Can Anaesth Soc J 23:1, 1976

75. Drummond JC, Brann CA, Perkins DE, Wolfe DE: A comparison of median frequency, spectral edge frequency, a frequency band power ratio, total power, and dominance shift in the determination of depth of anesthesia. Acta Anaesthesiol Scand 35:693, 1991

76. Thomsen CE, Christensen KN, Rosenfalck A: Computerized monitoring of depth of anesthesia with isoflurane. Br J Anaesth 63:36, 1989

77. Watt RC, Ehlers KC, Scipione PJ et al: Dimensional analysis of the electroencephalogram during general anesthesia. IEEE/Engineering in Medicine and Biology Society Eleventh Annual Conference, Seattle, Washington, November 9–12, 1989

78. Watt RC, Hameroff SR: Phase space analysis of hu-

man EEG during general anesthesia. Ann NY Acad Sci 504:286, 1988

79. Watt RC, Hameroff SR: Phase space electroencephalography (EEG): a new mode of intraoperative EEG analysis. Int J Clin Monit Comput 5:3, 1988

80. Lien CA, Berman M, Saini V et al: The accuracy of the EEG in predicting hemodynamic changes with incision during isoflurane anesthesia. Anesth Analg 74:S1, 1992

81. Kearse L, Saini V, DeBros F, Chamoun N: Bispectral analysis of EEG may predict anesthetic depth during narcotic induction. Anesthesiology 75:A175, 1991

82. Sebel PS, Bowles S, Saini V, Chamoun N: Accuracy of EEG in predicting movement at incision during isoflurane anesthesia. Anesthesiology 75:A446, 1991

83. Vernon J, Bowles S, Sebel PS, Chamoun N: EEG bispectrum predicts movement at incision during isoflurane or propofol anesthesia. Anesthesiology 77:A502, 1992

84. Rampil IJ, Mason P, Singh H: Anesthetic potency (MAC) is independent of forebrain structures in the rat. Anesthesiology 78:707, 1993

85. Rampil IJ, Laster MJ: No correlation between quantitative electroencephalographic measurements and movement response to noxious stimuli during isoflurane anesthesia in rats. Anesthesiology 77:920, 1992

86. Bennett HL, Arrcher S, Lin O. Jella S: F.A.C.E.: A Sensitive and Specific Monitor for the Adequacy ('Depth') of Anesthesia. Paper presented to the Second International Symposium on Memory and Awareness during Anesthesia, Atlanta, 1992

87. Bennett HL: The mind during surgery: The uncertain effects of anesthesia. ADVANCES, J Mind-Body Health 9(1):5–16, 1993

88. Chang T, Dworsky WA, White PF: Continuous electromyography for monitoring depth of anesthesia. Anesth Analg 67:521, 1988

89. Edmonds Jr HL, Paloheimo M: Computerized monitoring of the EMG and EEG during anesthesia. Int J Clin Monit Comput 1:201, 1985

90. Watt RC, Hameroff SR, Cork RC et al: Spontaneous EMG monitoring for anesthetic depth assessment. Proceedings AAMI 20th Annual Meeting, May 4–8, 1985

91. Engel AK, König P, Kreiter AK et al: Temporal coding in the visual cortex: new vistas on integration in the nervous system. Trends in Neuroscience 15:218, 1992

92. Koch C: Computational approaches to cognition: the bottom-up view. Neurobiology 3:203, 1993

93. Madler CH, Pöppel E: Auditory evoked potentials indicate the loss of neuronal oscillations during general anesthesia. Naturwissenschaften 74:42, 1987

94. Singer W: Synchronization of cortical activity and its putative role in information processing and learning. Annu Rev Physiol 55:349, 1993

95. Plourde G, Boylan JF: The auditory steady state response during sufentanil anaesthesia. Br J Anaesth 66:683, 1991

96. Plourde G, Picton TW: Human auditory steady-state response during general anesthesia. Anesth Analg 71:460, 1990

97. Evans JM, Bithell JF, Vlachonikolis IG: Relationship between lower esophageal contractility, clinical signs, and halothane concentration during general anaesthesia and surgery in man. Br J Anaesth 59:1364, 1987

98. Kuni DR, Silvay G: Lower esophageal contractility: a technique for measuring depth of anesthesia. Biomed Instrum Technol Sep/Oct:388, 1989.

99. Watt RC, Suwarno NO, Maslana GS et al: Esophageal contractility monitoring for anesthetic depth assessment. IEEE/Engineering in Medicine and Biology Society Tenth Annual Conference, New Orleans, Louisiana, November 3–7, 1988

100. Ghouri AH, Monk TG, White PF: Electroencephalogram spectral edge frequency, lower esophageal contractility, and autonomic responsiveness during general anesthesia. J Clin Monit 9:176, 1993

101. Estafanous FG, Brum JM, Ribeiro MP et al: Analysis of heart rate variability to assess hemodynamic alteration following induction of anesthesia. J Cardiothorac Vasc Anesth 6:651, 1992

102. Kato M, Komatsu T, Kimura T et al: Spectral analysis of heart rate variability during isoflurane anesthesia. Anesthesiology 77:669, 1992

103. Maslana ES, Watt RC, Navabi MJ et al: Beat to beat variability can indicate subtle differences in cardiovascular effects of anesthesia. Society for Technology in Anesthesia Annual Meeting, February 17–19, New Orleans, Louisiana, 1993

104. Larson M, Sessler DI: Isoflurane impairs the pupillary light reflex in humans. Anesthesiology 73:A408, 1990

105. Larson MD, Sessler DI, McGuire J, Hynson JM: Isoflurane, but not mild hypothermia, depresses the human pupillary light reflex. Anesthesiology 75:62, 1991

106. Tashiro C, Muranishi R, Gomyo I et al: Electroretinogram as a possible monitor of anesthetic depth. Arch Clin Exp Ophthalmol 224:473, 1986

107. Nishino T, Shirahata M, Yonezawa T, Honda Y: Comparison of changes in the hypoglossal and the phrenic nerve activity in response to increasing depth of anesthesia in cats. Anesthesiology 60:19, 1984

108. Nishino T, Honda Y, Kohchi T et al: Effects of increasing depth of anaesthesia or phrenic nerve and hypoglossal nerve activity during the swallowing reflex in cats. Br J Anaesth 57:208, 1985

109. Schils GF, Sasse FJ, Rideout VC: Automated control of halothane administration: computer model and animal studies. Anesthesiology 59:A169, 1983

110. Chilcoat RT, Lunn JN, Mapleson WW: Computer assistance in the control of depth of anesthesia. BR J Anaesth 56:1417, 1984

111. Nebot A, Cellier FE, Linkens DA: Controlling an anaesthetic agent by means of fuzzy inductive reasoning. Proceedings QUARDET '93: Qualitative Reasoning and Decision Technologies, Barcelona, Spain, June 16–18, 1993

112. Watt RC, Maslana ES, Navabi MJ: EEG spectral features provide basis for artificial neural network comparison of anesthetics. IEEE/Engineering in Medicine and Biology Society Fourteenth Annual International Conference, Paris, France, October 29–November 1, 1992

113. Watt RC, Navabi MJ, Scipione PJ et al: Neural network estimation of anesthetic dose using EEG spectral signatures. American Society of Anesthesiologists Annual Meeting, Las Vegas, NV, October 19–23, 1990

114. Watt RC, Maslana ES, Navabi MJ, Mylrea KC: Artificial neural networks: analytical tools for comparing anesthetics. American Society of Anesthesiologists Annual Meeting, New Orleans, LA, October 17, 1992

115. Watt RC, Samuelson H, Navabi MJ, Mylrea K: Pattern classification of EEG spectral signatures during anesthesia. IEEE/Engineering in Medicine and Biology Society Thirteenth Annual International Conference, Orlando, FL, November 1–4, 1991

116. Watt RC, Navabi MJ, Scipione PJ et al: Neural Network Estimation of Anesthetic Dose Using EEG Spectral Signatures. IEEE/Engineering in Medicine and Biology Society Twelfth Annual International Conference, Philadelphia, November 1–4, 1990

117. Watt RC, Gale AA, Kanemoto AC et al: Neural network classification of anesthetic levels using EEG spectral signatures. American Society of Anesthesiologists Annual Meeting, 1993

118. Sharma A, Wilson SE, Roy RJ: EEG classification for estimating anesthetic depth during halothane anesthesia. IEEE Engineering in Medicine and Biology Society 14:2409, 1992

119. Halsey MJ: Mechanisms of general anesthesia. In Eger EI II (ed): Anesthetic Uptake and Action. Williams & Wilkins, Baltimore, 1974

120. Allison AC, Nunn JF: Effects of general anesthetics on microtubules, a possible mechanism of anaesthesia. Lancet 2:1326, 1968

121. Lewis SA, Ivanov IE, Lee GH, Cowan NJ: Organization of microtubules in dendrites and axons is determined by a short hydrophobic zipper in microtubule-associated proteins MAP2 and TAU. Nature 342:498, 1989

122. Franks NP and Lieb WR: Selective actions of volatile general anaesthetics at molecular and cellular levels. Br J Anaesth 71:67, 1993

123. Davydov DS: The migration of energy and electron in biological systems. In Holden AV, Winlow 1 (eds): Biology and Quantum Mechanics. Springer Verlag, Berlin, 1982

124. Fröhlich H: The extraordinary dielectric properties of biological materials and the action of enzymes. Proc Natl Acad Sci 72:4211, 1975

125. Lawrence AF, Adey WR: Nonlinear wave mechanisms in interactions between excitable tissue and electromagnetic fields. Neurol Res 4:115, 1982

126. Fröhlich H: Long-range coherence and the actions of enzymes. Nature 228:1093, 1970

127. Scott AC: Davydov's soliton. Phys Rep 217:1–67, 1992

128. Hameroff SR, Watt RC: Do anesthetics act by altering electron mobility? Anesth Analg 62:936, 1983

129. Beck F and Eccles JC: Quantum aspects of brain activity and the role of consciousness. Proc Natl Acad Sci USA 89:11357, 1992

130. Hameroff SR: Ultimate Computing: Biomolecular Consciousness and Nanotechnology. North-Holland, Amsterdam, 1987

Neuroanesthesia Monitoring

18

Scott Podolsky
Audrée A. Bendo

Monitoring in neuroanesthesia must include all the routine monitors as well as more invasive monitors as appropriate for the particular patient and procedure. Beyond this, there are specialized monitors of neurologic function and physiologic status that are particularly useful during neurosurgical procedures. The different monitoring methods will be discussed within the context of their application to neurosurgical procedures.

MONITORING METHODS

Routine Monitoring

Monitoring by use of an electrocardiogram (ECG), noninvasive blood pressure cuff, pulse oximeter, end-tidal carbon dioxide ($ETCO_2$), precordial or esophageal stethoscope, and temperature probe are as necessary in neuroanesthesia as in any other anesthetic. The use of inspired oxygen analysis, airway pressure measurement, and spirometry are also required.

The routine monitors are required to determine a patient's physiologic status, but may have particular application to neurosurgical anesthesia as well. For example, decreases in $ETCO_2$ and oxygen saturation, increases in airway pressures, changes in heart sounds, and ECG changes are all used for detecting venous air embolism (see the section ''Detection of Venous Air Embolism'').

End-tidal CO_2 is monitored during neurosurgical procedures to measure hyperventilation. The difference between arterial carbon dioxide tension ($PaCO_2$) and the $ETCO_2$ must be determined for a given patient in a given position, then the $ETCO_2$ can be used with fair reliability to estimate the $PaCO_2$ throughout the operation.

Temperature monitoring is important because body heat is lost easily during a craniotomy. Hypothermia may prolong awakening from anesthesia and thus prevent early postoperative neurologic evaluation. In some situations, a decrease in core temperature may be useful, for example, when providing cerebral protection intraoperatively.[1,2]

Invasive Monitoring

Some type of invasive monitoring is necessary for most neurosurgical anesthetics. The particular monitoring implemented will depend on the type and extent of the procedure and the medical condition of the patient. Measurement of intraarterial blood pressure, arterial blood gases, central venous pressure (CVP) and urinary output is recommended for most major neurosurgical procedures (Table 18-1).

Intraarterial blood pressure monitoring should be used in any procedure or for any patient where beat-to-beat monitoring of blood pressure has value. In most neurosurgical patients, an arterial catheter is inserted before induction of anesthesia to continuously monitor blood pressure and to estimate cerebral perfusion pressure. When the arterial pressure transducer is at head level, cerebral perfusion pressure is calculated as the difference between mean arterial pressure and the CVP in pa-

509

tients without intracranial hypertension, or the intracranial pressure (ICP) in those with intracranial hypertension. With arterial pressure monitoring, the hemodynamic consequences of the pharmacologic agents administered during anesthesia are recognized instantly. It can also serve as an indicator of reduced intravascular volume or impaired venous return by showing respiratory variation with positive pressure ventilation. This is particularly useful for procedures in the prone position, where venous return may be compromised. In addition, the arterial catheter provides ready access for intraoperative measurement of arterial blood gases, hematocrit, serum electrolytes, and osmolality. Radial, femoral, or brachial arteries are suitable for short-term cannulation. After testing ulnar artery collateral blood flow, cannulation of the radial artery is preferred.

Measurement of cardiac preload and urinary output is important because neurosurgical patients often are dehydrated preoperatively and then subjected to intraoperative diuresis. A right atrial catheter reflects cardiac preload and is used to determine the preoperative fluid deficit and rate of intraoperative fluid infusion. In patients with intracranial hypertension, the CVP catheter should be inserted through an antecubital vein instead of the jugular or subclavian veins.[3] This avoids increasing ICP from the head-down position and neck-turning, which can decrease cerebral venous outflow. The position of the antecubital CVP can be verified by chest radiograph, transducer pressure and waveform, or P-wave configuration on the ECG. A CVP catheter should also be placed when venous air embolism is likely (see "Detection of Venous Air Embolism").

Urinary output is an indicator of perioperative fluid balance. Following the administration of osmotic or loop diuretics, a brisk diuresis is expected. A reduced urine output in neurosurgical patients may reflect either hypovolemia or release of antidiuretic hormone. A foley catheter should be inserted for any prolonged procedure and for all procedures requiring the use of diuretics.

A pulmonary artery catheter should be inserted when there is a risk for paradoxical air embolism and when a patient's underlying medical condition requires it. The use of a pulmonary artery catheter in the detection of air emboli is discussed in detail in the section "Detection of Venous Air Embolism."

Specialized Monitoring

Intracranial Pressure Monitoring

Since Lundberg's[4] report in 1960, continuous intracranial pressure monitoring has been used to guide the perioperative management of patients with head injury, ruptured intracranial aneurysm, brain tumor, cerebrovascular occlusive disease, and hydrocephalus. For example, during intracranial procedures, knowledge of ICP and arterial blood pressure allows precise titration of pharmacologic agents during induction and establishment of anesthesia, and guides positioning of the patient to avoid venous engorgement or bleeding.[5] Intracranial hypertension resulting from application of the bone flap or head dressing at the conclusion of surgery can also be observed and treated.[6] Postoperatively, ICP monitoring allows early detection and prompt treatment of brain swelling or hemorrhage. Another indication for intraoperative ICP monitoring is to detect intracranial hypertension in the multiple trauma patient during a nonneurosurgical procedure.[7]

There is no doubt that ICP monitoring can serve as an early warning system for impending disaster.[8–12] Whether or not outcome is improved by monitoring and controlling ICP is more difficult to prove.[8–10,13,14]

Lundberg[4] described three distinct pathologic waveforms: A waves (plateau waves), B waves (one-per-minute waves), and C waves (six-per-minute

TABLE 18-1. Monitoring for Major Neurosurgical Procedures

Routine
    Electrocardiogram
    Noninvasive blood pressure
    Pulse oximeter
    End-tidal CO_2
    Esophageal stethoscope
    Temperature
    Inspired O_2
    Airway pressure
    Spirometry
Invasive
    Intraarterial blood pressure
    Central venous pressure
    Urinary output
    Arterial blood gas analysis

waves) (Fig. 18-1). The A wave or plateau wave was seen in patients with elevated baseline ICP (>20 mmHg) and consisted of a further elevation of ICP from 50 to over 100 mmHg, varying in duration from 5 to 20 minutes before returning to baseline level. In subsequent studies, plateau waves were found to coincide with an increase in regional cerebral blood volume (rCBV) and a decrease in cerebral blood flow (CBF).[15–17] The increase in rCBV was thought to cause the ICP elevation.[16] It was proposed that vasodilation caused a rapid rise in ICP with obstruction of cerebral venous drainage resulting in the paradoxical increase in rCBV and decrease in CBF.[16]

The B and C waves were of lower amplitude and shorter duration. Lundberg and his colleagues[18] demonstrated an association between Cheyne-Stokes respiration and B waves and between Traube-Hering-Mayer blood pressure waves and C waves. The change in respiration and blood pressure and the ICP waves are thought to be the result of a common brainstem alteration. Both B and C waves were observed in association with a depressed level of consciousness. These waves, unlike A waves, were not useful in predicting outcome or managing patients.[4,15,18]

Techniques used to monitor ICP include a ventricular catheter, a subarachnoid bolt, and a variety of epidural transducers (Fig. 18-2). The ideal method of monitoring ICP has not yet been devised. An ideal transducer would be expected to record cerebrospinal fluid (CSF) pressure accurately with little or no risk of infection, hematoma, or brain damage. The ideal transducer should be small, implantable, easily calibrated in situ, sensitive, economical, and capable of functioning for many weeks impervious to the environment.

The intraventricular catheter is the standard method of monitoring ICP. This technique requires a small scalp incision and a burr hole through the skull. A soft, nonreactive plastic catheter is introduced into the lateral ventricle and

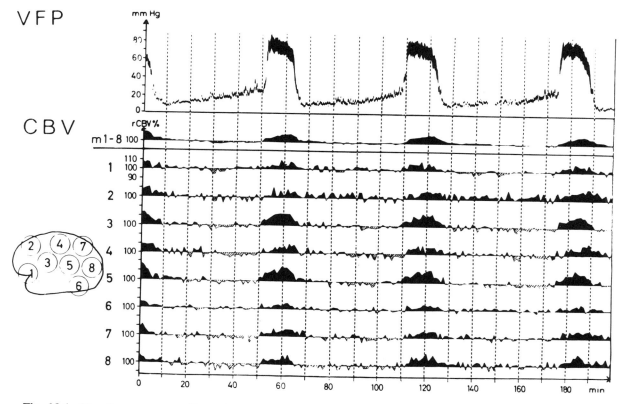

Fig. 18-1. Simultaneous recording of regional cerebral blood volume (rCBV) and ventricular fluid pressure during three consecutive plateau waves. (From Risberg,[16] with permission.)

connected with sterile tubing filled with saline to an external transducer. The intraventricular catheter measures CSF pressures reliably. It allows therapeutic CSF drainage and can also be used for compliance testing. There are, however, several potential problems with this technique. In a patient with severe brain swelling or a large mass lesion and small ventricles, it may be technically difficult to locate the lateral ventricle. Besides not being able to pass the catheter into the CSF, there is a possibility of brain tissue damage, hematoma, and infection.[19,20] Infection is a common complication of ventriculostomy and appears to be related to the length of catheterization (5 days or more), older age, and steroid administration.[19–21] Furthermore, this device depends on the transmission of ICP via fluid-filled tubes that can block and dampen or obliterate the recording.

The subarachnoid bolt is currently used as a method for monitoring ICP.[22] It is usually fitted into a burr hole made 2 to 3 cm anterior to the frontoparietal suture line, with the tip of the bolt passing through the incised dura. The advantages of the bolt are that it does not require brain tissue penetration or knowledge of ventricular position, and can be placed in any skull location that avoids major venous sinuses. There are several disadvantages to using this technique. The bolt cannot be used to lower ICP by CSF drainage or to test compliance reliably. As with the intraventricular catheter, the bolt is connected to a transducer with tubing filled with sterile saline. Not only can the tubing block, but brain substance can also obstruct the tip of the bolt, and in either situation, the recording may become damped or lost. Drilling side holes just proximal to the tip of the bolt compensates for this problem to some extent. Subarachnoid devices are easily inserted, but can malfunction if they are not coplanar to the brain surface or if they become loose. The major complication of this procedure is infection, commonly meningitis, osteomyelitis, or a localized infection, which has been shown to be related to the duration of monitoring, older age, and steroid administration.[19] Epidural bleeding and focal seizures, if the bolt is inserted too deeply, can also occur.

A variety of epidural transducers have been developed. The two primary types that are in use are a device that has a pressure-sensitive membrane, mounted close to or contacting the dura, and the Ladd epidural transducer, based on the principle of the Numoto pressure switch.[23,24] The main advantage to using an epidural transducer is the extradural placement. If infection occurs, it is separated from the brain by the dura. The disadvantages of monitoring with an epidural transducer

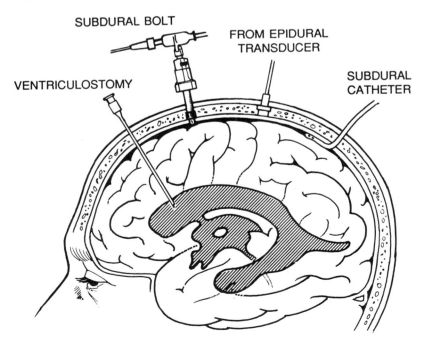

Fig. 18-2. Techniques used to measure intracranial pressure. (From Bendo et al,[58] with permission.)

SUBDURAL BOLT

FROM EPIDURAL TRANSDUCER

VENTRICULOSTOMY

SUBDURAL CATHETER

are technical problems in calibrating the transducer in situ, inability to perform compliance testing or to aspirate fluid to decrease ICP, and high cost of the equipment.

A relatively new development in ICP monitoring has been that of a miniaturized fiberoptic device (Camino Laboratories, San Diego, CA). This sensing device is mounted at the end of a 4-French fiberoptic bundle which can be inserted through a 2-mm burr hole. This monitor senses changes in the amount of light reflected off a pressure-sensitive diaphragm located at the tip of the fiberoptic catheter. Mean pressure can be displayed digitally or as a pressure waveform. With this device, it is possible to insert the tip of the catheter into the subdural, intraparenchymal, or intraventricular compartments. Since it is a solid-state monitor, the problems of infection, leaks, catheter occlusion, and drift that exist with fluid- or air-filled systems are minimized or avoided. From recent animal and human studies, it appears that pressure recordings obtained with the fiberoptic catheter are accurate and reliable.[25,26] Another advantage is that it allows direct measurement of brain tissue pressure, which may be important in edema formation and regional capillary blood flow. The main disadvantage to using this device is that it cannot be recalibrated in situ. In a recent study,[26] cumulative drift was analyzed. Since the cumulative drift became significant by the 5th day, the authors suggested that the monitor be replaced after 5 days. Another limitation of the fiberoptic device is that it cannot be used for CSF drainage or compliance testing unless it is used in conjunction with a ventriculostomy.

Noninvasive transducers have been designed to measure anterior fontanelle pressure in newborns and infants.[27,28] These devices record relative changes in fontanelle pressure which correlates closely with ICP. Accurate pressure recordings require coplanar application of the transducer.

All of the clinically available monitors have recognized advantages and disadvantages. Despite the problems associated with these devices, ICP monitoring provides useful information for evaluating the patient's condition, progress, and need for therapy. The primary risk to the patient is infection. It would seem, therefore, that the overall benefit to the patient far outweighs this risk.

Detection of Venous Air Embolism

Venous air embolism may occur whenever the operative site is elevated 5 cm or more above the heart. The likelihood of its occurrence increases as the distance of the wound above the heart increases. Therefore, patients operated on in the sitting position are particularly vulnerable to this complication with an incidence of venous air embolism of 25 to 35 percent. Entrainment of air can also occur during operations performed in the lateral, supine, or prone positions.[29]

Air may also pass directly through the pulmonary circulation or through right-to-left intracardiac shunts (e.g., probe patent foramen ovale) to the coronary and cerebral circulations, when right atrial pressure exceeds left atrial pressure. A reported 51 percent of patients develop right atrial pressure greater than left atrial pressure in the sitting position, and of these, 7 percent may experience paradoxical air embolism.[30]

There are several systems available for monitoring air emboli (Table 18-2). These systems vary in sensitivity and specificity. In theory, the more sensitive monitors provide early warning signs, whereas the less sensitive monitors may detect air emboli too late, but may be more specific. The monitors will be discussed in order of sensitivity from most to least sensitive.

Transesophageal Echocardiography

Transesophageal echocardiography (TEE) is the most sensitive monitor available for detecting venous air embolism.[31,32] When the probe is posi-

---

TABLE 18-2. Monitors Used for Detecting Venous Air Embolism

Most Sensitive

  Transesophageal echocardiography
  Precordial Doppler
  *Decrease in end-tidal CO_2
  Increase in end-tidal N_2
  Increase in pulmonary artery pressure
  *Increase in airway pressure
  *Decrease in oxygen saturation or arterial oxygen
    tension
  Increase in arterial carbon dioxide tension
  Increase in central venous pressure
  *Decrease in blood pressure
  *Decrease in pulmonary compliance
  *Change in heart sounds
  *Mill-wheel murmur
  *Cardiac arrhythmias

Least Sensitive

---

*Observed with routine monitors.

tioned at the level of the aortic valve to allow visualization of the right ventricular outflow tract, a bolus of less than 0.02 ml/kg of air and infusions of air from 0.001 to 0.01 ml/kg/min have been detected in animal studies.[33] The probe may be positioned to display both left and right atria or a four-chamber view.[31,34] Since the TEE visualizes air in left and right cardiac chambers, it can be used to detect paradoxical air embolism through a patent foramen ovale or other right-to-left shunt.[35,36]

Preoperative screening with precordial two-dimensional echocardiography during a Valsalva maneuver has been suggested as a method to identify patients at risk for paradoxical air embolism. However, such screening may have limited sensitivity for detecting a patent foramen ovale and is costly.[37] If a patent foramen ovale is detected preoperatively, a position other than sitting is recommended for surgery because of the risk of venous and paradoxical air embolism.

Doppler Ultrasound

The sensitivity of the precordial Doppler ultrasonic transducer for detection of venous air embolism is surpassed only by TEE.[32,38] Small volumes of air, as little as 0.25 ml, can be detected by using a precordial Doppler.[39,40] The Doppler transducer generates a continuous ultrasonic signal that is reflected by the movement of red blood cells and cardiac structures. When intravascular air enters the ultrasonic field, a loud turbulent noise is generated because the air/blood interface is a better acoustical reflector than red blood cells alone. The Doppler transducer should be positioned along the right parasternal border between the third and sixth intercostal spaces to maximize audible signals from the right atrium. Proper placement is confirmed by rapid injection of saline into the right atrial catheter.[41] The resultant turbulent flow changes the Doppler sounds to a high-pitched noise that is similar to the sounds produced by intravascular air.

When using the precordial Doppler, the reported frequency of air entrainment in neurosurgical procedures performed in the sitting position has been as high as 60 percent.[39,42] However, the incidence of clinically significant venous air embolism is much lower (25 percent).[39,42] The precordial Doppler ultrasound is a sensitive, noninvasive method for diagnosing air entrainment and should be used in all cases in which the site of the incision is higher than the heart. There are limitations to its use, however. Electrocautery interferes with the Doppler signal. Most units are equipped with cautery-suppression circuits that render the probe silent during surgical cautery. The disadvantage in this is that air entrainment can occur when Doppler sound has been silenced. In patients with abnormal chest wall configurations (e.g., increased anterior-posterior diameter), signals can become muffled or lost during inspiration. This obstacle can be overcome by using an esophageal Doppler probe. A transesophageal echocardiograph has also been developed with a Doppler sensor at the distal end of the probe. In a study comparing the precordial versus TEE Doppler, the precordial Doppler detected injected micro-air bubbles 10 percent of the time, whereas the TEE Doppler detected injected microbubbles 100 percent of the time.[32] When compared to the precordial Doppler, the TEE Doppler has advantages in that the sensor is placed under direct visualization and independent of external body habitus.

End-Tidal Carbon Dioxide and End-Tidal Nitrogen

End-tidal carbon dioxide ($ETCO_2$) monitoring is a useful and sensitive device for diagnosing venous air embolism.[43] End-tidal CO_2 monitoring complements the capabilities of the precordial Doppler by differentiating hemodynamically insignificant emboli heard with the Doppler from significant emboli. Doppler sounds without reduction in $ETCO_2$ usually indicate insignificant amounts of air. The entrance of air into the pulmonary circulation produces intense pulmonary vasoconstriction, which results in a ventilation-perfusion mismatch and is reflected by a proportional decrease in $ETCO_2$. The magnitude of the change in $ETCO_2$ is a guide to the size of the embolus, and the length of time during which the decrease persists reflects the continuation of an abnormal ventilation-perfusion relationship in the lung. A decrease in $ETCO_2$ can be nonspecific and must be differentiated from other causes, since, any significant decrease in cardiac output regardless of etiology will produce the same finding.

The use of mass spectrometry in the operating room provides measurement of exhaled concentrations of both CO_2 and N_2. As intravascular air in the pulmonary circulation crosses the capillary-alveolar membrane, it is exhaled, increasing the end-tidal nitrogen (ETN$_2$) concentration. End-tidal N$_2$ is considered a very sensitive monitor for diagnosing venous air embolism. In animal experiments, ETN$_2$ is considered less sensitive than changes in ETCO$_2$ following low-dose infusions of air and equally sensitive following bolus doses of air.[43-45] When a patient is ventilated with an air/oxygen mixture, the increase in ETN$_2$ with venous air embolism may not be evident. Additionally, other causes of increases in ETN$_2$ must be eliminated, for example, a leak in the breathing circuit or an incomplete seal around the endotracheal tube cuff.[46]

Pulmonary Artery Pressure

As embolized air is rapidly distributed to the pulmonary vascular bed, vascular resistance increases producing an increase in mean pulmonary artery pressure.[38,47] This sign occurs slightly later than the changes in Doppler sounds. Changes in PAP are less sensitive than either changes in end-tidal CO$_2$ or end-tidal nitrogen.[43-45] However, a change in pulmonary artery pressure correlates with the hemodynamic significance of the embolus because pulmonary artery pressure increases proportionally with the volume of air that enters the pulmonary arteries. The pulmonary artery catheter can also be used to detect patients at risk for paradoxical air embolism, that is, patients who develop a right atrial pressure greater than pulmonary capillary wedge pressure (PCWP).[30,48] When patients are moved from the supine to the sitting position, PCWP is reduced in a certain percentage, while right atrial pressure remains unchanged.[30] Thus, the normal interatrial pressure gradient is reversed and air entering the right atrium may pass through a patent foramen ovale into the left atrium. Therapeutic measures, such as fluid loading, designed to restore the normal interatrial pressure gradient, can also be assessed using the pulmonary artery catheter. The mean PCWP is not a reliable monitor for air embolism because the responses are dependent on the position of the catheter tip.[38]

Other Monitoring Methods

Many of the routine monitors are useful in detecting venous air embolism, but are less sensitive (Table 18-2). Of these, an increase in airway pressure is comparably sensitive and is a simple, inexpensive adjunct to other methods used to detect venous air embolism.[49] Decreasing oxygen saturation and changing heart sounds, that is, high-pitched sounds or a mill-wheel murmur as heard through an esophageal stethoscope, are later signs of air embolism. The least sensitive monitor for detecting air embolism is the electrocardiogram (ECG) showing cardiac arrhythmias as a very late sign.[38]

Central Venous Pressure Catheter

A CVP catheter should be inserted whenever there is a risk for venous air embolism. The use of a right atrial catheter for diagnosis and treatment of air embolism was introduced in 1966.[50] When the catheter is correctly positioned, entrained air can be aspirated from the right atrium. It is suggested that the optimal position for the tip of a single orifice catheter is 3.0 cm above the superior vena cava and the right atrial junction.[51] The position of the right atrial catheter may be confirmed by a chest film, by following the configuration of the P waves on the ECG, or by transducing a venous waveform. Figure 18-3 shows the electrocardiographic complexes associated with the catheter tip in various locations and the thoracic vertebral levels of the superior vena cava, right atrium, and right ventricle as seen on a chest radiograph. To confirm placement of the catheter tip using an ECG, a metal connector is inserted between the hub of the catheter and an intravenous saline solution. The chest lead of the ECG is connected to the metal connector with the other leads in their normal positions. All other electrical equipment is disconnected from the patient during this procedure. The catheter tip is advanced while monitoring the waveform on the ECG. The ECG is monitored on the lead V setting, if the chest lead is used, or the lead II setting, if the right arm lead is used. The P wave is inverted in the superior vena cava and biphasic at the superior vena cava-right atrial junction. This changes to a large biphasic wave in the right atrium, which becomes upright as the catheter advances past the midatrium (Fig. 18-3).

Multiorificed catheters are available and have been shown to be more effective than single-orificed catheters in air retrieval.[51,52] The optimal position for the tip of the multiorificed catheter is 0.5 cm beyond the sinoatrial node.[51] Because the ECG most likely arises from the proximal orifices, a predominantly negative rather than biphasic P wave should be sought during placement.[53,54]

It has been suggested that the addition of a balloon to the catheter tip improves air retrieval by causing the catheter to float into the air-blood interface.[55,56] Both the catheter position and the ability to aspirate from the catheter should be rechecked once the patient has been placed in the final position because catheters can migrate during positioning. In one study, when patients were placed in the sitting position, the catheter tip moved downward in 65 percent of patients.[57]

When compared to the CVP catheters, (both single lumen and multiorificed) catheters, the pulmonary artery catheter is not as effective in retrieving air.[52] The pulmonary artery catheter has a small single lumen leading to its right atrial orifice which makes air aspiration difficult. In addition, the position of the right atrial orifice is determined by the optimal position of the pulmonary artery catheter for pulmonary artery pressures, which may not be the most appropriate position for air retrieval.

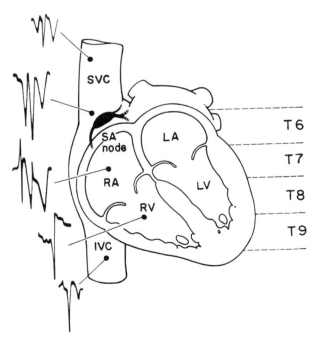

Fig. 18-3. Electrocardiographic complexes as seen when the tip of a fluid-filled catheter is used as an exploring electrode. SVC, superior vena cava; RA, right atrium; RV, right ventricle; IVC, inferior vena cava; SA node, sinoatrial node; T6 to T9, thoracic vertebral levels.

Electrophysiologic Monitoring

Electroencephalogram

The electroencephalogram (EEG) is used to monitor cerebral function during general anesthesia. The EEG waves recorded on the surface of the scalp are spontaneous electrical potentials generated by the pyramidal cells of the granular cortex. The EEG signal consists of graded summations of inhibitory and excitatory postsynaptic potentials. The EEG is sensitive to changes in anesthetic depth, temperature, and arterial tensions of carbon dioxide and oxygen. The EEG response to anesthetic agents can vary from cortical excitation through depression to isoelectricity.

The traditional EEG is a plot of voltage against time. Sixteen channels are usually recorded allowing analysis of activity of different regions of the brain. Because of the size and complexity of most EEG equipment, the need for trained personnel, and the difficulty in obtaining, interpreting and storing the raw EEG, its use in the operating room has been limited. Several signal processing techniques have been developed that improve the ability to interpret changes and evaluate trends and are more practical to use in the operating room.

The primary use of intraoperative EEG monitoring is the detection of cerebral ischemia during carotid endarterectomy procedures, cardiopulmonary bypass, or deliberate hypotension. A specific intraoperative application of the EEG is the localization of epileptic foci during surgery for intractable epilepsy. EEG monitoring is also used for intraoperative or perioperative assessment of pharmacologic interventions, such as barbiturate-induced burst suppression, and for the assessment of coma or brain death.

Evoked Potentials

Evoked potentials are used intraoperatively to monitor the integrity of specific sensory and motor pathways. Sensory evoked potentials (SEPs) evaluate the functional integrity of ascending sensory pathways, whereas motor evoked potentials test the functional integrity of descending motor pathways.

Sensory Evoked Potentials. Three SEP modalities are employed clinically: somatosensory, auditory, and visual. The waves of the evoked potentials are thought to represent potentials from specific neural generators. The individual peaks in the waveform are described in terms of polarity (negative, positive), poststimulus latency (msec), and peak-to-peak amplitude (μV or nV).

Somatosensory Evoked Potentials. Somatosensory evoked potentials are produced by stimulating a peripheral nerve, such as the median or ulnar nerves of the upper extremity or the common peroneal or posterior tibial nerves of the lower extremity, using small electrical impulses. The response to stimulation can be recorded by electrodes placed over the peripheral nerve, the lumbar spine, the brachial plexus, the cervical spine, and the scalp. Somatosensory evoked potentials are often used to monitor cerebral function and ischemia during cerebral procedures and spinal cord function and ischemia during instrumentation of the spine or thoracoabdominal surgery.

Auditory Evoked Potentials. Brainstem auditory evoked potentials are produced by stimulation of the cochlea using pulsed sound. The pathway tested starts with the ear and eighth nerve, then runs into the lower pons, ascending through each lateral lemniscus into the midbrain. Recording electrodes are placed near the ear and vertex. Following stimulation, a classic series of five to seven peaks are displayed that correspond to successive anatomic generators. Brainstem auditory evoked potentials provide information about the status of the auditory pathway and possibly, the integrity of adjacent brainstem structures. They are used intraoperatively during surgical procedures involving the cerebellopontine angle, the floor of the 4th ventricle, and the 5th, 7th, or 8th cranial nerves. They are also used to assess function in comatose patients.

Visual Evoked Potentials. Intraoperative visual evoked potentials are produced by flashing light that stimulates the retina. The optic nerves and chiasm are the main pathways measured. Recording electrodes are placed over the calcarine (visual) cortex in the occipital midline. Visual evoked potentials are very sensitive to anesthetic effects and are technically difficult to monitor intraoperatively. They are used, however, to monitor visual pathways during operations on tumors or aneurysms at or near the optic nerves and chiasm.

Compromise or injury of a neurologic pathway is manifested as an increase in the latency and/or a decrease in the amplitude of SEP waveforms. Accordingly, anesthetic, physiologic, and environmental factors capable of producing this pattern of alteration must be controlled when recording SEPs. All anesthetics that have been studied influence SEPs to some extent.[58] The sensitivity of SEPs to drug effects varies with the sensory modality being monitored. In general, SEPs of cortical origin (that is, the cortical component of the somatosensory evoked potentials and the visual evoked potentials) are more vulnerable to anesthetic influences than brainstem potentials (for example, brainstem auditory evoked potentials and the subcortical components of the somatosensory evoked potentials). To obtain satisfactory intraoperative SEP recordings, it is necessary to maintain constant anesthetic drug levels. Physiologic factors such as temperature, systemic blood pressure, and arterial tensions of oxygen and carbon dioxide that can alter SEPs, must be controlled during intraoperative recording.

Motor Evoked Potentials. Motor evoked potentials can be produced by direct (epidural) or indirect (transosseous) stimulation of the brain or spinal cord, using electrical or magnetic impulses.[59,60] Following transcranial stimulation, the signal descends through both the dorsolateral and ventral spinal cord and can be recorded from spinal cord, peripheral nerve, and muscle, using conventional electromyographic and evoked potential averaging techniques. An important indication for motor evoked potential monitoring is to assess spinal motor tracts during spinal cord surgery. The combination of somatosensory and motor evoked potential monitoring during spinal cord surgery allows assessment of both sensory and motor pathways. During intracranial procedures that involve large or complicated vascular lesions with potential compromise to the motor cortex or tracts, motor evoked potentials can also be used to guide the surgical resection.

Motor evoked potentials are very sensitive to anesthetics and require a controlled neuromuscular blockade when the electromyogram is recorded. Reliable responses have been recorded with a nitrous oxide-narcotic technique and with agents such as ketamine or etomidate.[61–63]

Measurement of Cerebral Blood Flow

Intraoperative measurement of cerebral blood flow occurs at only a few institutions because of its cost and relative complexity. The most commonly employed intraoperative method is the intraarterial injection of an inert radioactive gas, such as xenon-133. This method is an adaptation of the nitrous oxide technique of Kety and Schmidt.[64] With this method, the gas is dissolved in saline and injected into the carotid artery. A multiple (1 to 256) collimated scintillation counter is then placed over the skull to detect photons (ionizing radiation). The mean transit time of the freely diffusible inert tracer gas through the brain is measured with the scintillation counter, and total or regional blood flow is obtained. Other techniques that measure cerebral blood flow and metabolism include positron emission tomography and magnetic resonance imaging and have not found application in the intraoperative setting.

The transcranial Doppler is a noninvasive method that uses ultrasound techniques to determine blood flow through cerebral vessels. The ultrasonic waves are directed through the skull, and the change in frequency of the sound waves reflected off the moving red blood cells is used to determine the velocity of blood flow. Only blood flow velocity can be measured by this technique. Actual determination of cerebral blood flow cannot be made. To determine the actual blood flow, the diameter of the vessel in question would need to be determined, which is not possible at this time. Studies have shown a good correlation between blood flow and blood flow velocity in a particular patient.[65,66] An exception to this exists when vasospasm occurs. With vasospasm, blood flow velocity may increase through the severely narrowed artery, while blood flow decreases.[66,67]

SPECIFIC PROCEDURES

Intracranial Surgery

Supratentorial

Intracranial surgery involving the supratentorial region is performed for a variety of reasons, including tumor, infection, increased intracranial pressure due to hydrocephalus, arteriovenous malformation, aneurysm, head trauma or subarachnoid, subdural, or epidural hemorrhage. These procedures are usually performed in the supine or semireclining position, and often require the use of skull pins for immobilization and positioning of the head. Many of these patients have significantly increased intracranial pressure.

In patients with supratentorial mass lesions, ICP monitoring can be very useful during induction and positioning of the patient, at the conclusion of surgery, and postoperatively.[5,6] Many of the anesthetic agents that are routinely used have profound effects on intracranial pressure.[60] Head position, hypoxia, hypercarbia, coughing, laryngoscopy and intubation, application of the head holder pins, and surgical incision can all markedly increase ICP. The effect of maneuvers such as hyperventilation and drugs such as thiopental, diuretics, and steroids designed to lower intracranial pressure and improve intracranial compliance, can also be evaluated. When the cranium is opened, ICP becomes atmospheric, so that monitoring during surgery is not necessary. At the conclusion of surgery and during the postoperative period, ICP monitoring allows early detection and prompt treatment of neurologic deterioration.

The insertion of an ICP monitor for surgery is not without risks. ICP monitoring is an invasive procedure that can cause bleeding or infection.[19] When inserted under local anesthesia before anesthetic induction, the procedure can be uncomfortable for the patient. A discussion of the ICP monitors, risks, and benefits is in the section on ICP monitoring.

Most supratentorial craniotomies require an indwelling arterial catheter, CVP catheter, and Foley catheter in addition to the routine monitors. The exception to this is an otherwise healthy patient having a limited procedure, such as a burr hold for a ventricular drain or a ventriculoperitoneal shunt.

As stated previously, an indwelling arterial catheter is inserted in these procedures for continuous measurement of blood pressure, estimation of cerebral perfusion pressure and measurement of arterial blood gases. Hyperventilation is an important modality for controlling ICP, and both $PaCO_2$ and $ETCO_2$ should be monitored to ensure hyperventilation. After obtaining the $PaCO_2 - ETCO_2$ gradient for patient, continuous $ETCO_2$ monitoring can be used to trend the $PaCO_2$. It must be remembered, however, that anything that increases pulmonary physiologic dead space will increase this gradient making the $ETCO_2$ estimate of $PaCO_2$ inaccurate. In craniotomy patients, an increase in physiologic dead space may occur following fluid restriction, diuresis, hypotension, and positioning. Therefore, the $PaCO_2$ should be assessed hourly to accurately determine the $PaCO_2 - ETCO_2$ gradient.

A right atrial catheter is inserted to determine the preoperative fluid deficit and rate of intraoperative fluid infusion. Fluid restriction and the administration of large doses of diuretics, usually mannitol and/or furosemide, are used to control intracranial hypertension perioperatively, and therefore, the right atrial catheter is essential for measuring cardiac preload.

Perioperative fluid balance is also estimated by measuring urinary output. These patients are usually subjected to a diuretic-induced diuresis, but may also experience changes in urinary output as a result of their intracranial pathology. For example, posterior pituitary dysfunction from a variety of causes results in diabetes insipidus with its high output, poorly concentrated urine, and the syndrome of inappropriate antidiuretic hormone secretion (SIADH), occurring in the presence of intracranial tumors and head trauma, is associated with reduced urinary output.

Infratentorial

The operative management of posterior fossa lesions such as tumors, aneurysms, or hematomas poses significant surgical and anesthetic challenges because of the relatively confined space of the area bound by the tentorium cerebelli superiorly and the foramen magnum inferiorly. The posterior fossa contains the medulla, pons, cerebellum, major motor and sensory pathways, primary respiratory and cardiovascular centers, and lower cranial nerve nuclei. Because of the posterior fossa's small size, significant compromise to vital brainstem structures and cranial nerves can occur during surgery. Meticulous anesthetic technique and vigilant intraoperative monitoring are required to detect neurologic compromise.

Positions used for posterior fossa exploration are the sitting, lateral, prone, and park bench or three-quarters prone. Monitoring concerns are the same as for supratentorial procedures with some additions. Procedures performed in the sitting position are at greater risk for venous air embolism.[29,68] Therefore, monitors to detect venous air embolism should be applied as described previously in this chapter. Other problems associated with procedures performed in the sitting position include pooling of blood in the lower extremities with resultant hypotension and venous stasis and ischemia of the brain and upper cervical spinal cord. Because rapid reductions in blood pressure may occur as the patient is raised to the sitting position, intraarterial blood pressure must be carefully monitored during positioning. The transducer should be placed and zeroed at the level of the external auditory meatus (landmark for the circle of Willis) to determine the mean arterial pressure at that level and approximate the cerebral perfusion pressure.

A special consideration in posterior fossa procedures is surgical retraction or manipulation of the brainstem or cranial nerves resulting in compromise to respiratory and cardiovascular centers. The practice of permitting spontaneous respiration during posterior fossa procedures to identify encroachment on the brainstem has been replaced by monitoring the ECG and a continuous arterial blood pressure.

A hypertensive response has been demonstrated after cerebellar retraction or stimulation of the 5th cranial nerve, the periventricular gray area, and medullary reticular formation in the floor of the 4th ventricle.[69] Compression of the medulla and pons often results in sudden arterial hypotension. Bradycardia is the most common arrhythmia noted and can be seen with stimulation of the vagus nerve, the floor of the 4th ventricle and retraction near the brainstem. Other arrhythmias observed include atrioventricular nodal rhythm, atrioventricular dissociation, supraventricular and ventricular ectopic beats, and sinus tachycardia.[70] The surgeon should always be informed whenever there are hemodynamic or ECG changes. Usually, cessation of surgical manipulation or repositioning of retractors will return hemodynamic conditions and the ECG to baseline.

Electrophysiologic monitoring of sensory evoked potentials has been used to detect ischemia and compromise to the brainstem or cranial nerves. For example, brainstem auditory evoked potentials are monitored during surgery for acoustic neuroma to help preserve function of the 8th cranial nerve or during posterior fossa procedures to monitor brainstem ischemia. Depending on the tumor's location, somatosensory evoked potentials may also be used to detect brainstem compromise. During surgical positioning for posterior fossa exploration, cases of position-related brainstem and cervical spinal cord ischemia have been observed during monitoring with either brainstem auditory or somatosensory evoked potentials.[71,72] Electromyography is used during acoustic neuroma surgery to test 7th nerve function when the face is not accessible to palpation or visual assessment.[73]

Cerebrovascular Surgery

Cerebrovascular surgery includes the resection of aneurysms and arteriovenous malformations. These operations require careful control of blood pressure throughout the anesthetic, especially the induction of anesthesia, in order to avoid rupture and maintain cerebral perfusion pressure. To accurately observe the blood pressure during the induction of anesthesia, the arterial catheter should be inserted in the premedicated patient under local anesthesia. As undue pain and anxiety should be avoided in this patient population, an argument can be made to insert the catheter after induction of anesthesia and intubation of the trachea or during induction of anesthesia while the patient is manually ventilated with bag and mask.

During these operations, the patient may be subjected to deliberate hypotension and significant intravascular volume shifts (diuresis followed by volume loading). Sudden and massive blood loss may also occur. To optimally manage these patients intraoperatively, monitors of volume and hemodynamic status such as CVP or pulmonary artery pressures and urinary output, are usually inserted after the induction of anesthesia to minimize patient discomfort.

Intraoperative electroencephalography and sensory evoked potentials are used to assess the adequacy of cerebral perfusion during cerebrovascular surgery and to predict postoperative complications.[74–78] Electrophysiologic monitoring may detect ischemia resulting from vasospasm, surgical damage to a small vessel or major artery, brain retraction, and hypotension either pharmacologically induced or secondary to aneurysmal rupture. Sensory evoked potentials are a reliable indicator of ischemia provided that the vascular territory in question includes the sensory pathway being tested.[77,78] Somatosensory evoked potential monitoring has specific utility in guiding temporary or permanent clipping of vessels in the anatomic distribution of the somatosensory pathway.[78]

Until recently, intraoperative EEG monitoring with conventional 8 to 16 channels received little attention in these procedures because of problems with electrode placement in the operative area and on-line interpretation of the raw EEG. Computer-processed EEG monitors with 2 to 4 channels require fewer electrodes and have been used reliably in aneurysm surgery to detect cerebral ischemia.[75,76] EEG monitoring can also be used as a guide to dosing barbiturates or other agents to achieve burst-suppression or isoelectricity. A pharmacologically induced EEG burst-suppression may be used intraoperatively during resection of complex aneurysms or arteriovenous malformations or postoperatively following aneurysmal rupture.

Cerebral blood flow is not routinely monitored during general anesthesia for cerebrovascular surgery.[79,80] Following subarachnoid hemorrhage, the transcranial Doppler has been used to diagnose and monitor cerebral vasospasm.[67,81,82]

The postoperative care of patients following cerebrovascular surgery requires a continuation of intensive management of volume and hemodynamic status. The treatment of postoperative hypertension is critical to prevent the formation of cerebral edema or hematoma. Postoperative hypotension must also be avoided, and the patient's intravascular volume must be accurately assessed with either a CVP or pulmonary artery pressure catheter. A higher than normal intravascular fluid volume is recommended to prevent postoperative cerebral vasospasm. Both intravascular volume expansion and induced hypertension have been used to treat symptomatic vasospasm.[83,84] Such aggressive therapy usually requires the use of a pulmonary artery pressure catheter to measure pulmonary capillary wedge pressure and prevent complications. The major complications of this therapy are pulmonary edema and cardiac failure in patients at risk.

Carotid Endarterectomy

Carotid endarterectomy may be performed under regional or general anesthesia. Regardless of the type of anesthetic used, monitoring is directed toward detecting changes that develop in the cardiovascular and cerebrovascular systems. These patients usually have significant cardiovascular disease. Electrocardiographic monitoring using a five-lead system, with four electrodes on the extremities and a fifth electrode in the V_5 position (anterior axillary line in the fifth intercostal space) is recommended. With this system, leads II and V_5 can be simultaneously displayed to detect arrhythmias and myocardial ischemia. When only a three-electrode system is available, the modified V_5 leads, CM_5 or CB_5, can be used to detect myocardial ischemia. The central manubrium lead, CM_5, is obtained by placing the negative right arm electrode on the manubrium of the sternum, the positive left arm electrode in the V_5 position, and the ground (left leg) electrode in any convenient location. The central back lead, CB_5, offers good P wave morphology and ischemia detection and is accomplished by placing the negative right arm electrode over the center of the right scapula and the other electrodes in the same location as for the CM_5 lead.

Other cardiovascular monitors should include an arterial catheter and in select patients, CVP or pulmonary artery pressure catheters. An arterial catheter is inserted for continuous recording of blood pressure and intermittent determination of arterial blood gases. Continuous recording of blood pressure is beneficial, especially during the period of carotid cross-clamping, when maintenance of cerebral perfusion pressure is crucial. The systemic arterial pressure should be maintained near the upper limit of the patient's own normal blood pressure range. Continuous measurement of end-tidal CO_2 is extremely important in these patients in order to optimize cerebral oxygen delivery and cerebral metabolism. The $PaCO_2$ should be maintained at the patient's normal level throughout the surgical procedure and during the postoperative period. A central venous catheter is useful for infusion of vasoactive drugs. When placed, it should be inserted through an antecubital or subclavian approach. A pulmonary artery catheter is reserved for those patients with limited myocardial reserve associated with poor ventricular function or severe, uncorrected coronary artery disease.

Monitoring Cerebral Perfusion and Neurologic Status

Monitoring of neurologic status is critical during carotid endarterectomy procedures because these patients are at risk for intraoperative stroke due to emboli (plaque or air), cerebral ischemia, reperfusion injury, or carotid artery thrombosis.[85] Much neurologic monitoring has been devised to assess the adequacy of cerebral perfusion during the period of carotid artery cross-clamping. The adequacy of cerebral perfusion during clamping depends on collateral flow from the opposite carotid artery and/or the posterior circulation. Although the period of carotid cross-clamping is especially critical, cerebral perfusion should be assessed continuously throughout the anesthetic. The various monitoring devices used for this purpose include awake neurologic assessment, internal carotid artery stump pressure, raw and processed EEG, somatosensory evoked potentials, regional cerebral blood flow, and transcranial Doppler.

Awake Neurologic Assessment

Awake neurologic assessment is used during regional anesthesia and is the procedure of choice in settings where electrophysiologic monitoring is not available. Constant voice contact with the patient is maintained throughout the procedure. Although neurologic function may appear adequate at the time of carotid artery clamping, delayed signs of cerebral ischemia may occur when attention is directed elsewhere. Some method of evaluating motor function of the upper extremity is also used. For example, the patient may be asked to periodically squeeze a "clicker" or small toy that produces a sound.

Awake neurologic assessment allows selective placement of the bypass shunt during carotid cross-clamping. A trial occlusion of the carotid artery is performed and the patient's neurologic status followed. Changes in consciousness, seizures, visual disturbances, slurring of speech, and inappropriate restlessness all indicate cerebral ischemia in the awake patient.[86] If the patient tolerates the trial occlusion without developing any changes in neurologic status, the procedure proceeds without shunt placement. If signs of cerebral ischemia develop, a shunt is placed to restore carotid flow. Proponents of regional anesthesia point out that awake neurologic assessment is the ultimate test for the presence of cerebral ischemia. The time of onset of the neurologic deficit is apparent in the awake patient and may enable the specific cause of the deficit to be more easily determined and possibly corrected. However, unless the surgeon is quick and gentle, the patient may not tolerate surgery without significant sedation. Sedation decreases the specificity of this monitor, since decreases in sensorium may be caused by drugs, ischemia, or both.

Internal Carotid Artery Stump Pressure

Stump pressure, the pressure measured in the distal internal carotid artery when the common carotid is clamped, has been used as a measure of the adequacy of collateral flow at the time of carotid artery clamping. A stump pressure of greater than 50 mmHg has been hypothesized to represent adequate collateral circulation. It has the advantage of being easy and inexpensive to perform, requiring only that a needle or catheter be placed in the internal carotid artery above the clamp and connected via a length of tubing to a transducer. It was widely used in the past. Its disadvantage is that it is not an accurate measure of the true adequacy of cerebral perfusion. Stump pressure does not always correlate to measured regional cerebral blood flow or EEG changes.[87–89] In addition, the anesthetic agent employed can markedly influence the stump pressure reading by altering the relationship between stump pressure and cerebral blood flow.[87] If an agent that produces cerebral vasoconstriction is used, flow may be low even when stump pressure is above 50 mmHg. Conversely, if an agent that produces cerebral vasodilation is used, flow is more likely to be adequate when stump pressure is adequate. Thus, a high stump pressure may reflect a high cerebrovascular resistance without adequate collateral flow. Besides anesthetics, other factors such as PaCO$_2$, may alter the relationship between stump pressure and flow by causing changes in cerebrovascular resistance. Another disadvantage to using stump pressure is that it is not a continuous measurement, and therefore may not indicate changes occurring during the entire endarterectomy. Many clinicians no longer advocate the use of this technique.

Raw and Processed EEG

The conventional or unprocessed EEG is recognized as a sensitive indicator of inadequate cerebral perfusion. A 16-channel system is used and recordings are made continuously throughout the operative procedure. The appearance of EEG changes indicative of ischemia correlates well with low regional cerebral blood flow after carotid occlusion and with intraoperative neurologic complications. In a series of 1,145 carotid endarterectomies, no patient had a prolonged or fixed neurologic deficit without an associated EEG abnormality.[91] In another series of 392 carotid endarterectomies, the EEG was also found to be predictive of neurologic deficits occurring during surgery, and patients without significant EEG changes during surgery awoke without neurologic deficits.[92] In both of these series, EEG monitoring was used as a basis for selective shunt placement. The most commonly seen changes during carotid cross-clamping that are indicative of cerebral ischemia are ipsilateral attenuation of amplitude and progressive slowing.[93]

Despite the benefits of conventional EEG monitoring, its intraoperative use is limited because it requires trained personnel and cumbersome equipment. In many centers, computer-processed EEG monitors are used instead of conventional EEG. These monitors do not require extensive training to operate or interpret and can be easily mastered by the practicing anesthesiologist. Two methods of analysis used to process the EEG are power spectrum and aperiodic analysis. Power spectrum, using a computer to perform Fourier analysis, converts the EEG from a plot of voltage against time to a plot of power (amplitude squared) against frequency. With this technique, data are displayed in one of three formats: the compressed spectral array, the density spectral array, and the band spectral array. Power spectrum analysis has documented value as a monitor of cerebral ischemia.[94–96] Aperiodic analysis evaluates each EEG waveform in relation to its frequency, amplitude, and time of occurrence. The EEG signal is broken into the four component frequencies, with the amplitudes at each frequency in each hemisphere displayed. Aperiodic analysis of the EEG is also an effective monitor of cerebral ischemia.[97]

When implementing intraoperative EEG monitoring, awake controls should be obtained before induction of general anesthesia. Monitoring should be continuous throughout anesthesia and until the patient is awake. Bilateral data must be obtained. During carotid endarterectomy, bilateral changes may indicate anesthetic or systemic effects, whereas ipsilateral changes on the operated side are more likely consistent with surgical trauma or ischemia. Marked changes in anesthetic depth, systemic blood pressure, PaCO$_2$, and brain temperature must be avoided to distinguish between anesthetic and physiologic effects on the EEG and those attributable to ischemia or hypoxia.

Somatosensory Evoked Potentials

Cortical somatosensory evoked potentials (SSEPs) have been used to detect intraoperative cerebral ischemia during carotid procedures.[98–100] Ischemia to the cerebral cortex results in substantial changes in cortical SSEPs. In general, waveform alterations and amplitude attenuation begin at blood flows of less than 18 ml/100 g/min. The SSEP becomes systematically smaller and eventually disappears at about 15 ml/100 g/min.[101] Changes in SSEPs have been reversed with shunt insertion or raising the arterial blood pressure.[99] In one study, SSEP monitoring was found to be similar to conventional EEG in predicting postoperative neurologic deficits.[100] SSEPs require complicated computer-averaging techniques to extract the relatively small signal from the EEG and other background noise. However, the SSEP waveform is simpler and changes easier to interpret than changes in the conventional EEG. SSEP monitoring is continuous and could be performed by an anesthesiologist not responsible for conducting the anesthetic. Technical requirements and training in their application have made them less popular for monitoring during carotid endarterectomy procedures.

Regional Cerebral Blood Flow

Measurement of regional cerebral blood flow (rCBF) during carotid endarterectomy procedures is performed at only a few institutions because of the complexity and expense of the equipment. This measurement may be accomplished with either intravenous or intracarotid injection of a radioactive tracer and an array of detectors placed over the head. The technique described by Sundt and coworkers[90,91] recommends injecting 200 to 300 μCi of xenon 133 in 0.2 to 0.4 ml saline through a 27-gauge needle into the common carotid artery, following temporary occlusion of the external carotid artery. A scintillation probe placed over the motor strip on the ipsilateral side is then used to calculate clearance curves. From the initial slope of the curves, rCBF is determined. Blood flows are obtained prior to carotid occlusion, during occlusion, and after restoration of flow. If a shunt is placed, additional measurements are taken. These investigators were able to correlate rCBF measurements with continuous EEG monitoring.[91] Reductions in flow with carotid occlusion below a critical range created changes in the EEG. Occlusion flows of less than 15 ml/100 g/min usually produced EEG abnormalities consistent with ischemia, and some patients had abnormal EEG changes with even higher flows. The critical flow below which EEG abnormalities occur apparently

varies with the anesthetic used. A lower critical rCBF of 10 ml/100 g/min has been demonstrated with isoflurane anesthesia. In general, when a "critical rCBF" is obtained in a given patient, a bypass shunt is placed. Although this measurement may be repeated multiple times during surgery, it is not a continuous measurement. Cerebral blood flow measurements usually supplement a continuous monitor of cerebral function, for example, the EEG.

Transcranial Doppler

The transcranial Doppler has found application in the operating room relatively recently. This monitor uses the Doppler shift to measure blood flow velocity in the basal cerebral arteries, most commonly the middle cerebral artery. An assumption is made that blood flow velocity in the basal cerebral arteries reflects cortical cerebral blood flow. This assumption is true only if the measurement angle of the Doppler probe remains constant and the diameter of the conducting cerebral arteries does not change. Presumably, as long as blood flow velocity is maintained, cerebral blood flow should be adequate. This monitor has not been validated in a large series of cases against the EEG or cortical cerebral blood flow measurements. In addition, relatively little is known regarding the nature and degree of acceptable changes during carotid endarterectomy procedures.[102] Extensive laboratory and clinical work is needed before this device replaces other monitoring techniques during carotid surgery. This monitor is very attractive because it is easy to use, continuous and noninvasive. It will probably gain acceptance as an adjunct to electrophysiologic monitoring techniques with particular use in detecting plaque or air embolism.

In summary, many techniques have been suggested to determine the adequacy of cerebral perfusion during carotid endarterectomy. Stump pressure is of limited benefit. The unprocessed EEG and measurement of rCBF are valuable, but technical difficulties and equipment availability may preclude their use. Somatosensory evoked potentials are useful, but require technical assistance and experience in their application. Computer-processed EEG techniques are easy to use and apply by a nonelectrophysiologist and provide valuable information. Further studies are necessary to determine the precise role of the transcranial

Doppler. Awake neurologic assessment provides direct access to multiple levels of neurologic function, and in situations where electrophysiologic monitoring is not available, it is an alternative method of monitoring for cerebral ischemia.

Spinal Cord Surgery

The most common procedures on the spine include spinal fusion for scoliosis, vertebral fracture or spinal instability and operations for herniated intervertebral disk, including laminectomy, microdiskectomy, and chemonucleolysis. These operations are usually performed in the prone or occasionally the lateral position. The sitting position is used for some posterior cervical laminectomies, and the supine position is used for anterior cervical fusion. The process of turning the patient from the supine position to the prone or lateral position causes problems because one or more of the monitoring devices may be lost during this critical time. Not only are the cardiovascular compensatory mechanisms of the anesthetized patient significantly depressed, but the prone and lateral positions may further compromise circulation and ventilation. The problems encountered during procedures performed in the sitting position have been discussed previously in this chapter.

At the time the patient is turned, it is usually best to disconnect most lines leading from the patient to the various monitoring devices so that catheters and leads are not pulled out or off of the patient. If present, the indwelling arterial catheter should be retained and carefully protected during positioning to allow monitoring of blood pressure and heart rate. If an arterial pressure catheter is not present, the anesthesiologist should monitor the rhythm, strength, and character of the superficial temporal or carotid artery pulse while controlling the head and neck during the turn. All monitors must be reconnected immediately after turning, and the patient's vital signs, airway pressures, and CVP, if present, should be checked. If any problems are noted, the patient's position is readjusted until pressures are as normal as is possible.

For healthy patients undergoing laminectomy, the routine monitoring devices are often all that are needed. For more lengthy procedures during which extensive blood loss is expected, such as posterolateral decompression and spinal cord arteriovenous malformation, further measures for determining blood volume and hemodynamic status are necessary. This includes insertion of a central venous or pulmonary artery catheter, indwelling arterial catheter, and urinary catheter. The arterial catheter also provides convenient access for obtaining blood for laboratory tests. Since ventilation and oxygenation may be compromised by the patient's position, measurement of arterial blood gases is particularly useful. When replacing extensive blood loss with banked or cell-saver blood, acid-base status, electrolytes, and hematocrits should be measured frequently.

Thoracic laminectomies requiring a transthoracic approach are usually performed with a double-lumen endotracheal tube in order to collapse one lung and facilitate surgical exposure. All the precautions taken during thoracic operations with double-lumen tubes to monitor oxygenation and ventilation should be observed in these cases.

The patient with acute and chronic spinal cord injury requires extensive monitoring because of alterations in pulmonary and cardiovascular function.[103] Since fluid-electrolyte-volume management is critical, it is important to insert arterial, pulmonary artery, and urinary catheters before induction of anesthesia. Patients with recent cervical or high thoracic (T1 to T6) spinal cord lesions have an expanded vascular space secondary to sympathetic denervation during spinal shock. Large volumes of fluid may be infused in these patients without producing a significant rise in CVP and yet can cause pulmonary edema. To prevent the development of fulminant pulmonary edema, changes in pulmonary capillary wedge pressure should be used to guide fluid resuscitation and therapeutic interventions.[104] In addition, pulmonary artery catheters that measure mixed venous oxygen saturation may be particularly useful by providing continuous information on the amount of intrapulmonary shunting and tissue oxygen consumption.

Evoked potentials are used to monitor the integrity of the spinal cord during operations on the spine and spinal cord.[105,106] Somatosensory evoked potentials are used to monitor the integrity of the dorsal spinal cord, whereas motor evoked potentials are being used with increasing frequency to monitor the integrity of the dorsolateral and ventral spinal cord.[59,60,105,106] By monitoring somatosensory and motor evoked potentials during operations that entail a risk of mechanical or vascular injury to the spinal cord, both sensory and motor pathways can be evaluated during anesthesia.

CONCLUSIONS

Currently, neuroanesthesia monitoring is very challenging. Not only are all the cardiovascular monitoring systems used during neurosurgical procedures, but systems for evaluating neurologic function are being refined. Rapid advances in technology and computing power have allowed systems such as the EEG, evoked potentials, fiberoptic intracranial pressure, and transcranial Doppler to become more practical to use in the operating room. In the past, many of these systems were expensive, cumbersome, and technologically difficult to use; data interpretation required skills and training not possessed by many anesthesiologists. All of these problems are being solved by engineers and manufacturers making neurophysiologic monitoring increasingly possible and, finally, routine.

Because general anesthesia has its major effect on the central nervous system, the interpretation of neurophysiologic data should be made with this in mind. In addition, the anesthesiologist must facilitate intraoperative electrophysiologic monitoring by using those drugs that least alter the EEG and evoked potentials, by paying careful attention to technical details, and by keeping the pharmacologic and physiologic state of the patient relatively constant during critical monitoring periods.

The ultimate value of the various neurophysiologic monitors, as with all monitoring, will depend on the information obtained from the monitoring system and the criteria used to determine interventions or changes in technique. The anesthesiologist integrates the information obtained from all the monitoring devices and determines the best course of action for optimizing the patient's condition during surgery. Intraoperative neurophysiologic monitoring by providing the anesthesiologist with additional information, allows more comprehensive management of patients during general anesthesia.

REFERENCES

1. Astrup J, Sorenson P, Rabbek Sorenson H: Inhibition of cerebral oxygen and glucose consumption in the dog by hypothermia, pentobarbital, and lidocaine. Anesthesiology 55:263, 1981

2. Busto R, Dietrich WD, Globus MY-T et al: Differences in intra-ischemic brain temperature critically determine the extent of ischemic neuronal injury. J Cereb Blood Flow Metab 7:729, 1987

3. Smith SL, Albin MS, Ritter RR et al: CVP catheter placement from the antecubital veins using a J-wire catheter guide. Anesthesiology 60:238, 1984

4. Lundberg N: Continuous recording and control of ventricular fluid pressure in neurosurgical practice. Acta Psychiatr Neurol Scand 36:1, 1960

5. Shapiro HM, Wyte SR, Harris AB, Galindo A: Acute intraoperative intracranial hypertension in neurosurgical patients: mechanical and pharmacologic factors. Anesthesiology 37:399, 1972

6. Leech P, Barker J, Fitch W: Changes in intracranial pressure and systemic arterial pressure during termination of anesthesia. Br J Anaesth 46:315, 1974

7. Palmer MA, Perry JF Jr, Fischer RP et al: Intracranial pressure monitoring in the acute neurological assessment of multi-injured patients. J Trauma 19:497, 1979

8. Bowers SA, Marshall LF: Outcome in 200 consecutive cases of severe head injury in San Diego County: a prospective analysis. Neurosurgery 6:237, 1980

9. Byrnes DP, Ducker TB: Continuous measurement of intracranial pressure in 127 severe head injuries. p. 73–78. In Shulman K, Marmarou A, Miller JD et al (eds): Intracranial Pressure IV. Springer-Verlag, Berlin, 1980

10. Galbraith S, Teasdale G: Predicting the need for operation in the patient with an occult traumatic intracranial hematoma. J Neurosurg 55:75, 1981

11. Lobato RD, Rivas JJ, Portillo JM et al: Prognostic value of the intracranial pressure levels during the acute phase of severe head injuries. Acta Neurochir 28:70, 1979

12. Marshall LF, Smith RW, Shapiro HM: The outcome with aggressive treatment in severe head injuries. Part 1: The Significance of Intracranial Pressure Monitoring. J Neurosurg 50:20, 1979

13. Saul TG, Ducker TB: Effect of intracranial pressure monitoring and aggressive treatment on mortality in severe head injury. J Neurosurg 56:498, 1982

14. Uzzel BP, Obrist WD, Dolinskas CA et al: Relationship of acute CBF and ICP findings to neuropsychological outcome in severe head injury. J Neurosurg 65:630, 1986

15. Lundberg N, Cronqvist S, Kjällquist A: Clinical investigations on interrelations between intracranial pressure and intracranial hemodynamics. Prog Brain Res 30:70, 1968

16. Risberg J, Lundberg N, Ingvar DH: Regional cerebral blood volume during acute transient rises of the intracranial pressure (plateau waves). J Neurosurg 31:303, 1969

17. Matsuda M, Yondea S, Handa H et al: Cerebral hemodynamic changes during plateau waves in brain tumor patients. J Neurosurg 50:483, 1979

18. Kjällquist A, Lundberg N, Ponten U: Respiratory and cardiovascular changes during spontaneous variations of ventricular fluid pressure in patients with intracranial hypertension. Acta Neurol Scand 40:291, 1964

19. Rosner MJ, Becker DP: ICP monitoring: complications and associated factors. Clin Neurosurg 23:494, 1976

20. Mayhall CG, Archer NH, Lamb VA et al: Ventriculostomy related infections: a prospective epidemiologic study. N Engl J Med 310:553, 1984

21. Narayan RK, Pulla RS, Kishore MD et al: Intracranial pressure: to monitor or not to monitor? J Neurosurg 56:650, 1982

22. Vries JK, Becker DP, Young HF: A subarachnoid screw for monitoring intracranial pressure. J Neurosurg 39:416, 1973

23. Koster WG, Kuypers MH: Intracranial pressure and its epidural measurement. Med Prog Technol 7:21, 1980

24. Numoto M, Slater JP, Donaghy RMP: An implantable switch for monitoring intracranial pressure. Lancet 1:578, 1966

25. Ostrup RC, Luersson TG, Marshall LF, Zornow MH: Continuous monitoring of intracranial pressure with a miniaturized fiberoptic device. J Neurosurg 67:206, 1987

26. Crutchfield JS, Narayan RK, Robertson CS, Michael LH: Evaluation of a fiberoptic intracranial pressure monitor. J Neurosurg 72:482, 1990

27. Bunegin L, Albin MS, Rauschhuber R, Marlin AF: Intracranial pressure measurement from the anterior fontanelle utilizing a pneumoelectronic switch. Neurosurg 20:726, 1987

28. Rochefort MJ, Rolfe P, Wilkinson AR: New fontanometer for continuous estimation of intracranial pressure in the newborn. Arch Dis Child 62:152, 1987

29. Albin MS, Carrol RS, Maroon JC: Clinical considerations concerning detection of venous air embolism. Neurosurg 3:390, 1978

30. Perkins-Pearson NAK, Marshall WK, Bedford RF: Atrial pressures in the seated position. Implications for paradoxical air embolism. Anesthesiology 57:493, 1982

31. Cucchiara RF, Nugent M, Seward JB, Messick JM: Air embolism in upright neurosurgical patients: detection and localization by two dimensional transesophageal echocardiography. Anesthesiology 60:353, 1984

32. Muzzi DA, Lossaro TJ, Black S, Nishimura R: Comparison of a transesophageal and precordial ultrasonic Doppler sensor in the detection of venous air embolism. Anesth Analg 70:103, 1990

33. Furuya H, Suzuki T, Okumura F et al: Detection of air embolism by transesophageal echocardiography. Anesthesiology 58:124, 1983

34. Sato S, Toya S, Ohira T et al: Echocardiographic detection and treatment of intraoperative air embolism. J Neurosurg 64:440, 1986

35. Furuya H, Okumura F: Detection of paradoxical air embolism by transesophageal echocardiography. Anesthesiology 60:374, 1984

36. Cucchiara RF, Seward JB, Nisimura RA et al: Identification of patient foramen ovale during sitting position craniotomy by transesophageal echocardiography with positive airway pressure. Anesthesiology 63:107, 1985

37. Black S, Muzzi DA, Nishimura RA, Cucchiara RF: Preoperative and intraoperative echocardiography to detect right-to-left shunt in patients undergoing neurosurgical procedures in the sitting position. Anesthesiology 72:436, 1990

38. English JB, Westenskow D, Hodges MR, Stanley TH: Comparison of venous air embolism monitoring methods in supine dogs. Anesthesiology 48:425, 1978

39. Maroon JC, Albin MS: Air embolism diagnosed by Doppler ultrasound. Anesth Analg 55:399, 1974

40. Maroon JC, Goodman JM: Horner TG, Campbell RL: Detection of minute venous air embolism with ultrasound. Surg Gynecol Obstet 127:1236, 1968

41. Tinker JH, Gronert GA, Messick JM, Michenfelder JD: Detection of air embolism, a test for positioning of right atrial catheter and Doppler probe. Anesthesiology 43:104, 1975

42. Buckland RW, Manners JM: Venous air embolism during neurosurgery: a comparison of various methods of detection in man. Anesthesia 31:633, 1976

43. Drummond JC, Prutow RJ, Scheller MS: A comparison of the sensitivity of pulmonary artery pressure, end-tidal carbon dioxide, and end-tidal nitrogen in the detection of venous air embolism in the dog. Anesth Analg 64:688, 1985

44. Matjasko MJ, Petrozza P, Mackenzie CF: Sensitivity of end-tidal nitrogen in venous air embolism detection in dogs. Anesthesiology 63:418, 1985

45. Matjasko MJ, Hellman J, Mackenzie CF: Venous air embolism, hypotension and end-tidal nitrogen. Neurosurgery 21:378, 1987

46. Matjasko MJ, Gunselman J, Delaney J, Mackenzie CF: Sources of nitrogen in the anesthesia circuit. Anesthesiology 65:229, 1986

47. Marshall WK, Bedford RF: Use of a pulmonary artery catheter for detection and treatment of venous air embolism: a prospective study in man. Anesthesiology 52:131, 1980

48. Bedford RF, Marshall WK, Butler A, Welsh JE: Cardiac catheters for diagnosis and treatment of venous air embolism: a prospective study in man. J Neurosurg 55:610, 1981

49. Sloan TB, Kimorec MA: Detection of venous air embolism by airway pressure monitoring. Anesthesiology 64:645, 1986

50. Michenfelder JD, Terry HR Jr, Daw EF, Miller RH: Air embolism during neurosurgery: a new method of treatment. Anesth Analg 45:390, 1966

51. Bunegin L, Albin MS, Hesel PE et al: Positioning the right atrial catheter: a model for reappraisal. Anesthesiology 55:343, 1981

52. Colley PS, Artru AA: Bunegin-Albin catheter improves air retrieval and resuscitation from lethal venous air embolism in dogs. Anesth Analg 66:991, 1987

53. Tohans TG: Multiorificed catheter placement with an intravascular electrocardiographic technique. Anesthesiology 64:411, 1986

54. Warner DO, Cucchiara RF: Position of proximal orifice determines electrocardiogram recorded from multiorificed catheter. Anesthesiology 65:235, 1986

55. Bunegin L, Albin MS: Balloon catheter increases air capture. Anesthesiology 57:66, 1982

56. Diaz PM: Balloon catheter should increase recovery of embolized air. Anesthesiology 57:66, 1982

57. Lee DS, Kuhn J, Shaller MJ: Migration of tips of central venous catheters in seated patients. Anesth Analg 63:949, 1984

58. Bendo AA, Kass IS, Hartung J, Cottrell JE: Neurophysiology and Neuroanesthesia. p. 885–886. In Barash PG, Cullen BF, Stoelting RK (eds): Clinical Anesthesia. 2nd Ed. JB Lippincott, Philadelphia, 1992

59. Levy WJ, York DH, McCaffrey M et al: Motor evoked potentials from transcranial stimulation of the motor cortex in humans. Neurosurgery 15:287, 1984

60. Maccabee PJ, Amassian VE, Craaco RQ et al: Stimulation of the human nervous system using the magnetic coil. J Clin Neurophysiol 8:38, 1991

61. Ghaly RF, Stone JL, Aldrete A, Levy WJ: The effect of nitrous oxide on transcranial magnetic-induced electromyographic responses in the monkey. J Neurosurg Anesthesiol 2:175, 1990

62. Ghaly RF, Stone JL, Aldrete A, Levy WJ: Effects of incremental ketamine hydrochloride doses on motor evoked potentials (MEPs) following transcranial magnetic stimulation: a primate study. J Neurosurg Anesthesiol 2:79, 1990

63. Ghaly RF, Stone JL, Levy WJ et al: The effect of etomidate on motor evoked potentials induced by transcranial magnetic stimulation in the monkey. Neurosurgery 27:936, 1990

64. Kety SS, Schmidt CF: The determination of cerebral blood flow in man by the use of nitrous oxide in low concentrations. Am J Physiol 143:53, 1945

65. Bishop CCR, Powell S, Rutt D, Brows NL: Transcranial Doppler measurement of middle cerebral artery blood flow velocity: a validation study. Stroke 17:913, 1986

66. Murkin JM, Lee DH: Noninvasive measurement of cerebral blood flow: techniques and limitations. Can J Anaesth 38:7, 1991

67. Sekhar LN, Wechslow LR, Yonas H et al: Value of transcranial Doppler examination in the diagnosis of cerebral vasospasm after subarachnoid hemorrhage. Neurosurgery 22:813, 1988

68. Black S, Ockert DB, Oliver WC, Cucchiara RF: Outcome following posterior fossa craniectomy in patients in the sitting or horizontal positions. Anesthesiology 69:49, 1988

69. Artru AA, Cucchiara RF, Messick JM: Cardiorespiratory and cranial nerve sequelae of surgical procedures involving the posterior fossa. Anesthesiology 52:83, 1980

70. Whitby JD: Electrocardiography during posterior fossa operations. Br J Anaesth 35:624, 1963

71. McPherson RW, Szymanski T, Rogers MC: Somatosensory evoked potential changes in position related brainstem ischemia. Anesthesiology 61:88, 1984

72. Grundy BL, Procopio PT, Janetta PJ: Evoked potential changes produced by positioning for retromastoid craniectomy. Neurosurgery 10:766, 1982

73. Horner SG, Daube JR, Ebersolde MJ et al: Improved preservation of facial nerve function with use of electrical monitoring during removal of acoustic neuromas. Mayo Clin Proc 62:92, 1987

74. Jones TH, Chiappa KH, Young RR et al: EEG monitoring for induced hypertension for surgery of intracranial aneurysms. Stroke 10:292, 1979

75. Tempelhoff R, Modica PA, Rich KM, Grubb Jr RL: Use of computerized electroencephalographic monitoring during aneurysm surgery. J Neurosurg 71:21, 1989

76. Muizelaar JP: The use of electroencephalography and brain protection during operation for basilar aneurysms. Neurosurgery 25:899, 1989

77. Friedman WA, Kaplan BL, Day AL et al: Evoked potential monitoring during aneurysm operation: observations after fifty cases. Neurosurgery 20:678, 1987

78. Schramm J, Koht A, Schmidt G et al: Surgical and electrophysiologic observations during clipping of 134 aneurysms with evoked potential monitoring. Neurosurgery 26:61, 1990

79. Pickard JD, Matheson M, Patterson J, Wyper D: Prediction of late ischemic complications after cere-

bral aneurysm surgery by the intraoperative measurement of cerebral blood flow. J Neurosurg 53: 305, 1980

80. Barnett GH, Little JR, Ebrahim ZY et al: Cerebral circulation during arteriovenous malformation operation. Neurosurgery 20:836, 1987

81. Newell DW, Grady MS, Eskridge JM, Winn HR: Distribution of angiographic vasospasm after subarachnoid hemorrhage: implications for diagnosis by transcranial Doppler ultrasonography. Neurosurgery 27:574, 1990

82. Newell DW, Winn HR: Transcranial Doppler in cerebral vasospasm. Neurosurg Clin North Am 1: 319, 1990

83. Awad IA, Carter P, Spetzler RF et al: Clinical vasospasm after subarachnoid hemorrhage: response to hypervolemia, hemodilution and arterial hypertension. Stroke 18:365, 1987

84. Kassell NF, Peerless SJ, Durward QJ et al: Treatment of ischemic deficits from vasospasm with intravascular volume expansion and induced arterial hypertension. Neurosurg 11:337, 1982

85. Steed DL, Peitzman AB, Grundy BL, Webster MW: Causes of stroke in carotid endarterectomy. Surgery 92:634, 1982

86. Bosiljevac JE, Farha SJ: Carotid endarterectomy: results using regional anesthesia. Am Surg 46:403, 1980

87. McKay RD, Sundt TM, Michenfelder JD et al: Internal carotid artery stump pressure and cerebral blood flow during carotid endarterectomy: modification by halothane, enflurane, and Innovar. Anesthesiology 45:390, 1976

88. Kelly JJ, Callow AD, O'Donnell TF et al: Failure of carotid stump pressures. Its incidence as a predictor for a temporary shunt during carotid endarterectomy. Arch Surg 114:1361, 1979

89. Beebe HG, Pearson JM, Coatsworth JJ; Comparison of carotid artery stump pressure and EEG monitoring in carotid endarterectomy. Am Surg 44:655, 1978

90. Sundt TM Jr, Sharbrough FW, Anderson RE, Michenfelder JD: Cerebral blood flow measurements and electroencephalograms during carotid endarterectomy. J Neurosurg 41:310, 1974

91. Sundt TM Jr, Sharbrough FW, Piepgras DG et al: Correlation of cerebral blood flow and electroencephalographic changes during carotid endarterectomy: with results of surgery and hemodynamics of cerebral ischemia. Mayo Clin Proc 56:533, 1981

92. Messick JM Jr, Casement B, Sharbrough FW et al: Correlation of regional cerebral blood flow (rCBF) with EEG changes during isoflurane anesthesia for carotid endarterectomy: critical rCBF. Anesthesiology 66:344, 1987

93. McFarland HR, Pinkerton JA, Frye D: Continuous electroencephalographic monitoring during carotid endarterectomy. J Cardiovasc Surg 29:12, 1988

94. Rampil IJ, Holzer JA, Quest DO et al: Prognostic value of computerized EEG analysis during carotid endarterectomy. Anesth Analg 62:186, 1983

95. Chiappa KH, Burke SR, Young RR: Results of electroencephalographic monitoring during 376 endarterectomies: use of a dedicated minicomputer. Stroke 10:381, 1979

96. Myers RR, Stockard JJ, Saidman LJ: Monitoring of cerebral perfusion during anesthesia by time-compressed Fourier analysis of the electroencephalogram. Stroke 8:331, 1977

97. Spackman TN, Faust RJ, Cucchiara RF et al: A comparison of aperiodic analysis of the EEG with standard EEG and cerebral blood flow for detection of ischemia. Anesthesiology 66:229, 1987

98. Moorthy SS, Markland ON, Dilley RS et al: Somatosensory-evoked responses during carotid endarterectomy. Anesth Analg 61:879, 1982

99. Markland ON, Dilley RS, Moorthy SS, Warren C: Monitoring of somatosensory evoked responses during carotid endarterectomy. Arch Neurol 41: 375, 1984

100. Lam AM, Manninen PH, Ferguson GG, Nantau W: Monitoring electrophysiologic function during carotid endarterectomy: a comparison of somatosensory evoked potentials and conventual electroencephalogram. Anesthesiology 75:15, 1991

101. Branston NM, Symon L: Cortical EP, blood flow and potassium changes. p. 527. In Barber C (ed): Evoked Potentials. University Park Press, Baltimore, 1980

102. Halsey JH, McDowell HA, Gelman S: Transcranial Doppler and rCBF compared in carotid endarterectomy. Stroke 17:1206, 1986

103. Albin MS, Bunegin L, Gilbert J, Babinski MF: Anesthesia for spinal cord injury. p. 138. In Porter SS (ed): Problems in Anesthesia Neuroanesthesia. Vol 4. JB Lippincott, Phildelphia, 1990

104. MacKenzie CF, Shin B, Krishnapradad D et al: Assessment of cardiac respiratory function during surgery on patients with acute quadriplegia. J Neurosurg 62:843, 1985

105. Grundy BL: Monitoring of sensory evoked potentials during neurosurgical operations: methods and applications. Neurosurgery 11:556, 1982

106. Dinner DS, Luders H, Lesser RP et al: Intraoperative spinal somatosensory evoked potential monitoring. J Neurosurg 65:807, 1986

Monitoring Intracranial Pressure

19

David S. Warner
Martin D. Sokoll

Although intermittent short-term measurement of cerebrospinal fluid pressure was made as early as 1891 by Quincke,[1] the continuous measurement of intracranial pressure (ICP) is of more recent origin.[2,3] This technique, now practiced on a widespread basis, has provided an improved understanding of intracranial fluid dynamics and other aspects of intracranial disease processes.

A variety of acute brain insults, such as head trauma, tumor, subarachnoid hemorrhage, operative procedures, cerebrovascular occlusive disease, and other conditions, may result in increased ICP. That knowledge of ICP can serve as an early warning of impending disaster is well proven. What has not yet been proved is that this knowledge increased either quantity or quality of recovery from brain insult.

MEASUREMENT OF INTRACRANIAL PRESSURE

Basic Mechanisms

The intracranial compartment has a fixed volume in each individual. This volume is shared by the brain substance—cerebrospinal fluid—and blood. A change in volume of one of these is usually accompanied by a change in volume of the other two. Thus, when an increase in cellular mass occurs, the volume of cerebrospinal fluid and/or intracranial blood must be decreased to keep total volume constant. Since the volume of cerebrospinal fluid and intracranial blood volume that can be

replaced is limited, the result is an intracranial pressure-volume relationship (Fig. 19-1). This relationship consists of an initial flat portion that represents a region of "compensation," during which the increase in cellular volume (i.e., edema) or size of a space-occupying lesion is compensated for by a decrease in either cerebrospinal fluid volume, blood volume, or both and results in a very small change in ICP. When the latter two approach their maximum volume shift, an increase in cellular volume or lesion size results in a modest increase in pressure, producing a "knee" in this pressure-volume relationship. Further increases in cellular or lesion volume then produces a rapid increase in intracranial pressure called the phase of "decompensation." An increase in intracranial content is not limited to cellular volume, but may be due to an increase of cerebrospinal fluid volume, as in hydrocephalus, or other factors, such as subdural or epidural hematomas, intraparenchymal abscess, or trauma-induced edema. Whatever the cause of the increased volume, the only compensatory mechanisms available are a decrease in cerebrospinal fluid and/or intracranial blood volume.

The measurement of ICP and response of ICP to volumetric challenges can, to some extent, be useful in determining where the patient's position is on the intracranial pressure-volume curve.[4] This knowledge can be of importance, since the patient may be close to decompensation and yet show little change in clinical signs.[5,6]

The phase of decompensation, with its resultant rise in intracranial pressure, can have significant physiologic effects. Cushing[7] observed, in animal experiments, that an abrupt elevation of intracranial pressure caused a compensatory increase in blood pressure. He also described, in addition to systemic arterial hypertension, symptoms of bradycardia and irregular respiration (the so-called "Cushing triad").

The physiologic basis of these changes is probably twofold. First, increase in ICP with no change in blood pressure results in a decreased cerebral perfusion pressure. A sufficient decrease in cerebral perfusion pressure leads to cerebral ischemia. This then causes stimulation of the cardiovascular centers, resulting in an increase in blood pressure. Although Cushing originally described a concomitant bradycardia, tachycardia may also be seen. The mechanism underlying tachycardia may be related to a physiologic attempt to increase cardiac output. The second mechanism responsible for physiologic changes is transtentorial herniation resulting in pressure on medullary cardiovascular and respiratory centers.

Another benefit of monitoring ICP is the ability to calculate cerebral perfusion pressure (CPP). Perfusion pressure of an organ is usually defined as mean arterial blood pressure (MABP) minus venous pressure. For the brain, this can be expressed with satisfactory accuracy as MABP minus intracranial pressure[8–11]:

$$CPP = MABP - ICP$$

Knowledge of cerebral perfusion pressure can be of considerable importance. The normal level of cerebral perfusion pressure is in excess of 60 mmHg. As the level of cerebral perfusion pressure decreases below 60 mmHg, tissue perfusion becomes progressively more depressed and is likely to be inadequate at perfusion pressures of less than 40 mmHg.[12–14]

Previous Experience

Monitoring of ICP appears to have had its origin in 1951.[2] The first large series of patients to undergo continuous ICP monitoring was that of Lundberg.[3]

In his monograph on ICP monitoring, Lundberg described two types of waveforms seen in patients with increased ICP. The first, and most significant of these, is the A wave or plateau wave. It is seen in those patients with elevated or borderline elevated ICP and consists of a further elevation of ICP to levels of 50 to 100 mmHg that persists for a number of minutes before returning to baseline level. This type of pressure wave usually occurs in those patients with a poor neurologic outcome. The second type of pressure wave, the B wave, is of lower amplitude and shorter duration and does not have the poor prognosis associated with the A wave (Fig. 19-2). Since B waves usually last only a few minutes, with normal ICP between, it is obvious that continuous rather than intermittent monitoring of ICP is necessary to detect this pathology. Similarly, it is advantageous to measure pressure on the injured side of the brain rather than contralaterally or from the spinal subarachnoid space. This conclusion is based on the observation that if ICP is markedly elevated, there can be a clinically significant discrepancy in ICP when recorded at sites increasingly distant from the pathologic process.[15–17] Measurement of spinal cerebrospinal fluid pressure may be decreased by obstruction of the cerebrospinal fluid pathway as a result of medullary herniation. Under these circumstances, ICP is continuously and significantly higher than the spinal cerebrospinal fluid pressure.[18]

The patient with increased ICP, without direct monitoring of the pressure, may show surprisingly few symptoms before profound neurologic deteri-

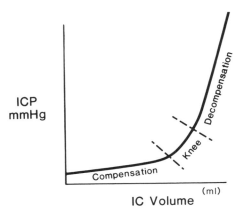

Fig. 19-1. Intracranial pressure-volume relationship. As intracranial pressure increases there is, at first, little change in pressure during the phase of "compensation." With further increase in volume, the pressure begins to increase, forming a "knee." Still further increases in volume cause a marked rise in pressure during the phase of "decompensation."

oration occurs.[5,19,20] The reason for rapid deterioration in the absence of preceding signs or symptoms is the suddenness with which intracranial herniation can occur. Knowing the directly measured ICP may allow the physician to anticipate and possibly prevent herniation. Since therapy is available for controlling ICP to some extent, knowledge of the pressure and the effect of therapeutic intervention should be useful in the care of patients.

When properly recorded with most techniques, ICP will show small fluctuations with each heartbeat. With proper amplification, the ICP recorded should be similar in shape, but lower in amplitude than the arterial pressure wave. Further, the waveform should reflect the respiratory cycle, particularly in patients undergoing positive pressure ventilation. Positive inspiratory pressure results in decreased cerebral venous outflow, with resultant increase in cerebral blood volume and an ICP increase in the range of 2 to 5 mmHg. The recording of a rounded pressure wave suggests that, for some reason, true ICP is not being recorded. An ICP waveform demonstrating characteristics of both the cardiac and respiratory cycles provides reassurance that the monitor has been properly placed and that an accurate value is being recorded. For this reason, it is important that the transducer be associated with a monitor allowing the waveform to be continuously assessed.

PROPERTIES OF THE IDEAL TRANSDUCER

The ideal transducer would have all the following properties:

1. The recording must accurately reflect ICP. Spinal cerebrospinal fluid pressure is not acceptable.
2. There should be little or no risk of infection. Minimizing the seriousness of an infection implies that the technique should be extradural.
3. Insertion of the device should produce no brain damage.
4. The procedures for insertion and removal must be simple.
5. If it is to be implantable, it must be small.
6. It must be drift-free with time and temperature and capable of being calibrated in situ.
7. It should allow freedom of patient movement.
8. It should have adequate sensitivity.
9. It should be impervious to the environment.
10. It should have extended usability (weeks).
11. It should not be too expensive.

CLINICAL USE

Head Injury

The use of ICP monitoring in the patient with head injury is well established.[21-23] What is less certain is the ICP level at which therapy should be

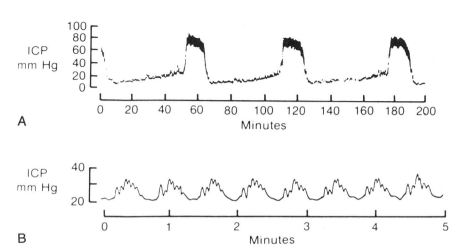

Fig. 19-2. **(A)** and **(B)** Types of intracranial pressure waves. Note differences in magnitude and duration of pressure elevations.

instituted.[24–26] An ICP value less than 10 mmHg is well within the normal range, but a pressure above 20 mmHg is seriously elevated. The border between normal and elevated ICP has not been well defined, particularly with reference to improving patient recovery. This is relevant because aggressive treatment of intracranial hypertension carries substantial risk and cost (e.g., neuromuscular blockade and hyperventilation, barbiturate coma, etc.).[27,28] There is agreement among many authors that aggressive treatment of intracranial hypertension should be commenced if ICP values are >25 mmHg. There is also evidence that reduction of the therapeutic threshold value to 15 mmHg increases both the number and the condition of survivors. Further, early aggressive treatment lessens the incidence of elevated ICP (25 mmHg or higher).[26] In other studies, survival is significantly related to low average ICP levels achieved at least in part by aggressive therapy.[3,29,30] What is probably most important in predicting outcome is the course of ICP values in the acute phase. Patients with persistently elevated ICP that remains refractory to therapy fare the worst.[29]

The necessity of monitoring ICP in all patients with head injury has been addressed by Narayan and colleagues.[29] They have compared the clinical course of patients with various neurologic signs and with findings on computed tomography (CT) scans. Those patients having either a low- or high-density lesion on CT scan had a high incidence (53 to 63 percent) of intracranial hypertension. Those having a normal CT scan had a lower incidence (13 percent) of elevated ICP. In the group with normal CT scans, three factors were associated with elevated ICP: (1) age over 40 years, (2) systolic blood pressure under 90 mmHg, and (3) unilateral or bilateral posturing. In contrast, patients with normal multimodality evoked potentials, without motor posturing, and with a Glasgow coma scale rating of 7 or more, tended to have normal ICP. Abnormal eye movements, abnormal pupil reactions, hypoxemia, and anemia were not significantly associated with intracranial hypertension.[29] Thus, those patients with abnormal admission CT scans merit ICP monitoring. Additionally, ICP monitoring may be indicated in patients having any two of the three characteristics described earlier, despite a normal CT scan.

The observation of ICP and its changes with time can also be used to evaluate patient progress after head injury and to determine the need for more or less therapeutic intervention.[31] Various therapeutic modalities may be begun sequentially to keep ICP below a predetermined level. Continuous monitoring of ICP allows the clinician to assess the effectiveness of each therapeutic step and to decide if more aggressive therapy is indicated.

Reye's Syndrome

Although not initially appreciated, it is now well accepted that uncontrolled increased ICP is one of the major factors in mortality from Reye's syndrome.[32–37] The syndrome is one of persistent vomiting and progressive encephalopathy without focal neurologic signs. It is usually possible to document a viral infection preceding onset of the syndrome. Abnormalities of the liver, kidney, heart, lungs, and pancreas may occur concurrent with the encephalopathy. The mechanism of development of encephalopathy is unclear. Very early in the course of the disease, ICP may be normal. With passage of time and increase in severity of the encephalopathy, the ICP is consistently seen to be elevated, though usually only for a few days. In severe cases, it may persist for as long as 3 weeks or more. Without control of ICP, the mortality rate of severe Reye's syndrome approaches 100 percent. If ICP can be controlled, the mortality rate is markedly decreased to 20 to 30 percent.[33] Jenkins and colleagues[32] demonstrated the necessity of not only monitoring ICP, but also of calculating cerebral perfusion pressure. A large percentage of survivors will have little or no neurologic deficit.

Brain Tumors

Although it is not frequently performed, Becker and coworkers[38] have maintained that monitoring ICP in patients with brain tumors gives clinically useful data. In their series of 50 patients, they noted that 2 patients had cerebral perfusion pressure values of less than 60 mmHg. In the same group, 18 patients had ICP values of 10 mmHg or less. In 23 patients, the ICP ranged between 11 and 39 mmHg, whereas 9 patients had ICP values in excess of 40 mmHg. Also, 9 patients exhibited plateau waves preoperatively. The anesthesiologist may observe the effect of anesthetic agents or therapy on ICP. Postoperatively, monitoring of ICP can give evidence of hemorrhage and/or edema.

Despite these concerns, intraoperative monitoring of ICP in patients with brain tumors is not widely performed. This may be due to information obtained from earlier studies, which allows the anesthesiologist to accurately predict the effect of anesthetic agents and techniques on brain bulk.[39–45] Also available is direct visual observation of brain bulk when the dura is opened. Further, there is little information to guide the decision-making process regarding a clinically meaningful anesthetic-induced increase in ICP.[44,46,47]

Other Conditions

It has also been suggested that ICP be monitored in patients with fulminant hepatic failure.[48] In Hanid's study,[48] 8 of 10 patients died; 6 of the 8 had ICP values in excess of 50 mmHg. The 2 patients who survived and 2 of those who died had peak ICP values of less than 50 mmHg. In this study, the terminal ICP increase occurred very rapidly. Although the patients' primary problem was hepatic failure, the final mechanism of death was probably increased ICP.

Many trauma patients are admitted to the hospital with multiple system injury. Frequently, head injury is combined with chest, abdomen, or extremity injury, which may need operative intervention. Palmer and coworkers[49] suggest that patients who are comatose and need emergency operations for hemodynamic stabilization should have ICP monitored during surgery. In some cases it may be indicated to place an ICP monitor in a head-injured patient who might otherwise not undergo monitoring but is now scheduled to undergo surgery for other problems (e.g., to repair a long-bone fracture). This patient, if awake, would be monitored by assessing the neurologic condition. During anesthesia this capability is lost and events such as impending herniation or accumulation of hematoma would go unheralded until very late signs (hypertension and/or dilated pupils) occur. Factors such as the patient's preoperative status as well as the length and type of planned procedure are important in making this decision. If acute increases in ICP occur during the operation, it may be necessary to discontinue the procedure and evaluate with CT scanning. In dire circumstances, exploratory trephines should be inserted.

A number of techniques using measurement of ICP to determine intracranial compliance (elastance) have been reported. The first of these consists of injecting increasing volumes of sterile saline into the intracranial space through the monitoring device and observing resultant changes in ICP and the rate at which it returns to the preinjection level.[4] If ICP returns to the preinjection level promptly, the patient is probably on the compensated portion of the curve. If a few seconds are required for the pressure to return, then the patient is either on the knee or decompensated portion of the curve. In addition to measurement of ICP, the pressure-volume index (PVI) may also be calculated[50,51]:

$$PVI = \Delta ICP/\text{volume injected}$$

The PVI is taken as the slope of a semilogrithmic plot of a pressure-volume curve generated by either injecting or withdrawing known volumes of cerebrospinal fluid into the intracranial compartment. The PVI has also been defined as the volume of cerebrospinal fluid necessary to increase ICP by a factor of 10 (i.e., in the normal individual $\approx$ 25 ml of cerebrospinal fluid would be expected to increase ICP from 6 to 60 mmHg). The PVI is thought to be a reflection of the compressibility of the intracranial vascular compartment.

Another technique for assessing compliance consists of a computerized analysis of the mean ICP measured for 10 seconds every 5 minutes compared to the standard deviation of this measurement. Regression analysis allowed the authors to plot a curve resembling an ICP-volume curve.[52] A method of determining intracranial compliance by observation of the pulse width of the recorded ICP has also been attempted.[53] Though some correlation of increasing pulse width with a similar increase in ICP could be found, the relationship is not clinically useful.

Long-term monitoring of ICP has also been reported as useful in the diagnosis of adult or normal-pressure hydrocephalus.[24,54–57] In these patients, intermittently measured ICP may be normal. Continuous monitoring, however, demonstrates elevations of ICP that occur principally during sleep. This diagnosis is essential because the uncontrolled disease process results in progressive impairment of cerebral function. The process appears to be terminated by closed ventricular drainage. Monitoring of ICP has also been useful in diagnosis and long-term follow-up of patients with pseudotumor cerebri.[58,59]

METHODS

A number of techniques are in use to monitor ICP, including the intraventricular catheter, the subarachnoid bolt, and a variety of epidurally or intraparenchymally placed transducers. In addition, measurement of anterior fontanelle pressure has been used to gain, more indirectly, information concerning ICP in pediatric patients.

Intraventricular Catheter

The intraventricular catheter technique was used first by Guillaume and Janny[2] and later by Lundberg.[3] The technique necessitates a small scalp incision and a twist drill burr hole through the skull. A styletted catheter of soft nonreactive plastic (Silastic) is then inserted into the lateral ventricle. The scalp incision is closed and covered with a sterile dressing. The ventricular catheter is connected to sterile tubing filled with a sterile saline solution and thence to an external transducer. This transducer may be mounted either on the patient's head or, more commonly, at the patient's bedside. The ventricular catheter usually gives a reliable indication of ICP.

There are many potential problems with the intraventricular catheter. To obtain accurate pressure readings, the system must be free of all air bubbles. Since the transducer is mounted externally, it must be kept zeroed at a particular reference point on the patient's head. Frequently, this reference is the external auditory meatus. If the patient's head is elevated or lowered, the transducer must be elevated or lowered to the same extent, with the zero point of the transducer again at the same point at the patient's head in order to have reproducible and reliable readings.

This system, with its external length of tubing, is subject to many artifacts that can result from striking or moving the external tubing. Virtually any manipulation of this tubing causes pressure waves against the transducer dome, which will be recorded. The recording system must be fluid-tight, since the loss of small amounts of fluid through leakage can reduce the ICP recorded.

In patients with an increased ICP and small ventricles, it can be technically difficult to locate the lateral ventricle. Once the lateral ventricle has been found, the catheter can later become obstructed with small bits of brain tissue or, as the result of even further increases in ICP, the side walls of the ventricle can collapse around the catheter with resultant obstruction.[10] To aid in preventing the latter, the CSF drainage reservoir is usually kept about 15 cm above head level. In contrast, if the ventricular catheter is being used to treat hydrocephalus, such as might occur after subarachnoid hemorrhage, care must be taken to not drain cerebrospinal fluid in an uncontrolled fashion for at least two reasons. First, there is a belief that rapid reduction in ICP might attenuate a tamponade against further hemorrhage and result in rebleeding from the aneurysm.[60] Second, if a rapid reduction of CSF volume occurs, the bridging veins between the convexity and dural sinuses may tear, leading to acute subdural hematoma formation. For this reason, a ventriculostomy is usually clamped during patient transport or surgical positioning.

Other problems related to the intraventricular catheter are damage to the brain during insertion and infection.[25,61] In experienced hands, the former should not be a significant problem. Infection in the form of ventriculitis is a well-known complication of long-term placement of an intraventricular catheter. The incidence of ventriculitis reported is variable, but to a great extent is directly related to the duration of time the catheter is in place.[25,61] Because of the recognized incidence of ventriculitis, most practitioners give prophylactic antibiotics to patients with intraventricular catheters in place.

The types, incidence, and factors contributing to complications of ICP monitoring via intraventricular catheters have been studied.[61,62] Among factors contributing to a higher complication rate were (1) an older age, (2) longer duration of monitoring, and (3) longer duration of steroid administration. The relationship to the use of prophylactic antibiotics is not clear.

The specific benefits of the intraventricular catheter as a method of monitoring ICP include the ability to remove cerebrospinal fluid from the ventricular space to help keep ICP within an acceptable range and the ability to recalibrate the transducer. All transducers tend to drift with prolonged use. The extent of drift, which is variable, but clinically significant, is usually most marked in the first 2 days. This shortcoming of current transducers has motivated some practitioners to precalibrate implanted transducers under sterile conditions for 2 to 3 days before use.[10]

Subarachnoid Bolt

The subarachnoid bolt is an alternative method for monitoring ICP.[38,63] The equipment consists of a stainless steel bolt through which a hole has been drilled lengthwise. A Luer-Lok connector is soldered to the head of this bolt (Fig. 19–3). The distal 2 to 3 mm of the bolt threads are removed. The bolt is fitted into a burr hole made 2 to 3 cm anterior to the frontoparietal suture line. The dura is incised and curetted up into the burr hole to avoid the presence of a dural flap, which might obstruct the tip of the bolt. The twist drill hole should be slightly smaller than the size of the bolt so that the bolt, when twisted into the skull, will seat securely. Once the bolt is in place, it may fill spontaneously with cerebrospinal fluid. If it does not, the bolt must be filled with saline and connected to sterile transducer tubing filled with sterile saline. Again, as with the intraventricular pressure apparatus, the transducer may be mounted either directly on the head or to the side of the bed. The tubing must be free of all air bubbles. It is extremely important with this monitoring technique that there be no fluid leaks at any of the junctions. To check this, the entire device should be assembled and connected to a manometer filled with fluid. Under these circumstances, there should be no decrease in the fluid level in the manometer as it is observed over a least 1 hour.

The brain substance may contact and obstruct the tip of the bolt giving artifactually low readings. To some extent, this can be compensated for by drilling side holds just proximal to the tip of the bolt. As with the intraventricular monitor, early transducer drift is a problem. With all intraventricular or subarachnoid pressure measuring devices, it is important to use a system that does *not* have an automatic flush, such as is commonly used for arterial pressure monitoring. The volume infused can be significant in a patient whose ICP is on the rising limb of the compliance curve, in addition to the added possibility for infection. From a practical standpoint, the subarachnoid bolt is

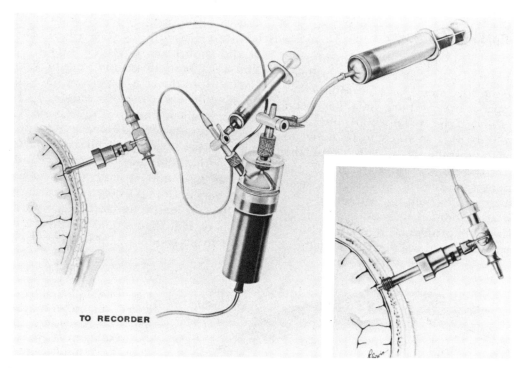

TO RECORDER

Fig. 19-3. Subarachnoid intracranial pressure bolt. The device is screwed into a twist drill hole in the skull. The dura is incised and curetted up into the hole. The insert shows that the tip of the bolt lies in the subarachnoid space.

most useful in adults. Although it has been used in infants and children, the thinness of the skull tends to make the bolt insertion unstable.

The incidence of complications with this device has been analyzed by Rosner and Becker.[61] In their series of 112 patients, there was an 18 percent incidence of complications (20 patients). All of these complications were the result of infection. Of these infections, 2 percent involved only the site of the bolt insertion, 1 percent were infections with subdural empyema, and 9 percent resulted in meningitis with a positive cerebrospinal fluid culture. Infection of the burr hole site, with or without positive cerebrospinal fluid culture, occurred in 7.2 percent of the patients. Five cases were thought definitely to be related to the monitoring device, and of the remaining 15 patients, 8 were thought to be possibly related, and 7 probably not related to monitoring. There was a direct relationship between duration of ICP monitoring and incidence of complications. In addition, those patients showing complications were older and had been receiving steroids longer than those who showed no complications. No deaths were directly related to the pressure monitoring device.

Epidural Transducers

Two primary types of epidural monitoring devices are in current use. In both cases, a transducer with a pressure-sensitive membrane is positioned in the epidural space after a burr hole has been drilled (Fig. 19–4). The pressure of the dura against the membrane is assumed to be equal to the pressure of the intradural contents against the inner surface of the dura. This is so, only if the transducing membrane is coplanar with the dura. Without coplanar application, the intradural pressures detected are modified by tension factors in the dura and become progressively less accurate.

The first type is known as the Ladd epidural transducing unit (Fig. 19–5). It is based on the principle of the Numoto pressure switch.[64] A small movable membrane mounted in a solid housing is placed in contact with the dura. Originally the apparatus involved a mirror positioned within the housing, which moved as the membrane moved in response to changes in epidural pressure. A system of fiberoptics allowed determination of the magnitude of mirror displacement. In response to this displacement, air was pumped into the housing at a sufficient pressure to realign the mirror. The pressure required to realign the mirror reflected the ICP. This system has recently been reconfigured to eliminate the optical components of the system (Steritek Intracranial Pressure Monitor, Steritek, Patterson, NJ). Instead, air is introduced into the housing at a pressure sufficient to displace a plenum allowing an exhaust vent to open. The pressure of air on the inflow side is directly related to the ICP.

The second type of currently available epidural pressure transducer is the Gaeltec (Medical Measurements, Inc. Hackensack, NJ). The theory of operation is identical to that employed by conventional arteriovenous strain gauge pressure transducers.[65] The pressure-sensitive membrane is overlaid on the transducer (Fig. 19–6). The back side of the transducer is vented to the atmosphere. Thus recalibration (zeroing) in situ is possible. The Gaeltec transducer is expensive but can be resterilized (ethylene oxide) for reuse.

The primary benefit of the epidural transducer is the extradural placement. Any infection that might occur would be separated from brain by dura.[10] An additional advantage of epidural catheters can be found in patients with coagulopathies (e.g., hepatic coma) where extradural placement is less likely to result in clot formation and exacerbation of ICP than would be the case when the parenchyma is penetrated for placement of a ven-

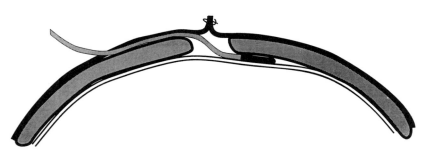

Fig. 19-4. Epidural pressure transducer. The transducer is placed with the pressure-sensitive surface coplanar to the dura. Care is taken to position the transducer so that it is not wedged between the dura and inner table of the skull to avoid artifactually high measurements.

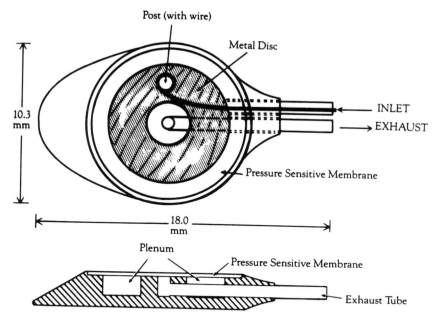

Fig. 19-5. The Steritek epidural ICP monitor. Designed to act as pneumatic flow switch, pressure will build up within the plenum of the sensor to overcome any outside pressure (ICP) against the membrane and reestablish airflow. (Courtesy of Steritek Medical Devices, Patterson, NJ.)

tricular or parenchymal pressure monitor. One shortcoming of epidural transducers is that ICP values are highly dependent upon accurate positioning of the transducer. We many times have seen apparently normal ICP waveforms (i.e., presence of cardiac and respiratory patterns), while the ICP recorded is unusually elevated. This probably results from ''wedging'' the transducer into the angle between the dura and the inner table of the skull. Repositioning of the transducer until a reasonable ICP is measured along with observation of stable values over a period of several minutes eliminates this artifact. Another shortcoming of the epidural technique is that volumetric testing of intracranial

compliance cannot be performed, nor can fluid be aspirated to decrease ICP in acute emergencies. The cost of the equipment is rather high.

Other Transducers

Recently, a miniaturized fiberoptic device has been developed to monitor ICP (Camino Laboratories, San Diego, CA). This system is composed of a 4 French fiberoptic bundle, which is inserted by means of a housing placed through a 2-mm burr hole. The fiberoptic bundle is inserted through the dura with the tip resting in the parenchyma. Subdural and intraventricular placements have also

Fig. 19-6. Gaeltec epidural ICP monitor. The monitor consists of a miniaturized strain gauge transducer with pressure-sensitive membrane positioned against the dura. This monitor can be zeroed in situ by injection of air, which exceeds ICP and lifts the membrane away from the transducer producing equal pressure across the strain gauge. (Courtesy Medical Measurements Inc. Hackensack, NJ.)

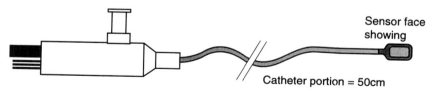

Showing assembled device with air injection port for confirming zero baseline.

Sensor face showing

Catheter portion = 50cm

been used. A light beam is directed from the sending fiber to a reflective movable diaphragm. The reflected light is transmitted through the receiving fiber to the amplifier connector, where the light energy is converted to an electrical signal. ICP can be presented either as a digital display or through an auxiliary monitor as the pressure waveform (Fig. 19–7). In animal models, recordings from this device have been compared to pressures derived from intraventricular catheters or subarachnoid bolts with excellent correlation.[66,67] In human studies, pressures recorded by this device closely followed intraventricular catheter pressures (within 2 to 5 mmHg).[17,66,68] On two occasions, the Camino catheter maintained persistent waveforms when those obtained from a bolt were dampened.[66]

In addition to the shortcomings noted previously, all of the discussed methods of monitoring ICP markedly limit patient mobility because they all require lead-wire connections to the recorder. For the comatose patient, this presents no problem, but for the alert patient this represents a considerable inconvenience. Even more important, the tubes and wires protruding from the skull may pose a significant danger to the confused or combative patient, either in terms of infection should the sterile system become contaminated or from mechanical injury.

A number of attempts have been made to devise totally implantable monitoring devices.[10,69,70] A glass transensor has been developed by Olsen and colleagues.[69] In this device, a pair of coaxial coils forms a resonant circuit whose frequency varies with the relative coil spacing. This system is completely implantable and requires no external connections, but an external inductively coupled oscillating detector is needed. This system measures episodic changes in pressure better than static pressure.

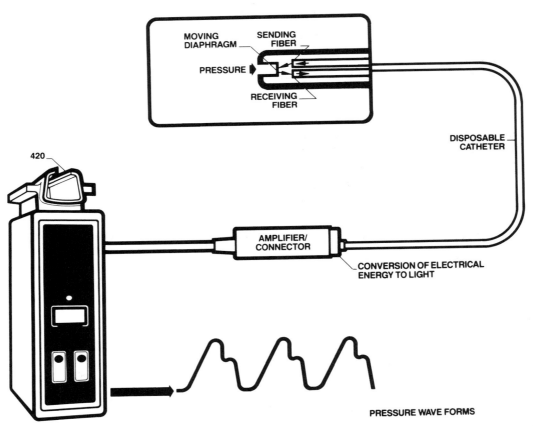

Fig. 19-7. The Camino intracranial pressure monitor. The sensing device is mounted at the end of a 4 French fiberoptic bundle. The tip may be placed in the subdural space, intraparenchymally or in the lateral ventricle. (Courtesy of Camino Laboratories, San Diego, CA.)

Rylander and colleagues[70] have measured ICP with an induction-powered oscillator transducer. The device is powered by an external radiofrequency field and induction coupling through the skin. This device appears to work well, but, with time, loses some of its sensitivity due to dural scarring. A somewhat similar system for recording ICP has been developed by Ko.[71,72] The external power source is again a radiofrequency generator. The transducer is a silicon piezoresistive bridge. Transducer drift with this system has been relatively small.

A number of transducers have been designed to measure anterior fontanelle pressure in newborns and infants.[73–76] These techniques have the benefit of being noninvasive. Coplanar application of the transducer is needed for accurate pressure recording. Although these devices do not record ICP, relative changes in ICP and fontanelle pressure correlate closely. Discussion continues regarding proper placement of these transducers.[77]

SUMMARY

The measurement of ICP can provide information of great use in evaluating the patient's condition, progress, and need or lack of need for therapy under many diverse conditions. Aside from the monetary cost of providing the monitoring equipment, the primary cost to the patient appears to be that of infection. With the intraventricular catheter, this can be a serious ventriculitis. With the subdural bolt, the usual infections reported are a small amount of osteomyelitis or a localized infection, which is usually easy to treat. With epidural transducers, infections, which are usually minor, are isolated from the brain by the dural membrane. Where monitoring of ICP is indicated, the benefit to the patient far outweighs the cost.

REFERENCES

1. Quinke H: Über Hydrocephalus. Verhandl Cong Inn Med 10:321, 1891
2. Guillaume I, Janny P: Manométrie intracranie et continue: intereact de la méthode et premiers résultats. Rev Neurol (Paris) 85:748, 1951
3. Lundberg N: Continuous recording and control of ventricular fluid pressure in neurosurgical practice. Acta Psychiatr Scand 36 (Suppl.): 149:1, 1960
4. Bouma G, Muizelaar J, Bandoh K, Marmarou A: Blood pressure and intracranial pressure-volume dynamics in severe head injury: relationship with cerebral blood flow. J Neurosurg 77:15, 1992
5. Marshall L, Toole B, Bowers S: The National Traumatic Coma Data Bank. Part 2: Patients who talk and deteriorate: implications for treatment. J Neurosurg 59:285, 1983
6. Constantini S, Cotev S, Rappaport Z et al: Intracranial pressure monitoring after elective intracranial surgery: a retrospective study of 514 consecutive patients. J Neurosurg 69:540, 1988
7. Cushing H: Some experimental and clinical observations concerning the states of increased intracranial pressure. Am J Med Sci 124:375, 1902
8. Miller J, Stanek A, Langfitt T: Concepts of cerebral perfusion pressure and vascular compression during intracranial hypertension. Prog Brain Res 35:411, 1972
9. Rowan J, Johnson I, Harper A et al: Perfusion pressure in intracranial hypertension. p. 165. In Brock M, Dietz E (eds): Intracranial Pressure. Springer-Verlag, New York, 1972
10. Langfitt T: Clinical methods for monitoring intracranial pressure and measuring cerebral blood flow. Clin Neurosurg 23:302, 1976
11. Beck D, Kassell N: Cerebral pressure module: technical note. Neurosurgery 5:267, 1979
12. Fitch W, MacKenzie E, Harper A: Effects of decreasing arterial blood pressure on cerebral blood flow in the baboon. Circ Res 37:550, 1975
13. Chan K, Miller J, Dearden N et al: The effect of changes in cerebral perfusion pressure upon middle cerebral artery blood flow velocity and jugular bulb venous oxygen saturation after severe brain injury. J Neurosurg 77:55, 1992
14. Robertson C, Contant C, Gokaslan Z et al: Cerebral blood flow, arteriovenous oxygen difference, and outcome in head injured patients. J Neurol Neurosurg Psychiatry 55:594, 1992
15. Miller J, Bobo H, Kapp J: Inaccurate pressure readings for subarachnoid bolts. Neurosurgery 19:253, 1986
16. Weaver D, Winn H, Jane J: Differential intracranial pressure in patients with unilateral mass lesions. J Neurosurg 56:660, 1982
17. Gambardella G, d'Avella D, Tomasello F: Monitoring of brain tissue pressure with a fiberoptic device. Neurosurgery 31:918, 1992
18. Langfitt T, Weinstein J, Kassell N, Simeone F: Transmission of increased intracranial pressure. I. Within the craniospinal axis. J Neurosurg 21: 989, 1964
19. Belopavlovic M, Buchthal A, Beks J, Journee H: Some principles of postoperative epidural pressure monitoring. Acta Neurochir 55:227, 1981

20. Rosner M, Becker D: ICP monitoring: complications and associated factors. Clin Neurosurg 23:494, 1976

21. Koster W, Kuypers M: Intracranial pressure and its epidural measurement. Med Prog Technol 7:21, 1980

22. Marshall L, Smith R, Shapiro H: The outcome with aggressive treatment in severe head injuries. Part II: Acute and chronic barbiturate administration in the management of head injury. J Neurosurg 50:26, 1979

23. Tindall G, Meyer G, Iwata K: Current methods for monitoring patients with head injury. Clin Neurosurg 22:98, 1975

24. Gucer G, Viernstein L, Walker E: Continuous intracranial pressure recording in adult hydrocephalus. Surg Neurol 13:323, 1980

25. Papo I, Caruselli G: Long-term intracranial pressure monitoring in comatose patients suffering from head injuries. Acta Neurochir 39:187, 1977

26. Saul T, Ducker T: Effect of intracranial pressure monitoring and aggressive treatment on mortality in severe head injury. J Neurosurg 56:498, 1982

27. Schalen W, Messeter K, Nordström C: Complications and side effects during thiopentone therapy in patients with severe head injuries. Acta Anaesthesiol Scand 36:369, 1992

28. Muizelaar J, Marmarou A, Ward J et al: Adverse effects of prolonged hyperventilation in patients with severe head injury: a randomized clinical trial. J Neurosurg 75:731, 1991

29. Narayan R, Kishore P, Becker D et al: Intracranial pressure: to monitor or not to monitor? J Neurosurg 56:650, 1982

30. Alberico A, Ward J, Choi S et al: Outcome after severe head injury: relationship to mass lesions, diffuse injury, and ICP course in pediatric and adult patients. J Neurosurg 67:648, 1987

31. Unterberg A, Kiening K, Schmiedek P, Lanksch W: Long-term observations of intracranial pressure after severe head injury: the phenomenon of secondary rise of intracranial pressure. Neurosurgery 32:17, 1993

32. Jenkins J, Glascow J, Black G et al: Reye's syndrome: assessment of intracranial monitoring. Br Med J 294:337, 1987

33. Kindt G, Waldman J, Kohl S et al: Intracranial pressure in Reye's syndrome. JAMA 231:822, 1975

34. Pfenninger G: Die montriniuerliche mitrakronielle Druküberwachung und neure Aspeckte su der Neurointensivpfleger beim Kind. Schweiz Med Wochenschr 109:1693, 1979

35. Pizzi F, Schut L, Berman W et al: Intracranial pressure monitoring in Reye's syndrome. Child Brain 2:59, 1976

36. Shaywitz B, Leventhal J, Kramer M et al: Prolonged continuous monitoring of intracranial pressure in severe Reye's syndrome. Pediatrics 59:595, 1977

37. Venes J, Shaywitz B, Spencer D: Management of severe cerebral edema in the metabolic encephalopathy of Reye-Johnson syndrome. J Neurosurg 48:903, 1978

38. Becker D, Young H, Vries J et al: Monitoring in patients with brain tumors. Clin Neurosurg 2:364, 1975

39. Adams R, Cucchiara R, Gronert G et al: Isoflurane and cerebrospinal fluid pressure in neurosurgical patients. Anesthesiology 54:97, 1981

40. Marx W, Shah N, Long C et al: Sufentanil, alfentanil, and fentanyl: impact on cerebrospinal fluid pressure in patients with brain tumors. J Neurosurg Anesth 1:3, 1989

41. Cottrell J, Patel K, Turndorf H, Ransohoff J: Intracranial pressure changes induced by sodium nitroprusside in patients with intracranial mass lesions. J Neurosurg 48:329, 1978

42. Cottrell J, Gupta B, Rappoport H et al: Intracranial pressure during nitroglycerin-induced hypotension. J Neurosurg 53:309, 1980

43. Jung R, Reinsel R, Marx W et al: Isoflurane and nitrous oxide: comparative impact on cerebrospinal fluid pressure in patients with brain tumors. Anesth Analg 75:724, 1992

44. Todd M, Warner D, Sokoll M et al: A prospective comparative trial of three anesthetics for supratentorial craniotomy: fentanyl/propofol, iosflurane/N₂O, and fentanyl/N₂O. Anesthesiology 78:1005, 1993

45. From R, Warner D, Todd M, Sokoll M: Anesthesia for craniotomy: a double-blind comparison of alfentanil, fentanyl, and sufentanil. Anesthesiology 73:896, 1990

46. Crosby G, Todd M: On neuroanesthesia, intracranial pressure, and a dead horse. J Neurosurg Anesth 2:153, 1990

47. Michenfelder J: [The 27th Rovenstein Lecture]. Neuroanesthesia and the achievement of professional respect. Anesthesiology 70:695, 1989

48. Hanid M, Davies M, Mellon P et al: Clinical monitoring of intracranial pressure in fulminant hepatic failure. Gut 21:866, 1980

49. Palmer M, Perry JJ, Fisher R et al: Intracranial pressure monitoring in the acute neurologic assessment of multi-injured patients. J Trauma 19:497, 1979

50. Gray W, Rosner M: Pressure-volume index as a function of cerebral perfusion pressure. Part 1: The effects of cerebral perfusion pressure changes and anesthesia. J Neurosurg 67:369, 1987

51. Gray W, Rosner M: Pressure-volume index as a function of cerebral perfusion pressure. Part 2: The effects of low cerebral perfusion pressure and autoregulation. J Neurosurg 67:377, 1987

52. Szewczykowski J, Dytko P, Kunicki A et al: A method of estimating intracranial decompensation in man. J Neurosurg 5:155, 1976

53. Wilkinson H, Schuman N, Ruggiero J: Nonvolumetric methods of detecting impaired intracranial compliance or reactivity. J Neurosurg 50:758, 1979

54. Leech P, Stokes B: On the uses of intracranial pressure monitoring. Med J Aust 2:285, 1976

55. Papada G, Poletti C, Guazzoni A et al: Normal pressure hydrocephalus: relationship among clinical practice, CT scan, and intracranial pressure monitoring. J Neurosurg 30:115, 1986

56. Friedland R: Normal-pressure hydrocephalus and the sage of the treatable dementias. JAMA 262:2577, 1989

57. Vanneste J, Augustijn P, Dirven C et al: Shunting normal-pressure hydrocephalus—do the benefits outweigh the risks?: a multicenter study and literature review. Neurology 42:54, 1992

58. Cooper P, Moody S, Sklar F: Chronic monitoring of intracranial pressure using an in vivo calibrating sensor: experience in patients with pseudotumor cerebri. Neurosurgery 5:666, 1979

59. DiLauro L, Tropelli F, Poli R et al: Recording of intracranial pressure and daily drainage in pseudotumor cerebri: a preliminary study. Surg Neurol 22:178, 1984

60. Pare L, Delfino R, Leblanc R: The relationship of ventricular drainage to aneurysmal rebleeding. J Neurosurg 76:422, 1992

61. Rosner M, Becker D: Monitoring: complications and associated factors. Clin Neurosurg 23:494, 1976

62. Mickell J, Reigel D, Cook D et al: Intracranial pressure: monitoring and normalization therapy in children. Pediatrics 59:606, 1977

63. Vries J, Becker D, Young H: A subarachnoid screw for monitoring intracranial pressure: technical note. Neurosurgery 39:416, 1973

64. Numoto M, Slater J, Donaghy R: An implantable switch for monitoring intracranial pressure. Lancet 1:578, 1966

65. Roberts P, Fullenwider C, Stevens F, Pollay M: Experimental and clinical experience with a new solid state intracranial pressure monitor with in vivo zero capability. p. 104. In Ishii S, Nagai H, Brock M (eds): Intracranial Pressure V. Springer-Verlag, Berlin, 1983

66. Ostrup R, Luerssen T, Marshall L, Zornow M: Continuous monitoring of intracranial pressure with a miniaturized fiberoptic device. J Neurosurg 67:206, 1987

67. Crutchfield J, Narayan R, Robertson C, Michael L: Evaluation of a fiberoptic intracranial pressure monitor. J Neurosurg 72:482, 1990

68. Chambers I, Mendelow A, Sinar E, Modha P: A clinical evaluation of the camino subdural screw and ventricular monitoring kits. Neurosurgery 26:421, 1990

69. Olsen E, Collins C, Loughborough W et al: Intracranial pressure measurement with a miniature passive implanted pressure transensor. Am J Surg 113:727, 1967

70. Rylander H, Taylor H, Wissinger J et al: Chronic measurement of epidural pressure with an induction-powered oscillator transducer. J Neurosurg 44:465, 1976

71. Ko W, Leung A, Cheng E et al: Intracranial pressure telemetry system I: hardware development. Biotelemetry Patient Monit 8:131, 1981

72. Leung A, Ko W, Spear T, Bettice J: Intracranial pressure telemetry system using semi-custom integrated circuits. IEEE Trans Biomed Eng 33:386, 1986

73. Bunegin L, Albin M, Rauschhuber R, Marlin A: Intracranial pressure measurement from the anterior fontanelle utilizing a pneumoelectronic switch. Neurosurgery 20:726, 1987

74. Friesen R, Thieme R: Changes in anterior fontanelle pressure during cardiopulmonary bypass and hypothermic circulatory arrest in infants. Anesth Analg 66:94, 1987

75. Rochefort M, Rolfe P, Wilkinson A: New fontanometer for continuous estimation of intracranial pressure in the newborn. Arch Dis Child 62:152, 1987

76. Vidyasagar D, Raju T: A simple noninvasive technique for measuring intracranial pressure in the newborn. Pediatrics 59:957, 1977

77. Bunegin L, Albin M: Pitfalls encountered in relating anterior fontanelle pressure to intracranial pressure. [Letter to the editor]. Anesth Analg 66:1196, 1987

Temperature Monitoring

20

Randall C. Cork

The practice of measuring body temperature was initiated in 1776 by the English surgeon John Hunter, who used a mercury-in-glass thermometer placed under the patient's tongue.[1] Recording patient temperature as part of the anesthetic record was first done by Harvey Cushing in 1895.[2] The monitoring of body temperature continues as an important aspect of anesthetic vigilance, but our methods have changed significantly since the times of John Hunter and Harvey Cushing. Even the simple medical ritual of taking someone's temperature has become another high-tech endeavor. An examination of this technology necessitates a basic clinical understanding of the physiology of temperature control. We shall begin with a discussion of physiology, and then go on to look at the special situations of hypothermia and hyperthermia with which the anesthesiologist must be prepared to contend. We shall then examine the monitoring devices now available and attempt to provide some clinical guidelines for intraoperative and perioperative temperature monitoring and maintenance.

PHYSIOLOGY

Body heat is one of the many pleasant physical manifestations of life. There is usually an equilibrium between the amount of heat generated by metabolism and the amount lost to the environment. When this equilibrium is disturbed, body temperature will either increase or decrease. With this alteration in body temperature, the risk of undesirable physiologic sequelae always increases. Body temperature is important—that is why it is called a vital sign.

Heat Production and Heat Loss

Heat production occurs by means of cellular metabolism, which can be affected by basal metabolic rate, muscular activity, sympathetic arousal, hormonal activity, and heat exogenously administered. Heat loss occurs by four specific physical phenomena (Fig. 20-1):

Radiation

Loss of heat by radiation occurs with release of infrared rays. Everything in the universe that is not at absolute zero temperature emits infrared rays. A body loses or gains temperature as a function of whether it is sending out or receiving the majority of infrared energy compared with other objects in the immediate environment. Most of the heat loss from a patient (<60 percent) occurs by this mechanism.[3] The amount of heat lost by radiation is affected by cutaneous vasodilation.

Conduction

Heat conduction to the operating room table, blankets, and other objects with which the patient is in contact represents only a small fraction of heat loss (<3 percent), because these objects rapidly warm up. This also holds true for heat conduction in a perfectly still environment to the air surrounding the patient.

Convection

Perfectly still environments are hard to come by. When warmed air moves away and is replaced by cool air, the subsequent heat lost by conduction to this cool air is called heat loss by convection. This accounts for about 12 percent of body heat loss in an operating room.

Evaporation

Water evaporation from the body results in heat loss. Evaporation from the skin surface and from the lungs is often referred to as insensible water loss. For every gram of water that is evaporated, 0.58 kcal of heat is lost, and at normal room temperature this amounts to about 25 percent of all heat loss.[4] This heat loss is even greater when the humidity is low. If the room temperature is greater than the body temperature—seldom the case in modern refrigerated operating rooms—heat is gained by conduction and radiation. Evaporation then becomes the only way in which the body can cool itself. That is why the body has a special gland, the sweat gland, which it uses for cooling.[5]

Newborns and Infants

The infant represents a special situation in temperature control because of differences from the adult in the way in which heat is produced and lost. The newborn does not shiver during the first few days of life unless exposed to very low temperatures (<15°C).[6] Newborns and infants use a method of heat production called nonshivering thermogenesis.[7] Newborns and infants have a special tissue called brown fat, located between the scapulae and around the large vessels. This tissue is sympathetically innervated and has a high content of mitochondria. When the infant is exposed to cold, sympathetic discharge causes these tissues to heat up. When this happens, as much as 25 percent of the cardiac output is diverted to the brown fat, so that the heat is distributed to the rest of the body.[8] Sick infants may have less brown fat; hypoxic infants cannot provide the mitochondria with enough oxygen for adequate heat generation.

Infants have less subcutaneous fat and 2 to 2.5 times the surface-area-to-mass ratio of adults.[9] With less insulation and proportionately more surface area, infants are more apt to lose heat by radiation, conduction, and convection (Fig. 20-2). Although newborns have six times as many sweat glands per unit area as an adult, their peak response to heat loss by evaporation of sweat is only one-third that of an adult.[10]

Control of these mechanisms of heat production and heat loss resides in the hypothalamus; warming or cooling the hypothalamus elicits the appropriate physiologic responses.[11] Anesthesia upsets thermal control in two ways: (1) direct inhibition of the hy-

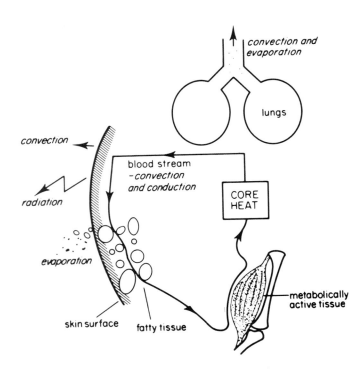

Fig. 20-1. Sources of heat production and heat loss. Heat is produced in metabolically active tissue to maintain core temperature. This heat is then dissipated through the body and into the environment by conduction, convection, evaporation, and radiation. (From Holdcroft,[1] with permission.)

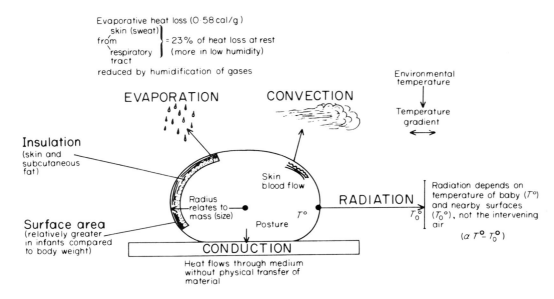

Fig. 20-2. Newborns and infants present a special risk of heat loss because of their higher ratio of surface area to mass. (From Brown and Fisk,[9] with permission.)

pothalamus results in less effective feedback control via this organ, and (2) peripheral vasodilation redistributes body heat and increases heat loss.[12-16] Since anesthesiologists cripple the body's ability to regulate its own thermal homeostasis, they must monitor the body temperature and take appropriate precautions to avoid wide deviations from normal temperature.

HYPOTHERMIA

Hypothermia is the most common temperature disorder resulting from anesthesia and surgery. Patients do not arrive in the operating room in a hypothermic state, but what we do to them there tends to make them so. *Res ipsa loquitur.*

Postoperative Incidence

We studied 198 men and women to look at the incidence, degree, and duration of hypothermia in adult patients arriving in the recovery room after anesthesia and surgery.[17] Patients undergoing craniotomies or open-heart procedures, those with coagulation defects or preoperative temperature elevations, and patients undergoing tympanoplasties were excluded from the study. This last restriction was employed because all temperature measure-

ments were made using tympanic membrane probes.[18] Temperature was measured within 5 minutes after admission to the recovery room and every 15 minutes thereafter. Presence or absence of shivering was also noted at these same times.

On admission to the recovery room, tympanic membrane temperatures averaged $35.6 \pm 0.1°C$ (mean ± SEM). About 60 percent of patients had temperatures of less than 36.0°C (Fig. 20-3). One

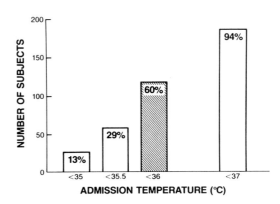

Fig. 20-3. Percentage of patients with core temperature (tympanic membrane) of less than 35.0, 35.5, 36.0, and 37.0°C on admission to recovery room. *Hatched bar* indicates percentage of patients with hypothermia. (From Vaughan et al.,[17] with permission.)

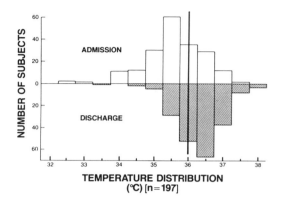

Fig. 20-4. Core temperature (tympanic membrane) on admission to recovery room and at discharge from recovery room. Left of the vertical black line indicates hypothermia (*T*<36°C). (From Vaughan et al.,[17] with permission.)

of many beneficial aspects of the stay in the recovery room was return to normothermia (Fig. 20-4). The majority (81 percent) of patients were normothermic upon leaving the recovery room. Nevertheless, in spite of an 82-minute average stay, 18 percent of patients were sent to the wards while still hypothermic. Older patients (≥60 years) were colder after anesthesia and surgery and remained colder for a longer period of time than did younger patients. No difference in core temperature was observed between the group of patients who had undergone regional anesthesia and the group who had undergone general anesthesia. Shivering was not related to hypothermia on admission to the recovery room or at 15 minutes, but at 30 and 45 minutes, hypothermic patients shivered significantly more than did normothermic patients (Fig. 20-5).

Causal Factors

One conclusion drawn from these data is that most of the normothermic patients who enter the operating room are hypothermic when they leave. We must also conclude that we do something in the operating room to cause patients to cool down. What are the specific agents of this effect?

1. The room is cold. Most operating rooms are kept at 18 to 21°C for the comfort of the sterile, heavily gowned operating team. Increasing the temperature produces perspiration and may increase chances of microbial transfer and seeding of wounds.[19] Morris and Wilkey[20] observed that patients lost heat in the operating room when the room temperature was under 21°C. They also observed that one of the things surgeons complain about is uncomfortably warm operating room temperature when it is over 17°C. They suggest that a reasonable compromise is to lower the room temperature to 17°C after the patient is draped.

2. The room can be windy. Use of laminar flow ventilation increases heat loss by convection 61

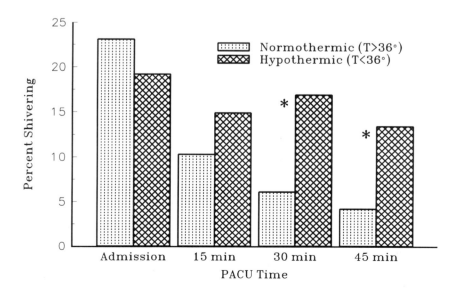

Fig. 20-5. Percent of patients shivering on admission to the Post Anesthesia Care Unit (PACU) was not a function of temperature. Percent normothermic (*T*>36°C) and percent hypothermic (*T*<36°C) differed significantly at 30 and 45 minutes after admission to the PACU (*$P = .05$).

percent and heat loss by evaporation 19 percent.[21]

3. Nonwarmed intravenous fluids given to patients cause hypothermia.[22]
4. The patient's body core is often exposed to the environment during the surgical procedure and, frequently, body cavities are exposed to cold irrigating solutions on repeated occasions.[23]
5. The direct effects of anesthetics and muscle relaxants ablate the body's feedback system for maintaining normothermia. The hypothalamus is anesthetized by general anesthesia,[15] and both spinal and general anesthesia produce extensive peripheral vasodilation, measurable by increases in skin temperature.[24] Redistribution of heat decreases core temperature with both general and regional anesthesia.[16] Although epidural anesthesia permits more heat production by the patient than does general anesthesia, the amount of heat loss is the same for both techniques.[25] The use of epidural narcotics results in less shivering and more hypothermia than the use of epidural local anesthetics alone.[26] Muscle relaxants impede thermogenesis by eliminating shivering.[27–29] Infants and geriatric patients are especially susceptible to these anesthetic causes of hypothermia.[19,30–32]

Physiologic Consequences

Most perioperative complications from hypothermia result from the altered physiology caused by hypothermia, but many additional postoperative dangers exist in the patient's own attempts at rewarming.

With hypothermia, the efficacy of many of our commonly used anesthetic agents is extended. Hallet[33] demonstrated reduced splanchnic blood flow and diminished liver function during hypothermia. Drugs that rely on liver metabolism for conjugation and excretion, such as morphine, have significantly prolonged half-lives.[34] Decreased glomerular filtration rate and renal blood flow increase the half-lives of drugs that depend on the kidney for clearance.[35] Prolonged *d*-tubocurarine neuromuscular blockade during hypothermia is due to delayed serum clearance (Fig. 20-6), as well as to delayed renal and biliary elimination.[29,36] Muscle relaxation lasts longer with pancuronium and hypothermia, due to the reduction in pancuronium metabolism (liver) as well as its elimination (liver and kidney).[28]

Hypothermia to 34.3°C more than doubles the duration of action of vecuronium (67 vs 29 minutes) and doubles the time to recovery of train-of-four twitch stimuli (23 vs 11 minutes).[37]

Bleeding is prolonged by hypothermia. In addition to the decreased activity of other coagulation factors, platelets are sequestered in the liver during hypothermia,[38] an effect which is completely reversed by rewarming.

Blood viscosity increases during hypothermia, raising the risk of decreased perfusion.[39] This risk can be compounded by the shift in the oxyhemoglobin dissociation curve to the left, resulting in less oxygen delivery to the tissues (Fig. 20-7).[1,40] Blood gas results must be adjusted for hypothermia, since increased oxygen solubility causes decreased PaO_2.[41]

Hypothermia is associated with increased mortality in trauma patients.[42] Postoperatively, hypothermia is associated with protein breakdown and nitrogen loss[43] as well as hypokalemia.[44]

Shivering and increased metabolism are used by the awakening patient to restore normothermia. Shivering increases tissue oxygen consumption by as much as 400 to 500 percent.[45] Also, an increased minute ventilation is required to provide the additional oxygen.[46] Cardiac output must also be increased to assure delivery of oxygen to the tissues. However, as the patient's temperature returns to-

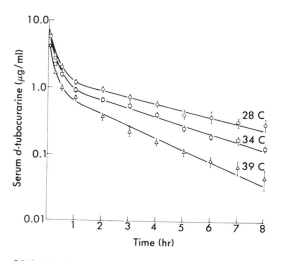

Fig. 20-6. Prolonged neuromuscular blockade after intravenous bolus of *d*-tubocurarine in cats of 28, 34, and 39°C. All groups significantly different ($P<.05$) after 3 minutes. (From Ham et al.,[27] with permission.)

ward normal, the peripheral vasoconstriction secondary to hypothermia becomes less marked, and rewarming shock may result. The capacitance of the circulatory system increases during rewarming, and volume administration may be necessary to prevent hypotension.[47]

Prevention

All these responses to hypothermia and rewarming are important to the anesthesiologist. Preventing hypothermia is by far the preferred choice over dealing with complications. Radiant heat lamps, warm blankets, warmer operating rooms, heated intravenous fluids and forced-air warmers provide us with the means to maintain normothermia. The use of closed-circuit anesthesia is also an effective means of maintaining the patient's body heat.[48] Passive heat/moisture exchangers, also called *artificial noses*, in the anesthesia circuit have been shown to be effective in maintaining patient temperature by minimizing evaporative heat loss.[49] Heated humidification prevents evaporative heat loss and has been shown to reduce recovery time in outpatients.[50] The use of reflective blankets for intraoperative heat conservation has proved useful when more than 60 percent of a patient's body surface can be covered.[51]

Once we take over the body's temperature main-

tenance functions, we must serve as the hypothalamus *in absentia*. This necessitates careful attention to the patient's temperature. We address this after a brief review of an increasingly rare but still dangerous aspect of increased intraoperative temperature.

HYPERTHERMIA

The problem of intraoperative hyperthermia used to be considered typical of the febrile patient, premedicated with atropine and anesthetized with diethyl ether in a humid environment.[52] We must still be vigilant with this problem, but malignant hyperthermia has taken its place in the minds of most anesthesiologists concerned about hyperthermia.

Malignant Hyperthermia

This disease is manifested by a hypermetabolic crisis that can be triggered by anesthetic agents and that can have a high mortality (70 percent) if not recognized and treated promptly.[53] The first case was reported in 1960 by Denborough and Lovell.[54] Since then we have learned a lot about recognizing and treating the disease. Following is a useful outline for quick review. This or something like it should be posted in any area which is used for anesthesia.

1. *Definition:* Malignant hyperthermia is a fulminant hypermetabolic crises triggered by certain anesthetics or adjuvants.
2. *Incidence:* Usually cited as 1 in 20,000, males more than females; familial autosomal dominant transmission with variable penetrance.
3. *Mortality:* Up to 70 percent without dantrolene treatment; with early dantrolene may be substantially reduced.
4. *Causative anesthetics/adjuvants:* Most frequently implicated are halogenated anesthetics and succinylcholine; no anesthetic should be presumed to be absolutely safe.
5. *Choice of anesthesia in susceptible individuals:* Sodium thiopental, propofol, nitrous oxide, narcotics (fentanyl, morphine), tranquilizers (droperidol, diazepam), nondepolarizing muscle relaxants, conduction or local anesthesia without epinephrine. Especially avoid halogenated anesthetics, cyclopropane, diethyl ether, and depolarizing muscle relaxants.

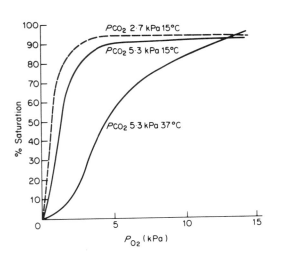

Fig. 20-7. Hypothermia shifts the oxyhemoglobin dissociation curve to the left, resulting in less unloading of oxygen to the tissues (2.7 kPa = 20 mmHg; 5.3 kPa = 40 mmHg). (From Holdcroft,[1] modified from Callaghan et al.,[40] with permission.)

6. *Prophylaxis:*
   a. Dantrolene: 5 mg/kg/24 hours p.o. or 2.5 mg/kg i.v. one-half hour preoperatively.
   b. Clean anesthesia machine and delivery circuit; flow oxygen through machine preoperatively; remove halogenated anesthetics from machine; fresh CO_2 absorbent in cannister or a nonrebreathing system.
7. *Clinical findings:* Variable course, tachycardia, tachypnea usually the presenting sign, *not* pyrexia.
   a. Early: increasing end-tidal CO_2, sometimes muscle rigidity (including isolated masseter spasm), tachycardia, tachypnea, unstable blood pressure, arrhythmia, cyanosis, profuse sweating, rapid temperature increase.
   b. Late: skeletal muscle swelling; left heart failure; renal failure; disseminated intravascular coagulopathy.
   c. Laboratory: respiratory and metabolic acidosis, hypoxemia, increased serum levels of K^+, Mg^{2+}, myoglobin, creatine phosphokinase, myoglobinuria.
8. *Monitoring:* Routine (malignant hyperthermia suspect): ECG, temperature, blood pressure, end-tidal CO_2, pulse oximeter. After presumed onset of malignant hyperthermia: arterial line for blood pressure and blood sampling for pH, P_{CO_2}, and electrolytes; central venous pressure; Foley catheter for urinary output.
9. *Supplies:* Have immediately available: Dantrolene for i.v. administration (36 amp), sodium bicarbonate (12 amp): iced saline ($12 \times 1,000$ ml bottles): furosemide; mannitol; procainamide; regular insulin, 50% glucose; ice chips, cooling blankets. Extracorporeal perfusion apparatus in hospitals with experience in its use.
10. *Treatment:*
    a. STOP ANESTHESIA AND SURGERY IMMEDIATELY. Continue with safe anesthetics if surgery cannot be stopped immediately.
    b. Hyperventilate with 100 percent O_2 at high-flow rates. Use new circuit as soon as possible.
    c. Administer:
       (1) Dantrolene: 2.5 mg/kg i.v. initial bolus with increments up to 20 mg/kg total.
       (2) Sodium bicarbonate: 1 to 2 mEq/kg increments guided by arterial pH and P_{CO_2}. Bicarbonate will combat hyperkalemia by driving potassium into cells.
    d. ACTIVELY COOL PATIENT. (If febrile)
       (1) Intravenous iced saline (not Ringer's lactate) 15 ml/kg every 10 minutes, for 3 administrations.
       (2) Lavage stomach, bladder, rectum, and peritoneal and thoracic cavities with iced saline.
       (3) Surface cool with ice and hypothermia blanket.
       (4) Extracorporeal circulation and heat exchanger (if facilities available).
    e. Maintain urine output: Mannitol 250 mg/kg i.v., furosemide 1 mg/kg i.v. (up to 4 doses each). Urine output greater than 2 ml/kg/h may help prevent subsequent renal failure.
    f. Procainamide for dysrhythmias: add 15 mg/kg to 100 ml NaCl and infuse over 10 minutes or until ventricular ectopy ceases. Do not use procaine hydrochloride, as it may cause seizures with this dose.
    g. Insulin for hyperkalemia: Add 10 units of regular insulin to 50 ml 50% glucose and titrate to control hyperkalemia. Monitor blood glucose and K^+ levels.
    h. Postoperatively: Continue dantrolene 1 mg/kg i.v. every 6 hours for 72 hours to prevent recurrence. Up to 10 percent of patients may have recurrence within first 8 hours postoperatively.
    h. Call 24-hour hotline: (209) 634-4917, provided by Malignant Hyperthermia Association of the United States (MHAUS). Ask for Index Zero.

Prediction

One aspect of malignant hyperthermia has to do with what we know about predicting the disease during the preoperative evaluation of the patient. There are three major predictors: (1) positive family history, (2) elevated plasma creatine phosphokinase (CPK) levels,[55] and (3) positive muscle biopsy.[56] Once a positive family history is elicited, an elevated blood CPK may be considered diagnostic without further testing. With a positive family history and a normal creatine phosphokinase on three separate occasions, a muscle biopsy should be considered.[53] Measurement of blood CPK alone is 70 percent reliable in estimating susceptibility.[57,58] Reliability is increased to more than 90 percent by obtaining a muscle biopsy for diagnosis.[53] In this way, a high-risk group for malignant hyperthermia can be defined, just as we have defined the very young and very old as high-risk groups for hypothermia.

TECHNOLOGY

The mercury-in-glass thermometer is gradually giving way to thermometers based on more advanced technology.

Thermistors and Thermocouples

Electrical thermometers are now commonly used for intraoperative temperature monitoring. The two most commonly used are the thermistor and the thermocouple.

Electrical resistance of the thermistor (Fig. 20-8) varies as a function of temperature. The principle of a thermocouple is that if a circuit is made up of two dissimilar metal elements, the current in the circuit will be directly proportional to the temperature difference between the two junctions of the dissimilar metals (Fig. 20-9).[59] The way this principle is implemented is that one of the junctions is always kept at a standard reference temperature (e.g., 0°C), while the other junction is located in the temperature probe. Manufacturers provide quite a variety of different probe types, which we will examine more closely in the following discussion of selecting monitoring sites.

Infrared Sensors

Infrared temperature detectors look like otoscopes and are used to measure the temperature of the tympanic membrane. Because tympanic membrane temperature is a very good index of

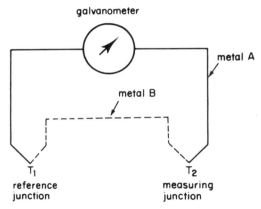

Fig. 20-9. Current, as measured by the galvanometer, is directly proportional to the temperature difference between the two junctions ($T_1 - T_2$) of the dissimilar metals (A and B) composing the circuit. (From Holdcroft,[1] with permission.)

core temperature (more about that later), these probes have been gaining in popularity, especially in recovery rooms and in operating rooms during regional anesthesia. Response time is less than 5 seconds, and a disposable plastic film cover reduces the risk of infection by cross-contamination between patients. Two disadvantages of using this type of probe are: (1) only intermittent spot checks can be made, and (2) the probe must be accurately aimed at the tympanic membrane. False low readings off the sides of the ear canal can be a problem.

Monitoring Sites

Until 1970 most studies involving temperature and anesthesia were conducted using rectal temperature. Whitby and Dunkin[60] suggested the use of nasopharyngeal or esophageal temperatures as more relevant to core temperature, and Benzinger[61] demonstrated that the rectal temperature has minimal thermal significance because the rectum is far removed from the heart and brain. In fact, Benzinger strongly recommends using tympanic membrane temperature as the best indicator of core temperature because tympanic membrane temperature is close to what the hypothalamus senses and attempts to regulate. Studies by Webb,[7] Wilson and colleagues[62] support Benzinger's preference for the tympanic membrane as the best index of core temperature. A significant objection to the use of the tympanic membrane temperature

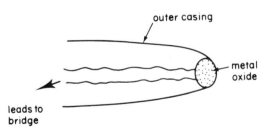

Fig. 20-8. A schematic of a thermistor temperature probe. (From Holdcroft,[1] with permission.)

probe is raised by Wallace and colleagues,[63] who report perforation of the tympanic membrane during anesthesia. Other monitoring sites that have also been employed are the forehead and axilla.[64] Great toe temperature has been recommended by Joly and Weil[65] because it is linearly correlated with cardiac output.

With the menagerie of different temperature probes available, two criteria from measurement engineering—accuracy and precision—may be applied to evaluate which of the temperature-monitoring sites best serve as indicators of core temperature. Accuracy quantitates the difference between a measurement and a true value, whereas precision quantitates the variability of this measurement, as compared with other available measurements.[66] We defined the temperature of the tympanic membrane as the true value for core temperature, and assessed the precision and accuracy of several commonly used sites for measurement of body temperature.[67] We monitored the temperatures of the nasopharynx, esophagus, rectum, bladder, axilla, forehead, and great toe of 56 patients

during anesthesia and surgery. A disposable esophageal stethoscope with a thermocouple was used to monitor esophageal temperature, and a Foley catheter with a thermocouple was used to monitor bladder temperature. Temperatures were recorded at the time the probes were placed and then every 15 minutes until the patient left the operating room.

Accuracy of temperature measurements at each site was assessed as the difference between measured temperature and the ''gold standard'' (tympanic membrane temperature). Precision was calculated as the correlation coefficient between the measured temperature and the tympanic membrane temperature at the same time.

Average temperatures at each site are shown in Figure 20-10 as a function of time from induction of anesthesia. Figure 20-11 illustrates the accuracy of the various temperature monitoring sites as compared with the tympanic membrane. Rectal, bladder, esophageal, and nasopharyngeal temperatures are the most accurate. Precision of temperature measurements as a function of duration of anesthesia is presented in Figure 20-12. Temperature

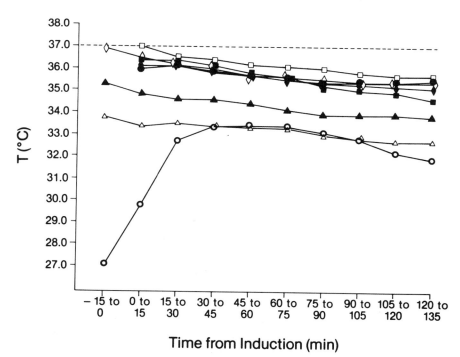

Fig. 20-10. Average intraoperative temperatures for 56 patients as measured by rectal (□), tympanic membrane (◇), bladder (■), esophageal stethoscope (◆), nasopharyngeal (●), axillary (▲), forehead (△), and great toe (○) probes. (From Cork et al.,[67] with permission.)

measurements with the nasopharyngeal, esophageal, and bladder probes are the most precise. The precision of temperature measurement with the rectal probe gradually improves with duration of anesthesia.

Monitoring of temperature at the nasopharynx, esophagus, or bladder appears to have the best combination of accuracy and precision as continuous measurements of core temperature. These sites are recommended when appropriate, rather than subjecting the tympanic membrane of the anesthetized patient to possible trauma.

Liquid Crystal Thermometry

The infrared detector represents a significant technologic advancement in our capabilities to monitor temperature, but another technologic innovation in temperature monitoring might tend to lead us astray. The liquid crystal thermometer is a liquid crystal adhesive strip that may be attached to the patient's forehead. The temperature is read from the adhesive strip as the color of the liquid crystal changes with temperature. This device has been recommended as a monitor for intraoperative hyperthermia[68] and as a continuous temperature monitor during anesthesia.[69]

We studied one of these liquid crystal devices, the Temp-A-Strip (Jelco Laboratories, Raritan, NJ), in 71 patients after anesthesia and surgery.[70] Tympanic membrane temperature was used as the gold standard for core temperature, and compared to Temp-A-Strip temperature at admission to the recovery room, and every 15 minutes for 1 hour (Fig. 20-13). The liquid crystal adhesive correlated poorly with tympanic membrane temperature. The best correlation was seen on admission to the re-

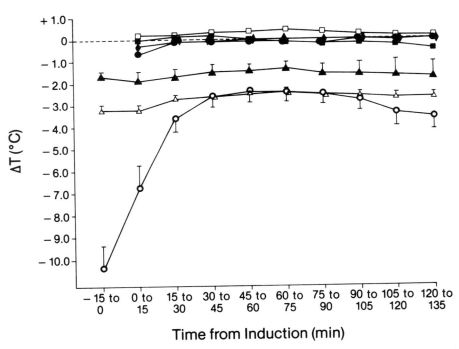

Fig. 20-11. Accuracy of temperature measurement sites as compared with tympanic membrane (TM) temperature. TM temperature is the *dotted line* at zero (0). Rectal (□), bladder (■), esophageal (♦), nasopharyngeal (●) temperatures are the most accurate. Mean axillary (▲) temperatures are 1.5° to 1.9°C below mean TM temperatures (*P* <.05), and mean forehead (△) temperatures are 2.4° to 3.2°C below mean TM temperatures (*P* <.05). Average great toe temperature (○) is 10.4°C below mean TM temperature at the start of anesthesia (*P* <.05), increases to 2.4°C below mean temperature after 45 minutes (*P* <.05), and drops to 3.6° below TM at 120 minutes (*P* <.05). (From Cork et al.,[67] with permission.)

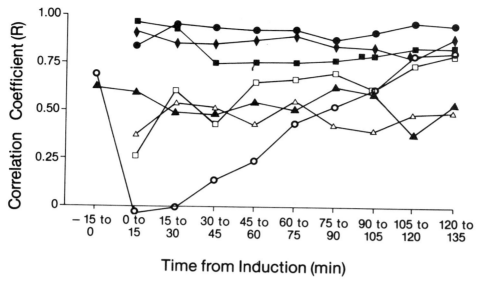

Fig. 20-12. Precision of bladder (■), esophageal (♦), and nasopharyngeal (●), forehead (△), rectal (□), axillary (▲), and great toe (○) temperature measurement sites as correlated with tympanic membrane temperature. Tympanic membrane temperature is not depicted but would be a line at unity (1.00). Precision is quantitated by correlation coefficients. Rectal temperature precision gradually improves from a correlation coefficient of .26 at 0.15 minutes to 0.81 at 120 to 135 minutes. Marked improvement in precision during anesthesia is exhibited by the great toe temperature, which improves from a correlation of −.04 with tympanic membrane temperature at the beginning of anesthesia to .82 after 2 hours of anesthesia. (From Cork et al.,[67] with permission.)

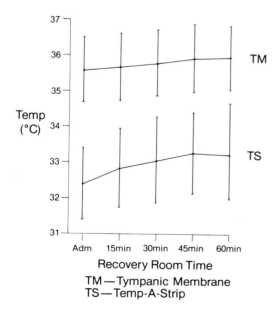

Fig. 20-13. Tympanic membrane (TM) and shell (liquid crystal adhesive strip, TS) temperature measurements taken simultaneously from admission to discharge in recovery room in 71 postsurgical adults. Values are means ± SD. (From Vaughan et al.,[70] with permission.)

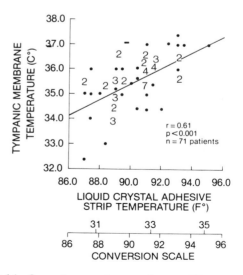

Fig. 20-14. Core (tympanic membrane, TM) and shell (liquid crystal adhesive strip, TS) temperature measurements taken on admission to recovery room from 71 postsurgical adults. Each number in scattergram represents number of points at that locus. (From Vaughan et al.,[70] with permission.)

**TABLE 20-1. Temperature of Forehead by Liquid Crystal
Thermometer Compared with Temperature of Tympanic
Membrane Thermometer**

Recovery Room Time (min)	TS Range (°F)	TM Range (°C)	Correlation Coefficient (r)
0	87.0–95.0	32.5–37.5	0.61
15	85.5–95.0	33.0–37.5	0.54
30	85.0–96.0	33.0–37.5	0.52
45	85.0–96.5	33.2–38.0	0.42
60	85.0–96.0	33.5–38.0	0.39
Discharge	87.0–96.5	33.5–38.0	0.39

Abbreviations: TM, tympanic membrane thermometer; TS, liquid crystal thermometer.
(From Vaughan et al.,[70] with permission.)

covery room (Fig. 20-14), and this was only $r = .61$. Table 20-1 shows that this correlation decreased with time. To examine the use of liquid crystal thermometry as a trend indicator, correlations of changes in tympanic membrane temperature with changes in Temp-A-Strip temperature were analyzed. Table 20-2 shows that these correlations were even worse than the correlations of absolute temperature readings. Liquid crystal thermometry is an excellent example of how the novelty and convenience of a new technology has blinded us to its lack of usefulness in clinical care.

PHILOSOPHY

After inhibiting the patient's own temperature control system, the anesthesiologist has the responsibility of performing as the hypothalamus *in absentia*. The anesthesiologist needs to take steps to prevent changes in body temperature, to monitor the temperature, and then to act on the information received from this monitoring to take whatever actions are necessary to maintain normal body temperature. High-risk groups need special attention. These include the very young and the very old at risk for hypothermia, as well as those who might have a genetic predisposition for malignant hyperthermia. The development of new technologies, such as the infrared detector, is providing us with new ways to monitor temperature. These technologies should be employed when appropriate. However, their efficacy in quantitative terms, such as accuracy and precision at whatever site measured, must be demonstrated.

**TABLE 20-2. Change in Temperature of Forehead by
Liquid Crystal Thermometer Compared with Change in
Temperature of Tympanic Membrane**

Recovery Room Time Period (min)	ΔTS[a] Range (°F)	ΔTM[a] Range (°C)	Correlation Coefficient (r)	Significance (P)
0–15	−2.5 to 4.0	−1.0 to 1.3	.04	.361
0–30	−4.0 to 4.0	−0.8 to 1.8	.11	.193
0–45	−4.0 to 6.0	−0.5 to 2.0	.25	.064
0–60	−4.0 to 5.0	−0.5 to 2.0	.36	.003
0–discharge	−2.0 to 6.0	−0.5 to 2.5	.47	.001

[a]Negative temperature changes indicate temperature decrease.
Abbreviations: ΔTM, tympanic membrane; ΔTS, liquid crystal thermometer.
(From Vaughan et al.,[70] with permission.)

REFERENCES

1. Holdcroft A: Body Temperature Control in Anaesthesia, Surgery, and Intensive Care. Baillière Tindall, London, 1980
2. Keys TE: The History of Surgical Anesthesia. Dover, New York, 1963
3. Guyton AC: Textbook of Medical Physiology. 4th Ed. p. 832. WB Saunders, Philadelphia, 1971
4. Hey EN, Katz G: Evaporative water loss in the newborn baby. J Physiol 200:605, 1969
5. Hemingway A, Price W: The autonomic nervous system and regulation of body temperature. Anesthesiology 29:693, 1968
6. Adamsons K, Gandy GM, James LS: The influence of thermal factors upon oxygen consumption in the newborn human infant. J Pediatr 66:495, 1965
7. Webb GE: Comparison of oesophageal and tympanic temperature monitoring during cardiopulmonary bypass. Anesth Analg 52:729, 1973
8. Heim T, Hull D: The blood flow and oxygen consumption of brown adipose tissue in the newborn rabbit. J Physiol 186:42, 1966
9. Brown TCK, Fisk GC: Anaesthesia for Children. p. 15. Blackwell, London, 1979
10. Foster KG, Hey EN, Katz G: The response of the sweat glands of the newborn baby to thermal stimuli and to intradermal acetylcholine. J Physiol 203:13, 1969
11. Hensel H: Neural processes in thermoregulation. Physiol Rev 53:948, 1973
12. Brennan HJ, Hunter AR, Hohnstone M: Halothane: a clinical assessment. Lancet 2:453, 1957
13. Hemingway A: The effect of barbital anesthesia on temperature regulation. Am J Physiol 134:350, 1941
14. Larson CP, Mazze RI, Cooperman LH, Wollman H: Effects of anesthetics on cerebral, renal, and splanchnic circulations. Anesthesiology 41:169, 1974
15. Theye RA, Michenfelder JD: The effect of halothane on canine cerebral metabolism. Anesthesiology 29:1113, 1968
16. Sessler DI, Moayeri A: Skin-surface warming: heat flux and central temperature. Anesthesiology 73:218, 1990
17. Vaughan MS, Vaughan RW, Cork RC: Postoperative hypothermia in adults: relationship of age, anesthesia, and shivering to rewarming. Anesth Analg 60:746, 1981
18. Benzinger M: Tympanic thermometry in surgery and anesthesia. JAMA 209:1207, 1969
19. Vaughan MS: Nursing treatment of hypothermia in adult recovery room postsurgical patients. p. 81. Doctoral dissertation. University of Arizona, Tucson, 1980
20. Morris RH, Wilkey BR: The effects of ambient temperature on patient temperature during surgery not involving body cavities. Anesthesiology 32:102, 1970
21. English MJM, Searle NR, Scott WAC: Heat loss and the thermal environment of the operating room. Anesthesiology 67:A162, 1987
22. Boyan CP, Howland HS: Blood temperature: a critical factor in massive transfusion. Anesthesiology 22:559, 1961
23. Stephen CR: Postoperative temperature changes. Anesthesiology 22:795, 1961
24. Forreger R: Surface temperatures during anesthesia. Anesthesiology 4:392, 1943
25. Stjernstrom H, Henneberg S, Eklund A et al: Thermal balance during transurethral resection of the prostate: a comparison of general anaesthesia and epidural analgesia. Acta Anaesthesiol Scand 29:743, 1985
26. Johnson MD, Sevarino FB, Lema MJ et al: Effect of epidural sufentanil on temperature regulation in the parturient. Anesthesiology 67:A450, 1987
27. Ham J, Miller RD, Benet LZ et al: Pharmacokinetics and pharmacodynamics of *d*-tubocurarine during hypothermia in the cat. Anesthesiology 49:324, 1978
28. Miller RD, Agoston S, Van der Pol F et al: Hypothermia and the pharmacokinetics and pharmacodynamics of pancuronium in the cat. J Pharmacol Exp Ther 207:532, 1978
29. Zaimis E, Cannard TH, Price H: Effects of lowered muscle temperature upon neuromuscular blockade in man. Science 128:34, 1958
30. France GG: Hypothermia in newborns: body temperatures following anaesthesia. Br J Anaesth 29:390, 1957
31. Harrison GG, Bul AB, Schmidt HJ: Temperature changes in children during general anaesthesia. Br J Anaesthesiol 32:60, 1960
32. Stephen CR, Dent SJ, Hall KD et al: Body temperature regulation during anesthesia in infants and children. JAMA 174:1579, 1960
33. Hallett EB: Effect on decreased body temperature on liver function and splanchnic blood flow in dogs. Surg Forum 5:362, 1954
34. Rink RA, Gray I, Reuchert RR, Slocum HC: Effect of hypothermia on morphine metabolism in isolated perfused liver. Anesthesiology 17:377, 1956
35. Moyer JH, Morris GG Jr, DeBakey ME: Hypothermia: effect on renal hemodynamics and on excretion of water and electrolytes in dog and man. Ann Surg 145:26, 1957
36. Ham J, Miller RD, Benet LZ et al: Pharmacocurarine during hypothermia in the cat. Anesthesiology 49:34, 1978
37. Heier T, Caldwell JE, Sessler DI, Miller RD: Mild intraoperative hypothermia increases duration of action and recovery time of vecuronium. Anesth Analg 70:51, 1990

38. Hessel E, Schmer G, Dillard D: J Surg Res 28:23, 1980

39. Rand WR, Lacombe, Hunt HE, Austin W: Viscosity of normal human blood under normothermic and hypothermic conditions. J Appl Physiol 19:117, 1964

40. Callaghan PB, Lister J, Paton BC, Swan H: Effect of varying carbon dioxide tensions on the oxyhemoglobin dissociation curves under hypothermic conditions. Ann Surg 154:903, 1961

41. Christoforides C, Hedley-Whyte J: Effect of temperature and hemoglobin concentration on solubility of O_2 in blood. J Appl Physiol 27:592, 1969

42. Juskovich G, Greiser W, Luterman A, Curreri W: Hypothermia in trauma victims: an ominous predictor of survival. J Trauma 27:1019, 1987

43. Carli F, Emery P, Freemantle C: Effect of perioperative normothermia on postoperative protein metabolism in elderly patients undergoing hip arthroplasty. Br J Anaesth 63:276, 1989

44. Boelhower R, Bruining H, Ong G: Correlations of serum potassium fluctuations with body temperature after major surgery. Crit Care Med 15:310, 1987

45. Bay J, Nunn JF, Prys-Roberts C: Factors influencing arterial pO$_2$ during recovery from anaesthesia. Br J Anaesth 40:398, 1968

46. Nunn JF: Applied Respiratory Physiology. p. 347. Butterworth, London, 1978

47. Blair E, Montgomery AV, Swan H: Post-hypothermic circulatory failure: physiologic observations on circulation. Circulation 13:909, 1956

48. Clark RE, Orkin LR, Rovenstine EA: Body temperature studies in anesthetized man, effect of environmental temperature, humidity and anesthesia system. JAMA 154:311, 1954

49. Haslam KR, Nielsen CH: Do passive heat and moisture exchangers keep the patient warm? Anesthesiology 64:379, 1986

50. Conahan TJ, Williams GD, Apfelbaum JL, Lecky JH: Airway heating reduces recovery time (cost) in outpatients. Anesthesiology 67:128, 1987

51. Bourke DL, Wurm H, Rosenburg M, Russell J: Intraoperative heat conservation using a reflective blanket. Anesthesiology 60:151, 1984

52. Guedel AE: Inhalational Anaesthesia. 2nd Ed. p. 110. Macmillan, New York, 1951

53. Gronert GA: Malignant hyperthermia. Anesthesiology 53:395, 1980

54. Denborough MA, Lovell RRH: Anaesthetic deaths in a family. Lancet 2:45, 1960

55. Isaacs H, Barlow MB: Malignant hyperpyrexia during anesthesia: possible correlation with subclinical myopathy. Br J Med 1:275, 1970

56. Kalow W, Britt BA, Terreau ME, Haist C: Metabolic error of muscle metabolism after recovery from malignant hyperthermia. Lancet 2:5, 1970

57. Britt BA, Endrenyi L, Peters PL et al: Screening of malignant hyperthermia susceptible families by creatinine phosphokinase measurement and other clinical investigations. Can Anaesth Soc J 23:263, 1976

58. Ellis FR, Clarke IMC, Modgill M et al: Evaluation of creatinine phosphokinase in screening patients for malignant hyperpyrexia. Br Med J 3:511, 1975

59. Hill DW: Electronic Measurement Techniques in Anaesthesia and Surgery. p. 366. Butterworth, New York, 1970

60. Whitby JD, Dunkin LJ: Temperature differences in the oesophagus. Br J Anaesth 40:991, 1968

61. Benzinger TH: Clinical temperature: a new physiological basis. JAMA 209:1200, 1969

62. Wilson RD, Knapp C, Traber DL, Priano LL: Tympanic thermography: a clinical and research evaluation of a new technic. South Med J 64:1452, 1971

63. Wallace CT, Marks WE, Adkins WY, Mahaffey JE: Perforation of the tympanic membrane, a complication of tympanic thermometry, during anesthesia. Anesthesiology 41:290, 1974

64. Kuzucu EY: Measurement of temperature. Int Anesthesiol Clin 3:435, 1965

65. Joly HR, Weil MH: Temperature of the great toe as an indicator of the severity of shock. Circulation 39:131, 1969

66. Grannis GF, Statland BE: Monitoring the quality of laboratory measurements. p. 2049. In Henry JB (ed): Clinical Diagnosis and Management by Laboratory Methods. 16th Ed. WB Saunders, Philadelphia, 1979

67. Cork RC, Vaughan RW, Humphrey LS: Precision and accuracy of intraoperative temperature monitoring. Anesth Analg 62:211, 1983

68. Lees DE, Schuette W, Bull JM et al: An evaluation of liquid-crystal thermometry as a screening device for intraoperative hyperthermia. Anesth Analg 57:669, 1978

69. Burgess GE, Cooper JR, Marino RJ, Peuler MJ: Continuous monitoring of skin temperature using a liquid crystal thermometer during anesthesia. South Med J 70:516, 1978

70. Vaughan MS, Cork RD, Vaughan RW: Inaccuracy of liquid crystal thermometry to identify core temperature trends in postoperative adults. Anesth Analg 61:284, 1982

Monitoring Renal Function

21

Alan S. Tonnesen

Monitoring of renal function in critically ill and perioperative patients continues to lag behind our ability to monitor cardiopulmonary function. Not only are most tests of kidney function performed intermittently, but the results frequently fail to reflect the current status of the patient's physiology. The primary reasons for monitoring of renal physiology are to make inferences regarding the status of the extracellular fluid and cardiovascular performance and to aid in detection and management of systemic problems such as hemolysis, rhabdomyolysis, diabetes insipidus, and ketoacidosis.

Under normal conditions, renal physiology is finely controlled to maintain water and electrolyte balance. It receives neurohumoral input from virtually every system relevant to control of blood pressure, blood volume, cardiac output, extracellular fluid volume, osmolality, sodium, potassium, calcium, phosphate, and magnesium concentrations. The volume and composition of urine thus give clues regarding vital physiologic processes.

Monitoring kidney function in order to detect early signs of dysfunction is crucial in patients at high risk for acute renal failure. Renal failure due to drugs or renal ischemia can be a disastrous complication in critically ill and perioperative patients. Although the manifestations of acute renal failure are often manageable when they occur as isolated events, when seen as an additional insult in the setting of multiple organ failure, there is considerable additional morbidity and mortality. In the face of additional organ system failure, the mortality rate associated with renal failure is doubled.

BASIC RENAL PHYSIOLOGY

Monitoring of the kidney is based on knowledge of basic renal physiology, including blood flow, filtration, and transport processes.

Renal Blood Flow

Renal blood flow is proportional to renal perfusion pressure and vascular resistance. Renal perfusion pressure is the mean systemic arterial pressure minus renal venous pressure. The renal venous pressure is not routinely monitored, but it is higher than the central venous pressure and higher than intraabdominal pressure. Patients with abdominal distension due to ascites, bowel edema, or other factors, who have elevated intraabdominal pressure may have inadequate perfusion pressure even when the mean arterial pressure appears to be adequate. Intraabdominal pressure can be monitored indirectly via the urinary bladder or stomach. To accomplish this the bladder catheter tubing is clamped, 100 ml of sterile saline is instilled retrograde, and a transducer is connected to the bladder via a needle inserted into the sampling port. The resulting waveform will show respiratory variation and rise upon abdominal palpation. The measured pressure, if higher than the central venous pressure, is substituted for renal venous pressure in the calculation of renal perfusion pressure. Alternatively, a catheter can be inserted into the inferior vena cava via the femoral vein and the venous pressure measured more directly.

Renal Vascular Resistance

Renal vascular resistance is controlled by the following factors: (1) the sympathetic nervous system, (2) angiotensin II, (3) autoregulation, (4) endothelial-derived relaxing factor, (5) endothelin, (6) prostaglandins, and (7) atrial natriuretic factor.

Sympathetic Nervous System

The sympathetic nervous system causes renal vasoconstriction (α-adrenergic) as well as releasing renin (β-adrenergic). It also inhibits sodium reabsorption (α-adrenergic) and causes renal vasodilation (dopaminergic). The sympathetic nervous system is also important in the moment-to-moment regulation of both blood pressure and renal vascular tone. The integrated activity of the sympathetic nervous system is responsive to changes in intravascular volume, blood pressure, cardiac output, and neuropsychological and metabolic abnormalities.

Angiotensin II

Angiotensin II is generated from angiotensin I, which is formed from angiotensinogen by the action of renin. Angiotensin II causes renal efferent arteriolar constriction, generalized systemic vasoconstriction, glomerular constriction, aldosterone release, thirst and sensitizes the adrenergic neurons to release more norepinephrine and suppresses further renin release. The rate-limiting step in generation of angiotensin II is the renin level. Thus, the regulation of renin controls the level of angiotensin II. Renin release is stimulated by renal arterial hypotension (decreased afferent arteriolar stretch), β-adrenergic receptor activation, and depressed sodium delivery to the distal tubule at the macula densa.

Autoregulation

Autoregulation refers to the relative constancy of blood flow over a wide range of perfusion pressures. Although renal blood flow is maintained down to a perfusion pressure of 50 to 60 mmHg in healthy kidneys, the lowest tolerable perfusion pressure (to maintain renal blood flow) is elevated in chronic hypertension. Autoregulation is severely impaired following ischemic injury, shifting downward and to the right. The precise processes responsible for autoregulation are not fully clarified, but appear to involve endothelial-derived relaxant factor and endothelin.

Endothelial-Derived Relaxing Factor

Endothelial-derived relaxing factor (nitric oxide or a closely related substance), is produced by endothelial cells. It is an extremely potent vasodilator. Upon contact with hemoglobin it is destroyed, resulting in an intravascular half-life of 1 to 2 seconds. This limits its systemic effects distant to the site of its production. It appears to be involved in maintaining normal autoregulation.

Endothelin

Endothelin is a family of potent vasoconstrictor molecules derived from the vascular endothelium. Unlike endothelial-derived relaxing factor, its intravascular half-life is sufficient to have systemic vasoconstrictive effects.

Prostaglandins

Prostaglandins are released when vasoconstrictive agents act upon the renal vasculature and serve to blunt any increase in vascular tone. In addition, they tend to lead to natriuresis and blunt the effects of vasopressin on the collecting tubules. They are also involved in the release of renin.

Atrial Natriuretic Factor

Atrial natriuretic factor primarily is produced in and released from the cardiac atrial myocytes in response to atrial stretch. The release of atrial natriuretic factor leads to diuresis and an increased glomerular filtration rate as well as vasodilation. This increased glomerular filtration rate is the result of afferent arteriolar dilation and preserved efferent arteriolar tone.

Glomerular Filtration Rate

Glomerular filtration rate (GFR) is determined by renal plasma flow, arterial pressure, and the ratio of afferent to efferent renal arteriolar resistance. In addition, the surface area available for filtration, the hydraulic conductivity of the glomerular apparatus, the pressure inside Bowman's space, and the oncotic pressure gradient between plasma and filtrate also contribute to maintenance of normal GFR. These relations are summarized by the modified Starling equation. Although renal plasma flow does not appear explicitly in the Starling equation, due to the high rate of filtration of plasma water, plasma proteins are concentrated as plasma traverses the glomerular capillary bed. This results in elevation of the capillary oncotic pressure.

$$GFR = Kf[(Pgc - Pt) - r(COPgc - COPt)]$$

Transport Mechanisms

Transport mechanisms predominantly reside in the basolateral (facing the capillary bed) membrane of the proximal and distal tubules and the thick ascending limb of Henle's loop. The primary active transport by Na-K-ATPase, located on the blood side of tubular epithelial cells, is responsible for most renal energy consumption and drives other forms of transport. The process of secondary active transport couples the concentration gradient for sodium generated by the Na-K-ATPase pumps to drive the transport of other substances, either cotransporters or countertransporters. Cotransporters are proteins located in the membrane, often the luminal membrane, which must be occupied by one or more sodium molecules and another specific molecule, such as glucose or chloride, resulting in both being transported in the same direction. Countertransporters function similarly, except that the sodium molecule and the other molecule are transported in opposite directions.

Absorption, or reabsorption, occurs when substances are removed from the filtrate and returned to the blood. During this process, organic acids and bases are transported by specific, separate, transport proteins located primarily in the proximal tubule.

Secretion is accomplished by a similar system (as in the absorptive process) operating in the opposite direction. The organic acid transporters are responsible for secretion of *p*-aminohippurate, penicillin, keto acids, and other acidic molecules.

Osmolality

Concentration (i.e., osmolality) of the urine is controlled by glomerular filtration rate and the vasopressin system. This process is further modulated by prostaglandins and factors that influence sodium pumping and the distribution of renal blood flow. Maximal concentration occurs only when each nephron segment performs its specific task. The involvement of so many aspects of kidney function results in concentration deficits in most acute renal diseases.

ACUTE RENAL FAILURE: PATHOGENESIS

The pathogenesis of acute renal failure in the critically ill or perioperative patient usually falls into one of three categories: ischemia, tubular toxins, or interstitial nephritis.

Ischemia

Ischemia (depressed renal oxygen delivery) causes renal failure when oxygen delivery fails to meet demands. Ischemic renal failure can be divided into three phases: (1) induction, (2) maintenance, and (3) resolution.

Induction

During the induction phase, renal blood flow, glomerular capillary pressure, and glomerular filtration surface area are depressed, resulting in an acute reduction in glomerular filtration rate. Simultaneously, reabsorptive functions are stimulated, resulting in oliguria. While oxygen delivery to the tubular cells meets the energy demands of sodium transport, tubular function is maintained and reabsorptive and secretory functions remain intact. This results in a concentrated urine with low sodium concentrations and a normal urinalysis. This phase is called "prerenal" dysfunction. If ischemia is severe enough, oxygen delivery falls below that required to maintain aerobic metabolism. Extraction of oxygen increases, resulting in a reduction of renal venous and cortical O_2 tension (Figs. 21-1 and 21-2). Tubular cellular energy reserves are exhausted (Fig. 21-3), intracellular acidosis occurs (Fig. 21-4), and transport functions begin to fail (Fig. 21-5). The failed transport functions are reflected in a rising urinary sodium concentration, and inability to concentrate the urine. Failure of sodium pumping also leads to cellular swelling and severe hypoxia ultimately causes necrosis. Necrotic cells shed into the lumen, causing formation of obstructive casts and the appearance of casts in the urine. The most metabolically

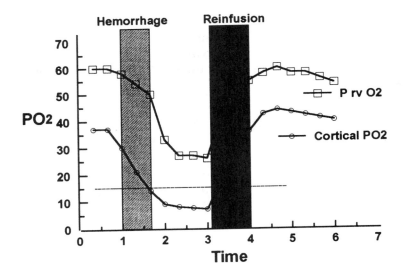

Fig. 21-1. During hemorrhage of 40 percent of blood volume to maintained a mean arterial pressure of 35 mmHg in pentobarbital anesthetized beagles, $PrvO_2$ and cortical PO_2 fell rapidly and were restored after reinfusion. $PrvO_2 = O_2$ tension (mmHg) in renal venous blood, cortical PO_2 = renal cortex tissue O_2 tension. (From Nelimarkka and Niinikoski,[4] with permission.)

active, and hence most susceptible, nephron regions are the proximal tubule and the thick ascending limb of the loop of Henle. The juxtamedullary region is characterized by a tenuous circulation in addition to being the site of a large proportion of the thick ascending limbs and terminal portions of the proximal tubule.

Maintenance

When the kidney passes from the phase of poor perfusion to cell necrosis, the maintenance phase of renal failure is entered (Fig. 21-6). Due to vascular injury, production of endothelial-derived relaxing factor (probably nitric oxide or a closely related agent) is impaired, leading to vasoconstriction. The loss of endothelium also makes the vasculature more sensitive to endothelin and other vasoconstrictor agents.

Resolution

Restoration of perfusion during the maintenance phase will fail to immediately improve renal function, although it is *crucial* for ultimate recovery. The ability to monitor oxygen delivery and consumption in addition to glomerular filtration rate on a moment-to-moment basis would be of great value in preventing or minimizing renal damage during stressful circumstances associated with poor renal perfusion.

Tubular Toxins

Toxic damage tends to affect the proximal tubule, resulting in loss of reabsorptive and secretory function and inability to concentrate the urine. Tubular damage results in secondary renal vasoconstriction and tubular obstruction. The ability to de-

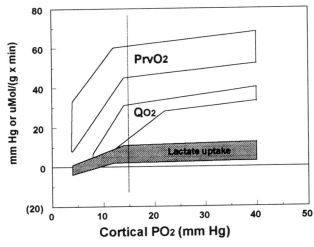

Fig. 21-2. When the cortical PO_2 reached a critical value, between 10 and 20 mmHg, renal O_2 consumption and $PrvO_2$ began to fall and lactate uptake declined. QO_2 = renal O_2 consumption ($\mu mol/(g \times min)$). Lactate uptake in $\mu mol/(g \times min)$. See legend of Figure 21-1 for description of experiment. (From Nelimarkka and Niinikoski,[4] with permission.)

tect early tubular dysfunction has the potential for guiding interventions designed to prevent the development of full-blown renal failure. Tubular dysfunction due to toxins usually takes days to manifest, thus intermittent testing on a daily basis should be sufficient for most toxins.

Hemoglobinuria and Myoglobinuria

Hemoglobinuria and myoglobinuria are frequently associated with acute renal failure. Several mechanisms are involved, including hemodynamic instability related to the causative event, activation of the coagulation and inflammatory cascades by cell membrane damage, precipitation of pigment in the tubule (due to a low glomerular filtration rate and increased water reabsorption), and possibly inactivation of endothelial-derived relaxing factor by the heme pigment. A common test for myoglobinuria is to detect heme pigment with a dipstick, followed by precipitation of myoglobin by ammonium chloride, centrifugation, and retesting of the supernatant with the dipstick. If the first test is positive and the second test is negative, it is presumed that myoglobin is present. However, this method is very nonspecific and should be abandoned. Turbidometric tests are readily available that use a specific antibody to myoglobin to give specific and quantitative measures of plasma and urine myoglobin levels.[1]

Interstitial Nephritis

Immune interstitial nephritis leads to tubular dysfunction and often eosinophiluria. The evidence of tubular dysfunction is normally more prominent than a reduction in glomerular filtration rate during the early phases of injury. Detecting the tubular dysfunction prior to a reduction in glomerular filtration rate could lead to earlier elimination of the offending agent. Monitoring of sodium balance, and urinary osmolality may detect earlier lesions.

ASSESSING RENAL FUNCTION: AVAILABLE TECHNIQUES

Clearance Methodology

Clearance methodology is the traditional method for measuring kidney function. The original techniques and principles have not been modified significantly since their description more than a half-century ago. More recently, plasma clearance techniques have been extensively explored because they avoid the need for urine collection. The "gold standard" clearance methodology continues to be continuous infusion of the markers until a steady state is achieved, coupled with timed urine collection.

All urinary clearance methods require collection of both urine and plasma with subsequent analysis of a marker of some aspect of kidney function.

Known, and preferably stable, plasma levels of this marker are necessary to estimate the arterial concentration available for filtration. Generally,

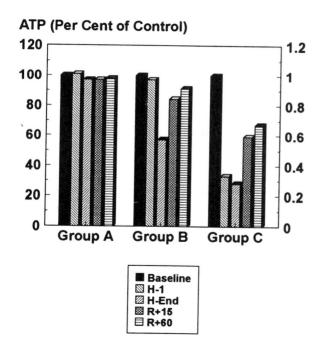

ATP (Per Cent of Control)

Legend:
■ Baseline
▨ H-1
▨ H-End
▨ R+15
▤ R+60

Fig. 21.3. Hemorrhagic hypotension (30 to 65 mmHg) was maintained in anesthetized rats for 30 to 45 minutes, while ATP and pHi were measured by nuclear magnetic resonance. Glomerular filtration rate was measured by inulin clearance. Group A had no changes in adenosine triphosphate (ATP) (shown as percent of control) during hypotension, Group B had reductions in ATP only during the last 10 to 15 minutes of hypotension and rapidly recovered, while Group C had reduced ATP for 25 to 35 minutes during hypotension and failed to recover to normal levels by 60 minutes after reinfusion. H1 is the first measurement during hypotension, H-End taken at the end of the hypotensive period, R+15 and R+60 were assessed 15 and 60 minutes after reinfusion of shed blood. (From Ratcliffe et al.,[3] with permission.)

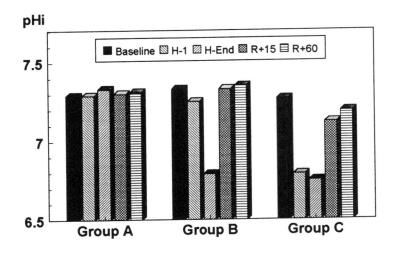

Fig. 21-4. Intracellular pH (pHi) fell transiently in rats who had transient ATP depletion and for prolonged periods in those who had prolonged ATP depletion. See Figure 21-3 for experimental description and legend. (From Ratcliffe et al.,[3] with permission.)

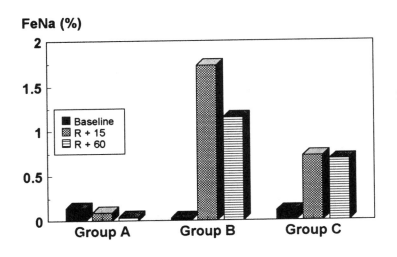

Fig. 21-5. FENa remained low in animals who maintained ATP levels despite hypotension, but rose dramatically in those whose ATP levels fell. See Figure 21-3 for experimental description and legend. (From Ratcliffe et al.,[3] with permission.)

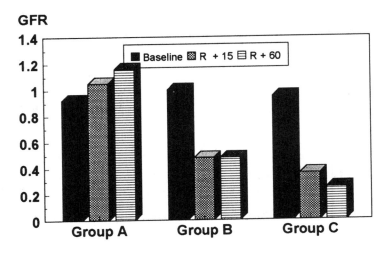

Fig. 21-6. GFR was well maintained in rats whose ATP remained normal, but fell significantly in those with transient reductions. Rats with prolonged ATP depletion suffered progressive loss of GFR over the hour after reinfusion. See Figure 21-3 for experimental description and legend. (From Ratcliffe et al.,[3] with permission.)

this has been necessary because of limitations on the frequency of plasma analysis. In fact, if the instantaneous plasma concentration could be measured, then one could estimate clearance into the urine in the absence of a stable plasma level. The remaining problem with interpreting urinary clearances during non-steady-state conditions is the delay between entrance of a marker into the filtrate and its appearance in the collected urine. The length of that delay is directly proportional to the volume between the nephron and the collection point and inversely to the rate of urine formation. If the urinary tract dead space and urine flow rate were known, then a time constant could be calculated. The urine collected after three time constants will be near equilibrium values. Unfortunately, data regarding urinary tract dead space are not available, but is estimated at 0.25 to 0.50 ml/kg ideal body weight. Alternatively, by continuous monitoring of the urinary concentration of the marker, it is possible to correct for the delayed appearance.

Utilizing this technique, urine flow rate errors result from incomplete bladder or upper urinary tract emptying at the beginning or end of urine collection. Although bladder catheterization probably improves the consistency of emptying, the larger the volume collected, the smaller the impact of volume errors: a 10-ml error is only 2.5 percent of a 400-ml collection but a 20 percent error in a 50-ml collection. Techniques used to minimize residual bladder urine include manual compression of the suprapubic area, injecting air to flush residual urine from the bladder or injection of known quantities of sterile water. When fluid is used to flush the bladder, the measured concentration of the substance must be corrected for dilution. The same technique of bladder emptying should be employed prior to the beginning of urine collection and at the end. Finally, sterile technique must be maintained at all times.

Plasma clearance techniques (single-shot techniques) utilize pharmacokinetic principles to describe the rate of clearance of the marker from the plasma. If the indicator is cleared only by the kidney, plasma clearance should be equivalent to renal clearance. This is substantially true for several agents. Major advantages of plasma clearance are that continuous infusion of the marker is not necessary and urine collection errors are eliminated. Because all known markers of renal function will distribute at least into the extracellular space, the effect of this distribution phase must be included in the analysis.

With this technique, certain assumptions must be made and clinical conditions must meet these assumptions to allow substitution of plasma for urinary clearance: (1) the substance is eliminated only by the kidney; (2) the phase of distribution has been completed, even if there is no other route of elimination; (3) the actual clearance fits a mathematical model of clearance. The model most commonly used is that of first-order elimination in which a constant fraction is eliminated per unit of time.

If one waits until the plasma clearance is on the stable log-linear down slope of the disappearance curve, then as few as one[2] to three samples will accurately reflect clearance. The available markers require 60 to 90 minutes for complete distribution within the extracellular space. Thus, although these techniques are useful in chronic situations, they have had little value for perioperative or critical care applications when changes in renal blood flow or function may occur over minutes.

Methods for Measurement of Renal Blood Flow

Total renal blood flow is 4 to 6 ml/g/min in the cortex, 1 ml/g/min in the outer medulla and 0.1 to 0.4 ml/g/min in the papilla. In comparison, most other tissues have flows of about 1 ml/g/min. As the metabolic rate of the kidney is not exceptionally high and is related to the active pumping of sodium, the extraction of oxygen is quite low. Most transport-related metabolic activity is confined to the proximal tubule and the thick ascending limb of Henle's loop. The quantity of sodium delivered to the pumping sites is directly proportional to glomerular filtration rate. During hemodynamic compromise, both glomerular filtration rate and renal blood flow decline, thus tending to maintain the energy supply:demand ratio. Only with severely compromised perfusion does tissue ischemia occur. This results in elevated O_2 extraction, depressed O_2 consumption, adenosine triphosphate (ATP) depletion, intracellular acidosis, and depressed lactate uptake or even production.[3,4] When ATP depletion occurs, even transiently, recovery of glomerular filtration rate and tubular transport functions may not occur.

Multiple methods of measuring renal blood flow have been developed; however, few have achieved success in the clinical setting. Methods presently available for measuring renal blood flow include (1) dye dilution, (2) microspheres, (3) arteriography or renal venography, (4) thermal dilution, (5) inert radioactive gas washout, (6) Doppler technology, and (7) clearance extraction.

Dye Dilution

Dye dilution has been performed by injecting indocyanine green dye into the renal artery and then sampling from the renal vein using conventional deconvolution of the concentration curve. The requirement for renal artery and venous catheterization with the potential for alteration in flow induced by the catheter and the injection itself relegate the technique to experimental situations only.

Microspheres

Radiolabeled microspheres have been used to assess renal blood flow in experimental situations. These microspheres are labeled with a radioisotope and the organ is dissected into representative portions (e.g., cortex, medulla) for radioactive counting. Therefore, this technique is only relevant for experimental situations in which the kidney is sacrificed for radioactive counting. The basis of this technique is that microspheres larger than 15 μm fail to pass through the capillary bed. Spheres 18 to 35 μm in diameter are trapped before reaching the glomerulus.[5] Trapping is incomplete for spheres less than 7 to 8 μm. Although this technique is suitable for assessing cortical blood flow, the degree of microsphere trapping in the medullary regions may not accurately reflect plasma flow.

Arteriography or Renal Venography

Arteriography or renal venography is sometimes used when acute renal failure may be due to a vascular accident. The procedure is invasive, expensive (in terms of both equipment and personnel), and may cause vascular damage. In addition, this procedure entails a large radiation exposure, and the potential toxicity of a large dose of contrast media. Its use is thus relegated for diagnostic purposes, not monitoring.

Thermal Dilution

Thermal dilution blood flow measurement via a catheter in the renal vein[6] has been developed. The catheter has a 180-degree bend near the tip with a thermistor at the tip and an injection port at the knee of the curve. The catheter is positioned in the renal vein and blood flow can be measured repetitively. Its advantages include the ability to rapidly measure blood flow without disturbing arterial flow. Disadvantages relate to the need for catheter placement and the potential that the catheter or rapid injection of indicator may disturb renal blood flow.

Inert Radioactive Gas Washout

The inert radioactive gas washout technique requires renal arterial catheterization with injection of radioactive xenon and external counting with a camera or probe. The resulting curve is mathematically analyzed into sequential log-linear curves representing mathematical compartments of progressively lower disappearance rates, presumably representing differing anatomic areas with varying blood flow rates. The requirement for arterial catheterization, the use of radioactive agents, and the inability to clearly associate the disappearance curves with anatomic areas has led to minimal use in recent years.

Doppler Technology

Doppler technology has advanced significantly during the past several years, and is likely to become an important part of the armamentarium in evaluating and possibly monitoring renal blood flow during pharmacologic and hemodynamic manipulations in the operating room and intensive care unit.

Furthermore, noninvasive Doppler studies can be utilized to evaluate the patency of the renal arteries and veins. However, quantitation of main renal arterial blood flow is not always reliable due to inability to accurately assess the angle of measurement. Using this technique the 95 percent confidence interval is ≤ 48 ml/m^2.[7] A Doppler probe, which can be implanted at the time of surgery and then released and removed, has been used to monitor perioperative renal blood flow in patients undergoing coronary surgery.[8]

Duplex Doppler ultrasound (a modification of

traditional Doppler technology) can be used to study interlobar artery flow repetitively. Using this technique, the pulsatility index (PI) correlates with resistance and mean velocity correlates with flow. The mean frequency shift correlates with blood flow and has been shown to increase following infusion of low-dose dopamine (Fig. 21-7).[9] In a study by Stevens and colleagues[9] evaluating the renal blood flow characteristics during acute renal failure, the PI was higher in patients with acute renal failure than those with transient dysfunction or normals[10] (Fig. 21-8). Likewise, Grigat and colleagues[11] demonstrated that the PI increased during episodes of renal transplant rejection.

Doppler technology can also be employed to measure renal blood flow distribution. Using injections of sonicated microbubbles with subsequent image detection via a Doppler probe placed on the surface of the kidney, renal blood flow can be determined. Aronson and coworkers[12] reported that the total blood flow, measured by an electromagnetic flow probe, correlated well with results obtained by the Doppler method. However, less success was reported when renal blood flow was varied using renal artery occlusion and dopamine agonist infusion.[13] This technique may prove useful intra-

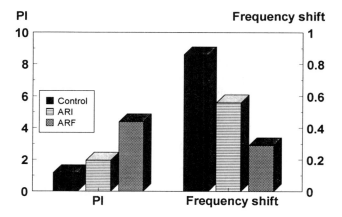

Fig. 21-8. Duplex Doppler ultrasound of an interlobar artery of 20 patients with acute renal failure (ARF), 14 with transient renal insufficiency (ARI), and 23 control subjects. PI = pulsatility index = peak systolic frequency shift minus end diastolic frequency shift divided by the mean frequency shift. PI is an index of distal resistance to flow: the lower the PI, the lower the resistance. The mean frequency shift is proportional to blood velocity multiplied by the cosine of the angle of insonation, which was believed to be zero degrees, whose cosine is 1.0. (From Stevens et al.,[10] with permission.)

operatively and in experimental animals, as an added benefit Doppler technology also has the ability to semiquantitatively determine blood flow to different regions of the kidney.

Clearance Extraction

The clearance extraction technique has been a widely employed method for estimating renal blood flow. Blood flow can be estimated from clearance methods if the venous concentration of the marker is measured, and the extraction ratio then determined as follows:

$$\text{Renal plasma flow} = \frac{\text{Clearance}}{\text{Extraction ratio}}$$

p-Aminohippurate (PAH) is the most frequently used agent when calculating renal blood flow via clearance techniques. For these calculations the volume of distribution of PAH is assumed to be 40 percent of body weight, but expands with time during continuous infusions. For determination of estimated renal plasma flow (ERPF), a low plasma concentration of PAH (0.02 mg/ml), which will not exceed the maximal rate of tubular transport (0.4

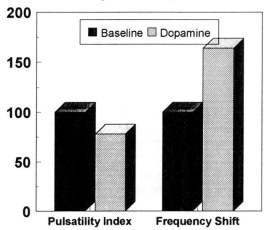

Per Cent Change After Dopamine

Fig. 21-7. Pulsatility index and mean frequency shift were measured in an interlobar artery before and 1 hour after starting dopamine infusion at 2 μ/kg/min in critically ill patients. There were no significant changes in mean arterial blood pressure or central venous pressure. PI decreased by 22 percent and frequency shift increased 64 percent. (From Stevens et al.,[9] with permission.)

to 0.6 mg/ml), is infused. By infusing a larger dose, calculated to achieve a plasma concentration of 0.45 mg/ml, the maximal rate of tubular transport can be calculated.[14] Use of a loading dose plus a constant infusion allows achievement of stable plasma levels earlier than a simple infusion.

Using PAH clearance, the following formula has been developed:

$$RPF = \frac{(Upah \times Vol)/(Ppah \times t)}{(Ppah - Vpah)/Ppah}$$

where Upah = urinary concentration of PAH, Ppah = arterial plasma PAH concentration, Vpah = renal venous PAH concentration, and Vol = volume of urine collected during time t.

The most frequently utilized clearance extraction technique clinically utilizes PAH, which is filtered and secreted by the proximal tubule. Its extraction from the plasma by the kidney averages between 80 and 90 percent. Thus, a large gradient exists between the arterial and venous concentrations. If one assumes a constant extraction ratio of 85 percent, then renal plasma flow can be calculated on the basis of clearance alone, by dividing PAH clearance by 0.85. Unfortunately, the extraction ratio has been shown to vary significantly during acute illness, making measurement of renal venous concentrations mandatory if renal plasma flow is to be calculated. Renal ischemia, sepsis, drug-induced vasodilation, and saline loading cause acute reductions in PAH extraction. The effect of changes in extraction on estimated renal plasma flow is shown in Fig. 21-9, which emphasizes why renal venous levels must be obtained if one wishes to estimate renal plasma flow. Changes in extraction ratio present a problem in interpretation when serial measurements are performed: Is the changing PAH clearance due to changing blood flow or changing extraction? If PAH clearance is viewed as reflecting a functional property of the kidney, then increasing PAH clearance will generally reflect improvement, a falling clearance deterioration. In fact, Hilberman[15] obtained data in postoperative patients consistent with this hypothesis.

Techniques for Measurement of Glomerular Filtration Rate

Presently available techniques for measurement of glomerular filtration rate (GFR) and plasma creatinine are quite imprecise.[16] With the variability inherent in these measurements, the minimal detectable difference in GFR and/or creatinine ranges between 20 and 30 percent (Table 21-1). In an attempt to find a more reliable method for determining GFR, new markers (i.e., molecules that can be used to estimate GFR) are presently being studied. Ideally, a marker of GFR should be eliminated only by the kidney and only by filtration. The marker should not be produced, metabolized, secreted, nor reabsorbed by the kidney; that is, all of the filtered substance should be excreted, and filtration should be its only source.

To assess GFR accurately these molecules must be freely filtered by the glomeruli. In addition, molecular weight and size (<1.5 to 2.0 nm) and electrical charge must be low enough to allow complete glomerular passage. Finally, protein binding should be weak or negligible so that all the marker in plasma is available for filtration. Clinically, a marker that can be easily analyzed, (especially noninvasively) and is nontoxic, has obvious practical advantages. Although radioactive markers are relatively easy to measure, and the actual dose of radiation approaches that of a chest radiograph, exposure of both the patient and staff to radiation limits their appeal.

Markers used to estimate GFR include inulin (the "gold standard"), ethylenediaminetetraacetic

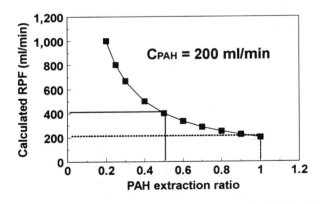

Fig. 21-9. The curve represents a measured CPAH of 200 ml/min. If the extraction ratio is 1.0, at point "A" the CPAH equals RPF. When the extraction ratio falls to 0.5 at point "B", the actual RPF is 400 ml/min even though the CPAH is still 200 ml/minute. RPF, renal plasma flow; PAH, = *p*-aminohippurate; CPAH, clearance of PAH, PAH extraction ratio is calculated by dividing the arteriovenous difference of PAH concentrations by the arterial concentration.

TABLE 21-1. Coefficient of Variation (CV) and Critical Differences (CD) of Glomerulofiltration Rate (GFR) and Plasma Creatinine (PCr) Measurements

Renal Function	Measurement	Intraindividual		Interindividual	
		CV (%)	CD (%)	CV (%)	CD (%)
Normal	GFR	7.5	20	15	42
Normal	PCr	11.0	31	15	42
Reduced	GFR	12.0	33		
Reduced	PCr	6.3	18		

(From Levey,[16] with permission.)

acid (EDTA), iothalamate, diethylenetriaminepentaacetic acid (DTPA), iohexol, creatinine, and urea.

Inulin

Inulin can be measured by plasma clearance or classic methods, but they are not interchangeable.[17] Chemical analysis of inulin requires complex sample preparation, making analysis of multiple samples tedious and time-consuming. This has led to the search for other methods of analysis and other filtration markers. Inulin can be made radioactive by incorporation of ^{14}C, thereby greatly simplifying analysis, but, at the same time, the cost is markedly increased and the patient is exposed to radioactivity.

To overcome these problems, enzyme methods have recently become available. With this method, a pharmacokinetic model can be used to calculate a leading dose and continuous infusion for measuring GFR.[14]

Ethylenediaminetetraacetic Acid

[51]Cr-labeled ethylenediaminetetraacetic acid (EDTA) compares favorably with inulin for measurement of GFR.[16,18] There have been problems with dissociation of the ^{51}Cr from the EDTA, giving a systematic error in the clearance measurements.[17] The clearance of the ^{51}Cr-EDTA is between 95 and 97 percent of simultaneously determined inulin clearance.

Iothalamate

Iothalamate and inulin clearance are equivalent[19–20,21–22] (Fig. 21-10). Analysis of radioiodinated forms of iothalamate is accomplished by standard techniques. Iothalamate can be tagged with radioactive iodine or it can be measured using high pressure liquid chromatography (HPLC).[23,24] As it is not protein-bound, it has been used in both classical clearance techniques and single-shot methods based on plasma clearance.

Diethylenetriaminepentaacetic Acid

Diethylenetriaminepentaacetic acid (DTPA)[18,25] clearance is also equivalent to inulin clearance (Fig. 21-10). Radioactive labeling with ^{99m}Tc allows rapid and accurate analysis. Plasma clearances can be performed with coefficients of variation of less than 10 percent.[26] Gadopentetate-dimeglumine-DTPA is measurable using a desktop nuclear magnetic resonance (NMR) spectrometer and has been

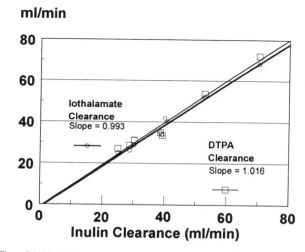

Fig. 21-10. The excellent correlations between inulin clearance and clearance of DTPA and iothalamate are shown. (From Barbour et al.,[25] with permission.)

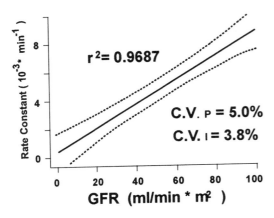

Fig. 21-11. The correlation between the rate constant for ^{99m}Tc-DTPA clearance by the noninvasive monitor and ^{125}I-iothalamate clearance and the 95% confidence limits are excellent. Radioactivity is monitored continuously by a counting device wrapped around the upper arm after intravenous injection of DTPA. CVp and CVi are the coefficients of variation for the population and individual, respectively. The rate constant is the slope of the log of activity versus time after correction for decay. (From Rabito et al.,[28] with permission.)

used to measure GFR without radiation. There was good agreement between the NMR and radioactive DTPA-measured GFR.[27] An exciting new application of an old method of measuring the clearance of ^{99m}DTPA after a single injection was recently reported. This newer method utilizes a detector apparatus, which is wrapped around the upper arm to detect radioactivity. The system automatically de-

termines the rate constant for the declining level of radioactivity as the tracer is excreted. This value is proportional to GFR (Fig. 21-11) and is updated every 9 to 59 seconds for 5-minute epochs. With this technique, the duration of effective monitoring is 12 to 24 hours, increasing as GFR falls. Using this system, Rabito and colleagues[28,29] were able to detect abrupt reductions of GFR within minutes of injection of radiocontrast in patients (Fig. 21-12). This dynamic, real-time analysis overcomes a major shortcoming of other variants of the single-shot technique, namely, the requirement to wait 90 to 240 minutes for equilibration to occur.[30]

Iohexol

Iohexol (Omnipaque 180) can be analyzed by x-ray fluorescence of the contained iodine in about 10 minutes following injection of the contrast agent.[31,32] Clearance calculated after injection 50 ml of contrast agent correlates reasonably well with simultaneous inulin clearance, $r = .86$. The major advantage of this technique is the lack of radioactivity and the simplicity of analysis. Before widespread acceptance, further work demonstrating a stable correlation with inulin or other standard clearance methodology is needed.

Creatinine

Creatinine has long been used as a marker of GFR. Creatinine levels are easily measured and do not require administration of an exogenous substance. The disadvantages of monitoring creatinine

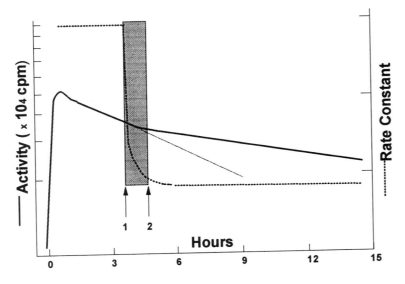

Fig. 21-12. Using the technique described in Fig. 21-11 to monitor GFR, angiography was performed between the times indicated by the shaded box and arrows 1 and 2. The solid curve represents the actual radioactive counts, the dotted line extending from the initial downward slope of the radioactive count line extrapolates the expected decline in counts had GFR remained constant, while the dashed line is the rate constant calculated from the rate of declining radioactivity. The change in the slope of the radioactive count curve shown during angiography is dramatically represented by the abrupt reduction in rate constant. (From Rabito et al.,[29] with permission.)

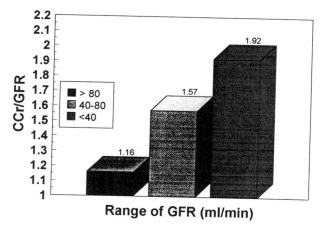

Fig. 21-13. The ratio of CCr to GFR as measured by inulin clearance in patients with glomerular diseases is shown for three ranges of GFR. The ratio increases progressively as the GFR falls. The numbers above the bar represent the mean value for that group. (From Shemesh et al.,[33] with permission.)

levels include an unknown rate of production and no assurance that the rate of production will be constant in critically ill patients. Creatinine[33,34] is freely filtered by the glomerulus, but nonfiltration elimination also occurs. Creatinine is secreted by the tubules. The amount of secretion increases as the plasma level rises, especially in cases of glomerular disease (Fig. 21-13). In cases of tubular necrosis, increases in creatinine secretion are less predictable. Creatinine secretion is impaired by cimetidine, trimethoprim, and probenecid.[35,36] Extrarenal elimination occurs by degradation of creatinine by intestinal microorganisms and has been best documented in chronic renal failure. As much as 66 percent of the creatinine may be eliminated

by nonrenal mechanisms in end-stage renal disease, causing creatinine clearance to overestimate true GFR (by an average of 30 percent).[36]

The analysis of creatinine is complicated by several interferants[37-42] (Table 21-2). Creatinine determined by enzymatic methods gives higher plasma creatinine (PCr) values than obtained by other methods, resulting in a lower creatinine clearance (CCr).[43] However, the enzymatic methods are less susceptible to interferants, such as bilirubin, acetone, cephalothin, and ethyl acetoacetate, than the Jaffe method, but still are not entirely independent of these.[44] Of clinical significance, furosemide infusions markedly lower the creatinine concentration, measured by the Jaffe colorimetric method.[45]

The plasma level of creatinine is directly proportional to creatinine intake plus production and inversely proportional to urinary excretion plus extrarenal disposition. Creatinine ingestion depends on intake of meat, which contains 3.5 to 5.0 mg of creatinine per gram, with plasma elevations of creatinine persisting for 8 to 12 hours following a meal. Creatinine production is proportional to muscle mass and in healthy persons with an estimated turnover of 1.6 to 1.7 percent per day. For men, the excretion of creatinine is $28.2 \text{ g} - 0.172 \times \text{age}$, and for women, $25 \text{ g} - 0.175 \times \text{age}$.[46,47] Using these relationships, Moran and Myers[48] derived a mathematical model, which accurately predicts the course of acute changes in GFR. These relationships are only valid when changes in extracellular volume and creatinine excretion are also measured. This analysis revealed that changes in plasma creatinine alone failed to accurately reflect GFR.[48] This supports the position that direct meas-

TABLE 21-2. Creatinine Interferants

Interferant		Enzymatic	Jaffe (ND)	Jaffe (ND)
Bilirubin	(330–435 umol/L)	↑↑	↓↓↓	↑↑
Glucose	(50 mmol/L)	↔	↑↑	↑↑
Cephalothin		↔	↓	↔
Acetone	(30 mmol/L)	↔	↑↑↑	↑↑
EAA	(800 mg/L)	↔	↓	↓↓

EAA, ethylacetoacetate; D, detergent present; ND, no detergent in the Jaffe measurements.
The directional changes in the measured creatinine caused by varying concentrations of the interferants shown in column 1 are shown by the arrows. Upward pointing arrows indicate falsely elevated creatinine, downward arrows indicate depression, and horizontal arrows indicate no consistent effect. The more arrows, the greater the effect.
(From Lindback and Bergman,[44] with permission.)

urement of GFR is the only reliable way to monitor patients with changing renal function.

Total creatinine elimination is the sum of extrarenal removal plus the amount filtered and the amount secreted. Extrarenal elimination occurs predominantly in sweat and from breakdown by intestinal organisms. The proportion of creatinine secreted rises as the plasma level increases, but falls with the onset of severe tubular loss. The difference between creatinine clearance and GFR and the ratio of CCr to GFR vary with the degree of renal dysfunction (Fig. 21-13). The sensitivity of an elevated plasma creatinine in detecting a reduced GFR is only 61 percent[16] (Fig. 21-14).

Clinically, measurement of serum creatinine is readily available, making it an attractive means of following kidney function. Serum creatinine monitored by the CUSUM technique on a daily basis in transplant recipients demonstrated 85 percent sensitivity and 94 percent specificity for detecting acute renal dysfunction.[49] For monitoring more chronic changes in renal function, a regression equation has been developed, which objectively identifies when the slope of the plot of time against 1/PCr changes.[50]

The formula of Cockcroft (shown below) predicts CCr most accurately in patients with normal function, while the Jeliffe formula does better in those patients with elevated PCr.[51] The Cockroft formula performs well in estimating GFR provided that the patient's renal function is stable. The age factor used here may not be accurate when the age is less than 30. Of note, ideal body weights should be used in the obese and those who have muscle wasting. Obviously, calculated clearances cannot be used to assess acute changes.[52]

$$CCr = \frac{(140 - Age) \times Wt}{PCr \times 72}$$

where CCr (creatinine clearance) is in ml/min, age is in years, Wt (weight) is in kg, and plasma creatinine (PCr) is in mg/dl. Multiply the result by 0.85 for females. However, creatinine excretion in the urine falls as renal function declines. This may be related to decreased meat intake, declining muscle mass, or increased extrarenal elimination. The net result is that plasma creatinine tends to overestimate true GFR.

Creatinine clearance (CCr) is a frequently measured variable of renal functions in critically ill patients. The clearance is the volume of plasma from which all creatinine would have to be extracted to account for the amount excreted. The amount of plasma cleared of creatinine models the process into two compartments: one from which all creatinine was removed, another from which none was removed. Unfortunately, due to the problems with creatinine analysis, the coefficient of variation for CCr is high, reportedly 27 percent.[53] The sensitivity of CCr in detecting a reduced GFR is only 75 percent.[16] Fortunately, short urine collection periods allow for repetitive measurement of CCr to monitor the effect of various interventions and correlate reasonably well with results calculated from longer collections[54] (Fig. 21-15).

Following an oral protein load, GFR increases but CCr increases more as a result of tubular creatinine secretion.[55] As a result, this quantitative increase in creatinine excretion may be a more reliable indicator of reduced renal reserve than the change in GFR.[56]

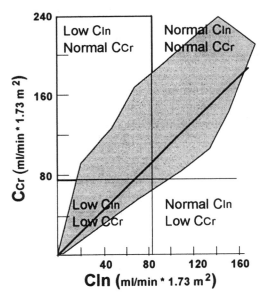

Fig. 21-14. The relationship between inulin clearance (CIn) and creatinine clearance (CCr) is shown for a group of patients. The cross hatched area contains the individual patient data points. It can be seen that many points in the distribution fall above the regression line, that is, CCr tends to overestimate CIn. The vertical line is the lower limit of CIn and the horizontal line the lower limit of CCr. The shaded upper left quadrant represents the area of false negativity of the CCr as a predictor of CIn. (From Shemesh et al.,[33] with permission.)

Despite these potential shortcomings, CCr is clinically useful tool. A CCr < 25 ml/min was a good predictor of subsequent renal dysfunction in patients who were hypotensive and required more than 10 units of blood during resuscitation from trauma. In addition, CCr was a better predictor than water clearance (CH_2O) or fractional excretion of sodium (FENa) for renal dysfunction in this patient population.[57,58]

Urea

Another frequently used clinical parameter of renal function is the blood urea nitrogen. Blood urea nitrogen (BUN) reflects the balance between protein breakdown and excretion. Urea nitrogen excretion accounts for the bulk of urinary nitrogen, approximately 85 percent. Of interest, urea contains 2 nitrogen molecules per molecule of BUN and the concentration is expressed as the nitrogen, not urea, concentration. Thus, the apparent molecular weight used in calculating the contribution of BUN to osmolality is 28, rather than 60. There is a modest correlation between GFR and BUN or urea nitrogen clearance, but several factors make BUN an undesirable measure of GFR. These factors—urine flow rate, protein intake, and catabolism—are not important determinants of creatinine excretion. The excretion of urea is accomplished by both filtration and reabsorption, the latter being inversely proportional to urine flow rate. Additionally, urea production rate is not as constant as creatinine production and is directly proportional to total protein turnover, including both intake and catabolism.

TRANSPORT FUNCTION

Basics of Renal Transport

The renal excretion of any substance is related to filtration, reabsorption, and secretion as expressed by the following equation:

$$Output = filtration - reabsorption + secretion.$$

An understanding of the basics of transport by different nephron segments allows inference about nephron function based on the composition of the urine.

Active transport, predominantly of sodium, is responsible for most of the oxygen consumption of the kidney and drives both secretion and reabsorption of other substances. Primary active transport is predominantly due to activity of the sodium pump, Na-K-ATPase. The pump is located in the basolateral membrane (which faces the interstitium) of the tubular cells. The action of this system produces a gradient for sodium between the lumen and the intracellular fluid and the interstitium. Secondary active transport is driven by these sodium gradients as well. Cotransport occurs when membrane receptors bind with specific molecules simultaneously with sodium, resulting in the molecule and sodium moving into the cell together. Countertransport occurs when sodium and the transported molecule move in *opposite* directions across the cell membrane.

Passive reabsorption is driven by the osmotic and oncotic pressure gradients produced by the processes of filtration and electrolyte transport. Passive movement occurs via the transcellular and paracellular routes.

Each of the various components of the renal system participates in the processes of absorption, active transport, and secretion. The proximal tubule absorbs 60 to 75 percent of filtered sodium and water. This sodium absorption drives reabsorption and secretion of other substances, such as glucose, phosphate, amino acids, β_2-microglobulin, amylase, potassium, and bicarbonate. The descending and

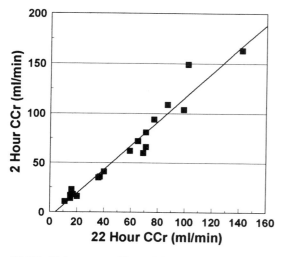

Fig. 21-15. Urine was collected from critically ill patients in 2 aliquots, one 2 hours in duration, the other from the remaining 22 hours of the day. Creatinine clearance (ml/min) was calculated. (From Sladen et al.,[54] with permission.)

thin ascending limbs of the loop of Henle perform little active transport, but their differing permeabilities are crucial to the development of a concentrated medullary interstitium. The thick ascending limb of the loop of Henle is another site of active transport with a high metabolic rate. It is responsible for further reabsorption of sodium and magnesium. Inhibition of transport in this segment by furosemide results in nearly complete failure to reabsorb that proportion of sodium that escapes more proximal absorption. This can result in fractional excretions of approximately 30 percent. Because the thick ascending limb is impermeable to water, sodium reabsorption contributes to the hypertonicity of the medulla and produces hypotonic tubular fluid. If the more distal nephron segments are not rendered permeable to water by vasopressin, this dilute fluid is excreted as urine. The distal convoluted tubule reabsorbs sodium and secretes potassium and hydrogen ions against large concentration gradients. Their secretion results from the production of a negative intraluminal charge, facilitating movement of hydrogen and potassium down the electrical gradient. The distal tubule is responsible for nearly all potassium in the urine because virtually all filtered potassium is reabsorbed in the proximal nephron.

Fractional Excretion

The processes of fractional excretion and fractional reabsorption are reciprocally related. The fractional excretion (see formula below) of any substance is its rate of clearance divided by the rate of glomerular filtration. For a substance that is filtered and neither secreted nor reabsorbed, the fractional excretion is 1.0. The fractional excretion of a substance exceeds unity only if secreted.

$$FEs = \frac{(Us \cdot \dot{V})/Ps}{GFR}$$

where FE is the fractional excretion, s represents any substance, Us is the urinary concentration of the substance, Ps is the plasma concentration of the substance, f = filtration marker, e.g. creatinine and $\dot{V}$ is the urine flow rate. When the equation for GFR is expanded and the *V* term is canceled:

$$FEs = \frac{(Us \cdot V)/Ps}{(Uf \cdot V)/Pf}$$

$$FEs = \frac{Us/Ps}{Uf/Pf}$$

Fractional Reabsorption

Fractional reabsorption represents the proportion of the amount filtered, which is reabsorbed. For example, with sodium, 99 percent is ultimately reabsorbed:

$$FRs = 1 - FEs$$

Electrolyte Excretion

Theoretically, the excretion of electrolytes can be estimated by measuring the electrical conductivity of the ionic content of the urine. The bulk of the ionic content is composed of sodium and potassium. Konig and Mackie[59] suggest that monitoring urine conductivity correlates with GFR ($r = .78$). Although some norms may be constructed for specific clinical situations, it seems unlikely that this will effectively monitor changes in renal function because changes in sodium intake and fractional reabsorption will also have major effects on sodium excretion.

Tubular Secretion

Overall, tubular secretion is measured by clearance of hippurate, which is secreted by the proximal tubule. This can be accomplished with a net extraction of about 85 percent. Hippurate clearance can be measured as plasma clearance using ^{131}I-labeled hippuran with a coefficient of variation of about 10 percent.[26]

Proximal Reabsorption

Various ionic determinations have been proposed as an indirect method for assessing the reabsorption capacity of the kidney. A crucial function of the kidney is to maintain Na balance. Na balance is normally achieved after 1 to 2 days on a constant Na intake. Although measurement of Na balance may be a useful technique in healthy or chronically ill, but stable, patients, the perioperative patient has many unmeasurable influences on sodium balance unrelated to kidney function.

Fractional excretion of sodium (FENa) or renal failure index (RFI) are often used to assess tubular function in the setting of oliguria or suspected acute renal failure. The RFI is similar to FENa:

$$RFI = \frac{UNa}{UCr/PCr}$$

FENa is usually measured in the oliguric patient in an attempt to differentiate "prerenal" oliguria or azotemia from intrinsic renal damage. FENa rises in acute renal failure due to tubular dysfunction, but only after creatinine clearance has fallen substantially.[58] However, patients in whom the pathophysiologically important lesion is glomerular in origin will have *low* FENa despite a *low* GFR. Patients with tubular dysfunction induced by diuretics (furosemide, glucose) will have high FENa, despite good renal function as reflected by GFR. This test was originally felt to be highly sensitive and specific for detecting intrinsic kidney dysfunction when the FENa was more than 1 percent.[60] Subsequent studies have failed to substantiate this claim.[61]

Both phosphate (PO_4) and glucose are reabsorbed by the proximal tubule. A rise in fractional excretion of PO_4 reflects proximal tubular dysfunction. Glucosuria results when glucose delivery to the proximal tubule (GFR × plasma glucose) exceeds the maximal rate of transport (approximately 300 mg/min). The rate of delivery of glucose is determined by the plasma level of glucose and the GFR. Certain critically ill patients, for example, burned and traumatized patients, have markedly elevated GFR at the same time as blood glucose is moderately elevated, resulting in glycosuria. Glucose transport (Tg) equals glucose filtration minus glucose excretion:

$$Tg(mg/min) = 0.01 \times GFR \times Pg - Ug \times \dot{V}$$

where Pg (plasma glucose) is in mg/dl, Ug (urine glucose concentration) is in mg/dl, and $\dot{V}$ is urine flow rate in ml/minute.

Most or all filtered bicarbonate is also reabsorbed in the proximal tubule. When drugs (e.g., acetazeolamide) or disease interfere with reabsorption in this segment, an excess of bicarbonate reaches the distal nephron. This results in an alkaline urine due to bicarbonate wasting and a hyperchloremic metabolic acidosis. Bicarbonate wasting occurs despite the fact that the distal convoluted tubule absorbs bicarbonate because this segment has low capacity, although it can produce a high concentration gradient.

Transport of β_2-Microglobulin

β_2-Microglobulin, with a molecular weight of 11.8 kDa, is freely filtered by the glomerulus and completely (99.9 percent) reabsorbed by the proximal tubule that metabolizes it.[53] It can be measured by radioimmunoassay or enzyme-linked immunosorbent assay (ELISA) with good reproducibility.[62] Normal production of 0.13 mg/(kg × h) leads to serum levels of 1.1 to 2.7 mg/L, with daily excretion of less than 370 μg/day. Proximal tubular damage leads to increased urinary excretion. Unfortunately, β_2-microglobulin is unstable in urine at room temperature if the pH is below 5.5, or below a pH of 6.0 at body temperature. In addition, enzymes from leukocytes destroy it. Thus, the patient's urine must be alkalinized prior to analysis. Because of urinary instability at physiologic conditions, its sensitivity in detecting tubular damage is limited. In contrast, α_1-microglobulin[53] is stable in urine despite low pH, and its production seems to be stable in multiple disease states. Therefore, it is preferred to β_2-microglobulin as an indicator of proximal damage.

URINE FLOW RATE AND CONCENTRATION

Measurement of Urinary Concentration

Measurement of urinary concentration is valuable in assessing kidney function, extracellular fluid volume and composition, and hemodynamic performance. The three measurements of urinary concentration in wide use are osmolality, specific gravity, and refractive index.[63]

Osmolality

Osmolality is a measure of the number of particles in solution in 1 kg of pure water, expressed as mOsm/kg H_2O. It is the preferred measure of urine concentration. Osmolarity is closely related, but it is the number of osmoles per liter of solution, and thus varies somewhat with temperature. Osmolality depresses vapor pressure and freezing point and elevates osmotic pressure and boiling point. When 1 mole of solute is dissolved in 1 kg of H_2O, freezing point falls by 1.858°C, vapor pressure drops by 0.3 mmHg, and osmotic pressure increases by 17,000 mmHg. Each particle contributes to osmolality. Thus, a nondissociating molecule, such as glucose, contributes 1 osm/mol, while dissociating molecules such as NaCl could theoretically contribute 2 osm/mol. However, at physiologic concentrations, dissociation is not complete, so each mole of NaCl contributes about 1.8 osm/mol.

Urine and serum or heparinized plasma, but not oxalated plasma, are acceptable specimens for measurement of osmolality, but must be thoroughly centrifuged to remove any particulate matter. The accuracy and reproducibility of the freezing point depression method is ± 2 mOsm/kg H_2O, and the vapor pressure method is ± 3 mOsm/kg H_2O. The freezing point depression method is considered to be more accurate and reproducible than the vapor pressure osmometer. Also, the vapor pressure method fails to account for volatile solutes such as ethanol, methanol, dissolved CO_2, and, presumably, volatile anesthetics.

Specific Gravity

Specific gravity is related to the weight of a solute in water. The physiologic range for specific gravity is up to 1.025. However, urine contains multiple solutes, each with its own relationship between molar concentration and specific gravity. Larger molecules, for example, protein, glucose, mannitol, and dextrose, contribute greatly to specific gravity, but because their molar concentration per unit of weight is low, they do not contribute proportionally to osmolality (Fig. 21-16). Therefore, the relation-

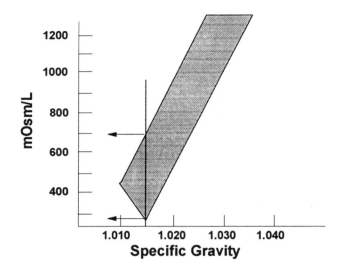

Fig. 21-17. The relationship between specific gravity and osmolality of the urine is shown. The shaded area represents the range of specific gravity and osmolality measurements. The vertical line at a specific gravity of 1.015 is associated with osmolalities ranging from approximately 300 (*lower arrow*) to 700 (*upper arrow*) mOsm/kg H_2O. (Adapted from Dunstan and Corcoran,[75] with permission.)

ship between osmolality and specific gravity exhibits wide variability (Fig. 21-17).

Errors in the measurement of specific gravity are common. Accuracy depends not only on true specific gravity, but also on surface tension, requiring that the surfaces of the measuring instruments must be completely cleaned. The float must not touch the side wall of the cylinder, and no bubbles may be allowed to cling to the stem. Each 1 g/dl of protein adds 0.003 units, and each 1 g/dl of glucose adds 0.004 units to the specific gravity.

Refractive Index

The total solids meter or refractometer estimates specific gravity from the refractive index, which, in turn, estimates osmolality. Each substance in solution contributes differently to specific gravity and refractive index. Glucose and protein in the urine may invalidate the relationship between refractive index and specific gravity. Thus, despite its convenience, it should be used only as a very rough guide to actual urine osmolality.

Free water clearance represents the difference between urine flow rate and osmolar clearance. It

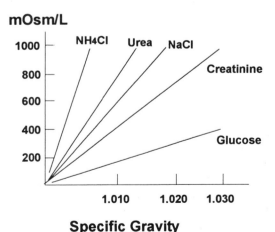

Fig. 21-16. Solutions containing a single solute demonstrate a good correlation between specific gravity and osmolality. However, as each line shows, in a complex solution such as urine, the relationship between specific gravity and osmolality will depend on the relative concentrations of each solute. (Adapted from Isaacson,[74] with permission.)

reflects the capacity of the kidney to generate a urine with an osmolality different from plasma, that is, dilution and concentration. A free water clearance of zero represents excretion of an iso-osmotic urine. Free water clearance approaches zero, 1 to 2 days prior to being able to diagnose acute renal failure. This occurs at about the same time that CCr declines.[57,58] Thus, although monitoring of free water clearance is easily performed, it does not appear to be a reliable predictor of renal dysfunction. Most patients in the operating room or intensive care unit are in circumstances that favor the production of concentrated urine. It will ordinarily be found at a value more negative than −0.3 ml/min.

Measurement of Urine Output

Urine output is one of the most commonly and easily measured parameters related to kidney function. Interpretation of the meaning of urine flow rate is more complex and requires knowledge of current hemodynamic and metabolic status. Of all the urinary parameters, it is the one that has an obvious change over short periods of time. Thus, despite problems with interpretation, it will continue to be monitored in the perioperative period. Measurement of urine output is most commonly performed by volumetric collection in a graduated collecting device. More recently, devices that measure the depth of urine using ultrasound in a collection device of known geometry have been marketed. Using microprocessor technology, the flow rate as well as cumulative output is displayed.

The evaluation of high urine output (polyuria) consists of searching for signs of intravascular and extracellular fluid volume expansion or depletion and measurement of solute concentration in the extracellular fluid. When hypovolemia or hypotension are present, vasopressin should be released, leading to a concentrated urine of minimal volume. When hyperosmolality is due to osmoles that fail to cross the blood brain barrier, vasopressin should be released. Glucose and urea cross the blood brain barrier easily. Thus, hyperosmolality due to these two substances does not cause vasopressin release. If one can document a reason for vasopressin release, then plasma osmolality and sodium are measured simultaneously with urine osmolality. If the urine is not maximally concentrated, then either insufficient vasopressin is being released or the kidney is not capable of responding to it.

Concentrating defects are suspected whenever hypernatremia develops or urine output remains high during clinical circumstances normally associated with oliguria. Hypotensive, hypovolemic or dehydrated patients should excrete a low volume of concentrated urine. If urine flow rate is not depressed, then suspect that there is tubular damage, abnormalities of renal blood flow distribution, inadequate vasopressin release, or the presence of a diuretic agent.

Oliguria is defined as inadequate urine output in relation to the output required to excrete water and solute derived from metabolic activity, that is, inability to maintain osmolar and water balance. The minimal acceptable urine output is that which will excrete all solute derived from intake of nutrients and electrolytes and metabolic production. Electrolytes are excreted in amounts equal to intake once a steady state is attained. The other major osmoles (urea, creatinine, ammonia) are derived from protein turnover. The greater the intake of exogenous or breakdown of endogenous protein or amino acids, the more urea will be produced. The majority of urea excretion occurs via the kidney. In health on a usual diet, approximately 12 mOsm solute/kg body weight are produced each day. Because the kidney can concentrate urine to about 1,000 mOsm/kg H_2O, or 1 mOsm/ml, then it follows that one needs to excrete 0.5 ml/kg/h.

Despite good theoretical grounds for relating urine flow rate to renal function, clear utility of monitoring urine output has been difficult to demonstrate. Urine output, specifically low urine output, failed to predict postoperative renal failure.[64] These patients underwent aortic reconstruction and had systemic and pulmonary artery occlusion pressures kept within normal limits. If urine output was less than 0.125 ml/kg/h, patients were treated with either Ringer's lactate infusion, or mannitol, or furosemide, or nothing. The BUN and creatinine concentrations did not vary among the groups, nor did they correlate with lowest or mean hourly urine output intraoperatively. Unfortunately, the criteria for defining renal dysfunction were not very sensitive. It would have been of interest to assess GFR by clearance of inulin or a substitute marker as well as tubular function in the various groups. Additionally, the maintenance of hemodynamics probably sustained renal cellular

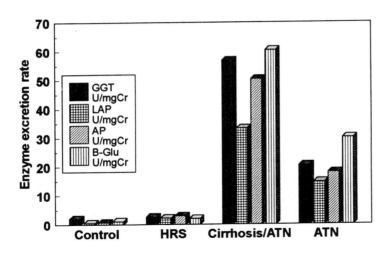

Fig. 21-18. Control patients ($n = 14$) had neither liver nor kidney disease; patients with hepatorenal syndrome (HRS) were ($n = 12$) cirrhotic patients with functional renal failure; patients with cirrhosis/ATN had acute tubular necrosis and cirrhosis ($n = 13$); ATN patients ($n = 7$) had ATN but no liver disease. GGT, gamma glutamyl transpeptidase; LAP, leucine aminopeptidase; AP, alkaline phosphatase; B-glu, β-glucuronidase; each normalized by dividing by creatinine excretion. HRS patients had increased excretion of LAP and AP compared to controls. Cirrhosis/ATN patients had markedly increased enzyme excretion compared with both control and cirrhotic patients. Their excretion rates were similar to patients with ATN without cirrhosis. (From Solis-Herruzo et al.,[70] with permission.)

energy supply sufficiently that recovery was rapid after the factors reducing GFR and urine output resolved.

Nevertheless, the occurrence of acute oliguria in the perioperative period represents a depression of GFR. In this setting, the reduction in GFR is primarily due to renal vasoconstriction. The reduction in filtration reduces the metabolic load on the nephron and is somewhat protective, but still reflects marginal renal perfusion.

Regulation of Kidney Function: Hormonal Effects

The renal regulatory hormones, vasopressin, renin, angiotensin II, aldosterone, and breakdown products of eicosanoids can be measured in plasma and urine. Vasopressin levels must be interpreted in conjunction regarding intravascular volume, hemodynamic performance, and state of hydration. Renin and angiotensin levels vary with hemodynamic performance, intravascular volume, and sodium balance. Aldosterone levels are assessed simultaneously with angiotensin II, sodium, and potassium concentrations and balance.

EVIDENCE OF TUBULAR DAMAGE: TESTS OF CELLULAR DAMAGE

Urinalysis

Urinalysis is a basic part of the assessment of kidney dysfunction. Microscopic examination of the centrifuged urinary sediment is a crucial test. Hematuria and proteinuria reflect glomerular damage. Granular and cellular casts and epithelial cells are found in acute tubular damage. White blood cells and white blood cellular casts are found in interstitial nephritis and pyelonephritis. Patients at high risk for renal failure should undergo urinalysis every 2 to 3 days, searching for signs of tubular damage.

TABLE 21-3. Specificities and Sensitivities of Various Tests in Differentiating Renal Tubular Damage from Functional Renal Failure in Cirrhosis (Hepatorenal Syndrome)

	GGT	LAP	AP	β-Glu
Sensitivity	0.92	0.92	0.92	0.92
Specificity	1.00	0.75	1.00	1.00
Correct	0.96	0.84	0.95	0.95

GGT, γ-glutamyl transpeptidase; LAP, leucine aminopeptidase; AP, alkaline phosphate; β-Glu, β-glucuronidase.
(From Solis-Herruzo et al.,[70] with permission.)

Eosinophiluria is present in immune interstitial nephritis. In a study by Nolan and colleagues[65] 10 of 11 patients with interstitial nephritis, but none of 30 cases of ATN, had eosinophiluria detected by Hansel's stain. Clinically, it is important to check for eosinophiluria in patients who develop renal dysfunction while receiving drugs, especially those with abnormalities of reabsorptive function that are more marked than the reduction of GFR.

Several small molecules are also found in the urine when kidney damage is present. β_2-microglobulin urinary excretion increases after kidney transplant due to rejection or cyclosporine therapy.[66,67] Return to the normal range was associated with healing.[67] However, questions about sensitivity, specificity and chemical stability in the urine have been raised (see earlier discussion) and α-microglobulin is a better marker.[68] Amylase is another small molecule that is filtered and fully reabsorbed by the proximal tubule. Measurement of the fractional excretion of amylase may be a useful marker of proximal tubular damage.[69] Retinol-binding protein[53] has a molecular weight of 21 and is freely filtered and completely reabsorbed. It is stable in urine, even at low pH, and is recommended over β_2-microglobulin as an indicator of tubular damage.

Adenosine deaminase-binding protein is a specific proximal tubular antigen with molecular weight of 120 kDa, which can be detected in the urine with specific monoclonal antibodies. It is stable in urine over a wide pH range.[53,68] It is reliably elevated in acute tubular necrosis and renal allograft rejection.

Enzymes present in the brush border of the proximal tubule include L-alanine aminopeptidase, β-galactosidase, angiotensin-converting enzyme, angiotensinase A, γ-glutamyl transpeptidase (GGT), dipeptidyl aminopeptidase IV, leucine aminopeptidase (LAP), and alkaline phosphatase (AP). Urinary excretion of these enzymes (which are too large to be filtered) reflects release into the ultrafiltrate by early ischemic or toxic tubular damage.[53,68,70,71] (Fig. 21-18; Table 21-3) SGP-240 protein is an immunologically detectable complex composed of alanine-aminopeptidase, γ-glutamyl transferase (GGT), and dipeptidyl peptidase IV.[71] LAP, alkaline phosphatase, and GGT excretion in the urine increase following radiocontrast media.[72]

Lysosomal enzymes include β-glucuronidase, and N-acetyl-β-D-glucosaminidase (NAG). NAG has

been used to detect tubular damage induced by aminoglycosides,[73] and radiocontrast agents.[72] However, there are problems with sensitivity, specificity, and chemical stability in the urine, which make the measurement of most value in research rather than routine clinical monitoring.[68]

Intracellular enzymes are released when cell damage is severe and are found in increased amounts in the urine. The lactate dehydrogenase (LDH) molecule is too large to be filtered by the glomerulus, thus urinary excretion is increased by tubular cell damage. The intracellular concentration is higher in more distal nephron cells. Lysozyme[53] has a molecular weight of 15 kDa and is nearly completely reabsorbed by the proximal tubule. Proximal damage causes excretion to increase.

REFERENCES

1. Parmley CL, Warters RD, Koch S et al: The relationship of serum creatine phosphokinase (CPK) to urine and serum myoglobin in the acutely traumatized patient. Crit Care Med 21(Suppl.):S240, 1993
2. Al-Uzri A, Holliday MA, Gambertoglio JG et al: An accurate practical method for estimating GFR in clinical studies using a constant subcutaneous infusion. Kidney Int 41:1701, 1992
3. Ratcliffe PJ, Moonen CTW, Holloway PAH et al: Acute renal failure in hemorrhagic hypotension: cellular energetics and renal function. Kidney Int 30: 355, 1986
4. Nelimarkka O, Niinikoski J: Renal venous oxygen tension as an indicator of tissue hypoxia in hemorrhagic shock. Crit Care Med 14:128, 1986
5. Aukland K: Methods for measuring renal blood flow: total flow and regional distribution. Ann Rev Physiol 42:543, 1980
6. Magrini F, Guo-Quing L: A critical improvement of the local thermodilution method for measuring renal blood flow in man. Cardiovascular Res 16:350, 1982
7. Avasthi PS, Greene ER, Voyles WF: Noninvasive Doppler assessment of human postprandial renal blood flow and cardiac output. Am J Physiol 252: F1167, 1987
8. Rabinovitz RS, Hartley CF, Michael LH et al: Implantable sensor for intraoperative and postoperative monitoring of blood flow: a preliminary report. J Vasc Surg 12:148, 1990
9. Stevens PE, Bolsin S, Gwyther SJ et al: Practical use of duplex Doppler analysis of the renal vasculature in critically ill patients. Lancet 1:240, 1989
10. Stevens PE, Gwyther SJ, Hanson ME et al: Noninva-

sive monitoring of renal blood flow characteristics during acute renal failure in man. Intens Care Med 16:153, 1990

11. Grigat KP, Leimenstoll G, Engemann R, Niedermayer W: Monitoring of renal allografts by duplex ultrasound. Transplant Int 2:102, 1989

12. Aronson S, Wiencek JG, Zarnoff JG et al: Assessment of renal blood flow in the dog with contrast ultrasound. Anesth Analg 70:S10, 1990

13. Aronson S, Wiencek JG, Feinstein SB et al: Assessment of renal blood flow with contrast ultrasonography. Anesth Analg 76:964, 1993

14. Schumann L, Wustenberg PW: An improved method to determine renal function using inulin and *p*-aminohippurate (PAH) steady-state kinetic modeling. Clin Nephrol 33:35, 1990

15. Hilberman M, Derby GC, Spencer RJ, Stinson EB: Sequential pathophysiological changes characterizing the progression from renal dysfunction to acute renal failure following cardiac operation. J Thorac Cardiovasc 79:838, 1980

16. Levey AS: Measurement of renal function in chronic renal disease. Kidney Int 38:167, 1990

17. Izzat NN, Rosborough JP: Renal function in conscious dogs: potential effect of gender on measurement. Res Exp Med 189:371, 1989

18. Rehling M, Moller ML, Thamdrup B et al: Simultaneous measurement of renal clearance and plasma clearance of ^{99m}Tc-labelled diethylenetriaminepentaacetate, ^{51}Cr-labelled ethylenediaminetetra-acetate and inulin in man. Clin Sci 66:613, 1984

19. Isralelit AH, Long DL, White MG, Hull AR: Measurement of glomerular filtration rate utilizing a single subcutaneous injection of 125I-iothalamate. Kidney Int 4:346, 1973

20. Ott NT, Wilson DM: A single technique for estimating glomerular filtration rate with subcutaneous injection of [^{125}I]iothalamate. Mayo Clin Proc 50:664, 1975

21. Adefuin PY, Gur A, Siegel NJ et al: Single subcutaneous injection of iothalamate sodium ^{125}I to measure glomerular filtration rate. JAMA 235:1467, 1976

22. Cohen ML, Smith FG Jr, Mindell RS, Vernier RL: A simple reliable method of measuring glomerular filtration rate using single, low-dose sodium iothalamate ^{131}I. Pediatrics 43:407, 1969

23. Dalmeida W, Suki WN: Measurement of GFR with nonradioisotopic radiocontrast agents. Kidney Int 43:725, 1988

24. Back SE, Krutzen E, Nilsson-Ehle P: Contrast media as markers for glomerular filtration: a pharmacokinetic comparison of four agents. Scand J Clin Lab Invest 48:247, 1988

25. Barbour GL, Crumb CK, Boyd CM et al: Comparison of inulin, iothalamate and ^{99m}Tc-DTPA for measurement of glomerular filtration rate. J Nucl Med 17: 317, 1976

26. Clifton GG, Anderson C, McMahon G et al: Monoexponential analysis of plasma disappearance of ^{99m}Tc-DTPA and ^{131}I-iodohippurate: a reliable method for measuring changes of renal function. J Clin Pharmacol 29:466, 1989

27. Choyke PL, Austin HA, Frank JA et al: Hydrated clearance of gadolinium-DTPA as a measurement of glomerular filtration rate. Kidney Int 41:1595, 1992

28. Rabito CA, Moore RH, Bougas C, Dragotakes SC: Noninvasive, real-time monitoring of renal function: the ambulatory renal monitor. J Nucl Med 34:199, 1993

29. Rabito CA, Fang LST, Waltman AC: Renal function in patients at risk of contrast material-induced acute renal failure: noninvasive, real-time monitoring. Radiology 186:851, 1993

30. Tauxe WN: Determination of glomerular filtration rate by single-plasma sampling technique following injection of radioiodinated diatrizoate. J Nucl Med 27:45, 1986

31. Lewis R, Kerr N, Van Buren C et al: Comparative evaluation of urographic contrast media, inulin, and ^{99m}Tc-DTPA clearance methods for determination of glomerular filtration rate in clinical transplantation. Transplantation 48:790, 1989

32. Back S-E, Krutzen E, Nilsson-Ehle P: Contrast media as markers for glomerular filtration: a pharmacokinetic comparison of four agents. Scand J Clin Lab Invest 48:247, 1988

33. Shemesh O, Golbetz H, Kriss JP, Myers BD: Limitations of creatinine as a filtration marker in glomerulopathic patients. Kidney Int 28:830, 1985

34. LaCour B: Creatinine and renal function. Nephrologie 13:73, 1992

35. Dubb JW, Stote RM, Familiar RG, Lee K, Alexander R: Effect of cimetidine on renal function in normal man. Clin Pharmacol Ther 24:76, 1978

36. Berglund F, Killander J, Pompeius R: Effect of trimethroprim-sulfamethoxazole on the renal excretion of creatinine in mad. J Urol 114:802, 1975

37. Wesslau C, Jung K, Schirrow R: Comparison of inulin and creatinine clearance determinations in anesthetized and conscious rats. Z Urol Nephrol 81: 395, 1988

38. VanLente F, Suit P: Assessment of renal function by serum creatinine and creatinine clearance: glomerular filtration rate estimated by four procedures. Clin Chem 35:2326, 1989

39. Datta P, Graham GA, Schoen I: Interference by IgG paraproteins in the Jaffe method for creatinine determination. Am J Clin Pathol 85:463, 1986

40. Young DS, Pestaner LC, Gibberman V: Effects of drugs on clinical laboratory tests. Clin Chem 21:1D, 1975

41. Narayanan S, Apleton HD: Creatinine: a review. Clin Chem 26:1119, 1980

42. Kroll MH, Olson D, Rawe M et al: Comparison of creatinine as determined with the Ames seralyzer and by three Jaffe-based methods. Clin Chem 31: 1900, 1985

43. Apple FS, Benson P, Abraham PA et al: Assessment of renal function by inulin clearance: comparison with creatinine clearance as determined by enzymatic methods. Clin Chem 35:312, 1989

44. Lindback B, Bergman A: A new commercial method for the enzymatic determination of creatinine in serum and urine evaluated: comparison with a kinetic Jaffe method and isotope dilution-mass spectrometry. Clin Chem 35:835, 1989

45. Murphy JL, Hurt TL, Griswold WR et al: Interference with creatinine concentration measurement by high dose furosemide infusion. Crit Care Med 17: 889, 1989

46. Walser M: Creatinine excretion as a measure of protein nutrition in adults of varying age. J Parenter Enter Nutr 11:73S, 1987

47. Bjornsson TD: Use of serum creatinine concentrations to determine renal function. Clin Pharmacokinetics 4:200, 1979

48. Moran SM, Myers BD: Course of acute renal failure studied by a model of creatinine kinetics. Kidney Int 27:928, 1985

49. Piccoli A, Rizzoni G, Tessarin C et al: Long-term monitoring of renal transplant patients by a CUSUM test on serum creatinine. Nephron 47:87, 1987

50. Rowe PA, Richardson RE, Burton PR et al: Analysis of reciprocal creatinine plots by two-phase linear regression. Am J Nephrol 9:38, 1989

51. Rhodes PJ, Rhodes RS, McClelland GH et al: Evaluation of eight methods for estimating creatinine clearance in men. Clin Pharm 6:399, 1987

52. Gault MH, Longerich LL, Harnett JD, Weslowski C: Predicting glomerular function from adjusted serum creatinine. Nephron 62:249, 1992

53. Flynn FV: Assessment of renal function: selected developments. Clin Biochem 23:49, 1990

54. Sladen RN, Endo E, Harrison T: Two-hour versus 22-hour creatinine clearance in critically ill patients. Anesthesiol 67:1013, 1987

55. Laville M, Hadj-Aissa A, Pozet N et al: Restrictions on use of creatinine clearance for measurement of renal functional reserve. Nephron 51:233, 1989

56. Hellerstein S, Hunter JL, Warady BA: Creatinine excretion rates for evaluation of kidney function in children. Pediatr Nephrol 2:419, 1988

57. Shin B, Mackenzie CF, Helrich M: Creatinine clearance for early detection of posttraumatic renal dysfunction. Anesthesiol 64:605, 1986

58. Brown R, Babcock R, Talbert J et al: Renal function in critically ill postoperative patients: sequential assessment of creatinine osmolar and free water clearance. Crit Care Med 8:68, 1980

59. Koning HM, Mackie DP: Is on-line monitoring of renal function possible? Int J Clin Monit Comput 6: 243, 1989

60. Espinel CH, Gregory AW: Differential diagnosis of acute renal failure. Clin Nephrol 13:73, 1980

61. Pru C, Kjellstrand CM: The FENa test is of no prognostic value in acute renal failure. Nephron 36:20, 1984

62. Parkin A, Smith HC, Brocklebank JT: Which routine test for kidney function? Arch Dis Child 64:1261, 1989

63. Rock RC, Walker WG, Jennings CD: Nitrogen metabolites and renal function. p. 669. In Tietz NW (ed): Fundamentals of Clinical Chemistry, 3rd Ed. WB Saunders, Philadelphia, 1987

64. Alpert RA, Roizen MF, Hamilton WK et al: Intraoperative urinary output does not predict postoperative renal function in patients undergoing abdominal aortic revascularization. Surgery 95:707, 1984

65. Nolan CR, Anger MS, Kelleher SP: Eosinophiluria: a new method of detection and definition of the clinical spectrum. N Engl J Med 315:1516, 1986

66. Bethea M, Forman DT: Beta 2-microglobulin: its significance and clinical usefulness. Ann Clin Lab Sci 20:163, 1990

67. Tataranni G, Zavagli G, Farinelli R et al: Usefulness of the assessment of urinary enzymes and microproteins in monitoring ciclosporin nephrotoxicity. Nephron 60:314, 1992

68. Tolkoff-Rubin NE, Rubin RH, Bonventre JV: Noninvasive renal diagnostic studies. Clin Lab Med 8: 507, 1988

69. Aderka D, Tene M, Graff E, Levo Y: Amylase-creatinine ratio: a simple test to predict gentamicin nephrotoxicity. Arch Intern Med 148:1093, 1988

70. Solis-Herruzo JA, Garcia-Cabezudo J, Diaz-Rubio C et al: Urinary excretion of enzymes in cirrhotics with renal failure. J Hepatology 3:123, 1986

71. Scherberich JE: Urinary proteins of tubular origin: basic immunochemical and clinical aspects. Am J Nephrol 10(Suppl. 1):43, 1990

72. Leander P, Allard M, Caille JM, Golman K: Early effect of gadopentateate and iodinated contrast media on rabbit kidneys. Invest Radiol 27:922, 1992

73. Langhendries JP, Battisti O, Bertrand JM: Aminoglycoside nephrotoxicity and urinary excretion of N-acetyl-beta-D-glucosaminidase. Biol Neonate 53:253, 1988

74. Isaacson LC: Urinary osmolality and specific gravity. Lancet 1:72, 1959

75. Dunstan HP, Corcoran AC: Functional interpretation of renal test. Med Clin North Am 39:947, 1955

Monitoring Metabolic Indices and Coagulation/ Hemostasis

22

Bruce D. Spiess

Blood samples obtained from a vein or artery can yield a great deal of clinically relevant information. Blood functions are extremely complex with both cellular and acellular components assuming importance. Proteins, electrolytes, fats, and many other nutrients are carried in an aqueous solution that we call plasma. Multiple different cell types perform functions in blood and some are present all the time, for example, erythrocytes, whereas others are present or concentrated only during disease processes. The cellular elements make blood a living fluid, carrying on metabolism and constantly changing or in equilibrium with other dynamic processes throughout the body. A number of potential tests can be carried out on blood samples. These tests, although useful, are limited for purposes of interpretation because, at best, they represent an estimate of a metabolic function only at one specific point in time. With these limitations in mind the following chapter is presented to acquaint the reader with some common blood tests.

Electronic and technological growth has given us the ability to obtain real-time continuous monitoring of many parameters. However, to date the process is not routinely available for either the measurement of major metabolic indices or coagulation. As a result, blood must be obtained from patients, preserved, transported, and tested in vitro at a distant laboratory site.

METABOLIC INDICES

Potassium

Potassium (K^+) is the key intracellular cation in all human excitatory cells and controls membrane excitability. Normally, tissues maintain a very steep gradient between intracellular and extracellular K^+ levels. Intracellular K^+ levels are 135 to 150 mEq/L and extracellular concentrations are 3.5 to 5.3 mEq/L[1] (Table 22-1). The sodium-potassium adenosine triphosphate (ATP) pump expends considerable energy to maintain this very steep gradient and its function. Total body stores of potassium are 3,200 mEq/70 kg in males and somewhat less, at 2,825 mEq/70 kg, for females.[2] Potentially greater than 90 percent of this is movable between intracellular and extracellular spaces. What is important is the relative intracellular to extracellular gradient. There is no easy way to measure that differential. Intracellular measurements, however, are not clinically available at this time. As a result, serum potassium is commonly measured. Normal levels are not an assurance that either total body stores are normal or that the intracellular to extracellular gradient is normal. The best illustration of this is when rapid intravenous replacement is being attempted, and, although it is relatively easy to raise serum potassium, the repletion of intracellular stores can lag significantly.

The electrocardiogram can be used as a physiologic reflector of myocardial potassium levels and gradients.[1,3–5] The appearance of peaked T waves or flattened T waves may be useful diagnostically; their clinical implications will be discussed further in the sections on hyper- and hypokalemia.

Plasma potassium is measured either using an ion-selective electrode or a flame photometer.[6] Ion-selective electrodes utilize specific membranes that are made semipermeable to the ion being tested. When the membrane material is selectively permeable to potassium, a potential is established that follows the Nernst equation:

$$E = 60 \log [K]o/[K]i$$

where o is extracellular concentration and i is intracellular concentration. A voltage logarithmically proportional to the gradient is then established. The valinomycin electrode provides a 5,000:1 selectivity for potassium to sodium.[7] Today it is the most commonly utilized technology, and it has replaced the older flame photometer.

The flame photometer utilizes changes in wavelength of light given off by a flame when lithium/cesium diluents are combined with plasma. Both sodium and potassium can be tested at the same time using these diluents. The flame photometer is perhaps less accurate, as it measures ions bound to proteins and fatty acids that would otherwise not be active in the aqueous phase of plasma.[6] For this reason, the semipermeable electrodes are the preferred method.

The act of obtaining blood specimens for measurement of potassium can also introduce considerable error. Erythrocytes contain the same intracellular concentration of potassium as most other tissues. Hemolysis caused by withdrawal through a very small needle, excessive negative pressure in the syringe of inappropriate handling of the sample such as overheating may cause excessively high measurements. Muscle activity in the extremity being utilized for blood sampling can also increase the serum potassium up to 2.7 mEq/L.[8] The mechanism for this is unclear but may have some relationship to intracellular calcium fluxes or increased potassium adenosine triphosphatase (ATPase) activity, and the effect of acidosis on potassium fluxes.

Hypokalemia

Hypokalemia, occurs frequently in the perioperative period[1,9,10] (Table 22-2). Its cause is most often iatrogenic; however, acute water intoxication can occur with Addison's disease (crisis) and acute states where antidiuretic hormone levels have increased. These events cause dilutional effects on serum potassium, and total body stores may be normal. In contrast, potassium-losing states can occur pathologically with any number of high urine output syndromes or with profound gastrointestinal losses. Emesis usually is noted for loss of sodium and acid, but significant amounts of potassium may be carried out as well. In addition, diarrhea results in the loss of high concentrations of potassium and bicarbonate.[11–13]

TABLE 22-1. Ionic Concentrations and Potentials in Mammalian Muscle Cells and Interstitial Fluid

	Interstitial Fluid	Intracellular Fluid	$[ion]_o/[ion]_i$	$E = 60 \log [ion]_o/[ion]_i$ (mV)
Cations				
Na^+	145 μmol/ml	12 μmol/ml	12.1	65
K^+	4 μmol/ml	155 μmol/ml	1/39	−95
H^+	3.8×10^{-5} μmol/ml	13×10^{-5} μmol/ml	1/3.4	−32
[pH]	[7.43]	[6.9]		
Others	5 μmol/ml			
Anions				
Cl^-	120 μmol/ml	3.8 μmol/ml	31.8	−90
$HCO3^-$	27 μmol/ml	8 μmol/ml	3.4	−32
Others	7 μmol/ml	155 μmol/ml		−90
Potential	0	−90 mV		

Abbreviations: o, extracellular; i, intracellular.
(Adapted from Woodbury,[137] with permission.)

In situations where patients have been recently started on therapy, drugs have been changed, or sudden aggressive intravenous therapy has been attempted, rapid potassium fluxes may occur. In such cases hypokalemia will be evident within the first 6 weeks of establishing therapy.[14,15] In a study by Lauer[14] of 50 patients receiving hydrochlorothiazide, the mean serum potassium was 4.3 mEq/L before beginning therapy. Only two patients had levels below 3.5 mEq/L 6 weeks later, and the mean returned to 4.1 mEq/L at 19 months of study.[14] Dietary supplementation is probably important, particularly if the patient is not receiving a potassium-rich diet, for example, elderly, chronically ill, undernourished, or poorly motivated patients.[16,17]

Chronic hypokalemia appears to be quite well tolerated.[9,10,16] There is little evidence to support any absolute number as a cutoff for elective anesthesia. The two most recent studies (with almost 500 patients between them) show no increased risk in this setting of chronic hypokalemia.[16,17] The incidence of ventricular arrhythmias does not linearly increase with progressive hypokalemia. However, some case reports do implicate hypokalemia as a cause of ventricular arrhythmia and potentially the cause of death.[18,19] The concomitant use of digitalis and hypokalemia appears to be the common theme in these cases. Rapid replacement of hypokalemia may actually increase the transmembrane difference in potassium and therefore may be detrimental. Potassium repletion should be done slowly so that intracellular repletion can occur. Daily intake should not exceed 250 to 500 mEq. Intravenous usage with high concentrations carries risks of tissue injury.[16,20] An infusion of potassium at a rate of 0.75 mEq/kg over 1 hour will increase the circulating potassium by 1 to 1.5 mEq/L.[21]

Monitoring of potassium concentration becomes very important in situations where rapid shifts may occur. Recent developments in certain surgical subspecialties (such as liver transplantation) have introduced some conditions where this may be anticipated.[22] Potassium-containing preservative solutions are used for these procedures. At the point of reestablishment of blood flow (to the transplanted organ) the preservative solution is flushed out into the peritoneal cavity. At this point large increases in K^+ occur and may result in hemodynamic sequelae. Later, once the organ begins to function, a potassium deficit may exist, as the new liver will act as a potassium sink (resulting in hypokalemia). Careful, frequent measurements of potassium will allow one to tailor therapy to the needs, so that severe hypokalemia does not occur. The development of this state can actually be used as a gauge that metabolic function is beginning. Another particularly critical time for the development of hypokalemia is immediately following cardiac surgery. Cardioplegia solutions, much like the transplant organ preservation solutions, are most often hyperkalemic. However, during the first several hours after reperfusion, the heart may be intracellularly potassium-depleted. If a severe diuresis has occurred during bypass, hypokalemia may exist, and a potential for arrhythmias may be created.

Hyperkalemia

Much like hypokalemia, there are no absolute rules that establish a "safe" level above which elective anesthesia cannot be performed. Once again,

---

TABLE 22-2. Potential Causes of Hypokalemia

I. Disturbances in potassium intake
  A. Decreased dietary intake
  B. Gastrointestinal disorders—villous adenoma, fistulas
II. Disturbances in potassium excretion
  A. Gastrointestinal—diarrhea, vomiting
  B. Renal
    1. Increased potassium excretion
      a. High potassium intake
      b. Mineralocorticoid excess
      c. Acute alkalemia
      d. Increased urinary flow rate (diuretics)
      e. Increased sodium delivery
      f. Acid-base balance
        1. Chronic respiratory acidosis
        2. Chronic metabolic acidosis
        3. Chronic metabolic alkalosis
      g. Hypomagnesemia
    2. Decreased potassium excretion
      a. Decreased dietary intake
      b. Decreased sodium delivery
      c. Mineralocorticoid insufficiency
      d. Acute acidemia
III. Disturbances in distribution
  A. Cell membrane integrity
  B. Hormones
    1. Insulin, aldosterone, catecholamines
  C. Osmolality
  D. Acid-base disturbances
    1. Four major acute acid-base disturbances
    2. Bicarbonate levels

(From Wong, et al.,[1] with permission.)

the electrocardiogram can be a very useful tool in assessing the effects of the measured serum level.[23,24] Prolongation of the PR interval, loss of sinus node activity, and peaked or elevated T waves are all hallmarks of elevated potassium levels. In addition, widened QRS complexes can occur. Often this is seen as a preterminal event. Although the serum potassium may not match what is being seen on the cardiogram, localized hyperkalemia or intracellular hypokalemia may exist such that the gradient is more severe than what the serum measurement alone signifies.

Hyperkalemia can be a common event and should actually be expected in certain situations much the same as hypokalemia. Particularly the use of certain medications, including beta-blocking drugs, ace inhibitors, and indomethacin, as these can all elevate serum potassium levels.[25,26] Ischemic tissue releases intracellular potassium and, as a result, patients with bowel ischemia, vascular compromise of a limb, crush injuries, and so on, may all present to the operating room with elevated potassium. Again the use of cardioplegia in cardiac surgery can be a major cause of elevated potassium. There is a move in some centers to utilize continuous cardioplegia with a resultant increase in total potassium load. With this regimen, it has been my experience to see serum potassium in those patients routinely elevated above 7 mEq/L and sometimes a great deal higher. Patients undergoing solid organ transplantation may experience severe sudden rises in potassium if the washout phase of preservative is not complete. This sudden rise has resulted in cardiac arrest in certain patients.[27]

The use of succinylcholine as an adjuvant drug for intubation carries a significant risk for elevation of the serum potassium.[28-30] In normal individuals given a routine intubating dose, the serum potassium acutely rises 0.5 to 1 mEq/L immediately after the depolarization. If hyperkalemia already exists, this effect will be additive. The most widely reported disasters with succinylcholine occur in situations where tissues are presensitized to the depolarization effects. Patients with relatively new neurologic injuries (<3 months) such that a significant amount of striated muscle is denervated are at risk. The denervated muscle responds with hypersensitivity and hyperplasia of receptor sites. In these situations depolarization is exaggerated and loss of intracellular potassium can be sudden and extreme with resultant cardiac arrest. Patients with

prolonged bed rest, muscle wasting, trauma, crush injury, and burns may behave in a similar manner. In these situations the electrocardiogram may aid in the diagnosis of clinically significant hyperkalemia.

Acidosis will serve to worsen hyperkalemia and therefore blood gas monitoring in conjunction with electrolyte monitoring is recommended in critically ill patients.[31] As hydrogen ions move intracellularly they are exchanged with potassium ions moving extracellularly. Lactic acidosis, coupled with tissue ischemia, can make hyperkalemia particularly difficult to deal with. Diabetic ketoacidosis, as well as respiratory acidosis, can contribute to hyperkalemia.

In certain clinical situations treatment of the cause of hyperkalemia can transiently worsen the situation. For example, the reestablishment of vascular flow to an ischemic leg may cause a washout of potassium, elevating total body potassium. Alkalinization of serum pH will drive potassium intracellularly much as acidosis will exchange hydrogen ion.[32] Sodium bicarbonate can be utilized for this purpose, but alkalinization like acidosis may be detrimental as well. Calcium can be used, as it changes transmembrane potential but does little or nothing to serum potassium.[33] The effects of hyperkalemia may be decreased by administering 1 to 4 calcium chloride (given with ECG monitoring). Unfortunately, this therapy is very short-lived, as the calcium is rapidly redistributed to other body stores. The use of insulin to move glucose intracellularly causes an obligatory movement of potassium intracellularly as well. Much of this occurs in the liver, and the practitioner can decide how much insulin is needed depending upon a patient's past history. Those who are not diabetic can tolerate 10 units of regular insulin for a load of 50 g dextrose. One should remember that in normal patients the capability for pancreatic production of insulin exits. Therefore perhaps only a glucose load may be required.

Potassium levels, both hyper- and hypokalemia, may be life-threatening. New technology is in the development stage that could give real-time continuous data. The use of fluorescent dyes (optodes) sensitive to individual ions are being perfected. Miniaturization of semipermeable membrane technology is also in development/early clinical utilization.[34,35] Whether such technology will be made to be indwelling perhaps placed through an arterial cannula or external but in contact with the blood circuit of the patient is yet to be determined.

Sodium

Sodium is the most abundant extracellular cation.[1] It is actively maintained at a level less than 5 mEq/L intracellularly by the sodium potassium ATPase pump that also pumps potassium intracellularly. The normal extracellular concentration of sodium should be between 135 and 145 mEq/L. Water and sodium are closely linked with sodium creating the major solute of serum osmolality. It freely moves through all extracellular spaces, a body compartment that makes up approximately one-third of the total body weight. Total body sodium therefore is partially responsible for the amount of extracellular water. Kidney regulation of sodium is of key importance to sodium homeostasis.[36] The kidney filters and reabsorbs 173 L water and with it 24,000 mEq sodium. Changes in glomerular filtration rate and tubular reabsorption of sodium modulate the end effect, which is sodium and free water clearance.[37]

The causes for sodium and free water derangement are numerous. Iatrogenic causes include fluid overload, excess sodium administration, and renal dysfunction secondary to a number of causes. Sodium and free water loads will be very well tolerated without major organ dysfunction as long as renal function is normal and other insults have not occurred, such as septicemia, hypoperfusion, or ischemia. Renal impairment with either high output syndromes or anuria are a complex subject that is not explored in this chapter. Perioperative renal failure is a particularly bad prognostic indicator for all surgeries.[38,39] Sodium fluxes in such patients warrant careful monitoring to assure that extracellular water and sodium are controlled.

Sodium, like potassium, can be measured by either flame photometry or ion-selective electrode techniques. The sodium electrode has a 300:1 selectivity for sodium over potassium and is very insensitive to hydrogen ion.[40] Future development of a miniaturized ion-selective electrode or optode technology is not yet available. Sodium changes are not as rapid as either potassium or other electrolyte changes. Also, minor changes in sodium concentration do not cause the myocardial irritability that can be seen with potassium changes. Therefore, there appears to be less need for real-time monitoring of serum sodium.

Perioperative sodium changes can occur in some specific situations. Treatment of metabolic acidosis with sodium bicarbonate may be limited by the fact that it is a hyperosmolar fluid carrying a heavy sodium load. It is possible to raise serum sodium acutely if repeated treatment with bicarbonate is utilized. Edema may be a result and, at least in pediatric patients, cerebral edema is a concern if excess bicarbonate is utilized. Other causes of perioperative hypernatremia include diabetes insipidus caused from resection of a pituitary adenoma or other neurologic resections.[41] Burn patients and potentially those with severe peritonitis can lose large amounts of free water and therefore hypernatremia is the result.

Hyponatremia as a result of free water administration using dextrose solutions without normal salt loads can occur. Irrigation solutions for a number of surgeries can be absorbed and cause dilutional hyponatremia. Transurethral resection of the prostate with glycine-containing irrigation solutions has been widely publicized as causing hyponatremia.[42] Other surgeries such as arthroscopies may result in a similar problem with hypokalemia. Hyponatremia can cause delayed awakening in the recovery room, coma, and/or seizures. Treatment with diuretics, normal saline, or hypertonic saline is a judgment based upon the degree of hyponatremia and the individual's clinical state.[43–46]

Calcium

Calcium is the most abundant cation present in the body, and it is mostly found tightly bound in bone mass.[1,47,48] Calcium has a vital role in many enzymatic reactions, including blood coagulation, neuromuscular contraction, smooth muscle tone, cardiac muscle contraction, and a myriad of hormone releases and functions.[48,49]

Calcium exists in the extracellular fluid in one of three forms. Movement of ions between these three forms occurs readily. It is either bound to serum albumin or globulin, diffusible by a nonionized chelate, or in a free ionized fraction (approximately 50 percent) of the serum level. The free ionized calcium is the form that can be physiologically active. Therefore it is very important when monitoring calcium to know what levels are being reported (i.e., free ionized vs bound).

Total serum calcium can be measured by the colorimetric *O*-cresolphthalein complexometric method.[50] With this technique, serum must first be separated from erythrocytes to prevent contamination from intracellular calcium.[51] Magnesium ions are then removed in a reaction with 8-quinolinol, and the calcium is allowed to react with *O*-cresolphthalein complexone. This reaction produces a purple color, and the proportion of that purple coloration is utilized to gauge the concentration of total serum calcium. This method is accurate and is linear over the range of 2.5 to 7.5 mEq/L (5 to 15 mg/dl).[52] The normal serum concentrations vary slightly with each laboratory, but are usually within the range of 4.5 to 5.3 mEq/L. Accurate reporting of serum calcium is dependent upon the close measurement of serum albumin because there is a 0.1 mmol/L decrease in total serum calcium for each 5 g/L decrease in albumin concentration.[53]

Ionized calcium can be measured with another ion-selective membrane electrode.[54,55] In the method, an organic liquid ion exchanger transports calcium ions across the sensing membrane. The ions change the voltage of the electrode as compared to a reference electrode, and voltage is logarithmically proportional to the calcium concentration.[56] A controversy exists with regard to the reporting of free calcium ions, and some believe that only a small fraction of these are actually active. Perhaps other ionized calcium atoms are bound by electrostatic forces and are not biologically active. The calcium electrode therefore measures only the free ions that can move from an active portion. To avoid changing the entire concept of ionic movement, the reciprocal of the activity coefficient for calcium ions is the value reported. Normal values for ionized calcium are usually 2.1 to 2.6 mEq/L (1.17 to 1.29 mmol/L).[53] Often practitioners become confused between how these values are reported and one should note whether it is mEq/L or mmol/L that they are reported in.

Like potassium, calcium changes can occur rapidly and do carry significant hemodynamic changes associated with them. Preoperative hypocalcemia is fairly rare as parathyroid hormone closely regulates calcium level. Bone acts as a major reservoir even if dietary intake is inadequate or gut absorption is impaired. Intraoperatively, hypocalcemia has been noted with rapid infusion of blood products.[57] Sodium citrate is utilized as a calcium chelating agent to prevent coagulation. Although most clinicians focus on the problem with red cell or whole-blood transfusions one should remember that significant citrate loads are carried in fresh frozen plasma, platelet, and cryoprecipitate transfusions as well. Acute hypocalcemia has been reported with infusions of 33 ml/kg-h in at least one report.[58] Patients with normal hepatic function appear to have some resistance to the effects of the citrate, as they can rapidly metabolize it and release free calcium. Those with hepatic failure, and particularly patients undergoing hepatic transplantation, are quite susceptible to the effects of hypocalcemia.[59] During the anhepatic period of liver transplantation, a time period when rapid hemorrhage occurs, there is no available hepatic clearance of citrate and ionized calcium levels can fluctuate wildly. At this time, systemic hypotension due to partial vasodilation and decreased cardiac output may occur. There is no way of discerning an appropriate infusion rate of blood products that warrant prophylactic calcium therapy. A high index of suspicion must be reserved for this as a cause of hypotension in the appropriate setting.

Postoperative hypocalcemia can be a complication of parathyroid surgery. Close postoperative monitoring of serum calcium levels is necessary. Like potassium deficiency, hypocalcemia can be reflected in the ECG, all of which is nonspecific.[60–62] Shortened Q-R intervals, tachycardia, and irritability are seen.[1] Alkaline pH increases the binding of calcium to albumin and can acutely lower ionized calcium levels. Severely low ionized calcium levels can lead to neuronal hyperexcitability and tetanus.

Hypocalcemia after cardiopulmonary bypass occurs in a significant number of patients.[63,64] The major causes appear to be hemodilutional effects and diuresis.

Hypercalcemia can be seen preoperatively from a number of conditions including, hyperparathyroidism, total parenteral nutrition, milk-alkali syndrome, and hypervitaminoses D and A.[65,66] However, malignancies causing acute bone destruction are the most common cause of preoperative hypercalcemia. Treatment of hypercalcemia involves increasing the clearance with diuretics, particularly loop diuretics such as furosemide and perhaps dialysis. Patients with long-standing or severe hypercalcemia may be volume-depleted due to increased renal free water loss and therefore volume assessment and reexpansion with saline may be necessary.

Magnesium

Magnesium is an often overlooked major metal ion catalyst that is found intracellularly. It regulates a number of enzymatic activities, and is important for ribosome stability and, therefore, protein production.[67] It has recently been shown to be important in maintaining myocardial rhythm stability. In addition, it is an excellent antiarrhythmic for the treatment of ventricular irritability.[68,69] Mechanisms similar to those causing hypocalcemia during cardiopulmonary bypass also contribute to hypomagnesemia.

As in calcium and potassium deficiency, the electrocardiogram (ECG) may reflect changes indicative of hypomagnesemia; however, these changes are not pathognomonic. Low-voltage T waves as well as decreased QRS complexes may be seen.[1,70–72] Shortening of the RR interval may also be seen. The risk of arrhythmias in patients taking digitalis is increased.[73]

Total body magnesium ranges between 22.7 and 35.0 mEq/L with approximately 1 percent being extracellular.[74] Serum magnesium levels should be between 1.44 and 1.95 mEq/L.[75] In the ionized form, 65 percent of it is biologically active and freely diffusible.[76]

Monitoring of magnesium today is carried out using atomic absorption spectrophotometry.[77,78] Serum is separated, and care must be taken to ensure that hemolysis does not occur because of the high intracellular concentration of magnesium. Lanthanum salts are used to remove phosphate ions and proteins. A light from a hollow cathode lamp at 285.2 nm is shown on the sample and absorption versus conductance is measured, thereby indicating the concentration of magnesium ions. This method is very precise and can be performed very rapidly. As a test it is not routinely performed because it is expensive and for most patients the yield is low.

Hypermagnesemia is most often the iatrogenic result of magnesium therapy for treatment/prophylaxis of preeclampsia/eclampsia.[79] Infusion and loading dosages should be targeted to have an effective plasma concentration of 4.8 to 8.4 mEq/L. During infusion of Mg^{2+}, close monitoring of serum levels is vital. Hypotension, depressed sensorium, muscle weakness, and bradycardia can all occur with acutely elevated magnesium. Because of the effects on the neuromuscular junction and depression of the level of consciousness, anesthetic requirements may be decreased and potentiation of nondepolarizing neuromuscular blocking agents may occur as well. If acute toxicity is encountered, treatment with calcium chloride may be helpful.

Glucose

Serum glucose is unlike any of the other biochemical measurements previously mentioned. It is a necessary substrate for cellular energy production in many tissues. Brain utilizes glucose exclusively for its energy requirements, and therefore in certain perioperative settings glucose monitoring is critical. Insulin controls cellular uptake of plasma glucose and therefore patients with diabetes have variable elevations of plasma glucose.[80,81] Preoperative screening and intraoperative monitoring of glucose is important for the appropriate perioperative management of diabetic patients. The frequency and method utilized for monitoring is dependent upon the individual patient's preexisting state, medications, and surgery planned.

One of the most common methods for measuring serum glucose levels is the oxygen electrode.[82] Glucose reacts directly with oxygen in the presence of the enzyme glucose oxidase and water to form gluconic acid and hydrogen peroxide.[83] The rate of oxygen utilization is directly proportional to the concentration of serum glucose and the electropotential of the electrode is changed as oxygen is utilized. This method is accurate to 2 percent error between 0 and 450 mg/dl. Differential anodic enzyme polarographic detection can also provide an automated method of determining serum glucose concentration.

Numerous less complex methods are presently available to be used in the hospital or in the home. Most of these methods employ the use of glucose peroxidase enzyme coupled with a dye indicator that reacts to the production of hydrogen peroxide.[84–86] Test strips impregnated with enzyme and dye can react over several reference ranges of glucose. The result can be obtained from visual comparison with a chart or from an electronic eye. Automated devices can simply utilize a drop of blood, which allows a plasma filtrate to pass through a semipermeable membrane and then come into contact with the reagent. Internal use of a reflectance meter can be used to give a direct readout of the glucose level. These devices have a very good accuracy rating when compared with other methods.

Miniaturization of glucose electrodes or optical probes is leading to development of devices that potentially could provide implantable closed circuit monitoring and dosing of insulin for diabetic patients.[87] Unfortunately, these devices are still in the investigational phase and are not presently available.

Intraoperative monitoring of serum glucose is warranted for diabetics, but it should be monitored in liver transplantation and during cardiopulmonary bypass as well. There is some evidence that if cerebral hypoxia exists, either from global hypoperfusion or from embolic phenomena that hyperglycemia may worsen the eventual neurologic deficits produced.[88] Some clinicians have advocated very tight control of glucose during cardiopulmonary bypass for this reason. Treatment of hyperkalemia with glucose and insulin infusions warrants close follow-up. In hepatic transplantation the liver is removed from circulation for a period of time. When it is reperfused it may be either poorly functioning or, occasionally, hypermetabolic. During the anhepatic phase of liver transplantation the liver is not available for regulating serum glucose levels.[22] Most often glucose rises as a response to the lack of uptake. The patient may be resistant to insulin therapy as well. Transfusion of banked blood products carries a significant glucose load as the preservative contains a large amount of dextrose. After the new organ begins to function, there may be an intracellular deficit of glucose and serum levels may drop. Rarely does hypoglycemia become a problem.

In the rare tumor resection for an insulinoma, frequent glucose determinations are required and may become lifesaving if tumor secretion is excessive.[89] Also patients receiving parenteral nutrition may have either high glucose levels or increased indigenous insulin production that can cause hypoglycemia when these fluid therapies are withdrawn.

Coagulation Monitoring

Coagulation is a very localized process occurring at the blood endothelial surface interface.[90] Blood is actively maintained in a liquid phase and shifted to a gel by a number of dynamic cellular and biochemical reactions. The interaction of forces to prevent, create, or lyse clot are ever-present and constantly changing within the microenvironment of the vessel lining.[91] A concept that coagulation is not a whole-body event but a localized issue phenomenon is key to the understanding of what blood coagulation monitoring can tell us about overall hemostatic function (Fig. 22-1). Blood samples drawn from a venous or arterial site are often remote from the site of actual biochemical event. Therefore they may not accurately reflect the dynamic activator and inhibitor responses that are going on. At best they give us very incomplete data from which inferences must be made about the organism's overall hemostatic function.

Historically, routine coagulation profile monitoring has utilized a group of screening tests. These may include the prothrombin time (PT), partial thromboplastin time (PTT or aPTT), thrombin time (TT), fibrinogen level (Fib), and the platelet count (PLT). Fibrin degradation product levels (FDP or FSP) and euglobulin lysis times (ELT) may in some institutions be included in a standard coagulation profile. A short review of coagulation function will facilitate the reader's ability to appropriately interpret these tests.

Blood is maintained in the liquid state by the release of substances from the endothelial cells onto their vascular surface.[92–95] The entire surface is coated with proteoglycan, a protein skeleton that carries a similar charge to plasma proteins and therefore repels them. It also provides an attachment for heparin molecules, which are constantly being grown and destroyed. The endothelial cell modulates local vascular tone by producing endothelial relaxant factor, nitric oxide.[94] This can defuse both into the smooth muscle as well as into plasma. Nitric oxide is a profound platelet inhibitor.[96–98] Prostacyclin is produced as well and also inhibits platelet contact activation. The thrombomodulin, protein S, protein C system forms a potent thrombin inhibition system as well. Endothelial cells also contribute to the activation of the fibrinolytic system.[99]

Once a vascular insult has occurred these inhibitory mechanisms are locally removed. Basement membrane exposed by trauma contains collagen, a potent stimulator of coagulation. The initiation of coagulation begins with von Willebrand factor binding to the collagen. Its multimetric constitution forms a glue to which platelets adhere.[100,101] Platelets become activated and then interact with other platelets to create a platelet plug. Protein cascade activity is stimulated simultaneously. For adequate coagulation to occur, the macromolecular complex of factor X, calcium, factor VIII, and factor V must come together on the surface of an activated platelet at one of the glycoprotein binding sites.[102] There is extensive feedback and cross-stimulation within both the intrinsic and extrinsic systems. The concept of these cascades as separate isolated biochemical processes is just not correct. Therefore analyzing them in isolation cannot possibly give a complete view of the complex activation and control mechanisms involved. Furthermore, it is becoming increasingly evident that platelets and immune cells actively communicate.[103–105] The activation of the coagulation system spreads reactions throughout the immune system and the end-product of that activation may be the formation of certain complement complexes.[106] These macromolecular complement complexes attack the endothelial cell linings and other surrounding tissues. Activity at the endothelial lining can promote coagulation as the inhibiting function of the endothelial surface is modified. These interactions are just beginning to be understood and our far-removed systemic blood sampling tells us little of the actual real-time localization and interaction.

Unfortunately, we are far from a real-time comprehensive coagulation monitor, and there is no one perfect coagulation monitor.

Coagulation Profile Monitoring

Activated Partial Thromboplastin Time

The activated partial thromboplastin time (aPTT) is a screening plasma test for the function of the intrinsic cascade and the final common pathway.[107] It is performed by centrifuging blood and separating the plasma, which is then placed in a warmed (37°C) fibrometer. A surface activator is added to provide some amount of Hageman factor (factor XII) acceleration. The activators utilized are cellite- or kaolin-type extracts of microparticle deposits. The activators utilized differ for various manufacturers, and they also have some variability between batches within specific activators. Therefore standards must be run on analyzers to determine the normal values for each machine. The aPTT is recorded as the time necessary for the formation of fibrin strands. Once initial fibrin for-

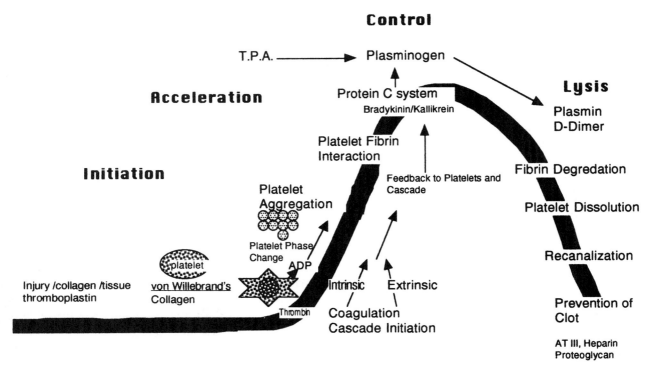

Fig. 22-1. The sine wave of coagulation occurs at the microenvironment of vascular injury. It represents a continuum of reactions from initiation to eventual clot lysis. (From Spiess,[90] with permission.)

mation has occurred, the aPTT test will give no further information regarding clot activity.

As a screening test the aPTT is very useful in monitoring the gross function of the intrinsic cascade. A functional final common pathway is necessary for normal test results. Abnormalities in thrombin or fibrinogen will also be reflected in a prolonged aPTT. Fibrinogen levels above 150 mg/dl are considered normal and levels much below (50–100 mg/dl) can prolong the aPTT without there actually being an isolated abnormality in the intrinsic cascade. Dysfibrinogenemia and fibrin degradation products or inhibitors can all prolong the aPTT due to inhibition of the final common pathway.

The intrinsic cascade is an enzymatic process of protein cleavages to eventually activate the macromolecular complex on the platelet surface. Serine proteases are enzymes manufactured in the liver that circulate in the plasma and when activated use each other as activator and substrate for stimulating further reactions. The heparin antithrombin III complex inhibits serine protease activity, particularly factor IXa and the action of thrombin. The aPTT therefore provides an excellent screening tool for monitoring low-dosage heparin therapy. The aPTT has a range of accuracy from 15 seconds to 120 or 140 seconds. Beyond that level reproducibility begins to be lost, and therefore when heparin levels are such that the aPTT is further prolonged it cannot be used to monitor coagulation.

Relatively low concentrations of the serine proteases are required for normal functioning of the intrinsic cascade. These proteins work as enzymes and are not consumable; therefore, levels of 20 to 35 percent only are required for normal aPTT values to be recorded. Hepatic disease may cause decreases in production and even states such as disseminated intravascular coagulation (DIC) do not cause direct consumption. In massive transfusion, dilution may effect the aPTT if more than 1.5 blood volume is replaced.[108]

The aPTT is often performed prior to surgery as a screening test. However, there are no data to indicate that any particular level of any abnormality in aPTT causes surgical bleeding. Hemorrhage or clot function is a complex process requiring the interaction of proteins and platelets. The formation of fibrin to hold platelets together can occur both from intrinsic cascade activity and from other mechanisms. Knowing an aPTT in isolation of other tests therefore provides rather limited information.

Prothrombin Time

The prothrombin time (PT) like the aPTT is a screening test for protein cascade function.[109] Unlike the aPTT, the PT primarily focuses on the activity of the extrinsic cascade. Like the aPTT, it is performed using isolated plasma that is artificially stimulated in vitro. Again plasma is placed in a fibrometer, and the activator added for this test is tissue thromboplastin. It may be derived from a number of sources but bovine brain extracted material is most common. The tissue thromboplastin activates factor VII, which in turn both activates the macromolecular complex on platelet surfaces and also provides an amplification step by partially activating some of the intrinsic serine proteases.[110] The fibrometer used for the PT determination senses turbidity changes using an electronic sensor of transmittance and therefore gives information only until the first strands of fibrin are formed. Like the aPTT, a normal functioning final common pathway is needed for the measurement to be valid. Dysfibrinogenemia and other inhibitors may prolong the PT.

The proteins involved in the extrinsic cascade are also hepatically produced and are dependent upon vitamin K for normal production. Patients that are vitamin K-deficient may show prolongations of their PT due to decreased levels of factors II, V, VII, and X. Coumadin or warfarin compounds given as oral anticoagulants produce their effect by partially inhibiting the production of these vitamin K-dependent proteins. Factor V, the labile factor, is a consumable protein, as is fibrinogen. Its levels may be of key importance in either massive transfusion or DIC. Like the aPTT there is no one level at which a patient is at risk for abnormal hemorrhage during surgery. Indeed the prolongation of the PT and aPTT should be looked upon as gradations, and those with at least twice normal values may have a significant tendency for easy bleeding, all other factors being equal.

The PT and aPTT may be artificially prolonged after cardiopulmonary bypass.[111] Therefore strict adherence to the normal values here with treatment of abnormal values may lead to overutilization of blood coagulation products. Recent work that has demonstrated that only levels greater than

1.5 to 1.8 normal are associated with increased clinical bleeding[111] and therefore require treatment. The exact reason for the elevated PT and aPTT after bypass may as yet be unknown, but it appears that an interaction of the heparin protamine complex and some of the substances used for activation may be involved. This is particularly true for the aPTT.

New technology is now available for bedside monitoring of the aPTT and PT.[112,113] A drop of whole blood is placed in a prewarmed plastic cartridge. That drop of blood sits in a well that has a convoluted capillarylike tube system leading from it. Blood enters the tube, mixes with activator reagent and then proceeds at a constant rate of speed to move through the tube by capillary action. Once coagulation is activated to the point of gel formation, a laser photometer detects that coagulation has occurred. The time in seconds that it takes for capillary action and coagulation does not directly correspond to that found with routine laboratory PT and aPTT tests.[112] Therefore the manufacturer has built correction factors into the system such that the display reading is the value in PT or aPTT that would have been derived if the plasma test had been done by routine methods.

This new whole-blood method has reasonable correlations with simultaneously conducted routine PT and aPTT tests.[112] In the setting of the postcardiac surgery patient the aPTT has more variability and less agreement. Once again this could be due to the interference of heparin-protamine complexes with the activators and the fact that the activator in the bedside monitor cannot possibly approximate that in the laboratory monitor. Recent work has suggested that using these monitors at the site of surgery in conjunction with a branching algorithm may reduce the use of blood products.[109]

Thrombin Time

The thrombin time is a screening test that measures the integrity of the final common pathway. Like the PT and aPTT, it is performed using a heated fibrometer and isolated plasma that is artificially activated.[107] The activator in this case is bovine thrombin, which simply stimulates the conversion of fibrinogen to fibrin. The thrombin time test use is used mainly to detect trace inhibitors of the final common pathway, and it is particularly sensitive to small amounts of heparin. Also, circulating D-dimer or dysfibrinogenemia will inhibit the thrombin time. It should be ordered in situations where some such phenomenon is suspected. The PT and aPTT will both be prolonged if a final common pathway defect is present and the thrombin time will only confirm that. The thrombin time is far more sensitive to the effects of "trace" amounts of heparin than either the aPTT or the activated clotting time (which is particularly insensitive to trace heparin). The thrombin time will give a normal determination even with greatly reduced fibrinogen concentrations. Values significantly less than 50 mg/dl must be encountered before the thrombin time is prolonged.

Reptilase Time

The reptilase time is much less often ordered but can be performed on plasma to discern abnormal functioning of fibrinogen from heparin. Reptilase, a snake venom, directly converts fibrinogen to fibrin and is not inhibited by the action of activated antithrombin III. It is performed in the manner of the other tests aforementioned. There is no routine situation where it would be utilized and, if required, may be in conjunction with a hematologist's extensive investigation of a complex coagulopathy.

Fibrinogen

Fibrinogen is the soluble precursor to the insoluble platelet-cementing glue, fibrin.[114] It is largely produced in hepatocytes and carried in the plasma; however, platelets contains fibrinogen as well in their alpha granules. The measured fibrinogen is made only on free plasma levels. Two major methods for determination are utilized. The older and less common method is a series of plasma dilutions utilizing thrombin time activations to determine the approximate concentration of fibrinogen. This technique may require five to ten plasma dilutions and, although automated, is somewhat inaccurate.

More recently radioimmunoassay techniques have been instituted, and they can be performed with great accuracy. Fibrinogen must be present in at least 150 mg/dl concentration for normal clot function. In the presence of heparin the dilution testing with the thrombin activation will be prone to give inaccurate results. Therefore the plasma may have to have heparin inactivated by passing it through a column containing heparinase bound to cephurose beads. With high concentrations of heparin, more than one pass through the column may be required to remove all the heparin, and this will introduce error into the technique.

Fibrin Split Products

Fibrin split products are the byproducts of either fibrinogenesis or fibrinolysis. These may be fibrinopeptides A or B, which are created during the initial stimulation of fibrinogen. The early fibrinolytic fragments X and Y are generally still capable of gel formation under proper stimulation. The final degradation product of fibrin is the D-dimer fragment, which has anticoagulant properties. Testing for these fragments is performed by dilutions of the isolated plasma with subsequent specific radioimmunoassays. Data can be reported either in ranges or in specific concentrations. For most clinical decision-making situations the ranges offered are all that are needed. The exact concentrations are much more important for research.

A positive presence of fibrin split products does not absolutely indicate that a patient is in either disseminated intravascular coagulation (DIC) or primary fibrinolysis. All it signifies is that some destruction of fibrinogen or fibrin has occurred somewhere in the body. Patients undergoing prolonged and relatively bloody surgery will have slow increasing elevations of their fibrin split products as clot is formed and eventually broken down. In cardiopulmonary bypass most patients will have positive fibrin split products results, as there is stimulation of plasminogen activation on bypass. Other cases where fibrin split products are common are in hepatic transplantation, neurosurgery, and prostatectomy. If DIC is suspected, the diagnosis should be made with multiple tests indicating a consumptive coagulopathy. The hallmarks of DIC are falling factor V and fibrinogen levels with concomitant decreases in platelet count. In addition, fibrin split products may be present if secondary lysis is occurring.

Factor Levels

As noted for fibrinogen, individual factor levels can be measured. Either plasma dilutions that are stimulated with variations of the PT and aPTT testing can be carried out or specific radioimmunoas-

say techniques are now available. The individual factor levels are of relatively little use for most clinical situations; however, in cases of severe hemodilution or suspected consumption they may be worth following. Individual specific deficiencies are most often known or suspected before elective surgery and certainly those patients with genetic deficiencies will most often have been worked up and followed by a hematologist. It is not cost-effective to do factor testing or even routine PT and aPTT screening for healthy patients undergoing routine surgery if they have a negative history.

Euglobulin Lysis Time

This is a test of plasmin activation and may be useful in assessing the function of the fibrinolytic system. Plasma must be centrifuged and separated. Further treatment of the plasma to separate the euglobulin fraction requires some extensive manipulation by technicians and a second centrifugation. The euglobulin fraction contains proteins without the globulin fraction. Most notably this includes fibrinogen, plasminogen, and plasmin. However, the inhibitors of plasmin and plasminogen activation are removed. The euglobulin fraction is stimulated to clot with thrombin and the time to eventual clot lysis is then monitored. Normal clot lysis should be in excess of 2 hours. The euglobulin lysis time is a good test of overall plasmin activation, but it should be understood that the lack of specific inhibitors may create some inaccuracies that do not directly reflect the clinical situation.

Platelets

Platelet number can be monitored easily by one of two methods. Either a blood smear can be made and the platelets can be counted manually under a high power microscope or they can be determined with a laser Coulter counter.[115] The automated method may be somewhat less accurate as any other particles of similar size will be counted as platelets. However, for critically low platelet counts the method of manual counting is most accurate. Clearly manual counting is more expensive and very labor-intensive. It cannot be done in situations where a large number of samples need to be processed. Platelet count does not connote normal platelet function. Particularly in postcardiopulmonary bypass, platelet function is most often impaired. Knowing the number does not infer that clot function will behave normally. Also a great number of pharmacologic agents affect platelet function. Aspirin has received a great deal of attention as a cyclooxygenase inhibitor that can inhibit platelet function by decreasing thromboxane release.[116] Multiple other drugs cause some element of platelet inhibition, including beta blockers, calcium channel blockers, nitroprusside, and cephalosporin antibiotics.[117]

Unfortunately, the monitoring of platelet function is incomplete in most operating rooms today. There are a number of potential ways to follow platelet function but all have their detractions. The bleeding time has been utilized as a screening test for platelet function abnormalities.[118,119] The Ivy bleeding time needs to be performed the same way every time preferably by a trained technician. Three small incisions (3 mm deep and 1.5 cm apart) are made on the volar aspect of the forearm. A spring-loaded template makes the incision quickly and to the same depth every time. A sphygmomanometer is inflated to 40 mmHg on the arm to maintain venous pressure. The inner aspect of the forearm is chosen because the skin here is not often exposed to chronic abrasion or callous formation. Once the skin incision has been made the technician will dab the incision with filter paper (No. 1 Whatman filter paper or equivalent) every minute. It is key to not wipe the incision but to only dab the wound. Wiping the incision will remove the platelet plug for which the test is evaluating the speed of formation.

Unfortunately the bleeding time has not proven to be predictive or cost-effective as a screening test for bleeding association with perioperative platelet dysfunction.[120] Several recent reviews have concluded that the bleeding time is not a good test for establishing perioperative hemorrhagic risk. One article reviewed 862 papers on the bleeding time.[120] A number of conclusions were drawn, most importantly, that a small skin incision on the forearm of a patient will not necessarily reflect the bleeding risk in other body cavities or perfusion beds. The skin of the forearm is exposed to heat and cold causing vasoreactivity, which may be different on the surface than in a deep body area. Also patients who perhaps are most in need of platelet function assessment, those who are critically ill in the intensive care unit, may be receiving vasoactive compounds which not only affect surface blood flow

but also either activate or inhibit platelet function. The bleeding time after cardiopulmonary bypass has had both positive and profoundly negative findings. In one early study of the bleeding time after cardiopulmonary bypass, correlations between abnormal tests and bleeding were very poor.[121] This was because the bleeding time was most often prolonged. In several recent studies it has had much better correlations with abnormal hemorrhage, but other whole-blood clotting tests have had even better sensitivity and specificity.[122]

In addition, to the previously mentioned problems, the bleeding time has some additional detractions. As an actual incision it does leave a small scar on the forearm. For some patients this is not a great problem, but for others it is one more reminder of their medical care. It is also costly due to the technician time and may be priced at $25.00 per test or higher. With over 1,000,000 bleeding times being performed per year one has to wonder if that is money well spent. Even in patients with preeclampsia/eclampsia the bleeding time, although sometimes used to decide the safety of proceeding with an epidural, has never been shown to be predictive of any increased risk for epidural bleed. Its use in that situation is strictly theoretical, and some practitioners obtain it for "legal reasons." Indeed there are no case reports of which this author is aware of epidural hematoma in preeclampsia/eclampsia or pregnancy, and use of the bleeding time is probably not the reason for that record.

Platelet Aggregometry

Other tests of platelet function do exist. Like the bleeding time they also have significant detractions. Platelets have multiple ways of being stimulated to change confirmation and adhere. Platelet aggregometry testing uses a battery of activators to test platelet responsiveness. Platelet-rich plasma is placed in a warmed platelet aggregometer. Photodetection of turbidity changes allows for the detection of decreased cloudiness of the platelet-rich plasma as platelet aggregates form and precipitate. Comparison with a reference sample of the patient's platelet poor plasma provides a control for the turbidity measurement. Various activators such as adenosine diphosphate (ADP), epinephrine, serotonin, thrombin, arachidonic acid, ristocetin, snake venoms, fibrin split products, and others can be used as platelet activation. The battery of platelet aggregometry is very labor-intensive and requires a number of hours to perform. Therefore it is quite expensive and furthermore it has no predictive value for the risk of perioperative hemorrhage. Obtaining such tests for patients clinically bleeding is impractical.

Platelet Retention

Platelet-rich plasma can be tested for surface activation adherence to a glass bead column. Simply passing platelet-rich plasma through such a glass bead column and comparing the platelet count before and after, yields a normal retention level of 75 to 90 percent. Platelets are activated by the abnormal surface and should form contact activation. This once again is unlike the in vivo activation as the in vitro column does not have von Willebrand's factor or the myriad of activators, inhibitors, and feedback loops present in the in vivo situation. There are no data to suggest that glass bead retention is predictive of perioperative hemorrhage.

WHOLE BLOOD COAGULATION

The Activated Clotting Time

The aPTT is the standard test utilized for low-dose heparin therapy. However, as heparin levels increase the activating substances utilized are insufficient to overcome the heparin-antithrombin III complexes and the aPTT is prolonged beyond a usable range. Hattersley[123] in the late 1950s developed a simple automated whole blood clotting test that can assess much larger doses of heparin. A surface activator, diatomaceous (Cellite) earth is placed in a glass test tube. At the bottom of the test tube is a small magnet that acts as a stirrer; 3 ml of blood is placed in the tube and inverted several times to provide adequate mixing with the activator. The tube is then placed in the ACT machine, which warms the tube to 37°C and gently rotates it. Once coagulation begins the small magnet becomes enmeshed in the clot and it then follows the spin of the tube around and enables a detection that clotting has occurred. Generally 5 percent activator is utilized in these tubes with the correct amount of blood injected. The reported value for the ACT is the time in seconds from when blood was placed in the tube until the first formation of

gel occurred. It is an adaptation of the Lee-White whole-blood clotting time, which is simply the time required for initial clot formation when blood is placed in a glass test tube. The Lee-White whole-blood clotting time is not clinically useful today other than a gross measurement of whether blood has been anticoagulated or previously undergone clot formation and lysis.

Another variation of the original ACT is now available. It uses a small plastic cuvette prewarmed in the ACT machine to 37°C. The cuvettes have a reservoir of activator and saline present in the bottom; 0.3 ml of blood is placed in the cuvette and the machine is initiated. A small mechanical arm gently lifts a small flag and plunger arrangement that not only mixes the blood with the activator but also works as a clot detector. When the viscosity of the whole blood becomes thick a gel is formed the rate of descent of the plunger is slowed. A photoelectric eye detects when the plunger no longer falls and therefore detects a clot.

Normal values for whole blood ACT should be between 95 and 140 seconds. Either of the previously described techniques for ACT determination can be utilized interchangeably. Bull and colleagues[124] demonstrated that the ACT has a straight line curve in individual patients and creates a reliable dose response curve from baseline to approximately 600 seconds. Above that level the curve becomes less reproducible. Each patient demonstrates his own unique dose response curve with at least a 3- to 4-fold variability in slope. Also heparin, being hepatically metabolized exhibits considerable variability in duration of effect. Therefore the conclusion has been drawn that even within the normal population there exists a 12-fold difference in ACT response to high-dose heparin therapy.[124]

There are a great number of influences that can affect the ACT.[125] Hypothermia prolongs the ACT, as does hemodilution. Platelet function abnormalities can prolong it and if severe enough thrombocytopenia can prolong or totally inhibit the test. Fibrinogen concentration as well as the presence of dysfibrinogenemia or inhibitors can artificially lengthen the test. There is no exact level of ACT that is universally accepted as the lower limit before proceeding to bypass and some institutions routinely run the levels quite low without untoward effects.[126] The kallikrein inhibitor, aprotinin can prolong Cellite ACT tests and the mechanisms and implications for bypass are unclear.[127] Routine use of this method of testing would dictate that a higher ACT should be achieved than if aprotinin was not present. Recommendations are not yet complete upon the levels that are safe for bypass in the presence of aprotinin but it would seem reasonable to expect considerably prolonged cellite ACT's. Furthermore, the heparin protamine complex can partially bind to the activator in the ACT and particularly excess protamine will coat the surface activator and artificially lengthen the result. No large study has evaluated the causes of very prolonged ACT values, but some of the above problems may be causes as well as technical difficulties with the machine, the inserts, activator, or the heating element.

The ACT, as stated earlier does have a linear dose response curve up until approximately 600 seconds.[128] We know that when the ACT drops below 300 seconds there is an increased risk of thrombin formation and platelet fibrin deposition. It then is reasonable that a window of safety and reproducible monitoring capability exists between 300 to 600 seconds.

Once heparin has been neutralized with protamine, the ACT should return to baseline or below. The presence of tissue thromboplastins have been implicated as one cause of low ACT value. As a result, suggestions have been made that the baseline ACT should be drawn sometime after median sternotomy has been performed to achieve the most accurate ACT value. The performance of the ACT before going onto bypass will detect patients with antithrombin III deficiency and also assure that mechanical and human error have not occurred. Close determination of the dose response curve by the ACT has been shown to decrease postoperative bleeding as compared to much more empiric anticoagulation therapy.

Other variations of the ACT technology have been developed including using thrombin as the activator. The Hepcon system (Medtronic Inc., Anaheim, California) utilizes a number of different preloaded cartridges with aliquots of protamine and surface activator (kaolin). By using these preloaded cuvettes an estimation of the circulating plasma heparin level can be made. This is actually done by a bioassay using back titration of the ACT with protamine. The machine also can do an individualized heparin dose response curve prior to administration of heparin. The Hepcon has been

utilized in most of the trials of aprotinin in the United States to follow heparin because of the interference with the cellite ACT. Once again there is no hard data that this technique affords safety when utilizing aprotinin.

Thromboelastography

The thromboelastogram was invented in the late 1940s by a German hematologist, H. Hartert. It has a very simplistic mechanism: It is a test of whole blood clot strength over time.[129] A polished metal cuvette (disposable plastic cuvettes are now available) is housed in a rotating seat that is heated to 37°C (Fig. 22-2). Suspended in that cuvette is a metal piston that is machined such that it does not touch the cuvette. Blood (0.35 ml) is placed into the cuvette and the piston is lowered into the blood. A small drop of oil is pipetted onto the top of the blood so as to prevent drying. If drying occurs at the surface of the blood the thromboelastogram will give a false reading of infinite clot strength.

Once blood is placed in the cuvette and the piston is lowered into place a surface contact activation of the whole blood occurs. Fibrin and platelet interactions proceed with an eventual gel being formed. The cuvette constantly rotates through a 4.5-degree arc, pauses for 1 second and then rotates back in the other direction. It should be noted that the cuvette does not make a circumferential turn but only turns in a slow arc repetitively. As gel forms a mechanical link is created between the wall of the cuvette and the piston. Because of the turning motion, the thromboelastogram is therefore constantly testing the viscoelastic properties or the shear modulus of the clot as it forms, matures and eventually lyses.

The thromboelastogram transfers the mechanical motion of the piston to a paper tracing that constantly proceeds at 2 mm/min. A torsion wire mechanism is utilized for the link to the tracing. The pen sweep deflection of this mechanism must be calibrated to maintain accuracy. Both the pen sweep and the torsion spring tension should be checked at regular intervals to maintain proper quality controls of the instrument. Recently a biologic assay utilizing fresh frozen plasma and calcium have allowed for a standardized check of the thromboelastogram output for a known biologic reagent.[130] This as well should be performed on a regular basis with adequate records to assure good quality control.

The thromboelastogram tracing produces a normal sausage shaped paper record. From that record a number of routine measurements can be made and are known as thromboelastogram parameters. Recently, a computerized model of the thromboelastogram has become available such that these measurements can be made automatically. The first measurement is the R value (reaction time) which is the amount of time from when the blood was placed in the cuvette until the amplitude of pen deflection equals 1 mm (a noticeable amplitude). The next measurement is from the time required from the end of the R value until the amplitude of pen deflection has equalled 20 mm. The 20-mm value is arbitrarily defined by the inventor but does give a measure of the speed of clot growth. This value is known as the K value (coagulation time). Both of these first two measurements

are reported in millimeters with the knowledge that the paper speed is at 2 mm/min. Another measurement of the speed of clot growth is the α angle, which is calculated as the acute angle formed by an assumptotic line to the outside of the growth curve of the thromboelastogram and the midline on the paper tracing. Both the K and the α angle measure similar coagulation events. The next measurement is the maximum amplitude and is exactly what its name describes. It represents the maximum clot strength generated. The last commonly measured parameter is the A60 or amplitude 60 minutes after the maximum amplitude (MA) has been measured. Both the MA and the A60 are reported in millimeters, which represents the width of the paper tracing.

The shear modulus measured by the thromboelastogram has an arithmetic paper representation, from 0 to 100 mm. However, these numerical values correspond to physical forces measured from 0

Instrument

Tracing

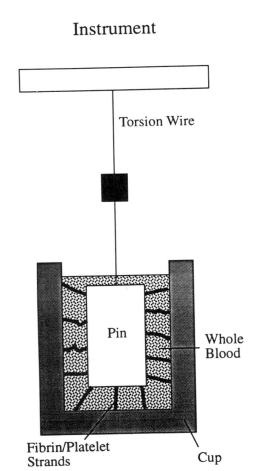

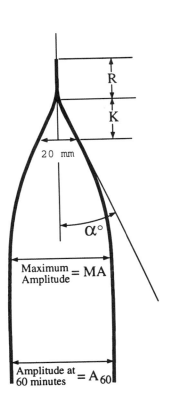

Fig. 22-2. Thromboelastography schematic of mechanism, tracing, and measurements. (From Chandler,[130] with permission.)

to infinite shear modulus. Therefore, although the thromboelastogram MA values reported vary according to millimeters, they represent the shear modulus applied to the clot. The actual equation that Hartert used in creating the thromboelastogram is

$$G = \frac{5,000A}{100 - A}$$

where G is shear modulus and A is the amplitude of the tracing. The units of the shear modulus are dynes/cm^2. Arbitrarily the midpoint of the scale, 50 mm, was chosen as where the majority of the normal populations clot strength should be measured at, and it actually works out that the shear modulus is 5,000 dyne/cm^2.[129]

Changes in MA translate into curvilinear changes in clot strength. For example, if the MA changes from 50 to 67 the clot strength has doubled. If it goes from 67 to 75 it has doubled again, and so on. Clinically it is important to realize that when values decrease considerably below 50 mm that may represent a clot strength that is a considerable factor less than normal.

Clot strength is influenced by a number of interactions but fibrinogen concentration and platelet activity (number and function) are the greatest contributors.[129] The thromboelastogram does not differentiate which precursor is deranged if overall clot strength is decreased. Recent work at our institution has shown that using a computer regression curve model an equation for predicting the MA can be developed if the fibrinogen and platelet count are known:

MA = (0.130 platelet count)

  + (0.081 fibrinogen concentration)

or

G = 22.3 (platelet count)

  + 11.8 (fibrinogen concentration) − 298

These equations are derived from simultaneous determinations during liver transplantation and assume that platelet function was normal.[129] If platelet function is abnormal they will not work and certainly in cardiopulmonary bypass that is a situation that is very common.

The thromboelastogram test has recently gained popularity in the anesthesia field for monitoring coagulation function during liver transplantation and cardiovascular surgery.[131–133] A schematic key has been published to help with site recognition of abnormal thromboelastogram tracings. The practitioner should be cautioned that site recognition and generalization of thromboelastogram abnormalities may not give accurate diagnoses of actual coagulopathies. A great number of medications and dysfunctions can affect the thromboelastogram. All the thromboelastogram parameters are interdependent parameters and therefore most often when one is changed they are all changed in some way. One cannot in any way claim that a depressed MA translates into a platelet defect or that a prolonged R value should be treated with FFP. These parameters should be viewed with a reflection on what they mean to whole blood clot dynamics. For example, a prolongation of the R value only indicates that there is some interference with initiation of clot formation. That may be due to trace or moderate amounts of heparin, Coumadin, other anticoagulants, circulating inhibitors, low factor concentrations, hypofibrinogenia, or even severely low platelet number or function.[134] The patient's clinical situation should be evaluated. If a patient has recently undergone cardiopulmonary bypass and the R value is prolonged, it may well indicate that some level of trace heparinization still exists. If a low MA is encountered, it may mean that platelet activity or function is depressed and/or that fibrinogen is diluted. In this situation, post-cardiopulmonary bypass, the more common event is a platelet dysfunction and one might be reasonable in trying a first line therapy of platelet transfusion if the patient is bleeding.

The thromboelastogram has been widely studied for its predictability for perioperative hemorrhage. Several studies in cardiopulmonary bypass patients have shown that the thromboelastogram is a useful predictor of cardiopulmonary bypass-related bleeding disorders.[129,131] These studies were conducted in a binary fashion. That is to say that the thromboelastogram and other routine tests were judged as normal and abnormal according to published criteria and chest tube bleeding was also judged as normal or abnormal. Percentages of matching results showed the TEG to be the best predictor of hemorrhage. A new study has focused upon sensitivity and specificity of the thromboelastogram and other coagulation profiles to aid in the management and diagnosis of cardiopulmonary bypass-related bleeding.[122] The thromboelastogram had the best sensitivity and specificity. In this study the bleeding time after bypass was sensitive but not specific. Coagulation profile data were far less acceptable in these specificity and sensitivity profiles. One large series has criticized the thromboelastogram for not having good correlation coefficients between actual chest tube bleeding and thromboelastogram parameters.[135] This is a widely criticized study and appears to be more a report of clinical activity. Perhaps correlations between chest tube output (a non linear data paradigm) and the actual shear modulus would have been more scientifically correct.

All the studies do agree that if the thromboelastogram is normal after cardiopulmonary bypass that a very high confidence can be placed on the diagnosis of surgical bleeding. The data for this are available from multiple sources and yield a greater than 90 percent confidence limit. In our institution the incidence of postoperative mediastinal reexploration has been dramatically reduced due to the institution of this test alone.

Much work yet remains to be done with the thromboelastogram and perioperative hemorrhage. It, like the coagulation profile, is not accurate as a screening tool to predict which patients will develop post-cardiopulmonary bypass hemorrhage. Perhaps if it is applied to other surgeries its use as a screening test will be widened. The practitioner must be cautioned again that one should understand the physical forces that the test is evaluating and not make blanket generalizations governing therapy based upon site recognition.

The Sonoclot

The Sonoclot is another whole-blood test for clot dynamics.[136] It is sometimes reported a s viscoelastic test but in reality it is strictly a viscometer. The mechanism by which the blood is tested has some similarities to that seen with the thromboelastogram. A plastic cuvette is housed in the body of the machine and warmed to 37°C. A small aliquot of blood is pipetted into the cuvette (0.36 ml) and a plastic probe is lowered into the blood. The Sonoclot probe vibrates vertically at 200 H through a very small movement. The electric motor that creates the motion will continue the movement, but it senses impedance to vibration by following the change in electric current necessary to continue the probe motion. The end result is a measurement of viscosity change over time as the clot goes through its formation, maturation, and lysis. Although there are correlations and changes in viscosity seen as clot strength increases, viscosity and clot shear modulus are not the same.

The Sonoclot develops a paper tracing known as the Sonoclot signature. It has a characteristic shape that has been described. Like the thromboelastogram there is a lag time from when blood is placed in the machine until the first clot formation begins. This is known as the lag time and is measured in minutes. The next phase of the Sonoclot signature is the primary wave and can be described both by its onset time, time to initial inflection, and slope. The secondary wave, like the primary wave can be also described by its onset and peak as well as its slope. Sometimes the peaks of the initial and secondary waves are labeled as T1 and T2 and are reported as times from the initiation of the test. Also the amplitudes of the two peaks can be reported. The final step of a normal tracing is a downward slope which if carried out long enough will either tail off to a 0 amplitude or level out for a period before eventual lysis.

The coagulation events that actually are contributing to these peaks, slopes, and plateaus are not well understood. The articles most often quoted regarding this technology do not given basic science explanations but some believe the primary and secondary upslopes are associated with primary and secondary platelet activation. This seems somewhat unlikely as that designation is an arbitrary one and platelets undergo such reactions as a graded response to a graded stimulus. Also it is unlikely that a large percentage of a given platelet population would be exactly synchronized to begin and end their levels of activation in phase with each other. At least this author is still left without good explanation as to what these slopes mean. The slopes are affected by different concentrations of platelet-rich or -poor plasma and therefore one can infer that the test is sensitive to platelet overall activity.

The final downslope has also been attributed to clot retraction or platelet retraction. Once again there are no conclusive studies that show that this is indeed what happens in the blood when the slope is decreasing. Fibrinolysis would conceivably produce the same change in overall viscosity and therefore when a falling final slope is seen the practitioner does not know what that signifies.

There are no published normal values for the

various inflection points or slopes. Although a number of institutions do use the Sonoclot during liver transplantation and cardiopulmonary bypass, the interpretation of tracings is specific to the experience of the user involved and when abnormalities are noted they can at least be partially corrected. A study did look at the agreement of the Sonoclot signature in predicting abnormal hemorrhage after cardiopulmonary bypass and found that it was almost as good as thromboelastogram. Clearly viscosity over time is a useful measurement for blood coagulation and perhaps it has some focus on platelet function but much further work needs to be done before this technology can be routinely applied in the operating rooms.

SUMMARY

Laboratory testing of blood obtained from venipuncture or arterial sample for the above-mentioned tests can provide clinically useful information. However, their limitations should be noted as well. At best these tests provide information at only one point in time. It is possible for there to be rapidly changing events that may occur such that the test data are outdated before it has even been returned from the laboratory. Also the methods in which blood is sampled, held, and transported are very important elements in accuracy of test results. Hemolysis is of paramount importance when electrolyte values are being assessed. Coagulation sampling needs adequate withdrawal from indwelling catheters to insure that heparin contamination does not occur. Also if a venipuncture is performed for many of the coagulation tests it is important to discard the first few milliliters of blood as they may contain tissue plugs from insertion, which can artificially activate both platelets and protein cascades. We have a long way yet to go in developing real time monitors for all these very important functions. Ideally, such monitors would be able to give patient data as changes occur. That technology may become available for some of the biochemical tests, but such is not yet even dreamed of for coagulation monitoring.

REFERENCES

1. Wong KC, Schafer PG, Schultz JR: Hypokalemia and anesthetic implications. Anesth Analg 77:1238, 1993

2. Vaughn RS, Lunn JN: Potassium and the anesthetist: a review. Anaesthesia 28:118, 1973

3. Fisch C: Electrocardiograph and vectorcardiograph. p. 116. In Braunwald E (ed): A Textbook of Cardiovascular Medicine. WB Saunders, Philadelphia, 1992

4. Braun HA, Surawicz B, Bellet S: T waves in hyperpotassemia. Am Med Sci 230:147, 1985

5. Whelton PK, Watson AJ: Diuretic-induced hypokalemia and cardiac arrhythmias. Am J Cardiol 58:5A, 1986

6. Flannery JM: Differences in electrolyte results as measured by direct potentiometry (ion selective electrode) and flame photometry. NOVA Biomed Semin, 1980

7. Proda L, Simon W: Determination of potassium concentrations of serum using a highly selective liquid membrane electrode. Clin Chim Acta 29:289, 1970

8. Skinner SL: A cause of erroneous potassium levels. Lancet 1:478, 1961

9. Vitez TS, Soper LE, Wong KC, Soper P: Chronic hypokalemia and intraoperative dysrhythmias. Anesthesiology 63:130, 1985

10. Hirsch IA, Tomlinson DL, Slogoff S, Keats AS: The overstated risk of perioperative hypokalemia. Anesth Analg 67:131, 1988

11. Gennari FJ, Cohen JJ: Role of kidney in potassium homeostasis: lessons from acid-base disturbances. Kidney Int 8:1, 1975

12. Wilkinson PR, Issler H, Hesp R: Total body and serum potassium during prolonged thiazide therapy for essential hypertension. Lancet 1:759, 1975

13. Kassirez JP, Harrington JT: Diuretics and potassium metabolism: a reassessment of the need, effectiveness and safety of potassium therapy. Kidney Int 11:505, 1977

14. Lauer MB: Clinical opinion. Anesth Analg 55:276, 1976

15. Morgan B, Davidson D: Hypokalemia and diuretics: an analysis of publications. Br Med J 280:905, 1980

16. Lawson DH: Adverse reactions to potassium chloride. Q J Med 43:433, 1974

17. Spino M, Sellers EM, Kaplan HL et al: Adverse biochemical and clinical consequences of furosemide administration. Can Med Assoc J 118:1513, 1978

18. Surawicz B, Lepeschkin E: The electrocardiographic pattern of hypopotassemia with and without hypocalcemia. Circulation 8:810, 1953

19. Brater DC, Morrelli HF: Systemic alkalosis and digitalis related arrhythmias. Acta Med Scand (Suppl.): 647:79, 1980

20. Goldstein G: Serum potassium levels and anesthesia. Curr Rev Clin Anesthesiol 1:170, 1981

21. DeFronzo BM: Intravenous potassium therapy. JAMA 245:2446, 1981

22. Spiess BD: Anesthesia. p. 182. In Williams JW (ed): Hepatic Transplantation. WB Saunders, Philadelphia, 1990

23. Ettinger PO, Regan TJ, Oldewurtel HA: Hyperkalemia, cardiac conduction and the electrocardiogram: a review. Am Heart J 88:360, 1974

24. Schwartz AB: Potassium-related cardiac arrhythmias and their treatment. Angiology 29:194, 1978

25. Goldzer RC, Goodlet EL, Rosner MJ et al: Hyperkalemia associated with indomethacin. Arch Intern Med 141:802, 1981

26. Jaffey L, Martin A: Malignant hyperkalemia after amiloride/hydrochlorothiazide treatment. [Letter]. Lancet 1:1272, 1981

27. Carmichael FJ, Lindop MJ, Faman MB: Anesthesia for hepatic transplantation. Anesth Analg 64:108, 1985

28. Gronert G, Theye RA: Pathophysiology of hyperkalemia induced by succinylcholine. Anesthesiology 43:89, 1975

29. Mazze BI, Escue HM, Houston JB: Hyperkalemia and cardiovascular collapse following administration of succinylcholine to traumatized patients. Anesthesiology 31:540, 1969

30. Tobey RE: Paraplegia, succinylcholine and cardiac arrest. Anesthesiology 32:359, 1970

31. Androgue HJ, Madias NE: Changes in potassium concentration during acute acid-base disturbances. Am J Med 71:456, 1981

32. Fraley DS, Adler S: Isohydric regulation of plasma potassium by bicarbonate in the rat. Kidney Int 9:333, 1976

33. Caralis PV, Perez-Stable E: Electrolyte abnormalities and ventricular arrhythmias. Drugs (Suppl.): 4 31:85, 1986

34. Drake HF, Treasure T, Smith B: Continuous display of potassium during cardiac surgery. Anaesthesia 42:23, 1987

35. Linton RAF, Lim M, and Band DM: Continuous intravascular monitoring of plasma potassium using potassium-selective electrode catheters. Crit Care Med 10:337, 1982

36. Slater JDH: The hormonal control of body sodium. Postgrad Med J 40:479, 1964

37. DeWardener HE, Clarkson EM: Concept of natriuretic hormone. Physiol Rev 65:658, 1985

38. Carrico CJ, Meakius JL, Marshall JC et al: Multiple organ-failure syndrome. Arch Surg 121:196, 1986

39. Knaus WA, Draper EA, Wagner DP et al: Prognosis in acute organ-system failure. Ann Surg 202:685, 1985

40. Sodium-Potassium Chemistry Module Manual: Astra™, Beckman Instruments, Inc., Bren, CA 1979

41. Maffly RH: Disorders of water, sodium and potassium. Sci Am 1982

42. Aasheim GM: Hyponatremia during transurethral surgery. Can Anesth Soc J 20:274, 1973

43. Arieff AI: Rapid correction of hyponatremia cause of positive myelinosis? [Reply to Letter]. Am J Med 71:846, 1981

44. Arieff AI: Hyponatremia, convulsions, respiratory arrest and permanent brain damage after elective surgery in healthy women. N Engl J Med 314:1529, 1986

45. Kleinschmidt-DeMasters BK, Norenberg MD: Rapid correction of hyponatremia causes a demyelination: relation to central pontine myelinosis. Science 211:1068, 1981

46. Nairns RG: Therapy of hyponatremia: does haste make waste? N Engl J Med 314:1573, 1986

47. Potts JJ Jr, Deftos LJ: Parathyroid hormone, calcitonin, vitamin D, bone and mineral metabolism. In Bondy PK, Rosenberg LE (eds): Metabolism: Diseases of Metabolism. WB Saunders, Philadelphia, 1974

48. Agus ZS, Wasserstein A, Goldfarb S: Disorders of calcium and magnesium homeostasis. Am J Med 72:473, 1982

49. Lytes KW, Drezner MK: The overview of calcium homeostasis in humans. Urol Clin North Am 8:209, 1981

50. Stern J, Lewis WHP: The colorimetric estimation of calcium in serum with σ-cresolphthalein complexone. Clin Chim Acta 2:576, 1957

51. Connerty HV, Briggs AR: Determination of serum calcium by means of orthocresolphthalein complexone. Am J Clin Pathol 45:290, 1966

52. Cali JP, Bowers GN, Young DS: A reference method determination of total calcium in serum. Clin Chem 19:1208, 1973

53. Muller-Plathe O, Lindemann K: Ionized calcium versus total calcium. Scand J Clin Lab Invest suppl 165:71, 1983

54. Drop LJ: Ionized calcium, the heart and hemodynamic function. Anesth Analg 64:432, 1985

55. Ross JW: Calcium-selective electrode with liquid ion-exchanger. Science 156:1378, 1967

56. Siggaard-Anderson O, Thode J, Fogh-Andersen N: What is "ionized calcium?" Scand J Clin Lab Invest suppl 165:11, 1983

57. Denlinger J, Nahrewald ML, Gibbs PS et al: Hypocalcemia during rapid blood transfusion in anesthetized man. Br J Anaesthesiol 48:995, 1976

58. Kahn RC, Jascott D, Carlon GC et al: Massive blood replacement: correlation of ionized calcium, citrate, hydrogen ion concentration. Anesth Analg 58:274, 1979

59. Marquez J, Martin D, Virji M et al: Cardiovascular depression of ionic hypocalcemia during hepatic transplantation in humans. Anesthesiology 65:457, 1986

60. Surawicz B, Gettes LS: Effects of electrolyte abnormalities on the heart and circulation. p. 539. In Conn HL Jr, Horwitz O (eds): Cardiac and Vascular Diseases. Lea & Febiger, Philadelphia, 1971

61. Tente JV, Davis LD: Effects of calcium concentration on the transmembrane potentials of Purkinje fibers. Cir Res 20:32, 1967

62. Seifern W, Flacke W, Alper MH: Effects of calcium on isolated mammalian heart. Am J Physiol 207:716, 1964

63. Johnston WE, Robertie PG, Butterworth JF et al: Is calcium or ephedrine superior to placebo for emergence from cardiopulmonary bypass? J Cardiothorac Vasc Anesth 6:528, 1992

64. Royster RL, Butterworth JF 4th, Prielipp RC et al: A randomized, blinded, placebo-controlled evaluation of calcium chloride and epinephrine for inotropic support after emergence from cardiopulmonary bypass. Anesth Analg 74:3, 1992

65. Mundy GR, Martin TJ: The hypercalcemia of malignancy: pathogenesis and management. Metabolism 31:1247, 1982

66. Weissman C, Askanazi J, Hyman AI, Weber C: Hypercalcemia and hypercalciuria in a critically ill patient. Crit Care Med 11:576, 1983

67. Schuster SM, Olson MS: Effect of magnesium chelators on the regulation of pyruvate oxidation by rabbit mitochondria. Biochemistry 11:4166, 1972

68. DiCarlo LA Jr, Morady F, deBuitleir M et al: Effects of magnesium sulfate on cardiac conduction and refractoriness in humans. J Am Coll Cardiol 7:1356, 1986

69. Shine KI: Myocardial effects of magnesium. Am J Physiol 237:H413, 1979

70. Surawicz B, Lepschkin E, Herrlich HC: Low and high magnesium concentrations at various calcium levels: effects on the monophasic action potential, electrocardiogram and contractility of isolated rabbit hearts. Circ Res 9:811, 1961

71. Kiyosue T, Arita M: Magnesium restores high K-induced inactivation of the fast Na channel in guinea-pig ventricular muscle. Pflugers Arch 395:78, 1982

72. Kraft LF, Kutholi RE, Woods WT, James TN: Attenuation by magnesium of the electrophysiologic effects of hyperkalemia on human and canine heart cells. Am J Cardiol 45:1189, 1980

73. Aikawa JK: Magnesium: its biological significance. CRC Press, Boca Raton, FL 1981

74. Widdouson EM, McLance RA, Spray CM: The chemical composition of the human body. Clin Sci 10:113, 1951

75. Wacker WEC, Parisi AF: Magnesium metabolism. N Engl J Med 278:658, 712, 1968

76. Alfey AC, Miller NL, Butkus D. Evaluation of magnesium stores. J Lab Med 84:153, 1974

77. Woo S, Cannon DC: Metabolic intermediates and inorganic ions. p. 133. In Henry JB (ed): Clinical Diagnosis and Management by Laboratory Methods. 17th ed. WB Saunders, Philadelphia, 1984

78. Willis JB: The determination of metals in blood serum by atomic absorption spectrophotometry. II. Magnesium. Spectrochim Acta 16:273, 1960

79. Finster M: Anesthetic considerations in pre-eclampsia and eclampsia. Refresher Courses Anesthesiol 14:8, 1987

80. Helgason CM: Blood glucose and stroke. Stroke 19:1049, 1988

81. Merritt WT, Gelman S: Anesthesia for liver surgery. p. 1991. In Rogers MC, Tinker JH, Covino BG, Longnecker DE (eds): Principles and Practice of Anesthesiology. Mosby Year Book, St. Louis, 1993

82. Clark LC Jr, Clark EW: Differential anodic enzyme polarography for the measurement of glucose. In Bircher HI, Burley DF (eds): Oxygen Transport to the Tissue: Instrumentation Methods and Physiology. Plenum Press, New York, 1973

83. Glucose Chemistry Module Manual: Astra™, Beckman Instruments, Inc., Bren, CA, 1979

84. Kubilis P, Rosenbloom AL, Lezotte D et al: Comparison of blood glucose testing using reagent strips with and without a meter (Chemistrips bG and Dextrostix/Dextrometer). Diabetes Care 4:417, 1981

85. Reeves ML, Forhan SE, Skyler JS, Peterson CM: Comparison of methods for blood glucose monitoring. Diabetes Care 3:404, 1981

86. Shapiro B, Savage PJ, Lomatch D et al: A comparison of accuracy and estimated costs of methods of home blood glucose monitoring. Diabetes Care 4:396, 1981

87. Soeldner JS: Symposium on potentially implantable glucose sensors. Diabetes Care 5:147, 1982

88. Lanier WL, Stangland KJ, Scheithauser BW: The effects of dextrose infusion and head position on neurologic outcome after complete cerebral ischemia in primates: examination of a model. Anesthesiology 66:39, 1987

89. Robin AP, Askanazi J, Cooperman A et al: Influence of hypertonic glucose infusions on fuel economy in surgical patients: a review. Crit Care Med 9:680, 1981

90. Spiess BD: Perioperative coagulation concerns: Function, monitoring, and Therapy. Vol. 4. No. 3. p. 1. In Barash PG, Cullen BF, Stoehting RK (eds): Clinical Anesthesia Updates. JB Lippincott, Philadelphia, 1993

91. Mann KG: Membrane-bound enzyme complexes in blood coagulation. Prog Hemost Thromb 7:1, 1984

92. Furlong B, Henderson AH, Lewis MJ et al: Endothelium-derived relaxing factor inhibits in vitro platelet aggregation. Br J Pharmacol 90:687, 1987

93. Ayuma H, Ishikawa M, Sakiyaki S: Endothelium dependent inhibition of platelet aggregation. Br J Pharmacol 80:411, 1986

94. Griffith TM, Edwards DH, Lewis MJ et al: The nature of endothelium derived relaxant factor. Nature 308:645, 1984

95. Mason RG, Sharp D, Chuang HYK et al: The endothelium: roles in thrombosis and hemostasis. Arch Pathol Lab Med 101:61, 1977

96. Furchgott RF, Zawadzki JV: The obligatory role of endothelial cells in the relaxation of arterial smooth muscle by acetylcholine. Nature 288:373, 1980

97. Mollace V, Salvemini D, Sessa WC et al: Inhibition of human platelet aggregation by endothelium-derived relaxing factor, sodium nitroprusside or Iloprost is potentiated by captopril and reduced thiols. J Pharmacol Exp Ther 258:820, 1991

98. Vanhoutte PM, Lüscher TF, Gräser T: Endothelium dependent contractions. Blood Vessels 28:74, 1991

99. Lazarchick J, Kizer J: Interaction of fibrinolytic coagulation and kinin systems and related pathology. p. 381. In Pittiglio DH, Sacher RA (eds): Clinical Hematology and Fundamentals of Hemostasis. FA Davis, Philadelphia, 1987

100. Nurden AT, Caen JP: Specific roles of platelet surface glycoproteins in platelet function. Nature 255:720, 1991

101. Rinder C, Bohnert J, Rinder HM et al: Platelet activation and aggregation during cardiopulmonary bypass. Anesthesiology 75:388, 1991

102. Kunicki TJ: Role of platelets in hemostasis. p. 181. In Rossi E, Simon TL, Moss GS (eds): Principles of Transfusion. Williams & Wilkins, Baltimore, 1991

103. Rinder CS, Gaal D, Student LA, Smith BR: Platelet-leukocyte activation and modulation of adhesion receptors in pediatric patients with congenital heart disease undergoing cardiopulmonary bypass. J Thorac Cardiovasc Surg 107:280, 1994

104. Rinder HM, Bonan J, Rinder CS et al: Activated and unactivated platelet adhesion to monocytes and neutrophils. Blood 78:1760, 1991

105. Rinder HM, Bonan J, Rinder CS et al: Dynamics of leukocyte-platelet adhesion in whole blood. Blood 78:1730, 1991

106. Wachtfogel YT, Kucich V, Hack CE et al: Aprotinin inhibits the contact, neutrophil, and platelet activation systems during simulated extracorporeal perfusion. J Thorac Cardiovasc Surg 106:1, 1993

107. Wyrick-Glatzel J, Gwaltney-Krause S: Laboratory methods in hematology and hemostasis. p. 402. In Pittiglio DH, Sacher RA (eds): Clinical Hematology and Fundamentals of Hemostasis. FA Davis, Philadelphia, 1987

108. Harrigan C, Lucas CE, Ledgerwood AM et al: Serial changes in primary hemostasis after massive transfusion. Surgery 98:836, 1985

109. Quick AJ, Stanley-Brown M, Bancroft FW: A study of the coagulation defect in hemophilia and in jaundice. Am J Med Sci 190:501, 1935

110. Sher PP: Prothrombin time (PT). Drug Ther 5:149, 1976

111. Despotis GJ, Santoro SA, Spitznagel E et al: Prospective evaluation and clinical utility of on-site monitoring of coagulation patients undergoing cardiac operation. J Thorac Cardiovasc Surg 107:271, 1994

112. Reich DL, DePerio M: Clinical validation of a bedside PT, PTT coagulation monitor. Anesthesiology 75:A430, 1991

113. Nuttall GA, Oliver WC, Beynen FM et al: The sensitivity and specificity of APTT and PT by portable laser photometer in predicting bleeding in CPB patients. Anesthesiology 75:A431, 1991

114. Clauss VA: Gerinnungsphysiologische Schnellmethode zur Bestimmung des Fibrinoges. Acta Haematol 17:237, 1957

115. Instruction Manual: Coulter Counter Model S-Plus II, October, 1981

116. Bashein G, Nessly ML, Rice AL et al: Preoperative aspirin therapy and reoperation for bleeding after coronary artery bypass surgery. Arch Intern Med 151:89, 1991

117. Baeuerle J, Mongan PD, Hosking MP: An assessment of the duration of cephapirin-induced coagulation abnormalities as measured by thromboelastography. J Cardiothorac Vasc Anesth 7:422, 1993

118. Harker LA, Slichter SJ: The bleeding time as a screening test evaluation of platelet function. N Engl J Med 287:155, 1972

119. Schwartz BS, Leis LA, Johnson GJ: In vivo platelet retention in human bleeding-time wounds: effect of aspirin ingestion. J Lab Clin Med 94:574, 1979

120. Rodgers RP, Levin J: A critical reappraisal of the bleeding time. Semin Thromb Hemost 16:1, 1990

121. McKenna R, Bachmann F, Whittaker B et al: The hemostatic mechanism after open-heart surgery. II. Frequency of abnormal platelet function during extracorporeal circulation. J Thorac Cardiovasc Surg 70:298, 1975

122. Essell JH, Martin TJ, Salinas J et al: Comparison of thromboelastography to bleeding time and standard coagulation tests in patients after cardiopulmonary bypass. J Cardiothorac Vasc Anesth 7:410, 1993

123. Hattersley PG: Activated coagulation time of whole blood. JAMA 196:150, 1966

124. Bull BS, Hughes WM, Brauer FS et al: Heparin therapy during extracorporeal circulation. II. The use of a dose response curve to individualize hep-

arin and protamine dosage. J Thorac Cardiovasc Surg 67:685, 1975

125. Gravlee GP, Case LD, Angert KC et al: Variability of the activated clotting time. Anesth Analg 67:469, 1988

126. Metz S, Keats AS: Low activated coagulation time during cardiopulmonary bypass does not increase postoperative bleeding. Ann Thorac Surg 49:440, 1990

127. Dietrich W, Spannagl M, Jochum M et al: Influence of high-dose aprotinin treatment on blood loss and coagulation pattern in patients undergoing myocardial revascularization. Anesthesiology 73:1119, 1990

128. Cohen EJ, Camerlengo LJ, Dearing JP: Activated clotting times and cardiopulmonary bypass. I: The effect of hemodilution and hypothermia upon activated clotting time. J Extracorp Technol 12:139, 1980

129. Tuman KJ, Spiess BD, McCarthy RJ et al: Comparison of viscoelastic measures of coagulation after cardiopulmonary bypass. Anesth Analg 69:69, 1989

130. Chandler W: The thromboelastograph and the thromboelastograph technique. Semin Thromb Hemost (in press)

131. Spiess BD, Tuman KJ, McCarthy RJ et al: Thromboelastography as an indication of post-cardiopulmonary bypass coagulopathies. J Clin Monit 3:25, 1987

132. Kang YG, Martin DJ, Marquez J et al: Intraoperative changes in blood coagulation and thromboelastographic monitoring in liver transplantation. Anesth Analg 64:888, 1985

133. Bigeleisen PE, Kang Y: Thromboelastography as an aid to regional anesthesia: preliminary communication. Reg Anesth 16:59, 1991

134. Shinoda T, Arakura H, Katakura M et al: Usefulness of thromboelastography for dosage monitoring of low molecular weight heparins during hemodialysis. Artif Organs 14:413, 1990

135. Wang JS, Lin CY, Hung WT et al: Thromboelastogram fails to predict postoperative hemorrhage in cardiac patients. Ann Thorac Surg 53:435, 1992

136. Saleem S, Blifeld C, Saleh SA et al: Viscoelastic measurement of clot formation: a new test of platelet function. Ann Clin Lab Sci 13:115, 1983

137. Woodbury JW: The cell membrane: ionic and potential gradients and active transport. p. 2. In Ruch TC, Patton HD, Woodbury JW et al (eds): Neurophysiology. WB Saunders, Philadelphia, 1965

Monitoring Neuromuscular Function

23

Marianna P. Crowley
Hassan H. Ali

Monitors of neuromuscular function have proven to be useful adjuncts to anesthesia involving the use of neuromuscular blocking drugs.[1] These devices permit administration of relaxants such that optimal surgical relaxation is achieved, and yet the block reverses spontaneously or is reversed reliably and quickly with pharmacologic antagonists. Drug dosage can be titrated to effect by monitoring the patient's response to nerve stimulation. This is particularly important because of the tremendous variability in the response to relaxants, as well as modification of that response by disease states or perioperative medication.

The desired endpoint for reversal of neuromuscular blockade is sustained adequate ventilation, especially in response to stresses such as vomiting, coughing, or partial airway obstruction. Before the development of devices now commonly used to evoke muscle response, clinical indices of adequate ventilation and muscle strength were used. They have included head lift for 5 seconds or more, vital capacity, inspiratory force, grip strength, tongue protrusion, and ability to open eyes widely, among others.[2] Most of these movements require a cooperative patient or are inappropriate to attempt while surgery is in progress. Methods of measurement have been developed that can assess the depth of neuromuscular block in an anesthetized patient in an objective manner. Importantly, the findings using these methods have been correlated with desired endpoints of ventilatory function.

NEUROMUSCULAR TRANSMISSION

Acetylcholine (ACh), the neurotransmitter at the neuromuscular junction, is synthesized in the nerve terminal and stored in synaptic vesicles, or quanta.[3] The supply of acetylcholine consists of two fractions: a small amount available for immediate release (the immediately available store) and a large supply from which the neurotransmitter cannot be directly released. Part of this latter fraction exists in vesicles and is more readily mobilized to replenish the immediately available store. The rest is not in vesicles and represents a reservoir from which quanta can be formed.[1] When an electrical impulse is applied to the nerve and reaches the nerve terminal, it releases acetylcholine quanta. Acetylcholine then traverses the synaptic cleft, combines with its receptors on the motor endplate, and causes a change in the motor endplate potential. If enough acetylcholine reaches the motor endplate, the membrane will depolarize, the depolarization will spread to the rest of the muscle fiber, and the fiber will contract. Muscle fiber contraction is an all-or-none phenomenon; that is, maximal contraction will ensue if stimulus intensity reaches a certain threshold. The force of contraction of the entire muscle is proportional to the number of muscle fibers activated. If the motor nerve is stimulated with enough intensity, all the muscle fibers supplied by it will contract and maximal contraction of the muscle will result. If stimulus intensity is increased beyond this point, it is described as supramaximal.[1]

During administration of relaxants, if a supramaximal level of stimulation is maintained, decreased force of contraction will reflect the degree of neuromuscular blockade.

After electrical stimulation, the nerve terminal must resynthesize acetylcholine and replenish its immediately available store. The amount of transmitter released on subsequent stimulation is related to the amount already released (transmitter depletion), the amount mobilized from less available stores, and facilitation of synthesis and mobilization by previous impulses.[1]

Repetitive nerve stimulation, especially at faster rates, triggers an increased rate of synthesis and mobilization of neurotransmitter.[4] This effect persists beyond the duration of stimulation and tends to offset acetylcholine depletion. Facilitation of synthesis and mobilization is of particular note during tetanic stimulation.[5]

TYPES OF NEUROMUSCULAR BLOCKADE

In clinical practice, neuromuscular blockade traditionally falls within one of three categories:

1. *Depolarizing block:* Produced by succinylcholine and decamethonium which depolarize the motor endplate, thereby preventing repolarization and the normal functioning of acetylcholine.
2. *Nondepolarizing block:* Produced by *d*-tubocurarine, pancuronium, metocurine, doxacurium, pipecuronium, rocuronium, vecuronium, atracurium, and mivacurium. The drugs compete with acetylcholine for its receptor sites, but do not cause depolarization of the motor endplate

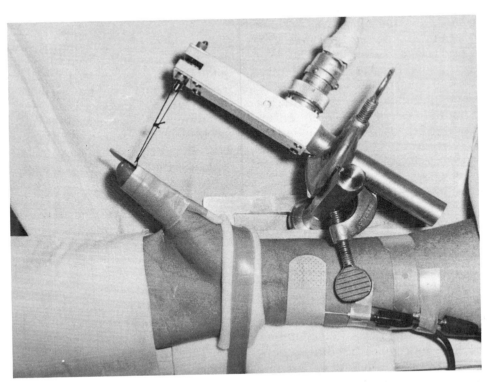

Fig. 23-1. Proper positioning of hand, thumb, stimulating needle electrodes, and transducer (Grass FT10) for recording of neuromuscular function. The thumb is abducted to place 100 to 300 g tension on the adductor pollicis. The direction of adduction is in line with the direction of displacement of the transducer cantilever. The thumb is splinted to ensure that only adduction is recorded. The stimulating needles are placed subcutaneously over the ulnar nerve at the wrist, 3 to 4 cm apart. (From Ali et al.,[1] with permission.)

membrane. This type of block can be antagonized by increasing levels of acetylcholine in the vicinity of the neuromuscular junction, as with administration of anticholinesterases.

3. *Phase II block (dual or desensitizing block):* Classically results after prolonged exposure to depolarizing drugs. The block then takes on gross clinical characteristics of nondepolarizing blockade,[6,7] although components of depolarizing block may persist.[8]

CLINICAL MONITORING OF EVOKED RESPONSES

The most satisfactory method for reliably monitoring neuromuscular function is the stimulation of an appropriate motor nerve and observation of the evoked response in the muscle supplied. This is done in one of two ways: by monitoring the mechanical force generated by the muscle, or its electrical response, the electromyogram (EMG). Similar patterns of nerve stimulation are used.

MECHANOMYOGRAPHY

The ulnar nerve-adductor pollicis muscle system is most commonly used for mechanical force measurement, although facial and lower extremity nerves (e.g., common peroneal or posterior tibial) may be substituted. The adductor pollicis muscle of the thumb is innervated solely by the ulnar nerve.[9] Electrodes are placed over the ulnar nerve at the wrist. Conductive surface electrodes, similar to electrocardiogram (ECG) electrodes, or subcutaneous needles are placed 3 to 4 cm apart. A supramaximal stimulus is applied, and thumb adduction is assessed.

Surface electrodes will usually be adequate, but when monitoring obese patients, needle electrodes may be necessary. Contact between the skin and electrode may be improved by rubbing the skin with alcohol or by applying friction with a towel. Slight alterations in placement may make a difference in evoked twitch height, as may changing polarity of electrodes.[10,11]

Monitoring should ideally be started before administration of any relaxants but after anesthesia is induced. Although tetanic stimulation is extremely painful, all other modes of stimulation are uncomfortable. Current suitable for stimulating nerves

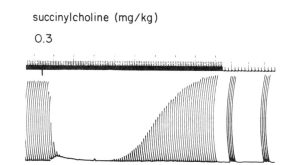

succinylcholine (mg/kg)

0.3

Fig. 23-2. Example of evoked mechanical twitch recording. At indicator, 0.3 mg/kg succinylcholine was given intravenously. Thumb and hand were positioned as shown in Figure 23-1. Time scale (in minutes) at top.

with needle electrodes usually lies between 5 and 8 mA. In order to achieve supramaximal stimulation with surface electrodes, at least 20 mA, and in many patients 50 to 60 mA is required.[12] The stimulus should be 0.2 msec in duration and should be square-wave in shape.[1]

Nerve stimulators should be capable of delivering at least a train-of-four and a single twitch, although 50 Hz tetanus is desirable as well. Single twitches should be delivered at 0.1 to 0.15 Hz, and trains-of-four should occur at 12-second intervals (see "Patterns of Stimulation" below).

In clinical situations, thumb adduction is evaluated visually or by touch. Usually for research purposes, more precise and objective measurements can be made by monitoring the tension developed in the muscle. The arm, fingers, and hand are immobilized to eliminate passive motion, usually with an arm board similar to the one shown in Figure 23-1. The thumb is attached to a strain gauge or appropriate force transducer preloaded with 100 to 300 g tension.[13] In response to nerve stimulation, the thumb movement activates the transducer, permitting conversion of contractile force into an electrical signal, which is amplified, and either displayed on an oscilloscope or recorded on a strip chart.[14] An example is shown in Figure 23-2.

ELECTROMYOGRAPHY

It is possible to monitor neuromuscular function by electromyography. EMG recording for the purpose of monitoring relaxant administration is currently primarily a research tool. Commonly, the ulnar nerve is stimulated, and the evoked compound electromyogram is recorded from the adductor pollicis,[15] abductor digiti minimi,[16] or first dorsal interosseous muscle of the hand.[17] Spontaneous EMG recording as an inexact index of muscle paralysis has also been recorded from the rectus abdominus muscle.[16]

Stimulating electrodes for EMG recording are placed as for mechanical recording. The active receiving electrode is placed over the motor point of the muscle to be studied and the indifferent electrode at the tendon of insertion. A larger ground electrode is placed between the two to reduce 60 Hz interference from the electrical equipment in the operating room. Supramaximal stimulation is applied, and the evoked compound action potentials are recorded.[18]

The EMG is a very fast response. At high-frequency stimulation (20 to 100 Hz) it cannot be recorded on a strip chart because pen inertia prevents separation of the individual action potentials. Action potentials are usually amplified, displayed on an oscilloscope, and then photographed. As an alternative, the EMG is recorded on frequency modulated analog tape and is later transferred to paper at slower speeds.[19] An example of an EMG recording is shown in Figure 23-3.

Recently computer technology has provided us with small, compact EMG monitoring equipment based on amplifying, filtering, rectifying, and integrating the raw EMG signal. This processing ability has made the EMG a clinically useful tool in the perioperative period. The data are instantly presented in both digital and graphic form. There is strong correlation between evoked mechanical and EMG responses if measured from the same muscle.[20]

ACCELEROMETRY

Accelerometers have been used in the aerospace industry for some time. Viby-Mogensen and colleagues[21] have recently used an accelerograph as a neuromuscular transmission monitor based on the concept of accelerometry. The rationale behind this concept comes from Newton's law, which states that

$$F = M \times A$$

where F stands for force, M for mass, and A for acceleration, and assuming that the mass is constant, then force will be proportional to acceleration. The transducer used for measuring acceleration is either a small piezoelectric ceramic wafer or a small aluminum rod with electrodes on both sides. When the electrodes are exposed to a force,

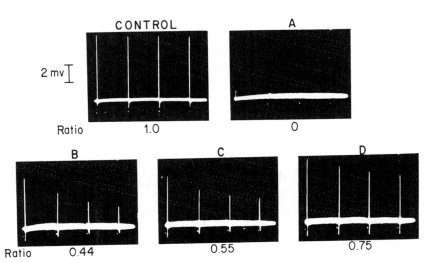

Fig. 23-3. Example of evoked EMG recording. Train-of-four stimulation (2 Hz for 2 seconds) was applied to the ulnar nerve. The compound EMG of the first dorsal interosseous muscle was photographed. Ratios indicate height of fourth response as a percentage of the first in each panel. (**A**) 50 minutes after 0.6 mg/kg *d*-tubocurarine, before reversal. (**B–D**) 5, 10, and 20 minutes after atropine, 0.03 mg/kg and neostigmine, 0.07 mg/kg. (From Ali et al.,[1] with permission.)

a voltage proportional to the acceleration is generated. This signal is amplified and can be measured. If the transducer is positioned such that the direction of force (that is, the thumb adduction) corresponds to the plane of acceleration, the voltage measured will be proportional to the force of thumb adduction. The accelerometer does not require a preload but a freely moving mass, the thumb. This can be achieved by immobilizing the wrist and fingers and leaving the thumb free. A close relationship has been shown between the train-of-four ratios measured by accelerometry of the thumb and evoked thumb adduction using a force transducer.[21]

PATTERNS OF STIMULATION

There are five commonly used patterns of stimulation for monitoring neuromuscular blockade: (1) single twitch: stimuli applied at 0.1 to 0.15 Hz; (2) train-of-four: stimuli applied at 2 Hz for 2 seconds (4 twitches 0.5 seconds apart) repeated every 12 seconds; (3) tetanus: stimulus at 50 to 100 Hz for 5 seconds; (4) posttetanic stimulation: single stimulus applied after tetanus, looking for posttetanic potentiation; (5) double-burst stimulation: two bursts of three stimuli each at 50 Hz, separated by 750 msec.

Single Twitch

The single twitch has been the most commonly used stimulus pattern. As both depolarizing and nondepolarizing muscle relaxants are administered in increasing dosage, the depth of block is defined as percent inhibition of the control response. As the block wears off, the twitch height returns toward baseline, defining the duration of action of the drug. Quantitation using the single twitch thus requires a control twitch height.

Stimulus frequencies from 0.1 to 1.0 Hz have been used. It has been shown that in the presence of nondepolarizing relaxants, the response to repeated stimuli will show increasing fade as the rate of stimulation is increased.[22] The faster the frequency of stimulation, the greater will be the apparent depth of neuromuscular blockade.[23] This fact has proved useful and is the basis for other stimulus patterns, but dictates that single twitches should be delivered at 0.1 to 0.15 Hz or slower.

At frequencies of 0.1 to 0.15 Hz, all desired levels

of clinical relaxation can be monitored without abolition of the twitch. Also at these slow stimulus rates, the presence of a twitch indicates that antagonism of the block with anticholinesterases should be successful.[23]

Train-of-Four

Ali and colleagues[17,24] first described the pattern of application of four successive stimuli to the ulnar nerve at a frequency of 2 Hz. At this frequency, the immediately available store of acetylcholine is depleted, and the amount released by the nerve decreases with each successive stimulus until the fifth or sixth, when it levels off under conditions of partial curarization.[9]

In the presence of nondepolarizing relaxants, the margin of safety is decreased such that some endplates fail to develop propagated action potentials, and some fibers consequently fail to contract in response to the lower acetylcholine output.[14] Twitch height and EMG are successively lower in amplitude as the first, second, third, and fourth responses in the train are elicited during nondepolarizing block.

With increasing degrees of block, the twitches in the train-of-four progressively fade starting with the fourth, and one by one eventually disappear (Fig. 23-4). The ratio of the height of the fourth re-

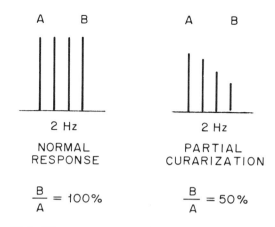

Fig. 23-4. Diagram representing responses to train-of-four stimuli at 2 Hz. (**Left**) Normal response before curarization. The height of B is equal to the height of A and the ratio of B to A expressed as a percentage is 100 percent. (**Right**) Partial curarization. The ratio of the height of B to A is 50 percent. (From Ali et al.,[1] with permission.)

sponse to the first has been defined as the train-of-four ratio. This ratio has been correlated with percent inhibition of the single twitch, or the first twitch in the train-of-four[17] (Fig. 23-5).

Decrease in height of the first twitch does not occur until the fourth twitch has decreased by 20 to 25 percent. As the block deepens, the fourth twitch disappears at 75 percent block of the first twitch during *d*-tubocurare-induced blockade. The third, second, and first twitches are abolished at 80 percent, 90 percent, and 100 percent block, respectively.[9] This may differ with the relaxant used particularly with the new intermediate and short-acting nondepolarizing relaxants.[25]

Train-of-four stimuli should be delivered no more frequently than every 12 seconds. A given first twitch will be unaffected by previous twitches and will serve as an accurate control only if 10 seconds have elapsed since any previous stimulation.[26] Trains of less than four responses or stimuli at slower frequency rates tend to sacrifice fade sensitivity. Higher frequency begins to result in tetanus, and muscle inertia complicates interpretation.[27]

The ratio of the fourth to the first twitch and absence of the fourth, third, or second twitches constitute independent entities. This pattern of stimulation can be applied at any time during nondepolarizing block and can provide quantitation of depth of block without the need for a control measurement before relaxant administration. Also, correlation of the depth of block with the number of responses frees the clinician from recording devices necessary to calculate a ratio.

During depolarizing neuromuscular blockade, the train-of-four ratio does not fade significantly. The height of all four twitches decreases simultaneously. However, the train-of-four ratio has proved useful in assessing neuromuscular block in patients who exhibit a prolonged response to depolarizing relaxants; it has been shown that train-of-four monitoring can be used to diagnose and follow a dual or phase II block.[8,9] A train-of-four ratio of 0.3 or less, in this situation, is diagnostic of the apparent nondepolarizing component that characterizes phase II block and reversal with anticholinesterases is often possible.[9] It must be noted, however, that any component of depolarizing block will not be reflected in the train-of-four ratio. This type of block will not reverse with antagonists and may in fact be made worse.[8]

Visual assessment of the evoked response to train-of-four stimulation can be used to determine the expected dose of relaxant for a given patient. The first visually perceptible sign of decrease in train-of-four ratio in the thumb occurs at approximately 40 percent train-of-four ratio if recorded.[8] Twice the relaxant dose producing this threshold fade produces 75 to 80 percent block of the single twitch or abolition of the third and fourth twitches in the train-of-four.[28] This degree of block reliably results in adequate abdominal muscle relaxation.[29,30] Three times the threshold fade dose produces 99 percent

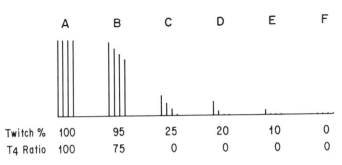

	A	B	C	D	E	F
Twitch %	100	95	25	20	10	0
T4 Ratio	100	75	0	0	0	0

Fig. 23-5. Correlation of the single twitch height at a frequency of 0.1 Hz (the first response in the train-of-four responses) and the train-of-four ratio (T_4, the calculated ratio of the height to the fourth of the first response in the train). **(A)** Control response. **(B)** When the single twitch is 95 percent of control, the train-of-four is 75 percent or less. **(C–E)** Disappearance of the fourth twitch; the third and fourth twitches; and the second, third, and fourth twitches in the train corresponds to 25, 20, and 10 percent single twitch height, respectively, and the ratio of the train-of-four is zero. **(F)** When all four responses in the train are abolished, the depth of block is the same as indicated by the absence of the single twitch. (From Ali et al.,[1] with permission.)

abolition of the twitch, which allows optimal conditions for intubation of the trachea. Thus, simple observation of the patient's evoked train-of-four in response to a small dose of nondepolarizer should allow accurate prediction of that patient's individualized dose requirement without risk of overdose.

Tetanus

High-frequency stimulation (≥ 50 Hz) results in a sustained tetanic contraction of the muscle. On EMG, tetanus can be recorded as individual action potentials. This is perhaps the most stressful method of stimulating the neuromuscular junction.[31] During tetanus, progressive depletion of acetylcholine output is balanced by increased synthesis and transfer of the transmitter from its mobilization stores.[9] There is thus an early decrease in acetylcholine output, which then levels off at the fifth or sixth action potential during partial curarization. With deepening neuromuscular block, there is a progressive loss of tetanic tension; nondepolarizing, but not depolarizing block. This results in fade of the tetanic response. This difference has classically been one distinguishing feature between the two types of block.[1]

There is some controversy over the optimal rate of tetanic stimulation. Fifty (50) Hz is a physiologic tetanic frequency in that, for example, maximal voluntary adduction of the thumb produces neural and muscular action potentials at a frequency equal to or slightly greater than 50 Hz.[32] Some workers have suggested that 100 or 200 Hz may be more stressful and thus more sensitive indicators of small degrees of neuromuscular blockade.[33] However, fade on tetanus at 100 Hz can occur in anesthetized patients in the absence of neuromuscular blocking drugs.[34,35] Stimulation at frequencies above 100 Hz approaches the refractory period of neuromuscular transmission.[31] For these reasons, interpretation of tetanic response at 100 Hz may be misleading. Tetanus at 50 Hz for 5 seconds is a physiologic tetanus; if sustained, it correlates well with acceptable levels of reversal as assessed by other methods.[35,36]

Posttetanic Potentiation

Mobilization and enhanced synthesis of acetylcholine continue during and after cessation of tetanic stimulation. Following the end of a tetanus, there is an increase in the immediately available store of acetylcholine and the quantal content.

Thus, after a tetanus, there is an increase in the amount of the transmitter released in response to nerve stimulation.[1]

Under normal conditions (i.e., no neuromuscular blockade), a single twitch evoked after cessation of tetanus may be stronger than the pretetanic control, as single muscle fibers may respond with greater strength of contraction due to increased calcium entry. This is a muscle effect and is not seen on EMG.[27] During nondepolarizing blockade with decreased sensitivity of the motor end plate, the posttetanic mechanical and EMG twitch are markedly facilitated as compared with pretetanic levels because of the larger amount of acetylcholine released. This has been termed posttetanic potentiation and is a hallmark of a nondepolarizing block.[1] The degree of potentiation is influenced by the depth of block, the duration and frequency of the tetanus, and the posttetanic interval[37] (Fig. 23-6).

Increased synthesis and mobilization of acetylcholine lasts at least several minutes and possibly as long as 30 minutes following tetanus.[7] Excessive or frequent use of tetanic stimulation distorts train-of-four and single-twitch responses in the direction of normality so that recovery from block may be overestimated.

Therefore, in assessing depth of neuromuscular blockade, tetanus should be used little, if at all, as subsequent monitoring may underestimate the degree of residual paralysis and most of the information derived from it can be obtained using the train-of-four stimulation.

Viby-Mogensen and colleagues[38] have described a way of using post-tetanic potentiation to evaluate the depth of non-depolarizing blockade so intense that there is no response to single twitch, train-of-four, or tetanic stimulation. Tetanus at 50 Hz for 5 seconds is applied followed by single-twitch stimulation at 1 Hz. The number of evoked posttetanic count (PTC) has been correlated with the time required for spontaneous recovery of the single twitch or train-of-four.[38] Thus the PTC should be useful in predicting an appropriate time to attempt reversal of nondepolarizing blockade as well as how successful reversal might be.

Double-Burst Stimulation

Double-burst stimulation (DBS) has been suggested as a method to manually detect fade easier than detecting fade after train-of-four or tetanic stimulation at 50 Hz for 5 seconds. DBS consists of two short bursts of three stimuli each at a frequency of 50 Hz. The two bursts are separated by 750 msec. The response to this pattern of stimulation is two single, separate muscle contractions. The response to the second burst of stimulation is less than the response to the first burst during partial nondepolarizing neuromuscular blockade. There is close correlation between fade ratios using train-of-four and double-burst stimulation.[39,40] The pattern of double-burst stimulation needs further clinical evaluation.

COMPARISONS OF PATTERNS OF STIMULATION

Train-of-four stimulation represents an advantage over single twitch in that it serves as its own control. This eliminates the need for a recorded pre-paralysis control twitch. Since tactile assessment of fade and abolition of successive twitches have been correlated with depth of block, train-of-four stimulation is useful without recording devices or transducers.

Comparisons have been made among various patterns of stimulation as to sensitivity in detecting blockade. During onset of neuromuscular blockade with nondepolarizing relaxants, the train-of-four response will be abolished before the single twitch (Savarese JJ, Basta S, Ali H, unpublished observations). As the block recovers, the train-of-four is more sensitive than the single twitch; that is, during spontaneous recovery the single twitch will reach control height when the train-of-four ratio is well below one.[36] At single-twitch height 90 percent of control, the train-of-four ratio may be only 55 to 60 percent.[41] This effect is much less important when a nondepolarizing block is reversed with anticholinesterases.[1] Nonetheless, recovery of single twitch to control may be somewhat misleading.

Various patterns of stimulation have been compared as to the number of acetylcholine receptors that must be occupied in order to detect blockade.[21] Because of the wide margin of safety of neuromuscular transmission, more than 70 percent of the cholinergic receptors must be occupied by relaxant before any mechanical weakness results.[42] Tetanus at 50 Hz will show fade at receptor occupancy greater than 70 percent. Although tetanus at 100 Hz will show fade at occupancy of less than 70 percent, there seems to be no need for this degree of sensitivity, and 50 Hz is an acceptable frequency. A train-of-four ratio of 70 percent or less correlates with receptor occupancy of 70 percent or greater, so that by receptor occupancy, train-of-four is a sensitive enough test for clinical use.[43] Single twitch, on the other hand, may be normal with 70 percent receptor occupancy and so has been called a less sensitive measure of neuromuscular blockade.

A 50 Hz tetanus is comparable in sensitivity to train-of-four. A 50 Hz tetanus will be well sustained for 5 sec if the train-of-four ratio is 0.7 or greater.[34,36] A 100 Hz tetanus has been found to show marked fade at a time when 50 Hz tetanus is well sustained. A train-of-four ratio of greater than 0.7 correlates well with acceptable clinical indices

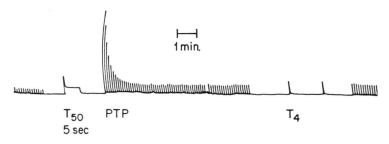

Fig. 23-6. Tetanic fade and posttetanic potentiation during partial nondepolarizing neuromuscular blockade produced by pancuronium in a patient during nitrous oxide-narcotic anesthesia. Twitches (0.15 Hz) and tetanus of the thumb were evoked via the ulnar nerve. At T_{50} tetanic stimulation was applied at 50 Hz for 5 seconds. Fade of the tetanic response and marked posttetanic potentiation (PTP) of the twitch stabilize after the period of potentiation at approximately twice the height of the pretetanic twitch. At T_4 train-of-four stimulation was carried out. Only the first response in the train is evoked at this depth of block (90 percent depression of the single twitch). (From Ali et al.,[1] with permission.)

of recovery. Tetanus at 100 Hz may be too sensitive a test; its use may lead to administration of antagonists that are not indicated and may be counterproductive.[34]

Taking all the foregoing into account, it seems that the train-of-four should provide the most reliably sensitive information, most easily obtained, and with least distortion of subsequent monitoring during neuromuscular blockade.

COMPARISONS OF MECHANICAL VERSUS ELECTRICAL RECORDING

There is controversy in the literature as to the usefulness of mechanical versus EMG recording.[15,17,30,44-46]

From a technical viewpoint, mechanical twitch evaluation in clinical practice has a tremendous advantage over EMG in that if train-of-four stimulation is used, all that is required is a nerve stimulator for tactile evaluation. If mechanical twitch tension is to be transduced, it requires specific criteria that make it impractical in the clinical setting.

In general, evoked mechanical and electrical responses run parallel, but there are differences. Mechanical twitch is less sensitive to small degrees of depolarizing block than the EMG. In contrast, with a nondepolarizing block, the EMG is less sensitive than the mechanical twitch. This means that during recovery from a nondepolarizing block, the EMG may reach control when substantial mechanical block persists.[15]

Posttetanic potentiation occurs in the normal state when assessed by mechanical twitch. This is not true with EMG monitoring. Since posttetanic potentiation is seen using both types of monitoring during nondepolarizing blockade, it has been stated that EMG evidence of posttetanic potentiation is diagnostic of a nondepolarizing block.[27]

Unlike mechanical twitch, the EMG is not affected by factors that change contractility of the muscle itself, so that in this respect the EMG is a more pure monitor of neuromuscular transmission. Fade is seen earlier during tetanus on EMG because muscle inertia is uninvolved and a shorter tetanus can be used to demonstrate fade. This is a particular advantage in awake patients because tetanic stimulation is painful.

CLINICAL CORRELATION

The various levels of relaxation achieved with the use of neuromuscular blocking drugs occur within reasonably well-defined limits of evoked responses.[1,28-30,46] Table 23-1 summarizes these data. Correlates are seen in Fig. 23-7.

Profound abdominal muscle relaxation can be achieved at 80 to 90 percent block in most cases under nitrous oxide-narcotic anesthesia[29,30] and at 75 percent block under potent inhalation anesthesia.[47] At 95 percent twitch suppression, jaw and laryngeal muscle paralysis is sufficient for smooth endotracheal intubation.[7]

Satisfactory reversal of nondepolarizing neuro-

TABLE 23-1. Correlation of Twitch Height, Clinical Relaxation, and Ventilation at Increasing Depths of Neuromuscular Blockade[a]

Twitch Height % of Control	Clinical Relaxation	Ventilation
100	None (train-of-four ratio > 70%, tetanus sustained at 50 Hz)	Normal
75	Poor, but head lift inadequate	Slightly to moderately diminished vital capacity
50	Fair	Moderately to markedly diminished vital capacity; tidal volume may be adequate
25	Good with potent inhalation anesthetics	Tidal volume diminished
10	Good with balanced technique	Tidal volume inadequate
5	Very good; adequate for tracheal intubation under light anesthesia	Some diaphragmatic motion possible
0	Excellent; very good for tracheal intubation	Apnea

[a]Clinical conditions found at various twitch heights, if the block were held constant at each level.

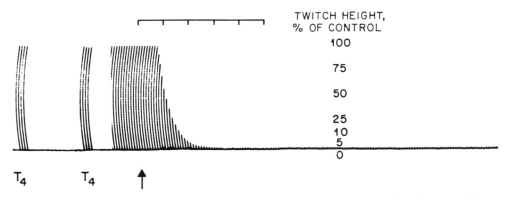

Fig. 23-7. A recording of evoked thumb adduction was made in a patient during nitrous oxide-narcotic-barbiturate anesthesia. The single twitch was evoked at 0.15 Hz. At T$_4$, train-of-four stimulation (2 Hz for 2 seconds) was carried out. Time scale (in minutes) at top. At the *arrow*, pancuronium, 0.1 mg/kg, was given intravenously, producing 99 percent twitch suppression. (From Ali et al.,[1] with permission.)

muscular blocking drugs is possible at 5 percent recovery and is greatly facilitated if twitch height has spontaneously reached 25 percent of control.[44,46,47] Respiratory muscles are less sensitive to neuromuscular blockade than peripheral muscles.[7] Compared with the tibialis anterior muscle, the diaphragm requires only one-half as many acetylcholine receptors free of relaxant to function.[48] Ventilatory parameters demonstrating acceptable minimal limits for recovery of paralysis have included a vital capacity of 15 to 20 ml/kg and inspiratory force of 20 to 25 cm H$_2$O. If the train-of-four ratio is greater than 70 percent or if tetanus is sustained at 50 Hz for 5 seconds, vital capacity and inspiratory force will be well within these limits.[1] At the same time, grip strength, tongue protrusion, and eyelid and jaw tone will be normal, and head lift will be well sustained for 5 seconds.[14,17,49]

It should be apparent that if relaxant is titrated to achieve one small twitch using train-of-four monitoring (i.e., to abolish the last three twitches), the anesthesiologist can be confident of adequate abdominal muscle relaxation and a good probability of reversibility. As the block dissipates, recovery of four twitches without perceptible fade indicates safe, acceptable criteria for extubation provided other clinical criteria are met.

REFERENCES

1. Ali HH, Savarese JJ: Monitoring of neuromuscular function. Anesthesiology. 45:216, 1976

2. Ali HH, Wilson RS, Savarese JJ et al: The effect of tubocurarine on indirectly elicited train-of-four muscle response and respiratory measurements in humans. Br J Anaesth 47:570, 1975

3. Hubbard J: Mechanism of transmitter release. Prog Biophys Mol Biol 21:35, 1970

4. Thesleff S: The mode of neuromuscular block caused by acetylcholine, nicotine, decamethonium and succinylcholine. Acta Physiol Can 34:218, 1955

5. Bowman W: Prejunctional and postjunctional cholinoceptors at the neuromuscular junction. Anesth Analg 59:935, 1980

6. Churchill-Davidson H, Christie T, Wise R: Dual neuromuscular block in man. Anesthesiology 21:144, 1960

7. Lee C: Dose relationship of phase II, tachyphylaxis and train of four fade in suxamethonium induced dual neuromuscular block in man. Br J Anaesth 47:84, 1975

8. Savarese JJ, Ali HH, Murphy JD et al: Train-of-four nerve stimulation in the management of prolonged neuromuscular blockade following succinylcholine. Anesthesiology 42:106, 1975

9. Lee C: Train of four quantification of competitive neuromuscular block. Anesth Analg 54:649, 1975

10. Berger J, Gravenstein J, Munson E: Electrode polarity and peripheral nerve stimulation. Anesthesiology 56:402, 1982

11. Gravenstein J, Paulus D: Monitoring Practice in Clinical Anesthesia. p. 178. JB Lippincott, Philadelphia, 1982

12. Kopman A, Lawson D: Milliamperage requirements for supramaximal stimulation of the ulnar nerve with surface electrodes. Anesthesiology 61:83, 1984

13. Donlon JV Jr, Savarese JJ, Ali HH: Cumulative dose-

response curves for gallamine: effect of altered resting thumb tension and mode of stimulation. Anesth Analg 58:377, 1979

14. Ali HH, Kitz RJ: Evaluation of recovery from nondepolarizing neuromuscular block, using a digital neuromuscular transmission analyzer: preliminary report. Anesth Analg 52:740, 1973

15. Katz R: Electromyographic and mechanical effects of suxamethonium and tubocurarine on twitch, tetanic and post-tetanic responses. Br J Anaesth 45:849, 1973

16. Gerber H, Johansen S, Mortimer T et al: Frequency sweep EMG and voluntary effort in volunteers after *d*-tubocurarine. Anesthesiology 46:35, 1977

17. Ali HH, Utting JE, Gray C: Quantitative assessment of residual antidepolarizing block. (Part I). Br J Anaesth. 43:473, 1971

18. Roberts D, Wilson A: Electromyography in diagnosis and treatment. p. 29. In Green R (ed): Myasthenia Gravis. Heinemann, London, 1969

19. Epstein RM, Epstein RA, Lee A: A recording system for continuous evoked electromyography. Anesthesiology 38:287, 1973

20. Ali HH, DeCesare R: Evoked EMG, integrated EMG (IEMG), and mechanical responses. Anesthesiology 71:A396, 1989

21. Viby-Mogensen J, Jensen E, Werner M et al: Measurement of acceleration: a new method of monitoring neuromuscular function. Acta Anaesthesiol Scand 32:45, 1987

22. Ali HH, Utting JE, Gray TC: Stimulus frequency in the detection of neuromuscular block in humans. Br J Anaesth 42:967, 1970

23. Ali HH, Savarese JJ: Stimulus frequency and dose-response curve to *d*-tubocurarine in man. Anesthesiology 52:36, 1980

24. Ali HH, Utting JE, Gray TC: Quantitative assessment of residual antidepolarizing block. (Part II). Br J Anaesth 43:478, 1971

25. Ali HH: Monitoring neuromuscular blockade. p. 827. In: Rogers M, Tinker J, Covino BG, Longnecker DE (eds): Principles and practice of anesthesiology. Vol. 1. Mosby Year Book, St. Louis, 1992

26. Lee C, Katz R: Neuromuscular pharmacology: a clinical update and commentary. Br J Anaesth 52:173, 1980

27. Epstein RA, Epstein RM: The electromyogram and the mechanical response of indirectly stimulated muscle in anesthetized man following curarization. Anesthesiology 38:212, 1973

28. Savarese JJ, Ali HH: Accurate prediction of metocurine dosage by clinical observation of "threshold fade" on train-of-four stimulation. p. 313. Abstracts of Scientific Papers, American Society of Anesthesiologists Annual Meeting, 1977

29. Dripps R, Eckenhoff J, Vandam L: Introduction to Anesthesia: The Principles of Safe Practice. 5th Ed. WB Saunders, Philadelphia, 1977

30. Katz R: Comparison of electrical and mechanical recording of spontaneous and evoked muscle activity. Anesthesiology 26:204, 1965

31. Lee A: Monitoring the neuromuscular junction. Int Anesthesiol Clin 19:85, 1981

32. Merton P: Voluntary muscle strength and fatigue. J Physiol 123:553, 1954

33. Waud B, Waud D: The relation between tetanic fade and receptor occlusion in the presence of complete neuromuscular block. Anesthesiology 35:456, 1971

34. Kopman A, Epstein R, Flashburg M: Use of 100 Hz tetanus and an index of recovery from pancuronium-induced non-depolarizing neuromuscular blockade. Anesth Analg (Cleve) 61:439, 1982

35. Stanec A, Heyduck J, Stanec G et al: Tetanic fade and post-tetanic tension in the absence of neuromuscular blocking agents in anesthetized man. Anesth Analg (Cleve) 57:102, 1978

36. Ali HH, Savarese JJ, Lebowitz PW et al: Twitch, tetanus and train-of-four as indices of recovery from nondepolarizing neuromuscular blockade. Anesthesiology 54:294, 1981

37. Unna K, Pelikan E, MacFarlane W et al: Evaluation of curarizing drugs in man. J Pharmacol Exp Ther 98:318, 1950

38. Viby-Mogensen J, Howardy-Hansen P, Chraemmer-Jørgensen B et al: Posttetanic count (PTC): a new method of evaluating an intense nondepolarizing neuromuscular blockade. Anesthesiology 55:458, 1981

39. Brull SJ, Connelly NR, Silverman DG: Correlation of train-of-four and double burst stimulation ratios at varying amperages. Anesth Analg 71:489, 1990

40. Engbaek J, Østergaard D, Viby-Mogensen J: Double burst stimulation (DBS): a new pattern of nerve stimulation to identify residual neuromuscular block. Br J Anaesth 62:274, 1979

41. D'Hollander A, Duvaldestin P, Delcroix C et al: Evolution of single twitch and train of four responses and of tetanic fade in relation of plasma concentrations of fazadinium in man. Anesth Analg 61:225, 1982

42. Paton W, Waud D: The margin of safety of neuromuscular transmission. J Physiol 191:59, 1967

43. Katz R: Neuromuscular effects of *d*-tubocurarine, edrophonium and neostigmine in man. Anesthesiology 28:327, 1967

44. Churchill-Davidson H: A philosophy of relaxation. Anesth Analg 52:495, 1973

45. Katz G, Katz R: Clinical considerations in the use of muscle relaxants. p. 313. In Katz R (ed): Muscle Relaxants. Exerpta Medica. American Elsevier, New York, 1975

46. Miller R: Monitoring of neuromuscular blockade. p. 127. In Saidman L, Smith N (eds): Monitoring in Anesthesia. Wiley, New York, 1978

47. Katz R: Clinical neuromuscular pharmacology of pancuronium. Anesthesiology 34:550, 1971

48. Waud B, Waud D: The margin of safety of neuro-muscular transmission in the muscle of the diaphragm. Anesthesiology 37:417, 1972

49. Brand JB, Cullen DJ, Wilson NE et al: Spontaneous recovery from nondepolarizing neuromuscular blockade: correlation between clinical and evoked responses. Anesth Analg 56:55, 1977

Automation and Anesthesia Information Management

William T. Merritt

24

The anaesthetic record should show one of the most detailed events in the patient's clinical life. The story should be complete from the first preoperative visit to the last postanesthetic visit.[1]

Given the frustrations and disappointments—and frequent fears—generated by computers, health professionals might prefer to delegate the challenge to someone else or, better yet, to stay away from computers altogether. However, the ubiquity of computer usage makes that approach unrealistic.[2]

From the earliest days of anesthesia "charts,"[3] the recording of observations has been rooted in a need to objectively acknowledge and explain events during anesthesia and surgery. The review of these written records provided material for discussion, research, and, ultimately, change of practice.

One hundred years later, most of the issues are still the same: the recording of observations, review and research when appropriate, and improvements in clinical care. However, during the past century our practice has changed dramatically. Due to advances in our understanding of physiology, anesthesiology, pharmacology, biomedical engineering, life support, and surgical techniques, surgery is now performed on older, younger, and sicker patients. Accompanying such advances has been a dizzying increase in data to be recorded from a growing array of electronic and manual patient monitors. Yet our anesthesia data is still captured at 5-minute time intervals. Even at this "slow" rate

of manual capture of data it is has been clearly demonstrated that we have considerable difficulty keeping up with the physiologic data we choose to document[4-8] unless an assistant is available solely for manual record-keeping purposes.[9] The intensity of data has simply outstripped our ability to manually record it in a way that is acceptable for peer review, for clinical research, and, unfortunately, for medical legal purposes.

In addition, the anesthesia record in most settings has evolved to contain considerable information useful for documentation and billing purposes. When such records are completed correctly, clerical staff are enabled to submit timely and accurate bills. Also, peer review personnel have an adequate picture of the care that was rendered. When data are missing, illegible, or inaccurate, valuable resources are expended in deciphering, contacting those involved, and correcting. In most areas then, the handwritten anesthetic record falls far short of the varied demands placed upon it.[10]

The competitive corporate world has committed to computerization of information management. The clinical medicine world is, by comparison, relatively far behind. The practice of anesthesia should not wait to be dragged into the area of computerized information management. To the extent that information management is a basis for advantage[11]—advantage in a competitive medical market—we cannot afford to be second best.

BRIEF HISTORY OF THE ANESTHETIC RECORD

The year 1994 marks a century of anesthesia record keeping. In 1894, Dr. E. A. Codman and Dr. Harvey Cushing, medical students at the Massachusetts General Hospital, conceived of "ether charts" as a means of learning more about the delivery of ether anesthesia and thereby improving outcome, which at the time they regarded primarily as reducing the tendency to vomit. There charts were simple, with a few comments about the patient and the procedure, the amount of ether administered, and the recording of pulse, respiration, and eventually temperature* (Fig. 24-1). They appeared unafraid to record the varied swings of the few physiologic variables they noted. And, yes, the interval of record was *5 minutes*. The inclusion of routine blood pressure measurements as part of the anesthetic record was recommended by Dr. Cushing in 1902![12]

---

*See Beecher.[3] Their records were apparently not placed with the patients' charts, since a number were donated to the Treadwell Library at Massachusetts General Hospital, from the private collection of Dr. Codman.

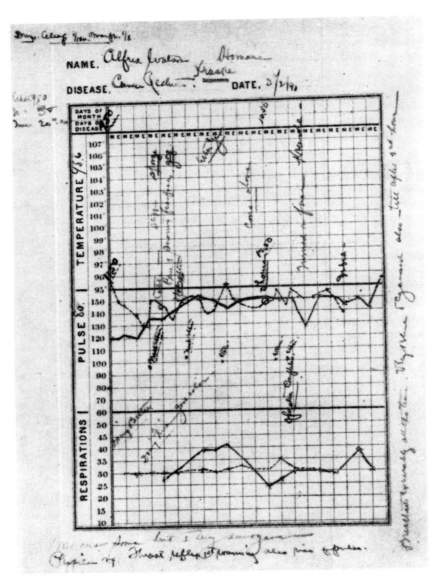

Fig. 24-1. An early anesthesia chart (circa 1891) of Harvey Cushing showing temperature, pulse, respiration, and various annotations regarding anesthetic, mucus, pupils, vomiting, etc. Appears to show an overlay of data when time ran out at right chart. (From Beecher,[3] with permission.)

Within a few years anesthetic records were kept over a wide geographic area including Canada,[13,14] New York City,[15] Alabama,[16] Ohio,[17] and England.[18] Over the ensuing decades there have been countless attempts to improve both on the anesthetic record and the management of the data it encompasses. Some of these efforts are worth noting.

Both in England and the United States these efforts are recounted in the early anesthesia literature.[19] At an early point, the American Society of Anesthesiologists decided that the unassisted manual compilation of data was inadequate, and it strongly supported the adoption of mechanized methods where possible.[20,21,22] They advocated the adoption of the Hollerith Punch Card Method,* a system that involved cards with holes (Fig. 24-2) punched into columns of numbers (associated with anesthesia text items at the top) and read from elaborate tabulators. This form of data collection led to a number of interesting related efforts at tackling the problems of managing anesthesia data. One early effort was referred to as the *Nosworthy* card, devised in England, that consisted of an 8-in. × 5-in. card: on the front side was a brief preoperative history, and on the back a small graphic representation of the anesthetic procedure. There were places for written comments, but around the edge of the front were a series of categories of information, including site of operation, physical state, and anesthetic agents. Within each of these categories the choices were written next to holes at the edge of the card. The choices were circled by hand, and, later, the holes were "removed" with a punch. When stacks of cards were placed together, the holes were aligned. If a knitting needle-type selector, was placed through a series of holes, and lifted, it would leave behind those cards that hand been "punched" at that hole (Fig. 24-3). Selection of simple data was considerably enhanced.[23] Others had experimented with a similar design,[24,25] but most efforts were toward a larger full-page type of format,[26,27] and one included recovery room data.[28] These larger *Keysort* records achieved a level of fre-

quent use[29] (Fig. 24-4). Similar systems were the basis for an elaborate statistical system for anesthesia, inhalation therapy, and therapeutic and diagnostic blocks,[30,31] specialty anesthetic records,[32] and even for the military anesthesiologist.[33,34] Recognizing that there was a mandatory medicolegal need for anesthetic records to accurately reflect the condition of the patient during the course of anesthesia, the Committee of Clinical Anesthesia Study of the American Society of Anesthesiologists devel-

---

*Herman Hollerith developed a unique card tabulation system for the 1890 U.S. census that was three times faster than manual methods. First read by "tabulators," and later by computers, such cards became the mainstay of data compilation for the first half of the twentieth century. Hollerith's company eventually evolved into IBM. See *Understanding Computers: Input/Output*, Time/Life Books, Chicago, 1986, p. 9.

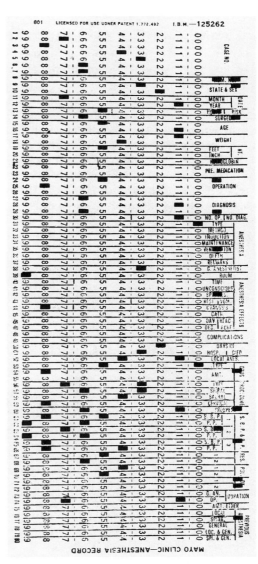

Fig. 24-2. An actual punch card from an anesthetic, which includes features of the anesthetic, the operation, and postoperative complications. (From Tovell and Dunn,[21] with permission.)

oped its own punchcard type of anesthesia record for the collation of anesthetic data.[35] This record contained both preoperative and postoperative information, as well as an account of the associated anesthetic. This system provided simple access to individualized data and was widely used, but it required ancillary personnel to decipher the anesthetic record and encode the data in a punchcard format.

What Is Wrong with the Written Anesthetic Record?

Many would argue that a written record suits them just fine, that its limitations are insignificant. Others have discussed, documented, or mused about its limitations for decades.

As mentioned above, even in the bygone era of limited, manually acquired anesthetic data, practitioners strove to include ever-increasing amounts of patient evaluation and intraoperative information on the anesthetic record. Their goal was to improve the ability to retrospectively answer outcome types of questions and thus help in the review of care. This led to elaborate designs of forms and sorting schemes, which were, by today's standards, limited in scope, personnel-intense, and cumbersome. Numerous authors (but not all[36]) have ac-

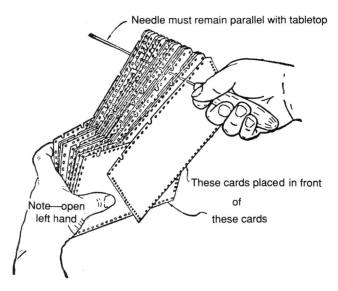

Fig. 24-3. Method of sorting cards and records with holes around the edges. When items are "punched," the card remains behind. (From Pender,[24] with permission.)

knowledged that the written record is nearly worthless when used as a tool to understand the events leading up to an anesthesia- or surgery-related intraoperative catastrophe.[37] Reviewers of anesthetic records have described inaccuracies in text entries[38] and serious deficiencies in requisite information,[4] a sad reality often used against the defendant anesthesiologist in the malpractice setting[5]— "The most common (frequency) and difficult (severity) barrier to successful defense in a malpractice claim in anesthesia is the poor or incomplete anesthesia record. The next most common barrier is the medical expert witness who reviews the poor anesthesia record and then proceeds to fill in the blank spaces with hypothetical "facts" and conjecture that always favors the proposition of the attorney who introduced the witness and the theory of the plaintiff's case."[39]

The phenomenon of "smoothing" of data has also been noted by several investigators interested in the differences between handwritten anesthesia records and automated ones. Typically, when values for systolic and diastolic pressure and heart rate are within a "normal," range there is little discrepancy between the two types of records, but as readings stray from these ranges, the magnitude of discrepancy increases; for example, high systolic and diastolic pressures and heart rates are lowered on the handwritten record, and low values are raised.[6,40,41] Table 24-1 shows that both arterial line and automated noninvasive blood pressure highest-systolic values are considerably higher and lowest-systolic values considerably lower on the automated record; thus, smoothing has taken place.

Additionally, the written anesthesia record is notorious for becoming soiled intraoperatively—the more invasive the surgery and anesthesia, the more likely the record will become soiled. Table 24-2 shows that during anesthesia for cardiopulmonary bypass, 36 percent of anesthesia records retrieved from the medical records department are soiled with blood, and another 15 percent are soiled with some other fluid. The values are nearly identical for major aortic aneurysm surgery, and considerably less for relatively noninvasive procedures such as laparoscopic cholecystectomy. We simply cannot keep our records clean; in an era of very noxious viruses, and the knowledge that even as fomites, viruses have some viability, this sort of information should cause concern.[42]

However, perhaps the most practical day-to-day

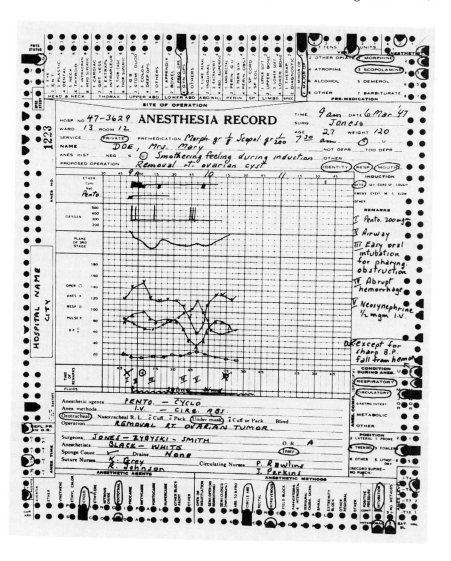

Fig. 24-4. The front side of a "Chicago Keysort" anesthesia record. The record is of a completed case that has been coded and punched. Notice various issues of anesthetic interest around the edges. The reverse of the same record shows preoperative and postoperative information dealt with in a similar manner. (From Conroy, et al.,[27] with permission.)

TABLE 24-1. Comparison of Highest and Lowest Systolic Pressure Values Obtained via an Automated Record with those on a Simultaneously Obtained Manual Record

	AL (mmHg; $n = 10$)	NIBP (mmHg; $n = 30$)
ΔHS (Manual HS—Automated HS)	−40.2 (SD 30.7)	−20.93 (SD 12.2)
ΔLS (Manual LS—Automated LS)	12.8 (SD 20.6)	7.8 (SD 8.5)

The highest systolic (HS) and lowest systolic (LS) pressure values recorded on an automated record (LifeLog, Modular Instruments, Malvern, PA) were compared with the values recorded on a simultaneously maintained manual record, ± 5 minutes. Arterial line (AL) and noninvasive blood pressure (NIBP) values are contrasted.

problems with the written anesthesia record are the difficulties of care review, and the tracking of personnel, pharmaceuticals, equipment, and supplies. The technology exists to computerize and streamline these tasks. The corporate/manufacturing world has adopted such technology, but like most of medicine, the clinical anesthesia world is considerably behind.

What is *good* with the written anesthetic record? It is relatively simple to use and easy to learn, permits considerable individual variation in style of completion, takes up very little operating room space, is low in maintenance, and is inexpensive—in short, it is quite "user friendly." Computerized systems that can duplicate many, if not all of these characteristics, will benefit in the process.

Computerization of the Anesthesiology Environment

Since the 1960s the anesthesiologists' environment has become increasingly dominated by equipment of a functionally computerized nature. We have seen an incursion into the operating room of intensive care unit equipment with subsequent development of specific monitors to accommodate the rapid physiologic changes seen in the operating room. EKG machines have gone from simple three-lead devices to five-lead machines with sophisticated computerized algorithms for determining heart

rate,[43] arrhythmias, ST-segment abnormalities, and respiratory rate.[44] "Manual" blood pressure measurement has given way to automated software-driven devices that measure systolic and diastolic pressure, arrive at a mean pressure,[45] determine heart rate, and permit the setting of a variety of limits with associated alarms. Invasive pressure monitoring has advanced from cumbersome fluid-filled transducer setups to small disposable units. Fiberoptic transducers for intracranial pressure monitoring,[46] transducer systems with dual blood gas and pressure functions, and transducer systems that permit analysis of respiratory variation and complex pressure recognition such as the pulmonary artery wedge pressure[47] are commonplace in the perioperative period. We have lauded the development of percutaneous oximetry and the ability to measure end-tidal carbon dioxide and respiratory gases. All of these advances and many others have depended upon advances in electronics, improved amplifiers and filters, a better understanding of physiologic biopotentials, miniaturization of design, but, most importantly, on the introduction of computer chip/software-driven processing of data. Some of these advances have even been incorporated into the FDA/ASA intraoperative monitoring standards. It is quite reasonable that in the not-too-distant future, most anesthesiologists will regard the computerization of both the intraoperative record and preoperative/postoperative patient history as essential to their practice.

TABLE 24-2. Contamination of the Anesthetic Record: Data Acquired from Visual Inspection of Records Saved in Patient Charts

Results	No. LABS ± SD	No. PRBCU ± SD	No. LINES ± SD
CABG: (209 cases 51% soiled)			
+ Blood (36%*)	9.2 ±2.8**	2.3 ±3	3.9 ±.8
− Blood (64%)	8.4 ±2.2	1.9 ±2.1	3.98 ±.8
AAA/TAA: (47 cases 51% soiled)			
− Blood (36%*)	6.5 ±2.7	6.1 ±3.8	4.3 ±.6
− Blood (64%)	5.3 ±3	4.9 ±5.2	4 ± 1
LAP CHOLE: (88 cases 15% soiled)			
+ Blood (1%)	2.5 ±2***	0	0
− Blood (99%)	.1 ±.6	.3 ±1	.8 ±.9

LABS, number of times blood was drawn for lab tests; PRBCU, number of packed red blood cell units administered; LINES, arterial, central venous and pulmonary artery lines inserted; CABG, coronary artery bypass graft; AAA, abdominal aortic aneurysm; TAA, thoracoabdominal aortic aneurysm; LAP CHOLE, laparoscopic cholecystectomy.
*$P<.01$ compared to lap chole; **$P<.03$ compared to −blood; ***$P<.01$ compared to −blood.
(From Merritt and Zuckerberg,[42] with permission.)

Anesthesiologists' Work Habits

Anesthesiologists engage in a variety of activities within the operating room. They must position patients on tables, place noninvasive monitors correctly, establish invasive monitoring, induce and maintain anesthesia. In addition to these technical tasks anesthesiologists observe, anticipate, and/or react quickly to physiologic demands created by the surgical procedure, administer medications and fluids, "monitor the monitors," and allow patients to emerge in a manner appropriate for their physical status and the nature of the surgical procedure performed. All the while, anesthesiologists assimilate patients status information from direct patient observations, review of the monitored vital signs, and verbal communication with the surgeon. When time permits, some of this information is manually recorded on the anesthetic record. A number of investigators have attempted to study how we go about performing these tasks.

Utilizing video recordings during anesthetic care, it has been consistently shown that record-keeping occupies from 6 to 15 percent of the anesthesiologist's time, with much of this activity occurring during quieter periods of the surgery.[48–52] Some consider manual record keeping as a distraction from patient care, while others view the manual recording of data as essential for "cerebralization" of events and trends. One study noted that anesthesiologists spent about 25 percent of their time involved in monitoring.[51] That study was repeated by the same investigators after a marked increase in task automation. In the subsequent study, it was found that the time spent observing patients, either directly or indirectly, had increased by nearly 2.5 times, to 59 percent.[52] If such research is accurate, the redirection of time previously spent in manual activities permits a considerable increase in indirect patient monitoring through visual inspection of electronic devices.[52] Automation of anesthesia record-keeping, however, may not decrease the amount of time spent attending to documentation of anesthesia care.[53] This is true partly because pen and paper may be slightly faster, but mostly because it becomes easier to enter a wide variety of comments that previously were not likely to be entered due to space limitations and the need to actually write down vital signs. The quality of the simultaneously trended data found in the good automated systems should greatly improve the anesthesiologist's understanding of a patient's anesthetic course, and as such becomes an indirect monitor of the patient's well-being.

Vigilance has been defined as "a state of clinical awareness whereby dangerous conditions are anticipated or recognized and promptly corrected."[54] Errors in the process of patient observation and vigilance have been cited as contributing to anesthesia-related mishaps.[55,56] Unfortunately, depending upon anesthesia workstation design, anesthesiologists may spend between 25 and 46 percent of their time in activities that physically direct them away from the patient.[49,50] It is important, as we continue our relentless search for better patients monitoring devices, that we physically place our anesthesia equipment in areas that facilitate direct visual patient observation (Fig. 24-5). This includes the positioning of the AIMS intraoperative components.

The Computerized Anesthesia Record: Some Early Experience

Various efforts at automation of anesthesiologists' tasks have been undertaken over the last 10 to 20 years. Each of these endeavors has provided

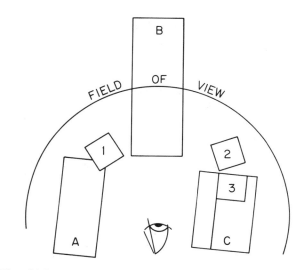

Fig. 24-5. Diagram representing the anesthesiologist's field of view intraoperatively. Since anesthesia activities are varied, it is important to keep the patient physically within view as much as possible. *A*, the anesthesia cart; *B*, the OR table; *C*, the anesthesia machine; *1*, *2*, and *3* represent potential sites for the monitor screen of an AIMS—each of which would facilitate continued direct patient observation.

insight into the issues inherent to the technology. Many however, have not stood the test of time.

A notable project was begun in the Department of Anesthesiology at Duke University in the early 1970s, and became known as the DAME system (*Duke Anesthesia Monitoring Equiement*).[57] Because of a dearth of monitoring instruments designed specifically for the operating room environment, the DAME program sought to develop an inhouse anesthesia monitoring capability that included not only a display of the directly monitored vital signs, but also the automated recording of those values (along with other entries that would otherwise be handwritten—drug and surgical events, etc.) for an anesthesia record printout, as well as storage for later review. The primary-monitor-data was captured in a digital Equipment Corporation (DEC) LSI 11/02 microcomputer which was integrated to a postoperative data manager (DEC PDP-11/23 minicomputer) via a network system also developed at Duke, called the DMXNET. The Data Manager had a 5 MB (megabyte) hard disk and 256 KB (kilobyte) or RAM (random access memory)! This system accommodated different software packages for varied types of patients, and the differing preferences of anesthesiologists. Data was backed-up every 90 seconds and eventually stored on a DEC PDP-11/60 computer with over 600 MB of storage. Drug and event entries were made by way of an elaborate light pencil/bar code system; this form of notation was also used to signify events such as transducer calibration. Along with the primary monitor screen, there was a computer video terminal and attached keyboard. There was a system of alarms and an uninterruptable power source (UPS).

The DAME system was installed as the only anesthesia monitoring system in ten new operating rooms in 1980. In spite of extensive preparation of users, the system failed; a look at some of the reasons for this failure is worthwhile. The machine was cumbersome, heavy, and not always able to be positioned in a optimal site for use by the anesthesiologist. Construction errors led to network outlets on the wrong side of the operating room. Physical characteristics of the electrocardiographic wiring were disliked by the users. The temperature channel was not used because users preferred a disposable device. The layout of the primary monitor screen was awkward. Bar codes, as the sole means for entry of drugs and events, were impractical. For example, some codes were too long and were often read incorrectly; the source pages containing the codes frequently disappeared or became soiled or otherwise damaged. Software glitches, monitor-processing crashes, and network difficulties frequently occurred. For these and other reasons more difficult to quantitate, an acceptable level of user acceptance never developed. Some anesthesiologists apparently even refused to have the device in their operating room. In spite of these unsurmountable problems, most users did like the automated blood pressure component of the monitor, and maintenance for the monitoring components of the system was less than for a commercial anesthesia monitoring system. Many of the innovative concepts attempted with this system, however, have remained valid, and have been adapted successfully by commercial vendors.

Numerous other efforts to develop a well-accepted automated anesthesia record system have been undertaken. Each has added the understanding of the technical and human factors likely to ensure success.

Some researchers have preferred to work on computer-*assisted* records, namely, selected items, especially vital signs, are entered automatically, while other entries (e.g., drugs and anesthesia care event notes) must be handwritten. One such system development at Emory University since the 1970s (computer-assisted anesthetic record [CARR]), utilized plotter-entered data over the preprinted anesthetic record. Initially printed horizontally (11 in. × 8.5 in.) and then redesigned to print vertically (8.5 in. × 11 in.), the completed record resembled a well-kept and accurate handwritten record. However, as new monitors and technologies came along it was increasingly difficult to "add" their output to the existing format. A touted feature was the ability to finish the record by hand should the computer/plotter "breakdown."[58]

A variation on the concept of partially automated-partially handwritten was the semiautomated anesthesia record keeper (SARC) developed by the Department of Anesthesia at the University of Florida (Gainesville) and the Datascope Corporation (Paramus, NJ). This system used a clipboard-based plotter that cleverly printed from behind the pre-printed page, allowing for handwritten notes to be made on that portion of the form not involved in the printing. One unique feature was that automated vital signs were printed vertically, allowing horizontal written entry of "drugs, events, notes, etc." which were thus time-aligned with the trended data (Fig. 24-6).[59] Both of these semiautomated systems processed data from the primary patient monitor directly to the printed form, without an intervening trend display screen.

A relatively simple system named NAPROS, reported from the Theodor-Kutzer-Ufer Hospital in Mannheim, Germany, used an XT/AT PC, and IBM Proprinter, and software written in the BASIC language. NIBP and anesthetic gas data were automatically entered, and presented in a vertical display. A keyboard was available to enter drugs, events, and comments. The system proved reliable, and was reasonably well accepted.[60] Other users of vertically aligned data, however, have found the vertical data display/time scale difficult to adjust to, especially when reviewing the printed record.[61]

In 1986 a system developed at the University Clinics in Aachen, Germany, was reported.[62] Called

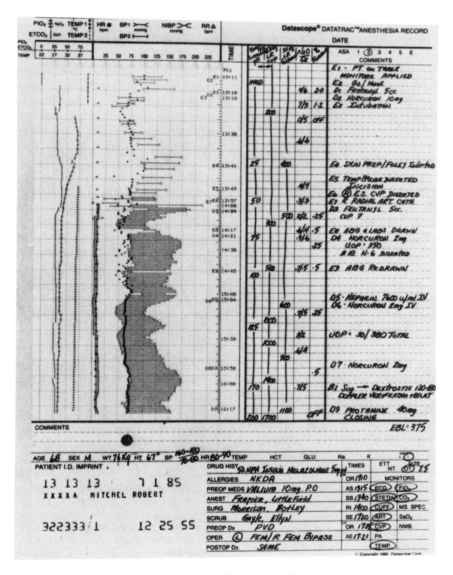

Fig. 24-6. An interesting semiautomated record with vertical display of trends, permitting horizontal written annotation, time-aligned with the trends. (From Paulus, et al.,[59] with permission.)

the Anesthesia Information System (AIS), it ran on the TSX-Plus operating system (S + H Computer Systems, Inc), which emulates a DEC RT-11. The AIS software was written in Pascal 2 (Oregon Software, Inc.), and an anesthesia decision support system used the PROLOG (PROgramming in LOGic) language (Interface GmbH, Munich). The only user interface/data entry method was a high resolution touch screen. Monitor format was standardized. Reported to be fairly easy to learn by "playing with the system," overall acceptance appears to have been good. The primary reasons for the positive acceptance were felt to be the simplicity of data entry (viz., touch screen) and the high quality of the paper printout. The system also included a SIMULATOR configuration for training purposes.[62]

The importance of accurate documentation in clinical situations has spurred the development of several systems. A system used during investigations of the cardiovascular effects of certain drugs consisted of an Apple II microcomputer, and a key board/light pen as the means of manual data entry.[63] An elaborate system has been assembled at the University of Washington to enable investigators to gather both digital and analog waveform data in a study correlating neuropsychological outcome with intraoperative EEG changes during cardiopulmonary bypass. Simpler and relatively slowly changing data (e.g., patient demographics, time, MAP, temperatures, stage of operation, etc.) were handled by a Commodore VIC-20 microcomputer. Analog arterial blood pressure waveforms and two channels of EEG were saved onto an 8-channel instrumentation tape system (HP 3968A). Such a system permitted the multiplexing of several digital and analog data sources on a single magnetic tape for later sophisticated manipulations (Fourier transformation, aperiodic analysis, etc.).[64] Another system designed for clinical research is capable of sequentially capturing data from up to 24 monitors utilizing an IBM AT compatible system running at 10 MHz, with only 640 k of random access memory (RAM) and a 20-MB hard disk. It incorporates 16 analog-to-digital channels and 8 serial communication ports. Waveform data are saved at 125 Hz, sufficient to capture most of the features of the EKG and arterial pressure waveforms. This system does not generate an anesthetic record, but has been used to study the acquisition of data in a variety of types of surgical cases.[65]

THE COMMERCIAL APPROACH TO AUTOMATED ANESTHESIA INFORMATION MANAGEMENT

A number of commercial products are marketed as anesthesia information management systems. Rather than exhaustively cover each system I am aware of, and possibly miss some newer entries into the market, four systems are presented in Table 24-3 with general comments and concerns offered for consideration in the text below. [The author has been a clinical consultant for Modular Instruments (LifeLog).] The operating room components of these systems are pictured as follows: LifeLog (Fig. 24-7), Arkive (Fig. 24-8), AIM (Fig. 24-9), and IdaCare (Fig. 24-10).

All such systems can be thought of as having two basic components: (1) the intraoperative record-keeper, and (2) the networked storage/retrieval data → information system. The clinical anesthesiologist tends to be most interested in the functions of the former. Department chairs, hospital, government and insurance administrators, and computer network specialists tend to be more interested in the latter. In addition, the intraoperative portion of the system is being developed from three perspectives: (1) as interdependent modular components, (2) as an integrated part of the primary anesthesia machine, and (3) as part of the primary patient monitoring system.

Operating System

Commercial systems span the gamut of current operating systems. Systems are available that are written for DOS, Apple/Macintosh, and IBM-OS/2.

Newer versions of MS-DOS, with continued downward compatibility, have evolved over the last decade or so, as newer Bus strategies (e.g., 80386 chips) have permitted 32-bit communications (e.g., extended ISA [EISA]).

---

*MS-DOS (Microsoft-Disk Operating System) was developed in 1981 to support a new 16-bit (the "width" of the data path, analogous to the number of lanes on a highway) microcomputer ISA (*I*ndustry *S*tandard *A*rchitecture) Bus system based upon "8088" chips and was downward-compatible with the older 8-bit format. (The Bus is the "nervous system" or "information highway" of a computer, carrying all communication signals through the system.)

Significant problems, however, still remain with MS-DOS for demanding computer activities. For example, MS-DOS based systems have historically had difficulty with higher-level graphics and user interface support, peripheral device support, internal data sharing, windowing, memory support, and multitasking (i.e., concurrent running of programs).[66] Newer versions of MS-DOS have an improved graphics "shell," expanded and extended memory support (necessary because of DOS limitations in the size of random access memory [RAM]), better text editing, better directory manipulation tools, permit better "undo" features, and employ much better HELP material. Various enhancements have also improved memory management, and the allocation of memory to function as RAM. Multitasking, however, can only be approximated. For example, TSR (Terminate and Stay Resident) functions allow one program to briefly "freeze" while another function is performed; a "heartbeat" interrupt permits the exiting of a foreground program so a background task can be performed—neither are truly concurrent activities. Other add-on capabilities can permit simulated multitasking via a "carousel" like process, that is, one can switch between programs, but only one actually runs at a time.

File management and data sharing have been troublesome features of the MS-DOS operating system that have been greatly improved by add-on

TABLE 24-3. Characteristics of AIMS[a]

Operating System	LifeLog[b] OS/2 2.1 (C++)	IdaCare[c] Macintosh 7.1	AIM[d] DOS (C-C++) (proprietary)	Arkive[e] DMTDOS (C) (proprietary)
CPU	80486/33/32 Bit RAM 10MB 3.5 Floppy 80 MB HD (Or user's own system)	Motorola 68040/25/32 Bit RAM 8 MB 3.5 Floppy 80 MB HD	80386/20/32 Bit RAM 4 MB 3.5 Floppy 80 MB HD	80386/33/32 Bit RAM 1MB 3.5 Floppy 40 MB HD
Data acquisition	Baud 300-19.2K Save = 10 s; 60 or 90 s medians Display/Print = 10 s; 60 or 120 s medians of 10 s	Baud 300-57K Print = resolution set locally	"RAW" = q 15 s Display = .25-20 min Print = 1,2.5,5,10,20 min	Baud 56–56K Display 1–30 min Print 1–30 min
Analog conversion	Yes	No	Yes	Yes
Analog waveform reconstruction	Yes	No	No	No
Annotative input	Touch Screen; i.e., Resistive Membrane Mouse Keyboard	Mouse Keyboard "Voice" ± Touchscreen	Trackball Keyboard	Pad of Fixed Keys Touch Screen Key Pad
UPS	Yes	Yes	Yes	Yes
Screen	Color SVGA 14-in. Touch 1024/768	14-in. Color 640/480	14-in. Color 640/480	6 × 7.5 Plasma Touch Arm Mounted 640/400
Network	Ethernet	Ethernet	Ethernet	Ethernet
Backentry/audit trail	Yes/Yes	Yes/Yes	Yes/Yes	Yes
Restart	Yes	Yes	Yes	Yes
Backup interval	q *x* min; rewrite	q 10 s update	≥ 15 s	q 2 min rewrite

[a]This is not an inclusive list of AIMS vendors, but along with the discussion in the text, illustrates important system level issues. (Data up-to-date for mid-1993.)
[b]Modular Instruments, Inc., 81 Great Valley Pkwy, Malvern, PA 19355.
[c]PAS, 1100 Ashwood Pkwy, Atlanta, GA 30338.
[d]CIS, 738 Airport Blvd., Ann Arbor, MI 48108.
[e]Diatek, 5720 Oberlin Dr., San Diego, CA 92121.

vendors and by later editions of DOS. Data transfer is facilitated by programs that operate in both text and APA (*All Points Addressable*) graphics modes; MS-DOS is designed to move text (ASCII) files around. This becomes an issue as graphics and video memory are manipulated, and would become of concern if graphics images (e.g., x-rays, ECG tracings, scans) were imported into an AIMS screen. Various enhancements can be utilized to get around this limitation, but the limitation remains.

The "Windows" approach to enhancing MS-DOS permits "cooperative" (executing programs *request their own operating time* from the central pro-

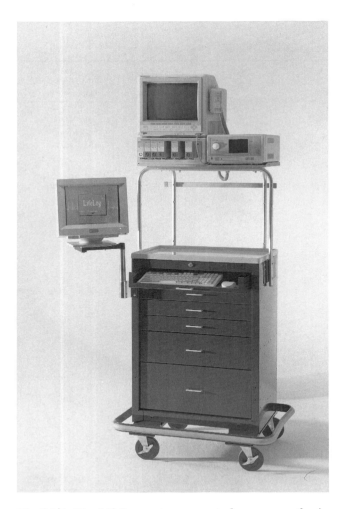

Fig. 24-7. The LifeLog system mounted on an anesthesia cart. Both pole mounted and user's-own-computer configurations are available. (Courtesy of Modular Instruments, Inc., Malvern, PA.)

cessing unit [CPU]) "multitasking" both of programs written specifically to run in Windows, as well as MS-DOS programs. Utilizing the advantages of a graphical user interface (GUI), with icons, buttons, and so on. Windows incorporates superior file manipulation characteristics and strengthens data-sharing functions. But largely because of the limitations of DOS, neither DOS nor Windows may be appropriate in an integrated hospital information management system.[67]

OS/2, however, is a conceptually and structurally a different system. It specifically supports multitasking via a "*preemptive*" process, that is, programs share the CPU during a timeslice dictated by the OS/2 operating system. By the use of "threads" to multitask its own internal functions, simultaneous activities are further enabled. OS/2 provides greater flexibility in data sharing through software written specifically to enhance this function. Utilizing "clipboards" (i.e., background notepads) both text and graphic (or APA) material can be transferred and integrated into other applications. Utilizing Dynamic Data Exchange (DDE), material that is updated in one application, is simultaneously updated at other relevant sites. As a full 32-bit operating system, OS/2 currently addresses up to 4 gigabytes of RAM, or "virtual" memory, using programs as large as 512 MB. Memory, file, and database management capabilities, graphical user interface, and networking capacity suggest an operating system with considerable potential to adapt to hardware and software innovations.

The Apple/Macintosh 32-bit system also handles real and virtual memory requirements well and has excellent graphical user interface and file management capabilities. Apple/Macintosh systems also have excellent networking abilities and permit dynamic data exchange of linked "editions" across programs and networks. The Multifinder multitasking capabilities of System 7 allows programs that are open but not active (i.e., working) to exist in a state of suspended animation; some background applications may actually be able to operate if they can function during intervals (fraction of a second) when the active program is not using the computer.[68] This issue would be important if an AIMS were ever called upon to perform a number of functions or operate a separate program (e.g., a word processor) while primary data collection was continuing in the background. Whereas IBM/Microsoft software/hardware tended to be "open," thereby encouraging expansion of both its software and hardware base, Apple/Macintosh has only recently strayed from its fairly "closed," stifling approach to direct system emulation.

Systems developed in Unix or Windows NT would also be expected to incorporate features that would permit adaptability to hardware and software integration and innovation.

This discussion of operating systems was meant to serve only as a caution that the underlying system supporting an AIMS will have far-reaching effects on the direction the system will be able to take over time. While there are good references for the uninitiated,[69] departments without inhouse computer/network expertise may well wish seek independent and unbiased consultation.

The Central Processing Unit

In many ways, the CPUs (the microprocessor chip [e.g., 80386, 80486] and memory) of the various systems are nearly identical. RAM, speed, bit transfer rate, and HD size are comparable. Many users will value flexibility when it comes to choosing this portion of their system.

Data Acquisition: Digital and Analog

Automated systems acquire monitored vital signs data automatically—by definition. This occurs over cabling from data outputs, usually on the back of newer primary patient monitors. These cables incorporate specific connectors adhering to interna-

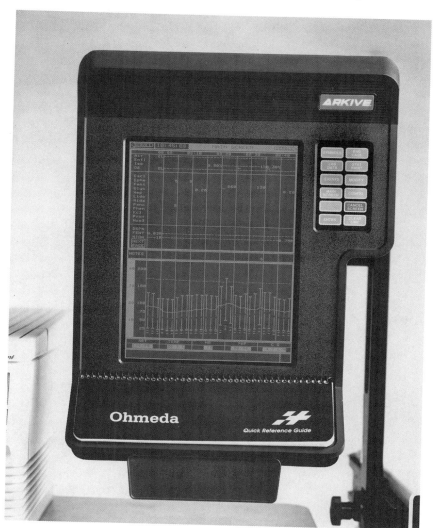

Fig. 24-8. The Arkive intraoperative panel touch monochrome screen with key pad. (Courtesy of Ohmeda, Madison, WI.)

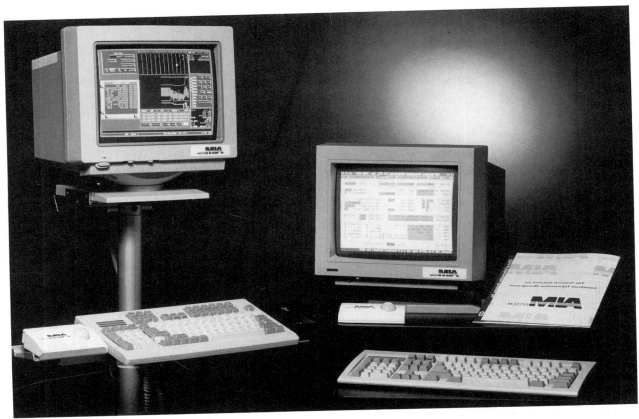

Fig. 24-9. Intraoperative and network workstations for the AIM system. (Courtesy of CIS, Ann Arbor, MI.)

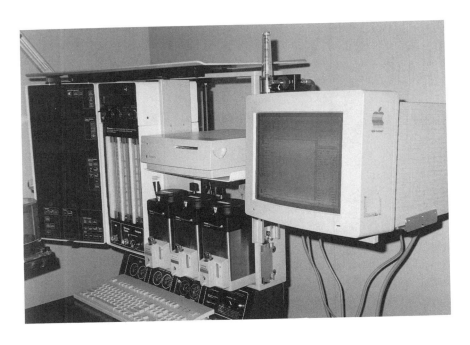

Fig. 24-10. Intraoperative components of the IdaCare system. (Courtesy of PAS, Atlanta, GA.)

tional data transfer standards, such as EIA-RS 232* and EIA-RS 422. Each pin on these connectors is reserved for a specific function—some for data transfer. Most primary monitors provide digital data (discrete numeric values represented by binary patterns of 0's and 1's) for processing by computers, since computers operate with binary digital data. Some provide both digital and analog, and some only analog outputs (i.e., voltage, varying continuously within a range of values).

To say that data is captured at a frequency that is faster than the output of the primary monitor may lead to confusion as to what is actually occurring. Before outputting digital data, the primary monitor gathers data as an analog signal, runs it through an analog to digital converter, and processes it. Some monitors "dump" their digital data episodically, usually every "x" (some multiple) seconds, but it can be continuous. Other monitors must be queried for their data—that is, the AIMS must request data form the primary monitor, again at some interval, for example, every 10 seconds. Data is "dumped" or transferred at a specific baud rate. A baud is a number of events or signal changes per second: for example, 2,400 baud (at 4 bits per event) is 9,600 bps (bits per second). Between "dumps," no data transmission occurs at all. A receiving monitor such as an AIMS unit captures this data via a protocol or "handshake" with the primary monitor that is configured when the two components are initially linked: for example, a noninvasive blood pressure machine transmitting at 600 baud and the AIMS receiving at 600 baud. The signal from a different device might transfer at 1200 baud, or 300, etc. There is then a rate at which data is transferred between monitors, and a frequency with which the automated anesthesia system actually stores a portion of that data.

When analog data is presented to an AIMS system, the AIMS system itself must convert it to digital format for processing and display on the AIMS monitor screen. Characteristics of the ADC (analog to digital computer) determine the quality of the data it passes along. The higher its resolving capacity or sampling rate, the more closely the digital numbers can be made to resemble the original analog signal. This is governed by the Nyquist prin-

ciple, which states that the sampling frequency should be at least twice the highest frequency component of the waveform being studied to permit reconstruction of a reasonable facsimile of that waveform.[70] In addition, it is also necessary to accurately represent the amplitudes of sampled analog waveforms, in a binary form; using a specified number of bits, the signal resolution can be determined. For example, if a dynamic range of 10 V (-5 V to $+5$ V) must be represented, for example, by 8 bits, the signal resolution is $1/(2^8 - 1)$ or 1.255 (0.39 percent) of 10 V, which equals 39 mV.

Meaningful digitalization of an analog signal, then, requires both an adequate sampling rate and the proper digital or binary representation of the signal amplitude. Some may ask whey this should be important for the clinical anesthesiologist: just use primary monitors that will provide digital data. But as familiarity with automation grows, various users may wish to periodically view the analog "facsimile" that can be reproduced from the digital data to document that the data has been properly sampled, or to save such waveforms for medicolegal, documentation, or research purposes. For this reason, evaluators of AIMS technology should require that the conversion of analog data is handled well.

The passive acquisition of data by AIMS is made more complex by the lack of an international standard for consistently patterned transmission of data from one device (e.g., primary monitor) to another (i.e., the AIMS). When the Medical Information Bus is finally agreed upon,[71,72] this process will be greatly facilitated. The IEEE P1073 Medical Information Bus Committee is proposing a standard for the bidirectional interconnection of medical devices and computers. P1073 is a family of standards for device communications based upon Open Systems Interconnection Basic Reference Model (OSI/RM) of the International Standards Organization (ISO).

Annotation Entry and Video Screen

The entry of data into the operating room components of an automated system has become one of the more vocal issues of AIMS technology. Most workers consider written notes as the most user-friendly, easiest to learn, and least time-consuming method of entering data; it is a "technology" perfected over thousands of years. Yet at some point

---

*Electronic industries Association-Recommended Standard. A number have been issued over the years, each with a specific number.

in the not too distant future, reasonably error-free—that is, high first-try recognition—pen-based computer recognition of free-text entries should become a practical reality, certainly the technology is under intense development.[73] Likewise, acceptably error-free voice recognition of standardized and free-text data will also play an essential role in the automated entry of anesthesia data items.[74] Unquestionably, voice entry will enable a level of annotation accuracy during the performance of sterile procedures and other preoccupied tasks that has heretofore been unlikely, if not impossible. This technology is developing and improving at a measurable pace.[75]

For the time being, the practical modes of data entry are three: touch screen, keyboard, and mouse/trackball. Touch screen and mouse/trackball provide an excellent means of selecting items from lists, and a keyboard is essential for entering free-text explanations that would be impossible from prepared lists. Each of these methods of data entry requires some adjustment of practice habits, especially for those who have limited to nonexistent computer experience. In addition, these data entry devices are at some risk of contamination from fluids and blood products—innovative modes for protecting them are available. The time spent entering data via these methods has not been well documented, but there is evidence that not only is time saved, but the superior quality of the recorded information has been noted.[76]

Others have attempted to use barcodes for the entry of drugs and events but found it cumbersome.[57] As part of a point-of-care system to document utilization of supplies, employing more recently developed technology, this may be more effective and practical.

General Issues

An increasing number of our monitors have short-term batteries, especially those used for transport purposes. Since operating rooms are on emergency power systems, why should an anesthesia record keeping system have its own battery? Primarily because record-keeping-system devices can become unplugged by feet, x-ray machines, and "helpful" assistants, and so on. And because emergency power systems may not activate immediately—at least data from those primary monitors with a battery will continue to be captured.

While all AIMS must be networked for optimal function, they must also work well in a stand-alone capacity. Networks will have predictably unpredictable dysfunctions, and it may take some time to sort things out; the system must "fall back" to its local hard disk seamlessly. In addition, it may be necessary to utilize an AIMS in an area that is not networked. Again, transferring patient data to the AIMS through the use of a "floppy disk sneaker-net" is essential. Backup of data, both to the local hard disk, and to the network, should be done with a frequency consistent with local (no national standards) interests, so that relatively insignificant amounts of data are lost in the event of a problem with a system.

Cases can end, and then unfortunately need to be resumed before the patient leaves the room; it is not really appropriate to start a new procedure—but to resume the original—done easily with another sheet of paper on the written record. This also must be done well with a computerized record.

While monitored data is automatically acquired, drug and annotative entries must still be individually entered. Even with an automated system, there will be many times when this must be done later and not simultaneously with an event. Such "batch-recorded" entries are entirely transparent in a written and must be permitted in an automated system. Changing data has always been a problem, since it can be argued to imply dishonest record-keeping. Yet errors are made, and time honored methods to change written data do exist. In an automated record, changes should be tracked using an "Audit Trail," both by timing and by the name of the person making the changes.

Printing of the intraoperative record is another area in which the systems are not too different. Laser printed records are certainly more elegant, but it may be desirable to have a dot matrix printer for draft or demonstration copies. Some institutions will want a printer available to each operating room, while others may be content to have them in the recovery area. Obviously printer quantity and networking must be up to the tasks demanded Figure 24-11 shows representative pages from an automated system.

Database Issues

The vendors of AIMS technology will need to develop their own preoperative and postoperative databases structures, or, where appropriate, accommodate those computerized systems already in place—these need not be mutually exclusive. Some departments will have in addition, a portion of the preoperative workup that is completed directly by the patient,[77,78] and this will need to be assimilated by the AIMS. An increasing number of departments will want to incorporate point-of-care (i.e., per patient, as it is used) tracking of anesthesia equipment, pharmaceuticals, and monitor use. However, ready implementation of this process is

---

ANESTHESIA RECORD
Johns Hopkins Hospital

Mi^2

Last Name: _____
First Name: _____
Middle Name: _____
Patient No: _____   Admission #: _____

ASA: 1 2 3 *4* 5 E   Height: 152.4 cm   60 in
                                Weight: 59.4 kg   131 lbs
  OR: 11
Site: GOR   Sex: F   DOB: 04/14/1932

Proc Date: Jul 30, 1993   Age: 61 yr ___ mo ___ day

                                                    Page 1 of 4

DIAGNOSIS:
    433.1 Occlusion/stenosis of carotid artery: LEFT
    434 Cerebral thrombosis: RECENT, IMPROVING, RIGHT SYMPTOMS

ANESTHESIOLOGISTS: SIGNATURES:
MERRITT, WILLIAM   00:00   _____
                                _____
                                _____
PROCEDURE: _____
    35301 Thromboendarterectomy, carotid artery: LEFT

SURGEONS:
                                _____
                                _____
                                _____

PRE-OPERATIVE
[■] Machine Checkout
[■] Patient to OR from: Ward
[■] Chart Reviewed
[■] Issues Discussed
[ ] Patient Condition
      Precluded Discussion

ANESTHESIA / METHODS USED
[■] General
[ ]   Change from Loc
[ ]   Change from Reg
[ ] Monitored Anes Care
[ ] Surg; Loc. Monitored
[ ] Obstetric
[ ] Diagnostic/Ther. Pain
[ ] Regional
[ ] Nerve Block
[ ] SA Block
[ ] Epid / Caud
[ ] Continuous
[ ]   Injects:
[ ]   Visits:
[ ]   Pump Used:
[ ] Cath Out Intact
[ ] Axial Narcotics Used
[ ] Hypotensive Anesthesia
[ ] Hypothermia

EQUIPMENT USED
[■] NIBP
[ ] BP Manual
[ ] Pulse Ox
[ ] ETCO2
[ ] ETCO2/Agent/N2/O2
[ ] Chest Steth
[■] Esoph Steth
[■] Temp: O
[■] EKG: 5
[■] In/Exp/O2
[■] NMB
[ ] RIS
[ ] Level One
[ ] Blood Warmer
[ ] Blanket Warmer
[ ] Warming Lights
[ ] Passive Humid
[■] Active Humid
[ ] Doppler

                     Ins/Mon
[ ] ICP
[■] CVP   X   X
[■] ALin   X   X
[ ] PA
[ ] Evok Poten   ___ ___
[ ] Pacing   ___ ___
[ ] Echo   ___ ___
[ ] _____
[ ] _____
[ ] _____

AIRWAY / VENTILATION
[■] Mask
[ ] Airway
[■] Oral
[ ] Nasal
[■] LScope: Miller 2
[ ] FO Intubation
[ ]   Oral Intubation
[ ]   Nasal Intubation
[ ] ETT
[ ]   DLETT
          Size: 7.5
          Secure at _____ cm
          Leak at _____
[ ] Awake
[ ] Rapid Sequence
[■] Attempts: 1
[■] BS=B
[ ] Difficult
[ ] Emer Trach/Cricothy
[ ] Siemens Vent
[■] Circuit
[■]   Circle
[ ]   Ped Circle
[ ]   Map D

PRE-OP MEDICATIONS
_____
_____
_____
_____

PROCEDURE TIMES
Scheduled Start   10:15
Anes Start   10:37
Patient in OR   10:37
Anes Ready   11:23
Surgeon Start   11:24
Surgeon Finish   12:45
Patient Leaves OR 13:00
Anes Finish   13:02
Scheduled Finish   12:15
Total Time   02:25
Attend. Anes Covering: 1 Rooms

PATIENT DISPOSITION
[■] Patient Transferred
        to: SICU   at 13:00

[ ] Spont Vent
[ ] Controlled Vent, O2
[■] FM O2
[■] EKG Monitor
[■] ART Monitor
[ ] O2 SAT Monitor
[ ] Patient Died in OR
[ ] Cancelled: _____

POST OP
[ ] BP: _____
[ ] Pulse: _____
[ ] Resp: _____
[ ] SAT: _____
[ ] Temp: _____

CASE SUMMARY:
    TRANSFERRED FROM DOCTOR'S HOSP AFTER MINI-STROKE AND IMPROVEMENT ON HEPARIN DRIP. HERE HAS HAD DOBUT/STRESS TEST = NEG; POOR VERTEBRAL FLOW; STRENGTH HAS IMPROVED, BUT STILL WITH SOME FINE MOTOR CHANGES, ? SPEECH CHANGES, AND SL. DIFF READING. BP TODAY 137/71 ON RT AND 108/62 ON LT.
    AWOKE READILY, AND EXTUBATED.

A

Modular Instruments Incorporated

Fig. 24-11. Representative printout from a commercial AIMS. Pages 1, 2, and 3 of an anesthetic for a 61-year-old female for a carotid endarterectomy. (**A**) Demographic, billing and case summary items. (**B**) Laboratory values and totals of drugs administered and losses measured. (**C**) The invasive arterial pressure, ECG and temperature trends (Marquette 7010), Rascal respiratory gas measurements, Nellcor SAT and HR. (Records generated by LifeLog (Modular Instruments, Inc, Malvern, PA, and an HP LaserJet IIP.) (*Figure continues.*)

complicated by the lack of a universal system for identifying medical supplies and equipment. Barcodes, which have enjoyed nearly universal success in the food industry, are being increasingly adapted to medical uses. The Health Industry Business Communications Council (HIBCC)* is promulgating a standard for medical industry barcoding, and in collaboration with IMS America's Health Care Division, is developing a Common Category Database† of medical industry equipment and supplies. Once this sort of equipment tracking becomes a universal practice, local development of barcode schemes will not be necessary. The physi-

---

*Address: 5110 North 40th Street, Suite 250, Phoenix, AZ 85018; (602)381-1091.

†IMS America, 660 W. Germantown Pike, Plymouth Meeting, PA 19462-0905; (215)834-5000.

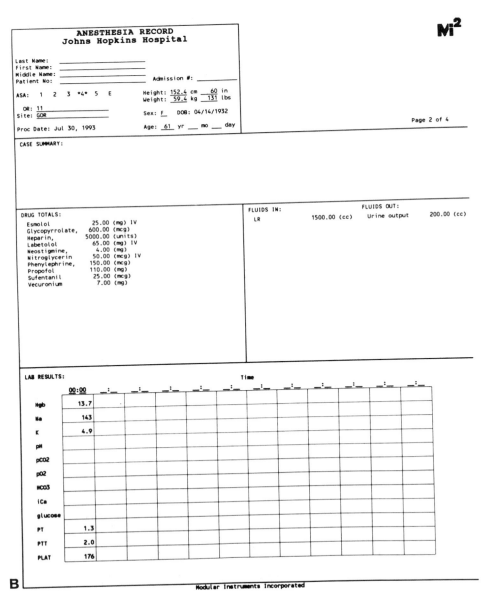

Fig. 24-11. (*Continued*)

cal location of the AIMS intraoperative unit suggests it as a logical site of entry of such data.

What Concerns Have Arisen Over the Automated Record

Cerebralization of Data

Automation of the anesthesia record separates the caregiver from the original "raw" data present on primary patient monitors. Many have expressed concerns that without the "oculocerebromanual" loop in the recording of data, effective cerebralization of patient data will not occur, or will occur in a manner not equal to current expectation. There is evidence, however, that vigilance is not affected by automation[53] and that the record of care is far superior, especially during the induction and emergence from anesthesia.[76,79,80]

What is ignored in these arguments are the data trends presented for view on some of the systems

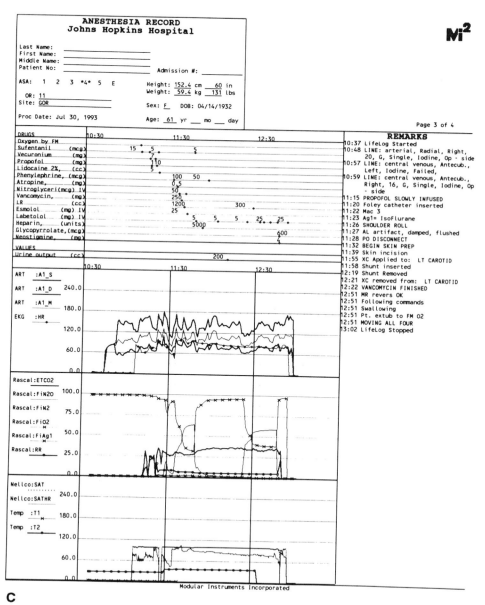

C

Fig. 24-11. (*Continued*)

currently available. Such data presentation should greatly enhance the practitioner's ability to deliver timely and effective clinical care. As systems progress into areas of "smart monitoring,"[81] for example, rate of change data,[82] recognition and alerting for abnormal values, intelligent alarms,[83] and analysis of trends, additional improvements in both our awareness and understanding of clinical events should occur. We have learned to adapt to a host of newly automated physiologic parameters in recent years—it is predictable that we will adapt and benefit from the nature of data presentation inherent in automated systems—albeit an untested hypothesis.

Artifact

This is a genuine phenomenon of medical measurement activities. By one means or another, some of the monitored values displayed as representing physiologic events are not accurate. To name a few sources, artifacts can arise from electrical interference, errors due to improper calibration, zeroing and leveling, and the mechanical effects of body motion, blood-drawing, and even the process of calibration, zeroing and leveling, and so on. There are several shades of meaning for the concept of artifact; all include an artificial quality of varied cause.

> **ar·ti·fact** - 1. a product . . . of artificial character due to extraneous (as human) agency [Webster's 9th New Collegiate Dictionary, 1990, Miriam-Webster, Inc, Springfield, MA]; 2. any artificial product; any structure or feature that is not natural, but has been altered by processing [Dorland's Illustrated Medical Dictionary, 24th Ed. WB Saunders, Philadelphia, 1965]; 3. an artificial or extraneous feature accidentally or unavoidably introduced into an object of observation and which may simulate a natural or relevant feature of that object. [Blakiston's Pocket Medical Dictionary, 4th Ed. McGraw-Hill, New York, 1980.]

Unfortunately, the term also seems to be a catch-all word for just about anything the anesthesiologist would rather not see either on the intraoperative monitor screen or on the printed record: for example, the physiologic swings seen during everyday clinical care. Since automated systems in general take data from primary patient monitors as it is displayed, artifact, if it is present, will come across to the record-keeping system. The AIMS can display and print the artifact, utilize a software algorithm or mathematical operation (e.g., median,

mean, etc.) to remove or obscure the artifact, or select the most likely "true" value from a predetermined hierarchy of similar redundant values, for example, one heart rate from several different sources. Regardless of the method chosen, artifact is a fact of life. Having it represented in the record-keeping system permits the reconstruction of the course of the anesthetic as it really happened, thereby reproducing the complexity of the tasks of observing, selecting data, and reacting. Artifactual data then, in my opinion, should not be deleted from the memory of a record-keeping system, but should remain available for review. The focus of artifact processing should lie with primary monitors.

Since much artifact is nonphysiologic, is should lead to little confusion when critically reviewing the course of an anesthetic. There can be times, however, when data are presented that is not distinctly nonphysiologic, for example, the pulse oximeter that has slipped from a proper position and reads a low saturation. A clinical event such as a low saturation leads to a search for the cause, mechanical vs physiologic, and a solution or a therapeutic intervention. Documentation is provided both by the improved values of the saturation and/or an explanatory note. This sort of occurrence should not be hidden, for it distinctly chronicles the perplexing events that frequently challenge the clinical anesthesiologist. In this light, some would argue that computer-captured artifact actually represents a signature of automation and as such represents a unique aspect of the record of our care.

To those who regard the written record as a "gold standard," it can be reasonably argued that handwritten anesthetic records are almost entirely artifactual,[38] largely due to both "smoothing"[41] and "batch-recording."[6] The record is an artifact of the "processor" who records the data. This fact is not lost on plaintiff's lawyers.[39]

Ease of Data Entry

Until the computerized entry of event-type data is at least as straightforward as is handwritten entry, many will not be impressed or satisfied. As mentioned above, systems available today permit annotative entries via keyboard, touch screen, mouse/trackball, and voice means. Some of these methods are more effective than others at varying periods during a surgical procedure. Each of these methods of data entry does require some practice and some users will prefer one mode over another. Whether any one method of data entry will supplant all other modes will depend upon issues such as ease of use and accuracy, and is yet to be decided. It is reasonable to assume that most users will prefer multiple methods of data entry as convenient alternatives to be used when appropriate.

User Acceptance

Computerization of business and medicine has been underway for some time; since the business community has traveled farther along this road than most clinical care settings, the medical world has much to learn from the corporate experience. One of the pitfalls of instituting an automated information system of any variety is the level of user support. It is quite clear that a high level of discontent will almost certainly compromise, if not derail, the efforts. Systems must "(1) meet the needs of projected users, (2) [be] . . . convenient and easy to use, and (3) fit the work patterns of the professionals for whom it is intended."[84] In short, overcoming such context sensitivity issues requires an understanding of the users' perceptions of whether the proposed system supports or interferes with the performance of their jobs as they define them. Grass-roots-level feasibility preparation helps to define the concerns of users and is complemented by post implementation evaluation. Some systems that are technically quite sound may only succeed when sufficient personnel turnover has weeded out those who disagree!

The federal government is intensely pushing the use of computers to assist in the measurement of quality, efficiency, and costs of patient care.[85] Some users may feel that data derived from a computerized system are desired largely for its potential to reveal patterns of care that will be dealt with in a punitive fashion. Since objective data make it easier to evaluate issues of practice, some aspects of detecting substandard anesthetic care may be made simpler. The process of care review and quality improvement is now part of the fabric of medical care in the United States, and it is important for anesthesiologists to take an active role in its maturation.

Costs

Computerization of the hospital environment has direct and indirect costs which at first can appear to be staggering. Few controlled data exist to demonstrate that these costs yield savings, but information is beginning to appear. In a randomized controlled clinical trial on an inpatient medical service, use of computerized order writing with various reminders of recent similar orders or tests has been shown to yield a savings of almost $900 per admission over controls using a paper order system, and to shorten the mean length of hospital stay by 0.89 days. The down side was an extra "5.5 minutes per patient" (during a 10-hour observation period) of data entry in the study group! Most would accept this small perturbation of practice to save "more than $3 million annually."[86] The costs of a nursing diagnosis QA audit program has been reduced by nearly 400-fold—from $82.50 per patient record, to $0.21—due to computerization of the screening process![87]

Anesthesia Information Management

Computerization of our record-keeping has been driven by the same goals as earlier efforts to incorporate preoperative and postoperative data with our intraoperative charts: better documentation, and a need to peer into the process and outcome of anesthesia to understand events and improve care. A prodigious amount of data is generated when automation assists in the organization of preoperative and postoperative data collection and the generation of an anesthetic record. But raw data reveals little about patterns of care, or the use of drugs and supplies, costs outcomes, and so on. Automated systems are being developed from the ground up employing an "object-oriented" structure, with the intent that large databases can be created and examined using tools (e.g., Structured Query Language [SQL]) that open up the database to interactive exploration. Many will utilize the relational database model. However, multidimensional databases may eventually offer a superior means to on-line transaction processing.[88] As the practice of anesthesia is examined using these recently described modalities, numerous areas of our care and working environment will be probed for insights into improving care, saving money, and fostering more efficiency. Listed in Table 24-4 are some expandable topics of potential interest to anesthesiologists that must be examined from both a local and national point of view (e.g., JCAHO, PRO). Such information is the sine qua non of an AIMS, and potential users must be certain that they

TABLE 24-4. Issues of Interest in an Anesthesia Database

Clinical
    Age/sex/ASA status
    Preoperative medical/surgical history (ICD-9)
    Preoperative medications/allergies
    Physical examination
    Laboratory/imaging evaluations
    Known anesthetic issues
    Surgeon
    Anesthesiologist
    Surgical procedure (CPT)
    Anesthesia drugs
    Monitoring/equipment
    Anesthesia/surgical events
    Early/late postoperative outcomes
Administrative
    Operating room scheduling
    Operating room efficiency
    Inventory management
    Communications

will reap the potential of the technology they are purchasing and/or developing.

Anesthesia workstations should be able to engage in "seamless" communication with other sources of useful patient data. Via a process known as "terminal emulation," information from differing computer systems and such disparate settings as laboratories (results for hematology, chemistry, microbiology, etc.), electrocardiography, and radiology (ECG results or tracings, standard film results or view, scan results or view, etc.), will become accessible at the AAIM workstation (i.e., both at the operating room and departmental level). In addition, the anesthesia system must be accessible from ward and outpatient area patient information management (PIM) workstations. Many of the standards for the computer links that make this possible, such as the HL-7 and similar standards, have been evolving for quite some time (Table 24-5). They will allow accurate and timely communication between various areas within the hospital, especially clinical laboratories, and the care provider.

In addition, proper communication between a hospital or practitioner patient data system and a subspecialty system such as the anesthesiologist's, requires a commonality of concepts, terminology, and definitions. Such requirements have influenced the multiple efforts at developing comprehensive PIMS. At the current time an effort is underway to establish a Unified Medical Language System (UMLS), which will incorporate concepts and terminology from multiple established medical databases. The Metathesaurus has been developed as part of this effort (Table 24-6). Standardization terminology and definitions for other clinical activities, for example, the physical examination, is also essential for proper interphysician communications. Even within anesthesiology there is a subcommittee of the Society of Technology for Anesthesia whose responsibility it is to standardize the nature of the anesthesia database. Also, there are

TABLE 24-5. Intersystem Communication Standards

HL-7	Health Level Seven communication protocol of the ISO
TCP/IP	Department of Defense protocols for interlinking dissimilar computers
Euclides-	European standard for clinical laboratory data exchange; collaborating with ASTM 1238
H.PR.I.M.-	French Laboratory consortium using ASTM 1238 communication standard
MEDIX P1157-	IEEE standard, similar to HL-7, to be compliant with ISO specifications
IEEE P1073-	Medical Information Bus (MIB) for standardization of communication between OR and ICU monitors and instruments
ASTM E1238-	Standard for transferring clinical laboratory data
ASTM E1239-	Standard for admission/discharge/transfer for PIMS
ASTM Committees	
ASTM E31.11-	Committee for Clinical Data Transmission
ASTM E31.12-	Committee for Medical Informatics
ASTM E31.14-	Committee for Laboratory Instruments
ASTM E31.15-	Committee for Medical Knowledge Representation
ASTM E31.16-	Committee for Digital Neurophysiological Data

ASTM, American Society for Testing Materials; ANSI-American National Standards Institute; IEEE, Institute of Electrical and Electronics Engineers; ISO, International Organization for Standardization; PIMS, Patient Information Management Systems; TCP/IP, Transmission Control Protocol/Internet Protocol.
(Adapted from McDonald and Hripcsak,[93] with permission.)

TABLE 24-6. Metathesaurus Meta-1
Numbers of Terms Included from Various Sources

MeSH[R]	195,409	15,510 preferred: 35,307 supplementary
DSM-IIIR	447	267 preferred terms
COSTAR	776	All unique concepts
ICD-9-CM	9,489	2,775 preferred terms
SNOMED	10,301	5,670 preferred terms
CPT	446	166 preferred terms
LCSH	5,106	7,000 preferred terms

MeSH, National Library of Medicine Medical Subject Headings; DSM-IIIR, Diagnostic and Statistical Manual of Medical Disorders, 3rd Ed, COSTAR, ambulatory patient record system of the University of Nebraska; ICD-9-CM, International Classification of Diseases, 9th Ed, *Clinical Modification*; SNOMED, Systematized Nomenclature of Medicine; CPT, Current Procedural Terminology; LCSH, Library of Congress Subject Headings.
(Adapted from Lindberg and Humphreys,[94] with permission.)

efforts to standardize the nomenclature and inventory structure of medical supplies, devices and pharmaceuticals using barcodes, undertaken by the HIBCC. Once such related activities are completed, not only will physicians, hospitals, insurers and industry be able to communicate more effectively, but large-scale national and international clinical studies will be enabled—a dream of physicians for generations.

Recently the Institute of Medicine (IOM) issued a report[89] defining a computer based patient record (CPR). The Computer-Based Patient Record Institute (CPRI) was established in early 1992. Interestingly, the mission of this organization is to "initiate and coordinate urgently needed activities to facilitate and promote the routine use of computer-based patient records throughout health care.[90] In 1992 and 1993 bills were introduced into Congress to address elements of a paperless medical record* and the Department of Health and Human Services has proposed the implementation of computerized patient record systems in hospitals by 1996.[91] Medical students are increasingly exposed to computerization of information resources.[92] This short of activity has major implications for anesthesiologists. It is imperative that we actively participate in the process of defining our needs and concerns about such technology as we automate our own practice.

What started out in the 1960s and 1970s as a desire to automatically record and print the course of an anesthetic as part of a paper patient record, has expanded through sophisticated desktop computer systems to include preoperative history and postoperative outcome and quality assurance data as part of an anesthesia information management system and a computerized patient record. It is quite possible that within the not too distant future we will see the establishment of national standards for data entry and the ability to perform process and outcome, pattern-of-care, and cost-benefit, clinical studies on a national scale.

---

*Senator C. "Kit" Bond (R-MO) introduced S.2878, the Medical and Health Information Reform Act of 1992, defining a clinical data set that hospitals would utilize to electronically streamline quality assurance and utilization review communications with Medicare Peer Review Organizations. Also Representative F. Stark (D-CA) introduced HR-4956, the Health Administration Simplification Act of 1992 which deals with standards of electronic billing. He introduced a similar bill in January 1993.

REFERENCES

1. MacDonald DAC: An anaesthetic record. Can Anaesth Soc J 8:177, 1961
2. Worthley JA, DiSalvo PS: Managing Computers in Health Care: A Guide for Professionals. 2nd Ed. p. 2. Health Administration Press Perspectives, Ann Arbor, MI, 1989
3. Beecher HK: The first anesthesia records (Codman, Cushing). Surg Gynecol Obstet 71:689, 1940
4. Dillon JB: The prevention of claims for malpractice. Anesthesiology 18:794, 1957
5. Bartimus J, Dymer M: Evaluating anesthesia negligence claims. Trial, May:38, 1992
6. Cook RI, McDonald JS, Nunziata E: Differences between handwritten and automatic blood pressure records. Anesthesiology 71:385, 1989
7. Logas WG, McCarthy RJ, Narbone RF et al: Analysis of the accuracy of the anesthetic record. Anesth Analg 66:S107, 1987

8. Thrush DN: Automated anesthesia records are they better? Anesth Analg 72:S296, 1991

9. Yagiela JA, Graef TR, Hooley JR: Computer-assisted validation of observer-recorded data in patients receiving intravenous sedation. Anesth Analg 74:S359, 1992

10. Gravenstein JS: The uses of the anesthesia record. J Clin Monit 5:256, 1989

11. Peters T: Liberation Management-Necessary Disorganization for the Nanosecond Nineties. p. 109. Knopf, New York, 1992

12. Cushing H: On the avoidance of shock in major amputations by cocainization of large nerve-trunks preliminary to their division: with observations on the blood-pressure changes in surgical cases. Ann Surg 36:321, 1902

13. O'Reilly C: Anaesthetic requirements. Can J Med Surg 1:154, 1897

14. Cassidy JC: Anaesthetic requirements. Can J Med Surg 1:176, 1897

15. Goldan SO: Intraspinal cocainization for surgical anesthesia. Phila Med J 6:850, 1900

16. Rogan BB: Remarks on the Administration of anaesthetics, with special reference to the technique of chloroform administration. Trans Med Assoc State Alabama. p. 481, 1901

17. McKesson EI: Nitrous oxide-oxygen anesthesia, with a description of a new apparatus. Surg Gynecol Obstet 13:456, 1911

18. Brown G: Notes on 300 cases of general anaesthesia combined with narcotics. Lancet 1:10056, 1911

19. Ayre P: The anaesthetic record. Br J Anaesth 18:180, 1943

20. Saklad M: A method for the collection and tabulation of anesthesia data. Anesth Analg 19:184, 1940

21. Tovell RM, Dunn HL: Anesthesia study records. Anesth Analg 11:37, 1932

22. Rovenstine EA: A method of combining anesthetic and surgical records for statistical purposes. Anesth Analg 13:122, 1934

23. Nosworthy M: A method of keeping anesthetic records and assessing results. Br J Anaesth 18:160, 1943

24. Pender JW: A combined anesthesia record and statistical card. Anesthesiology 7:606, 1946

25. Nosworthy MD: Anaesthetic record card. Anaesthesia 8:43, 1953

26. Conroy WA: Correspondence on a 8.5 × 11 inch record. Anesthesiology 8:204, 1947

27. Conroy WA, Cassels WH, Stodsky B: The Chicago Keysort anesthesia record. Anesthesiology 9:121, 1948

28. Livingstone HM, Wilner WK, Peters MP, Weygandt GR: A combined Keysort anesthesia and recovery room record. Anesthesiology 11:422, 1950

29. Sadove MS, Levin MJ: The Illinois E-Z Sort anesthesia record card. Anesthesiology 19:178, 1958

30. Saklad M, Gillespie N, Rovenstine EA: Inhalation therapy: a method for the collection and analysis of statistics. Anesthesiology 5:359, 1944

31. Saklad M, Sellman P: Statistical systems in anesthesiology. Anesthesiology 7:146, 1946

32. Ballantine RIW: An Anaesthetic record card for thoracic cases. Anaesthesia 5:44, 1950

33. Wangeman CP: An experiment in the recording of surgical and anesthetic data in military service: the adaptation of Hollerith punch cards, used at Second Army maneuvers, 1940. Anesthesiology 2:179, 1941

34. Wangeman CP, Martin SJ: The recording of surgical and anesthetic data in two army hospitals: the adaptation of Hollerith punch cards, used from July 1, 1941 to December 31, 1943. Anesthesiology 6:64, 1945

35. Crawford OB et al: A comprehensive simple anesthesia record. Anesthesiology 21:557, 1960

36. Campbell JE, Weiss WA, Rieders F: Evaluation of deaths associated with anesthesia: correlation of clinical, toxicologic and pathologic findings, Anesth Anal 40:54, 1961

37. Thrush DN: Automated anesthesia records and anesthetic incidences. J Clin Monit 8:59, 1992

38. Rowe L, Galletly DC, Henderson RS: Accuracy of text entries within a manually compiled anaesthetic record. Br J Anaesth 68:381, 1992

39. Gibbs RF: The present and future medicolegal importance of record keeping in anesthesia and intensive care: the case for automation. J Clin Monit 5:25, 1989

40. Shibutani K, Ogawa T, Oka S et al: Inaccuracy of arterial pressure and heart rate in the anesthesia record: a study of human factors. Anesth Analg 70:S369, 1990

41. Block FE: Normal fluctuation of physiologic cardiovascular variables during anesthesia and the phenomenon of "smoothing." J Clin Monit 7:141, 1991

42. Merritt WT, Zuckerberg AL: Contamination of the anesthetic record. Anesthesiology 77:A1102, 1992

43. Forbes AD, Jimison HB: A QRS detection algorithm. J Clin Monit 3:53, 1987

44. Weinfurt PT: Electrocardiographic monitoring: an overview. J Clin Monit 6:132, 1990

45. Ream AK: Mean blood pressure algorithms. J Clin Monit 1:138, 1985

46. Peura RA: Blood pressure and sound. p. 354. In Webster JG (ed): Medical Instrumentation, Application and Design. 2nd Ed. Houghton Mifflin, Boston, 1992

47. Ellis DM: Interpretation of beat-to-beat blood pressure values in the presence of ventilatory changes. J Clin Monit 1:65, 1985

48. Boquet G, Bushman JA, Davenport HT: The anaesthetic machine: a study of function and design. Br J Anesth 52:61, 1980

49. Drui AB, Behm RJ, Martin WE: Predesign investigation of the anesthesia operational environment. Anesth Analg 52:584, 1973

50. Kennedy PJ, Feingold A, Wiener EL et al: Analysis of tasks and human factors in anesthesia for coronary-artery bypass. Anesth Analg 55:374, 1976

51. McDonald JS, Dzwonczyk RR: A time and motion study of the anaesthetist's intraoperative time. Br J Anaesth 61:738, 1988

52. McDonald JS, Dzwonczyk R, Gupta B et al: A second time-study of the anaesthetist's intraoperative period. Br J Anaesth 64:582, 1990

53. Dzwonczyk R, Allard J, McDonald JS et al: The effect of automatic record keeping on vigilance and record keeping time. Anesth Analg 47:S79, 1992

54. Gravenstein JS, Weinger MB: Why investigate vigilance? [Editorial]. J Clin Monit 2:145, 1986

55. Holland R. Special committee investigating deaths under anesthesia: report on 745 classified cases, 1960–1968. Med J Aust 1:573, 1970

56. Cooper JB, Newbower RS, Kitz RJ: An analysis of major errors and equipment failures in anesthesia management: considerations for prevention and detection. Anesthesiology 60:34, 1984

57. Block FE, Burton LW, Rafal MD et al: Two computer-based anesthetic monitors: the Duke Automatic Monitoring Equipment (DAME) system and the MicroDAME. J Clin Monit 1:30, 1985

58. Frazier WT, Odom SH: Spatial organization of a computer-assisted anesthetic record. p. 67. In Gravenstein JS, Newbower RS, Ream AK, Smith NT (eds): The Automated Anesthesia Record and Alarm Systems. Butterworth, Boston, 1987

59. Paulus DA, van der Aa JJ, Mclaughlin G et al: Semi-automated anesthesia record keeping. p. 151. In Gravenstein JS, Newbower RS, Ream AK, Smith NT (eds): The Automated Anesthesia Record and Alarm Systems. Butterworth, Boston, 1987

60. Osswald PM: Development and practical use of a computerized anaesthesia protocol. p. 67. In Baillière's Clinical Anaesthesiology: Automated Anaesthetic Records, Vol 4. Baillière Tindall, London, 1990

61. Kalli K: Automated anaesthesia documentation: clinical evaluations in Helsinki University Central Hospital. In Baillière's Clinical Anaesthesiology: Automated Anaesthetic Records, Vol. 4. Baillière Tindall, London, 1990

62. Klocke H, Inform D, Trispel S et al: An anesthesia information system for monitoring and record keeping during surgical anesthesia. J Clin Monit 2:246, 1986

63. Prentice JW, Kenny GNC: Microcomputer-based anaesthetic record system. Br J Anaesth 56:1433, 1984

64. Bledsoe SW, Bashein G, Momii ST, Hornbein TF: A data acquisition system for clinical research. J Clin Monit 3:160, 1987

65. Schwid HA, Olson C, Wright P, Freund PR: Microcomputer-based data acquisition for clinical research. J Clin Monit 6:141, 1990

66. Henle RA, Kuvshinoff BW: Focus on MS-DOS. In: Desktop Computers. p. 337. Oxford University Press, New York, 1992

67. Clayton PD, Sideli RV, Sengupta S: Open architecture and integrated information at Columbia-Presbyterian Medical Center. MD Comput 9:297, 1992

68. Poole L: The New Look. Ch 2. In Macworld: Guide to System 7.1. 2nd Ed. IDG Books, CA, 1993

69. Henle RA, Kuvshinoff BW: Desktop Computers. Oxford University Press, New York, 1992

70. Geddes LA, Baker LE: Criteria for the faithful reproduction of an event. Ch. 16. In Principles of Applied Biomedical Instrumentation. Wiley-Interscience, New York, 1989

71. Figler AA, Stead SW: The medical information bus. Biomed Instrum Technol 24:101, 1990

72. Salvador CH, Pulido N, Quiles JA, González MA: Implementation of the IEEE medical information bus standard. IEEE Eng Med Biol June:81, 1993

73. Lewis PH: So far, the Newton experience is less than fulfilling. p. 10. In: The Executive Computer, NY Times *Business*, Section 3, September 26, 1993

74. Smith NT, Quinn ML, Sarnat AJ: Speech recognition for the automated anesthesia record. p. 115. In Gravenstein JS, Newbower RS, Ream AK, Smith NT: The Automated Anesthesia Record and Alarm Systems. Butterworth, Boston, 1987

75. Smith NT, Brien RA, Pettus DC et al: Recognition accuracy with a voice-recognition system designed for anesthesia record keeping. J Clin Monit 6:299, 1990

76. Edsall DW, Deshane P, Giles C et al: Computerized patient anesthesia records: less time and better quality than manually produced anesthesia records. J Clin Anesth 5:275, 1993

77. Tompkins BM, Tompkins WJ, Loder E, Noonan AF: A computer-assisted preanesthesia interview: value of a computer-generated summary of patient's historical information in the preanesthesia visit. Anesth Analg 59:3, 1980

78. Lutner RE, Roizen MF, Stocking CB et al: The automated interview versus the personal interview: do patient responses to preoperative health questions differ? Anesthesiology 75:394, 1991

79. Lerou JGC, Dirksen R, van Daele M et al: Automated charting of physiological variables in anesthesia: a quantitative comparison of automated vs handwritten anesthesia records. J Clin Monit 4:37, 1988

80. Ream AK: Automating the recording and improving

the presentation of the anesthesia record. J Clin Monit 5:270, 1989

81. Rennels GD, Miller PL: Artificial intelligence research in anesthesia and intensive care. J Clin Monit 4:274, 1988

82. Raemer D, Scott D, Topulos GP et al: Development of a monitoring-for-change algorithm for the Ohmeda modulus CD anesthesia machine. J Clin Monit 7:95, 1991

83. Westenskow DR, Orr JA, Simon FH et al: Intelligent alarms reduce anesthesiologist's response time to critical faults. Anesthesiology 77:1074, 1992

84. Anderson JG, Aydin CE: Theoretical perspectives and methodologies for the evaluation of health care information systems. p. 15. In Anderson JG, Aydin CE, Jay SJ (eds): Evaluating Health Care Information Systems: Methods and Applications. SAGE Publications, Thousand Oaks, CA, 1994

85. Palmer RH, Adams MME: Quality improvement/quality assurance taxonomy: a framework. In Grady ML, Berstein J, Robinson S (eds): Putting Research to Work in Quality Improvement and Quality Assurance, US Department of Health and Human Services, Agency for Health Care Policy and Research, July 1993, ACHPR Pub No. 93-0034.

86. Tierney WM, Miller ME, Overhage JM, McDonald CJ: Physician inpatient order writing on microcomputer workstations: effects on resource utilization. JAMA 269:378, 1993

87. Prophet CM: The patient problem/nursing diagnosis form: a computer-generated chart document. p. 326. In Safran C (ed): Proceedings of the Seventeenth Annual Symposium on Computer Applications in Medical Care (SCAMC). McGraw-Hill, New York, 1993

88. Stamen JP: Structuring databases for analysis. IEEE Spectrum 30:55, 1993

89. Dick RS, Steen EB et al: The Computer-Based Patient Record: An Essential Technology for Health Care. National Academy Press, Washington, DC, 1991

90. Toward a National Health Information Infrastructure. Report of the Work Group on Computerization of Patient Records to the Secretary of the US Department of Health and Human Services, April, 1993

91. U.S. Department of Health and Human Services. Initiatives Toward the Electronic Health Care System of the Future. White Paper, Washington, DC, 1992

92. Rootenberg JD: Information technologies in US medical schools: clinical practices outpace academic applications. JAMA 268:3106, 1992

93. McDonald CJ, Hripcsak GH: Data exchange standards for computer-based patient records. In Ball MJ, Collen MF (eds): Aspects of the Computer-Based Patient Record. Springer-Verlag, New York, 1992

94. Lindberg DAB, Humphreys BL: The Unified Medical Language System (UMLS) and computer-based patient records. In Ball MJ, Collen MF (eds): Aspects of the Computer-Based Patient Record. Springer-Verlag, New York, 1992

Monitoring in Unusual Environments

James V. Harper

25

Anesthesiologists deliver care in a number of locations distant from the operating room. This seems to produce discomfort among anesthesiologists because the specialty depends on very specific technology and devices to monitor and gauge a patient's well being. In some states, some or all the monitors used are mandated by law. In its 1993–1994 Standards the Joint Commission for the Accreditation of Health Care Organizations (JCAHO) has mandated that all patients being anesthetized receive the same level of care that is given to the patient in the operating suite. The technologic revolution of the last several years has contributed to an overall increase in both medical and anesthesia capabilities. This has resulted in more devices (i.e., pulse oximetry, various gas monitors including infrared analysis, Raman scatter, and mass spectrometry) available and deemed necessary to deliver anesthesia care safely and properly. This increased technologic capability is easily provided in the operating suite but is often difficult to provide or counterproductive in remote environments. This chapter considers some of the many remote environments to which anesthesiologists are summoned and suggests a rational approach to monitoring in remote environments.

GENERAL CONSIDERATIONS

When approaching anesthesia in a remote environment, it is useful to consider several factors:

1. *Type of anesthetic to be delivered.* Does the procedure require a general anesthetic or major conduction anesthetic or would some degree of sedation be adequate? Having the patient regularly respond verbally and appropriately to the question, "Are you O.K.?" provides important information concerning the airway, gas exchange, and level of consciousness. As will be seen, major anesthetics require a level of monitoring that in some cases will be difficult to obtain. It may be prudent to try to minimize the anesthetic intervention whenever possible—a sound practice in every case.

2. *Relative hazard level of environment.* The noise level of a first-generation lithotripter is unpleasant, but with ear protection the anesthesiologist can easily stay fairly close to the patient. However, it is not possible to stay close to a patient receiving of hundreds of rads during radiotherapy. Every standard of anesthesia care first postulates that an anesthesia provider be near the patient. When the procedure or environment precludes the caregiver's presence, modifications in technique are necessary.

3. *Distance of the patient from the anesthesiologist.* In a first-generation lithotripter (such as the Dornier) the patient is 2 to 3 ft away from the anesthesiologist in a water bath. In a cyclotron, the anesthesiologist is removed from the patient by 20 ft or more with intervening lead walls.

4. *Other factors.* Is the procedure affected by the anesthesiologist's monitors? This becomes a problem in magnetic resonance imaging. Are there physical constraints on the anesthesiologist's monitors? The waterbath lithotripter is hard on electronics and presents adhesive difficulties (ECG electrodes, etc.) Can the procedure be stopped? If a patient is in difficulty, can

the machine be stopped or must it complete its treatment?

The data given in Table 25-1 can be obtained from an anesthetized (or sedated) patient.

Although they vary in their level of specificity, most types of information are considered necessary to identify patient well-being in today's operating room. A few of the variables have only recently been subjected to objective measurement, and it is not clear how important to the practice of anesthesia these variables will become. The anesthesiologist of the 1950s attempted to measure all the variables with a hand on the bag (respiratory rate, quality), a finger on the pulse (heart rate, blood pressure, temperature), and an eye on the patient (oxygenation). The electrocardiogram (ECG), now considered necessary, was optional in the 1960s and in some institutions, the 1970s. Pulse oximetry has only been regularly available since about 1983, and quickly became standard of care. We cannot know what changes are portended for the future, except that the monitoring environment will become more complex. It is also important to remember that the anesthesiologist is constrained by law or practice guidelines to deliver a certain degree of anesthesia quality and use specific monitoring devices.

Witcher and colleagues[1] have proposed a minimum of monitors intended to prevent many common anesthetic mishaps. The monitors they propose are as follows:

Pulse oximeter
Capnography
Spirometer
Halometer (i.e., infrared with agent capability, mass spectrometry, etc.)
Automatic noninvasive blood pressure (ANIBP) monitor
Breathing circuit oxygen analyzer
Stethoscope
Electrocardiogram
Thermometer

They estimated that a suite so equipped would cost approximately $22,500. Others have also proposed Standards for Monitoring the anesthetized patient, both in specific institutions in the United States and internationally, and all include most, if not all of these devices.[2-6]

In the final analysis, it is likely that the most rational approach to delivering anesthesia in remote sites in the 1990s and beyond is to assemble a portable "package" of those devices needed for the safe practice of anesthesia and deliver them to a site. One could easily envision a portable anesthesia machine (on the order of the Ohmeda Excel, among others) equipped to ASTM F1161-88 standards (the specific standard published by the American Society for Testing in Medicine, 1916 Race St., Philadelphia, PA 19103-1187.) The actual standard is 34 pages long and includes many technical descriptions, including the recommended visual angles for the rotameters. One can take comfort in simply asking the manufacturer if their machine conforms (most modern machines do). Add to that a pulse oximeter, ECG, infrared (or other) gas monitor that has halogenated anesthetic capability, ANIBP, and temperature monitor, and roll the assemblage to wherever anesthesia needs to be delivered.

This "package" and a well-trained anesthesia provider will conform to any of the standards currently operational, and those proposed. More importantly, this "package" will enable the patient to have an anesthetic with as much safety as we can provide. One of the truest truisms of anesthesiology is that "compromise is possible with all *but* patient safety."[7]

The remainder of this chapter considers a few specific non-operating-room locations. The reader should assume that the above "package" is the ideal. The considerations here are to discuss problems present in meeting the Standards, and methods for approaching the Standard as closely as possible. The monitoring modalities are considered from the perspective of *cardiovascular*, which includes ECG, ischemia, arrhythmia, and blood pressure; *pulmonary*, which includes pulse oximetry, respiratory monitors, and halogenated anesthetics, and *temperature*. The last consideration, monitoring for disasters, briefly considers an environment with support facilities reduced to a minimum.

EXTRACORPOREAL SHOCK WAVE LITHOTRIPSY

Extracorporeal shock wave lithotripsy usually takes place in the operating suite, although location now varies.[8] "The remote location" aspect of this procedure was often the *location of the patient* during the procedure.

In the first-generation lithotripter (i.e., the Dornier HM-3), the patient lies on a couch suspended in a tank of water, which leaves the patient immersed up to the neck. This places the patient in an 18-in. wide moat that obstructs the anesthesiologist's access. The patient usually receives conduction (epidural)[9] or general endotracheal anesthesia,[10,11] although local infiltration anesthesia, with or without intercostal blocks, and sedation has been used.[12,13]

Much of this has changed with newer models of lithotripters. The new or nonwaterbath lithotripters, are really little different than the normal operating table, with the single exception of an inability to put the patient into the Trendelenburg position. In fact, some of the latest versions of lithotripters (piezo-electric)[14] are able to be used without anesthesia, only requiring very mild patient sedation.[15] Other models, (spark gap, electromagnetic), require local infiltration or deeper sedation.[16,17]

Another use for these devices is to break up gallstones. As a rule, the level of anesthesia required (and thus, monitoring) for gallstones is not different from that used for kidney stones.[18-20]

Cardiovascular Monitoring

An interference-free electrocardiogram (ECG) trace is particularly important in lithotripsy, since the machine fires on the R wave to minimize the arrhythmogenic propensities of the energy im-

TABLE 25-1. Data That Can Be Obtained from an Anesthetized (or Sedated) Patient[a]

Parameter	Absolute Necessity?	Device Used
Blood pressure	Yes	Sphygmomanometery
		Automatic noninvasive blood pressure monitor
		Arterial catheter
Heart rate	Yes	Palpation
		Auscultation
		Pulse oximetry
		Electrocardiogram
		Automatic noninvasive blood pressure monitor
Heart rhythm	Perhaps	Auscultation[b]
		Pulse oximetry[b]
		Electrocardiogram
Ischemia monitoring	Perhaps	Electrocardiogram
Abnormal beats	No	Electrocardiogram
Respiratory rate	Perhaps	Observation
		Auscultation
		Capnography
Respiratory quality	Yes	Observation
		Disconnect alarm (mechanical ventilation)
		Auscultation
		Capnography
		Pulse oximetry
Temperature	No	Hand contact
		Liquid crystal adhesive
		Intermittent measurement (sensor)
		Continuous measurement (sensor)
Level of anesthesia	No	Observation
		Esophageal tone
		Electroencephalograph
Inspired oxygen	Yes	Oxygen analyzer
		Mass spectrograph

[a]It is important that any discussion of minimum standards for monitoring in anesthesia assumes the presence of a member of the anesthesia team in attendance at all times.

[b]These devices will measure the "quality" of the rhythm. That is, regular versus irregular.

parted to the patient. It is best to use a 5-lead system (V_5 + 4 arm leads) and cover (in the immersion lithotripter, i.e., Dornier HM-3) each ECG electrode, 6 cm of lead wire and the connector with a clear, adhesive bioocclusive dressing (OP-Site, Tegaderm, etc.), which creates a somewhat waterproof barrier. This step is not necessary in the non-immersion lithotripters. The remainder of the ECG wires are routed up to the connector block, which is taped to the gantry, and the cable is subsequently connected to the monitor. Any method of monitoring blood pressure is adequate. Noninvasive automatic blood pressure machines are not interfered with by the lithotripter shock waves. Devices that use electronic sensors in the cuff should be checked for electrical safety if, as is likely in the older model device, they are to be immersed. Blood pressure cuff life is considerably shortened when immersed, and this may make disposable blood pressure cuffs attractive in this environment.

Pulmonary Monitoring

If the patient receives general anesthesia, the trachea will most likely be intubated. Halogenated anesthetics, end-tidal CO_2, and ventilatory volumes should be measured. The patient receiving major conduction anesthesia or local anesthesia plus sedation presents a problem. One is left with the option of eliciting patient responses to questions, (which can be difficult in the loud environment) or a more elegant technologic solution.

A mass spectrometer or infrared CO_2 monitor may be used by connecting the sampling tube to a cutoff O_2 delivery tube of a nasal cannula. This system will demonstrate a CO_2 waveform and respiratory rate. Goldman[21] has developed a system that allows oxygen to be delivered simultaneously through a nasal cannula using a 16-gauge angiocath for CO_2 monitoring. There are several commercially available devices that serve the same purpose. A pulse oximeter should always be used in these cases.

Most pulse oximeter sensors do not perform well when immersed in water. To obtain an acceptable signal, either the patient's hand can be suspended out of the water by a towel sling, or a nasal sensor may be used.

Temperature Monitoring

Any site for temperature monitoring will suffice, but some temperature probes, such as skin probes, cannot be immersed in water.

RADIATION THERAPY

Patients requiring anesthesia for radiation therapy are primarily children. Radiation is not painful per se, and the anesthesiologist's primary goal is to ensure patient immobility. This situation may change, as there is increasing interest in intraoperative radiation (radiotherapy to exposed organs) and uncomfortable total body irradiation,[22,23] which in the future may lead to a different patient population.

Regardless of the age of the patient, when anesthesia is administered, monitoring is required. The patient is separated from the anesthesiologist by several feet of a concrete and lead wall during therapy. The actual treatment periods are brief (usually less than 3 minutes) so adjustments to anesthesia delivery will not be necessary, but it is necessary to monitor the patient during the brief treatment periods. Each therapy area should have an audiovisual electronic monitor to provide remote audio and visual contact with the patient.[24]

Cardiovascular Monitoring

The standard ECG monitor performs well in this environment. If the audible volume is set at near maximum, the "beep" is easily heard over the audio pickup in the room. Most video monitors are not adequate to display the screen of the ECG monitor, so QRS-T configuration is not available, but only for the brief time of the actual treatment when the caregiver is forced to be out of the room. Automatic noninvasive blood pressure devices are useful in this situation. Alarms provide audible notification of a departure from baseline. A pressure measurement can be triggered as a last act before leaving the room for a treatment, and the pressure will be determined during the treatment.

Pulmonary Monitoring

The standard gas analysis monitors will serve in every case of the intubated patient. For the awake patient adaptations on sidestream monitors such as those referred to for lithotripsy would serve well. Again, the video monitor is not usually able to ascertain the actual measurements on the screen, but the audible monitors will reliably deliver the information needed to watch for catastrophe during the actual delivery of radiation. A sedated but awake patient can usually have his or her respiratory status monitored using verbal questions over the auditory system in the treatment room.

Most pulse oximeters are ideal for radiotherapy areas as they generate an audible tone that changes in pitch with varying oxygen saturations. These sounds are easily heard over the auditory pickup in the room and gives pulse information as well.

Temperature Monitoring

Temperature should be monitored if deemed necessary by the caregiver. There are no particular difficulties with temperature monitoring.

If one were involved in the design of a radiation oncology center, one could suggest the addition of a conduit with two 90-degree turns through a wall.[25] This would enable data to be transferred into the monitoring room via cable through the conduit, which would solve many problems.

MAGNETIC RESONANCE IMAGING

Since MRI is (so far) purely an imaging modality, anesthesia delivery is rarely necessary. However, patients unable to cooperate, such as semicomatose or claustrophobic adults, children, and seriously ill people, may require sedation and/or anesthesia. When anesthesia intervention is necessary for this modality, the situation becomes difficult. The patient is in a magnetic field, essentially a tube, with the head far from the anesthesia team. Visual contact with the patient's face is often through a prism or mirror. When the patient's head is enclosed by a "receive coil," there is even little room for a standard endotracheal tube and an RAE tube is necessary.[26] The tubelike nature of the device is likely to change in the future, as newer designs should resemble plates supported by pillars.

It is important to remember that the strong magnetic field created in this environment is not hazardous to the anesthesiologist (probably) but will be hard on his or her watch and credit cards. The environment is quite loud, and this presents difficulty for the patient, as well as for the anesthesia team, and is potentially harmful. The major problems created by the magnetic field are that (1) ferrous metal objects have the potential to become projectiles, (2) many monitoring devices can act as radiofrequency antennae and degrade the image, and (3) the function of specific devices (i.e., va-

porizers) can be adversely affected by the strong magnetic field.

Anesthesia machines have been developed specifically to function in the environment of the MRI scanner; one example is the Ohmeda Excel 210 MRI-compatible machine. The required modification is the substitution of nonferrous tanks for oxygen and nitrous oxide. This machine has vaporizers that can function properly in a high magnetic field.[27] This machine does not totally conform to ASTM F1161-88 standards, and as such represents a minor compromise in safety, but is acceptable. One unfortunate side effect of this failure to comply with the ASTM standard (because of constraints applied by the environment the machine is designed for, not because of any choice by the manufacturer) is that the machine is not suitable for use in the general operating suite. This may represent an unreasonable expense for an institution that needs the capability rarely.

Cardiovascular Monitoring

Most magnetic resonance imagers are equipped with electrocardiogram monitoring capability which is used for specific studies. The quality of these monitors is not at a diagnostic level. An ordinary ECG monitor may be used but there is a significant risk of burns (third-degree burns have been reported)[28] caused by induced currents in the wires attached to the electrodes. The magnetic field creates artifacts in the ECG, but there are microcomputer-based data acquisition devices that can remove the gradient impulses.[29] Currently, there is no safe effective way to monitor for ischemia using the ECG in the MRI environment. The ECG only provides the rhythm and rate of the heart. However, in an environment relatively safe for the anesthesia team, it is also useful to place a finger on the pulse (ankle or foot) or employ an esophageal stethoscope (with long tubing . . . and great difficulty hearing) during the actual scan to gather much of the same information.

A standard blood pressure cuff with rubber tubing will work well. Most automatic noninvasive blood pressure devices do not contain ferrous metals (fortunately). A Doppler apparatus may be used to sense the pulse without significant degradation of the scan.[30] An intraarterial catheter may be used, since disposable transducers have very little ferromagnetic material in them.[31] The data produced can be carried via cable to a monitor outside of the magnet or to one of the monitors that do well in the environment.[32]

Pulmonary Monitoring

There have been reports of the successful use of various capnographs and infrared monitors during MRI.[33] Aneuroid chest bellows (Coulbourn Instruments, Allentown, PA) have been used to detect chest-wall motion without signal degradation. Pulse oximetry has been used in this environment, but not without difficulties. Patients have been burned by induced currents,[34] and there are difficulties with signal degradation. Shellock described a fiber-optic cabled pulse oximeter in 1992, and adaptations of these are now widely available and used (one such is the Nonin model 8604 FO).[35]

Temperature Monitoring

It is probably not prudent to monitor the temperature in these patients by any of the usual modes. It is likely (although the usefulness and safety of these are unproven) that the liquid crystal adhesives will give sufficient information. To use any of our usual means will place another wire within the field, which will lead to another potential site for a burn.

ANESTHESIA DURING DISASTERS

An interesting unusual environment is the disaster or field environment. Acts of man or Mother Nature can render most or all of our technology useless. Without electrical current our monitors are soon rendered useless, and without piped gases or electrical current our ventilators soon fail. Yet, as witnessed in recent disasters, people are injured through acts of nature and lawlessness that seems to follow the disruption caused by the former.

The reader is encouraged to consider an environment without the conveniences now available to us in the modern operating theater. Without any electricity, one is reduced to reliance on the stethoscope, aneuroid blood pressure cuff, and ambu bag. If some of the older anesthesia machines were available, it would be possible to use volatile anesthetics, as these machines only need cylinder gases; there would be no place for modern machines as described earlier in this chapter. The only anes-

thetics usable in these circumstances would be intravenous or regional anesthetics. It would be possible to use high oxygen mixtures, as oxygen cylinders should continue to be available.

With a functioning generator, we could add battery-powered monitors. Grande[36] suggests that the single most useful monitor in this environment would be the pulse oximeter, and I agree. The heart rate or, most importantly, oxygen saturation is the best single source of physiological well-being information available. An ECG could well be the next best. In this environment the NIBP monitor would become a needless luxury, and is not typically amenable to battery operation. The Propaq by Protocol Systems is a very robust battery-powered monitor that provides all three of the above parameters with reasonable battery life. This monitor enjoyed great success during the recent hostilities in the Middle East, and may be the definitive monitor available for the extreme conditions that we are considering in this section. The gas monitors we use, with the exception of a polarographic oxygen sensor, would be too power-hungry and, as such, useless.

The purpose of this exercise was to encourage the reader to think about an irreducible minimum of monitors for anesthesia. Having considered that, it is useful to reflect on the necessity of the compromises we make for anesthesia techniques out of the operating suite. Lacking the overwhelming need created by a hurricane or a war, perhaps compromise is not necessary.

OTHER LOCATIONS

Anesthetic care rendered in locations remote from the operating/delivery suite should conform to the principles described in this chapter. These remote locations include, but are not limited to, the following:

Radiology suite (computed tomography scan, special procedures, etc.)
Cardiac catheterization area
Endoscopic care areas (gastrointestinal laboratory, etc.)
Cardioversion areas (patient rooms, emergency room)
Emergency room (trauma care, other procedures)

SUMMARY

Today there is no excuse for not having all of the appropriate equipment available for these procedures. As stated at the start of this chapter, some States (with more to follow) and many authors have defined the minimum Standard of Monitoring for anesthetized patients. The JCAHO requires that all patients who receive anesthesia receive the same standard of care. That is, what is acceptable in the operating room is acceptable, and required, in the gastrointestinal laboratory. A patient receiving anesthesia for a cardioversion or electroconvulsive therapy[37] should receive care at least at the same level as a patient who is having knee arthroscopy.

When the environment constrains our capabilities, compromises are necessary, but when the environment is neutral (e.g., radiology) we should give the same care as we do in the operating suite.[38]

Monitoring and delivery of anesthesia care in unusual environments require the anesthesiologist's ingenuity and willingness to adapt. If a few principles are adhered to, the experience will be safe for the patient and rewarding for the anesthesiologist. The driving force for compromise must be the constraints of the environment, and never convenience or cost. Every compromise made must be made with an eye to the ultimate goal: safety for the patient. With safety as the prerogative, intelligent choices will lead to satisfactory outcomes.

REFERENCES

1. Whitcher C et al: Anesthetic mishaps and the cost of monitoring: a proposed standard for monitoring equipment. J Clin Monit 4:5, 1988
2. Emmett C, Hutton P: Patient monitoring. Br Med Bull 44:302, 1988
3. McIntyre JW: A unified approach to providing general anaesthesia monitoring with special reference to developing countries. Int J Clin Monit Comput 7:147, 1990
4. Pullerits J: Anesthesia equipment for infants and children. Int Anesthesiol Clin 30:131, 1992
5. Rocke DA et al: Standards of practice in anaesthesia: intra-operative monitoring. S Afr Med J 81:403, 1992
6. Eichhorn JH et al: Anesthesia practice standards at Harvard: a review. J Clin Anesth 1:55, 1988
7. Prevoznik SJ: Personal Communication
8. Burns JR, Breaux EF, Crowe AD: Practical aspects of outpatient extracorporeal shock-wave lithotripsy. Urol Clin North Am 14:73, 1987
9. Cook RJ, Neerhut R, Thomas DG: Does combined epidural lignocaine and fentanyl provide better anaesthesia for ESWL than lignocaine alone? Anaesth Intens Care 19:357, 1991
10. Monk TG et al: Comparison of intravenous sedative-analgesic techniques for outpatient immersion lithotripsy. Anesth Analg 72:616, 1991
11. Monk TG, Rater JM, White PF: Comparison of alfentanil and ketamine infusions in combination with midazolam for outpatient lithotripsy. Anesthesiology 74:1023, 1991
12. Morgulis R et al: Alfentanil analgesia/sedation for extracorporeal shock wave lithotripsy: a comparison with general and epidural anesthesia. AANA J 59:533, 1991
13. Knudsen F et al: Anesthesia and complications of extracorporeal shock wave lithotripsy of urinary calculi. J Urol 148:1030, 1992
14. Bierkens AF et al: Efficacy of second generation lithotriptors: a multicenter comparative study of 2,206 extracorporeal shock wave lithotripsy treatments with the Siemens Lithostar, Dornier HM4, Wolf Piezolith 2300, Direx Tripter X-1 and Breakstone lithotriptors. J Urol 148:1052, 1992
15. Vandeursen H et al: Anaesthesia-free extracorporeal shock wave lithotripsy in patients with renal calculi. Br J Urol 68:18, 1991
16. Prystowsky JB, Nahrwold DL: Extracorporeal shock wave lithotripsy for biliary stones. Surg Clin North Am 70:1231, 1990
17. Pfister RC, Papanicolaou N, Yoder IC: Urinary extracorporeal shock wave lithotripsy: equipment, techniques, and overview. Urol Radiol 10:39, 1988
18. Vergunst H et al: Extracorporeal shockwave lithotripsy of gallstones: possibilities and limitations. Ann Surg 210:565, 1989
19. Ferrucci JT: Gallstone lithotripsy: a preview. Radiology 168:333, 1988
20. Frick TW et al: Electrohydraulic extracorporeal non-water bath shock-wave lithotripsy of gallstones: two years' experience. World J Surg 15:623, 1991
21. Goldman JM: A simple, easy and inexpensive method for monitoring ETCO2, through nasal cannulae. Anesthesiology 67:606, 1987
22. Ashayeri E et al: Anesthesia in intraoperative radiotherapy patients. J Natl Med Assoc 78:193, 1986
23. Freisen RH, Morrison JE, Verbrugge JJ: Anesthesia for intraoperative radiation therapy in children. J Surg Oncol 35:96, 1987
24. Casey WF, Price V, Smith HS: Anesthesia and monitoring for paediatric radiotherapy. J R Soc Med 79:454, 1986
25. Feingold A et al: Inhalation anesthesia and remote monitoring during radiotherapy for children. Anesth Analg 49:656, 1987

26. Peden CJ et al: Magnetic resonance for the anaesthetist. Part II: Anaesthesia and monitoring in MR units. Anaesthesia 47:508, 1992

27. Kross J, Drummond JC: Successful use of a Fortec II vaporizer in the MRI suite: a case report with observations regarding magnetic field-induced vaporizer aberrancy. Can J Anaesth 38:1065, 1991

28. Gangarosa RE et al: Operational safety issues in MRI. Magn Reson Imaging 5:287, 1987

29. Karlik SJ et al: Patient anesthesia and monitoring at a 1.5-T MRI installation. Magn Reson Med 7:210, 1988

30. McArdle CB et al: Monitoring of the neonate undergoing MR imaging: technical considerations: work in progress. Radiology 159:223, 1986

31. Rejger VS et al: A simple anaesthetic and monitoring system for magnetic resonance imaging. Eur J Anaesthesiol 6:373, 1989

32. Barnett GH, Ropper AH, Johnson KA: Physiological support and monitoring of critically ill patients during magnetic resonance imaging. J Neurosurg 68:246, 1988

33. Shellock FG: Monitoring sedated pediatric patients during MR imaging [Letter; Comment]. Radiology 177:586, 1990

34. Shellock FG, Slimp GL: Severe burn of the finger caused by using a pulse oximeter during MR imaging. [Letter]. AJR 153, 1989

35. Shellock FG, Myers SM, Kimble KJ: Monitoring heart rate and oxygen saturation with a fiber-optic pulse oximeter during MR imaging. AJR 158:663, 1992

36. Grande CM et al: Trauma anesthesia for disasters: anything, anytime, anywhere. Crit Care Clin 7:339, 1991

37. Kammerer W: Current anesthesia practice for electroconvulsive therapy. [Letter]. Anesth Analg 66:918, 1987

38. Gaines G, Rees DI: Anesthetic considerations for electroconvulsive therapy. South Med J 85:469, 1992

Special Monitoring Considerations in Cardiac Anesthesia

26

Mark N. Gomez

Alan F. Ross

John H. Tinker

As this is written, a clandestine cell is quietly planning a revolution in the conduct of cardiac anesthesia and surgery at our hospital. The group includes hospital administrators, directors of nursing, and the chiefs of cardiac anesthesia and surgery. Their goal is to present a unified front to third-party payors demanding negotiation of standard costs (read: cost containment) for all cardiac procedures. Everything is (or should be) negotiable: hospital charges, surgical instruments, suture, cardiopulmonary bypass equipment, and particularly, anesthesia monitoring practices. The working premise is that any monitor not firmly established as basic or necessary for safety reasons, or not cost effective on the basis of rigorous scientific analysis, is "fair game" in the press for cost containment.

The context of cost containment gives new meaning to the phrase "special monitoring considerations." In the absence of definitive outcome studies, *routine use* of certain monitors must give way to *selective use*, based on specific applications for each monitor. Yet, while selection may be guided by outcome and cost containment considerations, it is the patient who truly makes the ultimate investment. Above all, special monitoring considerations for cardiac anesthesia must emphasize those that significantly contribute to reasonable patient care for cardiac surgery.

THE PRELIMINARIES: BASIC MONITORING CONSIDERATIONS

Basic or standard monitors in cardiac anesthesia include those used in noncardiac anesthesia: esophageal stethoscope, electrocardiogram (ECG), blood pressure cuff, pulse oximeter, capnometer, and temperature probe. Additional routine and standard monitors in cardiac anesthesia are urinary output catheter and intra-arterial blood pressure monitoring catheter. It is worthwhile to review the special applications of these monitors for cardiac anesthesia.

ELECTROCARDIOGRAPHY

Intraoperative Myocardial Ischemia

The electrocardiogram (ECG) is commonly used for all anesthetic procedures as mandated by the ASA Standards for Intra-operative Monitoring. All anesthesiologists rely on ECG for diagnosis of arrhythmias, conduction disturbances, and myocardial ischemia. However, aspects of cardiac anesthesia require special considerations for this monitor. For example, consider the occurrence of intraoperative myocardial ischemia. In noncardiac procedures, this is relatively infrequent. Because the

651

lateral chest lead has been demonstrated to be most sensitive for detection of ischemia, a three-lead ECG "modified V$_5$," represents a convenient and effective monitoring strategy. However, in patients undergoing cardiac procedures, intraoperative myocardial ischemia is a distinct possibility necessitating more intensive surveillance. Electrocardiographically, ischemia is indicated by ST-segment abnormalities.[2] It may be confined to the inferior (leads 2, 3, and aVF), anterior (leads V$_2$ to V$_4$) or lateral (leads 1, aVF, V$_5$, and V$_6$) regions of the heart. Thus cardiac procedures routinely utilize a five-lead ECG system and routinely display two ECG leads (II and V$_5$) simultaneously.

ECG processing with ST-segment analysis is a recent addition to monitoring for intraoperative myocardial ischemia. It is debatable whether such software products actually increase detection of ischemic ECG changes. In contrast, a device with significant practical utility is a small printer that can make a paper copy of the monitored ECG. This allows direct comparison of the current ECG to that which occurred preoperatively or earlier in the case.

Rhythm Diagnosis

Rhythm diagnosis has special requirements in cardiac anesthesia. Even simple and common rhythm alterations may result in significant hemodynamic impairment in the cardiac patient. A good example is the occurrence of junctional rhythm in the patient with left ventricular hypertrophy. Such patients are very dependent on adequate ventricular filling. Therefore the loss of the atrial contribution (atrial "kick") can abruptly cause systemic hypotension which in turn can cause decreased myocardial perfusion. Thus, while junctional rhythm (a common arrhythmia during anesthesia) is often simply a curiosity for noncardiac patients, it can have important consequences for the cardiac patient (Fig. 26-1).

Cardiopulmonary Bypass

Cardioplegia

Cardiac procedures routinely utilize the ECG during cardiopulmonary bypass to provide (1) confirmation of successful cardioplegia administration and resultant electrical asystole; (2) detection of return of electrical activity, which would indicate the need for more cardioplegia, change in composition of cardioplegia, or other therapy; (3) differentiation of persistent electrical activity from ECG artifact. Circumstances in which "usual cardioplegia" practices might be inadequate and result in persistent ECG activity include (1) incompetent aortic valve such that pressure generated in the aortic root is insufficient for coronary perfusion; (2) incomplete cross-clamping of the aorta such that cardioplegia is "washed out" by flow from the aortic cannula; (3) left ventricular distension or hypertrophy causing inadequate cardioplegia flow to the subendocardium; and (4) dislocation of the cardioplegia cannula when retrograde cardioplegia is used.

Ventricular Fibrillation

It may be argued that ECG is not necessary to diagnose grossly inadequate cardioplegia, which may be detected by direct visualization of the fibrillating heart. However, persistent low-amplitude ventricular fibrillation may only be detectable by the ECG. If uncorrected, this may predispose to post-cardiopulmonary bypass ventricular dysfunction.[3] Ventricular fibrillation is especially troublesome in patients with aortic insufficiency. In these patients, prior to aortic cross-clamp application the beating left ventricle continues to eject blood which has regurgitated back across the incompetent aortic valve. When ventricular fibrillation occurs, this regurgitated blood cannot be ejected and may acutely distend the ventricle. In this situation the onset of ventricular fibrillation may be a sign of ventricular distension.

In certain procedures, ECG evidence of ventricular fibrillation is desirable. An example is an atrial septal defect repaired without use of cardioplegia. Here, an aortic cross-clamp is not used, so that perfusion of the heart continues during the operation. The heart cannot be allowed to contract, however, because of the risk of systemic air embolization. For this reason, ventricular fibrillation is purposely induced by application of electric current to the heart.

Electrocardiographic Interference

Electrocardiographic interference is common with initiation of cardiopulmonary bypass.[4] This electrocardiographic interference can mimic the appearance of ventricular fibrillation. Interference

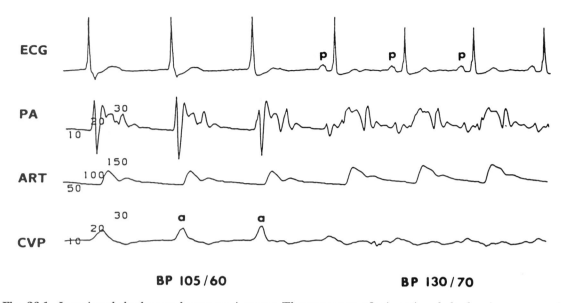

Fig. 26-1. Junctional rhythm and cannon A waves. The presence of a junctional rhythm is accompanied by cannon A waves in the central venous pressure tracing. The ECG at this time shows no P waves. The return of sinus rhythm is indicated by the presence of p waves in the ECG and loss of cannon A waves in the central venous pressure tracing.

is believed to be due to creation of static electricity at the pump head-tubing interface, or piezoelectric transduction due to compression of the pump tubing.[4] Differentiation of ECG artifact from ventricular fibrillation may be difficult. One strategy is momentary cessation of the bypass pump. Khambatta and colleagues[4] reported that spraying tap water via an atomizer onto the pump head to disperse the charge buildup was effective in 75 percent of cases.[4] However, there is risk of water damage to the electronic controls. Alternatively, Metz[5] created an electrical connection between the circulating perfusate and the grounded pump console housing, which led to charge dispersal and artifact elimination. If necessary, an electrical connection between the patient and the metal pump assembly

housing can also be made (Fig. 26-2). This creates a potential for microshock, and thus this connection should be broken when resumption of electrical activity of the heart is desired.[6]

Supraventricular Arrhythmia

During the management of patients undergoing cardiac surgery, the diagnosis of supraventricular arrhythmia from the basic ECG can be difficult. Specifically, if p waves are difficult to discern on the ECG, a rhythm could appear to be sinus, junctional, or even atrial flutter. In these situations, recording the atrial electrogram has been performed using an esophageal lead,[7] temporary atrial pacemaker wires,[8] or atrial leads from a pacing pulmo-

Fig. 26-2. ECG interference mimics ventricular fibrillation. When a connection is made between the patient and the metal hosing of the cardiopulmonary bypass machine (*arrow*), the electrical activity resembling ventricular fibrillation disappears.

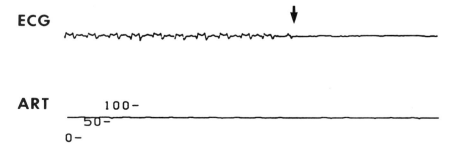

nary artery catheter.[9] These techniques, facilitate diagnosis because the amplitude of the p wave is now enlarged relative to the rest of the ECG (Fig. 26-3).

TEMPERATURE MONITORING

Procedures utilizing cardiopulmonary bypass require special considerations for temperature monitoring. Standard management of bypass involves the use of systemic hypothermia for the purpose of decreasing oxygen utilization, followed by systemic rewarming. Reliable temperature monitoring is critical, and both the patient and the cardiopulmonary bypass circuit are monitored. For the bypass circuit, it is now considered mandatory to monitor temperature of both the arterial perfusate (inflow to the patient) and venous return (outflow).[10] This permits the perfusionist to judge the progress of temperature exchange and maintain proper temperature gradients during heat exchange. For example, oxygen added to the bypass machine becomes less soluable when the blood is warmed. Perfusionists typically control the rate of temperature changes so as to prevent gaseous oxygen formation in the perfusate.

Because of variations in the vascular supply of body organs, perfusion of the arterial circulation with cooled or heated perfusate results in nonuniform temperature changes. Some tissues are slow to cool, and once cooled, are slow to warm (e.g., muscle, skin, fat). Distribution is further altered by temperature induced vasoconstriction or vasodilation. This uneven heat exchange process requires

that temperature be routinely monitored at *two* separate sites during cardiopulmonary bypass, such as nasopharyngeal and bladder-rectal sites. The richly perfused nasopharyngeal site quickly equilibriates to the temperature of the arterial inflow from the bypass machine. The temperature at the rectal-bladder site changes much more slowly (Fig. 26-4). Equilibration of temperatures occurs more uniformly as pump flows are increased with the administration of vasodilators.[11,12] Even at the point when these temperatures equalize, there may still be temperature gradients within the patient due to blood-flow differences among tissues.

The existence of these tissue temperature differences leads to confusion about the definition and measurement of "core temperature." Classically, core temperature refers to the temperature of ascending aortic blood.[13] A temperature probe placed in the lower third of the esophagus in proximity to the heart and aorta can be used to measure core temperature during cardiopulmonary bypass and will reflect arterial (perfusate) temperature. One caveat should be noted, however: if the pericardium is filled with ice (i.e., topical myocardial cooling) during cardiopulmonary bypass, temperature measured in the nearby esophagus could result in the underestimation of core temperature.

It is also useful to measure temperature at a more distal site as a means of assessing the progress (or lack of it) of cooling or rewarming in less well-perfused tissues. For example, in addition to esophageal temperature monitoring, many centers also monitor rectal temperature. Rectal temperature lags behind esophageal temperature both during

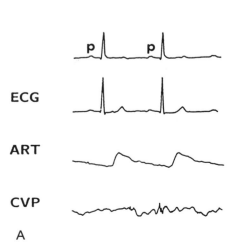

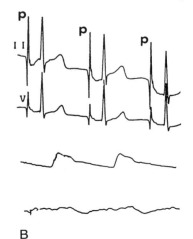

Fig. 26-3. The atrial electrogram. (**A**) A regular ECG tracing. (**B**) A tracing of the atrial electrogram. In both tracings the rhythm is sinus. The atrial p waves are made much more prominent by the atrial electrogram.

cooling and rewarming. Bladder temperature, via a thermistor-equipped Foley catheter can provide the same information as rectal temperature. Many centers have switched to this technique in an effort to reduce any potential for contamination from the rectal temperature probe.

Brain temperature during cardiopulmonary bypass can be assessed by either nasopharyngeal or tympanic temperature monitoring. Brain temperature is an important consideration when deep (25–20°C) or profound (below 20°C) hypothermia, with or without circulatory arrest, is anticipated. Both sites provide relatively reliable indications of brain temperature, but during rapid cooling or warming they will more closely reflect perfusate rather than brain temperature.[14,15]

INTRA-ARTERIAL PRESSURE MONITORING

Several aspects of invasive blood pressure monitoring deserve special consideration in the setting of cardiac anesthesia. These include (1) the site of invasive arterial blood pressure monitoring; (2) monitoring of blood pressure during cardiopulmonary bypass; (3) reversal of central-to-peripheral arterial pressure gradients after cardiopulmonary by-

pass; (4) assessment of blood pressure measurements during intra-aortic balloon counterpulsation.

Site of Arterial Pressure Monitoring

Virtually any accessible peripheral arterial site can be, and has been, used for blood pressure monitoring during cardiac surgery. Several generalizations regarding site of arterial blood pressure monitoring can be made: (1) in the absence of other considerations, the preferred site is the radial artery serving the nondominant hand; (2) cannulation distal to a cutdown (e.g., brachial cutdown for previous cardiac catheterization) may cause dampened waveforms or falsely low-pressure readings due to stenosis or vascular thrombosis[16]; (3) brachial and axillary arterial pressures reflect central aortic pressure more accurately than radial, ulnar, or dorsalis pedis pressures, particularly after cardiopulmonary bypass[17] (see below); (4) use of catheters in more proximal arteries (e.g., brachial, axillary) requires attention to the possibility that excessive flushing may push debris or air bubbles in retrograde fashion into the central aorta in the vicinity of the carotid arteries[18]; (5) anticipation of surgical "take-down" of the left internal mammary artery does not preclude cannulation of the left radial artery, particularly in a right-handed patient

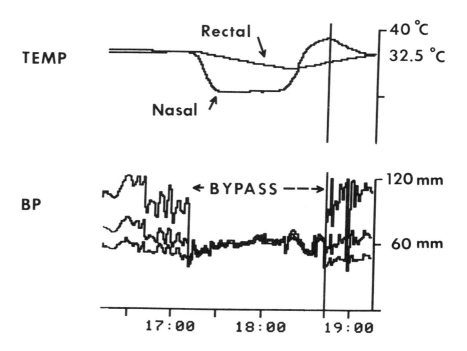

Fig. 26-4. Temperature gradients on bypass. Continuous recording of the nasal and rectal temperatures during cardiopulmonary bypass demonstrate the different rates at which these sites change temperature. The nasal temperature changes quickly, while the rectal temperature lags considerably behind. Note the temperature drop after the end of CPB, and that temperature finally equilibrate in the post-bypass period.

(a blood pressure cuff on the opposite arm can be used during the short time the left brachial artery is compressed by the retractor, although use of modern retractors such as the Ruhl-Tract rarely cause this problem). Our preferred cannulation sites, in decreasing order, are nondominant radial, dominant radial, nondominant brachial, femoral artery (either side). The axillary artery is avoided because systemic heparinization poses a risk for bleeding into the brachial plexus sheath.

Occasionally, during cardiac anesthesia and surgery two sites of arterial pressure monitoring are required. One such example is the repair of a thoracic aneurysm utilizing partial left-heart bypass for perfusion of the distal aorta beyond the cross-clamp. In this circumstance, the venous return to the left atrium is shared between the bypass circuit, which perfuses the lower body, and the left ventricle, which perfuses the upper body. When this occurs, the combination of a lower extremity and an upper extremity arterial pressure site facilitates management of the partial left-heart bypass.

Arterial Pressure on Cardiopulmonary Bypass

During cardiopulmonary bypass, the mechanical pump, which provides arterial circulation, generates very little in the way of a "pulse." For this reason, the blood pressure cuff cannot be used, and direct measurement of the mean arterial pressure (MAP) is accomplished using an intra-arterial catheter. There are a number of reasons why the mean arterial pressure varies during cardiopulmonary bypass. First, initiation of bypass involves hemodilution of the patient's blood with the pump prime. This reduces hematocrit and blood viscosity, thus contributing to a lower pressure. Next, systemic cooling results in vasoconstriction, which raises pressure, and, later, rewarming causes vasodilation and the subsequent lowering of pressure. With these various changes, the question arises as to what the mean arterial pressure *should be* during cardiopulmonary bypass.

First, one must consider that radial (or other) intra-arterial pressure reflects the pressure at which blood is being delivered to the brain. Furthermore, any estimation of cerebral perfusion pressure must include cerebral venous pressure, which must be subtracted from the arterial pressure.[19] In 1973 Stockard and coworkers[20] contended that the mean

arterial pressure should be >50 mmHg during moderate hypothermic (28 to 32°C) bypass. Longer periods of "hypotension" were related to a higher incidence of neurologic problems. However, Stockard's study included patients with preoperative syncopal episodes, patients for valve replacement, bubble oxygenators, and nitrous oxide as part of the anesthetic technique. Interestingly, Gordon and colleagues[21] calculated the Stockard "hypotensive index" in patients undergoing hypothermic bypass with hemodilution. Despite Stockard's prediction that calculated hypotensive indices would result in gross neurologic deficits, none could be documented postoperatively.

The characteristics of cerebral autoregulation during bypass are currently under investigation. It is clear that a multitude of factors contribute to organ perfusion. Until more complete understanding is available, it is prudent to maintain mean arterial pressures in a range demonstrated to be safe.

Some circumstances, however, deserve special mention. Consider the unusual case in which a fistula exists between the aorta and the right atrium. Here, a significant portion of the bypass pump flow is shunted back to the venous reservoir without perfusing the patient. A more typical case is aortic insufficiency with a vent in the left ventricle. Prior to aortic cross-clamping, blood from the bypass pump can regurgitate into the left ventricle and be returned to the bypass machine (via the left ventricle vent) without perfusing the patient. In each of these cases, the measured arterial pressure will be low. More important, the amount of blood flow that actually perfuses the patient will be the difference between the set flow of the pump (often 5 to 6 L/min) minus the shunt flow (1 to 2 L/min via vent). Therapy with vasoconstrictor drugs is ineffective because increased systemic resistance simply increases the amount of blood shunted back to the pump. The solution is cross-clamping of the aorta, which eliminates the shunt pathway.

Peripheral vascular resistance during bypass (PVR_B) can be described by the equation:

$$PVR_B = \frac{MAP}{pump\ flow}$$

because right atrial pressure is essentially zero. This allows some predictions for postbypass hemodynamics. For example, if pump flow is 5 L/min and mean arterial pressure is 40 mmHg, resistance on bypass is very low. Unless this resistance is altered, one can anticipate that immediately postbypass a cardiac output of 5 L/min generated by the patient will produce a relatively hypotensive mean arterial pressure of 40 mmHg. In this situation, before weaning from bypass, it seems logical to administer an α-adrenergic agonist to raise vascular resistance and achieve sufficient coronary perfusion. This is especially important for the hypertrophied left ventricle (e.g., aortic stenosis, hypertension).[22]

Bypass Pump Inflow Line Pressure

The perfusionist monitors the pressure in the arterial inflow line connecting the pump to the patient's arterial circulation. This line pressure is typically much higher than radial arterial pressure. The reasons for monitoring this pressure are as follows:

First, before actually going on bypass, pressure fluctuations in the inflow line should be similar to the patients arterial pressure to assure that arterial inflow line has been attached correctly to the pump. (In at least one case the arterial and venous lines to the pump were attached backward, resulting in death.)

Second, sudden increases in arterial inflow line pressure indicate arterial inflow line obstruction. A typical reason for this sudden pressure increase is the clamping of the arterial line by the surgeon without informing the perfusionist. Many pumps are equipped with a pressure sensor and automatic shut-off to prevent disruption of the pump tubing during inadvertent line occlusion. Another cause of high line pressure is aortic dissection by the arterial cannula. Here, high inflow line pressure may be accompanied by low patient (radial artery) pressure, and a tense-appearing aorta. Immediate discontinuation of bypass and resumption of the patient's own circulation may be critical for survival. Transesophageal echocardiography (if available) can be very useful to determine the extent of the dissection.

Radial Artery Versus Central Aortic Systolic Pressure

Normally, radial systolic blood pressure is higher, and radial diastolic pressure is lower, than corresponding pressures measured in the central aorta. These relationships occur as a result of decreased arterial compliance within the periphery and re-

flection and resonance of pressure waves within the arterial tree.[23] Although mean blood pressure is similar in both locations,[24] most physicians make clinical decisions based on systolic/diastolic measurements. Thus it is important that after cardiopulmonary bypass the relationship between central versus peripheral arterial systolic pressure is often reversed.[25] That is, the central aortic systolic pressure is now higher than that measured in the radial artery (Fig. 26-5). The radial catheter may "underestimate" central aortic pressure by 10 to 40 mmHg. Discrepancies in mean blood pressure tend to be smaller (5 to 15 mmHg) than those seen in systolic pressure. The mechanism of this change is not yet specifically defined, but evidence supports a vasodilatory or arteriovenous phenomena in the forearm or hand as being responsible.[10] Gravlee and associates[17] found that systolic pressure differences after cardiopulmonary bypass were not significantly influenced by duration of cardiopulmonary bypass, use of sodium nitroprusside or phenylephrine during the final 15 minutes of cardiopulmonary bypass, SVR, minimum cardiopulmonary bypass temperature, separation tempera-

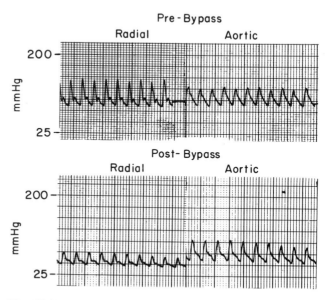

Fig. 26-5. Central versus peripheral systolic blood pressure measurements. In the pre-bypass period, systolic pressure measured in the radial artery is higher than in the central aorta. In the post-bypass period, the relationship has reversed so that the radial artery systolic pressure is now lower than the central aorta. (From Stern et al.,[25] with permission.)

ture, or duration of rewarming. It is unknown at what point during cardiopulmonary bypass radial-aortic pressure discrepancies develop, but most investigators report their resolution within 20 to 90 minutes after separation from cardiopulmonary bypass (Fig. 26-5).

Reversal of the central-to-peripheral pressure gradient is suspected when cardiac function appears satisfactory, yet blood pressure is low. Several actions can be taken: 1) palpation (by surgeon) of ascending aorta to estimate central BP; 2) measure central BP with a small needle (placed by surgeon) connected to transducer; 3) placement of a femoral arterial catheter. Some investigators advocate use of a long (50 cm) arterial catheter (either in the axillary or brachial artery) to monitor central blood pressure throughout the case.[26] However, flushing of such a long catheter theoretically could increase the risk of debris reaching the cerebral circulation. We prefer the previously discussed suggestions for this temporally limited problem.

Intra-Aortic Balloon Pump Counterpulsation

Proper timing of the intra-aortic balloon pump, allows inflation of the balloon in early diastole so as to augment aortic diastolic blood pressure and flow and thus improve coronary perfusion. Deflation of the balloon prior to systole reduces aortic pressure so as to facilitate left ventricular ejection (afterload reduction). Knowledge of intra-aortic balloon pump function (i.e., proper inflation and deflation timing) is necessary for correct assessment of the arterial pressure readings during intra-aortic balloon pump use. A typical error occurs in interpretation of systolic/diastolic pressure readings. For example, the monitor electronically chooses the highest number for "systolic" and the lowest number for "diastolic" pressure readings. However, during intra-aortic balloon pump use, the highest number often occurs with balloon pump inflation which is a *diastolic* event. The lowest number represents balloon deflation, a transient event occurring at the end of diastole (Fig. 26-6). Thus the true "diastolic pressure" must be somewhere between these numbers. The problem is that clinical decisions may be made on the basis of these electronic "systolic/diastolic" numbers. Thus the infusion of vasoactive agents to improve coronary flow makes little sense if one is simply treating balloon deflation pressure. In fact, it is likely that pressure during most of diastole is already higher than normal because of balloon pump inflation.

CENTRAL VENOUS PRESSURE MONITORING

Most authorities consider the establishment of *central venous access* to be standard in the practice of cardiac anesthesia, for at least two reasons. First, it provides a safe and reliable route for infusion of vasoactive (i.e., resuscitation) drugs and heparin. This function deserves emphasis. It is well described that various "vasopressor" drugs can cause serious necrosis of skin if administered through an infiltrated, peripheral intravenous catheter. However, administration of the systemic heparin dose into a peripheral intravenous catheter that has infiltrated may be catastrophic if unrecognized.

The second reason for central venous access is to monitor the central venous pressure (CVP) and it waveforms. Reliable CVP monitoring requires that the distal end of the catheter be located within a large intrathoracic vein or the right atrium.

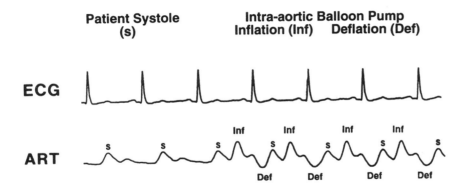

Patient Systole (s) **Intra-aortic Balloon Pump Inflation (Inf) Deflation (Def)**

ECG

ART

Fig. 26-6. Arterial pressure during intra-aortic balloon pump support. With initiation of intra-aortic balloon pump counterpulsation, the highest pressure corresponds to balloon pump inflation and the lowest pressure corresponds to balloon deflation. Both of these events occur during diastole.

Quantitative assessment of CVP, with a properly calibrated and zeroed transducer, system is useful for clinical evaluation of intravascular volume status, venous tone, and right ventricular performance. Assessment of waveform assists evaluation of some arrhythmias and right ventricular dysfunction complicated by tricuspid regurgitation. Finally, CVP measurement provides useful information pertaining to venous return to the cardiopulmonary bypass machine.

Central Venous Pressure and Intravascular Volume

The CVP is used to estimate intravascular volume because increased filling of the venous system will result in a rise in pressure. This relationship must be modified by the knowledge that the functional size and compliance of the venous system is not necessarily constant. For example, immediately following separation from cardiopulmonary bypass, the venous reservoir of the bypass machine typically is partially filled with blood. To facilitate return of this blood to the patient, nitroglycerin may be infused to dilate venous capacitance vessels and "make room" for the transfusion. Thus in this case, the CVP is decreasing at the same time that the intravascular volume is increasing.

Central Venous Pressure and Right Ventricular Function

The CVP waveform may provide additional information regarding right ventricular function and tricuspid valve regurgitation. As the severity of tricuspid insufficiency increases, the waveform of the CVP begins to resemble a right ventricular waveform (Fig. 26-7).[27] When this square-shaped CVP tracing is observed, right ventricular dysfunction is suspected. Two caveats should be noted. First, a true right ventricular pressure tracing can be observed if the "CVP port" of pulmonary artery catheter has been advanced into the right ventricle. The catheter should be withdrawn in this case to an appropriate distance. Second, the presence of a junctional rhythm will cause "cannon waves" in the CVP tracing that may resemble the tracing of tricuspid insufficiency. Inspection of the ECG rhythm will aid in this diagnosis.

If right ventricular dysfunction is suspected, accurate measurement of right artrial or CVP pressure is critical for guiding therapy. A typical mistake in such circumstances to focus on left ventricle filling (left atrial or pulmonary capillary wedge pressure) rather than the right. Left atrial pressure is often low because the dysfunctional right ventricle is unable to pump blood adequately, *not* because of hypovolemia. Nonetheless, a typical mistake is to infuse fluids that further distend the right ventricle and compromise its coronary blood flow. It is worth mentioning that this mistake can also be made during transesophageal echocardiography monitoring. In this case, the easily visualized left ventricle is seen to be "empty," which prompts vigorous fluid therapy. The less visible right ventricle is likely already distended and only worsens with fluid infusion. Finally, right ventricle failure is often accompanied by some degree of left ventricular failure. As a result, CVP monitoring alone will not provide enough information. When right and left heart filling pressures are expected to be different, measurement of each is indicated.

Cardiac Transplantation

Many centers routinely use only CVP monitoring in patients undergoing heart transplantation, with the pulmonary artery catheter being held in "reserve" for those cases complicated by severe pulmonary hypertension, right ventricular dysfunction, or low cardiac output. If pulmonary arteriolar dilators are considered in the approach to treating right ventricular dysfunction, then CVP monitoring alone is inadequate. In these patients extensive hemodynamic monitoring (i.e., pulmonary artery catheter, left atrial pressure, transesophageal echocardiography [TEE], or all the above) must be considered.

Central Venous Pressure and Cardiopulmonary Bypass

During cardiopulmonary bypass, the venous blood of the patient is directed to the bypass machine via plastic tubing in the right atrium (single cannula) or superior and inferior vena cavae (double cannulae). Because the venous blood flows down the tube by gravity, the CVP catheter in the right atrium often reads a negative pressure during cardiopulmonary bypass. The venous structures may intermittently collapse and momentarily stop venous return. In this case, the CVP pressure oscillates between a positive and negative number.

However, a sustained high positive CVP number may be indicative of an obstruction of the venous return to the bypass machine. In this circumstance, the perfusionist will have noted a fall in the venous reservoir volume and the patient's right atrium will be visibly distended. Some causes of poor venous return include: kinked venous return line, air lock in the venous tubing, and an overfilled venous reservoir due to excessive patient blood volume.

However, impairment of individual organ venous drainage may occur even with a non-elevated CVP tracing. For example, to enable anastomosis of vein grafts to the back of the heart, the apex of the heart is lifted upward. This may cause partial occlusion of the superior vena cava with resulting impairment of the venous drainage of the head. In this circumstance, the patient's head may appear plethoric with distension of superficial veins and abnormally brisk skin capillary refill. However, if the CVP port is distal to the obstruction, the CVP reading will be normal.

PULMONARY ARTERIAL PRESSURE MONITORING

The advent of the flow-directed pulmonary artery catheter has been described as a "quantum leap" in perioperative monitoring of patients undergoing complex surgical procedures.[28] Information obtained from the pulmonary artery catheter includes pulmonary artery pressures, cardiac filling pressures, cardiac output, and mixed venous oxygen saturation.[29,30] Using the pulmonary artery catheter allows us to make, for a given patient, therapeutic decisions with minimal physiologic uncertainty (i.e., with as much physiologic information as possible.) Does this mean that every adult undergoing cardiac surgery should have a pulmonary artery catheter placed? We believe the pulmonary artery catheter should be used selectively, based on the specific information required in light of the patient's underlying pathophysiology and the anticipated surgical insult. We acknowledge that in some patients the anticipated pulmonary artery catheter benefits do not justify its risks, or that the information it provides can be obtained by other, safer methods.[31,32] What special considerations help us rationally use the pulmonary artery catheter to optimize patient care without unduly offending the cost-containment sensibilities of all parties involved? These questions are explored.

Risks and Benefits of Pulmonary Artery Catheterization

The details of pulmonary artery catheter insertion, contraindications, pressure monitoring, thermodilution cardiac output measurement, and complications are discussed in detail in Chapter 5. However, the clinical benefits of the pulmonary artery catheter cannot be realized unless the risks to the patient are kept to a minimum.[33,34] This means a rigorous adherence to safety considerations (with

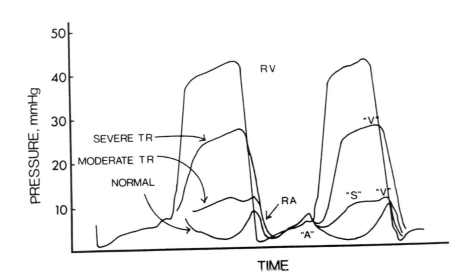

Fig. 26-7. Tricuspid insufficiency and right ventricular dysfunction. As the severity of tricuspid insufficiency worsens, the right atrial or CVP tracing begins to resemble that of the right ventricle. (Modified from Grossman,[27] with permission.)

specific reference to the area of cardiac anesthesia), some of which are discussed below.

Site of Catheterization

Many anesthetists favor an *internal jugular* (IJ) approach which facilitates intraoperative catheter manipulation. The right-sided internal jugular approach avoids the thoracic duct, but cannulation of the left internal jugular is an alternative. When using the left internal jugular approach, care is taken to limit the advancement of the dilator so as to prevent perforation of the innominate vein. In some surgical procedures, such as repair of aortic arch aneurysm, the left internal jugular site is undesirable because the innominate vein may be involved in the operation. The innominate vein is also at risk during reoperation procedures.

A *subclavian site*, preferred by many surgeons, is not favored perioperatively because of the possibility of tension pneumothorax. Further, when the sternum has been spread, a pulmonary artery catheter passed via the subclavian vein often becomes kinked rendering it useless. Pulmonary artery cath-

eterization can be successful via either external jugular or antecubital veins.

When the *external jugular vein* is to be used, a J wire can usually be passed into the superior vena cava, but the pulmonary artery catheter sheath may not be placed centrally.

Pulmonary artery catheters placed via the *femoral vein* are often present in patients who come from the cardiac catheterization laboratory. In such cases, before draping the patient, it should be determined that the catheter is in good position (i.e., is not in wedge position).

Catheterization of the Pulmonary Artery

In classic diagrams of passage of the catheter through the right atrium and right ventricle into the pulmonary artery, specific changes are noted to occur in the systolic and diastolic pressure measurements. However, in some cardiac surgical patients, a pronounced respiratory pattern causes large pressure variations simply because of inspiration and exhalation. In such cases, it is useful to examine the diastolic period of the tracing

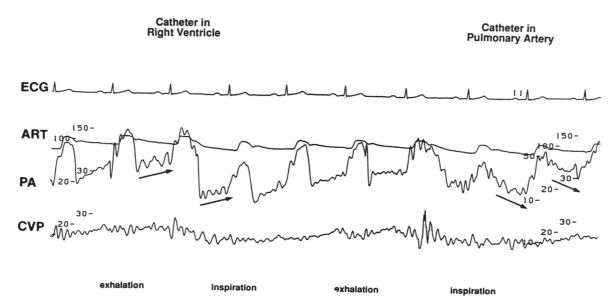

Fig. 26-8. Diastolic slope during pulmonary artery catheterization. The slope of the pressure tracing during diastole helps distinguish the right ventricle (*RV*) from the pulmonary artery (PA). In the RV, diastolic pressure rises (slopes up) as the ventricle fills. In the PA, diastolic pressure decreases (slopes down) as blood runs off into pulmonary vessels. Note that these distinguishing slopes are maintained in both inspiration and exhalation. In contrast, the diastolic pressure markedly fluctuates with respiration, rending it less useful for identifying location of the pulmonary artery catheter.

(Fig. 26-8). If the catheter is in the right ventricle, the diastolic pressure will be rising due to right ventricular filling. If the catheter is in the pulmonary artery, the diastolic pressure will be falling due to runoff of blood in the pulmonary artery.

Once a right ventricular pressure tracing is observed, many operators believe they now must rush the catheter through the right ventricle. This makes little sense. The center of the flowing stream of blood will have the highest velocity, and the greatest chance of propelling the balloon into the pulmonary artery. Passage through the right ventricle at a steady rate will be more likely to keep the balloon in the center of flow.

If, after several attempts, the catheter will not pass into the pulmonary artery, there are some "tricks." The patient can be taken out of Trendelenburg position and placed supine or even a little head-up, taking care not to induce hypotension. Warming of the catheter by the patient's blood may have caused the catheter to lose its preformed shape. Removal of the catheter (keep sterile) and injection of sterile iced saline through the distal pulmonary artery port will stiffen the catheter to its original shape. These tricks are especially useful in patients who have marked tricuspid regurgitation and a large right atrium.

There are few adults in whom a pulmonary artery catheter should be inserted beyond the 50-cm mark if the right internal jugular route is used. If, after a difficult passage, a definite pulmonary artery tracing is obtained, but an acceptable wedge pressure tracing does not appear until 55 or 60 cm, it is best to withdraw the catheter to the 50 cm position and wait 30 minutes or more. Usually the additional catheter length now looped in the right ventricle, will pass into the pulmonary artery and permit a wedge pressure to be obtained at the proper distance. Leaving the catheter at 55 to 60 cm may result in a wedged catheter during surgical heart manipulation. The extra length also theoretically increases the risk that a knot may be formed.

Recognition of Pulmonary Capillary Wedge Tracing

Clinicians utilizing the pulmonary artery catheter must be able to recognize both normal and abnormal wedge tracings. When the ventricular filling pressure has increased (either because of increased volume or decreased compliance), the normally small pressure fluctuations known as a, c, and v waves (atrial contraction, ventricular contraction, and atrial filling, respectively) become considerably more prominent[35] (Fig. 26-9). These pressure waves will be present even if the transducer is not correctly positioned at the level of the right atrium.

In circumstances of mitral insufficiency or significantly elevated left atrial pressure, the wedge tracing may superficially resemble the pulmonary artery tracing (Fig. 26-10). The inexperienced clinician may conclude that "the catheter cannot be wedged," when in fact, the catheter has been in a wedged position all along.[36] If these pressures of the wedged catheter are misinterpreted to be those of the pulmonary artery, the patient will not receive appropriate therapy. For example, a mean pressure of 20 mmHg is normal for the pulmonary artery and requires no treatment. However, a pulmonary capillary wedge pressure of 20 would indicate that aggressive treatment with inotropes, vasodilators, diuretics, and so on may be in order.

Pulmonary Artery Catheterization and Coronary Artery Bypass Surgery

Special considerations for pulmonary artery catheter use in patients undergoing coronary artery bypass surgery (CABG) include (1) prevention, detection, and treatment of myocardial ischemia[37] (i.e., cardioprotection) in the pre-cardiopulmonary bypass period; (2) detection of left ventricular distention during cardiopulmonary bypass; (3) assessment of ventricular function during and immediately after separation from cardiopulmonary bypass; and (4) as a secure route for emergency heparin administration in the event of right heart hemorrhage during reoperation.

Myocardial Ischemia

Myocardial ischemia in the pre-cardiopulmonary bypass period is reported to have an incidence of 10 to 50 percent, and it is associated with perioperative myocardial infarction in CABG patients.[38] The majority of episodes are not preceded by significant hemodynamic changes in blood pressure or heart rate.[38] An effective strategy for intraoperative cardioprotection is therefore a major goal for the anesthesiologist. This strategy includes the ability to detect myocardial ischemia reasonably early,

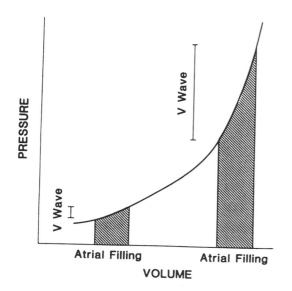

Fig. 26-9. Left atrial pressure-volume curve. On the left of this hypothetical left atrial pressure volume curve, the volume is low and compliance normal so the filling wave (V wave) is small. On the right, the left atrial volume is high and compliance is decreased. As a result the filling V wave is much more prominent. (From Ganz et al.,[35] with permission.)

the judicious use of anesthetic and vasoactive agents to prevent or treat ischemia, and the ability to monitor the efficacy of anti-ischemic therapy.[37]

Detection

Ischemia detection using the pulmonary artery catheter is based on the principle that ischemia reduces ventricular compliance and consequently raises left (or right) ventricular end-diastolic pressure.[29,39] Importantly, this compliance reduction represents an early, diastolic manifestation of ischemia. The pulmonary artery catheter allows assessment of left ventricular end-diastolic pressure via pulmonary capillary wedge pressure. An ischemia-induced increase in left ventricular end-diastolic pressure causes a detectable increase in pulmonary capillary wedge pressure, the appearance of increased A-C or V waves[40] in the pulmonary capillary wedge pressure waveform, or elevated pulmonary artery diastolic pressure (Fig. 26-11).

Recent studies suggest that the pulmonary artery catheter may not reliably detect mild, regionally isolated ischemia manifested by regional wall motion abnormalities. Such ischemia can be detected by other methods e.g., transesophageal echocardiography[41,42] (discussed below). Instead, the pulmonary artery catheter appears to be more useful for detection of global left ventricular dysfunction, as when intraoperative ischemia occurs in the setting of critical left main coronary stenosis, severe three-vessel

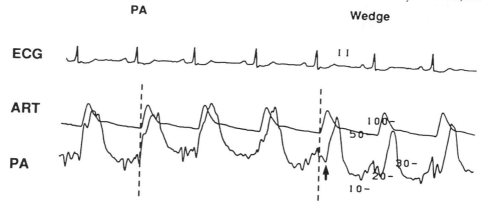

Fig. 26-10. Pulmonary capillary wedge pressure tracing, which resembles pulmonary artery pressure tracing. In circumstances of mitral insufficiency or other causes of elevated wedge pressure, the wedge tracing (wedge) superficially resembles the pulmonary artery tracing (PA). Distinction is facilitated by comparing the upstrokes of the arterial line (*ART*) and pulmonary artery (*PA*) pressure tracings. On the left, the upstrokes are approximately simultaneous (*dotted line*), indicating location of the catheter in the pulmonary artery. On the right, the upstroke occurs later (*arrow*) because it is that of the V wave, not the pulmonary artery.

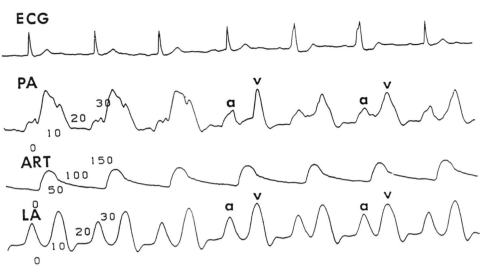

Fig. 26-11. Noncompliant left ventricle. When the pulmonary artery catheter (PA) is in wedge position, distinct a and v waves are seen. Simultaneous monitoring of left atrial catheter (*LA*) demonstrates that the wedge tracing is of reasonable fidelity. (From Ross et al.,[85] with permission.)

disease, or recent myocardial infarction. In these cases, ischemia is usually manifested as marked increases in pulmonary capillary wedge pressure and pulmonary artery pressure. Acute mitral regurgitation secondary to papillary muscle ischemia may also occur, and is often accompanied by a large V wave in the pulmonary capillary wedge pressure waveform. A decrease in cardiac output as measured by thermodilution, another function of the pulmonary artery catheter, confirms the suspicion of depressed left ventricular function secondary to severe ischemia.

Prevention

Another aspect of the cardioprotection strategy is prevention of ischemia.[37] Here the pulmonary artery catheter is used to maximize myocardial oxygen supply and limit oxygen demand.[43] For example, with critical coronary stenosis, coronary vasudilatory reserve may be expended simply to maintain resting coronary blood flow.[44] In this case, coronary blood flow is dependent on an adequate coronary perfusion pressure gradient. Because the coronary perfusion pressure distal to a coronary stenosis is substantially lower than aortic diastolic pressure, small changes in the left ventricular end-diastolic pressure may have significant impact on the gradient available for myocardial perfusion.[45] The pulmonary artery catheter facilitates therapy

(fluid restriction, nitroglycerin) which maintains a reasonably low pulmonary capillary wedge pressure (indicative of a low left ventricular end-diastolic pressure) so as to maximize the coronary perfusion pressure gradient. In other words, the pulmonary artery catheter functions to avoid the dangerous combination of low aortic pressure and high pulmonary capillary wedge pressure. The other goal of ischemia prevention is to limit myocardial oxygen demand.[46–48] Myocardial oxygen demand can be effectively reduced by volatile anesthetic agents,[49] or beta-adrenergic blocking agents (Fig. 26-12).

The Pulmonary Artery Catheter and Cardiopulmonary Bypass

An important related aspect of cardioprotection during cardiopulmonary bypass is prevention of left ventricular distention. Left ventricular distension may occur during ventricular fibrillation, cardioplegia administration, surgical operation, and reperfusion. Ventricular distention increases myocardial oxygen demand by increasing myocardial wall tension.[50] At the same time, subendocardial perfusion (blood or cardioplegia perfusate) is reduced secondary to increased intracavitary pressure.[50] This may result in myocardial injury and severe ventricular dysfunction. During cardiopulmonary bypass ventricular distention can be detected by (1) surgical palpation, (2) monitoring right and left atrial pressures, or (3) monitoring pulmonary arterial pressure. The most practical approach is to use the pulmonary artery catheter to continuously monitor right atrial and pulmonary artery pressures. As the left ventricle becomes distended, the pressure is transmitted backward through the mitral valve (rendered incompetent) into the left atrium, and the pulmonary circulation where it is measured by the pulmonary artery catheter. The right atrial port on the pulmonary artery catheter can be used to monitor for right ventricular distention caused, usually, by inadequate venous drainage. It should be noted that for the pulmonary artery catheter to detect left ventricular distention the mitral valve must be incompetent, as it almost always is when severe distention occurs. It has been reported, however, that severe left ventricular distention can occur with a competent mitral valve and not be accompanied by elevated pulmonary artery pressure.[51] Nonetheless, we believe that an effective strategy for cardioprotection includes vigilant pulmonary artery pressure monitoring during cardiopulmonary bypass, particularly in patients with poor or marginal left ventricular function and at centers where left ventricular venting (via right superior pulmonary vein, aortic root, or pulmonary artery) is not a routine practice.

Separation from Cardiopulmonary Bypass

The pulmonary artery catheter facilitates separation from cardiopulmonary bypass in several important ways.

First, some measure of ventricular filling is necessary during the separation process. Various methods of estimating left ventricular filling pressure include (1) monitoring pulmonary artery diastolic pressure, (2) intermittently measuring pulmonary capillary wedge pressure, (3) visual inspection of the heart, (4) palpation of the pulmonary artery, and (5) monitoring of the left atrial pressure directly by catheter or temporary needle. The pulmonary artery catheter provides a continuous monitor of ventricular filling that allows comparison to pre-bypass measurements, and extends into the postoperative period. Monitoring the central venous pressure has also been used, although this actually measures right ventricular filling pressure.

It has been argued that changes in the central venous pressure satisfactorily reflect changes in the pulmonary capillary wedge pressure as long as left ventricular dysfunction is not present.[52] The problem is that the relationship between central venous pressure and pulmonary capillary wedge pressure for one patient is not the same for another.[53] More importantly, however, normal ventricular function is not guaranteed by the preoperative ejection fraction, but rather is related many intraoperative factors including (1) preoperative ischemia, (2) adequacy of cardioplegia, (3) duration of aortic cross-clamping, (4) duration of ventricular fibrillation, and (5) quality of the coronary bypass grafts.

The pulmonary artery catheter also supplies data regarding the need for inotropic support. Early, during partial filling of the heart, an estimate is made of ventricular performance. For example, if the heart is able to generate a satisfactory blood pressure (e.g., 90 mmHg systolic) with a modestly filled left ventricle (pulmonary artery diastolic pressure = 5 to 8 mmHg) it is likely that no assistance will be needed. However, if systemic blood pressure is marginal (e.g., 60 to 70 mmHg systolic) and the left ventricle is sufficiently full (pulmonary artery diastolic pressure = 10 to 15 mmHg), it is likely that some inotropic support will be necessary (Fig. 26-13). After separation from bypass, meas-

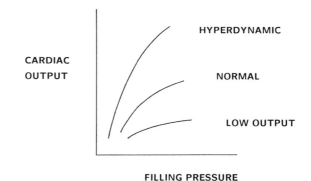

Fig. 26-12. Ventricular function described by Starling curves. Knowledge of ventricular function facilitates choice of therapy for ischemia prevention. The patient with low cardiac output and elevated filling pressure will benefit improved oxygen supply (e.g., nitroglycerin). In contrast, the hyperdynamic patient will benefit from control of oxygen consumption (e.g., beta-adrenergic blockade).

BEGIN PARTIAL BYPASS

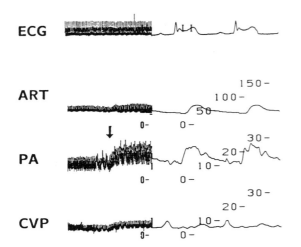

Fig. 26-13. Partial bypass and indication for inotropic support. At the *arrow*, partiai occlusion of the venous return line causes the heart to fill and eject blood. At a moderate pulmonary artery filling pressure, the generated systemic pressure is only modest. Inotropic support is needed. (From Ross et al.,[85] with permission.)

urement of cardiac output by thermodilution guides the administration of vasoactive agents.

Data obtained from the pulmonary artery catheter will also aid in providing optimal coronary perfusion during and after cardiopulmonary bypass.[54–56] Finally, the pulmonary artery catheter provides information which is useful in differentiating the potential causes of hypotension during separation from cardiopulmonary bypass (Table 26-1).

Pulmonary Artery Catheterization and Valvular Heart Surgery

In most centers, the pulmonary artery catheter is used more extensively in patients undergoing valvular heart surgery than in CABG patients. The decision to use the pulmonary artery catheter in patients undergoing valve surgery is based on the same principles of cardioprotection as discussed for CABG patients plus physiologic considerations of the individual valve lesion.

Aortic Stenosis

Patients with critical aortic stenosis have an abnormal myocardial oxygen supply/demand balance even when the coronary arteries are normal.[22] Coronary resistance vessels may be maximally dilated to supply the hypertrophied left ventricle. Decreased left ventricular compliance and elevated left ventricular end-diastolic pressure contribute to a marginally adequate coronary perfusion pressure. Further, because of the stenotic aortic valve, the heart is unable to compensate for systemic vasodilation by increasing cardiac output.

The key role of the pulmonary artery catheter for aortic stenosis is the assessment of adequate left ventricular filling. Because of left ventricular hypertrophy, a higher than normal left ventricular end-diastolic pressure is necessary for normal fill-

TABLE 26-1. Causes of Hypotension During Separation from Cardiopulmonary Bypass

	ART	PCWP	PAP	CVP	Cardiac Output[a]
Hypovolemia	Low	Low	Low	Low	Low
Vasodilation	Low	Normal	Normal	Normal	High
Left ventricular failure	Low	High	High	Normal	Low
Acute mitral insufficiency	Low	Very high	Very high	Normal to high	Low
Pulmonary vasoconstriction	Low	Low	High	High	Low
Right ventricular failure	Low	Low	Low	High	Low

[a]Note that cardiac output is high only in the circumstance of systemic vasodilation. The utility of cardiac output measurement is to monitor the effectiveness of therapy rather than be the key to diagnosis.

ART, arterial line; PCWP, pulmonary capillary wedge pressure; PAP, pulmonary artery pressure; CVP, central venous pressure.

ing, and patients with aortic stenosis are very sensitive to hypovolemia. If the elevated left ventricular diastolic pressure is sufficient to cause dyspnea in the preoperative period, some degree of diuresis may have been instituted. Such patients are at increased risk for hypotension because positive pressure ventilation may significantly decrease venous return. Measurement of left ventricular filling pressure (pulmonary capillary wedge pressure) and treatment of hypovolemia should take place before induction of anesthesia.

Mitral Stenosis

In patients with mitral stenosis, a gradient exists between the left atrium and the left ventricle. The left ventricle is relatively underfilled and the left atrium is overfilled. It is important to recognize that an elevated left atrial pressure is necessary to maintain adequate left ventricular filling. This is an issue when preoperative exertional dyspnea has been treated with diuresis. This therapy improves pulmonary congestion, but reduces the pressure gradient across the mitral valve. Reduction in venous return by anesthesia induction and positive pressure ventilation may further reduce left ventricular filling such that hypotension ensues. The pulmonary artery catheter is used to assess pulmonary capillary wedge pressure and treat hypovolemia prior to anesthesia induction. One caveat is that an elevated pulmonary capillary wedge pressure in mitral stenosis is not indicative of poor coronary perfusion gradient. In fact, the left ventricular end-diastolic pressure may be normal or even low in this situation.

Long-standing mitral stenosis may be accompanied by pulmonary vascular changes and subsequent right ventricular hypertrophy. During separation from bypass, marked pulmonary vasoconstriction may contribute to right ventricular dysfunction. Here the pulmonary artery catheter facilitates diagnosis of the problem, choice of optimal inotropic (e.g., pure beta-adrenergic agonist) and vasodilator agents, and assessment of efficacy of therapy.

Aortic Insufficiency and Mitral Regurgitation

Patients with regurgitant valvular lesions are susceptible to rapid and large increases in left ventricular end-diastolic pressure. Because mitral regur-

gitation, and to a lesser extent aortic insufficiency, are dynamic lesions, any physiologic insult that worsens valvular regurgitation (e.g., stress-induced vasoconstriction) will be reflected immediately by elevated pulmonary artery pressures. Continuous monitoring of pulmonary artery pressure during critical periods of induction and intubation may provide warning of impending problems.

In regurgitant lesions, vasodilator agents can markedly improve forward cardiac output.[57–59] The pulmonary artery catheter thus allows optimal vasodilator therapy. In the case of mitral insufficiency, large regurgitant pressure waves (V waves) may be visible in the pulmonary capillary wedge pressure tracing which disappear with vasodilator therapy (Fig. 26-14). If mitral insufficiency was due to ischemia, disappearance of these regurgitant waves would be a useful end point. However, in long-standing mitral insufficiency, the left atrium may become markedly dilated and compliant. In this case, significant mitral regurgitation can be present without manifestation of regurgitant V waves.[60] Differences in left atrial compliance are probably an important component of the reason why the height of regurgitant V waves has not been found to correlate with the severity of mitral regurgitation.[61–62]

TRANSESOPHAGEAL ECHOCARDIOGRAPHY

Occasionally, comparison is made between transesophageal echocardiography (TEE) and the pulmonary artery catheter.[63] Advocates of TEE emphasize that the measurement of filling *volumes* by echocardiography is superior to the measurement of *pressures* by the pulmonary artery catheter, because compliance is known to be nonconstant. Pulmonary artery catheter advocates emphasize that pressure *not* volume measurements are critical for determination of pulmonary vascular resistance and coronary perfusion pressure. Yet, in fact, these two sophisticated monitoring methods have quite different strengths and weaknesses. For example, the ability of the TEE to provide anatomic diagnosis is completely unique (Fig. 26-15). Instead of substitution of one method for the other, selective monitoring means that one or perhaps both monitors will be selected based on the circumstances of the patient and surgery.

CABG Surgery

Applications for TEE in CABG patients include (1) detection of myocardial ischemia; (2) evaluation of associated valvular lesions (e.g., ischemic mitral regurgitation; (3) detection of left ventricular distention during cardiopulmonary bypass; (4) evaluation of ventricular and valvular function during separation from cardiopulmonary bypass; (5) confirmation of placement of intra-aortic balloon pump.

Use of TEE for ischemia monitoring in CABG patients has been recently reviewed.[42] Intraoperative myocardial ischemia produces regional wall motion abnormalities detectable by TEE as changes in both wall thickening and excursion. Reductions in wall thickening are more sensitive for ischemia than changes in excursion. Also, severe acute regional changes in excursion, such as severe hypokinesis, akinesis, or dyskinesias, are more specific for ischemia than is mild hypokinesis. Regional wall motion abnormalities generally precede ECG changes, with the delay in ECG evidence being inversely proportional to the degree of ischemia.[64] In CABG patients new, persistent intraoperative regional wall motion abnormalities, particularly post-cardiopulmonary bypass, are predictive of perioperative cardiac morbidity.[65] Electrocardiography, on the other hand, via either 7-lead or Holter ECG, is not predictive.

The primary limitation of TEE for ischemia monitoring is that not all regional wall motion abnormalities indicate ischemia.[66,67] Nonischemic factors affecting regional wall motion, or its interpretation by TEE, include (1) chronic, fixed myocardial in-

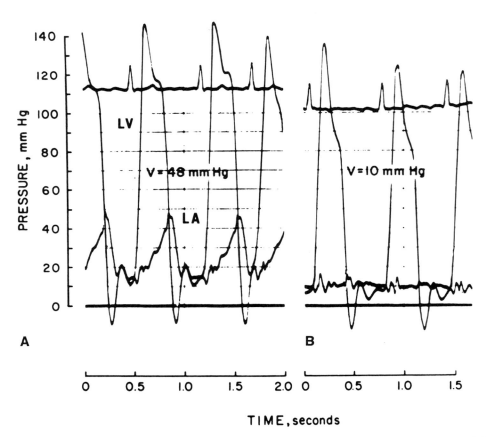

Fig. 26-14. Resolution of mitral regurgitation V wave with nitroprusside, showing left atrial and left ventricular tracings. (**A**) Before nitroprusside, a tall (70 mmHg) regurgitant wave is seen. (**B**) After nitroprusside, this regurgitant wave has considerably decreased. (Adapted from Harshaw et al.,[86] with permission.)

jury; (2) acute changes in loading conditions; (3) altered electrical activation of ventricular contraction; and (4) stunned myocardium with prolonged segmental dysfunction after reperfusion.[68] Additional limitations include difficulties in real-time interpretation of regional wall motion abnormalities, and the unresolved question of what constitutes adequate training for anesthesiologist echocardiographers.

Intraoperative TEE is becoming a useful tool for evaluation and management of associated valvular lesions in patients undergoing CABG surgery. For example, TEE has been used to assess the severity of ischemic mitral regurgitation. Because of poor survival statistics for patients with chronic, ischemic mitral regurgitation who undergo combined CABG and mitral valve repair or replacement, the ability to accurately assess the severity of mitral regurgitation at the time of surgery allows better patient selection and improved outcomes.[69] For example, patients with ischemic symptoms and moderate mitral regurgitation in the pre-cardiopulmonary bypass period can undergo CABG alone with operative mortality of 3 to 4 percent versus up to 28 percent for the combined procedure.[70]

The deleterious effects of left ventricular distention on myocardial perfusion and oxygen demand during cardiopulmonary bypass have been dis-

cussed. If the TEE probe is already in place, the short-axis view can be used intermittently during cardiopulmonary bypass to detect left ventricular distention (if the heart is not being retracted out of the pericardium). Use of TEE specifically for routine monitoring of left ventricular distention is probably not warranted.

Valvular Surgery

Doppler echocardiography is now widely used for evaluation and monitoring in patients undergoing valvular procedures, particularly reparative or reconstructive procedures. Successful valve repair surgery is associated with improved survival, better ventricular function, and fewer thromboembolic complications than prosthetic valve replacement.[71] Doppler echocardiography can be used to determine the nature and severity of valve dysfunction, the need for and feasibility of valve repair, and to facilitate planning of the surgical procedure. In the immediate post-cardiopulmonary bypass period, adequacy of repair, the presence of associated complications, and ventricular function can be easily assessed. Doppler echocardiography is particularly useful for identifying the underlying cause of

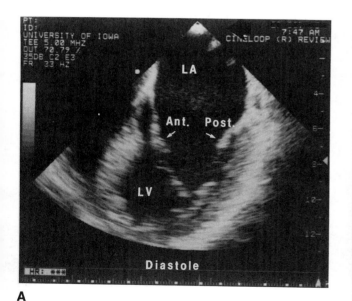

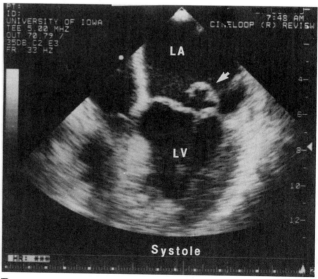

A **B**

Fig. 26-15. (A & B) Transesophageal echocardiography utilized during mitral valve repair. The clearly abnormal posterior leaflet of the mitral valve is seen prolapsing into the left atrium (LA). LV, left ventricle.

valve disease; this is important because the etiology (e.g., myxomatous degeneration versus ischemic heart disease) determines the need, feasibility, and type of repair. Also, the cause of residual valve dysfunction after repair can be identified by careful TEE examination. Although reparative techniques have been described for all valve positions, the mitral and tricuspid valves most commonly undergo repair. Doppler echocardiography-guided repairs may involve the valve annulus (e.g., tricuspid annuloplasty) or the leaflets and subvalvular apparatus (e.g., mitral chordal repair). Clearly TEE-guided surgery requires considerable expertise.

MONITORING OF BLOOD TESTS DURING CARDIAC SURGERY

Coagulation

Establishment of adequate anticoagulation is essential for cardiopulmonary bypass. Activated clotting time is used in most institutions, with baseline normal ranging from 75 to 120 seconds.[72] Heparin, in a dose 300 U/kg or 3 mg/kg, is given through a central line from which blood can be freely aspirated. At 2 to 4 minutes later, an activated clotting time should demonstrate adequate anticoagulation, which means >400 seconds at most centers. The activated clotting time that correlates with adequate anticoagulation is controversial.[73] Other methods, such as the automated protamine titration device, are available for monitoring anticoagulation but cost much more. In the absence of a clearly superior method, the activated clotting time remains a widely used, practical measure of anticoagulant status. One exception is the use of aprotinin (see Ch. 22).

Blood Gas

Prior to anesthesia induction, blood gas analysis in the stable cardiac surgery patient is probably unnecessary. However, the unstable patient or the prolonged hospitalized patient likely will benefit by analysis. Treatable conditions such as metabolic acidosis and hypoxemia may be identified.

During cardiopulmonary bypass, monitoring of arterial and venous blood gases assists in adjustments of the perfusion system (i.e., flow pressure,

O_2 flow, etc.). An area of recent controversy has concerned what blood gas values are appropriate during hypothermia.[74–77] In the past, it was felt that the blood pH and PCO_2 should be 7.4 and 40 at hypothermic temperatures. Because gas solubility increases as temperature falls, the partial pressure decreases if total gas content remains the same. Thus carbon dioxide was routinely added during hypothermic bypass. This method of management has been named *pH-stat* to indicate the goal of constant pH.

More recently, attention has focused on the maintenance of natural electrochemical neutrality at hypothermic temperatures. Thus, as temperature decreases, the dissociation of water into OH^- and H^+ decreases, thereby increasing the pH of the water. Similarly, blood in vitro will naturally show a decrease in PCO_2 as temperature decreases. Thus the pH change of blood follows the pH change of water as temperature falls. This management strategy is characteristic of poikilothermic animals, and is felt to provide a better environment for various enzyme functions. It has been named *alpha-stat* to emphasize the important buffer role of the α-imidazole ring of the histidine moiety in blood proteins. In this system *no* CO_2 is added on bypass (Table 26-2).

Before weaning from bypass, blood pH changes that developed during bypass should be normalized. Metabolic acidosis may make separation difficult due to increases in pulmonary vascular resistance, and reducing the effectiveness of inotropic drugs. In the post-bypass period, blood gas analysis may also be helpful. Unexpected hypoxemia may

TABLE 26-2. Carbon Dioxide Management on Bypass

Issue	pH-Stat	Alpha-Stat
Carbon dioxide adding during hypothermia?	Yes	No
pH/PCO_2 at 37°C	7.28/55	7.4/40[a]
pH/PCO_2 at 28°C	7.4/40	7.52/28

[a] The strategy of ''alpha-stat'' is to allow the pH and PCO_2 to change normally as the temperature decreases. When such blood is warmed to 37° in the blood gas analyzer, the pH and PCO_2 are 7.4 and 40. In contrast, the pH-stat strategy adds carbon diaoxide during hypothermia so that hypothermic blood has pH and PCO_2 of 7.4 and 40. When this blood is warmed to 37°C in the blood gas analyzer, the excessive CO_2 content causes pH and PCO_2 to be 7.28 and 55.

(From Ross et al.,[85] with permission.)

be due to atelectasis, low mixed venous P_{O_2}, or accumulated blood in the pleural space due to internal mammary artery dissection. A developing metabolic acidosis suggests poor tissue perfusion, and may indicate reduced cardiac output or excessive vasoconstriction. The marginal patient will benefit from more frequent blood gas and pH analysis to guide therapy.

Hematocrit

Because of marked fluid shifts, inevitable bleeding, and blood lost during surgery, patients' hematocrit will decrease following cardiac surgery. During hypothermic cardiopulmonary bypass, a hemodiluted hematocrit of 20 is frequently observed. However, a bypass hematocrit less than 20 percent may contribute to hypotension due to low viscosity. Excessively low hematocrits can be associated with decreased oxygen availability to the tissues resulting in anaerobic metabolism and metabolic acidosis.[78]

At the end of cardiopulmonary bypass, rather than relying on any specific number, the clinical circumstance will often make the decision regarding an "acceptable" hematocrit. For example, a hematocrit of 24 in a hyperdynamic patient who requires nitroprusside probably will not require transfusion. In contrast, a hematocrit of 26 in a patient with low cardiac output despite inotropic support may be too low. In this case, although cardiac output cannot be increased, the critical factor of oxygen delivery to the tissues can be improved with a higher hematocrit. The presence of ongoing bleeding significantly increases the need for transfusion.

Blood Glucose

Insulin-dependent diabetic patients will benefit from determination of blood glucose to prevent hypoglycemia as well as to avoid unnecessary administration of dextrose-containing intravenous fluids. Hyperglycemia is avoided because it has been demonstrated to worsen experimental ischemic central nervous system injury.[79]

Serum Potassium

Potassium levels normally decrease during hypothermic bypass, apparently due to increased catecholamine levels that drive the sodium-potassium pump to transfer K^+ into cells. High urinary output during bypass, whether due to hemodilution or to mannitol in the pump prime, may also contribute to potassium depletion. Finally the use of beta-adrenergic agonists during separation from bypass drives potassium into the cells, again contributing to low serum potassium levels. In the days before potassium-containing cardioplegia was routinely used, hypokalemia was a serious problem.

During administration of high-dose potassium cardioplegia, the hypokalemia formerly encountered routinely is rarely seen intraoperatively but still occurs postoperatively. Actually, there may be hyperkalemia, partly because of absorbed cardioplegia and partly because serum potassium is known to rise (come out of the cells) during rewarming. If asystole continues after the cross-clamp is removed, measurement of serum potassium is likely to demonstrate hyperkalemia. The best therapy is to wait for the potassium level to decrease by itself. In fact, there is evidence that a longer period of asystolic reperfusion is beneficial to the heart.[80] Temporary electrical pacing is usually effective even during hyperkalemia.

In contrast, rapid correction of serum potassium is unnecessarily dangerous. Giving insulin and dextrose to a nondiabetic patient is likely to be associated with severe hypokalemia and its attendent serious arrhythmias (premature ventricular contractions, ventricular tachycardia, and ventricular fibrillation). Large-dose furosemide administration may cause massive diuresis and require continuous crystalloid replacement. A gentler, more controlled method of potassium lowering is use of a hemofiltration (in essence a dialyzer) device by the perfusionist.[81] Finally, the use of a beta-adrenergic agonist, for example, epinephrine, can lower the serum K^+.[82]

SPECIAL CONSIDERATIONS OF PEDIATRIC CARDIAC SURGERY

Noninvasive Monitors

Monitors that can be applied include the ECG, pulse oximeter, blood pressure cuff, precordial stethoscope, and manual palpation of the pulse.

The pulse oximeter is particularly useful in patients who have reduced pulmonary blood flow or right-to-left shunts. In Fallot's tetralogy a falling saturation may be indicative of increased right to left shunting due to a "tet spell." The site chosen for pulse oximetry is important. Consider a patient with patent ductus arteriosus and elevated pulmonary vascular resistance. An oximeter placed on the right arm (preductal) indicates adequacy of pulmonary oxygenation and may show good saturation. In contrast, an oximeter placed on a lower extremity (postductal) reflects the degree of right to left shunting and may simultaneously show desaturation. In such cases, two pulse oximeter units should be used.

The site of blood pressure monitoring by cuff is important because of potential differences among the extremities. Patients with coarctation may have decreased pressures in the left arm as well as in the lower extremities. Patients with a prior Blalock-Taussig shunt may also have a variation between the arms (lower of the side of the shunt). Manual palpation of the pulse should routinely be employed during anesthetic induction. Although pulse palpation is a qualitative assessment, it provides early assessment and facilitates early treatment of problems.

Perhaps the most useful monitor in the induction period is the precordial stethoscope. Adequacy of ventilation is critical in patients with congenital heart disease. Patients with cyanotic lesions may not tolerate further decreases in arterial oxygenation. Also, the degree of right-to-left shunting can be markedly altered by changes in pulmonary vascular resistance[83,84] (increased by hypercarbia and hypoxic pulmonary vasoconstriction). The precordial stethoscope also is useful to assess cardiac function. A change from crisp to muffled heart tones may indicate an urgent necessity to stimulate the heart. The appearance or change in character of a heart murmur may indicate a change in the direction of quantity of blood flow.

Invasive Monitors

Arterial pressure monitoring is essential for most procedures. A percutaneous arterial line is preferable to a cutdown technique, which requires sutures around the vessel. If only one site is optimal for accurate monitoring (e.g., right arm in coarctation), the number of percutaneous attempts should be limited so as not to make subsequent cutdown difficult.

Central venous pressure monitoring can be achieved by percutaneous catheterization of the internal or external jugular vein, subclavian or femoral vein, or a long catheter via the antecubital vein. The use of double or triple lumen catheters allows central venous pressure monitoring, as well as drug infusions. When percutaneously catheterizing the internal jugular vein, it is important to use the carotid artery as a landmark. The color of the blood obtained from the presumed venous site should be compared blood from a known arterial site (radial arterial line). Patients with congenital lesions may well have desaturated arterial blood. Thus one cannot conclude that dark blood is venous unless it is compared to a reference sample (it will almost always be visibly darker than a known arterial sample drawn simultaneously). Oxygen saturation of both samples can be measured in the laboratory. The pressure can be transduced, but the fidelity of such a signal, especially after difficult cannulation, may be questionable (i.e., a dampened arterial trace may be misinterpreted as being venous). Intraoperatively, left and right atrial as well as pulmonary artery catheters can also be directly placed by the surgeon. Pulmonary artery catheters equipped with a venous oxygen saturation monitor can be quite helpful as change in mixed venous oxygen saturation reflect changes in cardiac output.

Other considerations in monitoring include the heparin flush system, which keeps catheters patent. A continuous flush system at 3 ml/h for an arterial catheter may contribute to fluid overloading in infants. We use a calibrated pump system to flush the lines in infants to minimize fluid administration.

SUMMARY

The preceding discussion represents a reasonable approach to selective monitoring for cardiac procedures. It makes sense that various monitoring techniques would be selected based on the patient's condition, the proposed procedure, incidence of complications, and cost of the technique. However, the experienced anesthesiologist recognizes that other considerations are involved. First is the element of uncertainty that accompanies every cardiac surgical procedure. A 1 to 5 (or more) percent *mortality* from coronary artery bypass surgery means that a number of patients will not survive. Which ones will these be? In addition, many patients will experience but survive an unexpected life-threatening problem such as: a severe protamine reaction causing pulmonary hypertension, an air bubble to the right coronary artery causing right ventricular failure, severe bleeding causing cardiac tamponade, or postoperative myocardial ischemia or infarction. Which ones will these be? The truth is that most of these potentially serious problems are unpredictable, yet occur with some frequency. The utilization of advanced cardiac monitoring makes possible early and accurate diagnosis.

The second consideration is acknowledgement that accuracy of clinical assessment is limited. For example, it had been demonstrated years ago that the assessment of cyanosis was difficult with the human eye alone. Yet the arrival of pulse oximetry was not welcomed by all clinicians. Many contended that it was just unnecessary. Most studies of cardiovascular clinical evaluation find a similar lack of accuracy. The etiology of hypotension (hypovolemia, vasodilation, cardiac ischemia) is a typical example. With monitoring devices, aspects of the cardiovascular system can be measured and appropriate therapy undertaken. Without monitoring devices, the clinician makes a best guess and "tries" a therapy (usually "give fluids"). The patient's response either supports or invalidates this first assessment, and facilitates a second approximation. Hopefully this process eventually identifies the correct therapy and the patient benefits. Occasionally however, even if the patient fails to respond, the original therapy is repeated again because the first trial was "not enough" (more fluids and Trendelenberg position). Unfortunately if incorrect, some patients will suffer from pulmonary congestion and worsened myocardial ischemia.

Overall, one must recognize that the processes of cardiac surgery and cardiopulmonary bypass present major alterations to patient homeostasis. The anesthesiologist has the ability to correct these disturbances. Appropriate selection and utilization of monitoring devices based on physiology, patient disease, and surgical procedure will provide optimal care at reasonable risk and cost.

REFERENCES

1. Knight AA, Hollenberg M, London MJ et al: Perioperative myocardial ischemia: importance of the preoperative ischemic pattern. Anesthesiology 68:681, 1988
2. Weiner DA, Ryan TJ, McCabe CH et al: Correlations among history of angina, ST-segment response and prevalence of coronary-artery disease in the coronary artery surgery study (CASS). N Engl J Med 301:230, 1979
3. Lell WA: Myocardial protection during cardiopulmonary bypass. p. 3. In: Kaplan JA (ed): Cardiac Anesthesia. 3rd Ed. WB Saunders, Philadelphia, 1993
4. Khamabatta HJ, Stone JG, Wald A, Mongero LB: Electrocardiographic artifacts during cardiopulmonary bypass. Anesth Analg 71:88, 1990
5. Metz S: ECG artifacts during cardiopulmonary bypass: an alternative method. [Letter]. Anesth Analg 72:715, 1991
6. Hindman BJ, Lillehaug SL, Tinker JH: Cardiopulmonary bypass and the anesthesiologist. p. 926. In Kaplan JA (ed): Cardiac Anesthesia. 3rd Ed. WB Saunders, Philadelphia, 1993
7. Kates RA, Zaidan JR, Kaplan JA: Esophageal lead for intraoperative electrocardiographic monitoring. Anesth Analg 61:781, 1982
8. Waldo AL, Machean WAH: Diagnosis and Treatment of Cardiac Arrhythmias Following Open Heart Surgery. Futura, New York, 1980
9. Zaidan JR, Freniere S: Use of a pacing pulmonary artery catheter during cardiac surgery. Ann Thorac Surg 35:633, 1983
10. Hindman BJ, Lillehaug SL, Tinker JH: Cardiopulmonary bypass and the anesthesiologist. p. 927. In Kaplan JA (ed): Cardiac Anesthesia. 3rd Ed. WB Saunders, Philadelphia, 1993
11. Noback CR, Tinker JH: Hypothermia after cardiopulmonary bypass in man. Anesthesiology 53:277, 1980
12. Stanley T, Jackson J: The influence of blood flow and arterial blood pressure during cardiopulmonary bypass on deltoid muscle gas tensions and body temperature after bypass. Can Anaesth Soc J 26:277, 1979
13. Stupfel M, Severinghaus JW: Internal body temperature gradients during anesthesia and hypothermia and effect of vagotomy. J Appl Physiol 9:380, 1956
14. Hindman BJ, Dexter F, Cutkomp J et al: Brain blood flow and metabolism do not decrease at stable brain temperature during cardiopulmonary bypass in rabbits. Anesthesiology 77:342, 1992
15. Davis FM, Barnes PK, Bailey JS: Aural thermometry during profound hypothermia. Anaesth Intens Care 9:124, 1981

16. Ryan JF, Raines J, Dalton BC et al: Arterial dynamics of radial artery cannulation. Anesth Analg 52:1015, 1973

17. Gravlee GP, Wong AB, Adkins TG et al: A comparison of radial, brachial, and aortic pressures after cardiopulmonary bypass. J Cardiothorac Anesth 3:20, 1989

18. Lowenstein E, Little JW, Hing HL: Prevention of cerebral embolization from flushing radial artery cannulas. N Engl J Med 285:1414, 1971

19. Stockard JJ, Bickford RG, Myers RR et al: Hypotension-induced changes in cerebral function during cardiac surgery. Stroke 5:730, 1974

20. Stockard JJ, Bickford RG, Schauble JF: Pressure-dependent cerebral ischemia during cardiopulmonary bypass. Neurology 23:521, 1973

21. Gordon RJ, Ravin M, Daicoff GR et al: Effects of hemodilution on hypotension during cardiopulmonary bypass. Anesth Analg 54:482, 1975

22. Marcus M, Doty D, Hiratzka L et al: Decreased coronary reserve: a mechanism for angina pectoris in patients with aortic stenosis and normal coronary arteries. N Engl J Med 307:1363, 1982

23. O'Rourke MF, Yaginuma T: Wave reflections and the arterial pulse. Arch Intern Med 144:366, 1984

24. Hamilton WF, Dow P: An experimental study of the standing waves in the pulse propagated through the aorta. Am J Physiol 125:48, 1939

25. Stern DH, Gerson JI, Allen FB, Parker FB: Can we trust the direct radial artery pressure immediately following cardiopulmonary bypass? Anesthesiology 62:557, 1985

26. Van Beck JO, White RD, Abenstein JP et al: Comparison of axillary artery or brachial artery pressure with aortic pressure after cardiopulmonary bypass using a long radial artery catheter. J Cardiothorac Vasc Anesth 7:312, 1993

27. Grossman W: Cardiac Catheterization and Angiography. 3rd Ed. p. 378. Lea & Febiger, Philadelphia, 1986

28. Reich DL, Kaplan JA: Hemodynamic monitoring. p. 276. In Kaplan JA (ed): Cardiac Anesthesia. 3rd Ed. WB Saunders, Philadelphia, 1993

29. Forrester J, Diamond G, McHugh T, Swan HJC: Filling pressures in the right and left sides of the heart in acute myocardial infarction. N Engl J Med 285:190, 1971

30. Ganz W, Swan HJC: Measurement of blood flow by thermodilution. Am J Cardiol 29:241, 1972

31. Bashein G, Johnson P, Davis K, Ivey T: Elective coronary bypass surgery without pulmonary artery catheter monitoring. Anesthesiology 63:451, 1985

32. Robin ED: The cult of the Swan-Ganz catheter. Ann Intern Med 103:445, 1985

33. Shah KB, Rao TLK, Laughlin S, El-Etr AA: A review of pulmonary artery catheterization in 6,245 patients. Anesthesiology 61:271, 1984

34. Matthay MA, Chatterjee K: Bedside catheterization of the pulmonary artery: risks compared with benefits. Ann Intern Med 109:826, 1988

35. Ganz P, Swan HJC, Ganz W: Balloon-tipped flow-directed catheters. p. 94. In Grossman W (ed): Cardiac Catheterization and Angiography. 3rd Ed. Lea & Febiger, Philadelphia, 1986

36. Barasch PG, Nardi D, Hammond G et al: Catheter-induced pulmonary artery perforation. J Thorac Cardiovasc Surg 82:5, 1981

37. Gomez MN, Duke PC: Prevention and treatment of intraoperative myocardial ischemia. Anesthesiol Clin North Am 9:591, 1991

38. O'Connor JP, Ramsay JG, Wynands JE, Kaplan JA: Anesthesia for myocardial revascularization. p. 613. In Kaplan JA (ed): Cardiac Anesthesia. 3rd Ed. WB Saunders, Philadelphia, 1993

39. Grossman W: Why is left ventricular diastolic pressure increased during angina pectoris? J Am Coll Cardiol 5:607, 1985

40. Kaplan JA, Wells P: Early diagnosis of myocardial ischemia using the pulmonary arterial catheter. Anesth Analg 60:789, 1981

41. Clements FM, DeBruijn NP: Perioperative evaluation of regional wall motion by transesophageal two-dimensional echocardiography. Anesth Analg 66:249, 1987

42. Bergquist BD, Leung JM: Perioperative monitoring of myocardial ischemia. Int Anesthesiol Clin 31:23, 1993

43. Hoffman JI, Buckberg GD: The myocardial supply: demand ratio: a critical review. Am J Cardiol 41:327, 1978

44. Hoffman JI: Maximal coronary flow and the concept of coronary vascular reserve. Circulation 70:153, 1984

45. Hoffman JI: Determinants and prediction of transmural myocardial perfusion. Circulation 58:381, 1978

46. Braunwald E: Control of myocardial oxygen consumption. Am J Cardiol 7:416, 1971

47. Chatterjee K, Parmley WW, Ganz W et al: Hemodynamic and metabolic responses to vasodilator therapy in acute myocardial infarction. Circulation 48:1183, 1973

48. Sonnenblick EH, Ross J, Braunwald E: Oxygen consumption of the heart. Am J Cardiol 22:328, 1968

49. Roizen MF, Hamilton WF, Yung JS: Treatment of stress-induced increases in pulmonary capillary wedge pressure using volatile anesthetics. Anesthesiology 55:446, 1981

50. Lell WA: Myocardial protection during cardiopulmonary bypass. p. 1033. In Kaplan JA (ed): Cardiac

Anesthesia. 3rd Ed. WB Saunders, Philadelphia, 1993

51. Roach GW, Bellows WH: Left ventricular distention during pulmonary artery venting in a patient undergoing coronary artery bypass surgery. Anesthesiology 76:655, 1992

52. Mangano DT: Monitoring pulmonary arterial pressure in coronary-artery disease. Anesthesiology 53:364, 1980

53. Lowenstein E: To (PA) catheterize or not to (PA) catheterize—that is the question. Anesthesiology 53:361, 1980

54. Tinker JH, Tarhan S, White RD et al: Dobutamine for inotropic support during emergence from cardiopulmonary bypass. Anesthesiology 44:281, 1976

55. Steen PA, Tinker JH, Pluth JR et al: Efficacy of dopamine, dobutamine, and epinephrine during emergence from cardiopulmonary bypass in man. Circulation 57:378, 1978

56. Mangano DT, Siliciano D, Hollenberg M et al: Postoperative myocardial ischemia. Anesthesiology 76:342, 1992

57. Chatterjee K, Paarmley WW, Swan HJC et al: Beneficial effects of vasodilator agents in severe mitral regurgitation due to dysfunction of subvalvular apparatus. Circulation 48:684, 1973

58. Grossman W, Harshaw CW, Munro AB et al: Lowered aortic impedance as therapy for severe mitral regurgitation. JAMA 230:1011, 1974

59. Harshaw CW, Grossman W, Munro AB et al: Reduced systematic vascular resistance as therapy for severe mitral regurgitation of valvular origin. Ann Intern Med 83:312, 1975

60. Pichard AD et al: Large V waves in the pulmonary wedge pressure tracing in the absence of mitral regurgitation. Am J Cardiol 50:1044, 1982

61. Grose R, Strain J, Cohen MV: Pulmonary arterial V waves in mitral regurgitation: clinical and experimental observations. Circulation 69:214, 1984

62. Fuchs RM, Heuser RR, Yin FCP, Brinker JA: Limitations of pulmonary wedge v waves in diagnosing mitral regurgitation. Am J Cardiol 49:849, 1982

63. Thys DM, Hillel Z, Goldman ME et al: A comparison of hemodynamic indices derived by invasive monitoring and two-dimensional echocardiography. Anesthesiology 67:630, 1987

64. Smith JS, Cahalan MK, Benefiel DJ et al: Intraoperative detection of myocardial ischemia in high-risk patients: electrocardiography versus 2-dimensional transesophageal echocardiography. Circulation 72:1015, 1985

65. Leung JM, O'Kelly B, Browner WS et al: Prognostic importance of postbypass regional wall-motion abnormalities in patients undergoing coronary artery bypass graft surgery. Anesthesiology 71:16, 1989

66. London MJ, Tubau JF, Wong MG et al: The "natural history" of segmental wall motion abnormalities in patients undergoing noncardiac surgery. Anesthesiology 73:644, 1990

67. Schnittger I, Keren A, Yock PG et al: Timing of abnormal interventricular septal motion after cardiopulmonary bypass operations. J Thorac Cardiovasc Surg 91:619, 1986

68. Konstadt S, Reich DL et al: Transesophageal echocardiography. p. 370. In Kaplan JA (ed): Cardiac Anesthesia. 3rd Ed. WB Saunders, Philadelphia, 1993

69. Rankin JS, Hickey M, Smith LR et al: Current management of mitral valve incompetence associated with coronary artery disease. J Cardiovasc Surg 4:25, 1989

70. Arcidi JM, Heberler RF, Craver JM et al: Treatment of moderate mitral regurgitation and coronary artery disease by coronary bypass alone. J Thorac Cardiovasc Surg 95:951, 1988

71. Czer LSC, Siegel RJ et al: Transesophageal and epicardial color-flow Doppler echocardiography: surgical repair of valvular, ischemic and congenital heart disease. p. 392. In Kaplan JA (ed): Cardiac Anesthesia. 3rd Ed. WB Saunders, Philadelphia, 1993

72. Bull BS, Korpman RA, Huse WM, Briggs BD: Heparin therapy during extracorporeal circulation. J Thorac Cardiovasc Surg 69:674, 1975

73. Young J, Kisker T, Doty D: Adequate anticoagulation during cardiopulmonary bypass determined by activated clotting time and the appearance of fibrin monomer. Ann Thorac Surg 26:231, 1978

74. White FN: A comparative physiological approach to hypothermia. J Thorac Cardiovasc Surg 82:821, 1981

75. Ream AK, Reitz BA: Temperature correction of P_{CO_2} and pH in estimating acid-base status. Anesthesiology 56:41, 1982

76. Williams JJ: A fresh look at an old question. Anesthesiology 56:1, 1982

77. Prough DS, Stump DA, Troost BT: Pa_{CO_2} Management during cardiopulmonary bypass: intriguing physiologic rationale, convincing clinical data, evolving hypothesis. Anesthesiology 72:3, 1990

78. Kawashima Y, Yamamoto Z, Manabe H: Safe limits of hemodilution in cardiopulmonary bypass. Surgery 76:391, 1974

79. Warner D, Smith M, Siesjp B: Ischemia in normo- and hyperglycemic rats: effects on brain water and electrolytes. Stroke 18:464, 1987

80. Teoh K, Christakis G, Weisel R et al: Accelerated myocardial metabolic recovery with terminal warm blood cardioplegia. J Thorac Cardiovasc Surg 91:888, 1986

81. Magilligan D, Oyama C: Ultrafiltration during cardiopulmonary bypass: laboratory evaluation and initial clinical experience. Ann Thorac Surg 37:33, 1984

82. Reid J, Whyte K, Struthers A: Epinephrine-induced

hypokalemia: the role of beta adrenoceptors. Am J Cardiol 57:23F, 1986

83. Burrows F, Klinck J, Rabinovitch M, Bohn D: Review: pulmonary hypertension in children, perioperative management. Can Anaesth Soc J 33:606, 1986

84. Hansen D, Hickey P: Anesthesia for hypoplastic left-heart syndrome. Anesth Analg 65:127, 1986

85. Ross AF, Gomez MN, Tinker JH: Anesthesia for adult cardiac procedures. p. 1668. In Rogers MC, Tinker JH, Covino BG, Longnecker DE (eds): Principles and Practice of Anesthesia. Mosby Year Book, St. Louis, 1993

86. Harshaw CW, Grossman W, Munro AB, McLaurin LP: Reduced systemic vascular resistance as therapy for severe mitral regurgitation of valvular origin. Ann Intern Med 83:312, 1975

Monitoring the Pediatric Patient

27

James M. Steven
Susan C. Nicolson

PHILOSOPHY OF MONITORING IN INFANTS AND CHILDREN

In 1985, Keenan and Boyon[1] reviewed cardiac arrests that occurred as a result of anesthesia in a large university hospital between 1969 and 1983. In their series, pediatric patients under 12 years of age had an incidence (4.7 per 10,000 anesthetics) of arrests that was threefold higher than that observed in adults. Three subsequent studies comparing the incidence of anesthetic cardiac arrest in children to that in adults revealed that children under 1 year of age suffered cardiac arrest three- to sevenfold more commonly (9.2 to 17.0 per 10,000) than adults.[2-4] The incidence of cardiac arrest for children over 1 year of age was the same or lower than that for adults. The respiratory system was the principal factor in the majority of these cardiac arrests.

Cohen and colleagues[2] examined the incidence of other adverse patient occurrences, both in the operating room and in the postanesthesia care unit. There was little difference between the rate of adverse events in the operating room for children compared with adults. In the postanesthesia care unit, not only was the incidence of adverse events higher in children (13 versus 5.9 per 10,000), but the profile of these events differed considerably. Children were more likely to have problems related to the respiratory system and were less likely to experience problems with ar-

rhythmias or hypotension. Tiret and coworkers[5] examined the complications related to anesthesia in more than 40,000 infants and children in France and concluded that the risk of complications was higher in infants than in children (4.3 versus 0.5 per 1000). Complications observed in infants occurred predominantly during maintenance of anesthesia and generally were the result of respiratory mismanagement. Circulatory failure was as frequent as respiratory complications in children over 1 year of age and events were equally distributed between induction, maintenance of anesthesia, and recovery.

Given the increased likelihood that morbidity and mortality will occur in pediatric patients during the perioperative period, it is prudent to emphasize the monitoring of cardiopulmonary parameters during this period.[6] In mapping out a strategy to monitor pediatric patients, it is important to remember that the clinician is the ultimate monitor. Technical devices are chosen to aid the practitioner and should not distract the care giver from monitoring the patient by using sight, sound, and touch.

This chapter describes the physiologic differences among infants, children, and adults as they relate to monitoring options. An understanding of these differences will aid both in selection of appropriate monitors for individual patients based on their specific needs and in the interpretation of data obtained from these monitors.

CARDIOVASCULAR SYSTEM

Noninvasive Monitoring

The use of noninvasive monitors, including electrocardiogram, blood pressure measurement, precordial stethoscope, pulse oximeter, and temperature measurement combined, with clinical observation, constitute essential patient monitoring in most situations. In healthy children, under certain circumstances, it is appropriate to limit monitoring to the clinician's observation, delaying the application of noninvasive monitors until loss of consciousness occurs. This permits a "steal" induction where the patient arrives in the operating room asleep and does not awaken before induction. This approach also increases the chance of a smooth induction in the child who arrives in the operating room awake and cooperative, but who may lose emotional control if the induction is delayed or if frightened by the application of monitors. Although most children will accept a precordial stethoscope and oximetry probe, the clinician must weight the benefit of delaying the application of any monitors against the risk of not having the monitoring established prior to induction.

Heart Tones

The acceleration and deceleration of blood and cardiac structures produces heart sounds whose intensity and character reveal valuable information about myocardial contractility. This information can be gleaned only by actively listening to the heart tones rather than passively noting their presence or absence. Crisp heart sounds accompany normal myocardial contractility. The snapping shut of the heart valves with each contraction produces the crispness. In order to appreciate the subtle changes in heart tones that accompany general anesthesia, it is important to "examine" the heart tones carefully prior to inducing anesthesia. The heart sounds lose their crispness, become muffled, and then sound distant in direct relationship to myocardial depression. Subtle changes in heart tones may be a clue to an impending disaster. Table 27-1 lists some conditions that change the quality of the heart tones.

Subtle changes in heart tones can indicate other changes in the patient's condition besides changes in cardiac inotropy and fluid status. Acute dilutional anemia may induce systolic flow murmurs. A large venous air embolus produces a characteristic churning "mill wheel" or crackling, bubbling sound (pansystolic murmur heralded by muffling of the first heart sound), as the air in the ventricle is reduced to minute bubbles during cardiac contraction. The appearance of a prominent (loud to booming) second heart sound may indicate the development of sudden pulmonary hypertension. Arrhythmias can also be detected.

Heart tones are monitored with a precordial or esophageal stethoscope (Fig. 27-1). These devices provide valuable information and should be considered an essential part of every anesthetic. If the stethoscope is optimally positioned on the child's chest (near the point of maximal cardiac impulse) both heart tones and breath sounds can be monitored. In intubated patients, an esophageal stethoscope (positioned in the midesophagus) can be used to auscultate heart and breath sounds. The larger-bore esophageal stethoscopes have a lower resonant frequency and produce louder sounds than the smaller-bore stethoscopes.[7]

In patients undergoing repair for esophageal atresia, an esophageal stethoscope cannot be used nor can a precordial stethoscope be placed in the usual chest position. A flat precordial stethoscope can be placed in the left axilla in these patients to monitor heart tones and to detect an intraoperative right main stem bronchus intubation (by loss of left-sided breath sounds). An esophageal stethoscope is relatively contraindicated in pediatric patients having tracheostomies and ventriculojugular cerebrospinal fluid shunt insertions.[8,9] Particular care should be exercised when inserting the esophageal stethoscope in patients with upper esophageal stenosis or diverticulae, as the esophagus may be abraded or perforated. In neonates and small infants, a relatively oversized esophageal stethoscope can cause airway obstruction by compressing the membranous posterior tracheal wall distal to

TABLE 27-1. Determinants of Heart Tone Quality

Condition	Change in Heart Tone
Deep anesthesia	Muffled to distant
Hypovolemia	Distant
Shock	Muffled to distant
Fluid overload	Crisp
Light anesthesia	Crisp

(From Mayer,[265] with permission.)

the tip of the endotracheal tube. Esophageal stethoscopes should be placed through the mouth rather than the nose to avoid trauma to the adenoids, which reach their maximum size when the patient is 3 to 5 years old.

When the esophageal stethoscope is removed (at the time of extubation) in the operating room, it should be replaced by a precordial stethoscope. Leaving the precordial stethoscope in place permits monitoring heart tones and breath sounds during transport of the patient to the postanesthesia care unit or other sites.

As summarized by Gravenstein and Paulus[10]:

The precordial or esophageal stethoscope is a sensitive, reliable and inexpensive device and an excellent adjunct to sophisticated monitoring systems that can be relied upon when other systems fail. . . . The stethoscope may be the single most important [monitoring] device because it allows us to monitor circulation and ventilation continuously without electronics, without lifting our eyes, and without hands!

Pulse

Palpation of the peripheral pulse gives information on the heart rate, rhythm, and pulse volume. The peripheral pulse can be monitored during administration of an anesthetic by palpation or through the use of a fingertip plethysmograph. When the pulse is diminished, examiners should be careful not to mistake their own pulse for that of the patient. Care must be taken when monitoring a child's pulse not to obliterate it by pressing too hard.[10]

Heart Rate

Relative increases in the proportion of the myocardial wall that is composed of fibrous elements renders the heart less compliant in the neonate and small infant as compared to adult patients.[11,12] As a result, acute reductions in heart rate in this population do not induce rapid compensatory increases in stroke volume. As a consequence, neonates and small infants exhibit proportionally greater reduction in cardiac output and systemic blood pressure with acute bradycardia, giving rise to the concept that they are "heart rate-dependent."

The normal heart rate is inversely related to the age of the child, approaching 200 beats per minute (bpm) in the neonate. The neonate's heart-rate response to a stimulus often appears out of proportion to the magnitude of the stimulus. Marked individual variation exists in the younger patient's heart rate. Table 27-2 lists the range of normal heart rates in children by age.

Bradycardia

Intraoperative bradycardia results from many stimuli. The most common causes of bradycardia during anesthesia are discussed in the following sections.

Potent Inhalational Agents. Inhalational agents produce bradycardia through direct myocardial effects. In the patient under 6 months of age, bradycardia may occur before the minimum alveolar concentration of the anesthetic has been achieved.

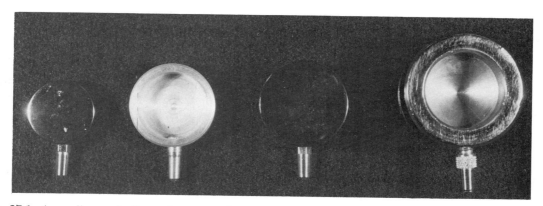

Fig. 27-1. A small sample from the many sizes and weights of precordial stethoscopes available. The smaller ones are necessary for use in neonates and mandatory for monitoring patients undergoing repair of esophageal atresia (see text).

Hypotension, defined as a decrease of 30 percent in the systolic blood pressure from preinduction levels, occurs in 70 percent of patients under 4 weeks of age, and 50 percent of infants up to 6 months.[13,14] Even at concentrations below the minimum alveolar concentration, potent inhalational agents blunt the baroreceptor response in young children, limiting their ability to increase heart rate in response to hypotension.[13-17]

Intravenous Succinylcholine. Bradycardia can occur with the first dose, but is more common and more marked with succeeding doses. It is diminished, but frequently not prevented, by atropine.[18] Bradycardia occurs less frequently and to a lesser magnitude with intramuscular succinylcholine.

Exaggerated Vagal Reflexes. Vagal bradycardia occurs in response to nasogastric suctioning and traction on extraocular muscles, abdominal viscera, the peritoneum, spermatic cord, and hilar structures of the lung. These reflexes occur due to the high ratio of vagal tone to sympathetic tone in the young.[12] Traction on the extraocular muscles can lead to cardiac arrest.[19]

Hypoxemia. In the neonate, unlike the adult, hypoxemia initially leads to bradycardia.[20] Oxygen delivery to the tissues must be increased in order to correct hypoxic bradycardia, although atropine administration may briefly mask it.

Tachycardia

Intraoperative tachycardia is far less significant in the pediatric patient than bradycardia. Some infants can sustain heart rates of more than 250 beats per minute for 10 to 12 hours without developing hypotension or heart failure.

The rapid heart rates in pediatric patients are difficult to count either by palpation or auscultation. Accurate monitoring of the heart rate in pediatric anesthesia is facilitated by use of the rate meter, which may derive its input either from an electrocardiograph (ECG) or a finger plethysmograph. Most automated blood pressure devices and pulse oximeters also determine and display heart rate.

Heart Rhythm

The most frequent arrhythmias in pediatric patients are bradycardia and tachycardia. These disturbances in the cardiac rhythm can be detected by the precordial or esophageal stethoscope, palpation of the pulse, pulse oximetry, or via the ECG. Premature ventricular contractions (PVCs), bigeminy, nodal rhythms and wandering pacemakers are less common. Although bradycardia may represent the initial response of the neonate to hypoxemia,[20-22] older infants will usually manifest an intervening period of tachycardia. Rolf and Cote[22] examined the relationship of hypercarbia to arrhythmias in over 400 infants and children and noted no arrhythmias in the 153 infants under 2 years of age, despite more frequent episodes of hypercarbia ($P_{ETCO_2} \leq 55$ mmHg for ≥ 60 seconds). Among children over 2 years, these investigators demonstrated arrhythmias in nearly 10 percent, 42 percent of which were associated with hypercarbia. On the other hand, the onset of arrhythmias is not a sensitive method for detecting hypercarbia, as only 28 percent of the older population who had hypercarbic episodes developed arrhythmias.

Cardiac Depolarization

The main difference in cardiac depolarization between the infant and adults results from the relatively thick right ventricle of the neonate. In the neonate the ratio of the weights of the left and right ventricles is close to 1:1 compared with 2–2.5: 1 in the adult.[12] This induces a moderate right axis shift in the neonatal ECG. In the infant the most pronounced R wave will be seen in standard lead III, as opposed to lead II, where it is found in the adult.

The ECG provides an ongoing monitor of cardiac rate, QRS configuration, repolarization, and

TABLE 27-2. Normal Heart Rates in Children

Age	Average (Normal Range), in bpm	
Newborn	125 (70–190)	
1–11 months	120 (80–160)	
2 years	110 (80–130)	
4 years	100 (80–120)	
6 years	100 (75–115)	
8 years	90 (70–110)	
10 years	90 (70–110)	
	Girls	*Boys*
12 years	90 (70–110)	85 (65–105)
14 years	85 (65–105)	80 (60–100)
16 years	80 (60–100)	75 (55–95)
18 years	75 (55–95)	70 (50–90)

(Adapted from Behrman and Vaughn,[266] with permission.)

rhythm, but not cardiac output. It is valuable in determining *why* there is a problem with peripheral perfusion, rather than *whether* there is a problem. In fact, this major limitation of ECG monitoring can be misleading. For example, a normal ECG may persist transiently despite the absence of cardiac output. In this circumstance, brain hypoxia may occur before the ECG shows significant abnormalities. Thus the ECG is not a satisfactory replacement for monitoring techniques that provide some indication of cardiac function such as auscultation, blood pressure measurement, and palpation of the pulse. ECG monitoring is valuable in detecting minor cardiac arrhythmias, such as nodal rhythms, where lack of an atrial contraction may impair ventricular filling, thereby producing modest reductions in stroke volume, cardiac output, and arterial blood pressure. ECG monitoring promotes rapid, accurate diagnosis and prompt treatment of arrhythmias. In the pulseless patient, the lack of a QRS complex on the ECG trace confirms cardiac asystole as the etiology of the hypotension.[23] Electrolyte disturbances during an anesthetic develop more rapidly in neonates and young infants than in adults: peaked T waves may indicate hyperkalemia; prolonged Q-T interval, hypocalcemia.

The full benefit of the ECG monitor will not be realized unless the ECG trace is analyzed for changes at regular intervals. As soon as the ECG leads are applied, a P-QRS-T complex should be printed on a strip chart or copied onto the anesthesia record. In interpreting the ECG trace, each component of the P-QRS-T complex should be analyzed separately for several factors:

1. Shape
2. Regularity and persistence or absence of each component
3. Location and axis of P, R, and T waves
4. Return to the isoelectric line
5. Evidence of artifacts
6. Corroborating reasons for any change in form

Myocardial ischemia is not a concern in most anesthetized pediatric patients, therefore a three-lead ECG system is adequate in the vast majority of cases. Interpretation of the pediatric ECG can be aided by placing the electrodes on the extremities rather than on the thorax. This will diminish movement of the ECG baseline caused by excursion of the thorax with respirations. The excursions are rather marked in the infant compared to the adult due to the high compliance of the infant thorax. If you wish to monitor respiration using impedance pneumography, the ECG leads must be placed on the thorax. A disadvantage of placing the ECG leads on the extremities is that 9 to 10 percent of the electrical current passing to ground through the electrodes during a electrical fault will pass through the heart. If all the electrodes are placed on the frontal or posterior surface of the thorax at the base of the neck, only 3 percent of the electrical fault current passes through the heart.[24] Only standard lead I is available with this electrode placement. Considerations of electrical fault currents may be of minimal importance when using equipment that is isolated and has, in addition, isolated patient leads.

Care should be taken to keep the electrodes off areas with bony protuberances. Miniature-size electrodes are available for young infants but are associated with an increased risk of electrosurgical burns.[25] Adult-size electrodes can be wrapped around the extremities of small infants. The adhesion of the electrode and the quality of the trace can be increased by carefully cleaning the skin beneath the electrode. When electrode placement results in contact with wet sheets, a short circuit to the operating table ground results, markedly degrading the ECG trace.

Peripheral Perfusion

The young infant, particularly the neonate, has the characteristic ability to give the appearance of satisfactory hemodynamics (i.e., adequate blood pressure, normal heart rate) only to suddenly develop hypotension and bradycardia. This may reflect the infant's ability to constrict their peripheral vasculature proportionally more intensely and to shunt blood to the vital organs more effectively than an adult. In the unanesthetized infant, the neurohumoral responses to hypovolemia results in a tachycardia. Volatile anesthetics, however, blunt baroreceptor responses even in the face of significant hypotension.[14–17]

Visual inspection of the extremities will provide clues to the magnitude of the vasoconstrictive response. An adequate vascular volume is associated with pink, warm limbs with brisk capillary refill and well-filled, visible veins. Inadequate peripheral perfusion due either to hypovolemia or cardiac failure is associated with mottled, cyanotic, cool limbs with delayed capillary refill and no visible veins.[23] Spreading of the cyanosis to the trunk is an ominous sign indicating hypotension and inadequate tissue oxygenation.

Other indicators of diminished peripheral perfusion are an increasing temperature gradient between core and surface, and damping of the digital plethysmograph or direct peripheral arterial waveforms. Determination of the systemic arterial pressure by noninvasive methods becomes increasingly difficult with decreasing peripheral perfusion.

Systemic Arterial Pressure

A compelling argument can be made that monitoring systemic arterial pressure is more important in infants than in adults. Infants demonstrate marked sensitivity to anesthetic agents, small circulating volume, and diminished cardiac reserve, particularly in the face of substantially increased metabolic demands. The higher minimum alveolar concentration requirements of the young infant means the infant's heart is exposed to greater myocardial depression than an adult's heart at a comparable anesthetic depth.[13,26] The myocardial depression observed in response to anesthetic concentrations substantially below the minimum alveolar concentration suggests increased myocardial sensitivity to volatile anesthetics as well. The absolute circulating volume in this population is extremely small in comparison to that of the adult, thereby creating a situation where small volumes lost to occult hemorrhage or fluid shifts can exert a significant impact on hemodynamics.

Unfortunately, a substantial historical precedent (bowing to the technical difficulties posed by the application of the Riva-Rocci method to infants) indicated that systemic pressure measurement was not necessary in this population. Heart tones were thought to be a satisfactory monitor of cardiac output. However, bradycardia is a late sign of inadequate cardiac output, occurring only after hypotension has produced myocardial ischemia or severe metabolic disturbance. Significant technical advances in the past 20 years have made noninvasive blood pressure monitoring feasible and therefore preferable for virtually all pediatric patients, in accordance with ASA monitoring standards.[27]

Alternative methods of measuring blood pressure in infants include the flush and needle-bounce techniques. In the flush method, the hand is compressed before the blood pressure cuff is inflated. The pressure at which a pink flush (signaling return of blood flow) appears during deflation of the cuff is taken as the systolic blood pressure. In the needle-bounce technique, the blood pressure cuff is slowly deflated, and systolic blood pressure is read at the point of maximum needle fluctuation. A large aneroid manometer is helpful with this technique. Both techniques provide subjective data and are therefore less desirable than any of the quantitative methods described subsequently. However, neither technique provides any information on mean or diastolic pressures.

Other techniques of measuring blood pressure that detect return of blood flow distal to an occlusive cuff include Doppler ultrasound flow detectors (e.g., Parks Electronics Laboratory, Beaveron, OR) (Fig. 27-2) or arterial wall motion detectors (e.g., Arteriosonde, Kontron Medical Instruments, Everett, MA). The systolic blood pressure is equal to the pressure in the cuff at the moment of return of blood flow or arterial wall motion. A fingertip plethysmograph can be used in a similar manner.[28] Diastolic and mean pressures are not reliably determined with any of these techniques.

Two other methods are employed by automated devices for noninvasive systemic arterial pressure determination: oscillometry and low-frequency sensors. The Infrasone (Puritan-Bennett Corp., Kansas City, MO) uses a filtered low-frequency microphone distal to an occlusive cuff in order to measure systolic and diastolic pressures. In addition, this monitor will calculate and display the mean arterial and pulse pressures. Although it has been shown to correlate well in adult studies, its accuracy in small children has been questioned.[29] Automated devices using the principal of oscillometry (e.g., Dinamap, Critikon, Tampa, FL) (Fig. 27-3) have become extremely popular. In infants and children, they have been shown to correlate well with both direct and Doppler measurements of systolic (first oscillation)[30] and mean (maximal oscillation)[31] arterial pressures. Unlike any other indirect technique, one need not meticulously locate the sensor over the distal artery in order for it to function accurately, and both the proximal and distal limbs may be used. All automated indirect systemic arterial pressure monitors exhibit poor correlation with direct diastolic pressure determinations in children.

Much has been written on the need to choose the appropriate size blood pressure cuff in order to obtain accurate blood pressure determinations. Traditional recommendations for cuff width were based on the length of the upper arm. More recent studies have demonstrated better accuracy when using formulas based on the cross-sectional area of the mid-upper arm (e.g., 50 percent of the circumference or 120 percent of the diameter).[31,32] A narrow cuff incompletely occludes the artery, resulting in premature return of flow and hence a falsely elevated blood pressure determination. The use of a cuff that is too narrow introduces larger errors than with cuff that is too wide.[31,32] Manufacturers of the Dinamap automated blood pressure devices recommend the use of the largest cuff that can be placed between the child's axilla and the antecubital fossa.

The normal systolic blood pressure of the neonate and young infant are directly related to age and body mass. The normal values and their ranges appear in Table 27-3.

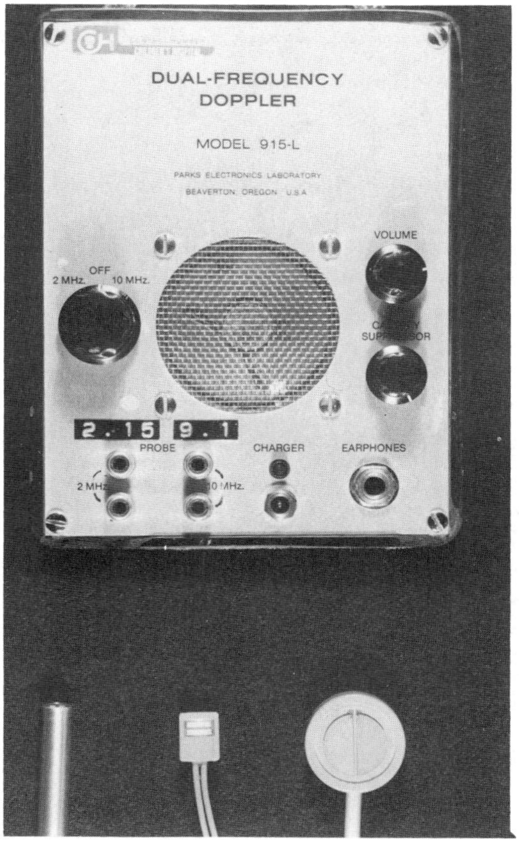

Fig. 27-2. A multipurpose Doppler device that detects the motion of red blood cells. From left to right, a pencil probe for tracing the course of a vessel and determining its patency, a small probe used primarily in determining systolic blood pressure, and the probe used for detecting cardiac air embolism. The probes each have an ultrasound transmitting and receiving crystal. The depth of focus of the crystals and their frequency varies according to the intended purpose of the probe. (Parks Electronics Laboratory, Beaverton, OR.)

Invasive Monitoring

In the management of selected critically ill children and children undergoing procedures where major changes in hemodynamics are anticipated, more information, obtainable only from invasive monitors, is needed to follow the patient's course, to institute therapy and to assess their response to the interventions. The decision to employ invasive monitors should be made after weighing the benefits derived from having the information against the risks associated with the insertion and use of these monitors.

Systemic Arterial Pressure

Visual analysis of the arterial waveform provides information on myocardial contractility, stroke volume, systemic vascular resistance, and circulating blood volume. The upstroke of the wave is dependent on the rate of left ventricular contraction (dP/dT) with a steep upstroke indicating a vigorously contracting myocardium. The stroke volume can be approximated by estimating the area under the systolic ejection phase of the arterial pressure waveform. A low dicrotic notch and steep downstroke indicate rapid diastolic runoff and a low peripheral vascular resistance. Respiratory variation of the arterial pressure waveform is a sensitive indicator of intravascular volume depletion in children with normal cardiac physiology.

Initially, application of intra-arterial pressure monitoring in the management of pediatric patients was limited by the technical difficulties of placing a catheter in small arteries. Increasing experience plus the availability of small-gauge Teflon catheters have led to more extensive utilization of this monitor.

Insertion Sites for Arterial Cannulae

The radial, ulnar, dorsalis pedis, posterior tibial, brachial, axillary, and femoral arteries and the umbilical artery in the newborn are the major access routes used in the pediatric patient. Table 27-4 lists the factors that influence vessel selection.

The individual artery has to be evaluated for quality of pulse, course of the vessel, and, if appropriate, collateral flow. A history of prior cannulation, both percutaneous and by cutdown, needs to be obtained. The incidence and type of complications should be considered when selecting the vessel. An understanding of the particular operative procedure can influence artery selection. Patients scheduled for cardiovascular procedures where an artery will be temporarily clamped or permanently ligated, or those who have had such a procedure in the past, require cannulation at an alternative site. In neonates who may exhibit right-to-left shunting across a patent ductus arteriosus, consideration should be given to positioning the catheter in a vessel that arises from the aorta proximal to the ductus.

The experience of the clinician with the various access routes weighs heavily in the decision as to which artery to cannulate. The success rate of percutaneous catheter placement in children weighing less than 5 kg is only 70 to 85 percent, and diminishes with size, even in experienced hands. Consid-

TABLE 27-3. Normal Blood Pressures in Children

| Age | Blood Pressure in mmHg (±95% Confidence Limits) | | |
	Systolic	Diastolic	Mean
Newborn[a]			
1 kg	47 (9)	27 (10)	35 (7)
2 kg	54 (9)	32 (10)	40 (7)
3 kg	62 (9)	37 (10)	45 (7)
4 kg	69 (9)	42 (10)	50 (7)
Males[b]			
0–9 yr	93 (18)	59 (18)	
10-19 yr	108 (20)	67 (18)	
Females[b]			
10–9 yr	96 (24)	62 (16)	
10–19 yr	105 (20)	64 (22)	

[a]Data from Versmold et al.[267]
[b]Data from Adams and Landaw.[268]

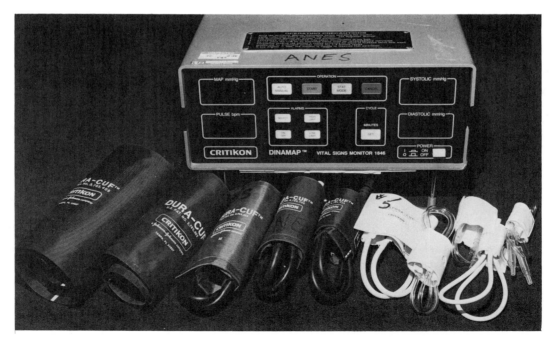

Fig. 27-3. An automated device for determining systolic, diastolic and mean blood pressures and heart rate using oscillometry. This instrument measures blood pressure noninvasively in nearly all pediatric patients from the neonate to the adult size adolescent. (Dinamap of Critikon, Tampa, FL.)

eration should be given to making the initial attempt via cutdown in these patients.

Indications

There are two major indications for insertion of an indwelling arterial cannula in the pediatric patient (Table 27-5). Patients with anticipated rapid or unpredictable pressure changes include children undergoing procedures with potential for rapid blood loss and fluid shifts of massive proportions and patients with labile hypertension. Children requiring the use of techniques that will deliberately lower the blood pressure and maintain it within a narrow range constitute another subset requiring continuous intra-arterial monitoring. In specific circumstances, indirect methods of blood pressure monitoring are inaccurate. Included in this category are patients requiring cardiopulmonary bypass and the small population of children in whom noninvasive methods do not provide reliable pressures. Although improvements in noninvasive blood pressure technology have virtually eliminated the latter group, low-birth-weight neonates and obese children occasionally require arterial cannulation for minor procedures because of an inability to obtain consistently reliable systemic arterial pressures by any other route.

Patients who require an $FIO_2 \geq 0.50$ to achieve an arterial PaO_2 of 100 mmHg, or perioperative mechanical ventilation, may benefit from an arterial catheter for serial blood gas determinations. Consideration should be given to placing an arterial catheter for serial $PaCO_2$ measurements in patients with increased intracranial pressure or elevated pulmonary vascular resistance whose therapy includes deliberate hyperventilation.

Types of Catheters

Clinical studies have documented that small-gauge, nontapered, radiolucent Teflon catheters are associated with the lowest incidence of throm-

TABLE 27-4 Factors in the Choice of Arterial for Cannulation

Suitability of artery for cannulation
Prior cannulations
Complication rate and nature of complications
Proposed surgical procedure
Presence of patent ductus arteriosus (PDA)
Experience and skill of clinician inserting catheter

TABLE 27-5. Indications for Indwelling Arterial Cannulae

Beat-to-beat monitoring of arterial pressure
   Rapid and/or unpredictable pressure changes
   Narrow limits of acceptable pressures
   Inaccurate indirect methods of measurement
   Unstable cardiovascular system

Serial sampling of arterial blood gases
   Infants with immature retinal vascularity for major intracavitary procedures
   Need for mechanical ventilatory support
   Deliberate hypocarbia

bosis and occlusion. A 22-gauge catheter can be used in peripheral arteries of all children.

Insertion Techniques

Catheters inserted percutaneously can be placed using the catheter over a needle apparatus or the Seldinger technique. When using the catheter over a needle apparatus, either the vessel may be transfixed (through-and-through technique) or the lumen can be identified on entry avoiding puncture of the posterior wall. The Seldinger technique involves identifying the vessel using either a 21- or 23-gauge butterfly or thin-wall needle and passing a 0.015- or 0.018-in. outer diameter, 15- or 20-cm flexible straight angiographic wire to aid in threading the catheter (Fig. 27-4). In experienced hands, the success rates of the two techniques are comparable.

Radial Artery

The radial artery is the preferred site of arterial cannulation in most children. Although most children have good collateral flow, an assessment of ulnar artery flow prior to radial cannulation is done by many. Either a modified Allen test or finger plethysmography can be used to determine the adequacy of collateral ulnar arterial flow. If either test indicates dominance of the radial artery in supplying the palmar arch, perhaps an alternative site should be selected for cannulation.[33,34]

The insertion site should be prepared using sterile technique. The wrist is dorsiflexed to an angle of 50 degrees and the hand and forearm secured to an armboard. Abducting the thumb stabilizes the artery at the wrist. The skin should be incised with a needle or scalpel blade to prevent burring of the catheter as it passes through the skin.

Complications of radial artery cannulae include distal ischemia, proximal embolization, and problems localized to the cannulation site. Frequent inspection of the hand should be made to detect ischemic changes. Flushing a radial arterial cannula occasionally results in blanching of the forearm. Frequent flushing with larger volumes may result in permanent damage to the skin and muscle of the forearm. Flushing may also result in retrograde arterial flow carrying air or particulate emboli to the central circulation. Edmonds and coworkers[35] demonstrated that as little as 0.3 ml of flush rapidly administered through a radial artery

catheter in an infant produced retrograde flow into the central circulation. Complications seen at the cannulation site include hematoma, hemorrhage, arterial spasm, infection, and obstruction to radial flow after removal of the catheter. Spasm can be minimized by continuous flushing of the catheter with heparinized saline and by splinting the forearm and hand on an armboard to minimize catheter motion within the vessel lumen. Injection of a small volume of 1 percent lidocaine intra-arterially occasionally relieves arterial spasm. Occlusion of the radial artery occurs in approximately 50 percent of children following removal of percutaneous catheters. Recanalization occurs within 14 days in nearly all patients with permanent obstruction be-

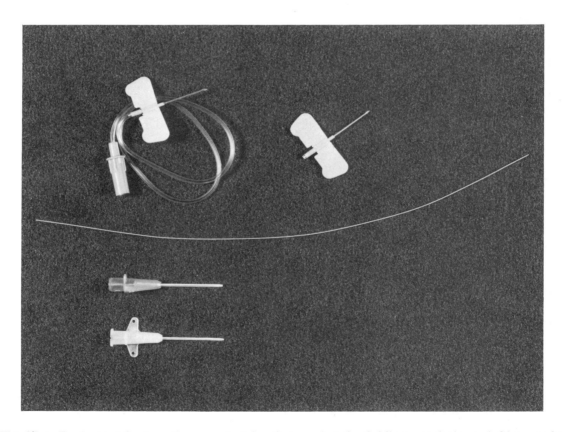

Fig. 27-4. Equipment for inserting an arterial catheter using the Seldinger technique. A 21-gauge butterfly needle (Abbott Laboratories, Inc., North Chicago, IL) is prepared by cutting off the extension tubing. After inserting the needle in the artery, the 20-cm (0.018-inch) diameter wireguide (Cook Inc., Bloomington, IN) is introduced into the artery and the needle removed. A 20- or 22-gauge Teflon nontapered catheter (Flash-Cath, Travenol Laboratories, Inc., Deerfield, IL) is then introduced over the wire and the wire removed. The catheter is sutured to the skin using the holes in the wings of the tapered catheter hub.

ing extremely rare.[36] The time for recanalization is longer and the incidence of permanent obstruction is higher when cutdown is required for insertion of the arterial catheter.[36] Arteriovenous fistula and carpal tunnel syndrome are rare late sequelae of radial artery cannulation.

Ulnar Artery

The ulnar artery is the other major arterial supply to the palmar arch. Difficulties in palpation and immobilization of the vessel make cannulation more difficult, especially in the small infant. Our experience indicates, however, that the ulnar artery is more predictable in its course and thus more readily cannulated percutaneously in children with trisomy 21. Complications are identical to radial cannulation.

Dorsalis Pedis Artery

In most clinical situations the dorsalis pedis artery serves as the first alternative to the radial or ulnar arteries. A disadvantage of this site is its particularly proclivity to intense vasoconstriction that precludes a pulsatile waveform or the ability to aspirate blood specimens. In addition, catheters in pedal arteries display an exaggerated waveform with significant (10 to 30 percent) increases in systolic pressures and reductions in diastolic pressures.[37]

The nature of the complications seen is similar to those for the radial artery. The propensity for central nervous system emboli from retrograde flushing of the catheter is virtually eliminated at this site by its distance from the aortic arch. The distance to the catheter from the head of the operating table often requires a longer length of high-pressure tubing, thereby increasing the likelihood of waveform artifact and the volume of solution needed to sample and flush the catheter.

Posterior Tibial Artery

The posterior tibial artery is an alternative pedal vessel that is subject to the same limitations as the dorsalis pedis artery. The artery can be cannulated in the groove posterior to the medial malleolus. The duration of catheter function compares favorably with that of the radial artery,[38] and complications are similar to those at other peripheral arterial sites.

Axillary Artery

The axillary artery may serve as a more reasonable alternative to the brachial artery when the arteries of the wrist are not accessible, since it has substantial collateral circulation. In a small series of 16 patients, Lawless and Orr[39] demonstrated the safety of this site in infants as young as 1 day. Distal arm noninvasive blood pressure determinations were not significantly altered by a proximal axillary artery catheter. Although this site poses the unique risk of brachial plexus injury and a substantial hazard from retrograde flush into the aortic arch, these complications were not noted in the report.[39]

Brachial Artery

Brachial artery cannulation is advised only when no other vessel is available, since no collateral arterial flow supplies the arm when brachial occlusion occurs following cannulation. However, we have been faced with many patients where it is the only available vessel and have had a complication rate no greater than with other vessels.

Umbilical Artery

Use of the umbilical artery in the neonate for pressure monitoring and obtaining serial blood specimens is controversial. Ease of cannulation must be weighed against the complications of this site. High placement, above the diaphragm in the thoracic dorsal aorta, and low placement, at L3, are the two sites recommended for tip position. Arterial blood gas specimens drawn from umbilical catheters distal to a patent ductus arteriosus may reflect right to left shunting at the ductal level.

Meticulous care should be taken to secure the catheter in place to avoid accidental removal with resultant hemorrhage. Several complications are unique to umbilical artery cannulation.[40] There is a high incidence of aortic thrombosis.[41] The incidence of renal artery thrombosis approaches 10 percent; of this group, 10 percent will develop renal artery hypertension.[42-44] Umbilical or hypogastric artery perforation can occur, especially following multiple attempts at insertion or if the catheter is inserted against resistance. Low catheter tip placement produces a high incidence of decreased lower extremity perfusion requiring either removal or reinsertion to a high position. In addition, the presence of an umbilical artery line is associated with a higher incidence of necrotizing enterocolitis.

Temporal Artery

Use of the superficial temporal artery for cannulation is controversial. An association between the temporal artery lines and ipsilateral cerebral infarcts with contralateral hemiparesis has emerged. Because of the proximity of the temporal artery to the origin of the internal carotid, cerebral embolization from the catheter ranks high in the differential diagnosis.[45,46] The location of the vessel makes the complication of skin slough particularly undesirable (e.g., the pinna of the ear may be sloughed).

Central Venous Pressure

The right atrial pressure reflects the preload of the right ventricle and provides an index of right ventricular function. Normal values for central venous pressure, measured at the junction of the vena cavae with the right atrium, are the same in infants, children and adults. Fluctuations with respirations and crying are more pronounced in younger patients.[47] The central venous pressure should be corrected to a normal intrathoracic pressure by subtracting the intrapleural pressure from the central venous pressure prior to interpretation and therapeutic intervention. The intrapleural pressure can be determined using either an intrapleural or an esophageal balloon catheter.

Application of central venous pressure monitoring to the management of pediatric patients has been limited by the technical difficulties of inserting the catheters. The recent availability of equipment of appropriate size has led to an increase in the use of this monitor.

Indications

There are three primary indications for the use of a central venous catheter in children: pressure determination, venous access, and administration of hypertonic solutions.

Pressure Measurement. Use of the catheter for central venous pressure monitoring is indicated in those patients in whom large fluid shifts are anticipated. Constant monitoring of the central venous pressure will permit early recognition of an abnormal circulating volume. Patients with fluid shifts who also require vasodilator therapy benefit from early detection of intravascular volume depletion to avoid the profound hypotension seen with the combined effects of vasodilator therapy and hypovolemia. Measurement of the central venous pressure is indicated in many patients with congenital heart disease undergoing cardiac surgery. Preexisting or resultant abnormalities in right ventricular function can be followed and the effect of therapy assessed. During cardiopulmonary bypass using bicaval cannulation, an acute rise in the central venous pressure noted in a catheter positioned above the superior vena caval drainage cannula provides information useful in the diagnosis of obstructed venous return from the head and neck. Catheters below the level of the superior caval cannula tape will not reflect superior vena caval pressures during bypass. Prompt recognition of occluded superior vena caval drainage will permit timely repositioning of the superior caval cannula or correction of other causes of obstruction and thus prevent the cerebral edema or intracranial hemorrhage seen with prolonged obstruction to venous return from the upper body.

Venous Access. A central venous catheter is a reliable large-bore access route to the central circulation. This route provides venous access in emergency situations as well as in other situations where peripheral access is inadequate. Resuscitative drugs can be infused via this route with assurance that they are entering the circulation in close proximity to the desired site of action. This is a major consideration in the small infant in whom the administration of substantial fluid volume for the purpose of flushing in medications is undesirable. Sclerosing agents, such as calcium chloride and many chemotherapeutic and antimicrobial agents, can be given without risk of skin slough.

Long-Term Parenteral Nutrition with Hypertonic Solution. An indwelling Silastic catheter in the central circulation permits delivery of hyperalimentation solutions to inpatients or outpatients. This indication applies to an increasing number of children. Central catheters also provide ready access and minimize discomfort for critically ill children requiring frequent venous specimens to follow abnormalities in their hemogram, electrolytes, and blood glucose.

Contraindications

Coagulopathy is a relative contraindication to the placement of any central line. Prior major neck surgery, extensive neck burns, and ventriculoatrial and ventriculoperitoneal shunts are relative contraindications to the use of the internal and external jugular veins. Tracheostomy poses difficulty in securing the catheter and maintaining a clean insertion site with either jugular or subclavian routes.[48]

Insertion Sites

Access can be achieved from a number of venous sites including the basilic, external jugular, internal jugular, and subclavian veins as well as the umbilical vein in the newborn. Table 27-6 lists the factors that influence the choice of cannulation site.

The suitability of a vein for cannulation includes the history of other percutaneous or cutdown attempts and their complications, if any. The prior experience of the clinician, including past success rate and types of complications encountered, weighs heavily in the decision. The choice of route depends, not only on the likelihood of successful venous cannulation, but on the probability of achieving proper catheter tip position rapidly and reliably. In small patients, the internal jugular and subclavian routes are the most likely to satisfy these objectives. The availability of a catheter of proper length is occasionally a limiting factor.

Catheter Tip Position

Over the past decade, numerous cases of perforation of the heart and great vessels by a central venous catheter have been reported in both children and adults.[49,50] Perforation by a stiff catheter or guidewire can occur at the time of catheter insertion. Delayed perforation, secondary to body movement or the contractile motion of the heart when the catheter is positioned in right atrium, presents hours to days following initial placement. Late perforations inflict serious morbidity and mortality. Catheter erosion within the pericardial reflection has been uniformly fatal. Catheter manufacturers have attempted to reduce the potential for perforation by improvements in catheter materials and in tip design. Clinicians who insert the catheters and those who care for patients with indwelling catheters need to be aware of the potential for late perforation. The following guidelines are recommended both to reduce the incidence of perforation and to promptly diagnose the perforation if it occurs:

Select a catheter of the proper length for each patient. The catheter tip should rest in the superior vena cava or at the superior vena cava-right atrium junction above the pericardial reflection. Ideally, the tip of the catheter is best positioned where it will be parallel with the wall of the vessel, avoiding contact with the vessel wall where it bifurcates or bends.

The position of the catheter tip should be confirmed by fluoroscopy or chest radiograph at the time of or immediately following insertion. Given that movement can advance the tip of the catheter, the position should be reassessed with serial radiographs.

Identify the cause in any catheter that is malfunctioning (e.g., dampening of venous waveform, disappearance of fluctuations in the waveform with respiration and absence of venous backflow).

Limit the pressure with which fluids are infused into the catheter.

If cardiovascular deterioration occurs in a patient with a central venous catheter in place, the possibility of perforation and cardiac tamponade should be considered in the differential diagnosis.

TABLE 27-6. Factors in Vein Selection for Central Cannulation

Patient
  Size of the patient
  Suitability of the vein for cannulation
  Prior cannulations
  Anticipated duration of cannulation

Clinician
  Prior experience with the technique

Technique
  Success rate including likelihood of proper catheter
    tip position
  Complication rate
  Nature of complications
  Availability of equipment for insertion

Insertion Techniques

The potential for paradoxical air embolus is real in children with right-to-left anatomic communications. Air can pass from right to left in children with a patent foramen ovale if right atrial pressure exceeds left. The possibility also exists for air embolization in children with left-to-right shunts during certain portions of the cardiac cycle. Strict bubble precautions should be taken to minimize even small amounts of air from embolizing to the brain or coronary arteries. Transducing central venous pressure permits prompt recognition of disconnections in the system that could lead to entrainment of air or to hemorrhage.

Basilic Vein

The advantage of the basilic vein approach is the fact that the vessel is peripheral and can be visualized or palpated. The major disadvantages of this vessel are the difficulty in achieving proper catheter position and the large dead space between the injection port and the central circulation.

Following successful identification of the vascular lumen, the advancement of the catheter may be difficult. External rotation and abduction of the arm as well as advancing the catheter with constant infusion of fluid through it may improve the likelihood of proper placement. The Drum Cartridge Catheter (Abbott Laboratories, North Chicago, IL) has resulted in an increased number of catheters being properly placed. In our experience with children over 20 kg the Drum catheter has resulted in successful central placement in more than 90 percent on the initial attempt using either the right or left basilic vein.

Immediate complications include arterial puncture, nerve injury, perforation of the vein with catheter advancement, malposition of the catheter tip, and hematoma. Arterial and nerve injuries are rare. Proximal vessel perforation occurs at a rate of about 1 percent.

Late complications include thrombosis, infection, and perforation. Adult experience with central catheters inserted via this route indicates that nearly all patients develop thrombosis within 24 to 48 hours of catheter insertion. In children, the reported rate of thrombosis is only 5 percent.[51]

Femoral Vein

Identification of the vascular lumen is most readily accomplished with a small-gauge thin-wall needle. The catheter is then inserted using the Seldinger technique.[52,53] Catheters of appropriate length are inserted with the tip resting in the inferior vena cava above the level of the diaphragm. Catheters in the inferior vena cava below the diaphragm are subject to fluctuations secondary to changes in intra-abdominal pressure. Assurance that the catheter is not intrahepatic is mandatory prior to infusion hyperosmolar or alkaline solutions.

Immediate complications include unintentional femoral artery puncture, transient arterial spasm, nerve damage, and hematoma. No extensive studies exist on late complications in children, but caval thrombosis with a fatal outcome has been reported.[51]

Umbilical Vein

Placement of a central catheter using the umbilical vein is possible in the newborn. The catheter should cross the ductus venosus to reside in the intrathoracic inferior vena cava. It should *not* be located within the liver (i.e., intrahepatic portal vein) where portal vein thrombosis or hepatic necrosis may result from injection of hypertonic or alkaline solutions.[51,54]

External Jugular Vein

At first glance, the external jugular approach to the central circulation would appear ideal. The advantages of avoiding blind venipuncture of deep veins must be weighed against the high incidence of noncentrally placed catheter tips and the high overall failure rate. The incidence of successful external jugular cannulation varies from 50 to 65 percent in children. Of the successful catheters placed, 14 to 33 percent of the catheter tips do not reside in the central venous structures.[55–57] Our experience with external jugular cannulation in 117 pediatric patients, ranging in age from 12 hours to 15 years, yielded a successful cannulation rate of 65 percent. The success of external jugular cannulation improves with increasing age of the patient. The success rate was 50 percent in children less than 5 years; 73 percent in children over 5 years. Of the successful cannulations, 11 resulted in catheter tips positioned in the extrathoracic veins on chest radiograph. The frequency of extrathoracic tip position was not related to the age of the patient.[54] The only acute complication is hematoma formation. Late complications are limited to infection and, rarely, thrombosis.

The patient should be positioned supine with a roll under the shoulders and the head turned away from the side of the puncture. The vein will be distended by 15 to 20 degrees of head-down tilt. Holding the lungs in inflation, manually if the patient is intubated or by asking a cooperative patient to perform a Valsalva maneuver, further distends the vessel. Catheterization should be attempted only when the vessel is palpated or visualized. A primary skin puncture minimizes formation of a skin plug and decreases the likelihood of catheter burring. Our experience indicates that using the Seldinger technique with a J wire the maximizes success rate. Humphrey and Blitt[56] postulated that the lower success rate in children can be explained in part by the mismatching of the child's vein size and the J wire curvature. The small diameter of the vein may not permit optimal use of the J wire when the radius of J curvature is larger than the internal diameter of the vessel.

Despite the lower incidence of complications, clinicians inserting central lines in children via the external jugular route should be aware of the probability of extrathoracic tip position. When catheter tip position is critical, it is essential to obtain a chest radiograph to confirm position.

Internal Jugular Vein

In 1969, English and coworkers[58] described the use of the internal jugular vein for central cannulation in a large series of adults and children. A success rate of 94 percent, with a low incidence of complications, was reported in 500 patients.[58] The technique quickly gained popularity in adults, but the clinicians caring for children, anticipating difficulties in safely and accurately placing the catheter, were hesitant to adopt this technique. Satisfactory results using this technique in children, reported in several series in the 1970s, paved the way for widespread pediatric use. The incidence of successful internal jugular cannulation varies from 77 to 100 percent in children.[59–63] Success rate appears to correlate with the experience of the clinicians inserting the catheter. Virtually all catheter tips were properly placed.

The incidence and types of complications vary with the approach and site of cannulation. In general, acute complications include carotid artery puncture, pneumothorax, Horner syndrome, and hematoma on either side, and injury to the thoracic duct when cannulating the left internal jugular. The incidence of carotid artery puncture is higher in children than in adults, reflecting the technical difficulty of dealing with small vessels in close proximity to each other. Our experience cannulating the internal jugular vein in 126 patients, ranging in age from 1 day to 18 years, revealed an overall incidence of carotid artery puncture of 8 percent. Carotid artery puncture occurred in 5.8 percent of patients less than 5 years of age, compared with 10.5 percent in children over age 5.[57] The lower incidence in the younger patients probably reflects the experience level of the clinician inserting the line. No permanent sequelae resulted from any carotid artery puncture. Late complications are limited to thrombosis and infection, both of which occur at a low incidence.

The approaches to the internal jugular vein can be classified as high or low, with the reference point being the level of the apex of the triangle formed by the sternal and clavicular heads of the sternocleidomastoid muscle and the clavicle. The high approach refers to inserting the needle at or above the apex, and the low approach below the apex. Techniques can also be classified as anterior, central, or posterior, depending on their relationship to the sternomastoid muscle. We prefer a high central approach to cannulation, based on the work of Coté and Jobes.[64] In comparing the high and low approaches in children, these workers demonstrated a significant increase in morbidity using the low approach without change in success rate.

The position of the patient for insertion is identical to that for cannulation of the external jugular vein. The patient's mastoid process and suprasternal notch are identified. The needle is inserted, at an angle of 30 degrees to the skin, on a line between these two landmarks at the level of the cricoid cartilage. The point of needle entry should lie just lateral to the carotid artery. A non-Luer lock syringe should be attached to a finder needle and constant negative pressure exerted, while slowly moving the needle tip. The internal jugular vein is a superficial structure. Penetration by a needle to a depth greater than 2 cm below the skin surface does not increase the likelihood of identifying the vessel but does increase the risk of pleural puncture.

Cannulating the internal jugular vein is a rapid, reliable means to the central circulation in children when appropriate measures are taken to recognize carotid artery puncture. There are difficulties in differentiating venous and arterial lumens in children more often than in adults. This is due to the smaller differences between arterial and venous pressures, the use of smaller-gauge finder needles, and in children with cyanosis, the similarity in color of venous and arterial blood. When the identity of the vessel is in doubt, we recommend transducing the needle or a small-gauge catheter to confirm the presence of a venous waveform and pressure prior to passing any large-diameter catheter.

Recent work has shown that two-dimensional ultrasound facilitates cannulation of the internal jugular vein in children.[65] This technique not only increases the chance of successful cannulation, particularly on the first attempt but reduces the time taken to aspirate blood from the vein. The Alderson study[65] was unable to demonstrate that the rate of carotid artery puncture was reduced with use of the ultrasound because of the small sample size.

Subclavian Vein

The infraclavicular approach to the subclavian vein in adults was first described in 1952 by Aubaniac.[66] Similar to experience with other approaches, a time lag of some 20 years elapsed between acceptance of the technique in adult and pediatric practice. The primary advantage of this approach is the fact that the catheter can be secured on the child's anterior chest wall, permitting free mobility of the head. For long-term parenteral nutrition, the mobility of the child's head is a real practical advantage. Successful insertion rates range from 81 to 96 percent in children.[67–70] A high percentage of catheters, particularly Silastic catheters, require repositioning to obtain proper placement. This manipulation can prolong the procedure time considerably. Acute complications include subclavian artery puncture, pneumothorax, hydrothorax, hemothorax, and hematoma. The incidence of arterial puncture is less than with the internal jugular route. Not only is the incidence of pneumothorax, hydrothorax, and hemothorax higher using the subclavian route, but the sequelae are more significant. Late complications are limited to infection and perforation.

When using the infraclavicular approach to the subclavian vein, the patient should be supine with 15 to 20 degrees or more of head-down position with a roll placed longitudinally in the interscapular region to allow the shoulders to fall posteriorly. The head should be in the midposition or turned to the side of the venipuncture. Rotating the head to the ipsilateral side results in the internal jugular vein meeting the subclavian vein at a more acute angle, favoring central catheterization. A palpable groove is formed where the clavicle and first rib cross. At this point, the needle is introduced bevel down at the inferior edge of the clavicle. Constant negative pressure applied to the needle improves early recognition of the lumen. In children the vessel is superficial and should be identified before advancing the needle beyond 1.5 cm.

Pulmonary Artery Pressure

The pulmonary artery pressure is very high in utero, but falls markedly with the initiation of ventilation and the increase in PaO₂ soon after birth. In the normal infant, adult pulmonary artery pressures are achieved within the first 2 weeks of life, with the major reduction occurring in the first 3 days of life.[12,71] Since Swan and Ganz[72] introduced the flow-directed balloon-tipped catheter in 1970, assessment of left heart hemodynamics via pulmonary artery and wedge pressures has been available. Application of the Swan-Ganz catheter to pediatric patients has been slow in evolving because of the difficulty with insertion, the lack of clearly defined indications, and the use of the directly placed pulmonary artery and left atrial lines.

Insertion Sites

All the venous access routes discussed for central venous pressure can be used to place a pulmonary artery catheter. Our experience indicates that placement is faster and more reliable using either the right internal jugular vein or the femoral vein. Technical difficulties of sheath insertion in a small neck require use of the femoral approach in patients weighing less than 15 kg. Table 27-7 lists guidelines for selecting the proper catheter for pediatric patients of all ages.

In patients weighing less than 30 kg, in patients with an abnormal musculoskeletal systems, and in children with low cardiac output, fluoroscopy aids in catheter placement. Pressure waveforms are

TABLE 27-7. Guidelines for Selection of Pulmonary Artery Catheters in Pediatric Patients

Age	Size (Fr)	Distance from RA port to tip of Catheter (cm)
Newborn–3 years	5	10
3–8 years	5	15
8–14 years	7	20
>14 years	7	30

used to place catheters in patients weighing more than 30 kg.

Indications

Table 27-8 lists the five major indications for insertion of a Swan-Ganz catheter in infants and children. Pediatric patients with global cardiac dysfunction may benefit from such a catheter to assist in directing complex fluid and pharmacotherapy. Pulmonary artery catheters may be useful in patients with complex congenital heart defects who have long-standing increased pulmonary blood flow and pulmonary hypertension and are undergoing surgical procedures where further alterations in hemodynamics are expected.[73] The effects of therapeutic interventions can be assessed by serial determinations of cardiac output. Occasionally a pediatric patient with an impaired myocardium requires a surgical procedure that results in acute changes in afterload. Examples are children with malignant hypertension requiring aortic cross-clamping and infants with arteriovenous malformations of the vein of Galen (i.e., great cerebral vein), where clipping of the malformation results in an acute increase in systemic vascular resistance. In these situations, a Swan-Ganz catheter permits assessment of the ability of the left heart to handle changes in afterload.

Complications of Swan-Ganz Catheters

This discussion is limited to complications unique to the use of catheters in children. Precautions must be taken to match sheath and catheter sizes to ensure an airtight seal to avoid air emboli and their sequelae. Paradoxical venous air embolism has also resulted from balloon rupture with release of air that travels from right to left via anatomic communications. The use of carbon dioxide to inflate the balloon eliminates this risk. Children with preexisting left bundle branch block may develop complete heart block on insertion of a pulmonary artery catheter. During insertion, Swan-Ganz catheters can disrupt suture lines on the right side of the heart. A previously placed catheter may also be sutured to the heart during surgery.[74] The information obtained from a pulmonary artery catheter is more frequently subject to error in infants and children than in adults. The presence of intra- and extracardiac communications may result in an aberrant catheter course, producing "wrong" pressures, spurious values for cardiac output, and an increased risk of systemic emboli. Close attention should be paid to distance on insertion with limits set depending on the size of the patient and the insertion site to prevent coiling, intracardiac tangles, and knots. The relatively large ratio of balloon diameter to right heart valve area and to the right ventricular outflow tract can result in structural damage or decreased right heart output when the balloon is inflated.

Left Atrial Catheters

Instead of a Swan-Ganz catheter, many pediatric patients have a left atrial catheter placed under direct vision at the termination of cardiac surgery. The line is inserted through a purse string suture in the right superior pulmonary vein and directed into the left atrium. Ease of insertion must be weighed against the incidence of catheter malfunction and the complications of removal through a closed chest. The mean left atrial pressure can be assumed to reflect left ventricular end-diastolic pressure in the absence of mitral valve disease.

Following right and left atrial pressures is useful in postoperative management. Simultaneous decreases in both pressures indicates either improved myocardial function or hypovolemia. The trend of the left atrial pressure is as helpful as the pressure itself. Progressive increases in both atrial pressures indicates decreasing myocardial performance, volume overload or tamponade. An abrupt increase in both pressures usually signifies a catastrophic event (e.g., myocardial ischemia or arrhythmias) while a precipitous decrease in atrial pressures usually accompanies hemorrhage of major proportion.

Complications unique to left atrial lines are bleeding after percutaneous removal,[75] catheter entrapment, and catheter embolus. The mediastinal

TABLE 27-8. Indications for Pulmonary Artery Catheter Placement

Cardiac dysfunction
  Global
  Disparity between left and right ventricular function
Pulmonary hypertension
Sampling mixed venous blood
Serial cardiac output determinations
Acute changes in afterload resulting in sudden
  alteration in left ventricular function

drain inserted at surgery should remain in place until the left atrial line is removed.

Cardiac Output

In the newborn, cardiac output may reach 400 ml/kg per minute. Left ventricular output exceeds right ventricular output due to the left-to-right shunts present in the neonate. By the end of the first week of life, these shunts have ceased and the output of the two ventricles is equal. During this period, cardiac output falls to between 150 and 300 ml/kg per minute, at which time systemic blood pressure is maintained by a compensatory peripheral vasoconstriction. Neonatal cardiac output, initially triple that of the adult, ultimately falls to twice the resting adult values.

Measurement of cardiac output enables assessment of the integrated performance of the circulatory system. Cardiac output, systemic and pulmonary arterial blood pressure, and atrial pressure measurements can be used to calculate the systemic and pulmonary vascular resistance, right and left ventricular stroke work, and stroke volume.

Three methods of invasive cardiac output measurement are commonly used in pediatric patients: (1) thermodilution using a thermistor in the pulmonary artery, (2) dye dilution, and (3) from the radial artery pressure curve.

Thermodilution

The thermodilution techniques are based on inducing a local change in blood temperature by injecting a measured volume of injectate at known temperature and measuring the change in temperature downstream. Specifically, after the baseline pulmonary artery blood temperature is measured, a known volume of cold injectate is administered through the proximal port in the right atrium or via a right atrial line, and the temperature change is determined by the pulmonary artery thermistor. The inert nature of the indicator (cold saline) in the thermodilution technique and the fact that arterial sampling is not required with each determination are advantages of this technique.

Thermodilution techniques measure right-sided cardiac output only. Measurement of pulmonary blood flow does not reflect systemic blood flow in patients with intracardiac communications. For example, a child with a ventricular septal defect who has left-to-right shunting will have an elevated right

heart output but normal to subnormal aortic blood flow. Balancing the risk of volume overload from the injectate versus inaccurate results from too small an injectate volume is a problem in small children needing frequent determinations. Progressive hypothermia needs to be avoided when using cold injectate. Systematic errors in the computer integration of the area under the curve occurs in infants with short circulation times.

Dye Dilution

The dye dilution technique uses the rapid injection of a known amount of indocyanine green dye into the central circulation. The dye passes through the right heart to the lungs and into the systemic arterial circulation. Blood is sampled via a constant rate pump from a peripheral arterial cannula and passed through a densitometer. Cardiac output can be calculated manually or can be determined with a computer by measuring the area under the curve of the dye concentration plotted against time. The dye is so rapidly removed by normal liver parenchymal cells that determinations may be repeated as frequently as every 2 minutes. The maximum dye dose is 2 mg/kg per day. Small aliquots should be used for each determination if multiple measurements are anticipated. Blood sampling can result in withdrawal of a significant blood volume occasionally requiring transfusion.

An advantage of this technique is that examination of the cardiac output curve when using dye dilution allows detection of residual or undiagnosed shunts. Right-to-left shunting will be manifest by earlier than normal appearance of dye. Curves in patients with large left-to-right shunts are prolonged and flat, reflecting recirculation of the dye. Small left-to-right shunts are accompanied by the appearance of a recirculation curve (hump) in the downslope of the primary curve.

Radial Artery Pressure Curve

Cardiac output can also be determined using the direct systemic arterial pressure. Since children do not have arteriosclerotic cardiovascular disease, the radial artery pressure curve can be used to accurately determine stroke volume. Cardiac output is calculated by multiplying stroke volume by heart rate. This can be done with each heart beat using computer-assisted analysis.[76] The technique is attractive in pediatric patients as it avoids the manipulation (injection or withdrawal) of any fluid volume. The applicability of this technique is enhanced by the ability to adapt the radial artery waveform in children as opposed to the aortic pressure waveform required in adults.

Noninvasive Cardiac Output Determination

Despite mixed results in clinical studies designed to evaluate their accuracy and precision in children, noninvasive methods used to quantify systemic cardiac output remain an area of ongoing interest and development. At present, noninvasive cardiac output devices employ one of two methodologies: Doppler flow determination or thoracic bioimpedance cardiography.

Doppler Cardiac Output

Doppler instruments are the most commonly employed and extensively studied devices for noninvasive cardiac output determination. When coupled with estimated or measured aortic cross sectional area and corrections based upon the incident angle of insonation (θ), Doppler velocity determinations can quantify flow.[77,78] Early investigations of this technique yielded encouraging results. During cardiac catheterization of 33 children ranging in age from 3 days to 17 years, Alverson and colleagues[79] demonstrated a correlation coefficient of 0.98 when comparing Doppler and Fick cardiac output determinations. Walther and colleagues[80] found a close correlation between flow measurements made in the ascending aorta and those in main pulmonary artery of preterm and term neonates.

Doppler determinations of cardiac output are subject to several limitations. Since the Doppler interrogation is customarily performed in the ascending aorta, coronary flow cannot be detected, thus resulting in a systematic under estimate of left ventricular output. Accurate Doppler evaluation of aortic blood velocity assumes laminar flow conditions. Therefore, disease of the aortic valve or other cardiovascular pathology that produces turbulent flow in the ascending aorta introduces an unpredictable error. In addition, cardiac anomalies that result in malposition of the aorta can create uncertainty with respect to the θ angle. Finally, malformations that result in circulatory patterns in which ascending aortic flow does not reflect systemic flow, most notably patent ductus arteriosus will generate misleading information. By mapping ascending aortic flow before and after closure of a patent ductus arteriosus in 18 preterm neonates, Alverson[77] elegantly demonstrated the increased left ventricular output that must occur in order to sustain sufficient bodily perfusion as a consequence of this left-to-right shunt (Fig. 27-5). Mean ascending aortic flow values fell from 343 ml/kg per minute to 252 ml/kg per minute following patent ductus arteriosus closure.[81] Hirsimaki and colleagues[82] classified the physiologic significance of the patent ductus arteriosus in healthy newborns on the basis of ascending aortic flow (i.e., 300 ml/kg per minute indicating moderate shunt, 266 ml/kg per minute a mild shunt, and 260 ml/kg per minute in the absence of any patent ductus arteriosus flow).[82]

Attempts to makes these measurements using Doppler probes in other sites have met with little success. Comparing transesophageal echocardiography derived Doppler data to thermodilution cardiac (i.e., pulmonary) output measurements in adults, Muhiudeen and associates[83] only demonstrated a weak correlation. In order to optimize the θ angle, they measured Doppler velocity in the main pulmonary artery and across the mitral valve. The latter bore virtually no relationship to thermodilution values ($r = .24$, $P \leq .11$, standard deviation ± 2 L/min), while the former exhibited a weak one ($r = .65$, $P \leq .01$, SD ± 1 L/min). In a study of 17 infants and children between 8 months and 17 years, transthoracic Doppler measurements of aortic flow correlated weakly with thermodilution as well, with 45 percent of paired determinations differing by more than 15 percent.[84] Doppler flow probes to determine cardiac output have also been incorporated onto tracheal tubes (Applied Biometric, Inc., Minnetonka, MN). Reports on the precision and accuracy of this device when used in adults have varied substantially.[85] The single case report of its use in a pediatric patient only reports Doppler-derived data in relation to other clinical signs of well-being rather than objective cardiac output determinations.[86]

Thoracic Bioimpedance

Thoracic bioimpedance or impedance cardiography employs the principle that the thoracic impedance changes with the intravascular volume changes that accompany cardiac systole. Integration of these changes provides an estimate of stroke volume that in turn permits the calculation of a series of hemodynamic variables. While the principle upon which it is based is qualitatively sound, the translation into a quantitative measurement is fraught with complex assumptions, the most vexing of which rests upon an estimate of thoracic volume, more precisely termed the volume of electrically participating tissue. While Mickell and coworkers[87] were able to establish reproducible baseline data (±5 percent) from this method over a wide range of children (2–60 kg) by pooling results from 100 studies, no attempt was made to relate these data to any other objective measure of cardiac output. During the 2-hour study period, averaged data collected over 5-minute spans in individual children deviated from baseline by as much as 44 percent. In a study of 24 children between 3.6 and 44 kg, O'Connell and coworkers[88] compared thoracic

bioimpedance to indocyanine green dye dilution. Despite a correlation coefficient of 0.94, the standard deviation over the range of children was 0.58 L/min, severely compromising the validity and clinical utility of these data in small patients. They also observed technical difficulties with bioimpedance in children exhibiting extreme tachycardia.

Transesophageal Echocardiography

Transesophageal echocardiography (TEE) serves three principal functions in the operating room or intensive care unit: anatomic diagnosis, physiologic assessment, and evaluation of a cardiovascular procedure. Several manufacturers are now producing probes with sufficiently large numbers of elements to enable biplane imaging in a probe small enough to use in infants weighing 3 kg or less.[89,90] Most investigators report good correlation of TEE with

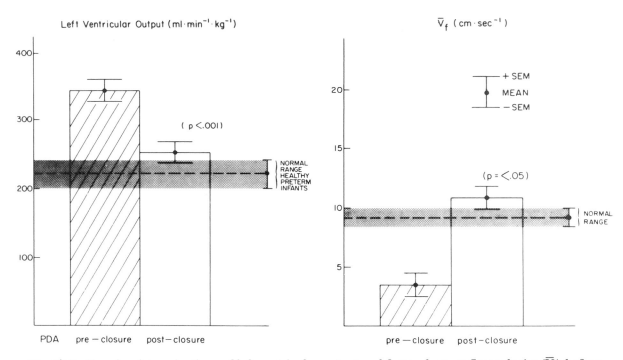

Fig. 27-5. Doppler determinations of left ventricular output and femoral artery flow velocity ($\overline{V}_f$) before and after closure of the ductus arteriosus. Note that despite substantial reduction in the output of the left ventricle after ductal closure, femoral flow velocity increases, implying an improvement in systemic flow. *Hatched areas* reflect age-adjusted normal values. Data are depicted as mean ± standard error. (From Alverson,[77] with permission.)

other diagnostic modalities.[90–92] Stümper and colleagues[93] described a series of 25 children in 60 percent of whom TEE provided new diagnostic information. The esophageal window provides superior resolution of the pulmonary veins and other posterior structures such as the left ventricular outflow tract when compared to transthoracic echocardiography. TEE also permits evaluation of atrioventricular valve anatomy and function. Deciphering the myriad forms of congenital heart malformation and drawing conclusions that may alter the surgical plan requires substantial training and ongoing experience and/or the close cooperation of a pediatric cardiologist to interpret anatomic studies.

As with adults, subjective physiologic evaluation of ventricular volume, regional or global abnormalities in ventricular shortening can be made. In order to evaluate the anesthesiologist's ability to detect intraventricular volume changes in small infants using the TEE, Reich and colleagues[94] conducted a blinded study of 11 infants between 3 and 15 kg, whom they deliberately phlebotomized to induce a 5 and 10 mmHg fall in systolic systemic arterial pressure. Despite the small magnitude of change in end-diastolic volume (5 and 13 percent, respectively), anesthesiologists experienced in TEE were able to detect these changes with 80 to 90 percent sensitivity and 80 percent specificity. TEE also permits the anesthesiologist to diagnose and treat pathophysiologic processes that are unique to congenital heart disease. Fyfe and coworkers[95] employed TEE both in the operating room and intensive care unit to devise optimal medical, surgical, and ventilatory management in a series of children after Fontan operation.

Although this technology permits instantaneous evaluation of a cardiovascular procedure, an understanding of the abrupt and dramatic physiologic changes that commonly occur during the immediate postbypass period require that echocardiographic findings be interpreted cautiously in this setting. Muhiudeen and colleagues[91] reported that early postbypass studies tended to overestimate atrioventricular valve regurgitation. In fact, the presence or absence of significant areas of obstruction or atrioventricular valve dysfunction must be analyzed in light of the rapidly changing loading conditions (e.g., intravascular volume, flow, and ventricular compliance) that have an impact on these processes.[96]

MONITORING THE RESPIRATORY SYSTEM

Noninvasive Monitoring

Breath Sounds

The movement of air within the airways produces vibrations, and thus sounds, with each breath. These sounds are characterized by a rising pitch during inspiration and a falling pitch during exhalation. Various abnormalities change the character, magnitude, and phase relationships of these sounds. One can often infer the location and the nature of pathology by characteristic changes in breath sounds. For example, the vibratory, high-pitched "crowing" that occurs during the inspiratory phase is called stridor. Stridor is the result of extrathoracic airway obstruction. If high-pitched ronchi were to occur during the expiratory phase, they would be characterized as wheezing. Unlike stridor, wheezing indicates the presence of intrathoracic airway obstruction. While this distinction may seem academic, these signs should bring to mind differential diagnoses and therapies that are quite different.

As with heart tones, in order to appreciate subtle changes in breath sounds, one must actively listen for them. The tools available to the anesthesiologist in the operating room, principally the precordial or esophageal stethoscopes, are limited in their ability to provide discriminating information. Nonetheless, one should maximize the information these devices provide by careful placement, active listening, and reducing interference such as that encountered by the bubbling of accumulated condensation in the breathing circuit. In the best circumstances, these stethoscopes reveal only gross changes, thus a detailed description of auscultatory findings is beyond the scope of this chapter.

Respiratory Rate

The frequency of breathing is inversely related to age. The resting respiratory rate of the neonate is 30 to 40 breaths per minute, decreasing throughout childhood to the adult rate of 12 to 16 breaths per minute. In conjunction with auscultation, the pattern of chest and abdominal wall movement is the best method of monitoring respiratory rate (f) and airway obstruction in the operating room. One may be misled by observing the reservoir bag in the anesthesia circuit as its volume may change in the absence of adequate gas exchange. With these techniques available, specific respiratory rate (i.e., apnea) monitoring by impedance pneumography is not generally necessary in the operating room. Such monitors are subject to false negative (e.g., poor lead placement, shallow respirations) and false positive (e.g., precordial/cardiac oscillations) respirations, and they require transthoracic placement of the ECG electrodes, which may violate the surgical field. Other monitoring devices that may be used in the operating room provide respiratory rate and apnea alarms in addition to their primary function. These include spirometers, capnometers, and mass spectrometers.

Tidal Volume

The resting tidal volume (V_T) is fairly constant over the pediatric age range, about 6 ml/kg, yet carbon dioxide production by small children is increased.[97] Thus their increased minute ventilation is achieved through a more rapid respiratory rate. When using mechanical ventilation in children, one may elect to provide a larger V_T at a lower f in order to reduce the fraction of dead space ventilation (V_D).

The measurement of a small V_T is subject to several sources of error, and thus can serve only as an estimate in most clinical situations. The flow sensors in clinical use fall into four basic categories: turbine, pneumotach, thermistor, and ultrasound. Only instruments employing the first three are available for use in the operating room and the intensive care unit. Anesthesia machines typically employ a spirometer of the turbine vane variety (e.g., Wright respirometer) in which a paddle vane rotates in proportion to the flow through it. These monitors are sensitive to mechanical friction and inertia especially at the low flow rates one would expect in children. However, minimal errors of 20 ml are not uncommon with this technology. This nearly equals the resting tidal volume of a normal 3.5-kg newborn. Pneumotachographs measure the pressure drop across a mechanical resistor, which is proportional to the flow through it. Several volume ventilators employed in the intensive care unit incorporate flow sensors of this type (e.g., Siemens Servo 900C). Such systems are subject to accumulated debris on the screen that commonly serves as the resistor as well as the nonlinear effects of tur-

bulence through the resistor. At low flows (<100 ml/s), these devices may have as much as 20 percent error. Hot-wire anemometers use the principle of convective cooling of a sensor as inspired air is drawn past it. Refinements in this methodology place it among the most accurate means of small volume detection,[98] although it is not incorporated into any anesthesia machine or ventilator in current use. Ultrasound transducers may be used to measure gas velocity from which flow can be calculated. This technique is currently confined to some of the spirometers used in pulmonary function testing.

The compression volume of the breathing circuits is the other large source of error in respiratory volume measurement. Even if one were able to measure V_T accurately, small infants ventilated at recommended volumes would be significantly hypoventilated unless one considers compression volume of the circuit. The compression volume, expressed in milliliters per centimeter of water, is the volume "absorbed" by the circuit as it is distended by positive pressure. It can be calculated by delivering a measured volume to the circuit with the patient connection and the popoff valve closed. The compression volume of anesthesia systems varies with the type of circuit (Mapleson D = 2–2.27 ml/cm H_2O, adult circle system 5 to 12 ml/cm H_2O) and whether a humidifier was used (an additional 1.5 to 3 ml/cmH$_2$O).[99] In infants the compression volume may exceed the desired V_T

As a result of these significant inaccuracies, respiratory volume monitors are of limited use in infants and small pediatric patients. The constant fresh gas flows through the valveless Mapleson breathing systems commonly used in small patients serves as yet another potentially large source of measurement error. Thus these monitors serve primarily to indicate trends in delivered volumes. This information should be considered only in conjunction with other sources of subjective (e.g., chest movement, auscultation) and objective data (e.g., inflating pressure, capnography, blood gas analysis). In this patient population, spirometers may have more value as monitors of respiratory rate and apnea if they are so equipped.

Peak Airway Pressure

The measurement of peak airway pressure has long served as an indication of V_T in infants and small children in whom actual volume measurements are plagued by technical difficulties. As with any pressure-volume relationship, this measurement is subject to assumptions that limit its accuracy. One assumption is that the circuit pressure precisely tracks the intrathoracic tracheal pressure. This relationship is influenced by several variables, most importantly the lumen and length of the tracheal tube and the gas flow characteristics during the inspiratory phase. The Hagen-Poiseuille law governing the resistance to movement through a tube dictates that the resistance is proportional to the length of the tube and inversely proportional to the fourth power of the radius. The lumen of a tracheal tube will have a dramatic influence on the resistance and therefore the pressure drop from the anesthesia circuit to the trachea. If a partial obstruction occurred (e.g., kink, tissue, or debris), the increase in resistance that follows assumes proportionally greater importance in small tracheal tubes. As the resistance increases, the pressure gradient increases. If inspiration is limited by peak pressure, then V_T falls, whereas if inspiration is volume limited, then the peak circuit pressure must rise. Although a properly placed esophageal balloon would be a more accurate indication of intrathoracic pressure,[100] in practice these devices are somewhat difficult to place precisely, and are therefore reserved for situations where this information is vital.

As with flow determinations, peak airway pressure provides another piece of data that contributes to an estimate of V_T. Airway pressure alone will not provide a reliable assessment of V_T. It must be integrated with the other pieces of subjective and objective data available in order to arrive at a reasonable estimate of V_T.

Minute Ventilation

Although the resting tidal volume of a neonate is comparable to that of an adult (~6 mg/kg), the metabolic rate is twice the adult value. The carbon dioxide production of an infant may approach 8 ml/kg per minute as opposed to approximately 3 ml/kg per minute in the adult.[97] In order to maintain normal $PaCO_2$, the infant's minute ventilation (V_E) must increase proportionally (220 ml/kg per minute versus 80–100 ml/kg per minute). Newborns balance the flow resistance and elastic properties of their lungs in such a way as to minimize respiratory work.[101] Despite an increase in dead-space ventilation, the newborn expends the least energy by maintaining V_T at 6 ml/kg per minute, while increasing respiratory rate. Carbon dioxide production diminishes gradually throughout childhood to reach adult levels by adolescence.[97]

Minute ventilation is measured by those devices that measure V_T. These units typically will average several breaths and multiply the average by the respiratory rate. Any errors inherent in the measurement of V_T are magnified by this calculation.

Integrated Pulmonary Function Analysis

By integrating volume delivery and inflating pressure data, the anesthesiologist is continually analyzing pulmonary mechanics. Should the pressure increase for a given V_T, this crude method cannot provide specific diagnostic information as to whether the problem reflects a kink in the tracheal tube, the accumulation of secretions or obstruction of the artificial or natural airways, or diminished pulmonary compliance. Using a laboratory simulation of the common intraoperative respiratory problems encountered in anesthetizing an infant, Brown and associates[102] demonstrated the diagnostic value of digital processing of flow-volume loops. The introduction of self-contained pulmonary mechanics diagnostic units permits display and analysis of the flow-volume and pressure-volume relationships that help to distinguish the various pathophysiologic processes. Seear and coworkers[103] compared the continuous linear regression analysis of an automated, noninvasive pulmonary mechanics device to traditional methods of pulmonary function testing (i.e., end-inspiratory hold and continuous flow techniques). The automated unit produced comparable values with a lower coefficient of variation than either of the other techniques. In the latter study, virtually all the episodes of increased resistance related to problems with the tracheal tube, while compliance changes reflected pulmonary parenchymal processes.

Inspired and Exhaled Gases

Oxygen

In 1986, standards for patient monitoring during anesthesia were published by Harvard Medical School[104] and the American Society of Anesthesiologists.[27] Both require the continuous use of an oxygen analyzer in the circuit of an anesthesia machine during the conduct of general anesthetics. These monitors are vital in pediatric anesthesia to ensure adequate, but not excessive, oxygen administration. It is generally held that neonates less than 44 postconceptual weeks may have immature retinas and therefore are at risk for retinopathy of prematurity.[105,106] The role of hyperoxemia in this multifactorial process remains controversial, particularly given the relatively brief exposure in the context of anesthesia and surgery.[107,108] Nevertheless, given case reports of retinopathy of prematurity, where oxygen exposure was limited to the operating room, oxygen administration should be carefully titrated in these infants.[109]

Oxygen analyzers in clinical use fall into three primary categories: paramagnetic, amphometric, and mass spectrometric. The latter is discussed in a subsequent section. Paramagnetic (Pauling) analyzers require a sample to be aspirated into a chamber for analysis and thus have largely given way to amphometric electrodes that can be placed directly in the circuit. Amphometric electrodes use electrochemical reactions to analyze oxygen, and fall into two classes; polarographic (i.e., Clark electrode) and galvanic (i.e., fuel cell). Polarographic sensors require an activating current to polarize the electrodes, warm-up time, regular membrane changes and may be slightly more sensitive to condensation of water on the membrane surface.[110] Galvanic analyzers use a spontaneous reaction, do not require warm-up or membrane changes, but periodic fuel cell replacement makes these units more costly over their lifetime. None of the amphometric or paramagnetic units has a sufficiently rapid response time to monitor tidal variations, although mass spectrometry can. The sensors should be placed in the circuit in a location most likely to reflect inspired oxygen concentration while minimizing their exposure to humidity and condensation.

Carbon Dioxide

Capnography is strongly encouraged by most published monitoring standards for anesthesia[27,104] and even conscious sedation.[111] The 1992 amendments to the ASA monitoring guidelines require confirmation of carbon dioxide in the expired gas when a tracheal tube is placed, unless extenuating circumstances preclude this analysis.[27] Capnometry is the instantaneous measurement of carbon dioxide in the breathing circuit, while capnography is

the continuous graphic display of this information. These devices provide unique insight into several areas of critical importance to the anesthesiologist. Capnometry is relatively limited as it is only able to quantify end-tidal and inspired CO_2, which, under ideal conditions reflect alveolar and rebreathed CO_2 concentration, respectively. Capnography, on the other hand, provides a display by which one can evaluate the validity of its numeric result as well as a wealth of additional information.

These instruments allow one to confirm tracheal placement of a tube, to assess the adequacy of ventilation, to recognize significant metabolic and cardiovascular events, and to diagnose faulty anesthesia delivery systems. In situations in which laryngeal structures are poorly visualized and breath sounds may be misleading (e.g., the small infant where sounds may be audible over the entire chest and abdomen), the detection of significant sustained CO_2 released into the circuit provides virtually incontrovertible evidence of tracheal intubation. As noted above, the calculation and measurement of minute ventilation for the small infant is fraught with physiologic variation[97] and technical difficulties. Capnography provides a means of accurately estimating the adequacy of a delivered minute ventilation, as well as evaluating Mapleson breathing circuits for rebreathing of exhaled gas to which they are prone. Exponential reductions in a formerly stable capnography pattern suggest a sudden reduction in pulmonary perfusion as might accompany severe hypotension, pulmonary embolus or, in the extreme, cardiac arrest.[112] Sudden increases in end-tidal CO_2 ($P_{ET}CO_2$) may signify an increased CO_2 production as occurs with temperature elevation, or an early sign of malignant hyperthermia.[113] Capnography monitors the anesthesia delivery system as well, revealing such equipment malfunctions as disconnections, floating unidirectional valves, exhausted CO_2 absorbers, and the rebreathing characteristics of Mapleson breathing systems.[112]

There are several instruments used for capnography, the general principles of which are discussed elsewhere in this text. The most common capnometers utilize infrared light absorption, and obtain samples in either a mainstream or sidestream fashion. Sidestream analyzers aspirate a sample from the circuit and transport it via a long, narrow bore tube to a distant analyzing chamber. They require only a very light airway adaptor, protect the delicate components of the analyzing chamber and enable shared systems (e.g., mass spectrometry). The disadvantages of sidestream systems include potential occlusion of the sampling tube, distortion or dilution of the exhaled gas wave as it is aspirated and transported to the analyzing chamber, and some delay in processing the information.[115] Mainstream analyzers use a sample chamber that is integrated directly into the circuit (Fig. 27-6). They have the advantage of providing virtually instantaneous analysis and avoiding transport of the sample. Such a system does, however, necessitate the addition of a delicate, vulnerable, and bulky sensor to the proximal airway connection, where it might easily serve as a fixation point to dislodge a small tracheal tube. The solid-state sensors that have been released recently weigh substantially less (Novametrix, Wallingford, CT). Although early mainstream sample chambers added as much as 17 ml dead space to the circuit, currently available models have reduced this volume to 0.6 ml.

The degree to which P_{ETCO_2} tension reflects Pa_{CO_2} is subject to many variables, some technical others physiologic.[112] The technical issues of primary importance in accurate measurement of al-

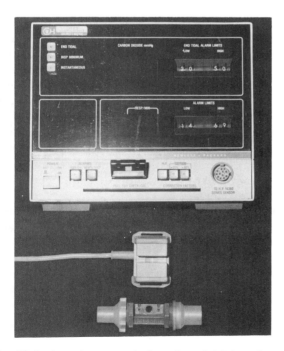

Fig. 27-6. A mainstream infrared end-tidal carbon dioxide monitor. The probe and the airway adapter containing a window are shown beneath the monitor. (Hewlett-Packard, Palo Alto, CA.)

veolar CO_2 tension include the volume and flow rate of exhaled gas,[112,115] the aspirating flow rate (sidestream analyzers),[112,115–117] the fresh gas flow rate, the respiratory rate,[118–122] the type of breathing circuit,[115,123] and the location in the circuit of the sampling chamber (mainstream analyzers) or lumen of the aspirating tubing (sidestream analyzers).[124–127] These variables are of particular importance in the small neonate whose small, frequent exhaled volumes are likely to become diluted by high fresh gas flows. Attempts to minimize the dilution of an aspirated sample of exhaled gas in small infants by lowering the aspirating flow rate have had a deleterious effect on the waveform and accuracy.[117] This occurs in part because lowering the aspirating flow rate slows the response time of the capnometer to the point that it exceeds the short respiratory cycle time in these infants. This process then superimposes the inspiration of one breath on the exhalation of the previous breath.[122] Unless the capnometer is specifically designed to operate at low flow, lowering the aspirating rate promotes waveform degradation in transit and slows the response time in the cuvette. Both of these problems will cause erroneous reductions in P_{ETCO_2} and increases in inspired P_{CO_2}. If the respiratory rate is sufficiently high (i.e., >40 breaths per minute), the response time of most capnometers will exceed the respiratory cycle time, and discernible inaccuracies in the waveform ensue, even at optimal aspirating flow rates.[119–121]

Although static in vitro models have suggested that proper placement of the sidestream sampling tube near the tracheal tube connection of the Bain circuit provides sufficient correlation[125] clinical studies in neonates and small infants appear to dispute that finding.[114,115,126] Badgwell and colleagues[114] have demonstrated that for infants weighing less than 12 kg an aspirating system that samples gas in the distal tracheal tube is necessary to avoid the exponential discrepancies in P_{ETCO_2} to Pa_{CO_2} gradients that develop in infants (Fig. 27-7). For this purpose these authors suggest using a small, coaxial catheter that slid into the tracheal tube lumen. Using this technique on a series of neonates and infants between 1 and 14 kg, they were able to show insignificant differences (mean 1.8 mmHg lower) between side-stream and flow-through capnometer, which, in turn, differed minimally (1 mmHg lower) from Pa_{CO_2}. Rich and associates[126] proposed an alternative solution for situations when a coaxial catheter is not available. They demonstrated that a needle placed 12 cm from the tip of a tracheal tube provides an aspirating port that samples gas the PCO_2 of which is within 1 to 2 mmHg that of the distal tip.

As mentioned previously, several physiologic variables will influence the accuracy with which $PETCO_2$ reflects $PaCO_2$. Most relate to alterations in ventilation:perfusion relationships or CO_2 production that are not unique to children. Children with congenital heart malformations are perhaps the most prevalent subset of patients who merit discussion in this chapter as they pose challenges in the interpretation of capnography. Burrows[127] has demonstrated that children with acyanotic cardiac malformations produce capnography data that are indistinguishable from normal children, even in the face of large left-to-right shunts. In a series of 27 children, nearly half of whom were hypoxic, Fletcher[128] described an inverse relationship between systemic arterial saturation and the arterial-end tidal CO_2 difference. At a systemic oxygen saturation of 60 percent, the arterial-end tidal CO_2 difference exceeded 10 mmHg. Since he combined children who were hypoxic on the basis of right-to-left shunt with those who had admixture of sys-temic and pulmonary venous return, the mechanism of this discrepancy was difficult to understand. Children with right-to-left shunts will have increased physiologic dead space leading to a progressive arterial-end tidal CO_2 difference. However, those with venous admixture might have normal or even increased pulmonary blood flow, and thus no significant change in dead space. Burrows[127] separated children who were hypoxemic into two groups: those with right-to-left shunts and those with venous admixture. He confirmed Fletcher's findings[128] that both groups exhibited significant arterial-end tidal CO_2 differences. Burrows proposed that the increased dead space created by right-to-left shunting represents the most important contribution to this process, but when the shunt fraction ($Q_s:Q_t$) exceeds 0.3, the carbon dioxide that bypasses the lung makes an important contribution to $PaCO_2$ thereby increasing the gradient.

Other Gases

The analysis of nitrogen and oxygen is typically provided along with that of nitrous oxide and volatile anesthetic agents. The analysis of oxygen near the patient connection provides confirmation of the accuracy of other oxygen analyzers. Quantifying the nitrogen present in the circuit is useful in determining adequate preoxygenation, detecting a leak in the delivery system, or, in combination with a sudden fall in $PETCO_2$, a venous air embolism. The analysis of anesthetic gases and vapors serves to illustrate the uptake and elimination of these agents, and to confirm the purity and the accuracy of the tanks and vaporizers, used to administer them. The quantity of residual anesthetic agent has importance in the evaluation of prolonged emergence from anesthesia.

The rate of uptake ($FE:FI$) of an anesthetic agent can be readily monitored by anesthetic gas analyzers with sufficiently rapid response times. The uptake and elimination of anesthetic agents has been shown to be significantly more rapid in the pediatric patient, especially the neonate.[132] This is true for nitrous oxide,[130–132] halothane,[129–132] and methoxyflurane,[130] although the differences are most striking with more soluble agents. The proposed mechanisms include increased alveolar ventilation (especially in relation to functional residual capacity) and an increased cardiac output, a larger percentage of which goes to the quickly saturated

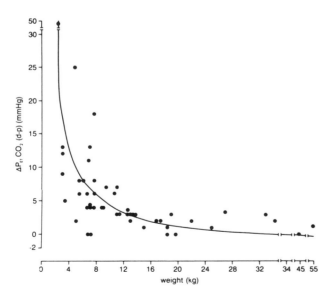

Fig. 27-7. Gradient between end-tidal CO_2 $PETCO_2$) determined in the distal and proximal ends of a tracheal tube. Note the potential for substantial inaccuracy in proximal measurements increases exponentially in children under 12 kg. (From Badgwell,[114] with permission.)

vessel-rich group.[130,131] Together they serve to increase mixed venous anesthetic concentrations and hence FE. Once the blood levels begin to rise, dose-dependent decreases in cardiac output and hepatic metabolism may contribute further.[130] Although the minimum alveolar concentration for young infants may be as much as 50 percent higher than the adult,[26,133,134] cardiovascular depression may occur in as many as 70 percent at that dose.[13,14] Knowledge of anesthetic uptake suggests that this myocardial depression that is observed with higher frequency in the young infant may represent, in part, increased myocardial anesthetic concentration.[139] Through anesthetic gas analysis, one can monitor the overall influence of these variables on a given patient and tailor an anesthetic accordingly.

The alveolar concentration at which children should awaken from an inhalational anesthetic (i.e., minimum alveolar concentration (MAC) awake) has not been determined. The MAC awake: MAC ratio has been shown to be over 50 percent in adults in whom no other preanesthetic medication or anesthetic agent is given.[135] The FE at which awakening occurs may be substantially lower in the more typical clinical situation in which there is no attempt to achieve equilibrium for each measurement as the anesthetic concentration is lowered.[135] The other confounding variables that typically accompany the routine pediatric anesthetic are the use of premedication, adjuvant anesthetic/analgesic agents and the variable influence of postoperative pain. In the authors' experience, the end-tidal anesthetic concentration at which a child will exhibit appropriate motor activity is less than 25 percent minimum alveolar concentration.

The techniques of multigas analysis that have found clinical application are based on properties such as ionized mass separation (i.e., mass spectrometry), ultraviolet and infrared light absorption, and absorption into lipophilic substances. Nitrous oxide and the volatile anesthetic agents all absorb infrared light and thus may be quantified using instruments similar to capnometers. Although the volatile anesthetics absorb infrared light at several wavelengths, the majority of manufacturers select a single wavelength at which they all absorb[120,136] in order to provide the most rapid response time.[137] As a result single-wavelength instruments cannot distinguish between agents, relying upon the clinician to identify the agent in use. Since each agent absorbs light to a different extent at the selected wavelength, individual algorithms are activated when the agent is identified by the clinician. Thus substantial errors can result if the agent delivered is not identified correctly (e.g., vaporizer filled incorrectly), or if there are two agents in the exhaled gas (e.g., halothane induction, isoflurane maintenance).[136] The magnitude of these errors depends upon the absorption differences between the agents at the selected wavelength. Single-wavelength agent analyzers are susceptible to other exhaled organic substances that might absorb infrared light (e.g., ethanol).[121,136] The Nellcor N-2500 (Nellcor, Inc., Hayward, CA) is the only infrared multigas analyzer employing four wavelengths thereby enabling it to accurately identify and quantify anesthetic agents used singly or in combination.[121]

Volatile anesthetics have significant hydrophobic properties, but readily permeate silicone. They produce concentration-related mechanical changes in the silicone that can be measured directly (Narcotest) or using a piezoelectric crystal (Engström multigas monitor for anesthesia or EMMA). Although the EMMA was quite accurate, its response time was relatively slow in comparison to current methodologies. It was also exquisitely sensitive to water vapor and nitrous oxide thereby requiring meticulous calibration and thus limiting its use. A variation on this method uses a piezoelectric crystal coated with a lipophilic compound (ICOR, Bromma, Sweden and Vital Signs, Inc, NJ). Changes in the oscillatory frequency of the crystal reflect anesthetic agent concentration.[138,139] This instrument provides accurate data within 3 minutes of cold start, and exhibits high signal:noise ratio.[139] But, because this property is common to all volatile anesthetics, neither of these monitors can identify individual agents in situations where they might be mixed or are unknown.

Mass spectrometry has become the standard to which other techniques of respiratory gas analysis are compared. These instruments ionize the gases and vapors, and separate them by mass in a high vacuum electric field. Molecules of identical mass (e.g., CO_2, N_2O) are identified by specific fragments that occur during ionization, while those with similar fragments (e.g., halogenated volatile anesthetics) are separated by the characteristic ratios of those fragments. In this manner, all gases and vapors of significance to the anesthesiologist can be specifically measured. These are sidestream analyzers, and are thus subject to distortion and dilution during sample transport as well as obstruction of the sampling tube. These monitors are sensitive to the water condensate that forms as humidified gases cool in the breathing circuit and sampling line. In light of the high cost of mass spectrometry, the expense of equipping each operation room with dedicated units becomes prohibitive in most settings. Thus the majority of systems currently in use are shared or multiplexed in order to diffuse the cost over 6 to 16 locations, thus reaching limits of excessive cost at the low end and unacceptable gaps in information at the high end. Processing delays, which are governed by the number of locations between which the system is multiplexed, are most significant in that they interrupt the continuous surveillance of capnography. The major providers of anesthesia mass spectrometers (Perkin-Elmer/Marquette, Milwaukee, WI and SARA/PPG, Pittsburgh, PA) now offer continuous, local (dedicated) infrared capnography as a supplement to a multiplex system.

A dedicated multigas analyzer utilizing the principle of Raman light scattering (RASCAL, Ohmeda, Madison, WI) employs an argon laser, which exhibits specific frequency shifts upon collision with a given molecule, the Raman effect.[140] A spectrum is produced the area under which is directly proportional to the concentration of the gas. As the scattering is the result of the laser interaction with covalent bonds, the instrument cannot detect single atoms that do not have these bonds (e.g., He). This device has the advantages of rapid response time (65 ms), distinct spectra for CO_2 and N_2O, and distinct peaks for each volatile anesthetic agent. Gas samples are obtained using a side-stream approach, and thus the monitors are susceptible to all the problems of that method. The instrument does not require the high vacuum that mass spectrometry does, nor is it sensitive to water vapor.

Oxygenation

Arterial oxygenation is a matter of consummate concern to all anesthesiologists, especially those whose practice includes significant numbers of children. Closed claim analysis of pediatric malpractice actions revealed 43 percent of the incidents were related to inadequate ventilation and oxygenation.[141,142] Children, in view of their high oxygen consumption, relatively small functional residual capacity and highly reactive airways are more likely to become hypoxemic during an anesthetic than an adult.[143,144] The frequency and severity of hypoxemic events relate directly to the severity of illness,[144] and inversely to age (i.e., $\leq$ 2 years) and the experience of the practitioner.[144,145] Neonates less than 44 postconceptual weeks may also be susceptible to retinopathy of prematurity if they become hyperoxemic.[106,109] Thus children, especially infants, constitute a population in whom the careful tracking of arterial oxygenation is of vital importance. In 1947, Comroe and Botelho[146] observed that even experienced health care providers are limited in their ability to recognize hypoxemia, a finding that has recently been confirmed in the conduct of pediatric anesthetics.[144]

In the 20 years since noninvasive systemic oxygenation monitoring has been available, a technological explosion has occurred that has made these devices virtually ubiquitous in operating rooms and prevalent in most other acute care settings. Spawned, in part by the unequivocal demonstrations that these monitors increase the frequency of detected hypoxemia,[144,147] they have gained universal acceptance. These devices have become incorporated into current anesthesia monitoring standards for both the operating room (1990) and the postanesthesia care unit (1992).[27] Yet the rarity of severe or catastrophic adverse outcomes makes the unequivocal benefit of oximetry virtually impossible to demonstrate, even in large studies.[147,148] Despite the report of pediatric closed claim reviewers that pulse oximetry and/or capnography could have prevented 89 percent of the cases ascribed to inadequate ventilation, it improved outcome in only one of seven such cases in which it was used.[142] Nevertheless, it seems logical, if unproven, that reductions in the frequency and magnitude of hypoxemic episodes perioperatively would likely have some benefit, particularly in infants in whom such events are more common. After ten years of experience with pulse oximetry, clinicians have become so convinced of the contribution that the data from this device makes to their management that they are reluctant to practice without it.[147]

Since the general principles of noninvasive monitoring of oxygenation are covered extensively elsewhere in this text, we shall focus on the application of these devices to pediatric patients, with particular attention to both the physiologic objectives and the limitations of data obtained from these monitors.

Cutaneous Oxygen Tension

In 1972, a miniature Clark polarographic oxygen electrode, similar to that used in vitro blood gas analysis, became available for skin application. When incorporated into a probe that heats the skin to 42 to 44°C, the cutaneous oxygen tension approaches arterial oxygen tension since the skin blood flow and permeability to oxygen are increased.[149,150] This correlation is better obtained in neonates where the epidermis is less keratinized and the cutaneous capillary bed more dense.[150] Despite theoretical concerns that skin heating changes O_2 dissociation and may even result in a P_{TCO_2} that is higher than Pa_{O_2},[150] clinical reports indicate that P_{TCO_2} monitors tend to underestimate Pa_{O_2} above 100 mmHg.[151,152] In fact, Rooth and colleagues;,[153] reported improved accuracy at increased Pa_{O_2} when the sensor temperature was elevated to 45°C. In older children and adults, as the keratinized layer thickens, the diffusion gradient for O_2, and hence the difference between Pa_{O_2} and P_{TCO_2}, becomes more significant.[154] In addition, these monitors are subject to the effects of any and all variables that influence skin perfusion, such as hypotension, hypothermia, and pharmacologic agents.[149,150]

Since this is the only noninvasive monitor that can provide information regarding significant hyperoxemia, the most natural application of the device would be to prevent hyperoxemia in a population vulnerable to retinopathy of prematurity.[149,155,156] Unfortunately, the correlation, especially outside the physiologic range of Pa_{O_2} (i.e., ≥ 100 mmHg), varies depending upon the individual conditions, and may well produce data that differs from the Pa_{O_2} by a substantial yet unpredictable amount.[149,151,152,155,156] In a group of 296 preterm infants, 500 to 1,300 g in size, Bancalari and colleagues[157] reported a reduced incidence of retinopathy of prematurity in the subset over 1,100 g when P_{TCO_2} monitors were employed.

Neonates who have elevated pulmonary vascular resistance due to pulmonary or cardiovascular diseases may exhibit a right-to-left shunt at the ductus arteriosus if it is patent. Under these circumstances, blood perfusing the head and eyes (i.e., preductal) will have a higher Pa_{O_2} than that to the lower body (i.e., postductal). If the objective of noninvasive monitoring of oxygenation is to reduce the risk of retinopathy of prematurity in a neonate with a right-to-left ductal shunt, a preductal site must be selected (e.g., right arm, upper right chest, head). However, in a study of 24 neonates with hyaline membrane disease in the first 24 hours of life, Pearlman and Maisels[158] made 10,000 pre- and postductal P_{TCO_2} determinations and found that 90 percent of the paired comparisons were within 15 mmHg and 99 percent were less than 30 mmHg. They concluded that the difference was rarely large enough to be of clinical significance.

From a practical standpoint the monitor is cumbersome. It requires calibration, warmup time of 10 to 20 minutes, meticulous skin preparation and placement of the probe. It is sensitive to electrosurgical interference and mechanical manipulation. Although it has been shown to be sensitive to halothane in vitro,[159] resulting in electrode depolarization and falsely elevated readings, this influence can be essentially eliminated by the use of a Teflon membrane or an electrode with a lower polarization voltage.[160,161]

Pulse Oximetry

In 1980, the first of a new generation of oximeters was introduced for clinical use. Like the oximeters described by Millikan[162] in 1941, these monitors measure photoabsorption at two wavelengths, 660 and 940 nm. While early oximeters measured total vascular bed absorption after increasing the volume of arterial blood with a heated probe, the current models employ microprocessors to subtract the nonpulsatile absorption from the signal, hence *pulse* oximeters. This enables these monitors to specifically determine the absorption of the pulsatile (AC) signal produced by the arterial vascular bed.[163] As a result, the instruments can be misled by excessive pulsations in the venous bed or by motion.

Although they use the same principle as in vitro co-oximetry, pulse oximeters use only two wavelengths and thus can assay only two forms of hemoglobin: oxyhemoglobin and reduced hemoglobin. The pulse oximeter calculates and displays a "functional" hemoglobin saturation [oxyhemoglobin/(reduced + oxyhemoglobin)], or the saturation of the hemoglobin available for oxygen binding. Co-oximeters use multiple wavelengths and thus can assay dyshemoglobins as well (e.g., carboxyhemoglobin, methemoglobin). They report "fractional" hemoglobin saturation [oxyhemoglobin/(reduced + oxyhemoglobin + dyshemoglobin)]. Since the pulse oximeter will not include dyshemoglobins in the denominator, falsely high determinations will result in clinical situations in which they are present in significant quantities.[163,164] One should not confuse dyshemoglobins (normal hemoglobin molecules bound to abnormal ligands) with hemoglobin variants (molecular variants of normal hemoglobin). The latter (e.g., fetal hemoglobin, sickle hemoglobin) are available for oxygen binding, usually with similar absorption characteristics, and hence are detected by the pulse oximeter.[165–167]

Clinical judgments made on the basis of SpO_2 data require some understanding of comparable investigations in normal children. Mok and associates[168] reported results of SpO_2 studies on 55 normal infants on four successive occasions between the first week of life and 6 months of age. During the first week of life, SpO_2 values were lower at all activity states—awake, feeding, sleeping. Feeding precipitated a significant fall in SpO_2 from mean values of 96 to 91 percent, while quiet sleep was associated with mean SpO_2 of 93 percent. Perhaps more important in establishing thresholds for action, the mean of the minimum values exhibited by the neonates at 1 week when awake, feeding, and sleeping were 92, 83, and 87 percent, respectively. These infants returned on three subsequent occasions for study; 4 to 8 weeks, 9 to 15 weeks, and 16 to 30 weeks. The results of these follow-up studies were comparable. Mean awake SpO_2 was 97 percent, while feeding resulted in a 1 to 2 percent fall, and sleeping values averaged 94 percent. The mean minimum SpO_2 in these older infants was 94, 91, and 89 percent while awake, feeding, and asleep, respectively. These values would require downward adjustment for children living at significant altitude above sea level.[169,170] In a series of 4- to 8-week old healthy term infants, Stebbens and coworkers[171] noted that 81 percent of the infants exhibited occasional fall in SpO_2 to ≤80 percent, usually associated with periodic breathing. The same investigators[172] conducting sleep studies on children 2 to 16 years of age found reductions in the prevalence and magnitude of these episodes with age. Among children 2 to 6 years old, 47 percent exhibited falls in SpO_2 to ≤90 percent, while this occurred in only 13 percent of those over 12.

Saturation values ≤80 percent occurred in only 6 percent of healthy children over 2 years.

The accuracy and response time characteristics of pulse oximetry are also related to the location of the sensor. Sensors placed on the head (e.g., ear, cheek, or even tongue) have demonstrated superior signal preservation under ambient or patient conditions that promote intense peripheral vasoconstriction.[173–175] These "central" sensors exhibit improved accuracy over those placed on the distal extremities.[176] The differences become even more marked under rapidly changing conditions.[175,177,178] Studying the interruption in mechanical ventilation in a group of 22 children with congenital heart disease, Reynolds and colleagues[178] detected desaturation at central sites more than 30 seconds earlier than peripheral sites. By the time the peripheral sensor detected a 5 percent reduction in SpO_2, the central sensor had fallen 30 to 40 percent. Resumption of ventilation resulted in detectable improvement in central SpO_2 within 12 seconds, while the peripheral sensor continued to fall for 30 seconds before beginning to return toward baseline. Severinghaus and Kaifeh[175] postulated that delays in peripheral response time are primarily related to diminished peripheral blood transit time, as well as differences in tissue/capillary composition, and vasoconstriction. Delayed recognition of an event that results in hypoxemia, or, perhaps even more concerning delayed appreciation that suitably effective measures have been taken engenders a situation in which increasingly aggressive measures designed to rectify the problem are undertaken often at some risk to the child.

Commercial pulse oximetry instruments are designed for maximal accuracy and precision at SaO_2 values over 80 percent. Manufacturers presume that once the SpO_2 falls below 85 percent, the clinician is taking whatever measures are necessary to rectify the problem. Therefore, there is some hazard in using these instruments as quantitative analyzers in children whose saturation would be expected to be below that range (e.g., cyanotic congenital heart disease). Most investigators report reasonable instrument precision at levels below 85 percent, and some even claim accuracy as low as 60 percent,[179,180] but the preponderance of studies of children with congenital heart disease reveal a progressive positive bias that typically falls within the range of 5 to 15 percent at 60 percent SaO_2[151,165,166,181–184] (Fig. 28-8).

The convenience, reliability, and freedom from special skin preparation and warming offered by pulse oximeters have enabled them to largely replace P_{TCO_2} monitors in the neonatal intensive care unit. In order to reduce the risk of retinopathy of prematurity in that population, oximeters must be adapted to a use for which they were not originally designed, detecting hyperoxemia. The inherent disadvantage that they face is that the oxyhemoglobin dissociation curve flattens above 96 percent, such that large changes in PaO_2 cause little or no change in SaO_2. If the threshold value for hyperoxemia is defined as 100 mmHg, the upper limit on an oximeter that provides maximal sensitivity (1.0) in detecting hyperoxemia varies between 89 and 95 percent, depending upon the manufacturer.[185–187] The physiologic obstacles imposed on oximeters employed for this objective must be balanced against the methodologic inadequacies that render P_{TCO_2} monitors inaccurate at values over 100 mmHg.[152]

The validity of pulse oximetry data is also subject to a variety of environmental, physiologic and pharmacologic challenges. They are susceptible to motion artifact, which poses significant difficulties in the pediatric postanesthesia care unit or intensive care unit. Although much less sensitive to changes in perfusion than transcutaneous probes, the pulse can be markedly attenuated during intense peripheral vasoconstriction. ECG interfacing helps identify weak signals and reject motion artifact (N-200, Nellcor, Hayward, CA). Certain medical dyes, notably methylene blue, indocyanine green and, to a lesser extent indigo carmine, will absorb light at the wavelength used to assess reduced hemoglobin

(660 nm) and thus falsely lower the oxygen saturation determination.[188] Electrocautery can produce interference which individual models have a varying ability to reject. Ambient lights as well as infrared warmers may produce interference with the photodetector that causes a loss of signal or result in a falsely low saturation determination.[189] Of more concern is a report in which a specific high-frequency operating room light interacted with the photodetector in such a way as to produce a falsely normal saturation despite clinical cyanosis.[190]

Apart from the hazards posed by any misleading data that they might generate, pulse oximeters are extraordinary safe instruments. Despite millions of yearly applications, injury reports are limited. Most relate to cutaneous burns caused by the use of incompatible probes with monitors of different manufacturers.[191] Rarely, electrical faults have been detected in probes.[192] Multiple-use clips have also been reported to cause pressure necrosis when applied to small infants for protracted periods.[193]

Invasive Monitoring

Arterial Blood Gas Analysis

The systemic arterial oxygen tension is lower in the neonate than in the older child and adult. During the first few hours of life, the PaO_2 is 50 to 70 mmHg in the full-term infant and approximately 10 mmHg lower in the premature infant breathing room air.[194] These values climb to those of the normal adult within the first month. The $PaCO_2$ is also slightly lower in the neonate, 31 to 37 mmHg.[194]

Fig. 27-8. Accuracy and precision of a pulse oximeter (Nellcor N-100) in chronically hypoxemic children with congenital heart disease. Data plotted as difference between simultaneous pulse oximetry (SpO_2) and co-oximetry (SaO_2) against the average of the two measurements reflect a mean positive bias ($d = +5.8\%$) for SpO_2 and a wide range (± 2 SD $= -3.8$ to 15.4 percent). (From Schmitt,[184] with permission.)

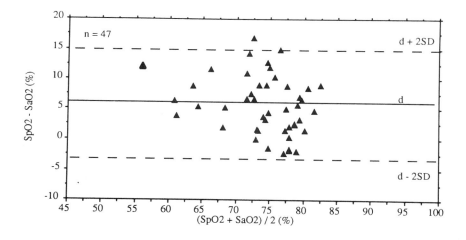

Most likely, this represents a compensatory mechanism for the mild metabolic acidosis that is present in these infants. These values approach normal within the first few months of life as well.

Miniaturization of both optical (SaO_2) and PO_2 electrode technology has enabled the transcatheter continuous invasive analysis of systemic oxygenation that may ultimately prove useful in managing children with volatile physiologies. Miyasaka[193,197] described a 100-μm filament capable of continuous PaO_2 determination through a 22-gauge catheter while still preserving the waveform and sampling functions of the catheter, although the prohibitive cost of such advances will limit their widespread application.

Metabolic Considerations

Serum glucose must be monitored closely in infants at risk for hypoglycemia as general anesthesia will completely mask its signs. Sick neonates are such a population whose glucose requirement may reach 6 to 12 mg/kg per minute. The glycogen stores in a full term infant are scant while those of the preterm are virtually nonexistent. The group at highest risk are preterm infants, those who are small for gestational age, and the infants of diabetic mothers. Once identified, hypoglycemia should be corrected with 0.2 to 0.4 g/kg dextrose (2 to 4 ml/kg D_{10}). Larger quantities may precipitate hyperinsulinemia and hypoglycemic rebound, while more concentrated solutions may precipitate an acute rise in serum osmolarity that has been postulated to increase the risk of intraventricular hemorrhage in the preterm infant.

Hypocalcemia may be seen in the same population at risk for hypoglycemia. In addition, the rapid administration of citrated blood products will bind calcium transiently and may precipitate significant hemodynamic changes. Serum ionized calcium determinations can be made on arterial blood and replacement therapy guided accordingly.

CENTRAL NERVOUS SYSTEM

Noninvasive Monitoring

Electroencephalography

Cerebral cortical activity in the neonate is very limited, and, prior to 35 week gestational age, it is discontinuous. The EEG pattern "matures" with age, and by 2 years of age it has assumed adult characteristics. While sporadic reports of investigational applications of EEG continue[198,199] typically in association with cardiac surgery utilizing cardiopulmonary bypass, widespread acceptance of EEG as an intraoperative monitoring technique has been severely limited by the cumbersome equipment, laborious lead placement, and data the significance of which remains largely obscure or controversial, either in terms of the anesthetic or brain well-being.

Evoked Potential Monitoring

Unlike EEG, evoked potential monitoring has become a valued adjunct to surgery involving the back and spinal cord since it was initially advocated in 1977 by Nash.[200] When the Scoliosis Research Society conducted a survey of a group of surgeons who had performed approximately 60,000 procedures to correct scoliosis over the previous 5 years, 78 percent relied upon somatosensory evoked potentials.[201] Although many variations have been reported, the fundamental elements of the technique require stimulation of a sensory nerve distal to the operative site and reception of a signal by cortically placed electrodes. The raw signal is processed and averaged in order to provide a waveform whose amplitude and latency are compared to baseline values. Reductions in amplitude by more than 44 percent or latency prolongation that exceeds 10 percent are generally accepted markers of spinal cord ischemia.[201] Survey participants reported, 1,000 false positive results (1.7 percent) in which somatosensory evoked potential changes was not associated with postoperative neurologic deficits. Among the 364 reported neurologic deficits (0.6 percent), 72 percent exhibited somatosensory evoked potential changes. The greatest concern relates to the 28 percent of those with neurologic deficits in whom somatosensory evoked potential changes were not detected, for a false negative rate of 0.17 percent. Nearly one-third of the patients who had false negative somatosensory evoked potentials suffered major or sustained deficits, although the majority of these patients did not have both amplitude and latency monitored. Concern over the false negative rate probably accounts for the observation that 70 percent of the surgeons who use somatosensory evoked potentials also used an intraoperative wake-up test as well.

Somatosensory evoked potential monitoring has been extended to any procedure in which spinal cord ischemia might occur (e.g., spinal tumors, cervical fusion, aortic surgery). Epstein and colleagues[202] reported no postoperative neurologic deficits or deaths in a series of 100 adults undergoing various cervical spine surgery procedures with somatosensory evoked potential monitoring. In the previous 218 patients having similar surgery at that institution, the incidence of postoperative quadriplegia was 3.7 percent and the death rate 0.5 percent. The sensitivity and specificity of somatosensory evoked potential monitoring for other surgical procedures may also vary. In an early study of 220 patients between 13 months and 77 years who underwent a variety of surgical procedures only half of which were scoliosis repair, Dinner and coworkers[203] reported four false negative studies (1.8 percent). The fact that 43 percent of the study group showed changes at some point in the procedure might reflect greater surgical risk or imperfections in the monitoring methods.

Apart from surgical manipulation, other elements of intraoperative management can alter somatosensory evoked potentials, most notably anesthetic agents and reductions in systemic arterial pressure. Volatile anesthetic agents tend to increase somatosensory evoked potential latency, while nitrous oxide exerts an influence primarily on amplitude.[204] The degree to which these agents interfere with somatosensory evoked potential signals seems to vary widely, with some authors advising against any vapor or gaseous agent,[205-207] while others suggest the signals are relatively impervious.[208] Some of this variability may relate to the positioning and type of sensing electrodes employed. Needle electrodes permit better signal detection than surface electrodes. Burke and associates[209] found electrodes placed in the epidural space highly resistant to the effects of volatile anesthetics. Sensing electrodes placed over the cervical spine detect cord impulse transmission despite significant cortical depression by anesthetic agents. In distinguishing disruption of spinal cord integrity from global cortical depression induced by anesthetic agents, it may prove useful to stimulate an alternate sensory pathway that enters the spinal cord above the surgical field (e.g., median nerve).

While some controversy remains regarding selection of anesthetic agents, the evidence that some degree of hypotension results in cord ischemia is incontrovertible.[205,210,211] These changes can occur with the modest reductions in systemic pressure often deemed valuable in minimizing blood loss during spinal surgery. The greatest risk occurs if spinal distraction is performed concurrent with hypotensive management. Booke and colleagues[210] described a 15-year-old child whose mean pressure had fallen from 80 to 56 mmHg and hematocrit to 20 percent, which, in association with rotatory correction of scoliosis, induced changes in somatosensory evoked potentials that were confirmed by a wake-up test. Restoration of systemic pressure and hematocrit resulted in resolution of the somatosensory evoked potential findings and a normal wake-up test. The extent to which induced hypotension is safe probably rests on other factors such as the degree of distraction. Grundy and coworkers[205] described a similar situation in which somatosensory evoked potential findings during distraction only resolved when they augmented the patient's blood pressure to a level 20 percent above the preoperative level.

Since somatosensory evoked potentials only examine sensory pathways, the risk of isolated motor pathway injury may account for some of the false negative studies. As a result, recent interest in cortically evoked motor responses has developed for selected, high-risk situations.[209,212,213] Stimulating electrodes are positioned over the motor cortex and sensing electrodes on the lower extremity. Prolonged latency serves to indicate ischemia of the motor pathways. Since surface electrodes can stimulate the corticospinal motor pathways only tangentially, this technique is much more sensitive to cortical depression by volatile anesthetics.[212] Although some have suggested the need to limit the use of muscle relaxants as well,[213] the typical cortically induced impulse is a far more potent stimulus of peripheral motor pathways than a peripheral nerve stimulator, thus muscle relaxants are often acceptable.[212] We have generally avoided volatile agents and nitrous oxide altogether in children requiring motor evoked potentials, using instead some combination of opioids, propofol, benzodiazepines, or ketamine. Burke and colleagues[209] obviates the need to restrict anesthetic agents by using a technique whereby the sensing electrodes for both somatosensory and motor evoked potentials are placed in the epidural space at levels above and below the surgical site.

Intracranial Pressure

A majority of investigators place the normal intracranial pressure in the neonate between 7 to 10 mmHg.[214] Crying and straining may increase the intracranial pressure to 44 mmHg. In a study of 12 preterm neonates, Friesen and colleagues[215] used a fiberoptic anterior fontanel pressure monitor (Ladd Research Industries, Burlington, VT) during awake tracheal intubation to demonstrate a mean increase in intracranial pressure from 8 to 24 cmH_2O.[215] This increase was completely ablated by the administration of any of four anesthetic agents in conjunction with pancuronium. The maximum anterior fontanel pressure he noted during awake intubation was 44 cmH_2O. Earlier investigators, however, noted increases in intracranial pressure to as much as 90 cmH_2O when infants were intubated without muscle relaxants or sedatives.[216] The neonatal intracranial pressure increases during childhood to the adult level of 5 to 15 mmHg in relation to the increase in systemic arterial blood pressure.

Invasive Intracranial Pressure Monitoring

Beyond the first few months of life, noninvasive determination of intracranial pressure is no longer possible. The three options most commonly employed for monitoring intracranial pressure beyond that period are subdural bolt, intraventricular catheter, and fiberoptic transducer. The latter (e.g., Camino catheter) can be placed virtually anywhere in the cranial vault: the epidural space, subdural space, ventricle, or even the brain parenchyma. Intraventricular catheters provide the most reliable and accurate data against which the others are compared. It also offers the ability to withdraw cerebrospinal fluid should that become necessary to treat elevated intracranial pressure. The major disadvantages are difficulty catheterizing the ventricle, hemorrhage during placement, and infection. Subarachnoid bolts are commonly used because they are less technically difficult and hazardous to place. Mendelow and coworkers[217] however, reported simultaneous recordings of intraventricular catheters and subarachnoid bolts that revealed systematic errors in which the bolt indicated pressures 16 mmHg lower than a ventricular catheter.

In the last five years, the fiberoptic transducers have become increasingly popular because of their versatility in placement. Recently, Schickner and

Young[218] have reported a series of adults, who demonstrated intracranial pressure values between 2 and 120 mmHg, in whom he compared Camino catheters placed in the brain parenchyma to ventricular catheters. Around 66 percent of the values from the fiberoptic system were higher than simultaneous measurements from the ventricular catheter. Taken together, the Camino transducer overestimated the ventricular pressure by a mean value of 9 mmHg.

MISCELLANEOUS MONITORING

Noninvasive Monitoring

Body Temperature

Hypothermia represents a major threat to the neonate and young infant since, compared to an adult, their body surface area is much larger with respect to mass (0.075 m^2/kg in the neonate versus 0.025 m^2/kg in the 70-kg adult). Normothermic neonates exposed to a skin-environmental temperature gradient of 10°C have to double their metabolic rate (from a Vo_2 of 4.5 ml/kg per minute to 9 ml/kg per minute) to support their core temperature.[219] Most operating rooms are kept at a temperature of 20 to 22°C (68 to 72°F), producing a skin-environment gradient of at least 15°C. Other hazards of hypothermia include respiratory depression (including apnea), cardiovascular depression and arrhythmias, and delayed emergence and prolonged depression of protective reflexes. Oxygen consumption may increase even further in the immediate postoperative period as the hypothermic pediatric patient tries to restore normothermia. The core temperature of patients should be monitored during administration of all but the shortest anesthetics (i.e., under 15 minutes).

Another concern in the pediatric patient is malignant hyperthermia, which has an incidence of 1:15,000 in children, compared with 1:50,000 adults. Children with diagnosed or occult musculoskeletal disorders that provoke an increased incidence of malignant hyperthermia often present for common pediatric surgical procedures (e.g, herniorrhaphy, strabismus repair, and orthopedic procedures).[220] Although hyperthermia may not represent the initial manifestation of malignant hyperthermia it serves as an important guide as to the efficacy of treatment. Given the proximity to major muscle groups, some have recommended axillary temperature monitoring when concern over the development of malignant hyperthermia is paramount.[221] In most patients, however, hypothermia is far more likely and therefore represents a more appropriate primary focus of body temperature monitoring.

The body temperature can be monitored through several orifices as well as on the surface. The most appropriate method of measuring temperature must be chosen for each patient. Sometimes more than one body temperature will need to be measured. Core temperature is most accurately reflected by esophageal temperature, then by brain (tympanic/nasopharyngeal), rectal, axillary, and least accurately, by skin temperature.

Esophageal Temperature

The esophagus reflects core temperature when the probe is in the distal fourth of the esophagus, since proximal esophageal temperatures are lower due to cooling by inspired tracheal gases.[222–226] Bissonnette and Sessler[222] confirmed this theory by showing that upper esophageal temperature increased above tympanic temperature if the inspired gas was actively warmed. Esophageal temperature monitoring is appropriate only in the intubated patient. Temperature probes are incorporated in most esophageal stethoscopes (see Fig. 27-1) and have the same precautions for use as other esophageal stethoscopes.

Rectal Temperature

The rectum reflects a stable core temperature but will lag behind during rapid changes in core temperature, such as active cooling on cardiopulmonary bypass.[225] Many factors decrease the accuracy of the rectal temperature.[227] The depth to which the probe is inserted influences the proportional effects of blood draining from the lower extremities and that from the viscera. When lodged in feces, a thermistor will exhibit significantly blunted response to rapid changes in core temperature. In situations in which one does not anticipate rapid changes in temperature and the environment is not so extreme as to dramatically lower the temperature of venous return from the legs, then a rectal thermistor provides a reasonable estimate of core temperature. Care must be taken inserting the probe in neonates, especially the pre-

mature, as it is possible to perforate the rectum with a large probe inserted too far. A rectal probe of the size typically used to monitor nasopharyngeal temperature serves to minimize this problem.

Nasopharyngeal Temperature

A probe can be inserted in the nasopharynx anteriorly and cephalad, seeking the olfactory place, or posteriorly to the nasopharyngeal mucosa in an area that reflects the temperature of the nearby carotid arteries. During cardiopulmonary bypass, nasopharyngeal temperature serves as an indicator of brain temperature. More precisely, it reflects the temperature of the blood that provides substantial perfusion to the brain.[228] Thermistors located in the nasopharynx suffer inaccuracies due to insufficient contact with nasopharyngeal mucosa to exclude ambient air, accidental displacement, and the convective influence of respiratory gases that escape around the tracheal tube.[229]

Tympanic Membrane Temperature

The tympanic membrane accurately reflects the temperature in the thermoregulatory center of the brain.[230,231] In determining the safety and efficacy of tympanic thermometry, one should recognize that at least three different methods have been reported. Early probes used thermocouples designed to contact the tympanic membrane directly. These probes gave rise to the initial reports citing a 1 to 3 percent incidence of bleeding and even tympanic membrane rupture.[231,232] Standard thermistor probes were subsequently designed to avoid direct contact with the tympanic membrane, but the accuracy and complications associated with these have not been described. In 1988, Shinozaki and colleagues[233] reported the use of infrared sensor technology for intermittent sampling of tympanic temperature. In comparing these data to pulmonary artery thermistors, the infrared tympanic determinations correlated closely (0.98), with minimal bias ($\leq 0.4°C$) and high precision ($\pm 0.2°C$). These devices are more readily accepted by conscious children than the rectal route, and, since they need not contact the tympanic membrane, traumatic injury of the canal or membrane has not been described. The major limitation of the currently available commercial infrared devices is their size. In these devices the speculum containing the sensor is too large to permit accurate measurement in infants under 3 months.[234,235]

Axillary Temperature

Axillary temperature is at least 1°C lower than core temperature, even when the probe is placed over the axillary artery. This site provides the best monitor of skeletal muscle temperature. To improve the correlation with core temperature, the probe may be covered with an insulator (e.g., foam adhesive pad), and the arm should be kept tightly adducted.

Skin Temperature

The skin does not accurately reflect core temperature unless it is measured over the liver with the probe insulated from the environment. Although this technique is used extensively on neonates in intensive care units, it is not suitable for most intraoperative monitoring. The skin temperature measured elsewhere on the body such as the forehead, is at least 3°C lower than core temperature and is subject to an even wider gradient during conditions resulting in vasoconstriction.[236,237] When liquid crystal thermography was applied to children, these devices consistently overestimated core temperature by more than 2°C.[238]

Inspired Gas Temperature

Unless actively warmed, there may be as much as a 20°C drop in temperature between the exit port of the humidifier and the T piece of the anesthetic system. The only safe way to deliver anesthetic gases to a patient at body temperature is to monitor the temperature of the gases at the patient connection (Fig. 27-9). This is even more important when using a heated wire in the fresh gas or inspiratory limb. Tracheitis from overheated gases has been reported.[239]

Operating Room Temperature

The operating room thermostat is part of the anesthetic equipment. Control of the room temperature is important in minimizing the skin-environment temperature gradient of the neonate and small infant. The operating room temperature and relative humidity should be monitored to minimize the heat loss of the child to the environment.

The operating room temperature can generally be lowered if the child's head and extremities are covered with plastic bags or waterproof drapes, and the operative field is covered with an adhesive plastic drape.[240]

Fluid Temperature

A further method of minimizing heat loss in the neonate and infant is to heat the intravenous fluids. Although this method is not very effective when the infusion rates are slow, because the intravenous fluids cool to the environmental temperature in transit from the heating unit to the patient, it is of benefit with rapid infusions. Blood stored at 4°C must be warmed before infusion to minimize its effect on body temperature. The temperature of the heaters used to warm fluids and blood must be monitored to prevent overheating, which can denature the proteins in the blood products.

Neuromuscular Function

The evaluation of neuromuscular function in infants and children requires an understanding of developmental physiology, developmental pharmacokinetics, and limitations children pose. At birth, muscle fiber composition, nerve conduction velocity and the motor end-plates are immature. Through repeated postnatal stimulation and myelinization, nerve conduction velocity increases and acetyl choline receptors (that were initially distributed diffusely over the entire muscle fiber) become concentrated at the motor endplate.[241] As a result, the immature neuromuscular system exhibits a characteristic myasthenic response to peripheral nerve stimulation: poorly sustained tetanus, posttetanic potentiation, and posttetanic exhaustion in the absence of muscle relaxants.[242] Premature neonates will develop fade at rates of stimulation as low as 20 Hz.[241] Electromyography demonstrates mature conduction and responses within 12 weeks of age.[243] Since the speed with which maturation progresses varies between infants, muscle relaxants must be carefully titrated in these first few weeks of life.

Objective monitoring of neonatal neuromuscular function serves two purposes (1) to define the time intervals over which an individual child requires repeat doses of muscle relaxant, and (2) to confirm the return of neuromuscular function adequate to support sufficient spontaneous ventilation and sustain a patent airway. Neuromuscular monitoring devices employ one of three basic methods to quantify the motor response to peripheral nerve stimulation: mechanomyography, electromyography, and accelerometry. Although perhaps the most common methods employed, visual and tactile assessment of peripheral nerve stimulation are notoriously inaccurate in children as they are in adults.[244,245] Recovery from neuromuscular blockade is typically quantified in terms of the T4: T1 ratio in response to a supramaximal train-of-four stimulus at 2 Hz and the magnitude of fade to a tetanic stimulus, usually 50 Hz for 5 seconds. Saddler and colleagues demonstrated that 0.44 was the mean measured train-of-four ratio at which cli-

nicians could no longer determine fade in children by tactile means.[245] Since a train-of-four ratio of 0.7 assures only minimally satisfactory neuromuscular function, a proportion of children extubated by this criterion alone will not possess sufficient strength to maintain a patent airway. These investigators improved the sensitivity of tactile analysis by employing "double burst stimulation," two 50-Hz stimuli of 60 ms duration separated by 750 ms. Clinicians detected fade in the second stimulus at a ratio of 0.67.

The application of mechanomyography requires a force transducer to quantify motor activity, usually of the adductor pollicis in response to ulnar nerve stimulation. Although these devices are accurate, they are cumbersome, requiring extensive,

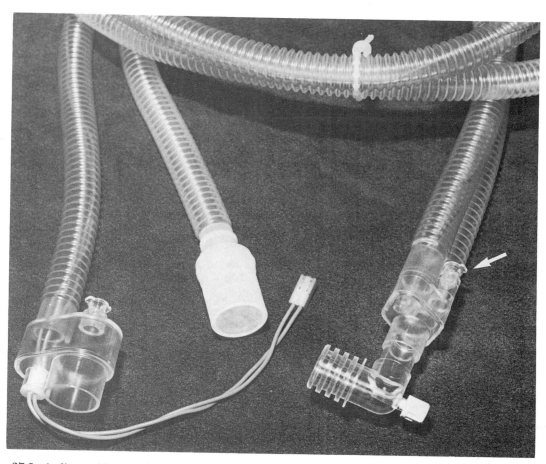

Fig. 27-9. A disposable circuit incorporating a port in the y-piece to monitor the temperature of the gases at the patient connection (*arrow*) (Isothermal Pediatric Circuit, Isothermal Systems Inc., Riverside, CA.)

preparation, calibration, and precise constant loading tension applied to the thumb.[246] While others have advocated simpler devices that transduce the depression of a syringe plunger,[247] there are no commercially available devices employing the principle.

Electromyographic monitors, that detect the composite action potentials of the contracting motor units, have recently become commercially available. These units require a minimum of three electrodes; stimulating, active (recording), and indifferent (reference). Meticulous preparation of the sites is vital. Kalli[248] identified several problems in electromyographic monitoring of small infants. Their small hand makes it difficult to avoid undesirable incidental stimulation of the median nerve and neighboring muscles. In infants under 12 weeks, baseline determinations are often abnormal as noted above. The best data resulted when the active electrode was located on the midpoint of the adductor pollicis and the indifferent electrode on another digit.[248] Even so, these monitors remain unreliable in producing interpretable data, particularly in small children, and they are plagued by variable comparisons to mechanomyography. In a study of adults in whom electromyography, mechanomyography, and pulmonary function tests were performed after subparalyzing doses of vecuronium, an electromyographic train-of-four ratio of 0.9 was required to achieve a mechanomyographic train-of-four ratio of 0.5.[249]

Accelographs employ a piezoelectric transducer attached to the thumb to measure acceleration in response to ulnar stimulation.[250,251] While the device has shown reasonably close comparisons with mechanomyography in adults,[251] it requires further investigation in children. The currently available clinical instrument is too large for infants.

In circumstances in which the ulnar nerve is not available for monitoring, other peripheral nerves may be stimulated if one remains cognizant of the differing sensitivities of various muscle groups. Posterior tibial stimulation of the flexor hallucis brevis usually reveals increased sensitivity to muscle relaxants and delayed recovery, while facial nerve stimulation of obicularis oculi is more resistant than adductor pollicis.[246] Laycock and colleagues[252] investigated the relative ED_{90} of pancuronium on adductor pollicis and the diaphragm of children 3 months to 10 years of age. Although the ED_{90} increased with age, the relationship of the two muscle groups remained relatively constant, with the ED_{90} ratios (diaphragm:adductor pollicis) between 1.64 and 1.75. In addition, local hypothermia of the extremity being monitored can lead to misleading prolongation of relaxant effect.[253]

While monitoring of peripheral nerve evoked potentials provides valuable, if qualified, information about the degree of neuromuscular blockade and the need for additional relaxant, none of the techniques possesses the proper combination of reliability, sensitivity, and specificity to judge sufficient recovery to maintain a patent airway. The latter requires additional clinical observation, such as negative inspiratory force, sustained leg lift,[254] or sustained head lift in children old enough to cooperate. In adults, a negative inspiratory force of -55 cmH_2O was necessary to assure competent airway muscle function,[255] while sustained leg lift in infants correlates with a negative inspiratory force of at least -35 cmH_2O.[254]

Blood Loss

The available blood loss (ABL) can be calculated from the estimated blood volume (EBV) and the starting hematocrit (Hct) by the following formula[256]:

$$ABL = \frac{EBV \times (Hct\ start - Hct\ end)}{avg\ Hct}$$

where avg hematocrit = (starting Hct + ending Hct)/2

EBV = 90–100 ml/kg for premature neonates

80–90 ml/kg for term neonates

75–80 ml/kg for infants 1 to 24 months

65–75 ml/kg for prepubertal children

For infants less than 3 months chronological age, the desired ending hematocrit should be higher to allow for the ongoing physiologic anemia, which reaches its nadir around 3 and 2 months for term and premature infants, respectively.

Visual monitoring of the patient, sponges, suction apparatus, drapes, and the floor is key to the assessment of blood loss, as most objective techniques are quite inaccurate. Patient signs of blood loss are listed in Table 27-9. Weighing sponges will quantitate the blood absorbed on them if they were not moistened prior to use and are weighed promptly after being discarded from the operative field. For convenience when weighing sponges, 1 ml of blood is assumed to weigh 1 g. The use of small-diameter, calibrated suction canisters will aid in the estimation of the blood suctioned from the surgical field.

The accuracy of blood replacement can be increased by transfusing the blood with a syringe. The relationship between losses and replacement is readily monitored if a chart is kept showing the running total in each category, namely, blood loss from suction, sponges, drapes, and total replacement fluids. Serial hematocrits from arterial or central venous specimens are helpful in monitoring loss and the adequacy of replacement.

Fluid Balance

Water losses due to evaporation from the neonate's relatively large surface area and to their higher metabolic rate render them especially vulnerable to dehydration. In addition, the neonate and infant have a higher total body water volume than the adult (70 to 84 percent in the neonate versus 55 to 60 percent in the adult).

Pediatric maintenance fluid requirement (after the first 5 days of life) is 100 ml/kg/24 h for the first 10 kg of body mass, 50 ml/kg/24 h for the next 10 kg, and 20 ml/kg24 h for body mass in excess of 20 kg. Even though the infant's fluid requirements are high when expressed in milliliters per kilogram, the milliliter per hour rate is low.

Pediatric fluid therapy can be monitored using small aliquots of fluid in intravenous infusion sets and syringe pumps and by meticulous tracking of fluid requirements. The deficit that occurs during the fasting period should be calculated. The state of the young child's hydration can be monitored pre- and intraoperatively using the signs and symptoms listed in Table 27-9.

Air Embolism

The opportunities for paradoxical venous air embolism appear to be greater in the neonate and infant than in the adult because the foramen ovale and ductus arteriosus are only functionally closed at this age. Probe-patent foramen ovale persists in 34 to 50 percent of children at age 5 years and even 25 to 34 percent of adults at age 21.[257,258] In addition, communications between the left and right sides of the heart at all levels can exist in children with congenital heart lesions.

All intravenous infusions should be carefully monitored for the presence of air bubbles. Infusion pumps containing monitors to detect the presence of air in the tubing are widely available. Syringes to inject drugs should be inspected for the presence of air before the drug is administered and, to prevent injection of the air lodged in the barrel of the syringe, the syringe should not be completely emptied. During operative procedures where the operative field is above the right atrial level (e.g.,

TABLE 27-9. Signs of Blood Loss in Pediatric Surgery

Mild (0–10%)	Moderate (10–20%)	Severe (>20%)
Visible loss: small	Moderate	Extensive
BP decrease: 5–15%	10–25%	>25%
Veins: less visible	Collapsed	Collapsed
CVP: decreased	CVP 0	CVP 0
Urine output: decreased	Marked reduction	Anuria
Conjunctival circulation: decreased	Conjunctivae pale	No conjunctival circulation visible
	Heart sounds muffled	Heart sounds distant
	Extremities cool	Generalized blanching
	Decreased respiratory effort	Gasping respirations or apnea
	Increasing relaxation	Flaccidity
	Weak peripheral pulse	Peripheral pulse not palpable
	Fontanelle depressed	Unobtainable BP
	Hematocrit reduced	Asystole
	Increased urine osmolality	Hypothermia
	Inncreased urine SG	Shock

Abbreviations: BP, blood pressure; CVP, central venous pressure; SG, specific gravity.
(Modified from Smith,[269] with permission.)

sitting posterior fossa craniotomies), early diagnosis of venous air embolism is enhanced by capnography, which reveals an acute fall in P_{ETCO_2}. Doppler ultrasound air embolism detectors are very sensitive, detecting even clinically insignificant air bubbles.[259] The onset of the mill wheel murmur can be noted by monitoring heart tones with a stethoscope. A right atrial catheter may aid in confirming the diagnosis and in aspirating the air.

Invasive Monitoring

Renal Function

The fetal kidneys begin to produce urine around the third gestational month. By term, the kidneys are able to perform normal tasks but do not counter the effects of severe dehydration, excessive water or solute load, trauma, or acidosis as well as mature kidneys. Although the infant's glomeruli are smaller than an adult's, the glomerular surface:body mass ratio is similar. The tubules are incompletely developed and may not extend into the renal medulla.

During the first week of extrauterine life, the neonate has a low glomerular filtration rate (24 ml/1.73 m^2 per minute versus 120 ml/1.73 m^2 per minute in the adult) and a low renal plasma flow (150 ml/1.73 m^2 per minute versus 600 ml/1.73 m^2 per minute in the adult). The tubular reabsorption mechanisms are also poorly developed. The neonatal kidney cannot concentrate urine above 600 mOsm/L in the presence of dehydration, nor is there a diuretic response to a water load during the first 48 hours after birth. By the end of the first week of life, the neonate can produce a dilute urine (50 mOsm/L—the same as in the adult), but water-load excretion is incomplete.[260]

Urine volume is limited by the low glomerular filtration rate and may be absent during the first 24 hours of life. Urine volume starts at about 25 ml/kg per day and rises to over 100 to 120 ml/kg per day by the end of the first week.[261] Urine osmolality decreases during this time from 400 to 500 mOsm/L to 100 mOsm/L.

The renal thresholds for glucose and bicarbonate are low in the neonate, the latter accounting for the mild metabolic acidosis (base deficit of 3 to 6 mEq/L) normally seen in neonates. These thresholds mature by age 2 years. The neonatal kidney is particularly inept at retaining sodium, especially in the premature kidney where sodium loss may be three times that of the term neonatal kidney. This predisposes the premature to hyponatremia. Excretion of a sodium load is also poor but reaches adult capacity by 1 year of age. The functional limitations of the neonatal kidney are largely corrected by the end of the first postnatal month and reach adult levels of function by the second year of life.

In the presence of a stable cardiac output and a systemic arterial pressure greater than the critical opening pressure required by the afferent arterioles of the glomerulus, urinary flow varies directly with the circulating blood volume unless it has been stimulated by osmotic or chemical diuretics.[262] Other factors influencing urine production include extracellular fluid volume, hormonal response to the stress of surgery and anesthesia, prior diuretic therapy, preexisting renal disease, hypothermia, and the loss of pulsatile flow during cardiopulmonary bypass. A minimum output of 0.5 ml/kg per hour, but preferably 1 to 2 ml/kg per hour (except in the newborn), indicates satisfactory renal function.[263]

Monitoring the urine for changes in color from light to straw yellow to brown or reddish brown will suggest the presence of red blood cells or free hemoglobin in the urine, indicating hemolysis (e.g., from a transfusion reaction or damage to red cells from suction during cardiopulmonary bypass) or the presence of myoglobinuria (e.g., from intravenous succinylcholine).

Urinary output can be monitored by transurethral or suprapubic catheterization of the urinary bladder. The incidence of urethral strictures is reduced by using Silastic Foley catheters. Measurement of urine output in the neonate is difficult for technical reasons. The use of low-dead space tubing (e.g., intravenous extension tubing), to connect the urinary catheter to low-volume graduated measuring container (e.g., a syringe) permits the measurement of very small volumes of urine.

A urinary bladder catheter will also prevent the development of a distended bladder, which can produce undesirable autonomic reflexes. A Foley catheter should be inserted when the use of diuretics is anticipated, when crystalloid replacement of third space losses is expected to exceed 50 percent of the estimated blood volume and when deliberate hypotension, hemodilution, or cardiopulmonary bypass is planned.

GUIDELINES FOR MONITORING THE PEDIATRIC PATIENT

The following outline summarizes the approach to monitoring the pediatric patient described in this chapter.

Healthy patients for minor surgery (superficial or less than 2.5 hours in duration)

Observation
Chest wall movement for adequacy of ventilation
Peripheral perfusion
   Nail bed color
   Skin color
Central perfusion by color of mucous membranes
Head, thorax, and abdomen for signs of airway obstruction
   Nasal flaring
   Use of accessory respiratory muscles
   Intercostal, sternal, and substernal retraction
   Abdominothoracic rocking
Face for signs of inadequate anesthetic depth
   Sweating
   Tearing
   Grimacing
   Pupillary dilatation
   Eye opening
Patient for movement indicating light anesthetic depth or neuromuscular blockade breakthrough
   Grimacing
   Swallowing
   Extremity movement
   Respiratory efforts
Peripheral pulse palpation
   Heart rate
   Heart rhythm
   Pulse volume
Precordial or esophageal stethoscope
   Breath sounds
   Heart tones
   Heart rate
   Heart rhythm
   Respiratory rate
Electrocardiography
   Cardiac depolarization
   Heart rate
   Heart rhythm
Noninvasive blood pressure
   Systolic blood pressure
   Diastolic blood pressure
   Mean blood pressure
Pulse oximeter
Mass spectrometry with continuous capnography
Patient temperature (if neonate or older child if operation > 15 minutes duration)
Inspired gas temperature
Circulating water mattress temperature
Fluid and blood temperature
Neuromuscular function
Inspired oxygen concentration
If controlled ventilation is used:
   Airway pressure
If a mechanical ventilator is used:
   Patient's tidal volume
   Minute ventilation
   Disconnect alarm

Healthy patients having major surgery (intracavitary of 2.5 to 4 hours duration) or *ill patients having minor surgery*

All monitoring employed in healthy patients with minor surgery
Blood loss
Fluid balance
Central venous pressure if:
   Estimated blood loss will exceed one estimated blood volume[7]
   Congestive heart failure is present
Urinary output if:
   The use of diuretic is anticipated
   Anticipated third space fluid replacement will exceed 50 percent of the estimated blood volume
   Hypovolemia exists or is anticipated
   Circulatory instability requiring extensive fluid resuscitation (>50 percent estimated blood volume)
   Blood loss is anticipated to exceed 15 to 20 percent of the estimated blood volume

Healthy patients having extended major surgery (greater than 4 hours duration) or *ill patients having major surgery*

All monitoring employed with major surgery
Direct systemic arterial pressure if:
   Anticipated estimated blood loss is > 50 percent of the estimated blood volume
   Cardiovascular system is unstable
   Potential for rapid blood loss exists (>10 percent of the estimated blood volume)
Pulmonary artery pressure if:

Fluid replacement and/or cardiovascular resuscitation are required in patients who are at high risk for cerebral or pulmonary edema (e.g., burns, increased intracranial pressure, and endotoxic shock)

Pulmonary hypertension is associated with right heart failure

Left heart failure exists

Arterial blood gases if:

Severe hypoxemia ($PaO_2 < 300$ mmHg on an FIO_2 of 1.0)

There is evidence for, or probable development of increased intracranial pressure

There will be a need for intraoperative hypocapnia (e.g., craniotomy)

Serial biochemical determinations if:

Third space fluid replacement will exceed 50 percent of the estimated blood volume

Acidosis or shock is likely to occur during the course of surgery

Massive blood transfusion are anticipated

There will be rapid alterations in serum glucose, (e.g., congenital hypoglycemia, insulinoma), calcium, (massive blood transfusion) or electrolytes (large third space fluid replacement, diuresis)

(The specimens can be obtained from any central venous or arterial catheter)

Cardiac output if:

There will be significant alteration in blood flow through an arteriovenous malformation during the surgery

There will be a need to determine the presence of intracardiac shunts during surgery

Modifying factors

An arterial catheter should be considered when:

A neonate <36 weeks postconceptual age will need supplemental O_2 ($FIO_2 > 0.21$) during an anesthetic (for serial determination of PaO_2)[264]

Manipulation of the arterial pressure is planned (e.g., deliberate hypotension or management of a pheochromocytoma)

Cardiopulmonary bypass is planned

Deliberate hemodilution is planned

Need for postoperative mechanical ventilation

There will be a need for serial arterial blood gas or biochemical determinations

A central venous catheter should be considered when:

Deliberate hypotension is planned

Deliberate hemodilution is planned

There is risk of air embolism (e.g., a craniotomy in the sitting position)

Cardiopulmonary bypass will be used

Rewarming after deep hypothermia

Anticipated blood loss is greater than the estimated blood volume[77]

Intracranial pressure monitoring should be considered when there is clinical evidence of, or potential for, increased intracranial pressure during or following the anesthesia and surgery

A urinary catheter will be needed when:

Deliberate deep hypothermia is planned

Deliberate hypotension is planned

Hemodilution is planned

Cardiopulmonary bypass is planned

CONCLUSION

The choice of monitors for a particular patient requiring anesthesia is a matter of clinical judgment. Nevertheless, guidelines are useful in helping one make that judgment. The guidelines presented here were initially developed by the Department of Anesthesiology and Critical Care Medicine at The Children's Hospital of Philadelphia in 1977 and have been modified with advances in practice and technology. They have served us well and continue to do so. Careful evaluation of the cost:benefit ratio for each monitor to be used during a particular anesthetic is always indicated. Never should the time spent placing a monitor be a factor in determining whether the monitor is appropriate for the patient. The overriding consideration must be the safety of the patient, and whatever is necessary to make the anesthetic safe needs to be done.

REFERENCES

1. Keenan RL, Boyon C: Cardiac arrest due to anesthesia. JAMA 253:2373, 1985

2. Cohen MM, Cameron CB, Duncan PG: Pediatric anesthesia morbidity and mortality in the perioperative period. Anesth Analg 70:160, 1990

3. Keenan RL, Shapiro JH, Dawson K: Frequency of anesthetic cardiac arrests in infants: effect of pediatric anesthesiologists. J Clin Anesth 3:433, 1991

4. Olsson GL, Hallen B: Cardiac arrest during anaesthesia: a computer-aided study in 250,543 anaesthetics. Acta Anaesthesiol Scand 32:653, 1988

5. Tiret L, Nivoche Y, Hatton, F et al: Complications related to anaesthesia in infants and children: a prospective survey of 40240 anaesthetics. Br J Anaesth 61:263, 1988

6. Keenan RL: Anesthetic mortality. Semin Anesth 11:89, 1992

7. Battersby EF: Monitoring during anesthesia for pediatric surgery. Int Anesthesiol Clin 19:95, 1981

8. Schwartz AJ: Esophageal stethoscopes not hazardous. Anesthesiology 48:382, 1978

9. Schwartz AJ, Downes JJ: Hazards of a simple monitoring device, the esophageal stethoscope. Anesthesiology 47:64, 1977

10. Gravenstein JS, Paulus DA: Clinical Monitoring Practice. 2nd Ed. JB Lippincott, Philadelphia, 1987

11. Friedman WF: The intrinsic physiologic properties of the developing heart. Prog Cardiovasc Dis 15:87, 1972

12. Perloff WF: Physiology of the heart and circulation. In Swedlow DB, Raphaely RC (eds): Cardiovascular Problems in Pediatric Critical Care. Churchill Livingstone, New York, 1986

13. Diaz JH, Lockhart CH: Is halothane really safe in infancy? Anesthesiology 51:S313, 1979

14. Friesen RH, Lichtor JL: Cardiovascular depression during halothane anesthesia in infants: study of three induction techniques. Anesth Analg 61:42, 1982

15. Barash PG, Glanz S, Katz JD et al: Ventricular function in children during halothane anesthesia: an echocardiographic evaluation. Anesthesiology 49:79, 1978

16. Gregory GA: The baroresponses of preterm infants during halothane anesthesia. Can Anaesth Soc J 29:105, 1982

17. Wolf WJ, Neal MB, Peterson MD: The hemodynamic and cardiovascular effects of isoflurane and halothane anesthesia in children. Anesthesiology 64:328, 1986

18. Craythorne NWB, Turndorff , Dripps RD: Changes in pulse rate and rhythm associated with the use of succinylcholine in anesthetized children. Anesthesiology 21:465, 1960

19. Chalon J: Causes of death during anesthesia. [Editorial]. Surv Anesth 26:257, 1982

21. Rigatto H, Brady JP, Verduzco RT: Chemoreceptor reflexes in preterm infants. I. The effects of gestational and postnatal age on the ventilatory response to inhalation of 100% and 15% oxygen. Pediatrics 55:604, 1975

21. Hickey PR: Cardiac dysrhythmias in pediatric patients during anesthesia and the role of oximetry and capnography. [Editorial]. Anesth Analg 73:686, 1991

22. Rolf N, Coté CJ: Persistent cardiac arrhythmias in pediatric patients: effects of age, expired carbon dioxide values, depth of anesthesia, and airway management. Anesth Analg 73:720, 1991

23. Lindop MJ: Monitoring of the cardiovascular system during anesthesia. Int Anesthesiol Clin 19:1, 1981

24. Leonard PF, Gould AB: Dynamic of electrical hazards of particular concern to operating room personnel. Surg Clin North Am 45:817, 1965

25. Finlay B, Couchie D, Boyce L: Electrosurgery burns resulting from use of miniature ECG electrodes. Anesthesiology 41:263, 1971

26. Nicodemus HF, Nassir-Rahimi C, Bachman L: Median effective dose (ED_{50}) of halothane in adults and children. Anesthesiology 31:344, 1969

27. ASA Directory of members: Standards for basic intraoperative monitoring. p. 709. American Society of Anesthesiologists. Park Ridge, IL, 1993

28. Wong DT, Volgyesi GA, Bissonnette B: Systolic arterial pressure determination by a new pulse monitor technique. Can J Anaesth 39:596, 1992

29. Reder RF, Dimich I, Cohen ML, Steinfield L: Evaluating indirect blood pressure measurement techniques: a comparison of three systems in infants and children. Pediatrics 62:326, 1978

30. Friesen RH, Lichtor JL: Indirect measurement of blood pressure in neonates and infants utilizing an automated noninvasive oscillometric monitor. Anesth Analog 60:742, 1981

31. Kimble KJ Darnall RA, Yelderman M, Ariagno RL: An automated oscillometric technique for estimating mean arterial pressure in critically ill newborns. Anesthesiology 54:423, 1981

32. Park MK, Kawabori I: Need for an improved standard for blood pressure cuff size. Clin Pediatr 15:784, 1976

33. Allen EV: Thromboangitis obliterans: methods of diagnosis of chronic occlusive arterial lesions distal to the wrist with illustrative cases. Am J Med Sci 178:237, 1929

34. Brodsky JB: A simple method to determine patency of the ulnar artery intraoperatively prior to radial artery cannulation. Anesthesiology 42:626, 1975

35. Edmonds JF, Barker GA, Conn AW: Current concepts in cardiovascular monitoring in children. Crit Care Med 8:548, 1980

36. Miyasaka K, Edmonds JF, Conn AW: Complication of radial artery lines in the paediatric patient. Can Anaesth Soc J 23:9, 1976

37. Park MK: Robotham JL, German VF: Systolic pressure amplification in pedal arteries in children. Crit Care Med 11:286, 1983

38. Spohr RC, MacDonald HM, Holzman IR. Catheterization of the posterior tibial artery in the neonate. Am J Dis Child 133:945, 1979

39. Lawless S, Orr R: Axillary arterial monitoring of pediatric patients. Pediatrics 84:273, 1989

40. Kitterman JA, Phibbs RH: Aortic blood pressure in the normal newborn: hazards of the umbilical artery catheter. Pediatrics 45:893, 1970

41. Neal WA, Reynolds JW, Jarvis CW: Umbilical artery catheterization: demonstration of arterial thrombus by aortography. Pediatrics 50:6, 1972

42. Baldwin CE, Holder TM, Ashcraft KW: Neonatal renovascular hypertension: a complication of aortic monitoring catheters. J Pediatr Surg 16:820, 1981

43. Bauer SB, Feldman SM, Gellis SS: Neonatal hypertension, a complication of umbilical artery catheterization. N Engl J Med 293:1032, 1975

44. Talbert JL: Intraoperative and postoperative monitoring of infants. Surg Clin North Am 50:787, 1970

45. Bull MJ, Schreiner RL, Garg BD: Neurological complications following temporal artery catheterization. J Pediatr 96:1071, 1980

46. Prian GW: Complication and sequelae of temporal artery catheterization in the high risk newborn. J Pediatr Surg 12:829, 1977

47. Haller JA: Monitoring of arterial and central venous pressure in infants. Pediatr Clin North Am 16:637, 1969

48. Michel L, McMichen JC, Bachy JL: Tracheostomy and indwelling central venous lines: a hazardous combination? Intens Care Med 5:83, 1979

49. Bar-Joseph G, Galvis AG: Perforation of the heart by central venous catheter in infants: guideline to diagnosis and management. J Pediatr Surg 18:284, 1983

50. Jay AWL, Kehler CH: Heart perforation by central venous catheters. Can J Anaesth 34:333, 1987

51. Burri C, Ahnefeld FW: The Caval Catheter. Springer-Verlag, New York, 1978

52. Hohn AR, Lambert EC: Continuous venous catheterization in children. JAMA 197:658, 1966

53. Seldinger SI: Catheter replacement of needle in percutaneous arteriography: new technique. Acta Radiol [Diagn] 39:368, 1953

54. Kitterman JA, Phibbs RH, Tooley WH: Catheterization of umbilical vessels in newborn infants. Pediatr Clin North Am 17:895, 1970

55. Dangel P: Technik der Infusions behandlung and der parenteral on Ernährung bei Neugeborenen und Säuglingen. Infusionsther Klin Ernaehr 2:34, 1975

56. Humphrey MJ, Blitt CD: Central venous access in children via the external jugular vein. Anesthesiology 57:50, 1982

57. Nicolson SC, Sweeney MF, Morre RA, Jobes DR: Comparison of internal and external jugular cannulation of the central circulation in the pediatric patient. Crit Care Med 13:747, 1985

58. English ICW, Frew RM, Pigott JF: Percutaneous catheterization of the internal jugular vein. Anaesthesia 24:521, 1969

59. Berlatzky Y, Freund H, Schiller M: Percutaneous internal jugular vein cannulation in pediatric surgical patients. Z Kinderchir 18:231, 1976

60. Hill DMB, Greefhuysen J: Percutaneous catheterization of the internal jugular vein in infants and children. J Pediatr Surg 12:719, 1977

61. Kransz MM, Berlatzky M, Ayalan A: Percutaneous cannulation of the internal jugular vein in infants and children. Surg Gynecol Obstet 148:591, 1979

62. Prince SR, Sullivan RL, Hackel A: Percutaneous catheterization of the internal jugular vein in infants and children. Anesthesiology 44:170, 1976

63. Rao TLK, Wong AY, Salem MR: A new approach to percutaneous catheterization of the internal jugular vein. Anesthesiology 46:362, 1977

64. Coté CJ, Jobes DR: Two approaches to cannulation of a child's internal jugular vein. Anesthesiology 50:371, 1979

65. Alderson PJ, Burrows FA, Stemp LI, Holtby HM: Use of ultrasound to evaluate internal jugular vein anatomy and to facilitate central venous cannulation in paediatric patients. Br J Anaesth 70:145, 1993

66. Aubaniac R: L'injection intraveneuse sousclaviculare: advantages et technique. Presse Med 60:1456, 1952

67. Eichelberger MR: Percutaneous subclavian venous catheters in neonates and children. J Pediatr Surg 16:547, 1981

68. Groff DB, Ahmed N: Subclavian vein catheterization in the infant. J Pediatr Surg 9:171, 1974

69. Poole JL: Subclavian vein catheterization for cardiac surgery in children. Anaesth Inten Care 8:81, 1980

70. Pybus DA, Poole JL, Crawford MC: Subclavian venous catheterization in small children using the Seldinger technique. Anaesthesia 37:451, 1982

71. Emmanouilides GC, Moss AJ, Duffie, E, et al: Pulmonary arterial pressure changes in human newborn infants from birth to 3 days of age. J Pediatr 65:327, 1964

72. Swan HJC, Ganz W, Forrester JS: Catheterization of the heart in man with the use of a flow directed balloon tipped catheter. N Engl J Med 283:447, 1970

73. Demen J, Wever JE: The use of balloon-tiped pulmonary artery catheters in children undergoing cardiac surgery. Intens Care Med 13:266, 1987

74. Schwartz AJ, Garcia FG: Entanglement of Swan-Ganz

catheter around an intracardiac suture. JAMA 237: 1198, 1977

75. Gold JP, Jonas RA, Lang P, et al: Transthoracic intracardiac monitoring lines in pediatric surgical patients: a ten-year experience. Ann Thorac Surg 42: 185, 1986

76. Goodman DE, Swedlow DB: Continuous cardiac output estimation in children. Crit Care Med 9:286, 1981

77. Alverson DC: Neonatal cardiac output measurement using pulsed Doppler ultrasound. Clin Perinatol 12:101, 1985

78. Berman W Jr, Lister G Jr, Pitt BR, Hoffman JI: Measurements of blood flow. Adv Pediatr 35:427, 1988

79. Alverson DC, Eldridge M, Dillon T, et al: Noninvasive pulsed Doppler determination of cardiac output in neonates and children. J Pediatr 101:46, 1982

80. Walther FJ, Van Bel F, Ebrahimi M: Duplex versus unguided pulsed Doppler measurements of right ventricular output in newborn infants. Acta Paediatr Scand 79:41, 1990

81. Alverson DC, Eldridge MW, Johnson JD et al: Effects of patent ductus arteriosus on left ventricular output in premature infants. J Pediatr 102:754, 1983

82. Hirsimaki H, Kero P, Wanne O et al: Doppler-derived cardiac output in healthy newborn infants in relation to physiological patency of the ductus arteriosus. Pediatr Cardiol 9:79, 1988

83. Muhiudeen IA, Kuecherer HF, Lee E et al: Intraoperative estimation of cardiac output by transesophageal pulsed Doppler echocardiography. Anesthesiology 74:9, 1991

84. Notterman DA, Castello FV, Steinberg C et al: A comparison of thermodilution and pulsed Doppler cardiac output measurement in critically ill children. J Pediatr 115:554, 1989

85. Siegel LC, Pearl RG: Noninvasive cardiac output measurement: troubled technologies and troubled studies. Anesth Analg 74:790, 1992

86. Jaimovich DG, Shabino CL, Nelson CB: Continuous cardiac output measurement by transtracheal Doppler technique in a pediatric patient with septic shock. Crit Care Med 20:707, 1992

87. Mickell JJ, Lucking SE, Chaten FC, Young ES: Trending of impedance-monitored cardiac variables: method and statistical power analysis of 100 control studies in a pediatric intensive care unit. Crit Care Med 18:645, 1990

88. O'Connell AJ, Tibballs J, Coulthard M: Improving agreement between thoracic bioimpedance and dye dilution cardiac output estimation in children. Anaesth Intens Care 19:434, 1991

89. Scott PJ, Blackburn ME, Wharton GA et al: Trans-oesophageal echocardiography in neonates, infants and children: applicability and diagnostic value in everyday practice of a cardiothoracic unit. Br Heart J 68:488, 1992

90. Shah PM, Stewart S III, Calalang CC, Alexson C: Transesophageal echocardiography and the intraoperative management of pediatric congenital heart disease: initial experience with a pediatric esophageal 2D color flow echocardiographic probe. J Cardiothorac Vasc Anesth 6:8, 1992

91. Muhiudeen IA, Roberson DA, Silverman NH et al: Intraoperative echocardiography for evaluation of congenital heart defects in infants and children. Anesthesiology 76:165, 1992

92. Weintraub RG, Sahn DJ: Pediatric transesophageal echocardiography: present and future. Anesthesiology 76:159, 1992

93. Stümper O, Elzenga NJ, Hess J, Sutherland GR: Transesophageal echocardiography in children with congenital heart disease: an initial experience. J Am Coll Cardiol 16:433, 1990

94. Reich DL, Konstadt SN, Nedat M et al: Intraoperative transesophageal echocardiography for the detection of cardiac preload changes induced by transfusion and phlebotomy in pediatric patients. Anesthesiology 79:10, 1993

95. Fyfe DA, Kline CH, Sade RM et al: The utility of transesophageal echocardiography during and after Fontan operations in small children. Am Heart J 122:1403, 1991

96. Hsu Y-H, Santulli T Jr, Wong A-L et al: Impact on intraoperative echocardiography on surgical management of congenital heart disease. Am J Cardiol 67:1279, 1991

97. Nightingale DW, Lambert TF: Carbon dioxide output in anesthetized children. Anesthesia 33:594, 1978

98. Gerhardt TO, Bancarlai E: Measurement and monitoring of pulmonary function. Clin Perinatol 18: 581, 1991

99. Coté CJ: Wasted ventilation measured in vitro with eight anesthetic circuits with and without inline humidification. Anesthesiology 59:442, 1983

100. Beardsmore CS: Improved esophageal balloon technique for use in infants. J Appl Physiol 49:735, 1980

101. Cook CD: Calculated pulmonary work in newborns versus respiratory rate. J Clin Invest 36:440, 1957

102. Brown K, Sly PD, Milic Emili J, Bates JH: Evaluation of the flow-volume loop as an intra-operative monitor of respiratory mechanics in infants. Pediatr Pulmonol 6:8, 1989

103. Seear M, Wensley D, Werner H: Comparison of three methods for measuring respiratory mechanics in ventilated children. Pediatr Pulmonol 10:291, 1991

104. Eichhorn JH: Standard for patient monitoring during anesthesia at Harvard Medical School. JAMA 256:1017, 1986

105. Merritt JC: Retrolental fibroplasia: a multifactorial disease. Anesth Analg 60:109, 1981

106. Phibbs RH: Oxygen therapy: a continuing hazard to the premature infant. Anesthesiology 47:486, 1977

107. Lucey JF, Dangman B. A reexamination of the role of oxygen in retrolental fibroplasia. Pediatrics 73:82, 1984

108. Purohit DM, Ellison RC, Zierler S et al: Risk factors for retrolental fibroplasia: experience with 3,025 premature infants: National Collaborative Study on Patent Ductus Arteriosus in Premature Infants. Pediatrics 76:339, 1985

109. Betts EK: Retrolental fibroplasia and oxygen administration during general anesthesia. Anesthesiology 47:518, 1977

110. Westenskow DR: Evaluation of oxygen monitors for use during anesthesia. Anesth Analg 60:53, 1981

111. American Academy of Pediatrics Committee on Drugs: guidelines for monitoring and management of pediatric patients during and after sedation for diagnostic and therapeutic procedures. Pediatrics 89:1110, 1992

112. Swedlow DB: Capnometry and capnography: the anesthesia diaster early warning system. Semin Anesth 5:194, 1986

113. Baunderdister L: End-tidal CO_2 monitoring. Anesthesia 39:1000, 1984

114. Badgwell JM, McLeod ME, Lerman J, Creighton RE: End-tidal PCO_2 measurements sampled at the distal and proximal ends of the endotracheal tube in infants and children. Anesth Analg 66:959, 1987

115. Schieber RA: Accuracy of expiratory carbon dioxide measurements using the coaxial and circle breathing circuits in small subjects. J Clin Monitoring 1:149, 1985

116. Evans JM: Correlation of alveolar PCO_2 estimated by infra-red analysis and arterial PCO_2 in the human neonate and rabbit. Br J Anesthesia 49:761, 1977

117. Gravenstein N: Capnometry in infants should not be done at lower sampling flow rates. [Letter]. J Clin Monit 5:63, 1989

118. Badgwell JM: Respiratory gas monitoring in the pediatric patient. Int Anesthesiol Clin 30:131, 1992

119. From RP, Scamman FL: Ventilatory frequency influences accuracy of end-tidal CO_2 measurements: analysis of seven capnometers. Anesth Analg 67:884, 1988

120. McPeak H, Palayiwa E, Madgwick R., Sykes MK: Evaluation of a multigas anaesthetic monitor: the Datex Capnomac. Anaesthesia 43:1035, 1988

121. Nielsen J, Kann T, Moller JT: Evaluation of three transportable multigas anesthetic monitors: the Bruel & Kjaer Anesthetic Gas Monitor 1304, the Datex Capnomac Ultima, and the Nellcor N-2500. J Clin Monit 9:91, 1993

122. Schena J, Thompson J, Crone RK: Mechanical influences on the capnogram. Crit Care Med 12:672, 1984

123. Badgwell JM, Heavner JE, May WS et al: End-tidal PCO_2 monitoring in infants and children ventilated with either a partial rebreathing or a nonrebreathing circuit. Anesthesiology 66:405, 1987

124. Badgwell JM, Heavner JE: End-tidal carbon dioxide pressure in neonates and infants measured by aspiration and flow-through capnography. J Clin Monit 7:285, 1991

125. Gravenstein N: Factors influencing capnography in the bain circuit. J Clin Monitoring 1:6, 1984

126. Rich GF, Sullivan MP, Adams JM: Is distal sampling of end-tidal CO_2 necessary in small subjects? Anesthesiology 73:265, 1990

127. Burrows FA: Physiologic dead space, venous admixture, and the arterial to end-tidal carbon dioxide difference in infants and children undergoing cardiac surgery. Anesthesiology 70:219, 1989

128. Fletcher R: The relationship between the arterial to end-tidal PCO_2 difference and hemoglobin saturation in patients with congenital heart disease. Anesthesiology 75:210, 1991

129. Brandom BW: Uptake and distribution of halothane in infants. Anesth Analg 62:404, 1983

130. Eger EI: The effect of age on the rate of increase of alveolar anesthetic concentration. Anesthesiology 35:365, 1971

131. Salanitre E, Rackow H: The pulmonary exchange of nitrous oxide and halothane in infants and children. Anesthesiology 30:388, 1969

132. Steward DJ, Creighton RE: The uptake and excretion of nitrous oxide in the newborn. Can Anaesth Soc J 25:215, 1978

133. Gregory GA: The relationship between age and halothane requirements in man. Anesthesiology 30:488, 1969

134. Lerman J: Anesthetic requirements for halothane in young children 0–1 month and 1–6 months of age. Anesthesiology 59:421, 1983

135. Stoelting RK: Minimum alveolar concentrations in man on awakening from methoxyflurane, halothane, ether and fluorexene anesthesia. Anesthesiology 33:5, 1970

136. Guyton DC, Gravenstein N: Infrared analysis of volatile anesthetics: impact of monitor agent setting, volatile mixtures, and alcohol. J Clin Monit 6:203, 1990

137. Walker SD: Anesthetic and respiratory gas measurements by infrared technology. Biomed Instrum Technol 23:466, 1989

138. Gedeon A: Anesthetic agent analysis using piezo-electric microbalance. Biomed Instrum Technol 23:493, 1989

139. Westenskow DR, Silva FH: Laboratory evaluation of the vital signs (ICOR) piezoelectric anesthetic agent analyzer. J Clin Monit 7:189, 1991

140. VanWagenen RA, Westenskow DR, Benner RE et al: Dedicated monitoring of anesthetic and respiratory gases by Raman scattering. J Clin Monit 2:215, 1986

141. Cooper J: An analysis of major errors and equipment failures in anesthesia management. Anesthesiology 60:34, 1984

142. Morray JP, Geiduschek JM, Caplan RA et al: A comparison of pediatric and adult anesthesia closed malpractice claims. Anesthesiology 78:461, 1993

143. Brooks TG, Gravenstein N: Pulse oximetry for early detection of hypoxemia in anesthetized infants. J Clin Monitoring 1:135, 1985

144. Coté CJ, Goldstein EA, Coté MA et al: A single-blind study of pulse oximetry in children. Anesthesiology 68:184, 1988

145. Kong AS, Brennan L, Bingham R, Morgan Hughes J: An audit of induction of anaesthesia in neonates and small infants using pulse oximetry. Anaesthesia 47:896, 1992

146. Comroe JH, Botelho S: The unreliability of cyanosis in the recognition of arterial anoxemia. J Med Sci 214:1, 1947

147. Moller JT, Johannessen NW, Espersen K et al: Randomized evaluation of pulse oximetry in 20,802 patients: II. Perioperative events and postoperative complications. Anesthesiology 78:445, 1993

148. Moller JT, Pedersen T, Rasmussen LS et al: Randomized evaluation of pulse oximetry in 20,802 patients: I. Design, demography, pulse oximetry failure rate, and overall complication rate. Anesthesiology 78:436, 1993

149. Barker SJ, Tremper KK: Transcutaneous oxygen tension: a physiologic variable for monitoring oxygenation. J Clin Monitoring 1:130, 1985

150. Lübbers DW: Theoretical basis of the transcutaneous blood gas measurement. Crit Care Med 9:721, 1981

151. American Academy of Pediatrics Task Force on Transcutaneous Oxygen Monitors: report of consensus meeting, December 5 to 6, 1986. Pediatrics 83:122, 1989

152. Fanconi S: Pulse oximetry and transcutaneous oxygen tension for detection of hypoxemia in critically ill infants and children. Adv Exp Med Biol 220:159, 1987

153. Rooth G, Huch A, Huch R: Transcutaneous oxygen monitors are reliable indicators of arterial oxygen tension (if used correctly). Pediatrics 79:283, 1987

154. Southall DP, Bignall S, Stebbens VA et al: Pulse oxi-meter and transcutaneous arterial oxygen measurements in neonatal and paediatric intensive care. Arch Dis Child 62:882, 1987

155. Monaco F: Continuous transcutaneous oxygen and carbon dioxide monitoring in the pediatric patient ICU. Crit Care Med 10:765, 1982

156. Rafferty TD: Transcutaneous Po_2 as a trend indicator of arterial Po_2 in normal anesthetized adults. Anesth Analg 61:252, 1982

157. Bancalari E, Flynn J, Goldberg RN et al: Transcutaneous oxygen monitoring and retinopathy of prematurity. Adv Exp Med Biol 220:109, 1987

158. Pearlman SA, Maisels MJ: Preductal and postductal transcutaneous oxygen tension measurements in premature newborns with hyaline membrane disease. Pediatrics 83:98, 1989

159. Severinghaus JW: Oxygen electrode errors due to polarographic reduction of halothane. J Appl Physiol 331:640, 1971

160. Gøthgen I, Jacobsen E: Transcutaneous oxygen and carbon dioxide monitoring in the pediatric ICU. Crit Care Med 10:765, 1982

161. Sugioka K, Woodley C: The use of transcutaneous oxygen electrodes in the presence of anaesthetic agents. Can Anaesth Soc J 28:498, 1981

162. Millikan GA: The oximeter, an instrument for measuring continuously the oxygen saturation of arterial blood in man. Rev Sci Inst 13:434, 1942

163. Yelderman M, New W: Evaluation of pulse oximetry. Anesthesiology 59:349, 1983

164. Barker SJ, Tremper KK: The effect of carbon monoxide inhalation on pulse oximetry and transcutaneous Po_2. Anesthesiology 66:677, 1987

165. Lebecque P, Shango P, Stijns, M et al: Pulse oximetry versus measured arterial oxygen saturation: a comparison of the Nellcor N100 and the Biox III. Pediatr Pulmonol 10:132, 1991

166. Praud JP, Carofilis A, Bridey F et al: Accuracy of two wavelength pulse oximetry in neonates and infants. Pediatr Pulmonol 6:180, 1989

167. Thilo EH, Andersen D, Wasserstein ML et al: Saturation by pulse oximetry: comparison of the results obtained by instruments of different brands. J Pediatr 122:620, 1993

168. Mok JY, McLaughlin FJ, Pintar M et al: Transcutaneous monitoring of oxygenation: what is normal? J Pediatr 108:365, 1986

169. Lozano JM, Duque OR, Buitrago T, Behaine S: Pulse oximetry reference values at high altitude. Arch Dis Child 67:299, 1992

170. Thilo EH, Park Moore B, Berman ER, Carson BS: Oxygen saturation by pulse oximetry in healthy infants at an altitude of 1610 m (5280 ft). What is normal? Am J Dis Child 145:1137, 1991

171. Stebbens VA, Poets CF, Alexander JR et al: Oxygen

saturation and breathing patterns in infancy. 1: Full term infants in the second month of life. Arch Dis Child 66:569, 1991

172. Poets CF, Stebbens VA, Samuels MP, Southall DP: Oxygen saturation and breathing patterns in children. Pediatrics 92:686, 1993

173. Coté CJ, Daniels AL, Connolly M et al: Tongue oximetry in children with extensive thermal injury: comparison with peripheral oximetry. Can J Anaesth 39:454, 1992

174. Jobes DR, Nicolson SC: Monitoring of arterial hemoglobin oxygen saturation using a tongue sensor. Anesth Analg 67:186, 1988

175. Severinghaus JW, Kaifeh KH: Accuracy of response of six pulse oximeters to profound hypoxia. Anesthesiology 66:677, 1987

176. OLeary RJ Jr, Landon M, Benumof JL: Buccal pulse oximeter is more accurate than finger pulse oximeter in measuring oxygen saturation. Anesth Analg 75:495, 1992

177. Kagle DM, Alexander CM, Berko RS et al: Evaluation of the Ohmeda 3700 pulse oximeter: steady-state and transient response characteristics. Anesthesiology 66:376, 1987

178. Reynolds LM, Nicolson SC, Steven JM et al: Influence of sensor site location on pulse oximetry kinetics in children. Anesth Analg 76:751, 1993

179. Boxer RA Gottesfeld I, Singh S et al: Noninvasive pulse oximetry in children with cyanotic congenital heart disease. Crit Care Med 15:1062, 1987

180. Fanconi S: Reliability of pulse oximetry in hypoxic infants. J Pediatr 112:424, 1988

181. Durand M, Ramanathan R: Pulse oximetry for continuous oxygen monitoring in sick newborn infants. J Pediatr 109:1052, 1986

182. Gidding SS: Pulse oximetry in cyanotic congenital heart disease. Am J Cardiol 70:391, 1992

183. Lynn AM, Bosenberg A: Pulse oximetry during cardiac catheterization in children with congenital heart disease. J Clin Monit 2:230, 1986

184. Schmitt HJ, Schuetz WH, Proeschel PA, Jaklin C: Accuracy of pulse oximetry in children with cyanotic congenital heart disease. J Cardiothorac Vasc Anesth 7:61, 1993

185. Bucher HU, Fanconi S, Baeckert P, Duc G: Hyperoxemia in newborn infants: detection by pulse oximetry. Pediatrics 84:226, 1989

186. Deckardt R, Steward DJ: Noninvasive arterial hemoglobin oxygen saturation versus transcutaneous oxygen tension monitoring in the preterm infant. Crit Care Med 12:935, 1984

187. Wasunna A, Whitelaw AG: Pulse oximetry in preterm infants. Arch Dis Child 62:957, 1987

188. Scheller MS: Effects of intravenously administered dyes on pulse oximetry reading. Anesthesiology 65:550, 1986

189. Brooks TD: Infrared heat lamps interfere with pulse oximetry readings. Anesthesiology 61:550, 1986

190. Costarino AT: Falsely normal saturation reading with the pulse oximeter. Anesthesiology 67:830, 1987

191. Murphy KG, Secunda JA, Rockoff MA: Severe burns from a pulse oximeter. Anesthesiology 73:350, 1990

192. Sobel DB: Burning of a neonate due to a pulse oximeter: arterial saturation monitoring. Pediatrics 89:154, 1992

193. Miyasaka K, Ohata J: Burn, erosion, and "sun" tan with the use of pulse oximetry in infants. Anesthesiology 67:1008, 1987

194. Koch G, Wendel H: Adjustment of arterial blood gases and acid base balance in the normal newborn infant during the first week of life. Biol Neonat 12:136, 1968

195. Peckmam GJ, Fox WW: Physiologic factors affecting pulmonary artery pressure in infants with persistent pulmonary hypertension. J Pediatr 93:1005, 1978

196. Rudolph AM: Fetal and neonatal pulmonary circulation. Am Rev Physiolol 41:383, 1979

197. Miyasaka K: Respiratory monitoring of the infant in anaesthesia and intensive care. Can J Anaesth 37:Scxxiv, 1990

198. Burrows FA, Volgyesi GA, James PD: Clinical evaluation of the augmented delta quotient monitor for intraoperative electroencephalographic monitoring of children during surgery and cardiopulmonary bypass for repair of congenital cardiac defects. Br J Anaesth 63:565, 1989

199. Rung GW, Wickey GS, Myers JL et al: Thiopental as an adjunct to hypothermia for EEG suppression in infants prior to circulatory arrest. J Cardiothorac Vasc Anesth 5:337, 1991

200. Nash CL Jr, Lorig RA, Schatzinger LA, Brown RH: Spinal cord monitoring during operative treatment of the spine. Clin Orthop Rel Res 126:100, 1977

201. Dawson EG, Sherman JE, Kanim LE, Nuwer MR: Spinal cord monitoring: results of the Scoliosis Research Society and the European Spinal Deformity Society survey. Spine 16:S361, 1991

202. Epstein NE, Danto J, Nardi D: Evaluation of intraoperative somatosensory-evoked potential monitoring during 100 cervical operations. Spine 18:737, 1993

203. Dinner DS, Luders H, Lesser RP et al. Intraoperative spinal somatosensory evoked potential monitoring. J Neurosurg 65:807, 1986

204. Perlik SJ, VanEgeren R, Fisher MA: Somatosensory evoked potential surgical monitoring: observations during combined isoflurane-nitrous oxide anesthesia. Spine 17:273, 1992

205. Grundy BL, Nash CL Jr, Brown RH: Arterial pressure manipulation alters spinal cord function during correction of scoliosis. Anesthesiology 54:249, 1981

206. Nuwer MR: Use of somatosensory evoked potentials for intraoperative monitoring of cerebral and spinal cord function. Neurol Clin 6:881, 1988

207. York DH, Chabot RJ, Gaines RW: Response variability of somatosensory evoked potentials during scoliosis surgery. Spine 12:864, 1987

208. Veilleux M, Daube JR, Cucchiara RF: Monitoring of cortical evoked potentials during surgical procedures on the cervical spine. Mayo Clin Proc 62:256, 1987

209. Burke D, Hicks R, Stephen J et al: Assessment of corticospinal and somatosensory conduction simultaneously during scoliosis surgery. Electroencephalogr Clin Neurophysiol 85:388, 1992

210. Brooke JS, Banta JV, Bunke FJ, Pelletier C: Somatosensory evoked potential monitoring during Cotrel-Dubousset instrumentation: report of a case. Spine 18:518, 1993

211. Mostegl A, Bauer R, Eichenauer, M: Intraoperative somatosensory potential monitoring: a clinical analysis of 127 surgical procedures. Spine 13:396, 1988

212. Edmonds HL Jr, Paloheimo MP, Backman MH et al: Transcranial magnetic motor evoked potentials (tcMMEP) for functional monitoring of motor pathways during scoliosis surgery. Spine 14:683, 1989

213. Tabaraud F, Boulesteix JM, Moulies D et al: Monitoring of the motor pathway during spinal surgery. Spine 18:546, 1993

214. Raju TN, Vidyasagar D, Papazafiratou C: Intracranial pressure monitoring in the neonatal ICU. Crit Care Med 8:575, 1980

215. Friesen RH, Honda AT, Thieme RE: Changes in anterior fontanel pressure in preterm neonates during tracheal intubation. Anesth Analg 66:874, 1987

216. Raju TN, Vidyasagar D, Torres C et al: Intracranial pressure during intubation and anesthesia in infants. J Pediatr 96:860, 1980

217. Mendelow AD, Rowan JO, Murray L, Kerr AE: A clinical comparison of subdural screw pressure measurements with ventricular pressure. J Neurosurg 58:45, 1983

218. Schickner DJ, Young RF: Intracranial pressure monitoring: fiberoptic monitor compared with the ventricular catheter. Surg Neurol 37:251, 1992

219. Adamsons K Jr, Gandy GM, James LS: The influence of the thermal factors upon oxygen consumption of the newborn human infant. J Pediatr 66:499, 1965

220. Britt BA, Kalow W: Malignant hyperthermia: a statistical review. Can Anaesth Soc J 17:293, 1970

221. Britt BA, Kwong FH, Endrenyi L: Management of malignant hyperthermia-susceptible patients. A review. In Henschel E.O. (ed): Malignant hyperthermia: current concepts. Appleton Century-Crofts, E. Norwalk, CT, 1977

222. Bissonnette B, Sessler DI: Passive or active inspired gas humidification increases thermal steady-state temperatures in anesthetized infants. Anesth Analg 69:783, 1989

223. Bloch EC, Ginsberg B, Binner RA Jr: The esophageal temperature gradient in anesthetized children. J Clin Monit 9:73, 1993

224. Hercus V, Cohen D, Bowring AC: Temperature gradients during hypothermia. Br Med J 1:1439, 1959

225. Stupfel M, Severinghaus JW: Internal body temperature gradients during anesthesia and hypothermia and effect of vagotomy. J Appl Physiol 9:380, 1956

226. Whitby JD, Dunkin LJ: Temperature differences in the oesophagus: the effects of intubation and ventilation. Br J Anaesth 41:615, 1969

227. Benzinger M: Tympanic thermometry in surgery and anesthesia. JAMA 209:1207, 1969

228. Hindman BJ, Dexter F, Cutkomp J et al: Brain blood flow and metabolism do not increase at stable brain temperature during cardiopulmonary bypass in rabbits. Anesthesiology 77:342, 1992

229. Whitby JD, Dunkin LJ: Cerebral, oesophageal and nasopharyngeal temperatures. Br J Anaesth 43:673, 1971

230. Benzinger TH: Clinical temperature: new physiological basis. JAMA 209:1200, 1969

231. Webb GE: Comparison of esophageal and tympanic temperature monitoring during cardiopulmonary bypass. Anesth Analg 52:729, 1973

232. Wallace CT, Marks WE, Adkins WY: Perforation of the tympanic membrane, a complication of tympanic thermometry during anesthesia. Anesthesiology 41:290, 1974

233. Shinozaki T, Deane R, Perkins FM: Infrared tympanic thermometer: evaluation of a new clinical thermometer. Crit Care Med 16:148, 1988

234. Chamberlain JM, Grandner J, Rubinoff JL et al: Comparison of a tympanic thermometer to rectal and oral thermometers in a pediatric emergency department. Clin Pediatr 30:24, 1991

235. Stewart JV, Webster D: Re-evaluation of the tympanic thermometer in the emergency department. Ann Emerg Med 21:158, 1992

236. Lees DE: Liquid crystal thermomotry. Anesth Analg 58:351, 1979

237. Lees DE, Schuette W, Bull JM: An evaluation of liquid-crystal thermometry as a screening device for intraoperative hyperthermia. Anesth Analg 57:669, 1978

238. Leon JE, Bissonnette B, Lerman J: Liquid crystalline temperature monitoring: does it estimate core temperature in anaesthetized paediatric patients? Can J Anaesth 37:S98, 1990

239. Klein EF, Graves SA: "Hot pot" tracheitis. Chest 65: 225, 1974

240. Bennett EJ, Patel KP, Grundy EM: Neonatal temperature and surgery. Anesthesiology 46:303, 1977

241. Goudsouzian NG: Maturation of neuromuscular transmission in the infants. Br J Anesthesia 52:205, 1980

242. Churchill-Davidson HC, Wise RP: Neuromuscular transmission in the newborn infant. Anesthesiology 24:271, 1963

243. Crumrine RS, Yodlowski EH: Assessment of neuromuscular function in infants. Anesthesiology 54: 29, 1981

244. Dupuis JY, Martin R, Tessonnier JM, Tetrault JP: Clinical assessment of the muscular response to tetanic nerve stimulation. Can J Anaesth 37:397, 1990

245. Saddler JM, Bevan JC, Donati F et al: Comparison of double-burst and train-of-four stimulation to assess neuromuscular blockade in children. Anesthesiology 73:401, 1990

246. Law SC, Brandom BW: Monitoring neuromuscular function in the pediatric patient. Int Anesthesiol Clin 30:147, 1992

247. Lyew MA, Pinto SR, Bevan JC: A simple device for monitoring neuromuscular blockade in children. Can J Anaesth 36:717, 1989

248. Kalli I: Effect of surface electrode positioning on the compound action potential evoked by ulnar nerve stimulation in anaesthetized infants and children. Br J Anaesth 62:188, 1989

249. Dupuis JY, Martin R, Tetrault JP: Clinical, electrical and mechanical correlations during recovery from neuromuscular blockade with vecuronium. Can J Anaesth 37:192, 1990

250. Jensen E, Viby Mogensen J, Bang U: The Accelograph: a new neuromuscular transmission monitor. Acta Anaesthesiol Scand 32:49, 1988

251. May O, Kirkegaard Nielsen H, Werner MU: The acceleration transducer: an assessment of its precision in comparison with a force displacement transducer. Acta Anaesthesiol Scand 32:239, 1988

252. Laycock JR, Baxter MK, Bevan JC et al: The potency of pancuronium at the adductor pollicis and diaphragm in infants and children. Anesthesiology 68: 908, 1988

253. Thornberry EA, Mazumdar B: The effect of changes in arm temperature on neuromuscular monitoring in the presence of atracurium blockade. Anaesthesia 43:447, 1988

254. Mason LJ, Betts EK: A clinical sign of neuromuscular blockage reversal in neonates and infants. Anesthesiology 52:441, 1980

255. Pavlin EG, Holle RH, Schoene RB: Recovery of airway protection compared with ventilation in humans after paralysis with curare. Anesthesiology 70: 381, 1989

256. Gross JB: Estimating allowable blood loss: corrected for dilution. Anesthesiology 58:277, 1983

257. Hagen PT, Scholz DG, Edwards WD: Incidence and size of patent foramen ovale during the first 10 decades of life: an autopsy study of 965 normal hearts. Mayo Clin Proc 59:17, 1984

258. Scammon RE, Norris EH: On the time of obliteration of the fetal blood passages (foramen ovale, ductus arteriosus, ductus venosus). Anat Rec 15: 165, 1918

259. Maroon JC, Albin MS: Air embolism diagnosed by Doppler ultrasound. Anesth Analg 53:399, 1974

260. Aperia A, Zetterstrom R: Renal control of fluid homeostasis in the newborn infant. Clin Perinatol 9: 523, 1982

261. Jones MD Jr, Gresham EL, Battaglia FC: Urinary flow rates and urea excretion rates in newborn infants. Biol Neonate 21:321, 1972

262. Furman EB, Roman DG, Lemmer LAS: Specific therapy in water, electrolyte and blood-volume replacement during pediatric surgery. Anesthesiology 42:187, 1975

263. Simpson JC: Monitoring during anesthesia for cardiac surgery. Int Anesthesiol Clin 19:137, 1981

264. AAP Guidelines for Perinatal Care. p. 212. American Academy of Pediatrics, Evanston, IL, 1983

265. Mayer BW: Pediatric Anesthesia: A Guide to Its Administration. JB Lippincott, Philadelphia, 1981

266. Behrman RE, Vaughan VC III: Nelson Textbook of Pediatrics. 13th Ed. p. 943. WB Saunders, Philadelphia, 1987

267. Versmold HT, Kitterman JA, Phibbs RH et al: Aortic blood pressure during the first 12 hours of life in infants with birth weights 610 to 4,220 grams. Pediatrics 67:607, 1981

268. Adams FH, Landaw EM: What are healthy blood pressures for children? Pediatrics 68:268, 1981

269. Smith RM: Anesthesia for Infants and Children. 4th Ed. CV Mosby, St. Louis, 1980

Monitoring in Obstetric Anesthesia

28

Michael A. Herzig
Gerard W. Ostheimer
J. Stephen Naulty

The obstetric patient presents a unique problem in monitoring: the necessity of simultaneously monitoring not one, but two physiologically inter-related patients. One must monitor the effects of an event on both the mother and the fetus, since an intervention that may produce an improvement in the physiologic status of the mother may be dele-terious to the fetus. This interrelationship provides the fascinating challenge of obstetric anesthesia.

In addition, profound maternal physiologic changes occur during pregnancy. Many alterations are observed in expected "normal" values of mon-itored variables, and responses of a pregnant pa-tient to anesthetic maneuvers and disease states may be different than a nonpregnant patient. Fi-nally, certain disease states found only in preg-nancy, such as toxemia of pregnancy, cardiomyopa-thy of pregnancy, intrauterine growth retardation, and placental insufficiency may require carefully applied and interpreted monitoring techniques for optimal outcome. This chapter attempts to discuss these physiologic alterations in obstetric patients and methods of monitoring these problems.

HISTORICAL ASPECTS

Many of the most significant advances in obstet-ric practice have been improvement of the ability of the obstetric practitioner to monitor the well-being of the laboring patient and her fetus. The history of this advance has been far from even, with periods of greater understanding of labor and its physiology alternating with periods of complete re-jection of these advances when complications and difficulties are recognized. For example, monitor-ing the progress of labor by vaginal examination was commonly employed in the seventeenth and eighteenth centuries, but when Semmelweiss de-scribed the association of manual examination and puerperal sepsis, this valuable technique was aban-doned for a hundred years.

Fetal monitoring has experienced a similar his-tory. Since the early part of the twentieth century it has been recognized that observation of the fetal heart rate could allow the obstetrician to predict with some reliability how the fetus was tolerating labor. This observation was further expanded with the advent of continuous electronic fetal monitor-ing in the 1960s and 1970s. Since that time, how-ever, complications and problems have been de-scribed as a result of such monitoring, and the technique is being questioned by many gravidae and practitioners. It can only be hoped that a ra-tional acceptance of the technique with its limita-tions (see below) will result, rather than an out-right rejection of a valuable technology.

PHYSIOLOGY OF PREGNANCY

The obvious reason to monitor the maternal-fetal unit in pregnancy is to maintain the mother and fetus in optimal condition. In order to do this one must know what "optimal condition" is. This statement is not as ridiculous as it might first appear, because the normal, "optimal," state of a pregnant patient is very different from that of the nonpregnant patient. Thus, we must discuss the physiologic alterations of pregnancy.

Pregnancy is characterized by three primary changes: (1) an alteration in the hormonal environment of the mother, (2) an alteration in the metabolic activity of the mother produced by the presence of an actively growing fetus, and (3) an alteration in uterine size and vascularity. These primary changes induce secondary changes in all maternal organ systems. We describe these changes and how they affect variables we wish to monitor.

Cardiovascular System

Cardiac output increases approximately 40 percent during gestation, with further increases during labor, and with a maximal increase of up to 80 percent above prepregnant values in the immediate postpartum period (Fig. 28-1).[1] This change in cardiac output is due to an increase in heart rate of 12 to 15 beats per minute (bpm) and an increase in stroke volume of 15 to 20 percent.[2] Total peripheral resistance decreases during pregnancy,

TABLE 28-1. Maternal Cardiovascular Alterations at Term

Variable	Change	Magnitude
Cardiac output	↑	40%
Stroke volume	↑	30%
Heart rate	↑	15%
Systolic blood pressure	↓	0–5 mmHg
Diastolic blood pressure	↓	10–20 mmHg
Total peripheral resistance	↓	15%
Central venous pressure	—	0%

(Modified from Skaredoff,[77] with permission.)

largely due to the low-resistance uterine circulation that acts as a parallel circuit in the vascular system. Normally, arterial blood pressure decreases only slightly because the increased cardiac output compensates for the decrease in peripheral vascular resistance (Table 28-1).[3]

The venous system is also greatly affected by pregnancy. The enlarging uterus produces compression of the inferior vena cava producing high venous pressures in the femoral and epidural venous systems, with a decreased venous pressure in the upper half of the body.[4] These changes are exaggerated when the parturient is supine. In this position the marked compression of the inferior vena

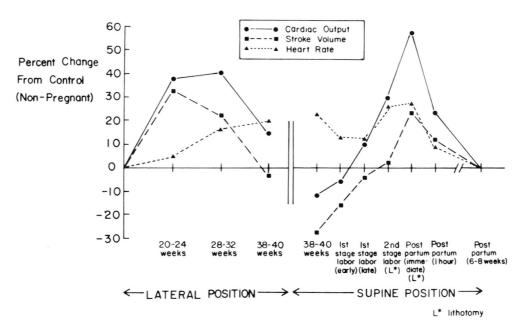

Fig. 28-1. Maternal cardiovascular alterations in pregnancy and parturition. (From Mangano,[78] with permission.)

cava by the gravid uterus leads to decreased right atrial filling pressure, decreased stroke volume, and decreased cardiac output, which produce large decreases in arterial blood pressure—the "supine hypotensive syndrome" (Fig. 28-2).[5]

The effects of uterine compression on the vascular system are not limited to the venous system. The aorta can be compressed by the gravid uterus, and arterial pressures and regional blood flows distal to the compression are reduced.[6] Since the uterine artery arises distal to the compression site, it is possible to produce decreased uterine blood flow, and hence "fetal distress," when the mother is supine. This effect is more difficult to detect than venous compression because upper extremity blood pressure declines with venous compromise but does not necessarily change with aortic compression. Multiple gestation and polyhydramnios make aortocaval compression more severe. In some situations monitoring both upper and lower extremity blood pressures is helpful. It is important to always be aware of the effects of position on monitored variables, and to avoid placing the parturient in the supine position. If maternal or fetal deterioration occurs, it is *always* important to check the position of the parturient to ascertain that her position is not the cause of the deterioration (as it frequently is). In addition, treating such a deterioration with fluids and vasopressors may be ineffective if aortocaval compression is not relieved.

Hematologic System

Blood volume increases gradually during pregnancy, reaching a maximum early in the third trimester[7] (Table 28-2). The rise in plasma volume is larger than the increase in red blood cell volume. This disparity produces a decrease in hematocrit, oxygen content,[8] and blood viscosity of approximately 10 to 15 percent.[9] Despite the altered plasma volume, there is no change in central venous pressure in the healthy gravida, and the response to an intravenous fluid load is normal.[4] The plasma oncotic pressure falls due to a decrease in plasma protein concentration.[10] This decrease places the parturient at greater risk of developing pulmonary edema after a pulmonary insult.

White blood counts usually increase during gestation and then increase further during parturition. The platelet count does not predictably

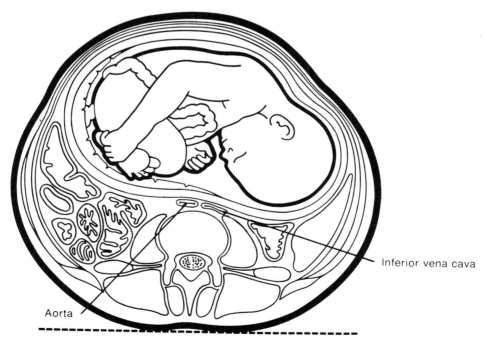

Fig. 28-2. The pregnant uterus compressing the aorta and the inferior vena cava (aortocaval compression). Patient in supine position. (From Ostheimer,[79] with permission.)

change significantly during pregnancy. Most clotting factors increase resulting in a hypercoagulable state.[11] It is not known if this increase in clotting factors predisposes to thrombus formation on intravascular catheters, but it is reasonable to assume that it does. Therefore, precautions should be taken to minimize thrombus formation, since pulmonary embolism is one of the leading causes of maternal mortality. Appropriately sized catheters should be employed and heparin-bonded catheters may be useful in preventing embolization. Catheters should be removed when no longer required for monitoring purposes.

Respiratory System

The increased oxygen consumption produced by pregnancy increases the demands on the respiratory system (Table 28-3). Minute ventilation is increased by 50 percent at term as a result of an increase in both respiratory rate and tidal volume.[12] Since dead space is unchanged in pregnancy, the increased minute ventilation represents a rise in alveolar ventilation resulting in a respiratory alkalosis. Respiratory changes seem to be stimulated in part by increased progesterone.[13] Arterial carbon dioxide tension falls to 30 to 35 mmHg. This allows arterial oxygen tension on room air to rise to 106 to 110 mmHg.[12] Arterial pH remains relatively unchanged because the kidneys excrete buffer base (largely bicarbonate) to compensate for the respiratory alkalosis.[14] However, if circulatory or respiratory inadequacy develops, this decreased buffer base will allow rapid development of systemic acidosis. Arterial oxygen tension may decline precipitously if gravidae are placed supine, secondary to decreases in cardiac output and functional residual capacity.

Renal System

The increased cardiac output in gestation is accompanied by a large decrease in renal vascular resistance. A large increase in renal blood flow is produced, which combines with the decrease in plasma oncotic pressure to produce an increased glomerular filtration rate and filtration fraction.[15]

The renal tubules are unable to completely compensate for the increased glomerular filtration of solutes, which results in a decreased renal "threshold" for glucose and amino acids.[16] Glucosuria is found in many parturients and the administration of large amounts of dextrose-containing intravenous fluids may produce an osmotic diuresis. Therefore, when monitoring urine output in pregnant patients, one should check frequently for glucosuria to ensure that one is not misled by large urine outputs due to an osmotic diuresis.

The renal collecting systems become dilated and exhibit reduced motility—the "hydronephrosis of pregnancy."[17] These conditions predispose to urinary tract infections. When urinary catheters are used in the parturient, scrupulous care must be taken to avoid introducing bacteria.

TABLE 28-3. Maternal Respiratory Alterations at Term

Minute ventilation	+50%
Alveolar ventilation	+70%
Tidal volume	+40%
Respiratory rate	+15%
Closing volume	Unchanged or slightly decreased
Arterial pH	Unchanged
Arterial PO_2	+10 mmHg
Arterial PCO_2	−10 mmHg
Airway resistance	−36%
Vital capacity	Unchanged
Inspiratory lung capacity	Unchanged
Functional residual capacity	−20%
Total lung capacity	Unchanged
Expiratory reserve volume	−20%
Residual volume	−20%
Oxygen consumption	+20%

(Modified from Skaredoff,[77] with permission.)

TABLE 28-2. Maternal Hematologic Alterations at Term

Variable	Change	Magnitude (%)
Blood volume	↑	35
Plasma volume	↑	45
Erythrocyte volume	↑	20
Blood platelets	—	0
Fibrinogen	↑	40
Fibrinolysis	↓	
BUN	↓	33
Plasma cholinesterase	↓	20
Total protein	↑	18
Albumin	↓	14
Globulin	—	0
SGOT, SGPT, LDH	↑	
Cholesterol	↑	
Alkaline phosphatase (produced by placenta)	↑	

(Modified from Skaredoff,[77] with permission.)

Peripartum Changes

Cardiovascular Changes

During parturition, the cardiovascular system must respond to the stresses of labor. Cardiac output may rise to 10 to 12 L/min during labor and reaches peak levels shortly after delivery (Fig. 28-1).[18] The mechanism by which this is accomplished is complex: hormonal changes, metabolic demands, and the effects of uterine contractions on preload and afterload are involved.

Hormonal Changes

During labor the pain of uterine contractions causes increased secretion of catecholamines by the adrenal medulla.[19] Plasma norepinephrine and epinephrine levels rise, producing an increase in heart rate and systemic vascular resistance. Systolic blood pressure during painful contractions may exceed 200 mmHg in previously normotensive women. This response can be attenuated by analgesic techniques.

Metabolic Demands

Oxygen consumption, which is elevated approximately 20 percent at term, increases further during labor. The magnitude of the increase depends on the frequency and severity of contractions, averaging approximately 15 percent.[14] Most women in labor develop a decreased venous oxygen saturation and a metabolic (lactic) acidosis, suggesting that the cardiovascular system can usually not meet this increased demand for oxygen delivery. Since buffer base is low during pregnancy, a severe acidosis may develop if the circulatory system is unable to meet the body's demand for oxygen (as is seen in patients with significant cardiac disease). The development of acidosis may be prevented by adequate epidural analgesia during labor.[20]

Uterine Activity

With every uterine contraction, profound changes are produced in both the arterial and venous vasculature. When intrauterine pressure exceeds venous pressure, the circulatory bed of the uterus acts as a Starling resistor, and perfusion ceases.[21] Since the uterus is in effect a low-resistance "shunt" in the peripheral vascular network, closing this shunt suddenly increases peripheral vascular resistance. This contributes to the rise in arterial pressure noted during contractions. Simultaneously, uterine contractions produce an autotransfusion that is estimated to be 300 to 500 ml. This results in a rise in central venous pressure, right atrial pressure, and a sudden increase in stroke volume.[22] Both ventricular preload and afterload increase during labor, and left and right ventricular stroke work also increase.

Postpartum Changes

In the immediate postpartum period, the uterus contracts and does not relax, producing the largest increase in ventricular work seen in labor. Cardiac output reaches a maximum in the immediate postpartum period, and the demands on the entire cardiovascular system appear to be maximal at this time (Fig. 28-1). Thus, if a patient has cardiovascular disease, this is the period in which she is most likely to decompensate. Therefore, any monitoring that is required antepartum should be continued for at least 12 hours postpartum.

Respiratory System

Respiration is profoundly altered during parturition. Hyperventilation is extremely common, and is frequently exacerbated by methods of pain relief that depend on "controlled breathing."[23] Arterial carbon dioxide tension may decline to 12 to 16 mmHg. This hyperventilation can have deleterious physiologic consequences. The oxyhemoglobin dissociation curve is shifted to the left, increasing the oxygen affinity of hemoglobin at a time when tissue oxygen demands are highest. The respiratory alkalosis that develops may result in uterine and cerebral vasoconstriction and decreased blood flow. Peripheral manifestations of hypocarbia, such as paresthesias and carpopedal spasm, are also common. This hyperventilation during contractions may alternate with periods of hypoventilation between contractions, which may occasionally produce hypoxemia.[24]

Summary

Profound physiologic alterations exist during pregnancy and parturition, and the immediate postpartum period. Knowledge of these changes is essential for interpreting data obtained by monitoring. Now we shall examine the use of monitoring techniques in normal and complicated obstetrics.

MONITORING IN ROUTINE OBSTETRICS

It is important to remember that at any time a "routine" or "low-risk" labor and delivery may become a life-threatening situation for the mother and/or the fetus, with little or no warning. Complications such as uterine rupture, amniotic fluid embolism, and prolapsed umbilical cord do occur with significant frequency in what appear to be low-risk gestations. Therefore, it would seem prudent to monitor all parturients at all times for early signs of such complications. This apparently self-evident idea, however, is far from self-evident to many parturients, childbirth educators, and even many physicians. The desire of many parturients for a "natural" childbirth experience (no matter what the risks), and the fear of technology and complications associated with monitoring (however rare or apparently trivial), has caused routine maternal and fetal monitoring and such elementary precautions as intravenous infusions to be abandoned in many centers. Maternal convenience and psychic comfort have been considered more important than maternal and fetal safety.

Questions of the cost-effectiveness of routine monitoring have also arisen. Studies of the utility and cost-effectiveness of routine monitoring are difficult to perform. They also require the investigators to make at least two crucial determinations: (1) the frequency of correctable complications detected by monitoring, and (2) the ultimate cost to society of failing to detect them. The conclusions reached in such studies are exquisitely sensitive to the magnitude of these determinations and, as might be expected, no definitive judgment has yet been reached about the economic utility of routine monitoring. Thus, the decision whether to use monitoring techniques in childbirth depends largely on the philosophy of individual childbirth centers. These range from absolute prohibition of routine monitoring (as at some "birthing centers," with occasionally tragic results[25]) to multichannel, computer-processed monitoring of all parturients (at great inconvenience and expense, and in the most "unnatural" environment).

The most rational approach is to avoid absolute dicta at either extreme. Education of parturients about the proper role of monitoring should be approached with the idea that all pregnancies are different and that no one approach can possibly cover all eventualities. Probably the most important monitor in labor is an experienced labor nurse, and staffing should be adequate in a labor area to allow all parturients close observation by such a nurse. By employing such observation, additional monitoring appropriate to the situation can be added.

At a minimum, the unanesthetized parturient should have her blood pressure measured at least every 30 minutes during labor. If hypertension develops, the frequency of measurement should increase because life-threatening hypertension can develop remarkably rapidly during labor.[25] Similarly the patient's urine should be monitored for protein at every voiding, and her reflexes checked periodically to detect the development of toxemia of pregnancy at an early, easily treatable stage. The parturient's body temperature should be measured on admission, and then every 2 hours after the fetal membranes have been ruptured, since chorioamnionitis is a common complication of prolonged labor. An occasional vaginal examination is important to assess the progress of labor and to detect such complications as vaginal bleeding. Fetal monitoring should be an integral part of monitoring during labor.

If the parturient receives analgesia or anesthesia for labor and delivery then the level of monitoring must intensify, in order that complications of these techniques can be detected before serious sequelae can occur.

Vaginal Delivery

During "medicated" vaginal deliveries, routine monitoring as outlined above should be extended to detect at an early stage the potential complications of the anesthetic technique employed.

Systemic Analgesia

All analgesic drugs commonly employed in labor (e.g., opioids, major tranquilizers, barbiturates, and inhaled anesthetics) are capable of producing severe depression of the central nervous system, with loss of protective airway reflexes. Since all parturients must be considered to be at risk for aspiration of gastric contents in such a situation, patients who receive such drugs must be carefully observed and their level of consciousness frequently assessed. These drugs are all respiratory depressants, and it is important to use a low threshold for monitoring for maternal and fetal hypoxemia and acidosis.

Epidural Analgesia

Monitoring for potential complications during epidural analgesia/anesthesia for labor should be continuous, or nearly so. This means that staffing should be adequate to allow sufficient vigilance to detect the three major complications of this technique: hypotension, unintentional intravascular injection, and unintentional subarachnoid injection.

Hypotension

Hypotension is by far the most common complication of epidural analgesia for labor. The incidence of hypotension can be decreased by such maneuvers as adequate hydration prior to the initiation of the block and avoidance of the supine position, but hypotension is still found in 10 to 20 percent of such anesthetics.[26] Early detection of hypotension is essential because prompt treatment is required to prevent serious complications, such as fetal acidosis and maternal cardiovascular collapse.[27] Therefore, blood pressure must be monitored frequently, particularly at the inception of epidural blockade. We recommend measuring blood pressure every 2 minutes for the first 20 minutes, then every 5 minutes for 20 minutes, then every 15 minutes thereafter if a continuous technique is employed. After subsequent bolus injections, the entire sequence should be repeated. An automated noninvasive blood pressure device is particularly helpful. Although hypotension is most likely to occur at the onset of the block, it may occur at any time. Hypotension in parturients almost invariably produces nausea, and a parturient who complains of nausea should have her blood pressure checked immediately.

Unintentional Intravascular Injection

Unintentional intravascular injection is a potentially catastrophic complication. The severity of this complication can be reduced to a minimum if no more than 3 to 5 ml of local anesthetic are injected at any one time. It is important to monitor the patient in between injections for early symptoms of

intravascular injection, which include tinnitus and circumoral numbness. If, however, a large volume of local anesthetic is accidentally introduced into an epidural vein, grand mal seizures, loss of consciousness, and cardiovascular collapse with severe and often intractable arrhythmias can ensue. Therefore, it is crucial that the labor floor be equipped to monitor cardiac rhythm and have the necessary equipment to perform cardiopulmonary resuscitation. Aortocaval compression by the gravid uterus can make external chest compressions ineffective. It is critical to maintain left uterine displacement. Elevation of the legs may be helpful in increasing venous return. Emergent cesarean delivery and open-chest cardiac massage must be considered if resuscitative efforts are ineffective. The delivery of fetus will help maximize venous return.

Unintentional Subarachnoid Injection

Unintentional subarachnoid injection of even small volumes of local anesthetic solution can produce extremely high levels of spinal anesthesia, with an attendant high likelihood of severe hypotension and bradycardia secondary to the complete sympathetic neural blockade. In addition, complete paralysis of the respiratory and pharyngeal musculature can occur. This is best avoided by careful monitoring of the results of a small test dose of local anesthetic—a dose sufficient to produce a manageable level of spinal anesthesia if this should occur, but not large enough to produce total subarachnoid block. Obviously, this dose varies with the local anesthetic chosen for the block, but usually ranges from 2 to 3 ml of the commonly employed local anesthetics. It is not enough to merely inject the small dose and immediately follow it with a large dose—it is vitally important to monitor the results of the injection. For example, the effects of the injection on blood pressure, motor activity, and sensory function must be observed. Any of these complications can occur, not only on the first injection, but on all subsequent injections. Therefore, all the above monitoring steps should be taken each time an epidural catheter is injected with local anesthetic with or without opioid. If a continuous infusion is selected, the dangers of a bolus injection are avoided, but it is still possible for the catheter to penetrate a blood vessel or enter the subarachnoid space. Vessel entry with a continuous infusion of local anesthetic should be suspected when the block becomes inadequate and sensory levels begin to recede despite an adequate rate of infusion. One should be very suspicious of such a catheter, and not inject a large bolus of local anesthetic to reestablish the blockade. On the other hand, a rapidly rising level of sensory analgesia during a continuous infusion should be seen as a sign of catheter entry into the subarachnoid space, and appropriate measures should be taken. It cannot be overemphasized that the most important monitoring technique during epidural anesthesia is frequent contact with the patient by knowledgeable personnel. This contact can be supplemented by the use of mechanical devices, such as automated blood pressure devices and apnea monitors, but never replaced by such devices.

Cesarean Delivery

During cesarean delivery, as for any other operation, monitoring should be performed as described elsewhere in this text. However, some features of cesarean delivery should be emphasized, depending on the type of anesthetic selected.

Regional Anesthesia

The same precautions as described for regional anesthesia for vaginal delivery should be employed when establishing the block. In addition, if epidural anesthesia is selected, both the mother and fetus should be monitored while the proper level of anesthesia is being established. This is important because the high thoracic levels required for satisfactory anesthesia during cesarean delivery can produce decreased uterine blood flow, especially if the patient has had inadequate intravascular volume expansion, or she experiences supine hypotension. Hypotension is relatively more common during regional anesthesia for cesarean delivery than during vaginal deliveries. This is due to the higher levels of sensory analgesia produced, with a consequent total sympathetic blockade and larger requirement for adequate intravascular volume expansion to maintain an adequate ventricular preload. The more rapidly the sympathectomy is produced, the more likely is the development of hypotension. Rapidly acting epidural local anesthetics, such as 2-chloroprocaine and pH-adjusted lidocaine, as well as spinal anesthesia are associated with a higher incidence of hypotension than slower acting anesthetics such as epidural bupivacaine.

Frequent monitoring of blood pressure during onset of these blocks is essential to observe the development of hypotension and initiate therapy. This is important because it has been demonstrated that better fetal acid-base and neurobehavioral scores are produced if fetal and maternal condition is maintained by the prompt use of a vasopressor, such as ephedrine, rather than instituting such treatment *after* hypotension has developed. The incidence of maternal nausea and vomiting is strongly related to the degree of hypotension. The significance of this observation is that if a patient undergoing cesarean delivery complains of nausea, an immediate blood pressure reading should be taken, because it is very likely that she has developed hypotension. This is particularly important during the early stages of spinal anesthesia, because the severe retching that can develop may produce higher levels of spinal anesthesia than desired, resulting in still greater hypotension and nausea. Such a sequence may produce total spinal anesthesia. Minimum monitoring equipment for regional anesthesia for cesarean delivery should consist of a pulse oximeter, a blood pressure cuff, and an electrocardiographic (ECG) monitor. As in vaginal delivery, however, it is vital that the anesthesiologist maintain verbal contact with the patient at all times, to assess her level of consciousness and detect the onset of nausea. An automated blood pressure device may be very useful in such procedures, to allow time to assess the level of anesthesia produced by the block and devote attention to monitoring and reassuring the patient. Obesity is common during pregnancy, and such devices may allow more accurate determinations of blood pressure in these patients.

General Anesthesia

Since all parturients are considered to be at risk for pulmonary aspiration of gastric contents, general anesthetic techniques used for cesarean deliveries are usually performed with rapid-sequence endotracheal techniques. Because many parturients are obese and the breasts are hypertrophied during pregnancy, intubation may be difficult in this population. Therefore, a most important monitoring step is to check correct placement of the endotracheal tube. This step may seem obvious, but in a large British study[28] the most common cause of maternal death during cesarean deliveries was incorrect placement of the endotracheal tube. In addition to auscultation in the axilla and over the epigastrium, end tidal carbon dioxide monitoring is mandatory to confirm correct endotracheal tube placement.[29] Since the typical rapid-sequence induction involves laryngoscopy under light general anesthesia, hypertension and arrhythmias are common. Therefore, it is important to monitor the blood pressure and ECG frequently following such inductions. For this purpose, an automated blood pressure device is extremely useful, particularly in patients with toxemia of pregnancy. Using such devices, antihypertensive therapy or deepening of the general anesthetic can be carried out promptly to prevent complications. It is also important to adequately assess respiration during general anesthesia for cesarean delivery. Hyperventilation in parturients produces decreased cardiac output and uterine blood flow, and thus may jeopardize the fetus. It has been demonstrated that a proper level of ventilation is difficult to predict in the parturient, but an average minute volume should be in the vicinity of 100 ml/kg/min.[30] The anesthesia machine should have some method of measuring the minute volume to allow determination of the proper level of ventilation. End-tidal carbon dioxide monitoring and pulse oximetry are extremely useful in the determination of proper minute volumes and oxygenation in the parturient. In addition to maintaining proper levels of arterial carbon dioxide, maintenance of adequate inspiratory levels of oxygen must be assured. An inspired oxygen concentration of at least 50 percent should be administered to produce optimal fetal oxygenation.[31] Although flowmeter settings can be used for this determination, it is better practice to actually measure the inspired oxygen concentration with any of the readily available devices used for this purpose.

MONITORING IN COMPLICATED OBSTETRICS

Toxemia of Pregnancy (Pregnancy-Induced Hypertension)

Pathophysiology

Toxemia of pregnancy is a disease state found only in parturients, which produces hypertension, proteinuria, and edema. The cause of this condition remains uncertain. Leading pathophysiologic theories involve vascular endothelial damage or an imbalance in thromboxane and prostacyclin production.[32,33]

Cardiovascular System

The initial response of the cardiovascular system in toxemia is an increase in cardiac output, accompanied by a moderate increase in systemic vascular resistance.[34] As the severity of the disease process increases, vasospasm becomes more marked. This produces a further rise in systemic vascular resistance, and cardiac output begins to fall.[35] Pulmonary capillary wedge pressure is normal or slightly decreased in the early stages of the disease, and only rises when afterload increases sufficiently to produce congestive heart failure.[35] In some patients, severe coronary artery involvement occurs, producing myocardial ischemia. In this group, severe congestive heart failure with pulmonary edema or myocardial infarction can occur. Cardiogenic shock may develop, with inadequate tissue perfusion, an increased arteriovenous oxygen content difference, and an extremely high total peripheral resistance. Aggressive therapy is required to reverse this condition, which is otherwise rapidly fatal.

Central Nervous System

The vasospasm, vasculitis, and increased capillary permeability found in toxemia have profound (albeit poorly understood) effects on the central nervous system (CNS). Multiple small intracerebral hemorrhages may be found throughout the brain and spinal cord, and cerebral edema may develop in severe cases. The symptom most commonly produced by CNS involvement is increased motor reflex activity, which, if severe, can lead to grand mal convulsions (eclampsia). Cerebral infarction and hemorrhage are the most common causes of death in toxemia of pregnancy, and efforts must be made to detect and treat incipient eclampsia at an early stage, before irreversible damage occurs.

Renal System

The kidneys are extensively involved in the disease process of toxemia. The vasculitis is especially prominent in the afferent arterioles and glomerular apparatus, and a picture similar to acute glomerulonephritis develops. Thick deposits of fibrin and complement are found on the glomerular basement membrane, and the glomerulus becomes "leaky." Protein escapes readily through the damaged basement membrane, producing the proteinuria and intravascular volume depletion typical of the disease. As the disease progresses, the afferent arteriole becomes "plugged" with similar deposits, and glomerular filtration rate and creatinine clearance decline. Oliguria then develops, and if the disease remains untreated, acute renal failure may occur. A baseline urea nitrogen and creatinine should be obtained to determine recent renal function. Remember that the normal nonpregnant value for blood urea nitrogen and creatinine is elevated when observed in the parturient.

Hematologic System

Many abnormalities are found in the blood in cases of toxemia. Plasma oncotic pressure is decreased as a result of protein losses from the kidneys,[36] but blood viscosity increases because of the obligatory loss of water from the vascular system and hemoconcentration which accompanies the proteinuria. This increased viscosity further aggravates the increase in afterload initiated by vasospasm, and further increases myocardial work.

Disseminated intravascular coagulation (DIC) may occur in toxemia, and is probably initiated by the vasculitis and complement activation typical of the disease. Severe involvement is not uncommon, and life-threatening hemorrhage may occur. It is difficult to predict which patients will develop this complication, but it is more common in patients with severe disease. It is important to know whether or not DIC is present in a patient in whom invasive monitoring is contemplated, because severe hemorrhagic complications could occur if this possibility is not recognized. Baseline coagulation screening consisting of a prothrombin time, partial thromboplastin time, and platelet count should be performed on patients with toxemia.[37]

Monitoring in Toxemia

The level of monitoring employed in patients with toxemia should be appropriate to the severity of the disease process. The challenges of the disease are manifold, as befits its nature as a multisystem disease. First, because the entire circulatory system is affected by the disease, the effects of the disease on all aspects of the circulation must be observed. Attention must be paid to intravascular pressures and the adequacy of cardiac output. The CNS manifestations and renal manifestations of the disease must be monitored. Careful attention must be paid to fluid management, because the limits between fluid overload and dehydration are extremely narrow, due to the coexisting renal and cardiac disease.

Mild Preeclampsia

Patients with mild preeclampsia have only slight elevation of the diastolic blood pressure, trace proteinuria, edema, and mild hyperreflexia. They require close observation because the disease process may worsen at any time and with frightening rapidity. They should have their blood pressure checked at frequent intervals, certainly no less frequently than every half-hour. Urine output should be measured, and if output decreases below 1 ml/kg/h, a urinary catheter should be inserted. Platelet count should be evaluated if regional anesthesia is being considered. If platelets are low or abdominal pain develops, serial coagulation studies should be obtained.[38]

Moderate Preeclampsia

Patients with moderate preeclampsia have 20 to 30 percent increases in both systolic and diastolic blood pressures, moderate proteinuria (1+ to 2+), edema, deceased urine volume, and significant hyperreflexia with mild clonus. They require extremely close observation for signs of development of complications such as DIC, acute renal failure, and life-threatening hypertension. At a minimum, these patients should have frequent blood pressure determinations, a urinary catheter, and coagulation tests. An automated noninvasive blood pressure device can be useful in such patients to detect the development of severe hypertension at an early stage. Since cardiac function in such patients is usually only mildly impaired, left ventricular performance is usually normal. For this reason, central venous pressure monitoring is usually adequate as a method of assessing cardiac filling pressure and (roughly) estimating the adequacy of fluid replacement.[38] However, if severe oliguria develops in the face of a normal or decreased central venous pressure, then the patient must be considered to have developed severe preeclampsia, and be monitored accordingly.

Severe Preeclampsia

Patients with severe preeclampsia have extensive and severe organ involvement in the disease process. They are extremely hypertensive, with blood pressures 50 percent greater than normal. As a result of the arteriolar spasm and increased myocardial wall tension and work, the heart becomes ischemic, and left ventricular dysfunction is frequently seen. Injudicious fluid therapy can easily provoke pulmonary edema, while oliguria is an almost invariable finding. DIC is common, as evidenced by decreases in the serum concentrations of many clotting factors, and may be further aggravated by the hepatic dysfunction typical of the more severe forms of toxemia. The HELLP syndrome may develop in these patients consisting of hemolysis, elevated liver enzymes, and low platelets. Furthermore, these patients evidence extreme hyperreflexia, and seizures may occur at any time. If cranial involvement is severe, the patients may be comatose, with signs and symptoms of increased intracranial pressure.

Obviously, close monitoring of such severely ill patients is a necessity. An experienced nurse should be with such patients at all times, and drugs and equipment for emergency airway management and seizure control should be readily available. An arterial catheter should be placed, since potent vasodilators such as nitroglycerin, trimethaphan, and nitroprusside may be necessary to treat the malignant hypertension. Probably the most difficult task in such patients is the determination of adequate fluid therapy. We have found that pulmonary arterial catheters are of considerable usefulness in monitoring the effects of fluid therapy in these patients. Right and left ventricular filling pressures are directly measurable, and the effects of various therapeutic maneuvers, such as the use of vasodilators, induction of general or regional anesthesia, and fluid infusions, are immediately evident. Cardiac output measurements are useful in these patients to assess the adequacy of cardiac function. Such monitoring is absolutely essential in these patients, and must be continued for at least 24 hours postpartum.

Maternal Cardiovascular Disease

The pregnant patient with cardiovascular disease presents a significant challenge to the skills and judgment of the obstetric anesthesiologist. The physiologic changes produced by pregnancy interact with the patient's underlying pathophysiology in many ways. This interaction usually represents an increased strain on an already compromised circulation, and cardiac decompensation is an ever-present threat. Monitoring techniques are essential and invaluable in these patients because they allow the practitioner to exactly ascertain the nature and severity of the underlying disease and its interaction with the pregnant state, concurrent therapeutic maneuvers, and anesthetic techniques. Without exact knowledge of the effect of such maneuvers, severe complications may occur. We will give examples of these interactions for specific cardiac lesions, and present some guidelines for the proper monitoring of these patients, but first, some general principles must be enumerated.

The care of pregnant patients with cardiovascular disease should not be undertaken if the equipment and skills necessary for invasive cardiopulmonary monitoring are unavailable in the institution. It is possible to care for most such patients without extensive invasive monitoring, but it is almost impossible to predict when (or whether) a given patient may require such intervention. This is because an apparently trivial and unexpected further insult (such as the acute development of toxemia of pregnancy, arrhythmias, or a prolonged, difficult labor) may cause rapid and unexpected cardiac decompensation with little or no warning.

A general principle to be followed in the management of these patients is the recognition that the care of parturients with cardiac disease requires a considerable investment in both time and staff. A nurse with experience in an intensive care environment must be with the patient at all times if invasive monitoring techniques are employed. This is mandatory because the techniques themselves, as described elsewhere in this text, carry the risk of complications. For example, pulmonary infarction from an improperly observed pulmonary artery catheter and exsanguination from a disconnected arterial line are two major complications that can be prevented by constant, close observation of the patient. This is often a difficult requirement to meet on a busy obstetric unit, which is designed and staffed for the care of normal, healthy parturients. Special "high-risk" labor rooms, located in close proximity to nursing stations and operating suites, are very useful in the care of such patients.

The same rigorous requirement must be true of the obstetric and anesthesia staff—they must be present and able to manage such a patient throughout the labor and puerperium. This represents a considerable investment in time and manpower. Merely inserting monitoring catheters and then abandoning the patient is a completely unacceptable method of managing these patients. It is particularly important to closely observe such patients during the postpartum period. Heart rate and cardiac output reach their maximum values at this time, and intravascular volume and total peripheral resistance rise abruptly. As might be expected, this appears to be the time when the stress on the cardiovascular system is most severe, and cardiac decompensation is most likely at this time. The tendency to relax one's vigilance after a difficult and trying labor and/or operative delivery is natural, but must be resisted!

It is important for the anesthesiologist to plan for (and monitor) the patient's recovery from the anesthetic. For example, epidural anesthesia is frequently employed in these patients, which produces sympathetic nervous system blockade. An abrupt restoration of sympathetic tone and pain sensation in the immediate postpartum period may precipitate cardiac decompensation. If this is thought to be likely, the epidural anesthetic (and the monitoring) should be continued into the postpartum period.

A final general principle must be stressed: the need for clear communication between all members of the team caring for the parturient with cardiovascular disease. Anesthesiologists should recognize that they probably are in the best position to integrate the input from the patient's cardiologist, obstetrician, and labor nurse and provide an overall plan for the care of these patients, because they have knowledge of and experience with acute obstetric and cardiovascular pathophysiology and pharmacology, and the monitoring and life-support techniques that are required to manage such patients. For example, obstetricians and labor nurses are generally oriented to the care of normal, healthy parturients undergoing uncomplicated childbirth. They may be completely unaware of, or forget, that "routine" obstetric techniques such as

prolonged Valsalva maneuvers during the second stage of labor must be avoided completely in patients with cardiac disease. With this knowledge, however, comes great responsibility: the anesthesiologist cannot abandon his or her central role in the care of these patients merely because the hour is inconvenient or because of other responsibilities. The anesthesiologist must be available to ensure that the patient's labor is as stress-free and painless as possible.

If these general principles are observed, then the care of parturients with cardiovascular disease becomes a matter of delineating the nature of the patient's disease, understanding the interaction of the pathophysiology of the specific lesion and pregnancy, and monitoring the patient to detect possible complications at an early, treatable stage.

Mitral Stenosis

Mitral stenosis is the most common cardiac lesion presenting in pregnancy.[39] The pathophysiology of mitral stenosis is easily worsened by pregnancy because the increased cardiac output and heart rate of pregnancy tend to elevate left atrial pressure and produce dilation of the left atrium. This predisposes these patients to the development of arrhythmias, such as atrial fibrillation; sudden cardiac decompensation and pulmonary edema may also develop. The situation is further complicated if the patient has been taking anticoagulants during her pregnancy, which increase the likelihood of both maternal and fetal hemorrhage.

The level of monitoring of these patients depends on the severity of the disease process. Previous history, cardiac catheterization data and consultation with the patient's cardiologist can be quite helpful, and should be sought prior to the patient's admission in labor. If the patient with a mild murmur has tolerated her pregnancy well until parturition, has not had a previous episode of atrial fibrillation or congestive heart failure, then invasive monitoring is not required, although her ECG should be monitored throughout labor. If there is any doubt about the patient's ability to withstand the increases in cardiac output and preload that occur during parturition, then arterial and pulmonary arterial catheters should be placed as soon as the decision to deliver the parturient is made. If the patient has been taking coumadin it should be stopped prior to labor and low-dose heparin substituted. Prevention of stress-induced increases in cardiac output and left atrial pressure are critical in poorly compensated patients with mitral stenosis, and adequate analgesia, preferably with a continuous epidural technique if the coagulation profile is acceptable, should be provided to minimize these stresses. Vasodilators should be administered if pulmonary arterial or wedge pressure suddenly increases. This is particularly likely if an emergency cesarean delivery under general anesthesia must be performed. The monitoring must be continued for at least 24 hours postpartum, or longer if the patient has required the use of vasoactive drugs in the postpartum period.

Mitral Regurgitation

Mitral regurgitation is the second most common cardiac lesion found in parturients.[40] Symptomatic complications of mitral regurgitation tend to occur later in life than the childbearing years. Unlike mitral stenosis, symptoms of mitral regurgitation may actually improve during gestation, because the decreased peripheral resistance of pregnancy favors "forward" flow and decreases the severity of regurgitant flow. During labor and delivery, afterload may suddenly increase and decompensation may occur. Therefore, one should not be lulled into complacency merely because the patient has tolerated her pregnancy without any difficulty. Patients with a history suggestive of left atrial enlargement or pulmonary hypertension or a left ventricular ejection fraction of less than 30 percent must be monitored aggressively, with both arterial and pulmonary arterial catheters. By monitoring cardiac output and arterial blood pressure one can calculate systemic vascular resistance and maintain it at low levels with vasodilators, if necessary. Observation of the pulmonary arterial pressure trace for the presence or absence of a V wave can also help quantify the amount of regurgitant flow. As in mitral stenosis, parturition should be as stress-free as possible, and the decreased peripheral resistance produced by epidural analgesia/anesthesia may improve forward flow. Anticoagulation should be managed in the same fashion as in patients with mitral stenosis.

Aortic Stenosis

Aortic stenosis affects approximately 0.5 to 3 percent of parturients,[41] but usually is not severe in this age group. Occasional patients have been de-

scribed with angina and syncope during pregnancy, suggesting a critical aortic stenosis (valve area less than 0.75 cm^2). Since these patients have a relatively fixed stroke volume, maintenance of an optimal heart rate is critical. Heart rates greater than 140 bpm in such a patient may produce severe myocardial ischemia, and bradycardia may produce syncope. Changes in afterload are poorly tolerated as is impaired ventricular filling due to aortocaval compression. Asymptomatic patients with noncritical stenoses do not require invasive monitoring, although ECG monitoring is recommended. Symptomatic patients should have arterial and pulmonary arterial catheters placed and utilized to maintain preload, afterload, heart rate, and cardiac output at optimal levels.[42]

Aortic Regurgitation

As in mitral regurgitation, patients with aortic regurgitation may actually improve during gestation because of the decreased peripheral resistance, and therefore a careful prenatal history should be obtained, as well as cardiac catheterization and ECG data. Aortic regurgitation is a rare finding during the childbearing years, but several cases have been reported in which sudden cardiovascular collapse was found when parturients with moderately severe lesions were placed in the supine position.[43] The authors postulated that the sudden aortic compression by the gravid uterus produced an abrupt increase in regurgitant flow, producing sudden left ventricular dilation and heart failure. The heart failure exacerbates the increased afterload, further increasing regurgitant flow and left ventricular dilation. Therefore, these patients should never be placed in the supine position, and if moderate to severe regurgitation is suspected, invasive hemodynamic monitoring should be employed.

Intra- or Extracardiac Shunts

The cardiac disease produced by either congenital (atrial septal defect, ventricular septal defect, patent ductus arteriosus, etc.) or acquired (shunt procedures for pulmonary atresia or tetralogy of Fallot) shunts depends on the magnitude and direction of the shunt flow. Most commonly, these lesions produce left-to-right flows of small magnitude, and cause little or no significant pathophysiology during the childbearing years. Patients with no history of cyanosis, growth retardation, or pulmonary hypertension, usually tolerate pregnancy well. However, if a patient has a history that suggests significant right-to-left shunting, then pregnancy, particularly labor and delivery, presents a considerable risk to the patient and a challenge to the anesthesiologist. Echocardiography and cardiac catheterization are quite helpful in delineating the exact nature and magnitude of the shunt. This is extremely important, because the maternal mortality of patients with right-to-left shunts or pulmonary hypertension with left-to-right shunts (Eisenmenger's complex) ranges from 30 to 50 percent,[44,45] and exact knowledge of the pathophysiology is essential in managing these patients.[46]

Monitoring these patients can present a considerable challenge, not only in the technical aspects of the insertion of monitors in the patient with intracardiac shunts, but in the interpretation of the results obtained by such monitoring. With complex intracardiac shunts, cardiac outputs obtained by indicator dilution techniques may be misleading, and the localization of intracardiac catheters may be impossible without the use of fluoroscopy. If it is possible, a catheter should be placed in the pulmonary artery both to allow assessment of pulmonary arterial pressures and oxygen saturations (therefore allowing one to calculate shunt fractions) and to allow the direct administration of vasodilators into the pulmonary artery. This may be necessary because acute pulmonary hypertension may provoke massive right-to-left shunting and cardiovascular collapse, and the only possible therapeutic maneuver is to decrease pulmonary vascular resistance. It has been suggested that administration of oxygen or instillation of vasodilators such as sodium nitroprusside directly into the pulmonary artery may be lifesaving in such cases.[47] However, insertion of pulmonary artery catheters in such patients is not without risk, since fatal arrhythmias have been provoked during insertion in such patients. Intraarterial pressure monitoring is also essential to detect decreases in aortic pressures that may lead to right-to-left shunting. In addition, it is critically important to monitor arterial oxygen saturation because hypoxemia can provoke sudden, irreversible pulmonary hypertension. This is a classic "vicious cycle" in which a small amount of right-to-left shunting provokes hypoxemia, which elevates pulmonary arterial pressures, which further increases the right-to-left shunt.

It is important to avoid introducing air into the circulation of these patients. This is of particular concern when managing these patients in labor because labor staff may not be aware of this problem. Air embolism has been reported during the insertion of epidural catheters,[48] and care must be taken during this procedure to avoid introducing air into the patient's circulation. Venous sinuses are frequently opened during cesarean delivery, and the possibility of systemic embolization of air or amniotic fluid must be entertained during cesarean delivery. Maneuvers that elevate venous pressure in the uterus, such as the reverse Trendelenburg position, should be employed in such patients during cesarean delivery to reduce this risk.

Primary Pulmonary Hypertension

Primary pulmonary hypertension, as the name suggests, is an idiopathic disorder produced by a progressive pulmonary arteritis, which produces extremely high pulmonary artery pressures and cor pulmonale. Hypoxemia is a typical feature of the end stages of this disease. It appears to be exacerbated by pregnancy, and the maternal mortality rate is approximately 50 percent.[49] Corticosteroids are commonly employed, but measures that reduce the pulmonary artery pressure are the only known effective therapy. Oxygen appears to be the most useful drug in these patients,[50] and monitoring of oxygen saturation during parturition appears to be useful. A pulmonary arterial catheter should be inserted in all these patients during labor, both to monitor pulmonary artery pressures and to allow the administration of vasodilators if pulmonary artery pressure becomes acutely elevated.

Peripartum Cardiomyopathy

Peripartum cardiomyopathy is a cardiac disease which is found only in parturients. The incidence has been estimated at 1 in 1,300 to 1 in 4,000 births.[51] It is idiopathic, and usually occurs in the immediate postpartum period. It is characterized by the sudden onset of left ventricular failure in a patient with no history of cardiac disease. A chest radiograph reveals cardiomegaly, and the electrocardiogram reveals a pattern of left ventricular hypertrophy with strain. These patients require immediate pulmonary arterial pressure monitoring, followed by diuresis and supportive measures. The maternal mortality of this disease has been reported to be 30 percent or more and is frequently refractory to therapy.[52,53]

β₂-Agonist Heart Failure

β_2-sympathomimetic drugs (e.g., terbutaline, ritodrine) have become popular for the treatment of premature labor.[54] They are quite effective for this purpose, but some parturients have developed pulmonary edema after the administration of these drugs. Risk factors for the development of pulmonary edema include preexisting cardiac disease, multiple gestation, anemia, overhydration, prolonged use of β-adrenergic agonists, hypokalemia, infection, and possibly concurrent use of magnesium.[55,56] Possible mechanisms include increased capillary permeability, fluid overload, and cardiac dysfunction. Patients developing pulmonary edema should be monitored with pulse oximetry and judiciously given diuretics.[57] If oxygenation remains poor then monitoring of central venous or pulmonary artery pressures can help guide further therapy.

Cardiac Surgery in Pregnancy

Medical management is usually associated with a lower maternal and fetal morbidity and mortality than cardiac surgery during pregnancy.[58] However, in some patients, with acute valvular dysfunction or refractory congestive heart failure in early pregnancy, cardiac surgery may be required. These patients should be monitored as indicated by the surgery to be performed and the pathophysiology of the disease process. However, it is necessary in this situation to monitor the fetus, if possible, as well as the mother. Werch and Lambert[59] found fetal heart rate monitoring to be a useful adjunct during cardiopulmonary bypass to detect inadequate uterine blood flow. During bypass, it is important to achieve a flow rate of approximately 60 ml/kg/min,[60] with further adjustments made to maintain a fetal heart rate greater than 100 bpm. If gestation has advanced beyond the first trimester, left uterine displacement should be employed to prevent aortocaval compression. Pulsatile perfusion may be useful in this situation to maintain near-normal uterine hemodynamics.[60]

Diabetes Mellitus

This disease is extremely common in gravidae, and the course of the disease is usually worsened by pregnancy. It is important to be aware of the complications of the disease, and monitor the course of the complications as well as the disease itself. Modern management of diabetes mellitus in pregnancy includes extremely tight medical control of the patient's blood glucose, in the belief that such control decreases the fetal consequences of the disease, particularly neonatal hypoglycemia and unexplained fetal demise.[61] Therefore, these patients should have their blood glucose maintained at 80 to 100 mg/dl, particularly in the immediate antepartum period. Modern methods of blood glucose measurement, such as glucose-oxidase Dextrostix combined with reflectance spectrophotometry, allow immediate determinations of blood glucose in the clinical setting. If even tighter control is necessary, devices that continuously measure blood glucose are available and can be interfaced with intravenous infusion pumps to administer insulin to maintain blood sugars in an extremely narrow range—the so-called "artificial pancreas." Because of the fetal complications of the disease, continuous fetal monitoring is also essential in these patients.

FETAL MONITORING

A large number of methods are currently available that allow the clinician to determine (more or less accurately) fetal maturity, biochemical functions, adequacy of placental function, and overall fetal "well-being." Obviously, the obstetric anesthesiologist should be aware of the results of such tests before an anesthetic intervention is planned and carried out. In this section, we shall discuss the more commonly employed forms of fetal monitoring (with an emphasis on intrapartum monitoring) and the anesthetic implications of this testing.

Antepartum Testing

A discussion of antepartum testing for genetic disorders, inborn errors of metabolism, and congenital anomalies is beyond the scope of this chapter.[62] Few have shown sufficient predictive value to be used as a generalized screening test. As ultrasonography has advanced, it has become the most widely used screening tool in obstetric practice. This technique allows the obstetrician to obtain almost immediate information about many fetal and in utero parameters and organ systems. There are many uses of this technique in obstetrics; we shall limit our discussion to peripartum use. This includes assessment of fetal age, weight, and rate of growth, and the diagnosis of obstetric complications such as placental and fetal anomalies.

Assessment of fetal maturity is of obvious utility in planning the optimal time for delivery. Ultrasound examination of the fetus is capable of very accurately determining fetal age by measuring various parameters of fetal size including the biparietal diameter of the fetal skull, crown-rump length, femur length, and gestational sac diameter. These size measurements correlate better with fetal age early in gestation. In addition, fetal weight can be estimated from ultrasound examination, although less precisely than (fetal) gestational age. Serial determinations can allow the diagnosis of intrauterine growth retardation to be made at an early stage. This information is useful to the anesthesiologist because special care must be taken to avoid decreases in uterine blood flow in premature or growth-retarded fetuses.

Placement anomalies, such as placenta previa and abruptio placentae, can be diagnosed at an early stage and with a high degree of accuracy with ultrasonography. As a result, the classic double setup examination for placenta previa has been virtually abandoned. In addition, recently, some ultrasonographers have been able to visualize placenta accreta. This information is of obvious value in modifying the anesthetic plans to accommodate the risk of significant blood loss or hysterectomy. Fetal anomalies, such as polyhydramnios, fetal hydrops and ascites, anencephaly, hydrocephalus, and renal anomalies can now be diagnosed in many cases with ultrasound. This allows appropriate antenatal and postnatal treatment to be planned and carried out.

Fetal Biophysical Profile

Technical advances in ultrasonography have led to refinements in the assessment of the fetus in utero. Recently, investigators have attempted to use ultrasound to evaluate the growth and development of the fetus. The fetal biophysical profile (BPP) evaluates fetal heart rate (nonstress test), fetal breathing movements, gross fetal movement, fetal tone, and amniotic fluid volume. Some investigators include the position and size of the placenta (placental grading). Unweighted scores of 0 to 2 are assigned for each evaluation. Some confusion has resulted from the exclusion of one or more evaluations in different studies. It is essential to know what assessments are included in the BPP at any particular institution. On a basis of 2 multiplied by the number of assessments, the maximum score may range up to 12. The perinatal care team needs to know the highest possible score (the denominator) and the assigned score (the numerator). Some institutions have deleted placental grading from their evaluations, whereas others have omitted the volume of amniotic fluid on the basis that it is a chronic and not an acute measure. Others have omitted the nonstress test or fetal heart rate evaluation.

Proponents of this "in utero" assessment feel that the fetal BPP is a useful tool for evaluating fetal status—particularly to follow up a nonreactive, nonstress test. Detractors state that the test needs to be standardized in order to make large-scale comparisons, since some investigators do not include one or two assessments and thereby change the denominator. Research in this area is active, but few conclusions can be drawn at present. Preliminary evidence indicates that the BPP is helpful in the serial assessment of high-risk pregnancies. Vintzileos and associates[63] found that the BPP was accurate in identifying the fetus with developing acidosis. The manifestations were a nonreactive, nonstress test and loss of fetal breathing. As acidosis advanced, fetal movements and tone decreased. As more investigations are performed using BPP, specific components may be found to be more predictive than others.

Amniotic Fluid Analysis

The leading cause of perinatal mortality in the United States is prematurity, and the leading cause of death in premature infants is respiratory insufficiency. The pathophysiology of this respiratory distress appears to be an inadequate amount of surface-active material (surfactant) in the alveoli of premature infants. This deficiency leads to collapse of alveoli secondary to the high surface tension, and the development of hyaline membrane disease. If adequate surfactant is present, hyaline membrane disease does not develop, and survival rates are quite high. Amniotic fluid can be obtained antenatally and assayed for the concentration of surfactant. Therefore, this test is of considerable usefulness in the timing of elective cesarean deliveries or the induction of labor. Its utility is further extended by the advent of effective drugs that are capable of inhibiting premature labor when the fetal lungs are thought to be immature (e.g., β_2-sympathomimetics). It has also been demonstrated that fetuses with low amniotic fluid surfactant activity may benefit from the administration of drugs that increase surfactant synthesis (e.g., glucocorticoids).

The actual tests used in the assessment of fetal lung maturity are designed to measure the activity of surface-active material (for example, the so-called "shake test") or a biochemical marker of surfactant synthesis. Biochemical methods appear to be the most satisfactory for accurate assessment. The primary components of surfactant are the phospholipids lecithin, phosphatidylinositol, and phosphatidylglycerol. Lung maturity is assessed by measuring the concentrations of these phospholipids in amniotic fluid and comparing them with the concentration of sphingomyelin (a phospholipid whose concentration changes very little with increasing fetal maturity) as an internal standard. The lecithin/sphingomyelin ratio (L/S ratio) is frequently used by itself as a measure of fetal lung maturity, but the accuracy of the determination is increased if the other phospholipids are also measured.[64] A L/S ratio of greater than 2.0 to 3.5 is generally considered to indicate a very low risk that the fetus will develop respiratory distress if delivered (Fig. 28-3).

Real-Time Fetal Monitoring

For all the fetal monitoring techniques discussed so far, the results are not available until some time after the test is performed. Real-time monitoring techniques give immediate information on the status of the fetus. These are the techniques that are most important in the management of labor, because parturition produces stresses on many maternal homeostatic mechanisms. The fetus is critically dependent on the mother for a supply of oxygen and nutrients and for the removal of metabolic wastes, and can be endangered during parturition by any disruption of placental or umbilical blood flow or oxygen content. These disruptions may be gradual, as in a placental abruption or placental insufficiency, or sudden, as in umbilical cord prolapse or uterine rupture. Thus, to adequately monitor the fetus, we must observe some change in a measurable parameter that indicates an adverse alteration in fetal homeostasis. In clinical practice today, this statement has come to mean an observable change that indicates a major (e.g., organ-threatening) interruption in fetal oxygen supply. The goal of intrapartum fetal monitoring is to detect these events before their effects lead to irreversible fetal damage. The fetal organ system most at risk when disruptions in homeostasis occur is the central nervous system, which begins to suffer irreversible damage after no more than 6

Fig. 28-3. Levels of lecithin and sphingomyelin in amniotic fluid at increasing gestational ages. An acute rise in lecithin at 35 weeks marks pulmonary maturity. (From Gluck et al.,[80] with permission.)

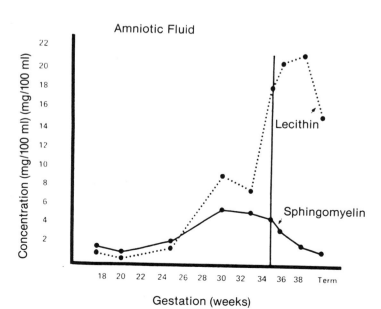

minutes of asphyxia. Fetuses that have been identified as high risk (premature or growth-retarded fetuses, infants of diabetic mothers, etc.) are able to tolerate asphyxia for even shorter periods of time. A useful fetal monitoring technique allows one to diagnose and act upon information suggesting fetal distress in a short period of time. Current monitoring techniques are not uniformly successful in this regard.

Many of the stresses of labor are capable of producing deterioration in fetal well-being. The most potent and ubiquitous of these causes is the cessation of placental perfusion that occurs each time the uterus contracts. In normal fetuses undergoing normal labor, this phenomenon is usually tolerated well because of the considerable reserve of placental function. With an abnormal fetus, placenta, or pattern of uterine contractions, this reserve may be inadequate, and progressive fetal hypoxemia and acidosis (respiratory and metabolic) will develop. In such situations, if fetal deterioration occurs, the physiologic effects will be first noted during or slightly after uterine contractions, since this is the time when fetal asphyxia is most severe. Therefore, it is important to stress at the outset of this discussion of fetal monitoring that uterine contractions must be measured simultaneously with any parameter chosen, if the asphyxia is to be detected before irreversible damage occurs. It is this "unmasking" of subtle abnormalities by the stress of uterine contractions (or other reversible stresses) that makes timely intervention possible.

Many methods of observation have been examined for utility in detecting this so-called fetal distress. Almost all are indirect measurements—that is, they depend on detecting the reaction of the fetus to asphyxia, rather than directly measuring fetal oxygenation. Thus, in order to understand these monitoring techniques properly, we must first discuss the reactions of the fetus to asphyxia. The response of the fetal cardiovascular system has been studied extensively, and we shall only discuss the rudiments of this information, focusing on changes in heart rates seen with various stresses.

The basis for fetal heart rate monitoring is the fact that in the absence of any stress, the fetal heart rate remains at a stable level (usually 120 to 150 bpm) with slight variations of 5 to 10 bpm. When the fetus is exposed to any of a wide variety of stresses, the fetal heart rate reacts in a manner that allows prediction of fetal status. Although this tech-

nique is far from perfect, it is currently the most clinically useful technique.

A number of transducer systems have been developed to allow the recording of fetal heart rate before and during parturition. These allow clinicians to measure heart rate in conjunction with uterine contractions. The fetal heart rate can be measured indirectly, using maternal abdominal ECG or ultrasonography. These methods are useful for prenatal measurements or in early labor, but can only yield approximate measures of instantaneous heart rate because of interference from maternal signals. Direct measurement of fetal heart rate, using electrodes placed directly on the fetus, produce much clearer input and are more useful in detecting short-term heart variability. Similarly, uterine contractions can be measured indirectly using belts fitted with strain gauges placed around the abdomen. While useful in routine monitoring, these indirect measurements can give only a rough approximation of the level of uterine activity, and are extremely sensitive to changes in maternal position. If it is necessary to accurately measure uterine activity, a pressure catheter can be placed through the cervical os and connected to a standard pressure transducer. Most commercially available heart rate monitoring systems allow both indirect and direct measurement of fetal heart rate and uterine activity, and the mode selected should be appropriate to the clinical situation. Monitors have recently appeared which allow telemetry of the acquired data, overcoming the objection of many mothers to the cumbersome hardware associated with continuous fetal heart rate monitoring.

The interpretation of fetal heart rate monitoring is a difficult task and cannot be presented completely in this discussion. For the anesthesiologist, a few basic principles should suffice. First, the baseline heart rate should be observed. A normal baseline fetal heart rate should be between 120 and 160 bpm, and there should be some variation in the heart rate from moment to moment, averaging 5 to 10 bpm. This baseline variability can better be observed using direct fetal ECG monitoring. There is strong evidence that the presence of normal heart rate variability represents normal central nervous system integrity including adequate oxygenation.[65] However, drugs (opioids, atropine, or local anesthetics) can temporarily decrease baseline variability without producing fetal hypoxia.[66]

Sustained increases in fetal heart rate (tachycardia) to greater than 160 bpm are associated with an increased incidence of fetal asphyxia and low Apgar scores. Occasionally, persistent tachycardias are found in conjunction with maternal hyperthermia.

Persistent decreases in fetal heart rate (bradycardia) to less than 100 bpm are strongly suggestive of a progressive fetal hypoxia/acidosis and a diminished fetal capacity to tolerate further insults. Previous knowledge of the fetal heart rate is essential since occasionally fetuses will present with congenital heart block and persistent bradycardias without acidosis. In the absence of prior history, however, persistent bradycardias are an ominous sign, and any technique that carries the possibility of further decreases in uterine blood flow should be avoided.

Next, the heart rate recording should be examined for transient increases of more than 15 bpm (termed accelerations), or decreases of the same magnitude (decelerations).

Accelerations

It must be remembered that the normal fetus is a nearly autonomous organism with an intact CNS, and as such is capable of responding to many external stimuli. The fetus normally responds to low-level aversive stimuli (e.g., loud noises, awakening from sleep, and changes in maternal positioning) with slight acceleration of the baseline heart rate. This responsiveness appears to be indicative of a normal fetus with an intact CNS, and forms the basis of modern antenatal fetal evaluation—the "nonstress" test.[67] In this test, indirect fetal heart monitoring is employed to assess the response of the fetus to stimuli. If a certain number of accelerations are observed in a specified time period, one can predict with some assurance that the fetomaternal unit is normal, with adequate reserves. If accelerations are not observed, then further testing, usually stimulation of uterine contractions with their attendant mild hypoxic stress, are performed (contraction stress tests).

Decelerations

The interpretation of fetal heart rate decelerations is the most difficult task in fetal monitoring. Several patterns of decelerations have been described to simplify this task, but it must be remembered that many results in fetal monitoring are false-positive (e.g., ominous fetal heart rate patterns without fetal compromise) or false-negative (normal fetal heart rate patterns in the presence of severe asphyxia). False-positive interpretations produce operative intervention when it is not required, and false-negative results lead to a lack of intervention and preparedness that can be fatal. Which type of error is more acceptable is questionable, and has produced considerable controversy in obstetrics.[68] In our view, the relative safety of modern operative obstetrics and anesthesia leads us to view the sequelae of false-negative results as more dangerous. It is important to be aware that the presence of these potential errors has called into question the entire technology of continuous fetal heart rate monitoring, and many studies have been performed to delineate its validity, with conflicting results.[68,69] The most reasonable conclusion that can be drawn from these studies seems to be that decelerations in the fetal heart rate are merely one indicator of fetal distress, and that this technology should be combined with other methods of fetal monitoring for greatest accuracy. With these cautions, we shall describe the most common deceleration patterns (Fig. 28-4).

Early Decelerations

Early decelerations (type 1) are the most common decelerations observed. The shape of the deceleration is smooth and gradual, and the maximal decline in fetal heart rate occurs no later than 20 seconds after the peak of the contraction. The heart rate returns to normal within 15 seconds of the end of the uterine contraction. These decelerations are thought to have a benign significance, and they can be reproduced experimentally with fetal head compression. If these decelerations occur early in labor, when head compression is not found, and are frequent and associated with profound bradycardia (a decline greater than 50 bpm) they may represent an early warning of incipient fetal compromise.

Late Decelerations

Late decelerations (type II) are characterized by a contour similar to early decelerations, but the timing of the deceleration in relation to uterine contraction is different. The maximum decline in fetal heart rate typically occurs later than 20 seconds after the peak of uterine contraction, and the recovery phase is prolonged. This pattern is associated with fetal acidosis and hypoxia secondary to uteroplacental insufficiency. Neonatal depression is found with high frequency in conjunction with these decelerations. Typically, the severity of the hypoxic insult correlates positively with the severity and duration of the deceleration—that is, the most severely acidotic fetuses exhibit severe, prolonged late decelerations.[70]

Variable Decelerations

Variable decelerations (type III), as the name implies, vary in severity and timing. They may be produced experimentally by cord compression, and are thought to represent a vagal response to the increased fetal blood pressure found in cases of umbilical cord occlusion. Their severity and frequency are correlated with the severity of the cord occlusion. Partial, intermittent cord compressions occurring at the end of labor are fairly common, being associated with such complications as loops of umbilical cord around the fetal neck. More severe cord compression is typically observed early in labor, and is associated with catastrophes such as umbilical cord prolapse and knotting of the cord. Prolonged variable decelerations in early labor must be considered as indicative of serious fetal compromise.

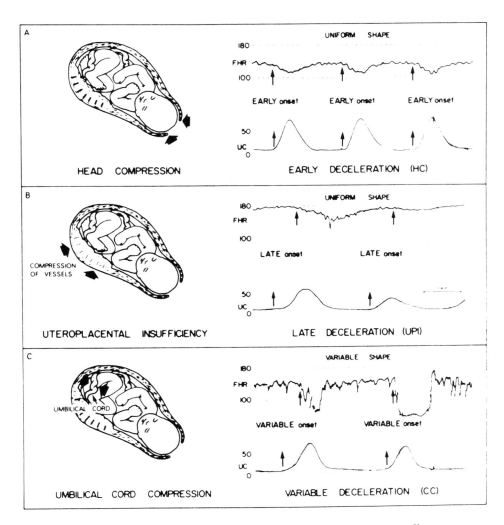

Fig. 28-4. Three FHR deceleration patterns of clinical significance. (From Hon,[81] with permission.)

Complications

Complications of fetal heart monitoring include infection of the fetal scalp, intrauterine infections, or trauma from improper insertion of monitoring devices.[71] Such complications are extremely rare, but are of concern to many parturients. Far more serious and common are the complications resulting from improper interpretation of the data acquired, as discussed above. In an effort to minimize these complications, other methods have been developed to monitor the response of the fetus to hypoxia.

Acid-Base Measurements

Measurement of fetal acid-base status has been suggested as a method to directly assess the presence of fetal hypoxemia. Saling, in 1962, showed that blood samples could be obtained from the fetal scalp in labor, and a scalp blood pH less than 7.20 was found in infants who were delivered in poor condition.[72] Many investigators have since confirmed his observations. It appears from primate experiments that a completely asphyxiated fetus will decrease its blood pH at approximately 0.1 pH unit per minute and increase its arterial carbon dioxide tension by 13 mmHg/min.[73] The resultant acidosis is both metabolic and respiratory in origin. Fortunately, total asphyxia is rarely encountered in clinical practice, and the partially asphyxiated fetus only gradually accumulates this combined acidosis. It is also important to recognize that fetal acid-base balance is directly affected by maternal acid-base status. For example, maternal acidosis, as may occur in prolonged labor or diabetic ketoacidosis, may depress fetal scalp pH in the absence of true fetal distress. Scalp sampling at present appears to be most useful in clarifying the results of fetal heart rate monitoring. Thus, when an ominous deceleration pattern is obtained or short term variability is diminished, fetal blood sampling should be performed. If a normal fetal pH (i.e., 7.25) is obtained, the labor can be allowed to continue. If the fetus is found to have a scalp pH less than 7.20, immediate intervention is clearly indicated.[74] In this manner, fetal scalp pH determinations can expand and clarify the information obtained from fetal heart rate monitoring.

Fetal Pulse Oximetry

Evidence of fetal asphyxia can be inferred from abnormal fetal heart rate patterns as just described. Recent reports of fetal pulse oximetry suggest that we may soon be able to more directly measure fetal oxygenation.[75,76]

SUMMARY

Monitoring has become an integral and essential component of modern obstetric practice. Monitoring techniques allow us to give better care to both mother and fetus if they are correctly employed. However, the evolution of monitoring technology has occasionally outstripped our knowledge of its limitations and complications. Information gained by the use of modern monitoring techniques is merely one element to be considered when formulating a clinical decision. Modern monitoring technology possesses an apparent precision and accuracy that can overwhelm clinical judgment. It cannot be used to take the place of a caring and concerned team at the bedside of the parturient. For this reason, such refinements as central, computerized processing of multiple monitored variables have been omitted from this discussion, because we feel they have only a limited place in the care of the parturient at present. With further development of monitoring technology, this may be possible, but we still must remember that our patients are experiencing one of the most intense and stressful human experiences, and they deserve all our support—not merely that which our machines can provide.

REFERENCES

1. Ueland K, Novy MJ, Peterson EN: Maternal cardiovascular dynamics. IV. The influence of maternal gestational age on the maternal cardiovascular response to posture and exercise. Am J Obstet Gynecol 104:852, 1969
2. Lees MM, Taylor SH, Scott DB: A study of cardiac output at rest throughout pregnancy. J Obstet Gynaecol Br Commonw 74:319, 1967
3. Bader RA, Bader ME, Rose DJ, Braunwald E: Arterial blood pressure and cardiac output in pregnancy. J Clin Invest 34:1524, 1955
4. McLellan CE: Venous pressures in pregnancy. Am J Obstet Gynecol 45:568, 1943
5. Kerr MG, Scott DB, Samuel E: Studies of the inferior vena cava. Br Med J 1:532, 1964
6. Bieniarz J, Crottogini JJ, Curachet E: Aortocaval compression by the uterus in late human pregnancy. Am J Obstet Gynecol 100:203, 1968

7. Ueland N: Maternal cardiovascular dynamics. VII. Intrapartum blood volume changes. Am J Obstet Gynecol 126:671, 1976

8. Pritchard JA: Changes in blood volume during pregnancy and delivery. Anesthesiology 26:393, 1965

9. Metcalfe J, Bartels H, Moll V: Gas exchange in the pregnant uterus. Physiol Rev 47:782, 1967

10. Blekta M, Hlavaty V, Trnkora M et al: Plasma proteins in pregnancy. Am J Obstet Gynecol 106:10, 1970

11. Hytten FE, Lind T: Diagnostic Indices in Pregnancy. p. 26. Documentia Geigy, Basel, 1973

12. Prowse CM, Gaensler EA: Respiratory and acidbase changes during pregnancy. Anesthesiology 26:381, 1965

13. Conklin K: Maternal physiological adaptations during pregnancy. Semin Anesth 10:211, 1991

14. Pernoll ML, Metcalf J, Korach PA: Ventilation during rest and exercise in pregnancy and postpartum. Resp Physiol 25:295, 1975

15. Dignam WT, Titus P, Assali NS: Renal function in human pregnancy. 1. Changes in glomerular filtration rate and renal plasma flow. Proc Soc Exp Biol Med 97:512, 1958

16. Berman LB: Renal tubular reabsorption in pregnancy. JAMA 230:111, 1974

17. Van Wagenen G, Jenkins RH: An experimental examination of factors causing ureteral dilation of pregnancy. J Urol 42:1010, 1939

18. Ueland K, Hansen JM: Maternal cardiovascular dynamics. III. Labor and delivery under local and caudal analgesia. Am J Obstet Gynecol 103:8, 1969

19. Shnider SM, Abboud TK, Artal R et al: Maternal catecholamines decrease during labor after lumbar epidural anesthesia. Am J Obstet Gynecol 147:13, 1983

20. Pearson JF, Davies P: The effect of continuous lumbar epidural analgesia upon fetal acid-base status. J Obstet Gynaecol Br Commonw 80:225, 1975

21. Lees MH, Hill JD, Ohsner AJ III et al: Maternal placental and myometrial blood flow of the rhesus monkey during uterine contractions. Am Obstet Gynecol 110:68, 1971

22. Ueland K, Hansen JM: Maternal cardiovascular dynamics. II. Labor and delivery. Am J Obstet Gynecol 103:1, 1969

23. Reid DHS: Carbon dioxide tensions during labour. Lancet 1:784, 1966

24. Huch A, Huch R, Lindmark G, Rooth G: Ventilatory patterns during labour. J Obstet Gynaecol Br Commonw 81:608, 1974

25. Anonymous: Karen's Death. SOAP Newsletter, Spring 1983

26. Marx GF, Macatangay AS, Cohen AV, Schulman: Prophylaxis of supine hypotension. NY J Med 69:819, 1972

27. Datta S, Alper MH, Ostheimer GW, Weiss JB: Method of ephedrine administration and nausea and hypotension during spinal anesthesia for cesarean section. Anesthesiology 56:68, 1982

28. Report on Confidential Enquiries into Maternal Deaths in England and Wales, 1952–1972. London, Her Majesty's Stationery Office, 1975

29. Brock-Utne, Downing JW, Seedat F: Laryngeal oedema associated with preeclamptogenic toxaemia. Anaesthesia 32:556, 1977

30. Burger GA, Datta S, Chantigian RA et al: Optimal ventilation in general anesthesia for cesarean delivery. Anesthesiology 59:A420, 1983

31. Moir DD: Anaesthesia for cesarean section. Br J Anaesth 42:136, 1970

32. Roberts JM, Taylor RN, Musci TJ et al: Preeclampsia: an endothelial cell disorder. Am J Obstet Gynecol 161:1200, 1989

33. Walsh SW: Preeclampsia: an imbalance in placental prostacyclin and thromboxane production. Am J Obstet Gynecol 152:335, 1985

34. Phelan JP, Yurth DA: Severe preeclampsia:peripartum hemodynamic observations. Am J Obstet Gynecol 144:17, 1982

35. Rafferty TD, Berkowitz RL: Hemodynamics in patients with severe toxemia during labor and delivery. Am J Obstet Gynecol 138:263, 1980

36. Benedetti TJ, Carlson RW: Studies of colloid osmotic pressure in pregnancy-induced hypertension. J Obstet Gynecol 135:308, 1979

37. Baker P, Collander CC: Coagulation screening before epidural analgesia in preeclampsia. Anaesthesia 46:64, 1991

38. Clark SL, Cotton DB: Clinical indications for pulmonary artery catheterization in the patient with severe preeclampsia. Am J Obstet Gynecol 158:453, 1988

39. Sugushita Y, Ito L, Ozeki K et al: Intracardiac pressures in pregnant patients with mitral stenosis. Jap Heart J 22:885, 1981

40. Ueland K: Cardiovascular disease complicating pregnancy. Clin Obstet Gynecol 21:429, 1978

41. Neilson G, Galea EG, Blunt A: Congenital heart disease and pregnancy. Med J Aust 1086:88, 1970

42. Easterling TR, Chadwick HS, Otto CM, Benedetti TJ: Aortic stenosis in pregnancy. Obstet Gynecol 72:113, 1988

43. Burwell CS, Metcalfe J: Heart Disease and Pregnancy. p. 102. Little, Brown, Boston, 1958

44. Arias F: Maternal death in a patient with Eisenmenger's syndrome. Obstet Gynecol 50:265, 1977

45. Greer DE, Evertson LF, Mathers JM, Porecco RP: Eisenmengern's syndrome and pregnancy. p. 79. Abstracts of the Annual Meeting, Am Coll Obstet Gynecol, Washington, DC, 1978

46. Pollack KL, Chestnut DH, Wenstrom KD: Anesthetic management of a parturient with Eisenmenger's syndrome. Anesth Analg 70:212, 1990

47. Midwall J, Jaffin H, Herman MV, Kupersmith J: Shunt flow and pulmonary hemodynamics during labor and delivery in the Eisenmenger syndrome. Am J Cardiol 42:299, 1978

48. Naulty JS, Ostheimer GW, Datta S et al: Incidence of venous air embolism during epidural catheter insertion. Anesthesiology 57:410, 1982

49. Blount SG, Vogel JHK: Pulmonary hypertension. Mod Concepts Cardiovasc Dis 36:61, 1967

50. Midwall J, Jaffin H, Herman MV, Kupersmith J: Shunt flow and pulmonary hemodynamics during labor and delivery in the Eisenmenger syndrome. Am J Cardiol 42:299, 1978

51. Demakis JG, Rahintool SH: Peripartum cardiomyopathy. Circulation 44:964, 1971

52. Homans DC: Peripartum Cardiomyopathy. N Engl J Med 312:1432, 1985

53. Gambling DR, Flanagan ML, Huckell VF et al: Anesthetic management and noninvasive monitoring for caesarian section in a patient with cardiomyopathy. Can J Anesth 34:505, 1987

54. Benedetti TJ, Hargrove JC, Rosene KA: Maternal pulmonary edema during premature labor inhibition. Obstet Gynecol 59:335, 1981

55. Benedetti TJ: Maternal complications of parenteral β-sympathomimetic therapy for premature labor. Am J Obstet Gynecol 145:1, 1983

56. Jacobs MM, Knight AB, Arias F: Maternal pulmonary edema resulting from betamimetic and glucocorticoid therapy. Obstet Gynecol 56:56, 1980

57. Wagner JM, Morton MJ, Johnson KA et al: Terbutaline and maternal cardiac function. JAMA 246:2697, 1981

58. Zitnik RS, Brandenburg RO, Sheldon R et al: Pregnancy and open heart surgery. Circulation 40:257, 1969

59. Werch T, Lambert HM: Fetal monitoring and maternal open heart surgery. South Med J 70:1024, 1977

60. Levy DL, Warriner RA, Burgess GE: Fetal response to cardiopulmonary bypass. Obstet Gynecol 51:112, 1980

61. Fadell HE, Hammond SD: Diabetes mellitus and pregnancy. J Reprod Med 27:56, 1982

62. Hobel OH, Hyrarinen M, Okada D, Oh W: Prenatal and intrapartum high risk screening. Am J Obstet Gynecol 117:1, 1973

63. Vintzileos AM, Gaffney SE, Salinger LM et al: The relationship between fetal biophysical profile and cord pH in patients undergoing cesarean section before the onset of labor. Obstet Gynecol 70:196, 1987

64. Hallman M, Kulovich M, Kirkpatrick E et al: Phosphatidyl-inositol and phosphitadylglycerol in amniotic fluid. Am J Obstet Gynecol 125:413, 1976

65. Parer JT, Livingston SG: What is fetal distress? Am J Obstet Gynecol 162:1421, 1990

66. Gaziano EP, Freeman DW, Bendel RP: FHR variability and other heart rate observations during second stage labor. Obstet Gynecol 56:42, 1980

67. Oh WJ: Antepartum cardiotachometry for fetal evaluation. South Med J 73:310, 1981

68. Council on Scientific Affairs, American Medical Association: Electronic fetal monitoring. JAMA 246:2370, 1981

69. Westgren M, Ingemarsson E, Ingemarsson L, Solum T: Intrapartum electronic fetal monitoring in low-risk pregnancies. Obstet Gynecol 56:301, 1980

70. Ball RH, Parer JT: The physiologic mechanisms of variable decelerations. Am J Obstet Gynecol 166:1683, 1992

71. Madames AE, David D, Cetrulo C: Major complications associated with intrauterine pressure monitoring. Obstet Gynecol 59:389, 1982

72. Saling E, Schneider D: Biochemical supervision of the featus during labour. J Obstet Gynaecol Br Commonw 74:799, 1967

73. Adamsons K, Behrmann R, Davies GS et al: Acid-base measurement in asphyxia. J Pediatr 65:807, 1964

74. Low JA, Cox MJ, Karchmar EJ et al: The prediction of intrapartum fetal metabolic acidosis by fetal heart rate monitoring. Am J Obstet Gynecol 139:299, 1981

75. Gardosi JO, Schram CM, Symonds EM: Adaptation of pulse oximetry for fetal monitoring during labor. Lancet 25:1265, 1991

76. Johnson NM, Johnson VA, Fisher J et al: Fetal monitoring with pulse oximetry. Br J Obstet Gynecol 98:36, 1991

77. Skaredoff MN, Ostheimer GW: Physiological changes during pregnancy: effects of major regional anesthesia. Reg Anesth 6:28, 1981

78. Mangano DT: Anesthesia for the pregnant cardiac patient. In Shnider SM, Levinson G (eds): Anesthesia for Obstetrics. Williams & Wilkins, Baltimore, 1979

79. Ostheimer GW: Regional anesthesia techniques in obstetrics. Winthrop-Breon Laboratories, New York, 1980

80. Gluck L, Kulovich MV, Borer RC et al: The diagnosis of the respiratory distress syndrome (RDS) by amniocentesis. Am J Obstet Gynecol 109:440, 1971

81. Hon EH: An Atlas of Fetal Heart Rate Patterns. Harty Press, New Haven, CT, 1968

Monitoring in the Critical Care Unit

29

H. Michael Marsh
Benjamin G. Guslits

In order not to be negligent, one must spend as much money to prevent an accident as the cost of that accident times its probability.

Judge Learned Hand

The monitoring needs of individual patients in critical situations are determined on the basis of utilities that could be expressed in maxims similar to that of the learned judge. The difficulty is to determine the probabilities of system dysfunction in each patient and to maximize the utility of monitoring by rational use of the available tools at our disposal.[1] We should only use monitors during those phases of illness when early detection and treatment or prevention of changes in the monitored physiologic or biochemical functions will improve our patient's chance for recovery, without increasing morbidity or overtaxing the economic system supporting the patient's treatment.

Our aim in this chapter is to discuss the process of monitoring in the intensive care unit, examining briefly its history, outlining the principles for choosing monitors, discussing practical solutions for each physiologic system, and finally discussing tools used for monitoring the overall function of an intensive care unit or hospital.

THE MONITORING PROCESS: BASIC PRINCIPLES

The Individual Patient

Physiologic monitoring implies the transduction (the conversion of a mechanical or chemical event into an electrical signal) of a physiologic or bio-chemical variable and its measurement on a calibrated scale (Fig. 29-1). The result may be either continuously presented or the measurement may be performed repetitively at time intervals that are usually determined by the time constant of decay, or time to dysfunction of the system, when the variable changes. For clinical monitoring to be useful to the patient, this measurement must be brought to cognition (either consciously by an observer or by activating a preset alarm by exceeding prescribed limits determined by an algorithm for the particular illness) and used in decision-making processes. Unless the measurement is attended to, either by human vigilance or mechanically, monitoring is not taking place, even if devices are attached to the patient.

Because of the duration of critical phases of illness in patients monitored in intensive care units, clinical monitoring can be thought of as encompassing variables where repetitive measurements are made hours apart, but where trends are followed and semicontinuous monitoring can be instituted if therapy dependent on this data is needed. This chapter concentrates primarily on semicontinuous or continuous modes of monitoring and discusses certain areas in more detail.

In the intensive care unit, the goals of monitoring are extended beyond the realms of simple safety monitoring that apply during intraoperative care.[2] The goals of ICU monitoring are, first, to detect trends that may indicate impending system dysfunctions, permitting timely activation of appropriate therapeutic regimens; and, second, to permit continuous adjustments in system support mechanisms, to maintain vital bodily functions within safe limits. In designing the system of monitors that will be used for a particular patient, it is vital to remain cognizant of the fact that the system should enhance the effectiveness of the critical care staff involved with that patient. The goal is not to replace these workers, but rather to amplify their senses and enhance their skills.[3]

The use of a large number of transduced variables in managing therapy for the critically ill patient with multiple system organ failure needing supportive care forces us to use automated alarms. This occurs because of the limited vigilance and attention span, and the tendency of data overload to exceed the ability of the human mind to comprehend and react to changes in multiple variables.[4] In anesthesia, failures of clinical vigilance are thought to contribute to a considerable proportion of preventable mishaps that result in death or permanent brain damage. Fatigue and distraction and a lack of mental preparedness for preventing deteriorations in a patient's condition with onset of a complication cannot be wholly overcome by sophisticated, automated monitoring systems.[5] Vigilance is task-specific and depends on training. The

bedside nurse must be trained fully in use of the equipment provided. The equipment must also be designed and placed to help the nurse.

Data overload can, to some extent, be overcome by combining several physiologic variables in a single parameter, which is then more easily followed to monitor a particular system or set of systems. Two examples can be used to illustrate this approach.

First, consider the use of end-tidal carbon dioxide tension ($P_{ET}CO_2$). $P_{ET}CO_2$ is determined by the alveolar CO_2 (P_ACO_2) and by the ventilation of the lung; it varies inversely with the level of alveolar ventilation ($\dot{V}_A$) and directly with carbon dioxide clearance ($\dot{V}CO_2$).

$$P_{ET}CO_2, P_ACO_2 = \frac{\dot{V}CO_2}{\dot{V}_A \cdot K} \qquad (1)$$

$\dot{V}CO_2$ is also determined by cardiac output ($\dot{Q}$) and the mixed venous ($C\bar{v}CO_2$) and arterial (C_aCO_2) carbon dioxide contents:

$$\dot{V}CO_2 = \dot{Q}(C\bar{v}CO_2 - C_aCO_2) \qquad (2)$$

In situations where $\dot{V}_A$, $C\bar{v}CO_2$ and C_aCO_2 remain unchanged, $P_{ET}CO_2$ varies directly with change in cardiac output.

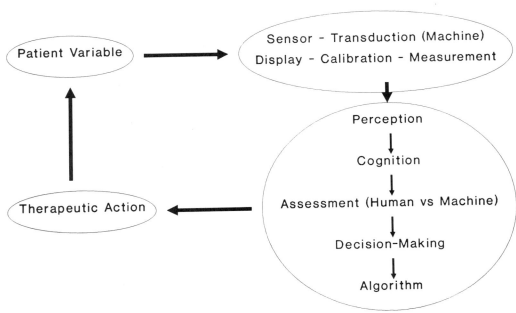

Fig. 29-1. The monitoring process. Unless this cycle is completed, monitoring is not occurring.

Next, let us consider the usefulness of mixed venous oxygen saturation ($S\bar{v}O_2$). From Fick's law we can derive the following expression:

$$S\bar{v}O_2 = SaO_2 - \left(\frac{\dot{V}O_2}{\dot{Q} \cdot CcO_2}\right) \qquad (3)$$

where changes in arterial oxygen saturation (SaO_2), oxygen uptake ($\dot{V}O_2$), cardiac output ($\dot{Q}$) and the blood's carrying capacity for oxygen (CcO_2) can all be followed by monitoring $S\bar{v}O_2$. The obvious disadvantage of this approach is that one cannot be sure which of the independent variables is responsible for a change in the dependent variable or parameter.

With these principles in mind, we can now approach the choice of monitors for an individual patient. It is wise to ask four sets of questions:

1. Which organ system(s) and which physiologic or biochemical variables need to be monitored?
2. What are the options available for monitoring these functions?
3. How are these data to be received, integrated, and used in clinical decision-making?
4. What is the likely cost, both in money and morbidity? Is the cost/benefit ratio acceptable, given the patient's status?

Whereas risk management committee activities at Harvard Medical School in 1985 led them to follow the Netherlands Health Council in developing minimal standards for basic intraoperative monitoring, later modified and approved by the House of Delegates of the ASA in October 1986 and last amended in 1990[2]; no such standard recommendations have been developed for the critical care unit. Rational choice of monitoring tools must then be made for each patient based largely on the answers presently available to these four questions. Ideally, the choice in individual situations would be guided by outcome data and not from current convention or a Delphic oracular process depending only on expert opinion. Very few good studies of the effects on outcome from ICU monitoring and therapy are available. It may only be by monitoring the outcomes from the whole ICU process that we can get some data useful in choice of parameters and processes of monitoring, that will help us to define minimal monitoring standards for the critically ill patient in the ICU of the future.[6]

The Intensive Care Unit

The basic aim for physiologic monitoring of the individual patient is to improve outcome, reduce morbidity, and reduce the cost of caring for the primary illness. This is done by speeding the clinical detection of events that may be either premorbid, for organ system failure, or immediately life-threatening. The aim for quality assurance programs for intensive care units as a whole, are similar to the aims for monitoring individual patients. The quality of care is indicated by the survival rates compared to similar patients treated in other institutions. Associated morbidity rates and cost must be kept low, but the process of care and the standards of maintenance of facilities and equipment must be at a high level. Quality assurance programs[7] use data from three major sources to examine the intensive care unit:

1. *Data relating to the structure and functional organization of the unit.* This information may be obtained as subjective assessments of the unit or may be made objective using sophisticated sociopsychological methodologies. General levels of staff satisfaction and work patterns in the unit are examined and monitored over time.
2. *Data relating to the process of care in the unit.* Satisfactory procedure guidelines must be established and compliance routinely audited. Thresholds for satisfactory performance are established over time, and deviations from usual performance are investigated and corrected.
3. *Data relating to the outcome for patients admitted to the unit.* Again, thresholds are established and deviations from usual performance investigated and corrected.

These processes are monitored by the Joint Commission for Accreditation of Hospitals and Organizations (JCAHO), a voluntary organization used by most hospitals in the United States.[7] Outcome studies using severity scoring systems are probably the best method for quality assurance in ICU practices nationwide.[8]

History

Physiologic monitoring in the intensive care setting has developed as the result of a number of changes in medical care since the early 1950s. The parallel developments of cardiac catheterization and cardiac surgery in the late 1940s, and of widespread application of mechanical ventilation after the poliomyelitis epidemic of 1952, together with the current Western pandemic of atherosclerotic vascular disease associated with cigarette smoking, and the consequent expansion of coronary and peripheral arterial bypass surgery, have stimulated the concept and practice of intensive care. The utilization of ECG monitoring for patients with myocardial infarction, the advent of blood gas measurement devices, flotation pulmonary artery catheterization, and newer concepts for pharmacologic management of shock, respiratory failure, sepsis, and multiple system organ failure have all stimulated development and widespread use of invasive monitoring tools in intensive care units. We are now in a phase where newer metabolic monitoring tools will broaden our horizons and older technology will be more rationally used.

APPROACH TO THE INDIVIDUAL PATIENT

The monitoring used for an individual patient admitted to an intensive care unit is determined by the system(s) involved by the primary illness, by the severity of physiologic disturbance, by the natural history of the disease, and by the patient's usual state of health, determined in part by age. Fixed routines, sometimes based on medicolegal considerations, usually result in some basic low level of monitoring for all intensive care unit admissions. Monitors will be augmented by protocol or individual decision as other systems become affected and need supportive care. Patients fall on a spectrum from low risk to high risk, the highest risk including those with organ failure who are receiving supportive therapy. One can then decide which physiologic variables need monitoring, which tools are available, what to do therapeutically for the patient using the data, and assess the costs in morbidity and money.

This section examines the physiologic variables easily monitored, relating these to systems and indicating some practical choices that can be made in the major disease categories with which patients present to the ICU. It is beyond the scope of this chapter to show exhaustively how these data are used and to consider all the cost factors.

The Low-Risk Patient

The low-risk patient may be defined using the severity scoring system of Knaus and others[9,10] where individual probabilities for death (R values) are calculated from age, acute physiology scores, chronic health evaluation, and an ICU admission diagnosis category. In the absence of any other systemic illness, a patient who has undergone a thoracotomy for resection of solitary lung nodule and who has an epidural catheter for narcotic administration may be an example of such a patient ($R < 0.5$). There is minimal immediate risk of dysfunction in other systems, and noninvasive monitoring should suffice.[11,12] An analog electrocardiogram with rate alarms, impedance apnea alarm, intermittent blood pressure and temperature measurements, and perhaps a pulse oximeter for a limited time (during sleep or for 24 hours only) and with a prescription for alarm limits are all or more than required. The number of events anticipated and the cost need to be carefully studied and standards developed.[13]

Some institutions have actually attempted to limit costs by having noninvasive respiratory care units set up,[14,15] and some low-risk surgical patients may be treated in this way. They may not require intensive care unit admission at all, but can be managed in stepdown areas. Considerable information is potentially available from noninvasive monitors, as has been known for some time.[16] Outcome studies need to be carried out in the face of different primary diseases to identify cost-benefit ratios.

The Intermediate-Risk Patient

As the limits of the physiologic reserve function are reached by body systems under stress, these systems approach failure and may need supportive therapy. The APACHE II-derived risk assessment ($0.5 < R < 0.75$) will increase,[10] and the need for intensified monitoring to identify impending or actual organ failure will increase. A 69-year-old man who has undergone an uncomplicated abdominal aortic aneurysmectomy, has a serum creatinine of 2 mg/dl, is intubated but alert, awake, and oriented, and who received 4 units of blood but seems hemodynamically stable is an example of such a patient.

Simple noninvasive monitoring now needs to be supplemented. In addition to the analog electrocardiogram with digital display of rate and rate alarms, an arrhythmia package and perhaps ST-segment monitoring may need to be added for elderly patients (>45 years of age) because of the risks of associated coronary artery disease. Regular and frequent checks of blood pressure must be made, and if an arterial line was not used in the operating room, automated cuff measurements with digital display should be the least that is done. Where no pulmonary artery catheter has been placed for surgery, central venous pressure should be measured and preferably electronically transduced. In patients with widespread vascular disease or very poor cardiac function, a pulmonary artery catheter is desirable because of the likelihood of either chronic pulmonary disease or pulmonary hypertension secondary to the heart disease. In these situations, the central venous pressure will not accurately reflect left heart function.

A urinary catheter with digital display of output and a built-in temperature probe to record bladder temperature is a useful addition. Where cardiac output is not available from a pulmonary artery catheter, noninvasive measurement of cardiac output can be helpful. Again, pulse oximetry may be useful for brief use, but is not considered essential for awake patients receiving only prophylactic mechanical ventilation.

Monitoring for intermediate-risk patients must be reviewed at least once in each 12-hour period and can usually be discontinued within 24 to 48 hours after surgery if no deterioration has occurred.

The High-Risk Patient

The high-risk patient has suffered organ failure, and monitoring should be expanded to cover the needs for managing the supportive care the patient needs to survive. The acute physiology score (APS) generated for APACHE II[10] is driven by deviation from normality of various physiologic and biochemical variables that reflect organ failure at the extremes of the scale (0–4) for the 12 variables used, and indicates the extent of organ failure present. This score alone, developed as a simplified APS, correlates well with survival.[17] Other studies of survival in situations of multiple systems organ failure have clearly shown that survival can be correlated with the number of organ systems in failure.[18] Patterns of response to stimuli such as septicemia have also been noted to change with time

in a predictable way, and may predict survivors and nonsurvivors.[18–21] So monitoring with intermittent assessment of these simplified APS scores therefore may be a useful prognostic tool as well as helping to guide therapy. However, individual patients suffering organ failure should have monitoring tailored specifically to the pattern of organ failure present.

Acute Respiratory Failure

In cases of acute respiratory failure, the extent of monitoring needed depends on the type and severity of respiratory failure. Where hypoxemic respiratory failure is present alone, pulse oximetry to guide FIO_2 may be sufficient.[22] Transcutaneous carbon dioxide tension monitoring may be added in infants and small children, but is not very helpful in adults.[23] One must then rely on intermittent blood gas measurements to detect progression of hypoventilation in adults.

If hypercarbic respiratory failure necessitating mechanical ventilation is present, end-tidal carbon dioxide concentration monitoring may be useful. However, the usual, essential monitoring for the patient on a ventilator for assisted respiration includes only expired minute ventilation and maximal airway pressures.[24] In this situation airway pressure is used as a disconnection or tube displacement alarm, and to some extent one relies on the presence of spontaneous ventilation as a backup and on the patient as an alarm mechanism should disaster occur. One can also derive respiratory system mechanics data, but this is rarely done. The paralyzed or heavily sedated patient may benefit from more intensive monitoring to provide redundant alarms.[25]

Preventing complications associated with mechanical ventilation depends, largely on choosing from the multitude of mechanical ventilatory support systems, the one that best provides adequate PaO_2 at the lowest FIO_2 (avoiding oxygen toxicity) and adequate $PaCO_2$ at a low $\dot{V}E$ and with safe mean airway pressures (MAP), avoiding barotrauma. This is achieved by monitoring SaO_2 with pulse oximetry and adjusting FIO_2, monitoring $PETCO_2$, (equation 1) and adjusting VT, f, and $\dot{V}E$ and monitoring airway pressures to avoiding very high maximal and mean pressures.

Because of interactions between the cardiac and respiratory systems, invasive circulatory monitoring may need to be used in patients in acute respiratory failure, to optimize oxygen delivery (DO_2) by reducing MAP or increasing CVP or adding inotropes to increase cardiac output ($\dot{Q}$), since

$$DO_2 = \dot{Q}(CaO_2) \qquad (4)$$

DO_2 can also be increased by increasing the arterial oxygen content (CaO_2) by increasing SaO_2 or hemoglobin concentrations. Because outcome studies for patients in acute respiratory failure suggest that associated organ failures have a large influence on outcome, additional systems will need monitoring, as outlined above.

Since the demonstrations by Dr. Zapol and colleagues[26,27] that nitric oxide administered in low (25–80) parts per million concentrations in the inspired gas may lower pulmonary arterial resistance, the use of nitric oxide in treatment of neonates and adults has been begun at a number of centers.[28] This remains experimental therapy in the United States, but a number of monitoring devices and pieces of equipment for safe delivery of this potentially very toxic gas are being developed. When NO is used, regular measurement of methemoglobin levels may become a useful monitor.

Acute Circulatory Failure

In using monitoring for the patient in acute circulatory failure, one must approach two sets of questions.

The first set of questions relates to the state of the circulation as a whole: Is cardiac output sufficient to maintain oxygen and nutrient flow to all tissues, preventing ischemic damage? Is regional flow well enough regulated that end organ damage will not occur—that is, are mean arterial pressure and resistance in this tissue matched optimally?

The second set of questions relates to the *state of the pump itself*: Is the coronary circulation adequate to the needs of the myocardium, or is pump dysfunction present because of poor coronary flow? Can anything be done to reduce myocardial oxygen demand and/or increase myocardial oxygen delivery?

Therapy must aim to balance these conflicting demands—on the one hand, the desire to increase cardiac output and/or myocardial flow, and on the other hand, the desire to reduce mean arterial pressure and/or heart rate. This subject has been reviewed recently.[29]

Monitoring must now be extended beyond the analog ECG with arrhythmia detection and ST monitoring to include two-dimensional esophageal echocardiography[30]; serial creatine kinase MB band and lactate dehydrogenase I/IV ratios are also estimated daily to assess myocardial survival. In approaching overall circulation, one must go beyond invasive pulmonary artery catheter pressure monitoring with every 4-hour cardiac output estimations to continuous fiberoptic $S\bar{v}O_2$ monitoring,[31,32] with intermittent indirect calorimetry for $\dot{V}O_2$, $\dot{V}CO_2$, and R estimations.

$$R = \frac{\dot{V}CO_2}{\dot{V}O_2} \qquad (5)$$

SaO_2 (pulse oximetry) and $S\bar{v}O_2$ estimations and intermittent $\dot{Q}$ estimations measured by thermodilution (or perhaps continuously modeled $\dot{Q}$ using Homer Warner's pulse contour method for cardiac output estimation) allow continuous $\dot{V}O_2$ estimation.

The usefulness of $S\bar{v}O_2$ alone as a monitored parameter (equation 3) has been outlined above. $\dot{V}O_2$ estimation is useful in assessing the circulation since, as DO_2 is reduced, a point is reached below which $\dot{V}O_2$ becomes dependent on DO_2.[33,34] This concept is particularly notable in septic shock when the threshold where $\dot{V}O_2$ becomes DO_2 dependent appears to be increased from about 300 ml/min/m^2—the usual value in the nonseptic adult—to values well above this (Fig. 29-2). This is known as *supply dependency of oxygen uptake*, and has now been demonstrated fairly convincingly in acute lung injury with adult respiratory distress syndrome and in multisystem organ failure.

Several factors could account for this increased level of supply dependency for oxygen in sepsis. First the metabolic rate in tissue may be increased by fever; second the inflammatory cascade may induce oxygen utilization for lysosomal or cytotoxic oxidative activity by white cells; third there may be an actually altered O_2 extraction ratio ($\dot{V}O_2/DO_2$). In addition, there may be cardiac depression secondary to the sepsis and reduced oxygen delivery which can further embarrass the supply of O_2 to the tissues. This altered oxygen extraction ratio could relate to the altered processes of microcirculatory flow and autoregulation in the tissues following the endothelial damage induced by the cascade reaction of interleukins and other cytokines induced by sepsis.[35] In this situation regional hypnoperfusion could lead to local hypoxemia and ischemia. Anaerobic metabolism may then lead to increased lactate levels.

Two studies have demonstrated[36,37] such supply dependence in patients on PEEP in acute respiratory failure. Attempts to demonstrate that increased DO_2 will move the septic patient to a lower extraction ratio and therefore over the knee of the theoretic curve (Fig. 29–2) have often been limited by the potential for mathematical coupling where VO_2 has not been measured from expired gas analysis but has been derived from the same cardiac output measurement as used for DO_2 calculations.[38,39] The presence of an altered O_2 extraction ratio in sepsis remains therefore somewhat controversial[40], above the point where blood lactate levels were normalized.

Acute Fluid-Electrolyte Imbalance and Renal Dysfunction

The patient in renal failure with acute electrolyte imbalance needs dialysis. These problems have been well reviewed recently.[41] The major risks during dialysis include acute circulatory disturbances, acute respiratory dysfunction, loss of consciousness, and seizures, the dysequilibrium syndrome, and complications from dialysis itself (bleeding tendency, infection, etc.). Thus, monitoring and nurse presence need to be intensified during episodes of dialysis.

Various continuous monitors for a variety of blood chemicals and pH that use ion-selective electrodes[42] or optodes (fiberoptic light sensing devices) with chromophores or fluorophores sensitive to pH, PO_2, PCO_2, Na^+, K^+, Ca^{2+}, and possibly also glucose have been or are being developed. The feasibility and clinical desirability of these products are now under study.[43] None has yet been accepted completely into ICU practice; thus, these devices largely remain experimental. Such indwelling devices are to be distinguished from flowthrough analyzers used for cardiopulmonary bypass.[44]

Metabolic Dysfunction

Managing the metabolic responses to stress and starvation requires knowledge of the components of these responses, the severity of the stress,[45] the preexisting state of nutrition, and the potential effects of the nutritional programs available.[46] Generally these situations are monitored by discontinuous (q12h, q24h, q48h, or longer) measurements. Measurement of serum albumin may be a useful prognostic index,[47] but there is no clear evidence that any form of treatment definitely improves outcome.

However, excessive calories and inappropriate fuel mixtures or totally inadequate nutrition are associated with poor outcome. Measurement of resting energy expenditure, using indirect calorimetry, is useful in tailoring caloric need to feeding regimens in the individual patient and should be provided as a monitoring tool for intensive care patients.[48] Indirect calorimetry can be performed using open circuit measurements estimating from inspired (FIO_2) and mixed expired ($F\bar{E}O_2$) oxygen fraction difference multiplied by mean expired ventilation ($\dot{V}E$) with corrections for inspired minute ventilation, based on fractional inspired and expired nitrogen concentrations. This method is accurate up to FIO_2 values of about 0.35 with standard equipment. At higher FIO_2, closed circuit methods that measure oxygen consumption ($\dot{V}O_2$) from a closed spirometer at an FIO_2 of 1.0 are preferable. Absence of circuit leaks is essential. When a pulmonary artery catheter is in place one can check $\dot{V}O_2$ by using the Fick principle:

$$\dot{V}O_2 = \dot{Q} \ (CaO_2 - C\bar{v}O_2) \cdot K \qquad (6)$$

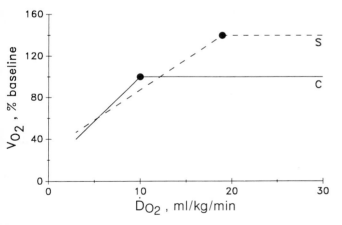

Fig. 29-2. The supply dependence of systemic oxygen uptake during sepsis. This conceptual diagram shows a control (*C*) and a septic (*S*) relationship for dogs exposed to endotoxin. Note that with the onset of sepsis, VO_2 increases to 140 percent of baseline, while the critical DO_2 (below which VO_2 is supply dependent) also increases from 8 to 10 ml/kg/min to 16 to 20 ml/kg/min. Similar relationships have been observed in humans.

To perform this measurement, blood samples from a systemic artery and from the pulmonary artery must be obtained and analyzed; oxygen content (CxO_2) is calculated as follows:

$$CxO_2 = Hb \times 1.34 \times SO_2 + PO_2 \times 0.0031 \quad (7)$$

where Hb is hemoglobin in g/dl, SO_2 is oxyhemoglobin saturation as a fraction, and PO_2 is oxygen tension in torr or millimeters of mercury. CxO_2 is then expressed in milliliters per deciliter. Cardiac output ($\dot{Q}$) can be obtained from thermodilution, and $K = 10$, to convert $\dot{Q}$ to deciliters per minute (resting energy expenditure can be roughly estimated as $7 \times V\dot{O}_2$, kcal/24 h). VCO_2 (carbon dioxide production) can be estimated at any FIO_2 using open circuit methodology, as follows, where $F\bar{E}CO_2$ is mixed expired fractional carbon dioxide concentration.

$$\dot{V}CO_2 = \dot{V}E \cdot F\bar{E}CO_2 \quad (8)$$

Bedside glucose estimates can be made using methods based on a glucose oxidase indicator reflectance meter. However, these have a variability which is in part observer-dependent, and quality assurance for this form of testing is mandatory. Lactate estimations have also been advocated as essential to intensive care unit monitoring,[49] but this is not universally accepted.

Severe depletion of body protein and caloric stores may result from prolonged starvation associated with hormonal and cytokine-mediated effects during critical illness. Nutritional support, although it does not usually lead to positive nitrogen balance, can increase protein synthesis, delaying loss of muscle bulk and strength and maintaining immune function. This has been recently reviewed.[50]

In summary, nutritional assessment should be conducted on admission to the ICU, taking into account hormonal and cytokine effects. When indications exist, nutritional support should be given. Indications for nutrition include (1) recent weight loss of 10–20 kg and moderate or severe stress, (2) recent weight loss of >20 kg, and (3) any severely stressed patient. External routes for administration of nutrition are preferable. After initiation of nutritional support, regular biochemical monitoring is indicated and for parenteral nutrition will include estimation of caloric need with indirect calorimetry in the maximally stressed patient. Otherwise, basal caloric needs can be predicted from the Harris-Benedict equation in patients up to moderate stress. Weight, fluid, and acid-base balances, plasma glucose and electrolytes to include calcium, magnesium, and albumin need to be followed. Hyperinsulinemia may become a problem during refeeding after stress or starvation and can cause severe electrolyte disturbances, which determine the need for close observation during this period. For enteral nutrition one can reduce to minimal monitors.

Coma

Monitoring for the comatose patient in the intensive care unit is determined largely by the cause of coma and the likelihood of progression of processes that may lessen the chance for cerebral recovery. The use of frequent observation and recording of the Glasgow coma scale by nursing staff should be supplemented by intracranial pressure measurement when cerebral edema is suspected. Thus, in cases of hepatic coma,[51] Reye syndrome, or when trauma or ischemia are the cause for coma, such measurement should be considered. Careful hemodynamic and blood pressure monitoring is also essential in such patients.

Hematologic Complications

Rapid methods for monitoring blood clotting functions are often necessary in the intensive care unit. Thromboelastography has proven useful for this purpose, since data are available in 15 to 20 minutes.[52] Use of the Sonoclot device may give similar results, while other, simpler measurements of blood clotting may suffice when monitoring heparin activity alone.

Infection Control

An important function in the intensive care unit is early detection, diagnosis, and treatment of infection. Equally important is the realization that many modalities of invasive monitoring carry a risk of infection to the patient. This risk increases exponentially after about 72 hours of indwelling for intravascular devices.

Various methods are under development to attempt to reduce the risk of infection from indwelling catheters. These range from the VitaCuff device (a silver-impregnated collagen implant placed subcutaneously at the skin entry point),[53,54] to heparin bonding to catheter plastic material, to attempts to impregnate catheter plastic with silver, to the use of antibiotic regimens for selective bowel decontamination. Constant vigilance, sterile placement techniques, use of Betadine skin site care, prevention where possible of transmigration of organisms from gut lumen or airway to bloodstream, reduction of urinary tract infection, use of an antacid regimen to reduce chances for bacterial overgrowth but still prevent gastrointestinal bleeding, and early removal of lines when possible all help limit line-related and indeterminate bacteremias secondary to monitoring.

Despite vigilance and recent advances in antimicrobial therapy, bacterial sepsis in the intensive care unit continues to produce substantial morbidity and mortality and to add to costs. The mortality rate from established sepsis has been estimated at 10 to 28 per cent in immune-competent patients and >30 per cent in the immunodeficient. Local cytokine production contributes to this process,[55,56] and it is possible that in the future, with use of specific blockers of the mediator process,[57] monitoring circulating levels of compounds that mediate septic shock may become part of our armamentarium. This remains experimental at the present time. However, attention to white blood cell counts, the immunocompetence of the patient, the bacterial and viral flora of each patient, and the flora and antibiotic sensitivity of the organisms in the unit is an essential component in ICU care.

Pharmacotherapy

Drug therapy requires a thorough understanding of the absorption, distribution, and clearance characteristics of each agent. Interactions between drugs are common in the ICU setting, and therapy is often limited by toxicity. Nutritional status and organ system function—in particular, hepatic and renal function—dramatically affect drug dosing and elimination.

Monitoring is critical to successful pharmacotherapy. Some agents, such as inotropes[58] and vasodilators,[59] are titrated to specific clinical goals, while others, such as anticoagulants,[60] require adjustment based on laboratory parameters. Still others, including antibiotics, antiarrhythmics,[61] anticonvulsants,[62] theophylline,[63] and cyclosporine are titrated to effect as well as to therapeutic concentrations. By appropriate drug monitoring, the lowest therapeutic dose can be provided, and toxicity can be minimized.

Pain and Pain Control

In 1987 a survey of recently hospitalized patients found that 58 per cent reported excruciating pain at some time during their stay. The incidence of pain is high in the ICU, but here pain is often difficult to assess and to monitor. Further adding to the pain are behavioral changes induced by the disease, including anxiety and reactive depression and profound physiologic disturbances, in part themselves caused by the pain.

Attempts to monitor pain in the conscious cooperative patient should include use of the visual analog pain scale and attention to physiologic sequelae from pain; sweating, hypertension, tachycardia, and splinting in muscle groups. Adequate pain relief to encourage spontaneous deep breathing, coughing, and movement is essential for maintenance of adequate pulmonary toilet and prevention of decubiti.

The unconscious or uncooperative patient may still suffer from pain and attempts to use physiologic sequelae to assess the adequacy of pain relief are essential. A recent text[64] has directed our attention to some of these problems in the critically ill patient.

APPROACHES TO MONITORING FUNCTIONS OF THE INTENSIVE CARE UNIT

Quality assurance programs demand monitoring for the overall intensive care unit. As outlined in the introduction, three sources of data are used.[7-10] This section discusses two major topics relating to these data. The first of these is automation of data management in the unit—a process basic to both individual monitoring, where computerized alarm systems and data arrays help overcome problems of lack of vigilance and data overload, and to quality assurance. The second topic is the use of severity scoring to predict outcome and the uses to which this data can be put, both in quality assurance and in individual patient management as an aid to decisions regarding admission, discharge, and the need for monitoring.

Computerized Database Management

The microcomputer is in widespread use in intensive care units. Bedside monitors and many other bedside devices use microprocessor-based functions for control and alarm loops. The concept of a hospital- or institution-wide information network,[65] with the patient record,[66] a laboratory information-inquiry system,[67] links to the business office for billing, utilization review and management operations, room occupancy, pharmacy, central service, respiratory therapy, operating room services, and links to the intensive care system is also well established. However, for reasons primarily of cost, centralized computer systems for the intensive care unit have been applied in relatively few centers, and there has been little commercial interest to develop such systems rapidly.

Computers were introduced to intensive care units in the 1960s, when M.H. Weil's group[68] in Los Angeles used a Xerox data systems Sigma 5 computer in a shock-trauma unit. Kirklin and Sheppard developed a computer monitoring system for cardiac surgical patients at about the same time at the Mayo Clinic, using an IBM System 7 with links to a large central computer for data storage.[69] Others followed, including Del Guercio, Siegel, Shoemaker, and Homer Warner's group.

While these systems are expensive, they are useful and serve to focus and discipline certain aspects of care. Such a system can be used to facilitate access to trended data and enable rapid decision making.[70] Outcome may also be improved using the computer because education and guidance provided by this means to various staff groups, where protocols are used for patient care, can be routinely enforced.[71]

OUTCOME PREDICTIONS

Knaus and Zimmerman[72] recently reviewed the prediction of outcome from intensive care. Briefly their argument is that outcome is determined by four patient-related factors—type of disease, physiologic reserves (in part determined by age and chronic health), severity of disease, and the individual's response to therapy—and by two treatment-related factors—the type of therapy available and the use or application of that therapy for the patient in question (its timing and process). These authors contend that by collecting information on patient risk factors, diagnostic class of disease, severity of disease, and physiologic reserve, one can arrive at a prognosis before instituting therapy.

This concept seems reasonable and is supported by studies of individual disease states such as acute myocardial infarction.[73] The increase in mortality rate with increasing organ system dysfunction in patients with acute respiratory failure and acute lung injury also supports this concept.[74] The APACHE II tool developed by these authors[10] is then one method for making prognoses. Again, this approach is supported by the widespread applicability of this tool and the similarity to other analyses such as that developed by Lemeshow and colleagues.[75] By contrast, Gonnella staging of disease and Medis/groups—tools adapted for overall hospital care and purporting to measure severity of illness—do not provide as good prognoses for intensive care unit patients.

Using APACHE II, the risk of death (*R*) is predicted from the expression[10]

$$\ln R/(1 - R) = -3.517$$
$$+ (\text{APACHE II score} \times 0.146)$$
$$+ 0.603 \qquad (9)$$
$$(\text{only if emergency surgery})$$
$$+ \text{a diagnostic weight category}$$

The APACHE II score is obtained from a score sheet combining the acute physiology score (the worst values for 12 variables during the first 24 hours in ICU; maximum score 59), the age (from 6 points for age greater than or equal to 75 years down to 0 for age less than or equal to 44 years), and chronic health points (maximum 5 points). The diagnostic category weight is obtained from a table of principal diagnostic categories leading to ICU admission.[10] The more positive the APACHE II score and the diagnostic category weight, the greater the risk.

This tool has been validated for group data predictions, having been used for 5,030 intensive care unit admissions in a multicenter trial performed in 1982 to 1983 in the United States[9] (Figs. 29-3 and 29-4). To make such predictions, a predicted group mortality rate (*P*) is generated using individual *R* values.

$$P = \frac{\Sigma R}{N} \qquad (10)$$

The use of this tool for prediction of individual risk is not yet as well founded. However, one can use the tool as a guide to help decisions regarding admission to ICUs. Low-risk patients are identified by

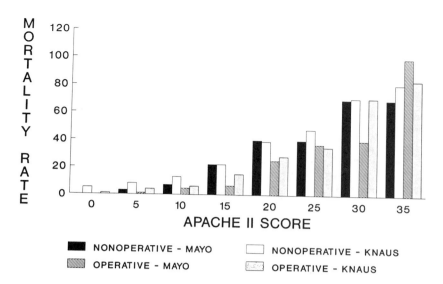

Fig. 29-3. The relationship between APACHE II scores and mortality rate for four groups of patients (two general medical/nonoperative and two general surgical/operative) obtained in 1982 to 1983 (Knaus,[9]) and in 1986 to 1987 (Mayo). Note the close similarity between the pairs.

their low scores, and the number of such admissions can be monitored over time.

In addition, the quality of care in intensive care units can be compared using the tool, defining quality as the ratio of actual to predicted deaths in defined diagnostic groups. Continued outcome analysis is essential to our knowledge of what is being achieved as therapies and routines change.

There has been an increasing amount of interest in these tools in recent times and a concerted review[76] has recently been published. There are errors in comparing intensive care unit outcomes with APACHE II, which may arise from the patient subset chosen in each different ICU, a form of selection bias, where the sample from the studied ICU does not match the original.[77,78] Lead-time bias may also occur, since the source of the patient matters in determining the natural history of the disease, APACHE II working best for freshly diagnosed and treated cases, not those referred from within a hospital. Imprecision in clinical diagnosis and data collection errors also occur. These issues have, in part, been addressed in APACHE III, a commercially developed database tool that still needs independent validation. This remains technology in evolution. Caution should be exercised in applying these tools to individual patient management at this time.[6,79,80]

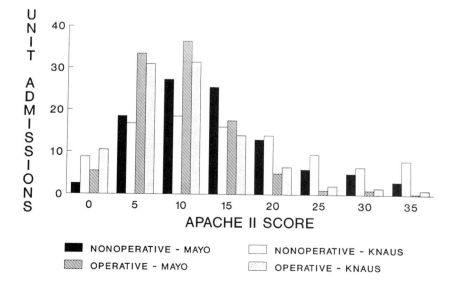

Fig. 29-4. The relationship between APACHE II scores and the percentage of intensive care unit admissions within each four-point range for the four patient groups shown in Figure 29-3.

REFERENCES

1. Schwartz S, Griffin T: Medical Thinking. Springer-Verlag, New York, 1986
2. Eichhorn JH: Effect of monitoring standards on anesthesia outcome. Int Anesthesiol Clin 31:181, 1993
3. Mora FA, Passariello G, Carrault G, LePichon J-P: Intelligent patient monitoring and management systems: a review. IEEE Eng Med Biol 12:23, 1993
4. Gravenstein JS, Weinger MB: Why investigate vigilance? [Editorial]. J Clin Monit 2:145, 1986
5. Nelissen RGHH, Meijler AP, de Jong JR et al: Is unified monitoring improving patient care? J Clin Monit 4:167, 1988
6. Teres D, Lemeshow S: Why severity models should be used with caution. Crit Care Clin 10:93, 1994
7. The Joint Committee on Accreditation of Health Care Organizations (JCAHCO): Monitoring and evaluation of the quality and appropriateness of care: a hospital example. JCAHO, Chicago, IL, 1988
8. Morgan CJ, Branthwaite MA: Severity scoring in intensive care. [Editorial]. Br J Med 292:1546, 1986
9. Knaus WA, Draper EA, Wagner DP et al: An evaluation of outcome from intensive care in major medical centers. An Intern Med 104:410, 1986
10. Knaus WA, Draper EA, Wagner DP et al: APACHE II: a severity of disease classification system. Crit Care Med 13:818, 1985
11. Block FE Jr: A proposed standard for monitoring equipment: what equipment should be included? [Editorial]. J Clin Monit 4:1, 1988
12. Gravenstein JS: Essential monitoring examined through different lenses. [Editorial]. J Clin Monit 2:22, 1986
13. Whitcher C, Ream AK, Parsons D et al: Anesthetic mishaps and the cost of monitoring: a proposed standard for monitoring equipment. J Clin Monit 4:5, 1988
14. Bone RC: The noninvasive respiratory care unit. [Editorial]. Am Rev Respir Dis 136:804, 1987
15. Spivack D: The high cost of acute heath care: a review of escalating costs and limitations of such exposure in intensive care units. Am Rev Respir Dis 136:1007, 1987
16. Powles ACP, Hershler R, Rigg JRA: A pocket calculator program for non-invasive bedside assessment of cardiorespiratory function. Comput Biol Med 10:143, 1980
17. Le Gall J, Loirat P, Alperovitch A et al: A simplified acute physiology score for ICU patients. Crit Care Med 12:975, 1984
18. Baue AE: Multiple, progressive or sequential systems failure. Arch Surg 110:779, 1975
19. Eiseman B, Beart R, Norton L: Multiple organ failure. Surg Gynecol Obstet 144:323, 1977
20. Fry DE, Pearlstein L, Fulton RL et al: Multiple system organ failure. Arch Surg 115:136, 1980
21. Siegel JH: Relations between circulatory and metabolic changes in sepsis. Ann Rev Med 32:175, 1981
22. Tremper KK, Barker SJ: Pulse oximetry. Anesthesiology 70:98, 1989
23. New W Jr, Barker SJ, Tremper KK: Pulse oximetry versus. $PtcO_2$ measurement. J Clin Monit 1:126, 1985
24. Hubmayr RD, Gay PC, Tayyab M: Respiratory system mechanics in ventilated patients: techniques and indications. Mayo Clin Proc 62:358, 1987
25. VanWagenen RA, Westenskow DR, Benner RE et al: Dedicated monitoring of anesthetic and respiratory gases by Raman scattering. J Clin Monit 2:215, 1986
26. Fratacci MD, Frostell CG, Tong-Yen C et al: Inhaled nitric oxide: a selective pulmonary vasodilator of heparin-protamine vasoconstriction in sheep. Anesthesiology 75:990, 1991
27. Frostell CG, Fratacci MD, Wain JC et al: Inhaled nitric oxide: a selective pulmonary vasodilator reversing hypoxic pulmonary vasoconstriction. Circulation 83:2038, 1991
28. Rossaint R, Falke K, Lopez F et al: Inhaled nitric oxide for the adult respiratory distress syndrome. N Engl J Med 328:399, 1993
29. Marsh HM, Abel MD: Postoperative management of adult cardiac surgical patients, p. 301. In Tarhan S (ed): Anesthesia and Coronary Artery Surgery. Year Book, Japanese Version, 1987
30. Smith JS, Cahalan MK, Benefiel DJ et al: Intraoperative detection of myocardial ischemia in high-risk patients: electrocardiography versus two-dimensional transesophageal echocardiography. Circulation 72:1015, 1985
31. Baele PL, McMichan JC, Marsh HM: Continuous monitoring of mixed venous oxygen saturation in critically ill patients. Anesth Analg 61:513, 1982
32. Norfleet EA, Watson CB: Continuous mixed venous oxygen saturation measurement: a significant advance in hemodynamic monitoring? J Clin Monit 1:245, 1985
33. Cain SM: Supply dependency of oxygen uptake in ARDS: myth or reality? [Review]. Am J Med Sci 288:119, 1984
34. Rackow EC, Asitz ME, Weil MH: Cellular oxygen metabolism during sepsis and shock. JAMA 259:1989, 1988
35. Kox WJ, Kox SN: Oxygen transport, consumption and cell metabolism in the critically ill. Int Pract Res 4:333, 1990
36. Powers SR, Mannal R, Neclerio M et al: Physiologic consequences of positive end-expiratory pressure (PEEP) ventilation. Ann Surg 178:265, 1973
37. Danek SJ, Lynch JP, Weg JG et al: The dependence of oxygen uptake on oxygen delivery in the adult

respiratory distress syndrome. Am Rev Respir Dis 122:387, 1980

38. Smithies M, Bihari DJ: Delivery dependent oxygen consumption: asking the wrong questions and not getting any answers. Crit Care Med 21:1622, 1993

39. DeBacker D, Berré J, Zhang H et al: Relationship between oxygen uptake and oxygen delivery in septic patients: effects of prostacyclin versus dobutamine. Crit Care Med 21:1658, 1993

40. Vallet B, Chopin C, Curtis SE et al: Prognostic value of the dobutamine test in patients with sepsis syndrome and normal lactate values: a prospective multicenter study. Crit Care Med 21:1868, 1993

41. Shires GT: Fluids, Electrolytes, and Acid Bases. Clinics in Critical Care Medicine. Vol. 15. Churchill Livingstone, New York, 1988

42. Drake HF, Treasure T: Continuous clinical monitoring with ion-selective electrodes: a feasible or desirable objective? Intens Care Med 12:104, 1986

43. Atwater BW, Parker JW, Chilcoat RT: Technological advances in pressure monitoring. In Vincent JL (ed): Update in Intensive Care and Emergency Medicine. Vol. 5. Springer-Verlag. New York, 1988

44. Bashein G, Greydanus WK, Kenny MA: Evaluation of a blood gas and chemistry monitor for use during surgery. Anesthesiology 72:123, 1989

45. Stoner HB: Interpretation of the metabolic effects of trauma and sepsis. J Clin Pathol 40:1108, 1987

46. Lakshman K, Blackburn GL: Monitoring nutritional status in the critically ill adult. J Clin Monit 2:114, 1986

47. Murray MJ, Marsh MB, Wochos DN et al: Nutritional assessment of intensive care unit patients. Mayo Clinic Proc 63:1106, 1988

48. Anderson CF, Loosbrock L, Moxness K: Nutrient intake in critically ill patients: too many or too few calories. Mayo Clin Proc 61:853, 1986

49. Vary TC, Siegel JH, Rivkind A: Clinical and therapeutic significance of metabolic patterns of lactic acidosis, p. 85. In Cerra FB (ed): Perspectives in Critical Care. Vol. 1. Quality Medical Publishing, St. Louis, MO, 1988

50. McMahon MM, Farnell MB, Murray MJ: Nutritional support of critically ill patients. Mayo Clin Proc 68: 911, 1993

51. Brajtbord D, Parks RI, Ramsay MA et al: Management of acute elevation of intracranial pressure during hepatic transplantation. Anesthesiology 70:139, 1989

52. Spiess BD, Tuman KJ, McCarthy PJ: Thromboelastography as an indicator of postcardiopulmonary bypass coagulopathies. J Clin Monit 3:25, 1987

53. Flowers RH III, Schwenzer KJ, Kopel PF et al: Efficacy of an attachable subcutaneous cuff for the prevention of intravascular catheter-related infection. JAMA 261:878, 1989

54. Maki DG, Cobb L, Garman JK et al: An attachable silver-impregnated cuff for prevention of infection with central venous catheters: a prospective randomized multicenter trial. Am J Med 85:307, 1988

55. Giroir BP: Mediators of septic shock: new approaches for interrupting the endogenous inflammatory cascade. Crit Care Med 21:780, 1993

56. Battafarano RJ, Dunn DL: Contribution of local cytokine production to the systemic host septic response. Crit Care Med 22:7, 1994

57. Fisher CJ, Slotman GJ, Opal SM et al: Initial evaluation of human recombinant interleukin-1 receptor antagonist in the treatment of sepsis syndrome. Crit Care Med 22:12, 1994

58. Notterman DA: Inotropic agents: catecholamines, digoxin, amrinone. Crit Care Clin 7:583, 1991

59. Curry SC, Arnold-Capell P: Nitroprusside, nitroglycerin, and angiotensin-converting enzyme inhibitors. Crit Care Clin 7:555, 1991

60. Guidry JR, Rascke RA, Morkunas AR: Anticoagulants and thrombolytics: risks and benefits. Crit Care Clin 7:533, 1991

61. Nolan PE, Raehl CL: Antiarrhythmic agents. Crit Care Clin 7:507, 1991

62. Dreifuss FE: Anticonvulsant agent. Crit Care Clin 7: 521, 1991

63. Truxit JD: Toxic effects of bronchodilators. Crit Care Clin 7:639, 1991

64. Hamill RJ, Rowlingson JC: Handbook of Critical Care Management. McGraw-Hill, New York, 1994

65. Bleich HL, Beckley RF, Horowitz GL et al: Clinical computing in a teaching hospital. N Engl J Med 312: 756, 1985

66. McDonald CJ, Tierney WM: Computer-stored medical records: their future role in medical practice. JAMA 259:3433, 1988

67. Morita K, Ikeda K: Evaluation of a microcomputer-based clinical laboratory data acquisition system linked with a minicomputer-based patient data management system. J Clin Monit 4:48, 1988

68. Wiener F, Weil MH, Carlson RW: Computer systems for facilitating management of the critically ill. Comput Biol Med 12:1, 1982

69. Pluth JR, Smith HC, Schultz GL: The computerized intensive-care unit: a comparative evaluation. Second Henry Ford Hospital Symposium on Cardiac Surgery, Section IV, Chapter 24, p. 152. 1977

70. Shortliffe EH: Computer programs to support clinical decision making. JAMA 258:61, 1987

71. Siegel JH, Cerra FB, Moody EA et al: The effect on survival of critically ill and injured patients of an ICU teaching service organized about a computer-based physiologic CARE system. J Trauma 20:558, 1980

72. Knaus WA, Zimmerman JE: Prediction of outcome from intensive care. In: Dobb G (guest ed): Clinics

in Anaesthesiology, Current Topics in Intensive Care. Vol. 3. WB Saunders, Philadelphia, 1985

73. Stadius ML, Davis K, Maynard C et al: Risk stratification for 1 year survival based on characteristics identified in the early hours of acute myocardial infarction. The Western Washington Intracoronary Streptokinase Trial. Circulation 74:703, 1986

74. Gillespie DJ, Marsh HM, Divertie MB et al: Clinical outcome of respiratory failure in patients requiring prolonged (>24 hours) mechanical ventilation. Chest 90:364, 1986

75. Lemeshow S, Teres D, Avrunin JP et al: Predicting the outcome of intensive care unit patients. J Am Stat Assoc 83:348, 1988

76. Schuster DP, Kollef MI: Predicting intensive care outcome. Crit Care Clin 30:1, 1994

77. Cowen JS, Kelley MA: Errors and bias in using predictive scoring systems. Crit Care Clin 10:53, 1994

78. Marsh HM, Krishan I, Naessens JM et al: Assessment of prediction of mortality by using APACHE II scoring system in intensive care units. Mayo Clin Proc 65:1549, 1990

79. Willats SM: The application of scoring systems in adult intensive care. Baillière's Clin Anesthesiol 4:253, 1990

80. Fakhry S, Muassaka F, Rutherford EJ et al: Prospective Comparison of Clinical Judgement and APACHE II. Score in Predicting the Outcome in Clinically Ill Surgical Patients. J Trauma 33:747, 1992

Monitoring Modalities of the Future

30

Judith L. Stiff
Amy Caplan

Monitoring techniques have undergone dramatic changes during the past 20 years as a reflection of the trends in available technology, most notably computerization, as well as trends in the concepts of what should be monitored in anesthesia and critical care. The original concept of monitoring during operations was that of frequent and repetitive monitoring looking at changes rather than isolated measurements. This was first evident in Snow's writings on ether and the changes in respiratory pattern, as well as patients' behavior as anesthesia with this agent was induced.[1] This concept was furthered by the development and use of the anesthesia chart, an ongoing record of one or more vital signs recorded simultaneously, a concept that has been transferred over to intensive care units (ICUs). For several decades the anesthesia record of blood pressure by auscultation and pulse by stethoscope or palpation, and perhaps respiration, remained the only frequent monitoring, although it is assumed that things such as color and pupillary signs were watched in an ongoing fashion. However, as operations became more complex and patients sicker when they were brought to the operating room, intermittent monitoring was not enough. Thus, there was a need to develop more truly continuous monitoring, second-to-second, not every 5 minutes, and with more emphasis on hard copy and the ability to retrieve data beyond that on the anesthesia record.

In addition to the emphasis on continuous monitoring, other trends have taken place over the past two decades. More exacting and complex information has become the standard of care in many situations. For example, oxygenation was, and still is to a certain extent, ascertained by watching the patient's color and vital signs. However, for patients with pulmonary disease, heart disease, or undergoing procedures that can impair ventilation, this may not be adequate, and reliance on arterial blood gas determinations has become important. These are only spot determinations, but in certain situations there is a need for more continuous information. Hence the development of transcutaneous oxygen electrodes and oximetry began. Even this was not enough, for the question remains of whether arterial oxygen pressure is reflective of oxygen content and whether that content meets the metabolic needs of tissues and organs. Thus, there are growing trends in looking at functional parameters, measures of the balance between tissue supplies and needs, on an organ level and even regionally within organs.

One problem with this approach is that many of the trends in monitoring have led to increasingly invasive techniques. Although the complication rates may be low, it is unacceptable to use invasive monitoring when it is not needed or when adequate noninvasive techniques are available. It is now necessary to concentrate on the development of noninvasive techniques, and, ideally, noninvasive techniques that possess the ability to tell if tissue metabolic needs in different organs are being met. However, there are no truly noninvasive techniques other than simple visual observations. Even electrocardiographic (ECG) monitoring involves passage of small currents through the body. Noninvasive, then, might be defined as subjecting the patient to low-energy forms of electromagnetic radiation, and/or placement of monitoring catheters or transducers externally or in body cavities open to the outside, such as the esophagus. Even some of these new modalities have not been thoroughly investigated as to their freedom from potential damaging effects to tissues and cells.

A further imperative in monitoring is to reduce cost. In choosing monitoring, the health care provider must be cognizant of costs: initial cost of instrumentation and cost per use, both in supplies and personnel. Although an expensive method will result in elegant information, a much cheaper method may give adequate enough information to provide safe and excellent patient care.

NONINVASIVE MONITORING OF CARDIAC AND CEREBRAL FUNCTION

Systolic Time Intervals

An early step toward noninvasive measurement of cardiac function was the development of the concept of systolic time intervals (STI). In the original method of measuring systolic time intervals, three simultaneous measurements are needed: electrocardiogram, phonocardiogram, and aortic arch pressure tracing, which is approximated by a carotid pulse tracing. There are two components of the systolic cycle (QS_2), the preejection period (PEP) and the left ventricular ejection time (LVET). QS_2 is the time from the beginning of the QRS complex to the closure of the aortic valve, or second heart sound. LVET begins at the first heart sound and the start of the upstroke of the carotid wave. PEP is determined by subtracting LVET from QS_2 (Fig. 30-1). When corrected for sex and heart rate, these measurements fall into a narrow range, and as left ventricular performance decreases in cardiac disease states, a pattern is seen consisting of an increase in PEP, a decrease in LVET, and constant QS_2. The ratio PEP/LVET does not need to be corrected for heart rate, and it rises with decreases in left ventricular performance. Increases in PEP/LVET have been found to parallel falls in stroke volume, cardiac output, and ejection fraction, and are sensitive measures; systolic time intervals becoming abnormal before the development

of symptoms or clinical signs. PEP/LVET is normally 0.35 ± 0.04, and impairment of function is considered to be mild for PEP/LVET of 0.44 to 0.52, moderate for 0.53 to 0.60, and severe for >0.60.

However, other factors may influence this ratio. It is decreased in patients receiving digitalis preparations and increased in those receiving β-blockers. Also, LBBB causes an increase in PEP/LVET. Interpretation of PEP/LVET in the absence of clinical information is a problem in valvular disease. In a patient with aortic stenosis or aortic insufficiency or both, PEP is decreased and LVET is increased, leading to a lower ratio and a false interpretation of "good" function. When cardiac decompensation begins, the ratio returns to a normal value in spite of poorer cardiac performance. STIs in a group of 56 patients with cardiac disease showed poor correlation with measures of cardiac function; however, when only patients with left ventricular disease were considered, PEP/LVET showed good correlation ($r = -.86$) with contractility index as calculated from dye dilution curves.[2] Similarly, it has been shown that in hypertensive patients without left ventricular hypertrophy, STI's cannot detect abnormal function, but the method becomes very sensitive to changes in function in patients with moderate to advanced left ventricular hypertrophy.[3]

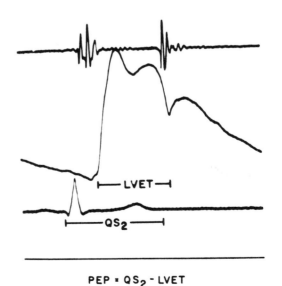

PEP = QS$_2$ - LVET

Fig. 30–1. Phonocardiogram, carotid arterial pulse, and electrocardiogram showing measurement of systolic time intervals. (From Lewis et al.,[94] with permission from the American Heart Association, Inc.)

STIs have not become widely applied because of a number of problems. They rely on some assumptions about the accurate determination of events such as the duration of systole, and in certain states of cardiac disease they may not be valid. As initially conceived, they required obtaining an accurate carotid pulse wave, which is quite unforgiving of artifact. However, echocardiographic determination of LVET, from the opening to the closing of the aortic valve, is more precise and can also be used to determine right ventricular STIs.[4] The use of densitometric photoelectric determination of the change in amount of blood in the pinna of the ear renders the system more resistant to movement artifact.[5] However, the greatest drawback is that STIs deal in a direction of change and perhaps a magnitude of change, but the desire is for information that deals in more absolute numbers, which are a more exact representation of the actual cardiac function. Using continuous wave Doppler and ECG, a new STI, the Q-V peak can be determined. Q-V peak is the time of Q wave to peak flow velocity. In patients undergoing cardiac catheterization who did not have LBBB, atrial fibrillation, valvular heart disease nor were taking cardioactive drugs other than nitroglycerin, the Q-V peak showed better correlation ($r = -.80$) with ejection fraction than other STIs.[6]

STIs have been used in preterm infants to follow response to dobutamine,[7] a situation where other methods of following cardiac function are difficult to achieve. They also have been used for fetal monitoring during labor, via a scalp ECG and transabdominal Doppler cardiogram.[8] In the fetuses that went on to have signs of asphyxia (umbilical artery pH < 7.20 and/or 5-minute APGAR < 7), PEP and PEP/LVET during labor were higher than those of normal fetuses. PEPs and PEP/LVETs greater than one standard deviation above normal had good predictive value for fetal asphyxia.

Traditional methods for STIs have been combined with impedance measurements. The *dZ/dt* waveform is used in place of the carotid pulse for the determination of LVET. An automated system with an algorithm for averaging over many cardiac cycles has been used during exercise testing and found to correlate well with STIs simultaneously measured using carotid pulse waves.[9]

STIs are inexpensive and relatively easily obtained. Their greatest drawback is that they deal in a direction of change and perhaps a magnitude of change. Usually the desire is for information in more absolute numbers and parameters of cardiac function that are more familiar.

Signal-Averaged Electrocardiography

Signal-averaged ECG is a technique using a mathematical analysis of electrocardiograms. All complex waves, such as ECGs, are the mathematical summation of multiple waves of varying amplitudes and frequencies. The mathematical analysis of these component waves has been studied as signal-averaged ECGs. Analysis of multiple (100–150) ECG complexes during sinus rhythm, excluding any noise or arrhythmias, can be done relative to time or frequency. Individual parts of the ECG, such as the beginning or the end of the QRS or the S-T segments, can be analyzed to detect any abnormal signals. One such abnormal signal is the late potential, a high-frequency, low-amplitude wave present at the terminal portion of the QRS complex. Late potentials are felt to be caused by aberrations of myocardial depolarization traveling through damaged myocardium.[10] The appearance of late potentials has been found to be a positive predictor of patients prone to sustained ventricular tachycardia following myocardial infarction.[11]

The signal-averaged ECG is a noninvasive, fairly rapid method of evaluating subtle changes in the ECG. It is presently used primarily in the study of postmyocardial infarction patients to recognize the tendency toward sustained ventricular tachycardia in an effort to prevent this malignant arrhythmia. The possibilities for uses of the signal-averaged ECG are varied and could possibly include the recognition of a predictor of ischemia, which is more sensitive than the analysis of S-T segments presently used. Signal-averaged ECG may someday be a part of routine intraoperative and intensive care monitoring.

Impedance Measurement of Cardiac Function

In 1940 Nyboer and colleagues[12] introduced a method they called radiocardiography. It has been reintroduced in the last decade as *impedance electrocardiography*. Impedance is the apparent resistance to the flow of alternating current. Thus if a small current is applied to the thorax and the resulting voltage is measured, the ratio of voltage over current equals impedance. The underlying theory assumes that the thorax is a relatively uniform conductor with a resistivity of ρ and that resistivity is due primarily to blood. This uniform conductor of length *L* has a steady-state mean impedance Z_0, and changes in impedance dZ/dt will be due to pulsatile variations in thoracic aortic blood flow. Comparison of dZ/dt waveforms with arterial pressure waveforms does show a similarity. The maximum value of dZ/dt is thought to reflect the peak aortic flow, and, when multiplied by the ventricular ejection time *T*, gives stroke volume. The formula for stroke volume (SV) according to Kubicek and colleagues[13] is

$$SV = \rho \cdot \left(\frac{L^2}{Z_0}\right) \cdot \left(\frac{dZ}{dt_{max}}\right) \cdot T$$

when *L* is the distance between electrodes.

Currents in the range of 200 μA to 4 mA at 40 to 100 kHz are applied using strip electrodes or electrodes opposite each other at the level of the neck and the lower rib cage. Another set of electrodes is applied in between to measure the voltage difference. In early applications, *T* was determined by phonocardiogram (Fig. 30-2).

A problem with this method has been the determination of the constants. It was assumed that the resistivity was influenced by the viscosity of blood and hence hematocrit and corrections needed to be made to ρ. However, Quail and Traugott[14] showed that over a wide range of hematocrits ρ remained constant. DeSouza and Panerai[15] investigated the effects of various respiratory maneuvers in humans and found that signal variability was greatest during normal breathing, less during apneusis, and least during postexhalation apnea; but the effects of variability could be minimized by signal averaging. Thus the derived value for stroke index is not truly beat-to-beat, but more nearly minute-to-minute. Impedance cardiography has been used in the operating room as a noninvasive means of comparing the hemodynamic effects of different drugs.[16] During cesarean section, impedance cardiographic stroke volumes have been compared to dye dilution determinations and found to be slightly lower, but they did correlate well ($r = .93$).[17]

The other constant *L* remains a greater problem. The Kubicek formula considered the thorax to be a cylinder. However, considering the placement of electrodes, the volume within them is closer to a truncated cone, the volume of which is related to height.

The Minnesota Impedance Cardiograph 304b (Surcom, Inc. Minneapolis MN) uses the Kubicek formula. Using this instrument to study over 100 patients without valvular heart disease who were

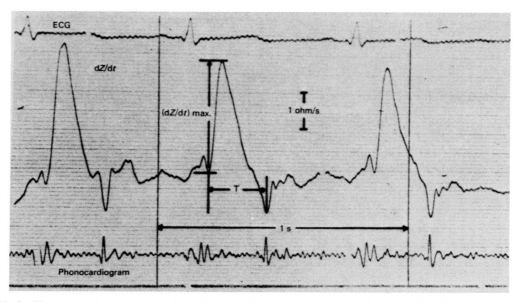

Fig. 30–2. Electrocardiogram, transthoracic impedance, and phonocardiogram showing measurements for calculation of stroke volume. (From Edmunds et al.,[95] with permission.)

scheduled to undergo MUGA studies, impedance ejection fraction correlates poorly when ejection fraction is low (<40 percent), but is better in more normal patients.[18] The instrument has also been used to look at hemodynamic changes caused by CO_2 insufflation during laparoscopy.[19]

Sramek and colleagues[20] determined the term defined as the volume of electrically participating thoracic tissue (V_{EPT}) to be $(0.17H)^3/4.2$ (where H is patient height), which replaces L^2 in the Kubicek formula. This modification dealt with the systematic overestimation of cardiac output for most patients. However, it did not deal with variations in body habitus. Bernstein[21] derived a factor δ that is a measure of deviation from ideal body weight. Thus, the formula becomes

$$SV = \delta \cdot \left(\frac{[0.17H]^3}{4.2} \right) \cdot \frac{(dZ/dt_{max})}{Z_0} \cdot T$$

The NCCOM-3 cardiovascular monitor (BoMed Medical Manufacturing Ltd., Irvine, CA) uses this formula for determination of stroke volume. However, to program V_{EPT}, the computer takes an L value that is determined by a nomogram for weight and height. The instrument determines T, the ventricular ejection time (VET) from the impedance curve and calls (dZ/dt_{max}) the ejection velocity index (EVI) and Z_0 the thoracic fluid index (TFI). In addition to stroke volume and cardiac output, this instrument displays other derived parameters of cardiac function. However, these derived measures depend upon assumptions of fairly normal cardiac function.

The stroke volume can be obtained beat-to-beat or an average of 12 beats. Electrocautery interferes with measurement. Conditions that lead to poor impedance signals include arrhythmias, tachycardia (HR > 150), and inability to achieve good application of the electrodes.

A comparison of impedance-determined cardiac outputs and thermodilution cardiac outputs in 16 critically ill patients in both an ICU and during surgery has been performed by Appel and coworkers.[22] For 391 paired determinations the correlation was $r = .83$. When five patients, in whom there were technical difficulties in either method, were eliminated, the correlation became $r = .90$. In a similar study Bernstein compared thermodilution cardiac outputs with impedance determined cardiac outputs in 17 patients with 94 paired measurements and found a correlation of $r = .88$. The greatest disparities were at low flows (less than 2 L/min), where impedance gives a higher value than thermodilution.

In a study of 56 critically ill patients, the overall correlation coefficient with bioimpedance to thermodilution cardiac output was $r = .61$ and bias of $-0.67 + 1.72$.[24] The authors speculate that poor electrode placement due to the dressing at the internal jugular site of insertion of the pulmonary artery catheter may have led to the poor correlation. In a smaller group of 17 critically ill patients, a correlation of .91 and a bias of $0.23 + .56$ has been found.[25] In 11 pregnant patients requiring a pulmonary artery catheter, Masaki,[26] found a correlation of .91.

In children, the determination of the constant L is difficult because of the changing thoracic cavity proportions as a child ages. In a study of children following repair of congenital heart defects or following multiple trauma, a thermodilution cardiac output was used to calibrate the bioimpedance cardiac output and back calculate L. Comparing this value to the manufacturer's suggested formula for adults (BoMed) showed that the formula would lead to a consistent under estimation in small children in this small sample (8 patients).[27] The manufacturer now has a table for L for small children based on weight.

Even though the absolute measurement of cardiac output may differ from thermodilution, impedance cardiac output measurements have been shown to be as consistent over time as other cardiovascular variables and affected little by minor electrode placement changes.[28] The values are fairly constant in a normal range of cardiac output, but at low cardiac output, impedance values are higher than thermodilution.[28] Thus, the method can be most useful as a method to look at change in cardiac output in response to interventions. Impedance cardiac output has been used to study the effects of blood and loss and position change in healthy volunteers,[29] and the response to pharmacologic and procedural stressors in critically ill children.[30] It also has been used to look at different volume loading protocols for cesarean section under epidural anesthesia.[31]

An important problem with this methodology is that it is not really known what is being measured, only that the value obtained correlates with stroke volume. The value for L must be correct or a great deal of systematic error is introduced. Thus, impedance measurements are useful in detecting change in cardiac function in an individual patient, but are less useful as an absolute measure. Measurements are technically easy to perform and inexpensive.

Radionuclide Scintigraphy Measurement of Cardiac Function

Radionuclear scintigraphy as a method of monitoring of cardiac function is actually somewhat invasive, in that a small amount of a radiopharmaceutical is injected by vein. However, in contrast to conventional contrast angiography, the amount of radioactivity is many times less. The method involves measuring the emission of electromagnetic radiation, which comes through the skin as gamma rays. The detector consists of a sodium iodide crystal with a small amount of thallium as an activator. The radiation first has to go through a collimater, which is made of lead with holes and which limits the field of view. A scintillation camera consists of a multicrystal detector, each crystal coupled with a collimater hole.

Two types of cardiac function studies are conducted with such an apparatus: First-pass studies of ventricular dimensions to determine ejection fraction, usually referred to as nuclear angiocardiography, and blood pool studies, which are gated studies or multiple-gated acquisition studies (MUGA). For studies over a period of time, a first-pass technique would require multiple injections of radiopharmaceutical, and consequently unacceptably high radiation doses. Blood pool studies require a nondiffusable substance to be injected and allowed to come to a steady state. In gated studies, a physiologic event acts as a trigger for recording, such as ECG events to signal systole and diastole. Ejection fraction is then calculated from the ventricular dimensions during systole and diastole using the formula

$$V = \frac{8A^2}{3\pi L}$$

This assumes that the accuracy of a three-dimensional value calculated from two-dimensional data is reasonable. Both first-pass and equilibrium radionuclide angiography with technetium 99m pertechnate have been used to study the effects of lumbar epidural anesthesia and subsequent volume loading in patients with and without stable angina.[32]

However, if the measurement consists merely of the fluctuations in radioactivity counts during the entire cardiac cycle, then a continuous trace of cardiac function can be obtained. After a correction for background count is subtracted, the top and bottom of the sinusoidal curve obtained correlates with the full and empty state of the left ventricle. As the whole curve moves up, the ventricle is emptying less, and as the top and bottom come closer together the ejection fraction has decreased. Thus, the nongated, nonimaging scintillation camera is the nuclear stethoscope or nuclear probe and yields a real-time continuous relative left ventricular volume. The data obtained by this technique correlate well with conventional first-pass scintillation techniques over a wide range of ejection fractions.[33] However, with asynchronous wall motion the correlation is poorer and the ejection fraction may be falsely high. This is due to the limited field of view and because positioning of the probe is accomplished by searching for the lowest background and best amplitude, hence missing the area of asynergy.[34] The nuclear probe has also been used to study patients undergoing coronary artery bypass operations during laryngoscopy and intubation.[35] The decrease in ejection fraction seen in these patients was mirrored by a rise in PCWP (Fig. 30-3).

Initially the application of this method in operating rooms and intensive care units was limited because the probe had to be attached to a mechanical arm or be hand held to maintain a stable position and required considerable user skill. Now there are two improved systems in which the detector is secured to the subject and, thus, have a wider range of use.

VEST (Capintech, Inc., Ramsey, NJ) is battery-powered and uses a thallium-activated sodium iodide crystal detector, which is secured to the subject by a plastic vest. The detector is positioned using a gamma camera. The vest also contains a two-lead ECG and a cadmium telluride detector to obtain background counts over the lung. With the addition of the ECG channels, changes in ejection fraction can be correlated with ST segments. Data collection is by cassette. During upright bicycle exercise in normal subjects and cardiac patients, the VEST measured EF has been shown to correlate well ($r = .87$) with values determined by gamma camera.[36] The VEST version of continuous radionuclide monitoring of cardiac function has been used for and is more adapted to ambulatory monitoring. It is not "on line," and data have to be retrieved for analysis.

Cardioscint (Oakfield Instruments, Oxford, UK) uses a cadmium telluride detector secured to the patient with a belt. It has no background count detector and has a one-lead ECG. Data collection is "on line," enabling the probe to be placed by looking for maximum counts. Prior to placement the probe can be used to determine background counts from a region where cardiac activity can barely be detected. In a study of 77 patients, with and without known cardiac disease, the Cardioscint values for ejection fraction correlated well with those determined by gamma camera ($r = .80$).[37] In three subjects with low ejection fractions, the probe could not determine adequate data; however, it was successful in other subjects with low ejection fractions. There were no difficulties in positioning the probe on women. Six patients then underwent a stepwise atrial pacing protocol with thermal dilution determination of stroke index at each step, and change in stroke counts by probe was compared to change in stroke index with an overall correlation of $r = .69$. Correlation was improved with deletion of data from one patient where there were probe stability problems.

This methodology is expensive because it uses a radiopharmaceutical. With training it is easy to use

and has promise as a cardiac monitor that is little affected by motion. Access to the thorax is needed and the length of time it can be used is limited by the decay and washout of the indicator.

Doppler Measurement of Cardiac Output

Doppler ultrasound measurement of cardiac output uses the frequency shift of an ultrasound wave when reflected from a moving substance. In the case of blood flow measurement, the reflectance is from erythrocytes. The simplest Doppler system merely detects the presence of a frequency shift and presents its occurrence in some analog form. In the apparatus most familiar in operating rooms and critical care areas, the analog is the audible signal of varying frequency one hears when using a Doppler instrument on the precordium or on a peripheral pulse. Both continuous-wave Doppler and pulsed Doppler systems for noninvasive measurement of cardiac output are commercially available.

Continuous-wave Doppler can be used to measure cardiac output by placement of a transducer in the suprasternal notch and aligning it with the ascending aorta. A continuous-wave technique looks at all returning echoes and hence all velocities along the length of the beam, so the transducer

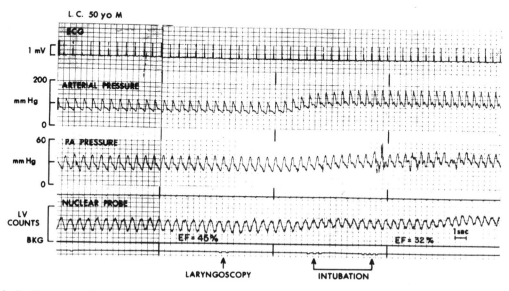

Fig. 30–3. Electrocardiogram, arterial pressure, pulmonary artery pressure, and left ventricular radioactivity counts recorded during laryngoscopy and intubation. BKG = background activity level. (From Giles et al.,[35] with permission.)

is placed to find the highest velocity (greatest frequency shift). By integration of the resulting velocity-time curve (Fig. 30-4), the mean velocity is determined. Mean velocity times cross-sectional area times the cosine of the angle of the beam with the axis of the aorta yields stroke volume. The angle can be assumed to be zero because for any angle less than 30 degrees, the cosine is very close to one. A continuous-wave system uses A mode or M mode Doppler measurement of the aortic root cross-sectional area, which is performed before taking the velocity measurements. It is assumed that the area of greatest velocity is at the aortic root.

Using this method, Nishimura and colleagues[38] compared continuous-wave Doppler cardiac outputs with thermodilution measurements. Correlation was .94 in medical patients and .85 in postoperative cardiac surgery patients. Rein and coworkers[39] found a correlation of .86 between continuous-wave Doppler and thermodilution outputs in children. This method is not applicable for patients with aortic valvular disease and measurements cannot be obtained in some patients, probably due to anatomic factors. It assumes that the aortic area is circular and remains constant during the cardiac cycle and that the velocity is being measured at the place where the cross-sectional area was determined. Cardiac outputs obtained by continuous-wave Doppler tend to be higher than those obtained by pulsed Doppler.[40]

Pulsed Doppler allows the velocity to be determined at a specific point along the beam because the reflected wave is sampled at a selected time after transmission. The selection of the amount of time allowed for the return of the echo determines the depth where the velocity is being measured. Pulsed Doppler systems are interfaced with ultrasonic imaging so that the source of the signal can be selected by visual control. Pulsed Doppler can also be used in locations other than the suprasternal notch to measure velocities in the great vessels and across heart valves.

Comparison of pulsed Doppler determinations of pulmonary artery and aortic cardiac outputs with indicator dilution or angiographic techniques in children with a variety of cardiac conditions showed good correlation for aortic outputs, but less satisfactory correlation was found on the pulmonary side.[41] Correlation was best for both outputs (r = .94) if the vessel area was determined by angiography, pointing out the importance of accuracy of this determination. Pulsed Doppler stroke volumes and those obtained by a direct Fick method in adults with valvular heart disease have been found to have a correlation of r = .91.[42]

Flow characteristics can be studied by pulsed Doppler. This makes the noninvasive determination of pulmonary artery pressure and resistance possible. Graettinger and associates[43] have presented a method for predicting these values in adults from the velocity characteristics obtained by Doppler. Applicability on any measurement of pulmonary artery outflow is limited by the inability to obtain adequate images in some patients. Pulsed Doppler has been used to follow the blood flow changes in the pulmonary artery and ascending aorta in normal neonates during their circulatory adjustments in the first day of life.[44]

Doppler methodology has been much enhanced recently by fast Fourier transform analysis of the Doppler frequencies and improved software. Accuracy and applicability to all patients often depends on transducer design.[40] It is inexpensive and easy to use at the bedside, but there is variability among operators. Although Doppler cardiac outputs show good correlation with other methods,

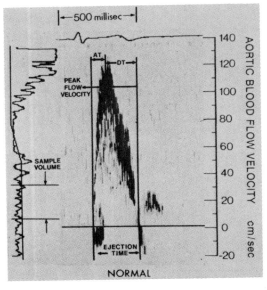

Fig. 30–4. Doppler blood flow velocity in the ascending aorta recorded from the suprasternal notch in a normal adult. Depth and axial length of sample volume are displayed to the left and measurements of velocity parameters are shown. (From Gardin et al.,[96] with permission.)

there are problems with their use as absolute measures because of the systematic error that can be introduced by inaccuracies in determination of cross-sectional area of the aorta or other vessels and probe placement problems. Thus, this methodology is more useful for following trends.

Transcranial Doppler

Pulsed Doppler systems are available for the non-invasive measurement of blood flow velocity (Vbf) in intracranial arteries (Transpect TCD, Medsonics, Inc., Fremont, CA). Transcranial Doppler (TCD) utilizes low frequency (1-2 MHz) ultrasonic signals which penetrate areas of the cranium and reflect off erythrocytes in the basilar arteries. Doppler shift principle and fast-Fourier transformation is used to calculate and display Vbf from which peak systolic, diastolic and mean velocities are determined. Spectrum analysis of the Doppler signal is displayed on an oscilloscope as a wave with time versus velocity. Vbf varies proportionately with cerebral blood flow (CBF) as long as vessel diameter remains constant. Autoregulation of CBF in response to changes in carbon dioxide or cerebral perfusion pressure occurs at the arteriolar level, leaving the arteries measured by TCD relatively stable.[45] There are three "windows" in the cranium which the Doppler signal can penetrate to insonate an artery. The temporal bone allows insonation of the middle cerebral artery (MCA) and the anterior and posterior cerebral arteries. The orbit gives access to the ophthalmic artery and the siphon area of the internal carotid, and the foramen magnum accesses the intracranial vertebral and basilar arteries. A head strap is available to transfix the probe facilitating multiple measurements for comparison.

The mean Vbf (systolic velocity − diastolic velocity/3 + diastolic velocity) has been measured intraoperatively in an effort to decrease the morbidity and mortality due to changes in CBF.[46] Electroencephalogram (EEG) and somatosensory evoked potentials monitor the consequences of decreased CBF. TCD has the ability to identify aberrations in CBF, possibly early enough for therapeutic intervention. During carotid endarterectomy (CEA), low Vbf in the ipsilateral MCA may indicate the need for a shunt to preserve adequate CBF. Correlation between mean Vbf and regional CBF during CEA was good during low flows, especially during cross-clamp. These periods of low flow also

correlated with suppression of the ipsilateral EEG.[47] Also during CEA, the detection of multiple air bubble emboli or prolonged evidence of solid emboli in the MCA was found to correlate positively with adverse neurologic outcome.[48] During cardiopulmonary bypass, TCD has been used to quantify MCA microemboli associated with different oxygenators and Vbf in the MCA during deliberate hypotension.[49,50]

Outside the surgical arena TCD has varied uses. The assessment of CBF and collateral flow in cases of intra- or extracranial artery stenosis is best accomplished by comparing bilateral flows. Cerebral vasospasm following subarachnoid hemorrhage has been classified using the peak Vbf in the MCA (flow velocity varies inversely with vessel diameter). Peak Vbf greater than 200 cm·sec^{-1} has been found to be a predictor of delayed cerebral ischemia.[51] Identification of arteriovenous malformations and the arterial supply is facilitated by studying the pulsatile properties of flow. Pulsatility Index (PI) = systolic velocity − diastolic velocity/mean velocity. A decrease in PI, primarily due to an increase in diastolic velocity, is an indicator of decreased resistance downstream. PI is also useful in the assessment of increased intracranial pressure (ICP). As ICP increases, perfusion pressure and Vbf decrease. The diastolic velocity decreases fastest leading to an increase in PI. Reversal of flow during diastole has been associated with eventual brain death.[46,51]

Transcranial Doppler has the advantage of being a noninvasive, portable and relatively inexpensive monitor of intracranial blood flow velocity. TCD does require adequate anatomy as the temporal "window" is absent in up to 20 percent of patients and insonation of basilar arteries is more difficult in women and the elderly. A high level of training is needed for proper examination and interpretation of data.[46] The absolute values determined by TCD are less valuable than the comparison of bilateral flows and the changes in flow that occur over time.

NONINVASIVE METABOLIC MONITORING

Infrared Spectroscopy

Many medical technologies deal with spectroscopic methods, that is, exposing a substance or a part of a patient's body to electromagnetic radiation and measuring the effect. Electromagnetic radiation may be transmitted, passed through with no effect, reflected, refracted, the ray bent, scattered, either unchanged or with a change in frequency; or absorbed, with release of heat, change of wavelength, or photochemical reaction. Whatever the process, in order to have a useful spectroscopic method, enough of the radiation must get into the tissue and must cause enough of a reaction that is unique and measurable. In the case of the older technology of x-rays, this form of radiation is high-energy, high-frequency such that it penetrates body tissue easily, much being transmitted to the film opposite, while some is scattered. However, newer technologies deal with low-energy, low-frequency radiation and are considered to be noninvasive. The problem consists of refining the methodology to enable a more poorly penetrating ray to yield discrete and reliable measurements.

Infrared and visible light radiation have been used for several decades to analyze chemical composition. Any organic molecule has a specific spectrum. In the infrared or visible wavelengths there will be one or more absorption bands, each representing a particular type and extent of bond formation within that molecule. Thus, spectrophotometric techniques were applied to identifying specific compounds in mixtures. If one looks at a specific portion of the spectrum (that portion that represents a known absorption band of a molecule) and there is no other compound present that has an absorption band close by, then changes in absorption will represent changes in the amount of that molecule present. Since a few selected wavelengths can be rapidly scanned, spectrophotometric analysis can give a dynamic picture of changes in the amount of specific molecules present. Initial studies of the metabolic demands and supplies of tissues have been conducted in the visible light wavelengths looking at changes in NADH, cytochromes, and oxygenated hemoglobin. However, visible light penetrates denser tissues poorly so these studies were undertaken on pieces of tissue or isolated organs or the brain via craniotomy windows.

Infrared light (700 to 1000 nm) can be useful for monitoring tissues and organs within the body because unlike visible light, these wavelengths penetrate fairly well, even through bone, and there are molecules of physiologic significance (hemoglobin and cytochromes) that have specific and discrete absorption bands. The oxidized form of cytochrome a,a_3 has one absorption band at 820 to 840 nm. Since the oxidation of cytochrome a,a_3 is the final reaction of the respiratory chain and accounts for 90 percent of all cellular oxygen utilization, measurement of this compound is useful in determining physiologic function within cells. Hemoglobin (Hb) has a weak absorption peak at 760 nm and its oxygenated form (HbO_2) does not; thus a rise or fall in HbO_2 can be detected. Using the 815 nm wavelength region which is the isobestic point of Hb-HbO_2, a value that is proportional to the blood volume can be obtained and used to correct the cytochrome and Hb signals for changes in blood volume. Thus, infrared monitoring has the potential for obtaining an integrated picture of cerebral oxygen supply and intracellular oxygen utilization, as well as determining cerebral blood volume changes to assess the overall function of the brain.

The method involves pressing a probe containing fiberoptic bundles against an area of the skull that has little or no overlying muscle or hair. The pressure must be firm enough to expel the blood. Monochromatic light is generated at the selected wavelengths. The receiving bundle is pressed on the opposite side of the head in the case of using a transmittance mode or adjacent in the case of using a reflectance mode, and the rays are passed through a photomultiplier for detection. The data are presented as the change in optical density (ΔOD) from the original baseline. Thus, as cytochrome a,a_3 becomes more oxidized, its absorption is increased and ΔOD will increase, and as more hemoglobin is carrying oxygen its absorption will decrease and ΔOD will decrease. If cerebral blood volume increases, absorption of Hb-HbO_2 at its isobestic point will increase so ΔOD will increase. The changes in cytochrome a,a_3 oxidation and hemoglobin oxygenation are usually accompanied by changes in cerebral blood volume (Hb-HbO_2), so this curve is subtracted from the other two curves and the subtraction is built into the recording circuit so that the difference curves are presented (Fig. 30-5).

Initial animal studies showed the expected changes in HbO_2, Hb-HbO_2, and cytochrome a,a_3 as measured by ΔOD's. In rats bilateral ligation of the common carotid arteries led to the expected decrease in cytochrome oxidation, accompanied by a blood volume decrease and a greater decrease in hemoglobin saturation. These changes were reversed by releasing the clamps within 20 minutes and the cytochrome overshot into a hyperoxidation state.[52] The protective effect of hypothermia during hypoxic hypotension in rats has been demonstrated by infrared spectroscopy.[53] Infrared measurements have shown that intracranial pressure (ICP) does not necessarily correlate with brain metabolism. In cats, when ICP was raised by infusion of mock cerebrospinal fluid, Hb increased and HbO_2 decreased, but when ICP then was lowered by hyperventilation, there was a further increase in desaturated Hb.[54]

Application to the larger human head requires an adequate light source and better detection. Using a photon counter and human volunteers, Jöbsis[55] showed that hyperventilation produced the expected decrease in Hb-HbO_2, a decrease in cerebral blood volume. Breathing 92 percent oxygen and 8 percent carbon dioxide resulted in an increased blood volume measurement and a slight

increase in the measurement of cytochrome oxidation. Hampson and associates[56] looked at normocapnic and hypocapnic hypoxia (SaO_2 down to 70 percent) in volunteers and found parallel increases in Hb and decreases in HbO_2 as saturation decreased, but the cerebral blood volume rose faster and the cytochrome a,a_3 decreased more slowly during normocapnic hypoxia. Ferrari and coworkers[57] compared infrared measurements to EEGs during compression of the carotid artery and found agreement when the EEG slowed. However, it appeared that the infrared measurements may be a more sensitive test for defective collateral circulation.

Validation of these measurements in humans is difficult, particularly in adults, because other methods for comparison are cumbersome. Also it is uncertain as to exactly how much of the brain infrared spectroscopy is measuring. However, in

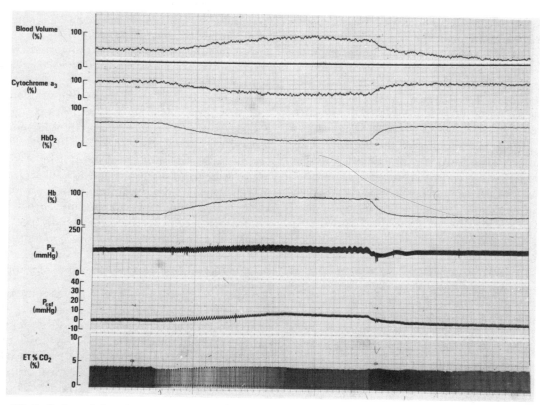

Fig. 30–5. Infrared absorption tracings in a dog showing the increase in cerebral blood volume, decrease in cytochrome a,a_3, decrease in oxygenated hemoglobin, and increase in deoxygenated hemoglobin during breathing of a hypoxic mixture [95 percent N_2, 5 percent O_2]. Lower tracings are of arterial pressure, cerebral spinal fluid pressure, and end tidal pCO_2.

neonates a validation study of the cerebral blood volume measurement has been done. Plethysmography of the neonatal head to determine change cerebral blood volume has been compared to infrared determination during brief jugular venous occlusion and found to produce fair agreement.[58]

The original work on this method was done on instruments designed by the investigators and some were the prototypes of what is now available for purchase. One instrument is the NIR1000 (Hamamatsu Phototonics KK, Hamamatsu City, Japan). It operates in a transmittance mode and has outputs for Hb, HbO_2, cerebral blood volume, and cytochrome a,a_3 and has been used predominently for monitoring of neonates. In 16 preterm infants with 50 episodes of hypoxia, all had rises in total cerebral Hb and falls in HbO_2 consistent with their decreases in oxygen saturation measured by pulse oximetry.[59] This instrument has also been used on fetuses during labor.[60] During normal contraction both HbO_2 and Hb fell, but with fetal decelerations Hb rose and HbO_2 fell more than during normal contractions. Using this instrument to measure cerebral blood volume in preterm and term infants, it was found that the cerebral blood volume response to carbon dioxide increases with gestational age.[61]

Another instrument is the INVOS 3100 (Somanetics, Troy, MI). It operates in the reflectance mode and uses the Hb and $Hb-HbO_2$ measurements, but converts them to a saturation which is called the approximate regional oxygen saturation (rSO_2). Since it represents mostly venous blood in the microvasculature, a normal value is around 73 percent. On the probe there is a separate receiver close to the light source that determines the shallow tissue (scalp and bone) contribution, which is subtracted out of the final signal. Using this instrument, rSO_2 was compared to estimated regional saturation calculated from arterial saturation, jugular venous saturation and published data for percentage of regional cerebral blood volume that is arterial.[62] Measurements made over the middle frontal gyrus in nine critically ill neurologic patients were correlated with the calculated value with $r = .74$. The same study also looked at normal subjects during normocapnic hypoxia (arterial oxygen saturation < 50 percent) and found the rSO_2 measurement to be as responsive to hypoxia as EEG monitoring.

A dual wave spectrophotometer that monitors percent (HbO_2 and total Hb is by NIMS Inc., Phil-

adelphia, PA.) The output is change in absorbance at 800 nm, which represents total hemoglobin and change in absorbance at 760 nm representing deoxygenated hemoglobin. It has been used to study neonates (< 1 month of age) undergoing cardiac surgery using deep hypothermic circulatory arrest[63] and also adults during brief periods of ventricular fibrillation during placement of automatic internal cardioverting defibrillators.[64] Using this monitor on preterm infants, it has been shown that preoxygenation will attenuate the response to endotracheal tube suctioning, decrease the fall in HbO_2 and rise in total Hb.[65]

A different application of near infrared spectroscopy is the evaluation of peripheral vacular disease. Using the Hamamatsu instrument, Cheatle and colleagues[66] compared 21 normal subjects with 17 patients with claudication. They propose that the responses to tourniquet ischemia and release can be used to monitor response to surgical or pharmacologic therapy.

Although this method appears to have clinical usefulness, some questions remain. Using transmittance mode instruments on neonates, the measurements would appear to relate to global change and the contribution of regional events is unknown. The reflectance instruments measure regionally, but the extent of that region is unknown. At this point it is not clear what extent of change in these measurements represent irreversible damage and when treatment should be instituted. This methodology is qualitative and cannot be used to compare individual patients. It is useful as a means of following an individual patient over time. Infrared instruments do reproducibly measure changes in brain tissue perfusion and metabolism, and the method is inexpensive and simple to use.

Magnetic Resonance Spectroscopy

Magnetic resonance (MR) technology is not new. In 1952, the Nobel Prize was awarded to Bloch and Purcell for their roles in its development. At that time, MR (called nuclear magnetic resonance (NMR) in the physical sciences) was used in analytical chemistry in the identification of the specific content of substances. As early as 1959, Singer[67] published his work on determining blood flow rates by MR. However, the real explosion of interest in MR for medicine began in 1973, with the publication of a paper on magnetic resonance imaging by Lauterbur.[68] There are two types of MR studies: imaging and spectroscopy. MR imaging (MRI) can define functional or dysfunctional areas, and spectroscopy has greater potential for true metabolic monitoring.

In the presence of an externally applied magnetic field, atomic nuclei with an odd number of protons or neutrons will "line up" or precess, that is, revolve about an axis parallel to the field. Applying a second or excitation field of radiofrequency will cause a shift of the alignment or precession, and as the nuclei return to their initial states they emit a signal of a precise frequency. The hydrogen nucleus has a single proton and because of its higher MR sensitivity and abundance in the body, it is the basis of (proton) MRI. By using a nonuniform magnetic field, such as one with its peak at a point or a line or in a plane, the location and concentration of specific resonant nuclei can be determined. However, the intensity of the emitted signal reflects more than the concentration of a specific atom. The rate at which the nuclei line up (T1), the spin lattice time constant, is determined by the strength of the magnetic field, temperature, viscosity, and interaction of the nuclei with the surrounding sample. T1 is short where water is closely bound to proteins such as in muscle or liver. The rate at which the energy emission decays (T2), the spin-spin time constant, is determined by interaction between nuclei. Therefore, by making the interval between successive applications of the second or radiofrequency field shorter, tissues with longer T1s will yield less signal, because the nuclei will have had less time to realign. Also, increasing the time interval between the application of the excitation field and measurement of the emission enhances the signal from tissue with a slower decay (T2). By using these variables, a very precise image can be built.

Nuclei other than hydrogen have potential for MR spectroscopy. [31]P is less abundant than hydrogen and has a lower MR sensitivity which makes it less ideal for imaging. However, it is useful for analysis of tissue using MR spectra of phosphorus compounds. A phosphorus spectrum of tissue will have peaks for sugar phosphate, inorganic phosphate, phosphocreatine, and adenosine triphosphate (ATP). Initial studies of phosphorus MR spectra were conducted on tissue preparations. With small topical surface coils and the development of superconducting magnets, study of major organs in

vivo is becoming possible (Fig. 30-6). In an in vivo rat heart preparation, the decline of phosphocreatine and ATP and the increase in inorganic phosphate following cardiac arrest has been shown.[69] Because of the need for adequate spatial localization of the ^{31}P signal, work had been limited to small animals. However, with the development of a depth-resolved surface coil, the technique is now available for the study of metabolism in human

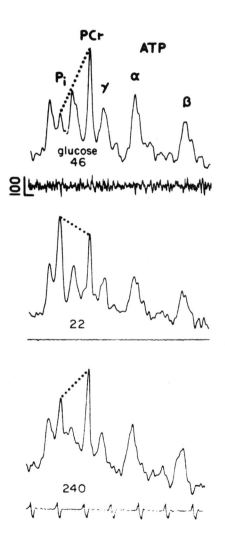

Fig. 30–6. [31]P nuclear magnetic resonance spectra of brain and EEG recordings in a rabbit during normal glycemia, hypoglycemia, and restoration of blood glucose. The phosphocreatine/inorganic phosphate ratio is reversed and adenosine triphosphate levels fall during hypoglycemia. (From Prichard et al.,[97] with permission.)

hearts.[70] Positioning of the coil is accomplished using conventional MRI.

As in cardiac applications, phosphorus MR can be used in the study of pathologic processes in the brain. Cady studied the brains of seven infants with abnormal neurologic assessments.[71] By looking at spectral peaks for phosphorus compounds, he found that in abnormal neonate brain, the phosphocreatine to inorganic phosphate ratios were low and increased in those babies whose clinical condition improved.

[13]C spectra also have potential value in metabolic monitoring. Unlike imaging techniques which can pinpoint the location of abnormal tissue, MR spectral analysis is nonspecific and can only refer to general location.

MR measurement of pH is possible because of the pH dependence of the resonance phenomenon. The pH change of the milieu of a molecule leads to different bond angles and occupation of orbitals as the resonant frequency changes. This change is called the chemical shift, and needs to be quantified by a titration curve in vitro prior to application in living tissue. The usual molecules used as pH "probes" are inorganic phosphate, ATP, or compounds containing PO_4 ions, although ^{13}C compounds can be used. However, there are some inherent problems. Molecules are compartmentalized in tissues and cells, for example in cytosol versus mitochondria. Therefore, there are a range of environments being measured.

RAPID TOMOGRAPHIC METHODS OF MONITORING

Rapid Computed Tomography (Cine-CT)

Tomographic imaging techniques such as computed tomography (CT), magnetic resonance imaging (MRI), and single photon emission computed tomography (SPECT) when initially developed accumulated data and assembled it slowly. Real-time monitoring applications were limited. However, within the past 10 years improvements in equipment and reconstruction of images have led to usefulness in these techniques in the care of critically ill patients.

Rapid CT or cine-CT has overcome the limitation of rotation of an x-ray tube by using a magnetically deflected electron beam, which not only vastly increases scanning speed, but also makes it possible to obtain multiple slices simultaneously. Coupled with scan reconstruction within a fraction of a minute, this technology becomes a useful monitoring tool.

Cardiac volume studies require peripheral injection of small amounts of contrast material. The volumes are calculated from planimetered data much the same as for angiography. However, because multiple slices are used, the geometric assumptions of angiography or two-dimensional echocardiography are overcome. Measurement of right and left ventricular volumes measured by cine-CT in closed chest dogs has been compared to simultaneous volumes by thermodilution or electromagnetic flow probes.[72] Correlation for left ventricular stroke volume was found to be .99 and for right ventricular stroke volume, .98 at various levels of stroke volume perturbated by dobutamine, sodium pentobarbital, sodium nitroprusside, or coronary artery occlusion.

Another application is the use of cine-CT to follow changes in cardiac wall thickness. This technique leads to good definition of endocardial and epicardial wall edges. A study in dogs before, during, and after left anterior descending coronary artery occlusion showed significant decrease in systolic thickness of the anterior wall during the 60-second occlusion.[73]

Cine-CT has been shown to have application in the dynamic evaluation of stridor in children, possibly avoiding bronchoscopy in laryngomalacia and tracheomalacia.[74] It has also been shown to be useful in evaluation of the site and extent of obstruction in sleep apnea.[75]

Magnetic Resonance Imaging

Magnetic resonance imaging (MRI) now has the capacity for measurement of left ventricular volumes and ejection fraction and thus becomes another minimally invasive means of measurement of left ventricular function. To determine volumes and thus ejection fraction by MRI, the pulse sequence is synchronized with a point in the cardiac cycle. Multislice acquisition can be obtained from a single cardiac cycle, each successive one with a slight delay to make each occur at a comparable point in the cycle. However, the complete image is built up over several cycles. The analysis of the image is similar to angiography, tracing the left ventricular borders and determination of the volume from an algorithm. A problem with this methodology is proper gating such that the images do represent the exact moment of end diastole and end systole. Until recently, MRI data acquisition was time-consuming (30 to 60 minutes). Dilworth and coworkers[76] compared MRI with angiography and found correlation coefficients of .75 for LVEDV (left ventricular end diastolic volume), .90 for LVESV (left ventricular end systolic volume), and .76 for LVEF (left ventricular ejection fraction). Recent developments in MRI technology allows much faster acquisition of data, up to 20 images per heartbeat, leading to real-time imaging of cardiac function. Because of the shortened time for data acquisition, the MRI can become less expensive per study and be better tolerated by patients.

Magnetic resonance imaging of the brain is becoming increasingly important in neurologic critical care in the diagnosis and following of acute events. It has some specific advantages over CT scanning as there is an absence of bone artifact, making visualization of the posterior fossa and of subdural and subarachnoid hemorrhage more precise.[77] MRI has the ability to detect acute ischemia. In an animal model, ischemia caused by carotid artery ligation was detected within 3 hours.[78] In patients with acute strokes, MRI is more sensitive than CT in identifying the lesion.[79]

Blood flow can be studied by MR, using a plane perpendicular to the flow of the vessel and the specific volume containing the vessel. Proper sequencing of applications of the radiofrequency pulse and the time delay between excitation and measurement of emission allow calculation of flow. For example, nuclei that move across the imaged volume faster than the excitation pulse is reapplied would emit no signal. Thus, the intensity of the emitted signal for a given sequencing will decrease with increasing blood velocity. The images are processed into an angiogram.

Paramagnetic contrast agents (chelates of gadolinium) are used in certain applications for image enhancement and some blood flow studies. Although this makes MRI more invasive, these agents appear to be safer than traditional radiographic contrast materials. MRI coronary angiography has been compared with conventional angiography and found to have a sensitivity of 90 percent and specificity of 92 percent for 50 percent or greater stenoses.[80]

Magnetic resonance imaging requires very expensive and very technologically demanding equipment. Its advantage lie in its noninvasiveness and superior diagnostic ability when applied in cases where other technology is inadequate. In the case of angiography, MRI angiography may well become the less expensive technique.

Single Photon Emission Computed Tomography

Single photon emission computed tomography (SPECT) is scintigraphy with a rotating detector and reconstruction of images. Since spatial resolution depends on counts cubed, imaging time can be long (e.g., 20 minutes for thallium tomography of the heart). However, SPECT offers certain advantages over planar scintigraphy; most important, it eliminates overlapping segments and thereby increases sensitivity. It does require larger doses of radionuclide. Like planar cardiac radionuclide studies, current SPECT cardiac studies use thallium-201 (^{201}Tl) for identification of individual coronary lesions and technetium 99m pyrophosphate (^{99m}TcPYP) for detection of acute myocardial infarction, particularly nontransmural infarction. In a group of 57 patients with coronary artery disease demonstrated on angiography, adenosine-thallium SPECT had 83 percent sensitivity and 94 percent specificity.[81] Most false negatives were in patients with single-vessel disease.

SPECT has been used to measure left ventricular volumes with ^{99m}Tc and compared to volumes determined by planar angiography with a correlation of $r = .89$.[82] SPECT, like other tomographic methods of measurement of ventricular volumes, offers the advantage of being less invasive than angiography and overcomes geometric assumptions made by a planar method. However, for all tomographic methods as well as angiography, the patient must be moved to the equipment. Technetium is also used for SPECT studies of the brain and these studies have been shown to be more sensitive than MRI in identifying focal lesions in a group of head injured patients.[83] SPECT studies are sensitive for early detection of cerebral ischemia.[84] It has also been shown to be sensitive in detecting morphologic changes in the brains of infants following extracorporeal membrane oxygenation.[85]

SPECT is used to monitor CBF. Using intravenous injection or inhalation of ^{133}Xe, Sugiyama and colleagues[86] followed CBF in patients with ischemic stroke due to middle cerebral artery occlusion. The same technique has been used to determine the effect of using a calcium antagonist in patients with ischemic areas due to stroke.[87] Because of its limited spatial resolution, this method is not suitable for quantitative determination of flow; however, it does follow the qualitative course for individual subjects and can easily discriminate between low- or no-flow and high-flow states and can be useful in directing therapy.

Tomography is a very rapidly advancing field. The various techniques can produce elegant images, including translating a gray scale to colors. The initial equipment is very expensive, but with high usage, costs for individual studies are reasonable.

ARTIFICIAL NEURAL NETWORKS

A current direction in monitoring is the development of "smart" systems for alarms or directing therapies. Artificial neural networks (knowledge based systems) have great potential for use in situations where complex pattern recognition or interpretation is needed. The pattern to be analyzed could be a constellation of signs and symptoms, such as in the presentation of acute myocardial infarction, a physiologic signal needing interpretation, such as an arterial waveform, or a set of signals, such as the inputs from various monitors of ventilation leading to an alarm condition with diagnosis of the problem.

An artificial neural network is first designed based upon expert knowledge of the situation. The network is set up on a computer with input nodes, layers of intermediate nodes, interconnected and having paths leading to all possible output nodes. The connections can feed forward or feed back. The network is then supplied with inputs of situations with known solutions in order to assign the weighting factors at the various intermediate nodes. After the network has been "trained" by these known inputs, it is tested in a set of situations where the answer is known. When the network has been sufficiently refined to a high level of sensitivity and specificity, it is ready for use.

For example, an artificial neural network has been designed for the diagnosis of myocardial infarction for use in the emergency room.[88] Inputs include risk factors, symptoms, physical findings, ECG findings, and response to nitroglycerin. It has

been found to have a sensitivity of 97.2 percent and specificity of 96.2 percent, which outperformed physicians. The advantage of a neural network is that it is not susceptible to factors that bias human judgment, such as fatigue or the recall of recent events. Another application of artificial neural networks is in processing of electronic signals. A network has been designed to reject corrupted arterial pressure waveforms.[89]

An artificial neural network has been set up and tested for the diagnosis of ventilation problems in intubated and machine ventilated patients in the operating room.[90] It is a three-layered (input, intermediate, and output), feed-forward network, which uses 52 inputs from the anesthesia machine monitors (Modulus CD, Ohmeda, Madison, WI). Based on the inputs it diagnoses 20 faults. After "training," it was tested on dogs. Fault conditions were set up, and the network reached the proper diagnosis in 83 percent of cases. This "intelligent alarm" system in a simulated operating room situation was compared with conventional alarms in aiding diagnosis of conditions of cuff leak, airway obstruction, open expiratory valve, inspiratory leak, exhalation hose disconnect, airway disconnect, and airway leak. Anesthesiologists diagnosed conditions faster with the "intelligent alarm" system than with the conventional anesthesia machine alarms.[91]

A further problem in setting up "intelligent alarm" systems is that input information often is not binary, yes-no, or normal-abnormal. A knowledge-based system for hemodynamic monitoring in cardioanesthesia has been described.[92] A "fuzzy" value such as normal systolic blood pressure is represented by a range. For each input there is a value between 0 and 1, indicating to what extent the value is compatible with the normal range. The system uses automatically acquired data and manually entered drug administration and intraoperative events. Outputs consist of a description of the hemodynamic state and suggested therapies.

A clinical algorithm for treatment of high-risk surgical patients, based on hemodynamic and oxygen transport parameters has been developed.[93] This, then has the potential to become the basis of an artificial neural network. This is a more difficult task, for here the outputs (suggested therapies) must be judged against a wide range of outcomes: organ failure, prolonged recovery, morbidity. Any network needs to be shown to be superior to conventional management, given the same information. If the network shows better output, but demands input of a pulmonary artery catheter when it would not be placed under conventional management, then is it an improvement?

The potential benefits of artificial neural networks are many: rapid resolution of problems, sorting of complex data, reduction of human time, and elimination of human bias. For simpler tasks the development is not difficult. However, for more complex monitoring situations, the development of these knowledge-based systems is very complex and, of course, this leads to the question, how much can artificial intelligence be used to replace human judgment? It does seem certain that anesthesiology and critical care are areas where artificial neural networks will find increasing applications.

CONCLUSION

An ideal monitoring modality of the future would be one that is noninvasive, not too costly, and provides continuous, real-time data about organ function or the metabolic state of tissues. The more complex technologies such as magnetic resonance and single photon emission computed tomography have the greatest potential for the very sophisticated metabolic level of monitoring, but are costly and bulky, requiring a separate installation with the patient being transported to the monitor for single or repeated measurements. Less complex modalities are less costly, more portable, and often much easier to operate with results that are more readily interpreted. However, the data obtained may not be "absolute" or may have a consistent "error" relative to more "standard" conventional monitoring methods. These kinds of measurements may be very useful in following individual patients over time, or evaluating the effects of therapy. Certainly there are many situations where change in a variable is all that is needed for evaluation.

A monitoring technique, whether continuous or intermittent, to be most useful must present the data obtained in a rapid manner. With microprocessors virtually any monitoring modality can be made into a real-time system. Currently, many monitoring systems display several real-time parameters simultaneously, allowing the user to integrate the data more easily and act upon it. The next generation of monitoring will be that of integrated systems. Linking data via artificial neural networks will bring about "smart alarms" and "artificial intelligence," which will suggest diagnoses and can suggest therapies. This will certainly save time for the health care provider in reaching a judgment about patient management because all the relevant data and possible conclusions will be presented in a readily interpreted visual display. A further step may be that integrated monitoring will not only reach a diagnosis and suggest a therapy, but will also implement the therapy. A simple example of this would be a feedback loop that automatically changes the rate of a drug infusion in response to the change of a monitored variable.

In any development in monitoring, the goals should remain clear. Any new modality should be directed at obtaining

More accurate information

Information at a more basic level (organ or tissue function)

Information by less invasive means

Information by less expensive means

Continuous information to replace intermittent information

Real-time information to replace retrieved information

Information at the bedside

New monitoring that does not accomplish one or more of these goals should be rejected.

REFERENCES

1. Snow J: On the Inhalation of the Vapour of Ether in Surgical Operations. John Churchill, London, 1847
2. Ahmed SS, Levinson GE, Schwartz CJ, Ettinger PO: Systolic time intervals as measures of the contractile state of the left ventricular myocardium in man. Circulation 46:559, 1972
3. Hamada M, Hidwada K, Kokubu T: Clinical significance of systolic time intervals in hypertensive subjects. Eur Heart J 11(Suppl. I):105, 1990
4. Hirschfeld S, Meyer R, Schwartz DCM et al: Measurement of left and right systolic time intervals by echocardiography. Circulation 51:304, 1975
5. Spodick DH, Haffty BG, Kotilainen PW: Noninvasive monitoring of physiologic data: recording systolic time intervals. Med Instrum 12:343, 1978
6. Ohte N, Hashimoto T, Narita H et al: Noninvasive evaluation of left ventricular performance with a

new systolic time interval, the Q-V peak, and comparison with established systolic time intervals. Am J Cardiol 66:1018, 1990

7. Stopfkuchen H, Queisser-Luft A, Vogel K: Cardiovascular responses to dobutamine determined by systolic time intervals in preterm infants. Crit Care Med 18:722, 1990

8. Lewinsky RM, Sharf M, Degani S, Eibschitz I: Prediction of pregnancy outcome by combined analysis of the fetal electrocardiogram and systolic time intervals. Am J Perinatol 9:348, 1992

9. Sheps DS, Petrovick ML, Kizakevich PN, Craige E: Continuous noninvasive monitoring of left ventricular function during exercise by thoracic impedance cardiography—automated derivation systolic time intervals. Am Heart J 103:519, 1982

10. Breithardt G, Cain ME, El-sherif N et al: Standards for analysis of ventricular late potentials using high-resolution or signal-averaged electrocardiography: a statement by a task force committee of the European Society of Cardiology, the American Heart Association, and the American College of Cardiology. J Am Coll Cardiol 17:999, 1991

11. Nalos PC, Gang ES, Mandel WJ et al: The signal-averaged electrocardiogram as a screening test for inducibility of sustained ventricular tachycardia in high risk patients: a prospective study. J Am Coll Cardiol 9:539, 1987

12. Nyboer J, Bagno S, Barnett A, Halsey RH: Radiocardiograms—the electrical impedance changes of the heart in relation to electrocardiograms and heart sounds. J Clin Invest 19:773, 1940

13. Kubicek WG, Karnegis JN, Patterson RP et al: Development and evolution of an impedance cardiac output system. Aerospace Med 37:1208, 1966

14. Quail AW, Traugott FM: Effects of changing haematocrit, ventricular rate and myocardial intropy on the accuracy of impedance cardiography. Clin Exp Pharmacol Physiol 8:335, 1981

15. DeSouza WM, Panerai RB: Variability of thoracic impedance cardiograms in man. Med Biol Eng Comput 19:411, 1981

16. Christensen JH, Andreasen F, Kristofferson MB: Comparison of the anaesthetic and haemodynamic effects of chlormethiazole and thiopentone. Br J Anaesth 55:391, 1983

17. Milsom I, Forssman L, Biber B et al: Measurement of cardiac stroke volume during cesarean section: a comparison between impedance cardiography and the dye dilution technique. Acta Anaesthesiol Scand 27:421, 1983

18. Miles DS, Gotshall RW, Quinones JD et al: Impedance cardiography fails to measure accurately left ventricular ejection fraction. Crit Care Med 18:221, 1990

19. Johannsen G, Andersen M, Juhl B: The effect of general anaesthesia on the haemodynamic events during laparoscopy with CO_2 insufflation. Acta Anaesth Scand 33:132, 1989

20. Sramek BB, Rose DM, Miyamoto A: Stroke volume equation with a linear base impedance model and its accuracy, as compared to thermodilution and magnetic flowmeter techniques in humans and animals. Proceedings of the Sixth International Conference on Electrical Biopedance. Zadar, Yugoslavia, 1983

21. Bernstein DP: A new stroke volume equation for thoracic electrical bioimpedance: theory and rationale. Crit Care Med 14:904, 1986

22. Appel PL, Kram HB, Mackabee J et al: Comparison of measurements of cardiac output by bioimpedance and thermodilution in severely ill surgical patients. Crit Care Med 14:933, 1986

23. Bernstein DP: Continuous noninvasive real-time monitoring of stroke volume and cardiac output by thoracic electrical bioimpedance. Crit Care Med 14:898, 1986

24. Wong DH, Tremper KK, Stemmer EA et al: Noninvasive cardiac output: simultaneous comparison of two different methods with thermodilution. Anesthesiol 72:784, 1990

25. Clancy TV, Norman K, Reynolds R et al: Cardiac output measurement in critical care patients: thoracic electrical bioimpedance versus thermodilution. J Trauma 31:1116, 1991

26. Masaki DI, Greenspoon JS, Ouzounian JG: Measurement of cardiac output in pregnancy by thoracic electrical bioimpedance and thermodilution. Am J Obstet Gynecol 161:680, 1989

27. Introna RPS, Preutt JK, Crumrine RC, Cuadrado AR: Use of transthoracic bioimpedance to determine cardiac output in pediatric patients. Crit Care Med 16:1101, 1988

28. Jewkes C, Sear JW, Verhoeff F et al: Non-invasive measurement of cardiac output by thoracic electrical bioimpedance: a study of reproducibility and comparison with thermodilution. Br J Anaesth 67:788, 1991

29. Wong DH, O'Connor D, Tremper KK et al: Changes in cardiac output after acute blood loss and position change in man. Crit Care Med 17:979, 1989

30. Mickell JJ, Lucking SE, Chaten FC, Young ES: Trending of impedance-monitored cardiac variables: method and statistical power analysis of 100 control studies in a pediatric intensive care unit. Crit Care Med 18:645, 1990

31. Wennberg E, Frid I, Haljamae H et al: Comparison of Ringer's lactate with 3 percent dextran 70 for volume loading before extradural caesarian section. Br J Anaesth 65:654, 1990

32. Baron JF, Coriat P, Mundler O et al: Left ventricular global and regional function during lumbar epidural anesthesia in patients with and without angina pectoris: influence of volume loading. Anesthesiology 66:621, 1987

33. Berger HJ, Davies RA, Batsford WP et al: Beat-to-beat left ventricular performance assessed from the equilibrium cardiac blood pool using a computerized nuclear probe. Circulation 63:133, 1981

34. Strashun A, Horowitz SF, Goldsmith SJ et al: Noninvasive detection of left ventricular dysfunction with a portable electrocardiographic gated scintillation probe device. Am J Cardiol 47:610, 1981

35. Giles RW, Berger HJ, Barash PG et al: Continuous monitoring of left ventricular performance with the computerized nuclear probe during laryngoscopy and intubation before coronary artery bypass surgery. Am J Cardiol 50:735, 1982

36. deYang L, Bairey CN, Berman DS et al: Accuracy and reproducibility of left ventricular ejection fraction measurements using an ambulatory radionuclide left ventricular function monitor. J Nucl Med 32:796, 1991

37. Broadhurst P, Cashman P, Crawley J et al: Clinical validation of a miniature nuclear probe system for continuous on-line monitoring of cardiac function and ST-segment. J Nucl Med 32:37, 1991

38. Nishimura RA, Callahan MJ, Schaff HV et al: Noninvasive measurement of cardiac output by continuous wave Doppler echocardiography: initial experience and review of the literature. Mayo Clin Proc 59:484, 1984

39. Rein AJJT, Hsieh KS, Elixson M et al: Cardiac output estimates in the pediatric intensive care unit using a continuous-wave Doppler computer: validation and limitations of the technique. Am Heart J 112:97, 1986

40. Wilson N, Goldberg SJ, Allen HD et al: Does transducer selection affect aortic arch velocities? Am Heart J 113:878, 1986

41. Goldberg SJ, Sahn DJ, Allen HD et al: Evaluation of pulmonary and systemic blood flow by 2-dimensional Doppler echocardiography using fast Fourier transform spectra analysis. Am J Cardiol 50:1394, 1982

42. Loeppky JA, Hoekenga DE, Greene ER, Luft UC: Comparison of noninvasive pulsed Doppler and Fick measurements of stroke volume in cardiac patients. Am Heart J 107:339, 1984

43. Graettinger WF, Greene ER, Voyles WF: Doppler predictions of pulmonary artery pressure, flow, and resistance in adults. Am Heart J 113:1426, 1987

44. Takenaka K, Waffarn F, Dabestani A et al: A pulsed Doppler echocardiographic study of the postnatal changes in pulmonary artery and ascending aortic flow in normal term newborn infants. Am Heart J 113:759, 1987

45. Aaslid R, Lindegaard K-F, Sorteberg W, Nornes H: Cerebral autoregulation dynamics in humans. Stroke 20:45, 1989

46. Caplan LR, Brass LM, DeWitt LD et al: Transcranial Doppler ultrasound: present status. Neurology 40: 696, 1990

47. Halsey JH, McDowell HA, Gelman S, Morawetz RB: Blood velocity in the middle cerebral artery and regional blood flow during carotid endarterectomy. Stroke 20:53, 1989

48. Spencer MP, Thomas GI, Nicholls SC, Sauvage LR: Detection of middle cerebral artery emboli during carotid endarterectomy using transcranial Doppler ultrasonography. Stroke 21:415, 1990

49. Lundar T, Lindegaard K-F, Froysaker T et al: Cerebral perfusion during nonpulsatile cardiopulmonary bypass. Ann Thorac Surg 40:144-150, 1985

50. Padayachee TS, Parsons S, Theobold R et al: The detection of microemboli in the middle cerebral artery during cardiopulmonary bypass: a transcranial Doppler ultrasound investigation using membrane and bubble oxygenators. Ann Thorac Surg 44:298, 1987

51. DeWitt LD, Weschler LR: Transcranial Doppler. Stroke 19:915, 1988

52. Wiernsperger N, Sylvia AL, Jöbsis FF: Incomplete transient ischemia: a nondestructive evaluation of in vivo cerebral metabolism. Stroke 12:864, 1981

53. Palladino WG, Proctor HJ, Jöbsis FF: Effect of hypothermia during hypoxic hypotension on cerebral metabolism. J Surg Res 34:388, 1983

54. Proctor HJ, Cairns C, Fillipo D et al: Brain metabolism during increased intracranial pressure as assessed by niroscopy. Surgery 96:273, 1984

55. Jöbsis FF: Noninvasive infrared monitoring of cerebral oxygen sufficiency and hemodynamic parameters. p. 223. In Popp AJ (ed): Neural Trauma. Raven Press, New York, 1979

56. Hampson NB, Camporesi EM, Stolp BW et al: Cerebral oxygen availability by NIR spectroscopy during transient hypoxia in humans. J Appl Physiol 69:907, 1990

57. Ferrari M, Zanette E, Giannini I et al: Effects of carotid artery compression test on regional cerebral blood volume, hemoglobin oxygen saturation and cytochrome-c-oxidase redox level in cerebrovascular patients. Adv Exp Med Biol 200:213, 1986

58. Wickramasinghe YABD, Livera LN, Spencer SA et al: Plethysmographic validation of near infrared spectroscopic monitoring of cerebral blood volume. Arch Dis in Childhood 67:407, 1992

59. Livera LN, Spencer SA, Thorniley MS et al: Effects of hypoxaemia and bradycardia on neonatal haemodynamics. Arch Dis Childhood 66:376, 1991

60. Peebles DM, Edwards AD, Wyatt JS et al: Changes in

human fetal cerebral hemoglobin concentration and oxygenation during labor measured by near-infrared spectroscopy. Am J Obstet Gynecol 166: 1369, 1992

61. Wyatt JS, Edwards AD, Cope M et al: Response of cerebral blood volume to changes in arterial carbon dioxide tension in preterm and term infants. Pediatr Res 29:553, 1991

62. McCormick PW, Stewart M, Goetting MG, Balakrishnan G: Regional cerebrovascular oxygen saturation measured by optical spectroscopy in humans. Stroke 22:596, 1991

63. Kurth CD, Steven JM, Nicolson SC et al: Kinetics of cerebral deoxygenation during deep hypothermic arrest in neonates. Anesthesiology 77:656, 1992

64. Smith DS, Levy W, Maris M, Chance B: Reperfusion hyperoxia in brain after circulatory arrest in humans. Anesthesiology 73:12, 1990

65. Shah AR, Kurth CD, Gwiazdowski SG et al: Fluctuations in cerebral oxygenation and blood volume during endotracheal tube suctioning in premature infants. J Pediatr 120:769, 1992

66. Cheatle TR, Potter LA, Cope M et al: Near-infrared spectroscopy in peripheral vascular disease. Br J Surg 78:405, 1991

67. Singer JR: Blood flow rates by nuclear magnetic resonance measurement. Science 130:1652, 1959

68. Lauterbur PC: Image formation by induced local interactions: examples employing nuclear magnetic resonance. Nature 242:190, 1973

69. Grove TH, Ackerman JJH, Radda GK, Bore PJ: Analysis of rat heart in vivo by phosphorus nuclear magnetic resonance. Proc Natl Acad Sci USA 77:299, 1980

70. Bottomley PA: Noninvasive study of high-energy phosphate metabolism in human heart by depth-resolved ^{31}P NMR spectroscopy. Science 229:769, 1985

71. Cady EB, Dawson MJ, Hope PL et al: Non-invasive investigation of cerebral metabolism in newborn infants by phosphorus nuclear magnetic resonance spectroscopy. Lancet 1:1059, 1983

72. Reiter SJ, Rumberger JA, Feiring AJ et al: Precision of measurements of right and left ventricular volume by cine computed tomography. Circulation 74:890, 1986

73. Farmer D, Lipton MJ, Higgins CB et al: In vivo assessment of left ventricular wall and chamber dynamics during transient myocardial ischemia using cine computed tomography. Am J Cardiol 55:560, 1985

74. Frey EE, Smith WL, Grandgeorge S et al: Chronic airway obstruction in children: evaluation with cine-CT. AJR 148:347, 1987

75. Stein MG, Gamsu G, deGeer G et al: Cine-CT in obstructive sleep apnea. AJR 148:1069, 1987

76. Dilworth LR, Aisen AM, Mancini J et al: Determination of left ventricular volumes and ejection fraction by nuclear magnetic resonance imaging. Am Heart J 113:24, 1987

77. Bydder GM, Steiner RE: NMR imaging of the brain. Neuroradiology 23:231, 1982

78. Manu I, Levy RM, Crooks LE, Hosobuchi Y: Proton nuclear magnetic resonance imaging of acute experimental cerebral ischemia. Invest Radiol 17:345, 1983

79. Edelman RR, Warach S: Magnetic resonance imaging. N Engl J Med 328:708, 785, 1993

80. Manning WJ, Li W, Edelman RR: A preliminary report comparing magnetic resonance coronary angiography with conventional angiography. N Engl J Med 328:828, 1993

81. Verani MS, Mahmarian JJ, Hixson JB et al: Diagnosis of coronary artery disease by controlled coronary vasodilation with adenosine and thallium-201 scintigraphy in patients unable to exercise. Circulation 82:80, 1990

82. Caputo GR, Graham MM, Brust KD et al: Measurement of left ventricular volume using single-photon emission computed tomography. Am J Cardiol 56:781, 1985

83. Newton MR, Greenwood RJ, Britton KE et al: A study comparing SPECT with CT and MRI after closed head injury. J Neurol Neurosurg Psychiatry 55:92, 1992

84. Holman BL, Devous Sr MD: Functional brain SPECT: the emergence of a powerful clinical method. J Nucl Med 33:1888, 1992

85. Park CH, Spitzer AR, Desai HJ et al: Brain SPECT in neonates following extracorporeal membrane oxygenation: evaluation of technique and preliminary results. J Nucl Med 33:1943, 1992

86. Sugiyama H, Christensen J, Olsen TS, Lassen NA: Monitoring CBF in clinical routine by dynamic single photon emission tomography (SPECT) of inhaled xenon-133. Stroke 17:1179, 1986

87. Vorstrup S, Anderson A, Blegvad N, Paulson OB: Calcium antagonist (PY 108-068) treatment may further decrease flow in ischemic areas in acute stroke. J Cereb Blood Flow Metab 6:222, 1986

88. Baxt WG: Use of an artificial neural network for the diagnosis of myocardial infarction. Ann Int Med 115:843, 1991

89. Pike T, Mustard PA: Automated recognition of corrupted arterial waveforms using neural network techniques. Comput Biol Med 22:173, 1992

90. Farrell RM, Orr JA, Kuck K, Westenskow DR: Differential features for a neural network based anesthesia alarm system. Biomed Sci Instrument 28:99, 1992

91. Westenskow DR, Orr JA, Simon FH et al: Intelligent alarms reduce anesthesiologist's response time to critical faults. Anesthesiology 77:1074, 1992

92. Scheke T, Langen M, Popp HJ et al: Knowledge-based decision support for patient monitoring in cardioanesthesia. Int J Clin Monitor Comp 9:1, 1992

93. Shoemaker WC, Patil R, Appel PL, Kram HB: Hemodynamic and oxygen transport patterns for outcome prediction, therapeutic goals, and clinical algorithms to improve outcomes: feasibility of artificial intelligence to customize algorithms. Chest 102: 617S, 1992

94. Lewis RP, Ritgers SE, Forester WF, Boudoulas H: A critical review of systolic time intervals. Circulation 56:147, 1977

95. Edmunds AT, Godfrey S, Tooley M: Cardiac output measured by transthoracic impedance cardiography at rest, during exercise and at various lung volumes. Clin Sci Mol Med 63:109, 1982

96. Gardin JM, Bunn CS, Childs WJ, Henry WL: Evaluation of blood flow velocity in the ascending aorta and main pulmonary artery of normal subjects by Doppler echocardiography. Am Heart J 107:310, 1984

97. Prichard JW, Alger JR, Behar KL et al: Cerebral metabolic studies in vivo by ^{31}PNMR. Proc Natl Acad Sci USA 80:2749, 1983

Index

Page numbers followed by f *indicate figures; those followed by* t *indicate tables.*

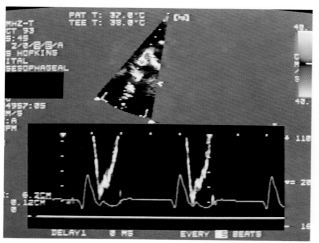

Plate 11-1A.

Plate 11-1B.

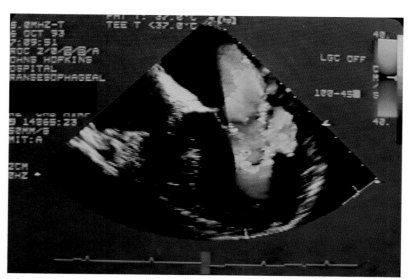

Plate 11-2.

Plate 11-1. The distinction between laminar and turbulent flow. **(A)** Laminar flow across the mitral valve is shown in this transesophageal echocardiography (TEE) study. Laminar flow produces a smooth envelope with a clear space beneath it. **(B)** Turbulent flow across a prosthetic mitral valve produces a curve that is filled to a large extent because of the movement of blood in a disorganized fashion.

Plate 11-2. Color Doppler flow image. In the color scale to the right, red indicates blood moving toward the transducer and blue indicates blood moving away from the transducer. Velocity is represented by the brightness of the color, and high velocity flow is displayed as small echogenic dots.

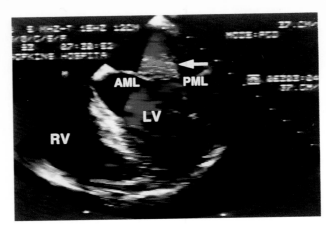

Plate 11-3A.

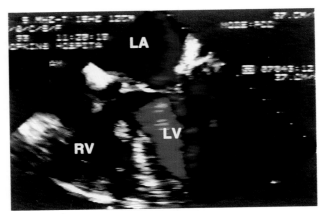

Plate 11-3B.

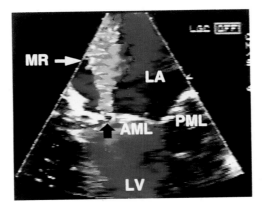

Plate 11-4.

Plate 11-3. (A) Color Doppler image showing mitral regurgitation seen as a mosaic of color at the arrow (see also Fig. 11-38). RV, right ventricle; LV, left ventricle; AML, anterior mitral leaflet; PML, posterior mitral leaflet. **(B)** Color Doppler image of mitral valve after repair. LA, left atrium.

Plate 11-4. A hole in the anterior leaflet of the mitral valve secondary to endocarditis, resulting in a jet of mitral regurgitation (MR) in the middle of the leaflet (seen at the black arrow). This was repaired by suturing the perforation. LA, left atrium; AML, anterior mitral leaflet; PML, posterior mitral leaflet; LV, left ventricle.